# Atlas of Small Animal Diagnostic Imaging

# Atlas of Small Animal Diagnostic Imaging

**Edited by**

**CLIFFORD R. BERRY, DVM, DACVR (DI)**

Clinical Assistant Professor, Diagnostic Imaging
Department of Molecular Biomedical Sciences
College of Veterinary Medicine
North Carolina State University
Raleigh, NC, USA

Courtesy Professor of Diagnostic Imaging
College of Veterinary Medicine
University of Florida
Gainesville, FL, USA

**NATHAN C. NELSON, DVM, MS, DACVR (DI AND EDI)**

Clinical Professor, Diagnostic Imaging
Department of Molecular Biomedical Sciences
College of Veterinary Medicine
North Carolina State University
Raleigh, NC, USA

**MATTHEW D. WINTER, DVM, DACVR (DI)**

Veterinary Consultants in Telemedicine
Cambridge, UK
Department of Small Animal Clinical Sciences
College of Veterinary Medicine
University of Florida
Gainesville, FL, USA

**WILEY** Blackwell

*Registered Office*
John Wiley & Sons, Inc., 111 River Street, Hoboken, NJ 07030, USA

For details of our global editorial offices, customer services, and more information about Wiley products visit us at www.wiley.com.

Wiley also publishes its books in a variety of electronic formats and by print-on-demand. Some content that appears in standard print versions of this book may not be available in other formats.

*Library of Congress Cataloging-in-Publication Data*
Names: Berry, Clifford R., editor. | Nelson, Nathan, 1972- editor. | Winter, Matthew D. (Matthew Damian), editor.
Title: Atlas of small animal diagnostic imaging / edited by Clifford R. Berry III, Nathan Nelson, Matthew D. Winter.
Description: Hoboken, NJ : Wiley, 2023. | Includes bibliographical references and index.
Identifiers: LCCN 2022027172 (print) | LCCN 2022027173 (ebook) | ISBN 9781118964408 (cloth) | ISBN 9781118964422 (adobe pdf) | ISBN 9781118964415 (epub)
Subjects: MESH: Diagnostic Imaging–veterinary | Animal Diseases–diagnostic imaging | Animals, Domestic | Diagnosis, Differential | Atlas | Case Reports
Classification: LCC SF757.8 (print) | LCC SF757.8 (ebook) | NLM SF 757.8 | DDC 636.089/60754–dc23/eng/20230103
LC record available at https://lccn.loc.gov/2022027172
LC ebook record available at https://lccn.loc.gov/2022027173

Cover Image: © Clifford R. Berry and Elodie Huguet
Cover Design by Wiley

Set in 9.5/12.5pt SourceSans Pro by Straive, Pondicherry, India

Printed in Singapore
M097522_200123

*In general, this textbook is dedicated to those radiologists who have gone before us and shown us the "light" for the acquisition and interpretation of radiographs. They have shown us the "art and science" of diagnostic imaging. Some of those would include Drs Norman Ackerman, Timothy O'Brien, David Hager, Ronald Burk, and the many others who are memorialized on the veterinary radiology website (https://acvr.org/in-memoriam/). We would be remiss not to also dedicate this text to the next generation of veterinary radiologists and diagnostic imagers who can build on some of these foundations and provide new materials and insights to the "art and science" of diagnostic imaging in veterinary medicine. We trust that your futures in veterinary imaging are as fruitful and rewarding as the careers that we have had so far in this field.*

*– Kip*

*This book is dedicated to my wife and love of my life, Brigitt, who has put up with this veterinary radiology stuff all our adult lives. There will be a special place in heaven for her with her patience. To God be the Glory (John 3:16)!*

*– Nate*

*To Laura, Claire, Paul, and Sylvia, my bright lights in a dark room.*

*– Matt*

*To my wife, Brandy. Without her love, support, and twinkling spirit, none of this would be possible.*
*To my children, Mia and Damian, who make me the proudest person on the planet.*
*To my entire family, who have supported me always.*
*To all veterinarians and veterinary paraprofessionals that give of themselves day in and day out – you are Superheroes.*

# Contents

# Contributors

**CLIFFORD R. BERRY, DVM, DACVR**
Clinical Assistant Professor, Diagnostic Imaging
Department of Molecular Biomedical Sciences
College of Veterinary Medicine
North Carolina State University
Raleigh, NC, USA

**ROBSON GIGLIO, DVM, MS, PHD, DACVR**
Assistant Professor, Radiology
College of Veterinary Medicine
University of Georgia
Athens, GA, USA

**FEDERICO R. VILAPLANA GROSSO, LV, DECVDI, DACVR**
Clinical Associate Professor, Diagnostic Imaging
Department of Small Animal Clinical Sciences
College of Veterinary Medicine
University of Florida
Gainesville, FL, USA

**SILKE HECHT, DVM, MS, DECVDI, DACVR**
Professor, Diagnostic Imaging
Department of Small Animal Clinical Sciences
College of Veterinary Medicine
University of Tennessee
Knoxville, TN, USA

**SEAMUS HOEY, MVB, DECVDI, DACVR (DI AND EDI)**
Lecturer/Assistant Professor
School of Veterinary Medicine
University College Dublin
Veterinary Science Centre
Dublin, Ireland

**ELODIE E. HUGUET, DVM, DACVR**
Clinical Assistant Professor, Diagnostic Imaging
Department of Small Animal Clinical Sciences
College of Veterinary Medicine
University of Florida
Gainesville, FL, USA

**ELIZABETH HUYNH, DVM, MS, DACVR**
Veterinary Radiologist
VCA West Coast Specialty and Emergency Animal Hospital
Fountain Valley, CA, USA

**MARTHA M. LARSON, DVM, MS, DACVR**
Professor of Radiology
Department of Small Animal Clinical Sciences
VA-MD College of Veterinary Medicine
Virginia Tech
Blacksburg, VA, USA

**NATHAN C. NELSON, DVM, MS, DACVR (DI, EDI)**
Clinical Professor, Diagnostic Imaging
Department of Molecular Biomedical Sciences
College of Veterinary Medicine
North Carolina State University
Raleigh, NC, USA

**CINTIA R. OLIVEIRA, DVM, DACVR**
VetsChoice Radiology
Madison, WI, USA

**ERIN PORTER, DVM, DACVR (DI, EDI)**
Clinical Associate Professor, Diagnostic Imaging
Department of Small Animal Clinical Sciences
College of Veterinary Medicine
University of Florida
Gainesville, FL, USA

**SANDRA TOU, DVM, DACVIM (INTERNAL MEDICINE AND CARDIOLOGY)**
Veterinary Cardiologist
Department of Clinical Sciences
College of Veterinary Medicine
North Carolina State University
Raleigh, NC, USA

**MATTHEW D. WINTER, DVM, DACVR**
Chief Medical Officer
Vet-CT
Orlando, FL, USA
Clinical Associate Professor, Diagnostic Imaging
Department of Small Animal Clinical Sciences
College of Veterinary Medicine
University of Florida
Gainesville, FL, USA

# Acknowledgments

We would like to acknowledge our colleagues, residents, interns, and students who have asked the right questions and helped us to shape our interpretation paradigms for diagnostic imaging. A special shout out to the radiologists at the University of Florida, Michigan State University, and North Carolina State University for their insights and help in our formulation of Roentgen abnormalities, tying things together, and prioritizing differentials. Of course, our programs would not be complete without the veterinary imaging technicians who go above and beyond the call of duty daily to ensure quality studies without compromising patient care. A special shout out to the technicians at the University of Florida, Michigan State University, and North Carolina State University, especially Danielle Maruagis, Bobbie Davis, Mary Wilson, and Theresa Critcher. The residents over the years have always pushed us to be better and we greatly appreciate that.

We want to acknowledge the incredible patience of the editors and staff at Wiley Blackwell, especially Merryl Le Roux and Erica Judisch, who have not relented in their efforts to help us and have believed in this project from the beginning.

We want to acknowledge Elodie Huguet, DVM, DACVR, for doing the textbook cover and the section pages for us. She is incredibly gifted in art and gave us great images to work with for these areas. We greatly appreciate you and your talents, Elodie.

Thank you.

Why another diagnostic imaging textbook? There are many excellent textbooks on veterinary imaging that have been published previously and are still moving forward, with historical editions being replaced with new ones. We felt that this text should be first and foremost an introduction to diagnostic imaging, although most of the text deals primarily with radiology. But more importantly, this textbook was meant to be an atlas so that we could show not necessarily the "classic" cases but some average cases and how the same disease can look differently depending on the stage of the disease at the time when the images are made. Being an atlas, this textbook is not a comprehensive overview of all the different diseases that one may find in the literature, but should serve as an approach for "common things occurring commonly." And when there is overlap between different disease presentations on the radiographs, formulating a prioritized differential diagnosis list is given precedence. It is hoped that the book will serve as a foundation upon which the reader can add layers of information (science) and clinical experience (art) over the course of their career in veterinary medicine.

It would be impossible to present all the potential images that a patient will present with any given disease process, whether dealing with multicentric lymphoma or elbow dysplasia. Again, this atlas will form a foundational pillar upon which other pillars can be built. We recognize that "pattern recognition" is a lower-order learning technique, but it is critical for building the foundation of interpretation of diagnostic images that occurs each time a new set of images is made.

As with all published works, there will be mistakes in this book. We have tried our best to minimize those mistakes, but take the ultimate responsibility for errors.

We wish you the best in your future endeavors and hope that this textbook can play some role in the diagnostic imaging part of your veterinary medicine career.

**CLIFFORD R. BERRY (KIP)**

**NATHAN C. NELSON (NATE)**

**MATTHEW D. WINTER (MATT)**

# About the Companion Website

This book is accompanied by a companion website.

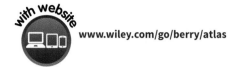 www.wiley.com/go/berry/atlas

The website includes figures from the book as downloadable PowerPoint slides and Radiology templates (Appendices I, II, III).

# Introduction and Physics

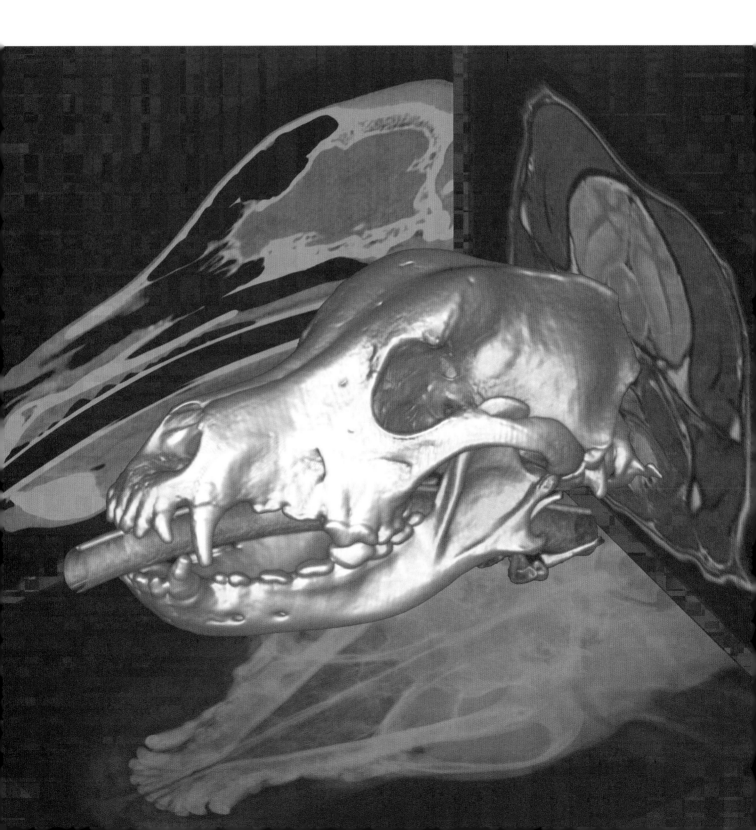

# CHAPTER 1

# The Science, Art, and Philosophy of Radiographic Interpretation

**Matthew D. Winter**

Department of Small Animal Clinical Sciences, College of Veterinary Medicine, University of Florida, Gainesville, FL, USA

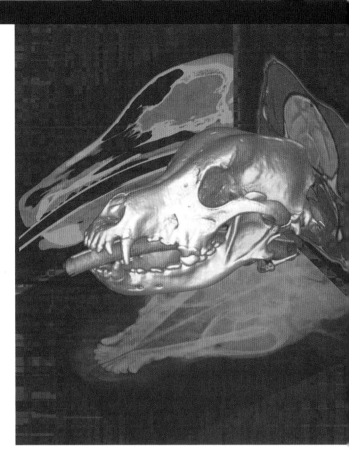

## Introduction

Diagnostic imaging is an art and a science. The science of diagnostic imaging is didactic information that is learned during veterinary training. The art is the experiential learning that takes place over the course of a lifetime as one interprets radiographs and the ability to extract information from an image. As one studies radiographs, one moves from a lower order of learning (pattern recognition) to a higher level of interpretation where different aspects of the interpretation process impact the final conclusions. Then, the interpretation is filtered through the clinical information relevant to the patient at hand.

Interpretation of a radiograph should be directed by a paradigm. An interpretation paradigm is a map that guides you along a path of thorough and complete evaluation of a radiograph. The paradigm is an essential tool to use for evaluation of all radiographic studies, and examples are provided in each section. This chapter presents an approach to and overview of the philosophies shared by the editors of this textbook regarding radiographic interpretation.

## Why Radiographs?

Why bother with radiography, or diagnostic imaging in general? Specifically, radiography is relatively fast and readily available as a diagnostic imaging test. The procedures for most standard examinations are well defined, and expectations for the capabilities of the modality are relatively well understood. In the realm of diagnostic imaging tests, it is also inexpensive and noninvasive, a rapid test to perform. Therefore, it is a great tool to monitor and stage disease and evaluate anatomy. We also use radiographs to document the results of patient management, to figure out if a treatment is working or not. And of course, when possible, we use radiographs to actually diagnose disease.

*Atlas of Small Animal Diagnostic Imaging*, First Edition. Edited by Clifford R. Berry, Nathan C. Nelson, and Matthew D. Winter.
© 2023 John Wiley & Sons, Inc. Published 2023 by John Wiley & Sons, Inc.
Companion website: www.wiley.com/go/berry/atlas

Most often, imaging is used to decrease the level of uncertainty about a diagnosis. In most cases, we do not end up with a definitive diagnosis, but we do use the imaging findings as well as any other information to narrow the list of probable diseases. We do this by gathering data. If we think of each individual finding as a test, with each of those tests as having a particular value, then when we add them together, we should hopefully paint a picture or pattern of disease. So, think of each finding as a piece of a larger pattern. As we fit more and more of these diagnostic puzzle pieces together, the pattern becomes more clear. As that pattern emerges, hopefully we can recognize that it is consistent with a specific disease, or perhaps a subset of diseases. The result should be a shorter list of potential or probable pathologic processes (differential diagnoses), and we can direct our next steps accordingly.

## Imaging Findings as Tests

As mentioned, tests can be characterized by their value, and that value is best described by sensitivity, specificity, and accuracy as tested against a normal and abnormal population of animals. If we think of each radiographic finding as a test, we realize that each finding can be associated with a certain number of true and false positives as well as true and false negatives when compared to a gold standard [1]. The gold standard would be the test considered to be the best available to diagnose a given disease. That said, the test may be relatively unavailable, too expensive, or perhaps very invasive, and therefore cannot always be done. The sensitivity or specificity for each and every finding for each and every disease are not always known, but we do have data for some of this, and we often can extrapolate. We also have our clinical experience and diagnostic acumen to draw on, which continue to grow over time. As more and more clinical research is done, we get new information on the value of findings as tests through science. Perhaps most importantly, the combination of findings can be most powerful as a diagnostic tool, and can further increase the sensitivity, specificity, and accuracy of radiography as a diagnostic tool for a given disease.

It is important to recognize that some individual findings may be very nonspecific, and that they are not exact for any particular disease and can be features of many different, completely unrelated diseases [1]. This means that, individually, they do not contribute to the reduction of uncertainty that we hope to attain. However, when we combine multiple findings, the added value of each finding narrows our scope in the "cone of certainty" (Figure 1.1).

For example, an unstructured interstitial pulmonary pattern that is moderate in severity and hilar in distribution could result in a large list of potential differential diagnostic considerations from multiple etiologies. If we combine this finding with other radiographic changes, such as left-sided cardiomegaly, elevation of the carina on the lateral images, widening of the caudal bronchi on the ventrodorsal image and enlargement of the pulmonary veins in a dog, our differential list narrows very quickly to pulmonary edema secondary to

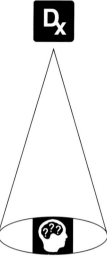

**Cone of certainty**
Specific diagnosis

Non-Specific Change

**FIGURE 1.1** The "cone of certainty." A nonspecific change at the mouth of the funnel does not help narrow the list of differential diagnoses. However, a series of findings added together improves our degree of certainty, narrowing the list of diagnoses at the tip of the cone. There are few diseases for which imaging findings are pathognomonic. However, a series of findings with varying degrees of value can result in a short and prioritized list of differential diagnoses that aid in decision making, clinical progress, and improved patient care.

left-sided cardiac disease. Depending on other signalment and physical examination findings (small breed dog with a grade IV/V pansystolic cardiac murmur), our differential list narrows even more to mitral valve degenerative disease (endocardiosis) with secondary left heart failure.

This is why one of the most important and fundamental interpretation skills is learning to describe abnormal radiographic anatomy in an organized and systematic fashion. Being systematic and organized helps us to recognize patterns that might otherwise elude us.

## Describing Abnormalities: Roentgen Signs

The fundamental language of radiographic interpretation is the *Roentgen signs*. These are the six features that we describe for every organ or body system that we evaluate: *location*, *size*, *shape*, *number*, *margin*, and *opacity*. The definitions as well as some terminology for use in description of abnormalities are listed in Table 1.1. Figure 1.2 is a radiograph that contains all radiographic opacities.

*Opacity* is the term we use to characterize the relative radiographic density of an organ or structure. The relative physical density of a structure and the atomic number of its components will dictate how many x-rays are stopped, or attenuated, within

**TABLE 1.1   Roentgen signs, definitions, and terminology.**

| Roentgen sign | Definitions | Abnormal descriptive terminology |
|---|---|---|
| Size | The relative extent or dimensions of an organ or object on the image. This can be an absolute measurement in mm or cm, or may be a ratio formed by comparison to a standard (i.e., vertebrae, pelvic diameter). The description should always be relative to the expectation of normal for a given species and breed | Enlarged<br>Increased in size<br>Small<br>Reduced in size<br>Distended<br>Dilated |
| Shape | The external shape or contour of an organ or object. Most organs have a narrow range of normal shapes. Intestines are tubular, kidneys are, well, kidney shaped, etc. | Round or rounded<br>Oval<br>Rectangular<br>Triangular<br>Fusiform<br>Broad-based<br>Amorphous |
| Number | A value representing quantity or amount. In its simplest form, we might identify that there are 2 kidneys, 7 lumbar vertebrae, or 10 pulmonary nodules. But we also might use this to characterize the specific quantity of cardiac chambers or liver lobes enlarged or affected by disease | Value (i.e., 3 pulmonary nodules)<br>Increased in number (compared to normal or a prior study)<br>Decreased in number<br>Numerous |
| Margin | The edge or border of a structure or organ. | Smooth<br>Well-defined<br>Ill-defined<br>Regular<br>Irregular<br>Sharp<br>Normal or abnormal contour |
| Location | Place or position. Most organs have a normal, expected position that can be altered by disease. In many cases, the position of an organ may be altered by an adjacent abnormality. Recognizing this is key to understanding the lesion. Knowledge of radiographic anatomy is of the utmost importance. Remember that "Anatomy is Power!" | Normal<br>Displaced (dorsally, ventrally, laterally, to the left, etc.) |
| Opacity | The relative ability to attenuate x-rays. There are five radiographic opacities. Relative differences in the soft tissue opacity of organs are often related to physical density or thickness | Gas, fat, soft tissue/fluid, mineral/bone, metal |

the x-ray beam as it passes through a patient. Gas has a small physical density and does not attenuate x-rays. Therefore, things that contain gas are black, or less opaque on a radiograph. We see this in the lungs and the gastrointestinal tract. We should note the presence of gas where it is unexpected. Fat is more dense than gas and attenuates more x-rays. Therefore, it appears gray on radiographs. Soft tissue attenuates even more x-rays than fat, and has the same density as fluid. It is important to realize that soft tissue structures (e.g. aortic walls) and fluid (e.g. the blood within the aorta) cannot be distinguished radiographically. As with gas, it is always important to document the presence of fluid in a space in which it does not belong or is excessive (pleural space, peritoneal space, retroperitoneal space, subcutaneous tissues).

Next on the opacity continuum is mineral. Bone is probably the most recognizable mineral opacity on a radiograph, but recall that many processes result in accumulation of abnormal

mineral, including but not limited to dystrophic mineralization, metastatic mineralization, uroliths, nephroliths, etc. At the end of the continuum is metal. Metal attenuates, or stops, all x-rays, and therefore appears white (radiopaque) on a radiograph. Examples are barium, microchips, surgical plates, and some foreign bodies.

In addition to describing abnormal opacities, one may also identify the relative uniformity of an organ or structure by using terms such as *homogeneous* or *heterogeneous*. The presence of variable opacities in a structure that is normally uniform can be described in terms of heterogeneity. Recognizing heterogeneity in a normally homogeneous structure can be an important finding.

While the above process is described in the context of radiographic interpretation, this tool set is similar for all imaging modalities. The Roentgen approach is still the method by which abnormalities should be characterized, though we modify the terminology around the Roentgen sign of *opacity*, which

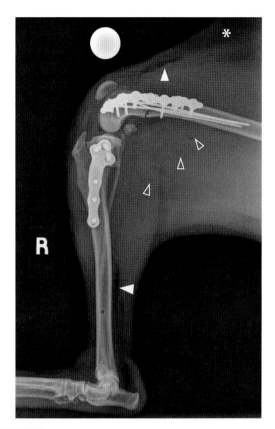

**FIGURE 1.2**   Postoperative lateral radiographic image of the right crus of a dog that contains all radiographic opacities. Gas is evident outside the patient, but also notice the subcutaneous gas cranial to the femur and caudal to the distal tibia (arrowheads). Gas is also superimposed/within the musculature caudal to the crus (open arrowheads). Fat is present in the subcutaneous tissues (asterisk). The musculature of the limb is soft tissue opaque. The variable shades of soft tissue are related to thickness. The femur, tibia, fibula, tarsal and metatarsal bones are mineral opacity. The implants are metal opaque.

| TABLE 1.2 | Relative consistency (optical density on the image) by modality. | |
| --- | --- | --- |
| **Modality** | **Characteristic** | **Terminology** |
| Radiographs | Opacity | Gas, fat, soft tissue, mineral, metal |
| Ultrasound | Echogenicity | Hyperechoic, hypoechoic, anechoic |
| Computed tomography | Attenuation/density | Hyperattenuating/ hyperdense |
| | | Hypoattenuating/ hypodense |
| Magnetic resonance imaging | (Signal) Intensity | Hyperintense, increased signal intensity |
| | | Hypointense, decreased signal intensity |
| Nuclear medicine | Radiopharmaceutical Uptake Activity | Increased/decreased radiopharmaceutical uptake |

abnormalities. Your knowledge base and clinical acumen will help you determine the value of each finding. Connecting the abnormal findings to abnormal pathophysiologic mechanisms is the next step, allowing you to generate differential diagnoses and, ultimately, your next clinical step.

represents the relative signal or consistency of an object as defined by its ability to attenuate x-rays. Other imaging modalities also characterize the consistency of tissue relative to the signal that they generate (Table 1.2).

Using this tool set is predicated on our understanding of normal radiographic anatomy, and the many normal breed and species variations that exist. You can imagine that a dachshund and Great Dane will differ dramatically from one another, yet still be normal for the breed. Each of these Roentgen signs can be normal or abnormal and, depending on the type of abnormality we describe, can help paint a picture of disease. This tool set also requires careful and intentional application. It is very easy and tempting to skip portions of the process, which can result in clinical errors. Following a regular, standardized, and consistent approach to image evaluation will ensure that you are thorough, and that you understand your findings.

The standard approach begins with the interpretation paradigm, or map, that guides you through the anatomy present in the image. This map ensures that you do not skip any portion of the process, and you use the appropriate tools to describe

# General Interpretation Concepts

There are a few concepts that will come up regularly as we review images. In Figure 1.3 the image on the left has a plastic container and two surgical gloves filled with water. One glove is suspended over the box, while the fingers of the other glove are immersed in the container. On the right, the same two water-filled gloves are there, and you'll notice that some of the fingers overlap. Remember, water is soft tissue/fluid opaque, therefore these items should attenuate the same number of x-rays and therefore have the same opacity. However, you'll notice that not all of these areas have the same exact opacity. In the upper left of the first image (Figure 1.3A), you see that in the region of the image where the glove and the container overlap, the opacity is greater than the container alone. In the right image (Figure 1.3B), where the fingers overlap, you see that the opacity is greater, and that the palms of the gloves are more opaque than the individual fingers. This is because there is a difference in the physical thickness of these regions, and that difference translates to a difference in x-ray attenuation. The thicker part attenuates more x-rays than the thinner part, despite the fact that both are fluid. When multiple soft tissue opaque structures are superimposed on one another, the overall attenuation of x-rays is additive, and is called *summation*.

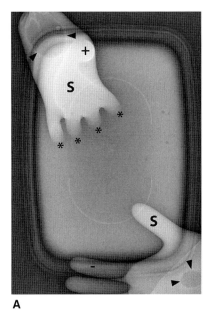
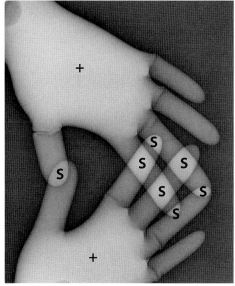

A                                      B

**FIGURE 1.3**   Radiographs of a plastic container and two surgical gloves filled with water (**A**) and of two surgical gloves in which the fingers have various degrees of superimposition (**B**). In both gloves, there are small gas bubbles (black arrowheads). In (**A**), note that the thumb in the lower right of the image and the palm of the glove in the upper left are more opaque than the water in the container due to summation (S). The index finger of the glove in the lower right (-) is less opaque than the thumb and the palm of the same glove. Some of this can be explained by summation, but some is also a result of differences in the physical thickness of these structures. The margins of the fingers of the glove in the upper left are almost completely lost in the container. These margins are border effaced as they are immersed in the water. Both the fingers and the water in the container have the same opacity. The thumb of the glove in the upper left (+) is also very opaque. This thumb is viewed "end-on", as if pointing down at the container, creating even greater summation in this orientation. The margins of this thumb remain visible, as it is not immersed in the water. In (**B**), note that in the regions in which the fingers of the two gloves overlap, the overall opacity is increased compared to the individual fingers alone (S). This is another example of summation. Note that the margins of these digits are all well defined. While there is summation, there is gas surrounding each digit, highlighting the margins. There is no border effacement here. Also, the palms of each glove (+) appear slightly more opaque than the digits. This is due to the greater physical thickness of the palms compared to the digits. There is more water for the x-rays to penetrate, therefore more x-rays are attenuated, creating a more opaque region despite the fact that this is the same material (water).

Also note that the fingers that are immersed in the water-filled container are not visible. This is because the fingers are surrounded by the same opacity, and the margins of the fingers have become *border effaced*. This means that the margins of two structures of the same opacity, when in contact with one another, cannot be differentiated as separate structures (called *border effacement*). This is why you will not see hepatic veins or portal veins in the liver, why you will not differentiate fluid in the urinary bladder or intestines from the wall of those structures, or why you cannot see the individual chambers of the heart on a plain radiograph. These changes are seen commonly on radiographs, so make sure that you have an understanding of these radiographic concepts.

# Organizing Information/ Abnormalities

It is important to organize data to assist in pattern recognition. The process of organization can be divided into four parts: the description of abnormalities, the conclusion or summary statement, the differential diagnosis list, and next steps. The first step, the description, is the process of using Roentgen signs to evaluate anatomic abnormalities noted in the image. The second step, the conclusion, consists of interpreting the findings individually and in the context of other abnormalities and recognizing patterns. In the third step, we construct a list of probable diseases that have pathophysiologic mechanisms that could explain the imaging abnormalities or that fit the pattern observed.

There are a large number of possible radiographic presentations for a disease process. Although this text is an atlas, it cannot present all possibilities, just common examples of them. Part of the reason for this is the timeline of the disease process. The image created during radiography represents a snapshot in the timeline of a disease process. When are we taking the image relative to the severity of disease? Other factors such as individual variations in response to disease (dealing with a biological system) as well as the severity of disease are important factors.

In the final part, one must strategically select next steps that might help to arrive at a definitive or final diagnosis, or list possible treatment options for the disease process that is the primary consideration based on the signalment, physical examination, and other tests done in assessing the patient.

In the description, you will use Roentgen signs to identify and describe any abnormalities on the image. Be sure to use all available projections and ensure there is a complete study (technique and position are critical).

In the next section, you draw conclusions based on your observations. For example, you may have described a soft tissue bulge in the region of the left atrium and lateral displacement of the principal bronchi on the ventrodorsal/dorsoventral image. Your conclusion on this could be "left atrial enlargement." If you also described a bulge or enlargement in the region of the left ventricle and an increase in apical to basilar length of the heart with dorsal displacement of the carina, you might also conclude that there is "left ventricular enlargement." If you indeed have both, you might draw a broader conclusion of "left-sided cardiomegaly." This broader conclusion will feed into the next step, defining your differential diagnoses.

For differential diagnoses, one must reflect on the conclusions, and list the most probable diseases that might explain the conclusions or summary statements by trying to tie all the concluding statements together as one disease process. To continue with the above example, you would list the most probable diseases that could cause left-sided cardiomegaly, with consideration of the patient's signalment. If this is a 12-year-old toy poodle, you would likely list myxomatous degeneration of the mitral valve as the primary differential diagnosis. If this is a 6-month-old lab, you might consider congenital dysplasia of the mitral valve primarily. If this is a 10-year-old German shepherd, you might consider endocarditis. And if this is an 8-year-old domestic shorthair cat, you might consider feline cardiomyopathy in all its various forms, which you might prioritize based on likelihood and prevalence. Other diseases may also be on your list, and the prioritization of this list should be filtered through all the other information available at the time of interpretation. As new data is presented, always review the differential list. New information could serve to eliminate or reprioritize your differentials.

As you consider your differentials, remember that the goal is to reduce the level of uncertainty. However, you do not want to inadvertently or erroneously eliminate diseases that should remain in contention as possible causes of the patient's disease pattern. One way to accomplish this is to consider broad categories of disease first and then decide if any can or should be eliminated. This process is incredibly important as it keeps us from excluding diseases that we might dismiss due to any of our biases.

One scheme is the DAMN IT V mnemonic. Each letter stands for one or more general disease categories that might account for the constellation of data that you have before you (Table 1.3). For those potentially offended by this scheme, you might choose to use CITIMITVAN, which functions in the same way (Table 1.4). Always evaluate these lists as you generate differentials to be sure that a disease process is not overlooked. Equally, try to eliminate categories for which a disease

| TABLE 1.3 | Acronym for different disease etiologies (DAMN IT V). |
|---|---|
| D | Degenerative/developmental |
| A | Anomalous (congenital)/autoimmune |
| M | Metabolic |
| N | Neoplastic/nutritional |
| I | Inflammatory/infectious/iatrogenic/idiopathic |
| T | Trauma/toxic |
| V | Vascular |

| TABLE 1.4 | Acronym for different disease etiologies (CITIMITVAN). |
|---|---|
| C | Congenital |
| I | Inflammatory |
| T | Trauma |
| I | Infectious |
| M | Metabolic |
| I | Idiopathic/iatrogenic |
| T | Toxic |
| V | Vascular |
| A | Autoimmune |
| N | Neoplasia/nutritional |

in the specific patient is highly unlikely, improbable, or even nonexistent.

Within each of these broad categories, consider specific disease types that might explain your imaging findings and conclusions. In our cardiac example, we considered congenital, degenerative, and infectious etiologies for left-sided cardiac enlargement, and would prioritize them based on the information we have about the patient, including species, breed, and age. Always run through this list to be sure you do not unintentionally exclude diseases that may explain the patient's history, clinical signs, and imaging findings.

Finally, you need to determine your *next steps*. These may be additional diagnostics, or may consist of therapeutic options. In our example, echocardiography might be the next best step in truly determining the underlying pathology and creating a treatment plan. This will obviously differ depending on the diseases that we identify or suspect. To continue the example, if the patient is in left heart failure and has clinical signs related to the radiographic changes identified, one should always stabilize the patient prior to other diagnostic tests that might add to respiratory stress and compromise the patient further.

# Pitfalls of Interpretation

Many interpretation pitfalls have been characterized. Some are called different names by different specialists. Awareness of the major pitfalls can be important in their avoidance. While the following list is not exhaustive, it serves as a reminder of the more common pitfalls and biases that you may encounter as you continue on the journey toward becoming a radiologist. These are biases that should be avoided. One way to do this is to present the case and radiographic images to a colleague without the clinical information (history and signalment) to hear their interpretation and conclusions. This will help to eliminate some of the biases presented below.

## Framing Bias

Framing bias is a particularly common error. The problem presented in the clinical history may erroneously or incompletely implicate a particular system that influences both the evaluation and interpretation process [2]. A patient is presented for acute vomiting, and the owner suspects that the dog ate something that they can no longer find. We are programmed to look for the foreign body, and we may be sensitized or biased to identify something abnormal in the gastrointestinal tract. The problem may be elsewhere, and if the clinical context we were given was a bit different, we may have directed our search differently. This is why some radiologists choose to review the history and clinical findings after their first review of a study.

## Confirmation Bias

We are often guilty of confirmation bias, which is simply looking for evidence that supports what you already know, or think you know [2]. It is human nature to see only what we actively look for; who does not prefer to have their opinions or ideas validated rather than refuted? When our awareness is raised by new knowledge, whether that is a new journal article identifying a novel finding or an addition to our process that forces recognition of previously ignored features, we hopefully increase our ability to diagnose diseases.

## Satisfaction of Search

Satisfaction of search bias is also common. It is the tendency to halt the search for abnormalities once one has been found [2]. Often patients have more than one abnormality, and while not all abnormalities may be related to the clinical complaint, additional findings may further support a diagnosis. Alternatively, additional findings may implicate an occult process that has not yet declared itself clinically. The radiologist's goal is always to provide a complete diagnostic assessment of the study at hand.

## Availability Bias

Availability bias is probably less common but still prevalent. Also known as heuristic bias, this error occurs when we allow easily recalled experiences to have a large influence on our thinking. It makes us consider diseases that we know about and recall easily, even if they do not apply specifically to a particular case [2].

## Inattention Bias

Inattention bias is also called a location-related error. It is the inability to recognize an abnormal finding within the study because it does not appear in the purposefully evaluated area, or is at the periphery of the study [2]. This is a particular risk when one does not follow an interpretation paradigm, which can help ensure that the entire image is examined thoroughly.

# Conclusion

Diagnostic image interpretation is exciting, challenging, and fun. This chapter has introduced the concepts on which to build a successful interpretation paradigm for evaluating all forms of imaging. Interpretation paradigms will be presented for each of the sections in this book (musculoskeletal, thorax, and abdomen). These paradigms should be used as a starting point for ensuring complete evaluation of the radiographic images. The formulation of conclusions or summaries, differentials and next steps is a critical piece of the puzzle when interpreting radiographic studies. Remember that this process involves continuous learning strategies, and journal clubs/evaluations should be a routine part of the practice of a veterinarian.

# References

1.  Scrivani, P.V. (2002). Assessing diagnostic accuracy in veterinary imaging. *Vet. Radiol. Ultrasound* 43: 442–448.

2.  Gunderman, R.B. (2009). Biases in radiologic reasoning. *Am. J. Roentgenol.* 192: 561–564.

# CHAPTER 2

# Physics of Diagnostic Imaging

**Elizabeth Huyhn[1], Elodie E. Huguet[2], and Clifford R. Berry[3]**

[1] VCA West Coast Specialty and Emergency Animal Hospital, Fountain Valley, CA, USA
[2] Department of Small Animal Clinical Sciences, College of Veterinary Medicine, University of Florida, Gainesville, FL, USA
[3] Department of Molecular Biomedical Sciences, College of Veterinary Medicine, North Carolina State University, Raleigh, NC, USA

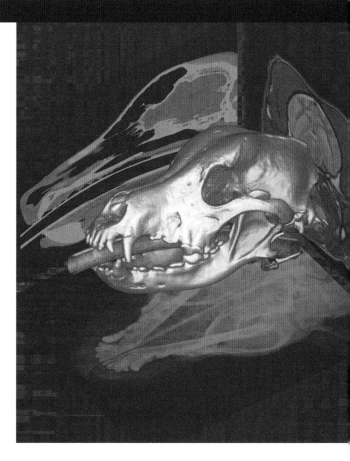

## Overview: Uses and Advantages

Radiography is an imaging technique that uses x-ray attenuation within veterinary patients to obtain two-dimensional images of internal organs and to assess for the presence or absence of disease. Radiography in veterinary medicine can be subdivided into projectional radiography, computed tomography (CT), and fluoroscopy.

Projectional radiography utilizes electromagnetic or ionizing radiation to obtain static two-dimensional images of a three-dimensional patient (body part), which in and of itself presents projection artifacts that have to be properly interpreted as normal or abnormal. Common uses for projection radiography in veterinary medicine include thoracic, abdominal, musculoskeletal, and contrast imaging (Figure 2.1).

Computed tomography uses ionizing radiation reconstructed by a computer to create multiple transverse images of the patient based on the various physical densities compared with the normal attenuation of water (called a Hounsfield unit or HU).

Fluoroscopy also utilizes ionizing radiation to obtain dynamic, real-time images (usually limited by a frame rate of 30 frames/second) that are viewed over time. This modality is used to observe the movement of contrast through the esophagus, cardiac structures, or different vessels, as well as diagnosing dynamic diseases such as a collapsing trachea.

Contrast radiography can be used in projectional radiography, computed tomography, and fluoroscopy to supplement information gained from these modalities. Types of contrast radiography include positive contrast and negative contrast. Common positive contrast agents used include barium sulfate paste or liquid or iodine (i.e., nonionic, iodinated positive contrast medium). In radiography, positive contrast is metallic,

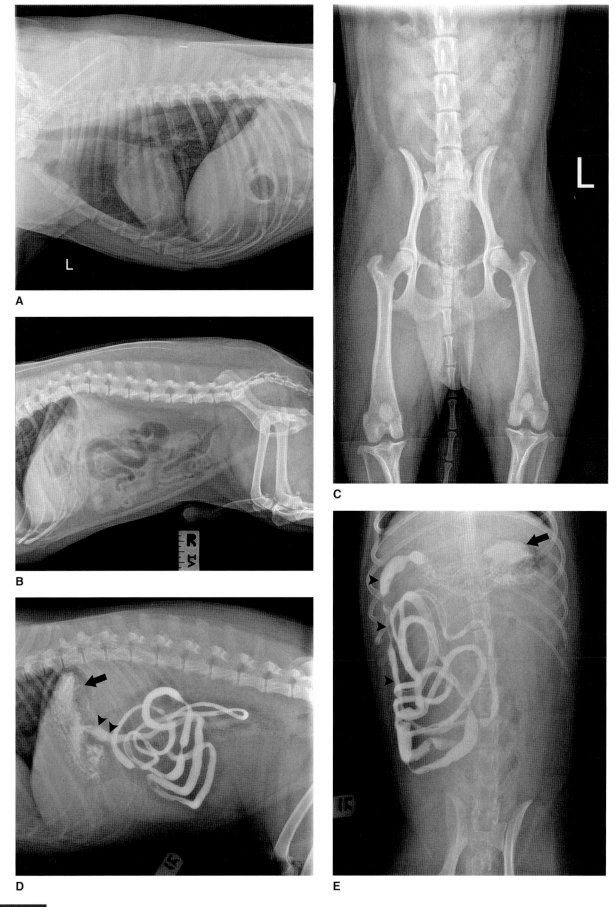

**FIGURE 2.1** (**A**) Left lateral thoracic radiograph in a normal dog. (**B**) Right lateral abdominal radiograph in a normal dog. (**C**) Ventrodorsal pelvis radiograph in a normal dog. (**D**) Right lateral abdominal radiograph after barium positive contrast administration in a normal dog. (**E**) Ventrodorsal abdominal radiograph after barium positive contrast administration in the same patient. Note the positive barium contrast in the stomach (black arrow), duodenum (black arrowheads), and some segments of the jejunum.

so it increases the visibility of the organ or vessel within which it is introduced (Figure 2.1). Negative contrast agents typically used are room air or carbon dioxide which is gas opaque (radiolucent) on the image (Figure 2.2). Double-contrast studies can be done using a combination of positive and negative contrast media to give optimal detail of a mucosal surface such as the urinary bladder (Figure 2.3) [1].

Digital projectional radiography is used as a common first-step modality in diagnostic imaging as it is relatively affordable and can be obtained quickly. Digital radiography has an increased dynamic range which implies that the anatomy has varying density values that can be visualized. Using a broad scale contrast display, all the anatomy can be seen in the radiographic image within the displayed range of optical densities. The displayed densities can be adjusted according to the contrast and brightness of the image. The contrast and brightness of the image are attained through window width and window level. If changes to the window width are made,

the contrast of the image will change; when the window width narrows, there is increase in the displayed contrast. If changes to the window length are made, the brightness of the image will change.

# Basics of X-Ray Interaction in Matter

To understand how radiographs are made, it is important to recognize how photons interact with matter. Photons can interact with matter via (i) coherent scattering, (ii) photoelectric effect, (iii) Compton scattering, (iv) pair production, and (v) photodisintegration [2]. Pair production and photodisintegration have no relevance to diagnostic radiology so they will not be reviewed further.

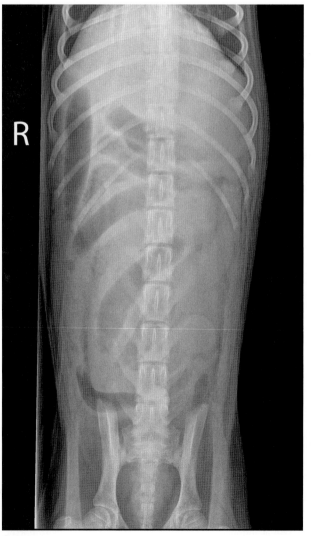

**A**

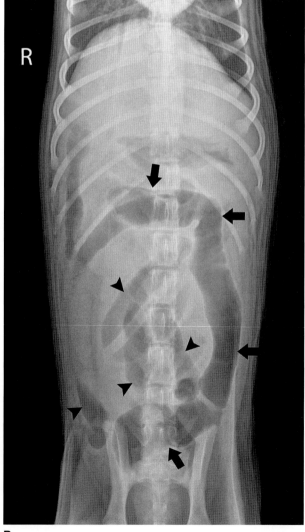

**B**

**FIGURE 2.2** (**A**) Survey ventrodorsal abdominal radiograph. (**B**) Ventrodorsal abdominal radiograph after a pneumocolon. Note the distinguishing margins of the colon (black arrows) in relation to the fluid- and gas-dilated segments of the small intestine (black arrowheads).

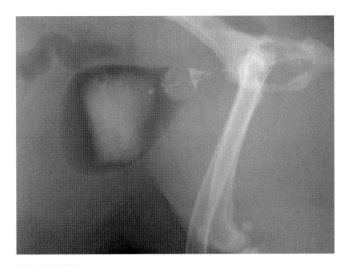

**FIGURE 2.3**  Double contrast medium cystogram outlining the inner mucosal wall with negative contrast medium (room air) and there is a central pool of positive iodinated contrast medium for the evaluation of cystoliths, clots, masses, etc.

## Coherent Scattering (Figure 2.4)

Coherent scattering is not useful in the production of a radiographic image. When a photon interacts with an object with subsequent directional change, the object does not absorb the photon but rather scatters it, and consequently degrades the image and increases personnel exposure if present within the x-ray room at the time of exposure. The goal of all radiographic procedures would be "hands free" imaging, where all personnel are out of the x-ray room at the time the exposure is made.

## Photoelectric Effect (Figure 2.5)

Photoelectric effect is the most important type of photon interaction that produces a radiographic image. The photon striking the patient is completely absorbed by an inner k-shell electron without scatter. The photons that are not absorbed or attenuated create the radiographic image. Differential absorption is based on the physical density, patient thickness, atomic number (Z), and the energy (kVp) of the x-ray beam.

## Compton Scattering (Figure 2.6)

When a photon interacts with a peripheral shell electron of an atom, this electron is ejected, and the photon is then scattered in any direction at a lower energy. The probability of a Compton reaction increases with increasing photon energy. If Compton absorption predominates in a reaction, the radiographic image will have poor contrast, degrading the image. Compton scattering will also increase personnel exposure.

# Radiation Safety

Basic principles of radiation safety should always be practiced when making radiographic images (Table 2.1). All levels of ionizing radiation should be considered dangerous and the ALARA (As Low As Reasonably Achievable) principle should be observed at all times [3].

The three major principles of ALARA are time, distance, and shielding. Time is important to reduce the time of exposure.

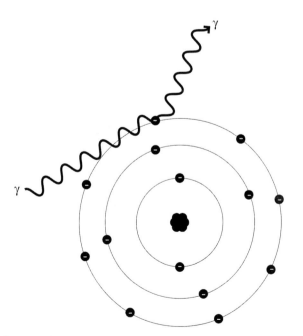

**FIGURE 2.4**  Coherent scatter. Note the incoming photon (γ) is absorbed then immediately reemitted with minimal direction and energy change. This photon may result in radiographic film fog and is only significant at very low diagnostic x-ray energies.

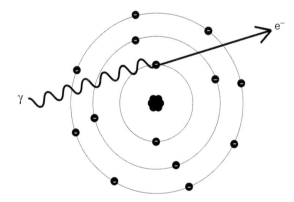

**FIGURE 2.5**  Photoelectric effect. Note the incoming photon (γ) interacting with the orbital electron in the inner shell. The orbital electron (e-) becomes dislodged (the energy of the incoming photon must be greater than or equal to the electron's energy). The incoming photon gives up all its energy and the ejected electron is now a photoelectron. The photoelectron can interact with other atoms which results in increased patient dose, contributing to biological damage. When the orbital electron is dislodged, the vacancy is filled by an electron from the outer shell. Once the vacancy is filled, that electron releases its energy in the form of a characteristic photon. Emission of characteristic photons continues until the atom becomes stable.

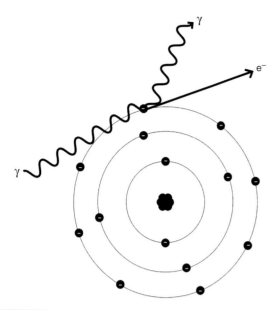

**FIGURE 2.6** Compton scatter. Note the incoming photon (γ) is partially absorbed in an outer shell electron, which absorbs enough energy to break the binding energy, and then becomes ejected (e⁻). The ejected electron is a Compton electron. The incoming photon (γ) continues on a different path with less energy as scattered radiation. The scattered photon can interact with other atoms via photoelectric effect or Compton scattering.

| TABLE 2.1 | Principles of radiation safety for veterinary medicine. |
| --- | --- |

1. The use of "hands free" exposures (all personnel out of the x-ray room at the time of x-ray exposure of the patient) should be the goal of every practice.

2. Sandbags, sponges, tape, and positioning devices should be used to accomplish "hands free" exposures. Adequate sedation or general anesthesia should be used when appropriate.

3. Collimate the primary beam to the area of interest, recognizing that the smaller the collimated field, the greater the reduction in x-ray scatter.

4. All personnel operating the equipment should be properly trained in usage of the equipment, proper anatomic positioning, technique, and transfer of images to different workstations and work environments (i.e., telemedicine).

5. If personnel are in the room at the time of the exposure, then:
   - always wear lead apron, gloves, and thyroid shields
   - always wear radiation detection badges to monitor exposure and adhere to strict guidelines for rotating personnel in radiology to minimize exposure to any one individual
   - never have any part of the personnel in the primary x-ray beam even if wearing lead (lead only protects against scatter radiation, not the primary beam)
   - personnel must be over 18 years of age
   - pregnant personnel should never be used for holding patients for x-ray studies.

Note: all states will have different regulations related to radiation safety and it is incumbent upon the end user to determine these rules and laws for the individual practice.

However, personnel excluded from the x-ray room during an exam include those younger than 18 years old and pregnant individuals. All personnel involved with radiography should wear a radiation detection badge and appropriate shielding (gloves, apron, thyroid shields) when making exposures. If the distance is doubled between the personnel and radiation source, the radiation exposure is reduced by a factor of four (called the inverse square law). The most effective personal shielding for radiation personnel is lead-impregnated aprons, gloves, thyroid shield, and eyeglasses. Lead aprons and gloves are designed exclusively to protect against scattered radiation and must never be placed in the primary beam because they do not attenuate high-energy x-rays [3, 4].

# Digital Radiography

Digital imaging is the current standard of care for diagnostic radiography, replacing analog film-screen combinations that have been used for decades in human and veterinary medicine [5, 6].

Digital detectors fall into two broad categories: computed radiography (CR) and digital radiography (DR). The DR category is really a misnomer as CR is a form of DR. In CR, an imaging plate (also called the PSP or photostimulable plate) and cassette are placed on the tabletop or in the table tray for radiographic exposures. After an exposure is made, the CR cassette is processed through a reader and the reader then produces an image based on the digital information stored in the imaging plate. This information is then erased and reloaded into the cassette for the next exposure. In DR (direct or indirect), photon-sensitive hardware within the digital plate directly interacts with the photons that are not attenuated by the patient.

The digital systems (DR) available currently include hardwired and wireless indirect, direct or CCD (charge coupled device) types of detectors. A full explanation of these is beyond the scope of this text, but needless to say, digital radiography is here to stay and has replaced the older analog systems.

# Limitations

The primary limitation of projectional radiography is the superimposition of organs causing summation or border effacement (flattening of a three-dimensional object into a two-dimensional image). Orthogonal projections are made to help create a three-dimensional image in the interpreter's brain. Radiography is a great first step to diagnosing and treating diseases in veterinary patients. When referring to digital radiography, the main disadvantage in relation to film-screen radiography is decreased spatial resolution, but enhancement techniques are used to improve the perceived spatial resolution of an image.

# References

1. Wallack, S. (2003). *Handbook of Veterinary Contrast Radiography.* San Diego, CA: Veterinary Learning Systems.
2. Bushberg, J.T. (2012). *The Essential Physics of Medical Imaging.* Philadelphia, PA: Wolters Kluwer/Lippincott Williams & Wilkins.
3. Centers for Disease Control and Prevention (2015). ALARA – As Low As Reasonably Achievable. www.cdc.gov/nceh/radiation/alara.html.
4. Thrall, D.E. and Widmer, W.R. (2018). Radiation protection and physics of diagnostic radiology. In: *Textbook of Veterinary Diagnostic Radiology,* 7e (ed. D.E. (e.) Thrall). St Louis, MO: Elsevier.
5. Robertson, I.D. and Thrall, D.E. (2018). Digital radiographic imaging. In: *Textbook of Veterinary Diagnostic Radiology,* 7e (ed. D.E. (e.) Thrall). St Louis, MO: Elsevier.
6. Widmer, W.R. (2008). Acquisition hardware for digital imaging. *Veterinary Radiology and Ultrasound,* 49: s2–s8.

# CHAPTER 3

# Computed Tomography and Magnetic Resonance Imaging

**Elodie E. Huguet[1], Elizabeth Huyhn[2], and Clifford R. Berry[3]**

[1] Department of Small Animal Clinical Sciences, College of Veterinary Medicine, University of Florida, Gainesville, FL, USA

[2] VCA West Coast Specialty and Emergency Animal Hospital, Fountain Valley, CA, USA

[3] Department of Molecular Biomedical Sciences, College of Veterinary Medicine, North Carolina State University, Raleigh, NC, USA

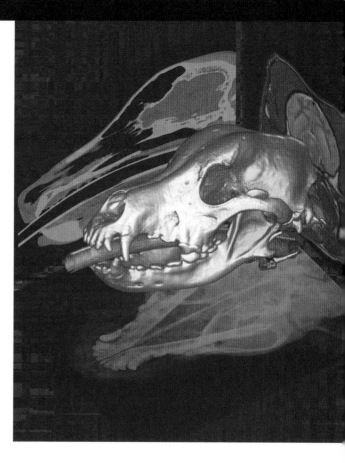

## Overview

The use of cross-sectional imaging modalities, such as computed tomography (CT) and magnetic resonance imaging (MRI), has changed the landscape of diagnostic imaging in veterinary medicine over the past several decades. This chapter will provide an overview (not meant to be comprehensive) of the basics in acquisition and interpretation of these cross-sectional imaging techniques.

## Computed Tomography

### Overview: Uses and Advantages

Computed tomography is a diagnostic imaging modality that creates transverse images of a patient without superimposition of other anatomic structures. The field of view can be selected to give detailed transverse images of the internal organs and areas of interest. The transverse images made during a CT study can also be reconstructed into sagittal, dorsal, and oblique imaging planes and also used to create three-dimensional images of the anatomy of interest.

Computed tomographic exams are usually done in anesthetized or heavily sedated patients to prevent motion artifact, unnecessary repeated examinations and consequently reexposure to ionizing radiation for the patient and possibly personnel. With recent advances in technology, a CT can be done relatively quickly, which is beneficial for a veterinary patient under general anesthesia. CT is often the best imaging modality for detecting a variety of neoplasms since the images allow confirmation of the presence of subtle abnormalities that are potentially not seen on radiographs. CT can also determine size and location for surgical and radiation therapy planning.

## Contrast

Iodine-based contrast media are categorized according to osmolarity (high, low, or iso-), ion formation ability (ionic or nonionic), and the number of benzene rings within the chemical structure (monomer and dimer) [1]. The most commonly used contrast medium for CT in the United States is nonionic, iodinated contrast medium such as iohexol (Omnipaque®) or iopamidol (Isovue®).

Nonionic, iodinated contrast agents cause less discomfort and fewer adverse reactions compared with ionic agents. Adverse reactions to nonionic iodinated contrast medium are rare. When nonionic iodinated contrast medium is given intravenously, adverse reactions include but are not limited to twitching, sinus tachycardia, supraventricular tachycardia, and hyperventilation [2]. When this medium is given intrathecally, adverse reactions include alterations in heart rate and respiratory rate, prolonged apnea, muscle fasciculations, muscle rigidity, seizures, and worsening of neurologic condition [3].

## Basic Physics

Similar to radiographs, CT also exhibits variable absorption of x-rays depending on the physical density of the tissues being imaged. The unit used to express CT values is standardized from the physical densities of tissues compared with water and is called the Hounsfield unit (HU). HUs are obtained from a linear transformation of measured attenuation coefficients. An attenuation coefficient is quantified as the measure of how easily a density of material can be penetrated by an x-ray beam. It quantifies the weakening of the beam when it passes through the material. The linear transformation of the attenuation coefficients is based on the subjectively assigned densities of air and pure water. The radiodensity of distilled water and air at standard temperature and pressure is 0 HU and −1000 HU, respectively. On a CT image, the scale can run from −1000 HU for air to ≥2000 HU for dense osseous structures (Figure 3.1).

The CT image is divided into an array of pixels in the x-y imaging plane. The pixel, short for picture element, is the basic unit of the displayed 2D image. Each pixel represents a voxel, or volume element, which is a 3D volume of tissue described by x, y and z dimensions. Each voxel attenuates the x-ray beam based on the average density of the tissue contained within it. Based on this attenuation, a gray scale value is assigned to the representative pixel in the image.

Window level (WL) is the CT number or HU at the midpoint of the gray-scale display window. The WL is set at the attenuation of the structure being assessed. For example, if bone is being assessed, the WL must be high (Table 3.1). Window width (WW) determines the contrast of an image, with narrower windows resulting in greater contrast [4]. The WW is selected based on what is being compared. If the attenuation of the structures being compared is widely variable, the WW is wide. If the attenuation of the structures being compared is similar, the WW is narrow (Figure 3.2).

## MPR Reconstructions and 3D Renderings

Initial CT images are acquired in the transverse or axial plane using a volumetric data set; in other words, anatomy is scanned in the x-y plane in relation to the bore of the CT machine

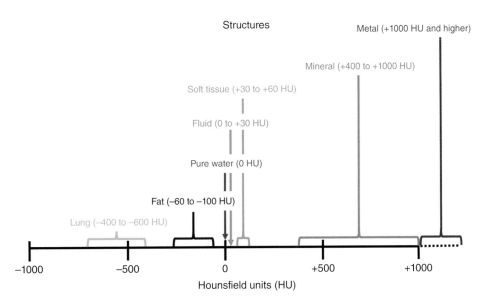

**FIGURE 3.1** Hounsfield units (HU) scale. Note the HU range for different anatomic structures.

| TABLE 3.1 | Window width and window level in Hounsfield units (HU). | |
|---|---|---|
| **Structures of interest** | **Window width (HU)** | **Window level (HU)** |
| Lung | 1500 | −400 |
| Soft tissue | 400 | +50 |
| Bone | 1600 | +500 |

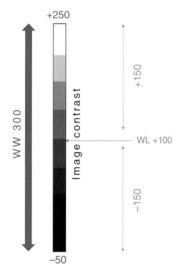

**FIGURE 3.2** Example of window width (WW) and window level (WL). Note that arbitrarily the WL is set at 100 HU and the WW is 300 HU, there is 150 HU above and 150 HU below the gray scale (150 + 150 = 300). In this case, greater than +250 HU will be hyperattenuating (toward the white part of the image contrast scale) and less than −50 HU will be hypoattenuating (toward the black part of the image contrast scale).

(z-axis of the patient). These sets of initial axial images contain information in three dimensions and are used to reconstruct images to be displayed in different planes (Figure 3.3). In veterinary medicine, sagittal and dorsal plane reconstructed images are typically made from the volumetric data set of axial images at the CT computer prior to review of the data set. This data set (raw data) typically consists of axial images with a section thickness of ≤1 mm, preferably with an overlapping interval as the spatial resolution of the sagittal or dorsal plane images is usually reduced compared to the axial plane [5]. The in-plane pixel dimensions approximate the x-y-axis resolution, but the slice thickness limits the z-axis resolution. Sagittal and dorsal multiplanar reformatted (MPR) images combine the x- or y-axis dimensions of the CT image with image data along the z-axis, and therefore a mismatch in spatial sampling and resolution occurs during reconstruction with significantly thick slices (3, 5, or 10 mm slice thickness) [4].

Multiplanar reformations enable images to be displayed in a different orientation from the original one. These multiplanar reformations include maximum-intensity projection (MIP) (Figure 3.4), minimum-intensity projection (MinIP) (Figure 3.5), surface rendering (Figure 3.6), volume rendering (VR) (Figure 3.7), and virtual endoscopy (Figure 3.8).

Maximum-intensity projection enables the evaluation of each voxel (volume element within the image) along a line from the viewer's eye through the volume of data and to select the maximum voxel value, essentially transforming a two-dimensional image into a three-dimensional image with increased conspicuity of the most attenuating structures, such as bone and contrast medium [6]. MIP is helpful when assessing the pulmonary parenchyma for pulmonary metastatic disease. The relative attenuation of a pulmonary metastatic nodule is increased compared to normal aerated pulmonary tissue, thereby increasing its conspicuity on MIP images.

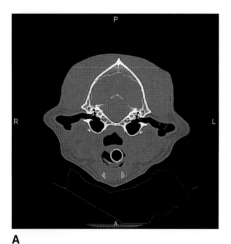
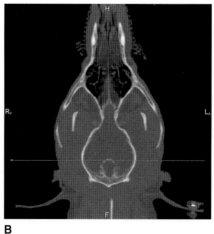
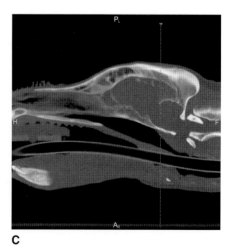

**A**      **B**      **C**

**FIGURE 3.3** Skull CT of a dog in bone algorithm. **A:** Transverse plane of the skull at the level of the tympanic bullae. **B:** Dorsal plane of the skull at the level of the cribriform plate. Note the dotted line demarcating the region where the transverse plane intersects from Figure 3.3a. **C:** Sagittal plane of the skull along the midline. Note the dotted line demarcating the region where the transverse plane intersects from Figure 3.3a.

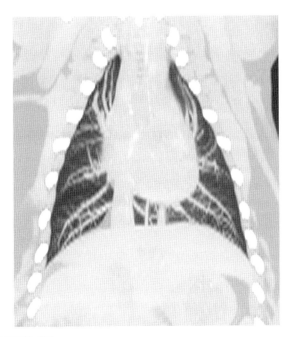

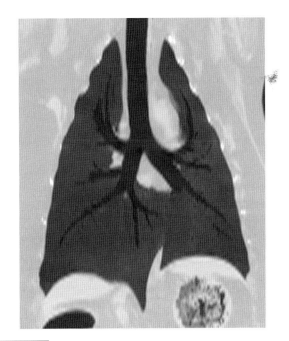

**FIGURE 3.4**   Maximum-intensity projection (MIP) of the thorax in a dog in the dorsal plane at 32 mm slice thickness. Note the increased conspicuity of the hyperattenuating tissues of the bone, heart, and pulmonary vasculature after contrast medium administration.

**FIGURE 3.5**   Minimum-intensity projection (MinP) of the thorax in the same dog as Figure 3.4 in the dorsal plane at 32 mm slice thickness. Note the increased conspicuity of the hypoattenuating tissues of the bronchi and pulmonary parenchyma.

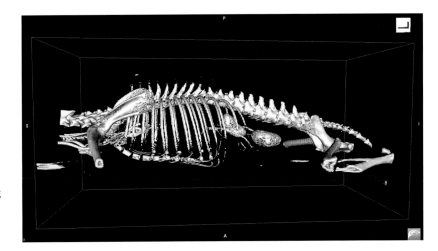

**FIGURE 3.6**   Surface rendering. Hyperattenuating values are selected for this surface rendering with visualization of the osseous structures and organs with contrast medium enhancement.

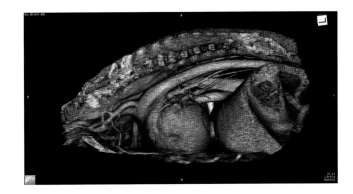

**FIGURE 3.7**   Volume rendering (VR) image of the thorax of a dog using Horos®, an open *source* media image software (Horos™, https://horosproject.org/). Note the visualization of the heart and thoracic vasculature mimicking a lateral thoracic radiograph.

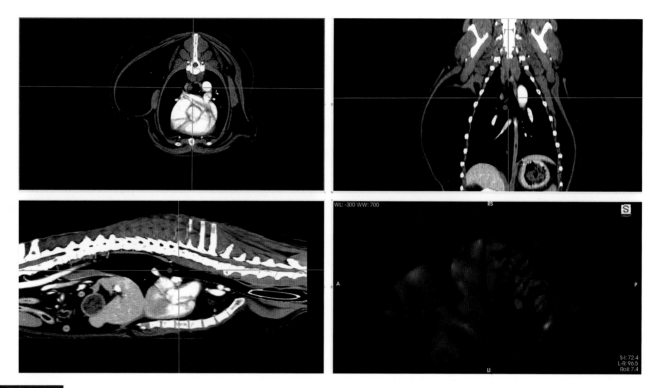

**FIGURE 3.8**    Virtual endoscopy of the carina of a dog using Horos. Note that the top left image is a transverse plane, the top right image is a dorsal plane, and the bottom left image is a sagittal plane, all denoting the pink caliper and green cross-hairs to delineate the carina as the region of interest. The bottom right is the image produced using the three planes to create a 3D intraluminal image of the carina, mimicking a tracheoscopy/bronchoscopy image.

Minimum-intensity projection images are multiplanar slab images produced by displaying the lowest attenuation value through an object toward the viewer's eye, which is the opposite to MIP [7]. For MinP images, the most hypoattenuating structures are represented and are useful in detecting subtle pulmonary changes and otherwise hypoattenuating lesions.

Surface rendering is a process in which apparent surfaces are determined within the volume of data and an image representing the derived surfaces is displayed [6, 8].

Volume rendering takes the entire volume of data, sums the contributions of each voxel along a line from the viewer's eye through the data set, and displays the resulting composite for each pixel of the display [6, 8]. To optimize the anatomic structures, VR enables modulation of WW and level, opacity, and percentage classification, and enables the interactive change of perspective of three-dimensional rendering in real time [6].

Virtual endoscopy is a computer simulation of an endoscopic perspective obtained by processing volumetric data [6]. Virtual endoscopy can be used to assess hollow viscus organs noninvasively, such as the respiratory tract and gastrointestinal tract.

## Gated Studies

Electrocardiographic gated CT examinations are done on patients with aortic arch or other cardiovascular pathology. The benefits of gated cardiac CT include the removal of motion artifact with high temporal and spatial resolution in patients with variable heart rates. Two methods of cardiac gated CT

exist: (i) prospective EKG-triggered sequential CT scanning and (ii) retrospective EKG-gated spiral scanning [9].

Prospective EKG-triggered sequential CT scanning synchronizes the motion of the heart to acquire data in the diastolic phase. In the diastolic phase, cardiac motion is very minimal. Retrospective EKG-gated spiral scanning synchronizes the movement of the heart by using a simultaneously recorded EKG tracing. The advantage of retrospective over prospective is that retrospective provides an isotopic, three-dimensional data set of the cardiac volume without intervals and misregistration of data because it acquires information during all phases of the cardiac cycle [9].

## Safety

Safety guidelines for personnel operating the CT are similar to those used in routine radiography and based on the basics of radiation safety and protection as outlined in Chapter 2. Compared to MRI, CT acquisition times are much shorter, so the patient can be either heavily sedated or undergo general anesthesia for diagnostic CT imaging.

## Limitations

Some limitations of CT include the high cost of purchasing and maintaining a CT machine. The inner workings of a CT machine are complex, thus requiring a specialist who is

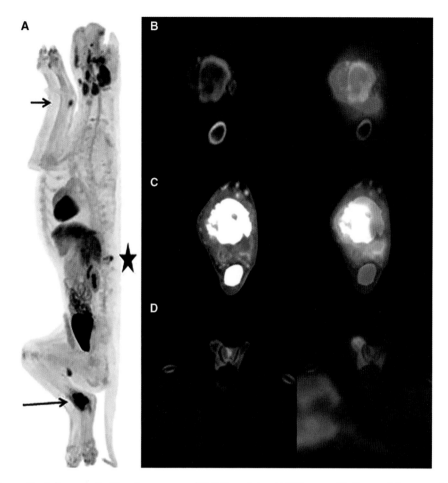

**FIGURE 3.9** PET-CT in a patient diagnosed with osteosarcoma. (**A**) Oblique lateral MIP image with the cranial aspect of the patient at the top and the dorsal aspect on the right side of the image. It shows a primary osteosarcoma lesion in the left tibia (long black arrow), a metastatic lesion to the left radius (short black arrow), and a metastatic lesion to the articular process of L1 vertebra (star). In the soft tissues adjacent to the left tibia, there is a hot spot, indicating hypermetabolism of the left popliteal lymph node. (**B**) Transverse CT image in a bone window, showing osteolysis and periosteal proliferation of the primary tibial neoplasm. The image to the right is a fused PET-CT image at the same location showing the hypermetabolic activity of the neoplasm. (**C**) Transverse CT image in soft tissue window showing soft tissue swelling with contrast enhancement surrounding the mass. The image on the right is a fused PET-CT image at the same location showing hypermetabolic activity of the bone and soft tissue abnormalities. (**D**) Transverse CT image in a bone window showing osteolysis and expansion of the articular process of L1 and sclerosis of the pedicle. The image on the right is a fused PET-CT image at the same location showing the hypermetabolic activity in the articular process. *Source:* Courtesy of Elissa K. Randall, DVM, MS, DACVR.

designated to operate the machine. Another disadvantage of the CT images in relation to other modalities is that the spatial resolution is poorer than film and dental radiographs, which limits assessment of details. Additionally, CT is best used to assess osseous structures than soft tissue structures when compared to MRI. However, for angiographic studies, CT provides the best spatial resolution and anatomic detail when compared with MRI.

## PET-CT

Positron emission tomography-CT is a combined modality using the technology of CT and nuclear scintigraphy (Figure 3.9). The combined method uses small amounts of radiopharmaceuticals to evaluate organ and tissue function by overlaying the nuclear scintigraphy image over a more anatomically detailed CT image. This allows veterinarians to evaluate specific organ anatomy and tissue function at the same time.

# Magnetic Resonance Imaging

## Overview

The use of MRI in veterinary medicine has grown in response to the increased availability and speed of MRI systems [10–13]. Based on the detected response of nuclei within atoms to a strong magnetic field created by the MRI unit, images of normal anatomic structures and pathology can be produced with good contrast and anatomic resolution. MRI can be used to image a wide range of body systems and is most used to evaluate structures of the central and peripheral nervous system. In some cases, MRI may provide a useful assessment of the cardiovascular and musculotendinous structures.

Specific paramagnetic contrast agents may be administered to increase the conspicuity of cardiovascular structures and soft tissue pathology. Gadolinium contrast medium is used in veterinary medicine and consists of gadolinium ions bound to variable brand-dependent chelating agents, which counteract the toxic effects of gadolinium. Gadolinium contrast medium is injected intravenously and excreted through the renal system. In patients with renal insufficiency, gadolinium contrast medium should be used with caution. Some MR sequences, such as phase contrast MR-angiography or time-of-flight, may be used to increase the signal intensity of the vasculature without using contrast agents.

In order to decrease motion artifacts associated with respiration or cardiac contractions, the acquisition of MRI sequences can be synchronized to the respiratory or cardiac cycles using different gating techniques. The images may then be reviewed and correlated to the phase of the respiratory or cardiac cycle during which the images were prospectively acquired.

Magnetic resonance imaging is noninvasive and does not use ionizing radiation, so it has favorable safety benefits for patients and veterinary personnel. Due to the increased time required to acquire MRI images and the inherent sensitivity of MRI to motion, general anesthesia is necessary to optimize the quality of MRI images. MRI systems used in veterinary medicine commonly range between 0.2 and 3 tesla. MRI systems of lower field strengths have made MRI more affordable and easier to integrate in veterinary practices. However, trade-offs of low-field MRI systems include loss of image resolution and longer scan and anesthesia times.

An understanding of the physics of MRI is important for interpretation of MRI images. The brightness or signal intensity of different tissues in the body is dependent on their response to different changes in a magnetic field generated by the MRI unit. A detailed explanation of these principles is beyond the scope of this text but we aim to provide an understanding of the fundamental physical principles and characteristics of commonly used MR pulse sequences.

## Basic Principles

The different parts of the MRI system are illustrated and described in Figure 3.10. When an electric current is transmitted through a wire loop or coil configuration, a magnetic field is created perpendicular to its axis in accordance with *Faraday's law*. The strength of the magnetic field is directly proportional to the applied current and is maintained by reducing the resistance of wires through cooling to near absolute zero temperatures. The act of conducting an electric current through this mechanism is known as superconductivity and is effectively achieved with liquid helium (approximately −270 °C boiling point).

Specific atoms within the body, such as the proton, have a specific magnetic field generated by the rotation of proton nuclei about their axis. The magnetic moment of a nucleus is a vector

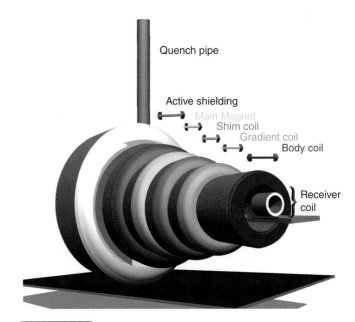

**FIGURE 3.10** Schematic drawing of the different components of the MRI system (main magnet). See text for details.

measurement of the direction and strength of this magnetic field. The most abundant and important nucleus used in MRI is hydrogen ($H^+$). Under normal circumstances, the magnetic moments of these hydrogen atoms are randomly orientated within tissues. When the magnetic field of a hydrogen atom is exposed to the magnetic field created by the MR system, the magnetic moments align with the stronger externally applied magnetic field. The magnetic moments of hydrogen atoms in the body will align in a similar longitudinal plane (z-axis) as the magnetic field; some will align in the same direction as the magnetic moment of the external magnetic field, while others will oppose the direction of the external magnetic field. The *net magnetization vector* represents the difference in direction of these magnetic moments.

When a radiofrequency (RF) pulse with a particular strength and duration is applied, the hydrogen nuclei will be excited, and the net magnetic vector will move away at a particular angle from the longitudinal plane of the external magnetic field. Concurrently, the net magnetic vector will continue to precess in a plane transverse to the external magnetic field. As the net magnetic vector precesses in a transverse plane, it will generate a RF signal into the receiver coil. The strength of the MR signal is proportional to the degree of magnetization present in the transverse plane. When the RF pulse ceases, the net magnetization vector realigns into a longitudinal plane, parallel to the external magnetic field, through a process called T1 recovery. Simultaneously, the net magnetization vector spirals inward as the angle of the net magnetization vector decreases, resulting in a loss of transverse magnetization, or T2 decay. Variations in T1 relaxation and T2 decay times exist in different tissues and in order to demonstrate contrast between normal anatomy and pathology, these differences are exploited.

Image contrast is dependent on the repetition time (TR) and echo time (TE) of a RF pulse sequence. The TR is measured in milliseconds (ms) and represents the time interval between two consecutive RF pulses. In comparison, the TE is the time interval between the RF pulse and the peak signal intensity of the RF energy released during relaxation, also measured in milliseconds (ms). Different contrast is generated between fat and water due to their different T1 recovery and T2 decay times. The T1 recovery and T2 decay time are prolonged in water when compared to fat (Table 3.2). Therefore, images acquired with a short TR and short TE are T1 weighted with increased signal in tissues containing water (Figure 3.11). On the other hand, images acquired with a long TR and long TE are T2 weighted with increased signal intensity in fat (Figure 3.12). When a long TR and short TE is selected, fat cannot be contrasted from water; therefore, the signal intensity generated is instead dependent on the proton density, or number of hydrogen nuclei, in tissues (Figure 3.13).

T2* decay occurs when traverse magnetization is dephased due to magnetic field inhomogeneities. Dephasing with T2* decay occurs at a faster rate than with T2 decay. While small, variations in the magnetic field contribute to T2* decay and may be exacerbated by the presence of ferromagnetic objects, such as implants.

The two principal types of MR pulse sequence acquired are spin-echo (SE) and gradient-echo (GRE). Small variations in these two MR pulses produce a wide array of MR sequences, some with characteristics beneficial for the recognition of normal anatomic and pathologic structures. Within a single TR, both proton density and T2 weighted can be generated to reduce the acquisition time.

| TABLE 3.2 | Repetition time (TR) and echo time (TE) to create T1, T2, and proton density contrast. | |
| --- | --- | --- |
| | **TR** | **TE** |
| T1 weighting | Short | Short |
| T2 weighting | Long | Long |
| Proton density | Long | Short |

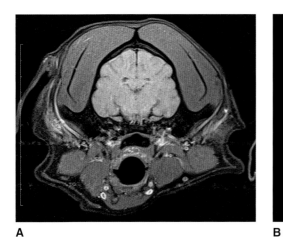
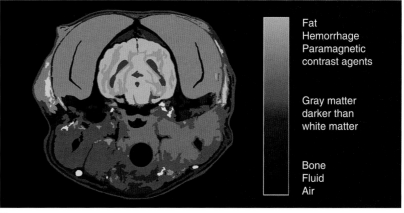

**A**　　　　　　　　　　　　　　　　**B**

**FIGURE 3.11** T1-weighted image (**A**) and schematic drawing (**B**) of a transverse image from a normal canine brain. In the schematic drawing, notice the intensities of the different structures relative to each other.

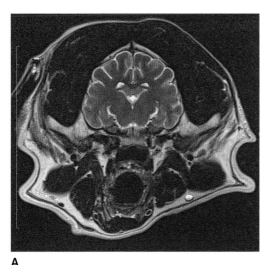
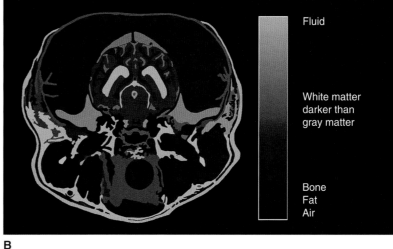

**A**　　　　　　　　　　　　　　　　**B**

**FIGURE 3.12** T2-weighted image (**A**) and schematic drawing (**B**) of a transverse image from a normal canine brain. In the schematic drawing, notice the intensities of the different structures relative to each other.

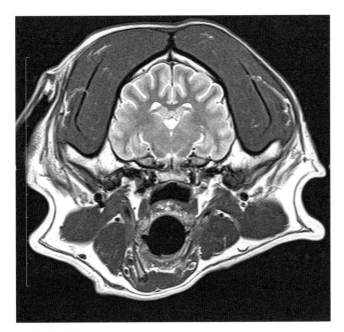

**FIGURE 3.13**    Proton density (PD)-weighted transverse image of a canine brain.

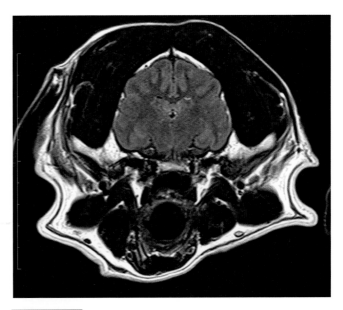

**FIGURE 3.14**    FLAIR image from a normal canine brain where the fluid is attenuated using an inversion recovery sequence.

**Spin-Echo Sequences**    In SE sequences, transverse magnetization is created by an initial 90° RF pulse, which is succeeded by dephasing after cessation of the RF pulse. Dephasing occurs as T2* decay. To rephase the magnetic moments, a 180° rephasing RF pulse is applied so that magnetic moments with a lower precessional frequency lead faster magnetic moments, which eventually "catches up." The recovery of in-phase magnetization in the transverse plane results in signal detection at peak intensity within the receiver coil.

In *fast or turbo spin-echo* sequences, multiple 180° RF pulses are applied in succession within a TR to repeatedly rephase the magnetic moments and generate maximum signal within the receiver coil. The number of successive 180° RF pulses is referred to as the *echo train length* and greatly reduces the acquisition time.

*Inversion recovery* sequences are acquired by applying an initial 180° RF pulse instead of a 90° RF pulse to align the magnetization vector in an opposite direction within the longitudinal plane. The magnetic moments are then allowed to relax until a 90° RF pulse is applied to create heavily T1-weighted images with nulling either fat or water. Signal is maximized in the transverse plane by applying an additional 180° rephasing RF pulse. The time interval between the 180° RF pulse and the 90° RF pulse is known as the inversion time (TI). In the *short tau inversion recovery* (STIR) sequence, fat is nulled by applying a 90° RF pulse at a TI when fat has only transverse magnetization. The magnetic moment of hydrogen atoms in fat recovers full longitudinal magnetization, resulting in no signal detection. Similarly, *fluid attenuated inversion recovery sequences* (FLAIR) are acquired after the application of a 90° RF pulse once water has recovered full transverse magnetization (Figure 3.14). The TE is then adjusted to detect transverse magnetization while

water has only longitudinal magnetization, thereby having no signal.

**Gradient-Echo Sequences**    In GRE sequences, transverse magnetization is generated by a RF pulse often with a flip angle of less than 90 degrees, thereby having both longitudinal and transverse magnetization. Once the RF pulse ceases, T2* decay occurs rapidly and results in a signal called the *free induction decay* (FID). By applying another magnetic field with a gradient in the transverse or phase direction, the magnetic moments with a slower precessional frequency speed up and the faster magnetic moments are slowed, so that the magnetic moments rephase which results in maximum signal intensity in the transverse plane. By reversing the gradient, the magnetic moments can be dephased in a similar fashion.

Because GRE sequences use gradients to rephase and dephase transverse magnetization, T2* decay or field inhomogeneities have a considerable impact on the acquired image, as evidenced by the presence of magnetic susceptibility artifact. The paramagnetic properties of hemosiderin in blood cause magnetic susceptibility artifacts, which are useful when trying to differentiate hemorrhage from other types of fluid.

One of the main advantages of GRE sequences is the decreased scan time, mostly attributed to faster rephasing of transverse magnetization with the use of gradients, instead of a 180° RF pulse. T1 and T2* weighting can be acquired with particular flip angles and timing parameters described in Table 3.3. Specific T1 and T2* weighting parameters are described in Table 3.4.

Based on the motion of water in tissues, the rate of diffusion of water can be differentiated with *diffusion-weighted imaging* (Figure 3.15A). In tissues with restricted water motion, such as those subject to ischemic damage, a high signal intensity will appear on the image. When water is unrestricted, the signal intensity will be decreased. *Apparent diffusion coefficient* (ADC)

| TABLE 3.3 | Signal intensity of tissues in T1-weighted and T2-weighted images. | |
|---|---|---|
| **Signal intensity** | **T1-weighted** | **T2-weighted** |
| High | Fat* | Fluid |
| | Hemorrhage | |
| | Paramagnetic contrast agents, such as gadolinium | |
| | Neurotransmitters in the pituitary | |
| Medium | Gray matter darker than white matter | White matter darker than gray matter |
| Low | Bone | Bone |
| | Fluid | Fat |
| | Air | Air |

* When using Fast Spin Echo or Turbo Spin Echo techniques, fat has high signal intensity on T2 weighted images due to J-coupling.

| TABLE 3.4 | Flip angle, repetition time (TR), and echo time (TE) to create T1 and T2* gradient-echo contrast. | | |
|---|---|---|---|
| | **Flip angle** | **TR** | **TE** |
| T1 weighting | Large | Short | Short |
| T2* weighting | Small | Long | Long |

mapping is often used in conjunction to remove T2-weighted contrast on ADC maps and create an image with signal intensities opposite to those seen on diffusion-weighted images (Figure 3.15B). When interpreted in conjunction with diffusion-weighted images, ADC maps can help determine the chronicity of an ischemic event.

## Image Formation

Using gradients, the signal intensities are located in space along two axes in the phase and frequency encoding directions. In the three-dimensional space the images are acquired, and the third axis serves as the slice selection gradient to determine the thickness and track the position of a slice along its axis. The signals detected are digitalized by encoding the frequencies detected in a two-dimensional graph, known as *K space*. The frequencies in K space are arranged so that centrally located frequencies have a high signal intensity and low contrast resolution, whereas peripherally located frequencies have a low signal intensity and high contrast resolution. The frequencies are then extrapolated from K space to form an image via a process call *Fourier transformation*.

## Safety

While MRI does not generate ionizing energy, the RF pulse used to shift the vector of nuclei transfers energy to the patient and can be measured as the specific absorption rate (SAR). The SAR represents the rate at which this energy (watts) is distributed into a certain tissue mass (kilograms). The SAR is exponentially related to the MRI field strength, so that it is equal to the field strength squared ($B_o^2$) when all other variables are maintained constant. For example, if the field strength is doubled, the SAR is increased by a factor of four. When exposed to elevated SAR levels, thermal injuries have been reported in human patients. The prevalence of these effects remains uncertain in veterinary patients.

While the magnetic field created by the MRI system has tremendous diagnostic utility, the magnetic field acts as a large magnet capable of attracting ferromagnetic objects. The strength of the magnetic field created by the MRI unit will attract

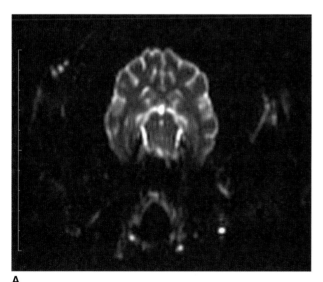

**A**

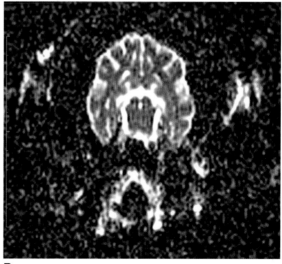

**B**

**FIGURE 3.15**   Diffusion-weighted image (**A**) and calculated ADC map (**B**) of the midbrain from a normal dog.

ferromagnetic objects at extremely high speed, exposing patients and personnel to the risk of projectile injuries. Therefore, it is important that all ferromagnetic objects are properly labeled as MRI unsafe and kept away from the MRI room. MRI may be contra-indicated with particular surgical implants, which may experience motion and torquing induced by the external magnetic field. The movement of surgical implants can induce tissue trauma with possible fatal consequences. Therefore, patients and personnel should always be carefully screened for internal and external ferromagnetic objects prior to entering the MRI room.

# References

1. Beckett, K.R., Moriarity, A.K., and Langer, J.M. (2015). Safe use of contrast media: what the radiologist needs to know. *Radiographics* 35: 1738–1750.
2. Scarabelli, S., Cripps, P., Rioja, E., and Alderson, B. (2016). Adverse reactions following administration of contrast media for diagnostic imaging in anaesthetized dogs and cats: a retrospective study. *Vet. Anaesth. Analg.* 43: 502–510.
3. Fatone, G., Lamagna, F., Pasolini, M.P. et al. (1997). Myelography in the dog with non-ionic contrast media at different iodine concentrations. *J. Small Anim. Pract.* 38: 292–294.
4. Bushberg, J.T. (2012). *The Essential Physics of Medical Imaging*. Philadelphia, PA: Wolters Kluwer/Lippincott Williams & Wilkins.
5. Dalrymple, N.C., Prasad, S.R., Freckleton, M.W., and Chintapalli, K.N. (2005). Informatics in radiology (infoRAD): introduction to the language of three-dimensional imaging with multidetector CT. *Radiographics* 25: 1409–1428.
6. Neri, E., Vagli, P., Odoguardi, F. et al. (2005). *Multidetector-Row CT: Image Processing Techniques and Clinical Applications*. New York: Springer.
7. Ghonge, N.P. and Chowdhury, V. (2018). Minimum-intensity projection images in high-resolution computed tomography lung: technology update. *Lung India* 35: 439–440.
8. van Ooijen, P.M., van Geuns, R.J., Rensing, B.J. et al. (2003). Noninvasive coronary imaging using electron beam CT: surface rendering versus volume rendering. *Am. J. Roentgenol.* 180: 223–226.
9. Bertolini, G. and Angeloni, L. (2017). Vascular and cardiac CT in small animals. In: *Computed Tomography* (ed. A. Halefoglu). www.intechopen.com/chapters/56129.
10. Bushberg, J.T., Siebert, J.A., Leidholdt, E.M. Jr., and Boone, J.M. (2012). *The Essential Physics of Medical Imaging*, 3e. Philadelphia, PA: Lippincott Williams & Wilkins.
11. Thrall, D.E. (2018). *Textbook of Veterinary Diagnostic Radiology*, 7e. Philadelphia, PA: WB Saunders.
12. Westbrook, C. and Talbot, J. (2018). *MRI in Practice*, 4e. Hoboken, NJ: Wiley.
13. Bitar, R., Leung, G., Perng, R. et al. (2006). MR pulse sequences: what every radiologist wants to know but is afraid to ask. *Radiographics* 26: 513–537.

# CHAPTER 4

# Ultrasonography

**Elizabeth Huyhn[1], Elodie E. Huguet[2], and Clifford R. Berry[3]**

[1] VCA West Coast Specialty and Emergency Animal Hospital, Fountain Valley, CA, USA
[2] Department of Small Animal Clinical Sciences, College of Veterinary Medicine, University of Florida, Gainesville, FL, USA
[3] Department of Molecular Biomedical Sciences, College of Veterinary Medicine, North Carolina State University, Raleigh, NC, USA

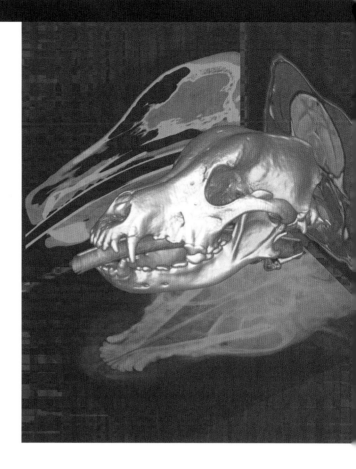

## Overview: Uses and Advantages

Ultrasound is a valuable and noninvasive modality used for the identification and diagnosis of small animal diseases. With advanced training and a good understanding of cross-sectional anatomy, ultrasound can also be used to thoroughly evaluate anatomic structures and abnormalities based on their acoustic impedance. In an emergency room setting, ultrasound is routinely used for the Thoracic or Abdominal Focused Assessment with Sonography in Triage (TFAST or AFAST), for the identification and tracking of abnormal fluid collections. The portability of today's ultrasound equipment allows for cage-side evaluation of veterinary patients. However, this is not the ideal environment for complete abdominal ultrasound evaluations to be done. Using a darkened, quiet room where dogs and cats can be laid on their backs or in lateral recumbency for the scan is important.

Ultrasound can be used to assess all abdominal organs and the heart. The use of echocardiography to assess the cardiovascular structures will be discussed in the cardiovascular chapter.

Ultrasound can provide information related to size, shape, position, margin or contour, echogenicity, and echotexture of the organ being evaluated. Other uses of ultrasound include Doppler ultrasound, elastography, and use of ultrasound-specific contrast agents.

## Basic Physics and Principles of Ultrasound in Diagnostic Imaging

Ultrasound consists of high-frequency sound waves (MHz or 1 000 000 Hz), with the normal human hearing range being between 2000 and 20 000 Hz. Ultrasound waves are thus not

*Atlas of Small Animal Diagnostic Imaging*, First Edition. Edited by Clifford R. Berry, Nathan C. Nelson, and Matthew D. Winter.
© 2023 John Wiley & Sons, Inc. Published 2023 by John Wiley & Sons, Inc.
Companion website: www.wiley.com/go/berry/atlas

audible to the human ear. The ultrasound waves are generated by nonionizing, mechanical compression and relaxation of a special *piezoelectric crystal* inside the transducer that creates a mechanical wave which then travels through the tissues. The sound wave can be generated and recorded at a specific frame rate, depending on the features that are engaged (abdomen typically has a frame rate of 40–80 frames per second compared with echocardiography which will have frame rates of greater than 100 frames per second), allowing the evaluation of static and dynamic structures.

The ultrasound wave will travel through and interact with tissues in a number of different ways. Echoes (reflected ultrasound waves) are created based on the specific intrinsic property of tissue through which the sound wave is passing. This property is called *acoustic impedance* (Z = physical density of the tissue × the speed of sound in the tissue; defined in units of Rayl [gm/m$^2$ s]). These mechanical sound waves return to the ultrasound probe, where they are detected and converted from mechanical into electrical energy and then changed into an anatomic image. This pulse–echo technique results in the transducer "listening" for returning pulses 99% of the time and generating outgoing (sending) pulses 1% of the time.

The ultrasound beam is created by a series of piezoelectric crystals arranged in a curved, linear, or annular format. The first two arrangements are found in transducers used for the abdomen and small body parts. The last is used specifically for echocardiography where crystals do not act in unison but can act independently. This results in the ability to do spectral continuous wave Doppler ultrasound where independent crystals send US waves 100% of the time and different crystals receive and process incoming echoes 100% of the time (see Doppler section of this chapter for more details).

## Interaction of Sound Waves in the Tissues

The ultrasound transducer creates pressure variations in the form of ultrasound waves which travel through the tissues, with resultant interactions being based on variations in physical properties within the tissue and between tissue boundaries. These sound waves have a characteristic speed, frequency, and wavelength with a relationship represented by the following equation:

*Wavelength λ (m) = speed of sound in tissues [c (m/s)]/ frequency [f (MHz)]*. The speed of sound propagating in soft tissues is an average speed of sound and ultrasound machines will use 1540 m/s as the average speed of sound in tissues. The propagation speeds of sound vary for different tissue types as listed in Table 4.1. The frequency corresponds to the number of cycles, or complete waveform of the US wave, per second. Ultrasound imaging transducers used in veterinary medicine have a frequency ranging between 1 and 20 MHz (1 megahertz [MHz] defined as $1 \times 10^6$ cycles per second or Hz).

| TABLE 4.1 | The propagation speeds of sound waves in different tissues. |
|---|---|
| **Tissue** | **Propagation speed of sound (m/s)** |
| Gas | 331 |
| Fat | 1450 |
| Liver | 1549 |
| Kidney | 1561 |
| Brain | 1541 |
| Blood | 1570 |
| Bone | 4080 |

Multiple acoustic variables affect the way sound waves travel in tissues, including pressure, physical density of the tissue, and relative speed within the tissue as well as elastic motion of the tissues themselves. As previously stated, reflection of ultrasound waves within and between tissues is based on differences in *acoustic impedance*. The acoustic impedance increases if the physical density of the tissue and/or the propagation speed of the US sound wave increases. This increase in different acoustic impedances will then result in more ultrasound waves being reflected toward the transducer.

When the ultrasound waves travel in tissues, there are five potential interactions: *reflection, refraction, scattered, absorption* or no interaction and therefore the wave is *transmitted* further into the tissues.

- *Reflection*: occurs when there are differences in acoustic impedance and the ultrasound wave is reflected back toward the transducer (Figure 4.1). If there are no differences in acoustic impedance, then the ultrasound waves are propagated further into the tissues (called *transmission*). Reflectors perpendicular to the incident beam of the ultrasound waves are the best whereas incident ultrasound waves interacting with acoustic boundaries that are parallel to ultrasound beam are poor reflectors. The larger the differences in acoustic impedance, the greater the number of ultrasound waves reflected. For example, there are large differences in acoustic impedance between soft tissues ($1.65 \times 10^6$ Rayls) and bone or mineral ($7.8 \times 10^6$ Rayls) that will result in reflection of all sound waves without transmission of waves to a depth below the soft tissue–mineral interface.

- *Refraction*: refraction differs from reflection in that sound waves being transmitted into bordering tissues with a different acoustic impedance will undergo a change in direction (Figure 4.2). These sound waves may eventually return to the transducer and provide misinformation regarding the position of a tissue in relation to another. This results in refraction artifacts on the image. The degree of displacement or refraction of the sound wave is directly proportional to the propagation speed of the second tissue through which the sound wave travels.

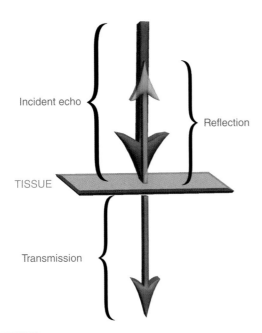

**FIGURE 4.1**  Schematic diagram of the interaction of ultrasound waves at different acoustic interfaces (tissue) whereby some of the incident US waves are reflected toward the transducer and will be used to create an image at depth.

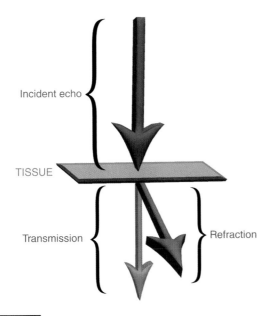

**FIGURE 4.2**  Schematic diagram of the interaction of ultrasound waves at different acoustic interfaces (tissue) whereby some of the incident US waves are refracted and continue into the tissue. These US waves may never contribute to the image.

- *Scattering*: when the sound wave encounters irregular surfaces, heterogeneous tissues, or objects equal to or smaller than the size of its wavelength, it can be redirected in many directions (Figure 4.3). Some of these sound waves may return to the transducer and result in loss of resolution. In comparison, specular reflections occur when sound waves encounter a smooth and flat interface and are returned to the transducer without a change in direction and therefore recorded accurately as to depth.

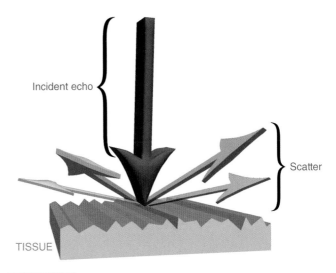

**FIGURE 4.3**  Schematic diagram of the interaction of ultrasound waves at different acoustic interfaces (tissue) whereby some of the incident US waves are scattered in different directions other than being reflected toward the transducer and will not aid in image creation.

- *Absorption*: sound waves attenuated in tissues may be converted into heat, and therefore may not contribute to the final image. Most of the sound waves attenuated in tissues are absorbed. The heat generated consequently contributes to some of the risks associated with ultrasonography and will be discussed later in this chapter.

# Transducer Elements and Characteristics

Piezoelectric crystals within the ultrasound transducer have the unique characteristic of converting an applied voltage into a pressure, or mechanical energy, and vice versa. The mechanical energy created is in the form of high-frequency sound waves which are then returned to the probe and converted into an electrical signal containing information used to create an image.

In addition to the piezoelectric crystals, the transducer consists of the following elements (Figure 4.4).

- *Damping material*: located behind the piezoelectric element to absorb scattered ultrasound energy and decrease the amplitude and spatial pulse length of the ultrasound pulses to increase the spatial resolution of the ultrasound beam. The damping block removes weak echoes, and therefore reduces noise. By doing so, the sensitivity of the ultrasound probe to weak diagnostic echoes is also reduced.
- *Matching material*: reduces the impedance of the transducer element to increase the transmission of ultrasound pulses from the probe into the patient. Without this layer, most of the ultrasound pulses would be reflected at the surface of the ultrasound probe and lost as heat.

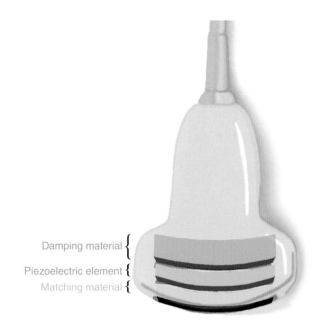

**FIGURE 4.4** Schematic diagram of the ultrasound transducer with different layers of matching material, the actual piezoelectric crystals, and damping material.

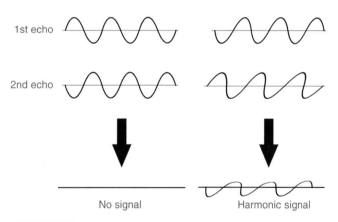

**FIGURE 4.5** Harmonic signal creation within the tissues whereby US waves double their frequency. The machine then "listens" for the higher frequency harmonic signal. Harmonic imaging provides better spatial resolution but at the expense of depth.

Patient preparation is also important to optimize the transmission of sound waves into tissues. The patient should be shaved to maximize contact of the transducer with the skin. Additionally, coupling gel should be applied to remove any air between the transducer and patient, which may impede the transmission of sound waves into the tissues.

Ultrasound transducers with a wide bandwidth are used to generate a range of variable and adjustable frequencies to adjust the image resolution and depth. Additionally, ultrasound transducers with a wide bandwidth permit *harmonic imaging*, which uses higher frequency pulses for the creation of nonsinusoidal ultrasound echoes to enhance image quality (Figure 4.5). Ultrasound transducers with a higher frequency generate images with a higher resolution but have a lower spatial pulse length and do not travel as far within the tissues,

decreasing the imaging depth. Conversely, lower frequency transducers have a lower resolution but improved ability to penetrate tissues.

Linear and sector array transducers are commonly used in veterinary medicine and have advantages and disadvantages described in Table 4.2 (Figure 4.6).

# Image Formation

As previously discussed, sound waves returned to the transducer are converted back into an electrical signal and contain information used to create an image. The information contained within the electrical signal includes the location of origin and intensity of the returning sound wave. The intensity of sound waves in a particular region is assigned a corresponding gray-scale value, with brighter (or more hyperechoic) pixels representing regions of increased intensity and darker (or more hypoechoic) pixels representing regions of decreased intensity.

## Artifacts

Artifacts are incorrect representations of tissues on the image. The misinformation associated with artifacts originates from the attenuation or propagation characteristics of certain sound waves based on their physical characteristics. Therefore, structures on the ultrasound image may be false, absent, misplaced or have an altered structural appearance or echogenicity. Some of the commonly encountered artifacts include the following.

*Shadowing* is seen when tissues that are highly attenuating or strong reflectors reduce or in some cases fully hinder the passage of sound waves into deeper tissues. Subsequently, those tissues are falsely more hypoechoic (Figure 4.7). Inversely, *acoustic enhancement* is observed when sound waves pass through weakly attenuating structures, resulting in stronger sound waves propagating through deeper tissues. Therefore, those tissues are more hyperechoic in appearance (Figure 4.8).

*Reverberation* artifacts commonly occur when sound waves are reflected by gas, mineral, and metal. These materials are strong reflectors, resulting in the return of high-intensity sound waves to the transducer. At the level of the transducer, there is partial return of those sound waves into the tissues, which once again reflect from the same strong reflector. The sound waves ricochet between the strong reflector and transducer to create parallel lines in the far field of the strong reflector on the image (Figure 4.9).

The *mirror image* artifact occurs when the sound waves encounter a strong reflector, such as the diaphragm, and are then reflected toward a structure, such as the liver. The ultrasound beam is then redirected toward the strong reflector, where it is again reflected and returned to the transducer. The delayed return

**TABLE 4.2** Different types and characteristics of ultrasound transducers.

| Types | | Characteristics | Beam path diagrams |
|---|---|---|---|
| Linear probes | Linear array transducer | Ultrasound pulses are generated at different linearly arranged locations within the ultrasound probe to create parallel arrays, which produce a rectangular image (Figure 4.6b) | |
| Sector probes | Phased array transducer | Ultrasound pulses are generated from a single point within the ultrasound probe and diverge to fan out into the tissues and create a sector image (Figure 4.6d) | |
| | Convex array transducer | Ultrasound pulses are generated at different locations along the convex surface of the ultrasound probe to generate diverging arrays and create a sector image (Figure 4.6f) | |

of the sound wave to the transducer results in duplication of the structure on the other side of the strong reflector (Figure 4.10).

As previously discussed, *refraction artifacts* are seen when sound waves being transmitted into bordering tissues with a different acoustic impedance undergo a change in direction. When returned to the transducer, these sound waves are laterally mispositioned on the image (Figure 4.11). The degree of displacement or angle of refraction of the sound wave is directly proportional to the propagation speed of the second tissue through which the sound wave travels, so that tissues with a lower acoustic impedance or density are more laterally displaced on the image.

Weak sound waves, known as *side or secondary lobes*, commonly propagate from the transducer in directions angled away from the primary beam. Also originating from the transducer, *grating lobes* represent similar but stronger divergent sound waves. Most often, these divergent sound waves go undetected, unless they are reflected from a strong reflector, particularly when imaging weakly attenuating regions, such as the urinary bladder (Figure 4.12). Evaluation of body regions in two planes helps to differentiate these artifacts from pathology. Additionally, harmonic imaging improves lateral resolution and reduces image artifacts, like reverberations, and side or grating lobes.

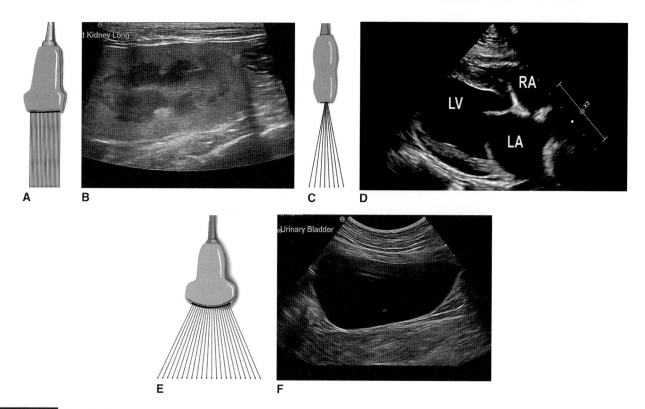

**FIGURE 4.6** (**A,C,E**) Schematic representations of a linear, phased array and convex transducers. (**B,D,F**) Actual ultrasound images acquired with those specific transducers.

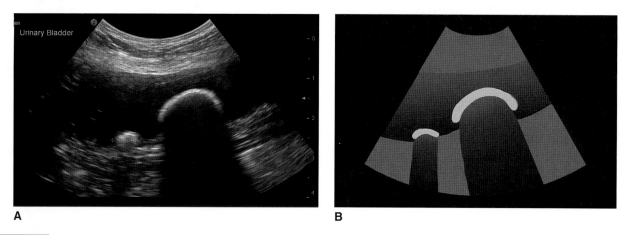

**FIGURE 4.7** Ultrasound image (**A**) and representative schematic (**B**) documenting multiple stones in the urinary bladder with a "clean" shadow deep to the calculus.

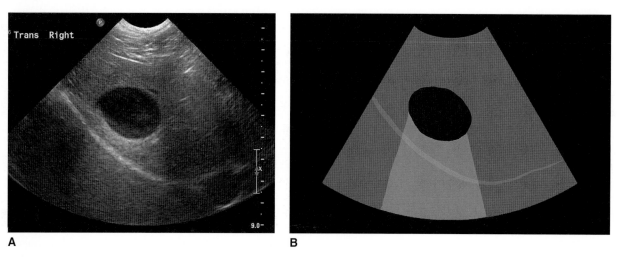

**FIGURE 4.8** Ultrasound image (**A**) and representative schematic (**B**) documenting through transmission where there is decreased attenuation (reflection, refraction, and scattering) of the ultrasound beam and thereby more ultrasound waves available for reflection deep to the cystic structure (in this case, the gall bladder).

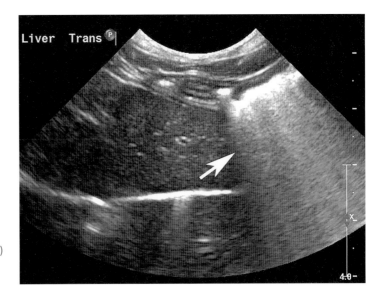

**FIGURE 4.9** Ultrasound image of the liver (left side of the image) and the stomach with gas in the lumen (right side of the image) where the gas results in a reverberation artifact (white arrow).

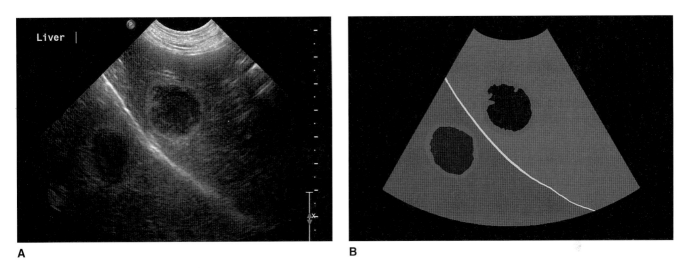

**A**

**B**

**FIGURE 4.10** Ultrasound image (**A**) and representative schematic (**B**) documenting a mirror image artifact where the ultrasound waves interact with the lung–diaphragm interface (hyperechoic line deep to the liver), reflected to the gall bladder and then back to the diaphragm–lung interface and then back to the transducer. The artifactual image is placed deep to the diaphragm–lung interface as if there was a gall bladder in the thorax.

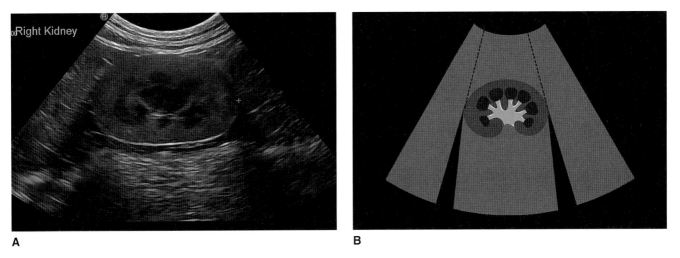

**A**

**B**

**FIGURE 4.11** Ultrasound image (**A**) and representative schematic (**B**) documenting a refraction artifact at the edge of the curved surface of the kidney whereby the ultrasound beam diverges away from the curved surface creating a black triangle deep to the curve.

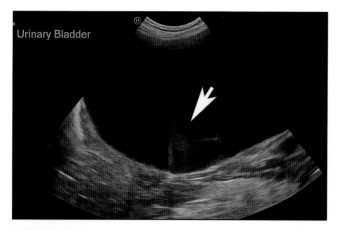

**FIGURE 4.12** Ultrasound image where there is urinary bladder echogenic material (white arrow) that is consistent with a side lobe artifact from the secondary ultrasound lobes and information outside of the primary ultrasound beam.

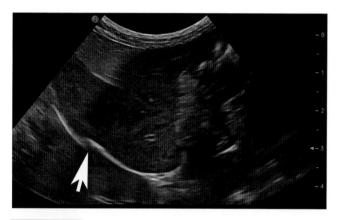

**FIGURE 4.13** Speed propagation error along the diaphragm–lung interface. There appears to be a defect at this level in the diaphragm (white arrow). This is because there is fat in the falciform ligament so that the US waves travel at a slower speed than throughout the adjacent liver. This delays the return trip and the echoes are placed deeper in the tissues (speed of sound in fat is 1450 m/s whereas speed of sound in liver or soft tissues [average speed assumed by the US machine] is 1540 m/s).

*Speed propagation error* occurs when tissues with a different density or acoustic impedance alter the propagation speed of a sound wave (Figure 4.13). Since the speed of sound in soft tissues is assumed to be 1540 m/s, the increased or decreased speed of the wave results in tissues being displayed respectively closer or deeper to the transducer on the image in comparison to their actual location.

*Aliasing* occurs with Doppler imaging when maximum velocities exceed the sampling frequency. Subsequently, the velocity is incorrectly recorded on the opposite site of the graphical display. Adjusting sampling frequency, also known as the pulse repetition frequency (PRF) or scale, will allow more accurate display of the recorded velocities, as determined by the Nyquist limit. Decreasing the depth of the sampling window will also increase the PRF and reduce aliasing. Improper adjustment of the PRF may cause misinterpretation of aliasing as turbulent blood flow.

# Doppler Ultrasound

The systemic vasculature is a routine part of a comprehensive ultrasound examination. This is best achieved with the use of Doppler ultrasonography. Currently, four different Doppler techniques are routinely used to assess for the presence or absence of blood flow, as well as to characterize the velocity, type of flow and relative flow with respect to the transducer and the angle of interrogation. Those techniques are color, power, pulsed, and continuous wave Doppler and are described in Table 4.3.

# Ultrasound-Specific Contrast Agents

Ultrasound contrast agents can be administered safely to enhance the echogenicity of tissues and increase the conspicuity of lesions. Ultrasound contrast media contain microbubbles stabilized in a liquid suspension with different impedance characteristics. The difference in impedance between the microbubbles and the liquid suspension generates detectable echoes. These echoes generated by contrast agents are usually much higher than the surrounding tissues and are distorted into a nonsinusoidal waveform, resulting in harmonic frequency echoes with high contrast resolution.

# Ultrasound Safety

While ultrasonography has the potential to create some biologic effects, the risk is low. The absorption of sound waves in tissues results in conversion to heat. This thermal effect is dependent on the intensity and frequency of a sound wave. Some tissues, such as moving blood, have a greater cooling ability. In comparison, highly attenuating structures, such as bone, retain heat. The duration of tissue exposure to ultrasound energy should also be taken into consideration, although this is much more negligible with the use of pulsed-wave ultrasonography as the transducer is not transmitting sound waves approximately 99% of the time.

Nonthermal biologic effects may also be experienced with ultrasonography due to the mechanical properties of sound waves resulting in increasing pressure and torque within tissues. Small vapor-filled structures cavities within tissues may expand and contract in response to the applied pressure of sound waves (cavitation). When higher energy sound waves are used, these cavities may release energy, cause torque within tissues and result in a biologic effect, such as cell death. While these risks are known, they are generally so small at diagnostic intensities that the effects may be insignificant.

**TABLE 4.3   Properties and limitations of the four most common Doppler techniques.**

| | Properties | Limitations |
|---|---|---|
| Color Doppler | Identification and color-coded representation of blood flow direction and velocities | Susceptible to motion (e.g., panting) |
| | | Best measurements obtained at less than a 60° angle of incidence[a] |
| | | Aliasing artifact where color maps are reversed when the velocity threshold is exceeded. Map options (called variance) can recognize aliasing as a different color (ex. displayed as green and not red or blue) |
| Power Doppler | Documents only the presence or absence of blood flow. More sensitive to flow in smaller vessels. No aliasing limitations | No characterization of flow direction or velocity |
| | | Insensitive to abnormal patterns of blood flow, such as turbulent blood flow |
| | | Susceptible to motion (e.g., panting) |
| Pulsed-wave Doppler | Graphical (spectral display) depiction of the velocity of blood measured in a region of interest within a selected vessel by using a sampling gate set at the desired depth. The velocities are then displayed against time | Must maintain an angle of incidence <60°[a] |
| | | Susceptible to motion (e.g., panting) |
| | | Aliasing artifact if velocities exceed 2 m/s |
| Continuous-wave Doppler | Similar graphical or spectral representation of blood velocities as pulsed-wave Doppler, except continuous-wave Doppler can detect high-velocity blood flow (>6 m/s) without aliasing | No sampling gate to localize recorded region. Instead, records blood flow anywhere within single line array (range ambiguity) |

[a] If the ultrasound beam is perpendicular to the flow of blood, no flow will be detected. This is in accordance with the Doppler shift frequency equation (Doppler frequency $(f_d) = [2 \times f_o \times V \times \cos \theta]/c$). fo, fundamental frequency; V, velocity of blood flow in the sample of interrogation; $\cos \theta$, incidence angle of the Doppler interrogation with the vessel in question; c, the average speed of sound in tissues or 1540 m/s.

# Further Reading

1.  Bushberg, J.T., Siebert, J.A., Leidholdt, E.M. Jr., and Boone JMl. (2012). *The Essential Physics of Medical Imaging*, 3e. Philadelphia, PA: Lippincott Williams & Wilkins.

2.  Drost, W.T. (2018). Physics of diagnostic ultrasound. In: *Textbook of Veterinary Diagnostic Radiology*, 7e (ed. D.E. Thrall). Philadelphia, PA: WB Saunders.

3.  Kremkau, F.W. (2014). *Sonography: Principles and Instruments*, 9e. St Louis, MO: Elsevier Saunders.

4.  Mattoon, J.S., Sellon, R.K., and Berry, C.R. (ed.) (2021). *Small Animal Diagnostic Ultrasound*, 4e. Philadelphia, PA: Elsevier Saunders.

# CHAPTER 5

# Nuclear Scintigraphy

**Elizabeth Huyhn[1], Elodie E. Huguet[2], and Clifford R. Berry[3]**

[1] VCA West Coast Specialty and Emergency Animal Hospital, Fountain Valley, CA, USA

[2] Department of Small Animal Clinical Sciences, College of Veterinary Medicine, University of Florida, Gainesville, FL, USA

[3] Department of Molecular Biomedical Sciences, College of Veterinary Medicine, North Carolina State University, Raleigh, NC, USA

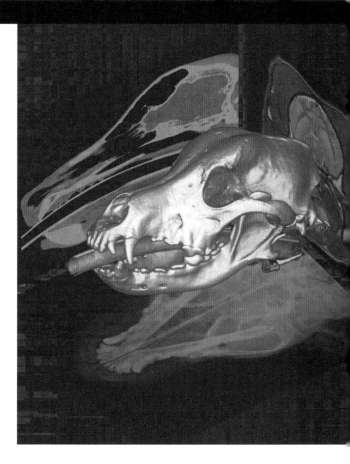

## Overview

Nuclear scintigraphy uses radioactive labels called radionuclides that are linked to an active marker for a specific physiologic process in the body, called a *radiopharmaceutical*, which is injected into the patient. The physiologic marker delivers the radioactive label to an area of interest to the clinician. Employing a special detector called a *gamma camera*, the gamma rays emitted from the radionuclide are counted, and can be related to organ function.

## Basic Physics

A radiopharmaceutical injected into the patient consists of two components: (i) a radionuclide that emits gamma radiation and (ii) a pharmaceutical that will target the radionuclide to the physiology of interest. A variety of radionuclides are available but, commercially, technetium ($^{99m}$Tc) is favored because (i) it has a half-life of approximately 6 hours which will allow sufficient time for images to be obtained but avoid excessive radiation exposure to the patient and handlers; (ii) it emits gamma radiation at energies such that the electromagnetic emissions are sufficiently able to escape from the body and is in the detectable range for gamma cameras; (iii) it has a simple chemistry so that it can be bound to a variety of pharmaceuticals to target different physiologies within the body, and (iv) when injected as sodium pertechnetate, it acts like iodide and is taken up by the salivary and thyroid glands.

## Uses and Advantages

Although nuclear scintigraphy is not used commonly due to the accessibility of other advanced imaging techniques, there are specific applications that are still indicated for imaging using scintigraphy. These applications of nuclear scintigraphy in veterinary medicine can include glomerular filtration rate studies, shunt detection, liver function, bone metabolism, thyroid function, and mucociliary function.

The benefit of glomerular filtration rates (GFR) studies is to detect renal dysfunction before renal azotemia is apparent, as diseased kidneys do not regulate GFR well. Types of GFR studies include (i) the imaging studies where the regions of interests (ROI) are placed over the kidneys and (ii) plasma clearance studies where the ROI is placed over the heart. The imaging studies can determine the individual kidney GFR data whereas the plasma clearance studies provide global GFR data. After the ROIs are placed over the respective anatomy, counts are made over time and a chart is produced (Figure 5.1).

Portal scintigraphy can be used for congenital or acquired portosystemic shunt (PSS) detection and is considered a noninvasive procedure. In patients with PSS, the radiopharmaceutical bypasses the liver and goes to the heart first and later accumulates in the liver. Two techniques can be used for PSS detection: the radiopharmaceutical can be administered transrectal or transsplenic. For the transsplenic technique, radiopharmaceutical is injected into the splenic parenchyma parallel to the long axis of the spleen (Figure 5.2). PSS patterns observed in this study include portoazygous, single portocaval, splenocaval, and internal thoracic shunts. Single shunts can be distinguished from double or multiple shunts. The termination of the shunt and number of vessels can also be determined.

To determine liver function, a hepatic perfusion index (HPI) can be performed (Figure 5.3). This is done to compare the arterial and portal blood supply to the liver. In a patient with normal HPI, the liver curve progresses from the arterial to the portal phase. In a patient with a PSS or hepatic neoplasia, there is flattening of the liver curve on the portal phase which indicates decreased perfusion of the liver or increased arterial blood supply, such as in cases of hepatic neoplasia.

Bone scintigraphy is considered the most sensitive diagnostic imaging modality to detect areas of active bone turnover, which is nonspecific, and may overestimate the extent of osseous involvement. In areas of active bone turnover such as osseous neoplasia, osteomyelitis, osteoarthropathy, open physes in normal young animals, etc., there is increased radiopharmaceutical uptake (Figure 5.4).

Thyroid scintigraphy is beneficial to determine the function and anatomic information of the thyroid lobes (Figure 5.5). In abnormal thyroid scans, there could be decreased radiopharmaceutical uptake which may indicate primary hypothyroidism, secondary hypothyroidism, thyroid hormone replacement therapy, thyrotoxicosis, or excessive exogenous iodine. Alternatively, there could be increased radiopharmaceutical uptake which may indicate adenomatous hyperplasia, adenoma multinodular adenoma, thyroid carcinoma, or increases in thyroid-stimulating hormone as seen in limited iodine diets or methimazole administration.

Mucociliary function can be easily determined using nuclear scintigraphy. In this procedure, a small droplet of radiopharmaceutical is placed at the tracheal bifurcation. The cranial movement of the radiopharmaceutical is imaged over time as its progresses toward the oral cavity in normal patients. In patients with an abnormal mucociliary function, there is no movement or delayed radiopharmaceutical movement.

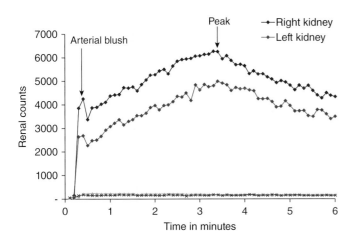

**FIGURE 5.1** Quantitative renal scintigraphy chart denoting the right (blue line) and left (red line) kidneys in relation to the renal counts over time in a normal patient. Renal counts are calculated by drawing regions of interest over the kidneys and noting the accumulation of radiopharmaceutical over time. In a normal patient, the arterial blush is seen early in the curve. The peak renal activity for both right and left kidneys is at the highest point, which is 3 minutes. *Source:* Courtesy of Daniel GB, Berry CR, Textbook of Veterinary Nuclear Medicine.

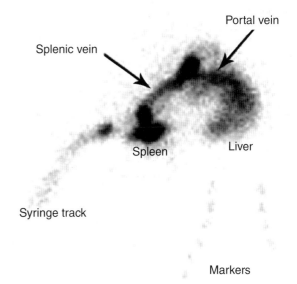

**FIGURE 5.2** Transsplenic portal scintigraphy in a normal dog. The cranial aspect of the patient is to the right of the image and the dorsal aspect is at the top of the image. Note the increased radiopharmaceutical uptake in the spleen. The curvilinear track caudal to the spleen is the small amount of radiopharmaceutical left in the syringe after injection. The dots ventral to the liver are markers to delineate the region of the liver. *Source:* Courtesy of Daniel GB, Berry CR, Textbook of Veterinary Nuclear Medicine.

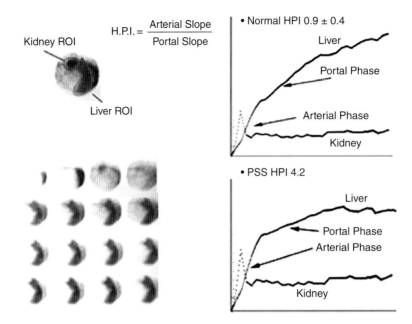

**FIGURE 5.3** Hepatic perfusion index (HPI) in a dog. This is done to evaluate patients with portosystemic shunts that have decreased portal blood supply relative to hepatic arterial blood supply to the liver. Note the collimated images of the liver and kidney with regions of interest (ROI) drawn around them over time after $^{99m}$Tc-sulfur colloid is administered intravenously. In a patient with normal HPI (0.9 ± 0.4), there is an upward progression of the liver HPI. In a patient with a portosystemic shunt or hepatic neoplasia, note the flattening off at the level of the portal phase of the liver HPI, denoting decreased perfusion to the liver in patients with a portosystemic shunt or increased arterial supply in patients with hepatic neoplasia. *Source:* Courtesy of Daniel GB, Berry CR, Textbook of Veterinary Nuclear Medicine.

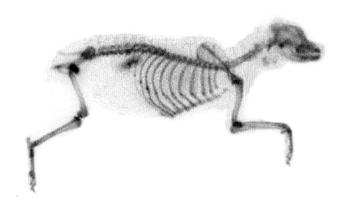

**FIGURE 5.4** Bone scintigraphy of a dog using $^{99m}$Tc-MDP (Medronate®, methylene diphosphonate). The cranial aspect of the dog is to the right of the image and the dorsal aspect is at the top of the image. Note the normal uptake of the radiopharmaceutical throughout the skeletal structures. Additionally, as $^{99m}$Tc-MDP is excreted by the kidneys, note the uptake in the region of the kidneys, superimposed over the last set of ribs. *Source:* Courtesy of Daniel GB, Berry CR, Textbook of Veterinary Nuclear Medicine.

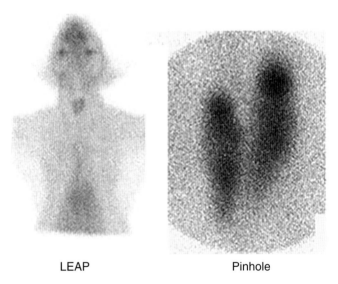

LEAP                    Pinhole

**FIGURE 5.5** Thyroid scintigraphy of a cat in dorsal recumbency. The image on the left uses a low-energy all-purpose (LEAP) collimator which includes the majority of the patient's anatomy and the image on the right uses a pinhole collimator to increase the conspicuity of the thyroid lobes. Note the symmetry and homogeneous radiopharmaceutical uptake of both thyroid lobes in this normal patient. *Source:* Courtesy of Daniel GB, Berry CR, Textbook of Veterinary Nuclear Medicine.

# Safety

The primary radiation safety concerns pertaining to nuclear scintigraphy include radiation exposure to personnel, radiation exposure to owners or handlers, and radioactive contamination of the environment from urine, feces, and/or glandular secretions. After injection of the radionuclide, the patient is monitored using a Geiger–Müller (GM) survey meter for instantaneous dose readings at the surface of the patient, in the location where the highest amount of radioactivity would be, like in the heart for radiotracers that do not localize to target organs rapidly [1]. A second reading is done at a

1 m distance. These measurements are recorded and a radiation sign with this information, type of radiation, and amount of radioactivity injection is posted on the patient's cage or stall door.

The amount of restriction placed on an individual licensee is determined by the state and nuclear regulatory agency at the time of evaluation and establishment of the original nuclear medicine licensure. The factors that must be considered include the radionuclide used, the type of study done, the time the patient is expected to be within the hospital after the procedure, the possible routes of excretion or contamination, release criteria for the patient, and possible public exposure after the procedure. Each license determines the specific radionuclide for which the individual is licensed and the total radioactivity of that particular radionuclide that the licensee is limited to having on the premises at any given time.

## Limitations

Limitations of nuclear scintigraphy include an extensive duration for obtaining a study. The duration of the scintigraphy is dependent on the half-life of the radionuclide used. Another limitation of nuclear scintigraphy is the associated health risk to the personnel involved in handling and imaging the patient. Additionally, nuclear scintigraphy, like other imaging modalities, is not fool proof, meaning that it should be used in conjunction with physical examination, history, and additional diagnostics to appropriately treat a patient.

## Positron Emission Tomography

Positron emission tomography (PET) imaging uses fluorodeoxyglucose (FDG), a glucose analog, as its radiotracer and is considered one of the most significant diagnostic imaging tools in human medicine. Most PET studies today are combined with computed tomography (CT) studies in order to better locate areas of abnormal cell activity [2]. The advantages of PET include the ability to obtain functional data, the ability of the radiotracer to distribute based on cellular function of an organ or structure, and the short half-lives of positron emitters. This minimizes the radiation dose to the subject because the decay is rapid and allows for repeated studies in a reasonable time frame [3]. A disadvantage of PET is that the images exhibit low spatial resolution [4]; however, these studies can be fused with high-resolution anatomic data from magnetic resonance imaging (MRI) and CT.

Spatial resolution refers to the number of pixels that construct a digital image. Images with higher spatial resolution are composed of a larger number of pixels than those of lower spatial resolution. Other disadvantages include the high cost of the equipment, tracers, and cyclotron, and the short-half-lives of the positron emitters, which can limit transportation of doses over long distances.

Fluorodeoxyglucose accumulates in areas of the body that are most metabolically active [5, 6]. After FDG is injected into the patient's bloodstream and allowed to accumulate for a short time, the PET scanner then creates images that show the distribution of the radiotracer throughout the body, which helps determine if abnormalities are present. For example, highly active cancer cells show higher levels of uptake of FDG, whereas brain cells affected by dementia consume smaller amounts of glucose and show lower FDG uptake [6].

Functional rather than structural factors define the images obtained using PET. A radiopharmaceutical tagged with positron-emitting radionuclide is administered to the patient, and the PET detector maps the distribution of the radioactivity. The resulting image is a three-dimensional map of radiopharmaceutical distribution of location and intensity. Because accumulation of the radiopharmaceutical is dependent on cellular function, PET conveys information regarding physiologic and metabolic processes in the body [5, 6]. PET can be used to provide complementary information to anatomic images and vice versa. Recently, PET/CT combination scanners have been released in the human market so that image registration between imaging modalities is not an issue.

The main veterinary clinical application of PET is in oncology [7]. It helps characterize lesions, differentiates recurrent disease from treatment effects, stages tumors, evaluates extent of a disease process, and monitors response to therapy. Additionally, PET is useful for detecting lymph node involvement of canine lymphoma and cutaneous mast cell tumor [8].

## References

1. Zuckier, L.S., Boardman, B., and Zhao, Q.H. (1998). Remotely pollable Geiger–Müller detector for continuous monitoring of iodine-131 therapy patients. *J. Nucl. Med.* 39: 1558–1562.
2. Krause, B.J., Schwarzenböck, S., and Souvatzoglou, M. (2013). FDG PET and PET/CT. *Recent Results Cancer Res.* 187: 351–369.
3. Poon, D., Burns, P., Murray, D. et al. (2010). PET for pets: PET/CT imaging of veterinary patients. *J. Nucl. Med.* 51: 1028.
4. Moses, W.W. (2011). Fundamental limits of spatial resolution in PET. *Nucl. Instrum. Methods Phys. Res. A* 648 (Supplement 1): S236–S240.

5. Lee, M.S., Lee, A.R., Jung, M.A. et al. (2010). Characterization of physiologic 18F-FDG uptake with PET-CT in dogs. *Vet. Radiol. Ultrasound* 51: 670–673.

6. Hansen, A.E., McEvoy, F., Engelholm, S.A. et al. (2011). FDG PET/CT imaging in canine cancer patients. *Vet. Radiol. Ultrasound* 52: 201–206.

7. Lawrence, J., Rohren, E., and Provenzale, J. (2010). PET/CT today and tomorrow in veterinary cancer diagnosis and monitoring: fundamentals, early results and future perspectives. *Vet. Comp. Oncol.* 8: 163–187.

8. LeBlanc, A.K., Jakoby, B.W., Townsend, D.W., and Daniel, G.B. (2009). 18FDG-PET imaging in canine lymphoma and cutaneous mast cell tumor. *Vet. Radiol. Ultrasound* 50: 215–223.

# Musculoskeletal

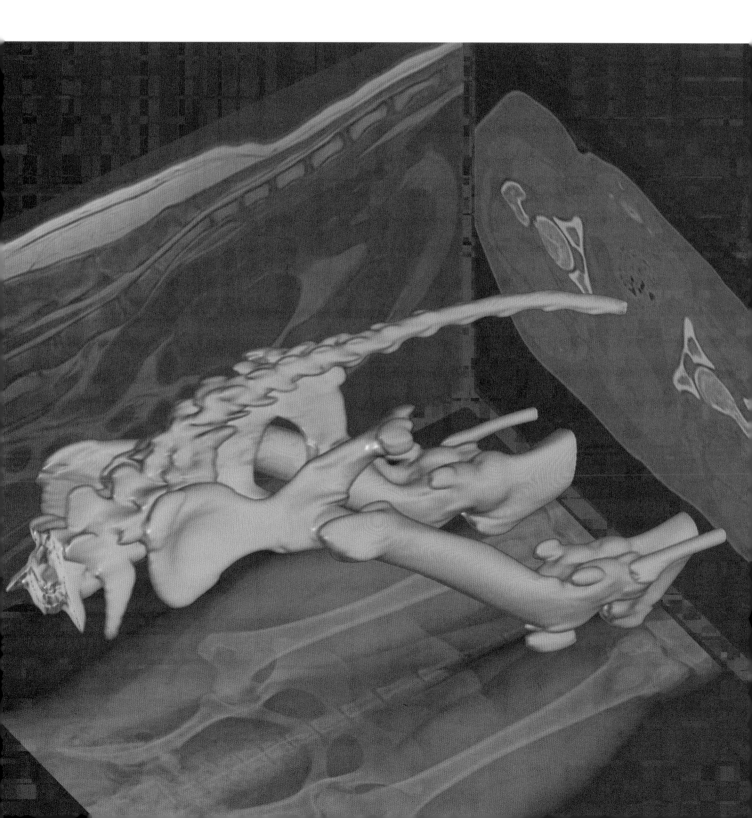

# CHAPTER 6

# Anatomy, Variants, and Interpretation Paradigm

Nathan C. Nelson

Clinical Professor, Diagnostic Imaging, Department of Molecular Biomedical Sciences, College of Veterinary Medicine, North Carolina State University, Raleigh, NC, USA

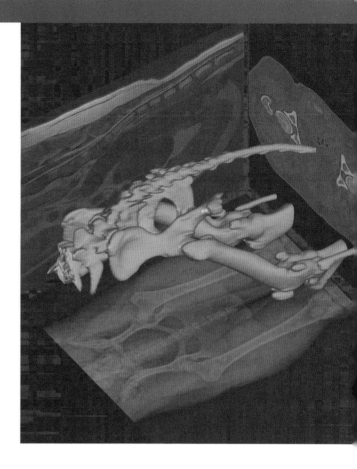

## Overview

Osseous anatomy is well suited for radiographic evaluation. The high mineral content within bones imbues them with improved x-ray attenuation ability compared to surrounding soft tissue structures. This differential attenuation results in high radiographic contrast between osseous and soft tissue structures. Pathology that alters bone density or bone margination is therefore readily recognized. For that reason, radiographs are typically the initial screening test when musculoskeletal disease is suspected.

While osseous structures are relatively easy to identify, radiographs are much more limited in their ability to evaluate the soft tissue components of the musculoskeletal system. Given their similar density and constitution, muscles, tendons, ligaments, and vascular structures share the same opacity. Where these soft tissues contact one another, no distinct margin is identified. This so-called "silhouette sign" often prevents more exact determination of the nature of the soft tissue disease, instead resulting in a generalized, nonspecific swelling on radiographs. Direct imaging of soft tissue musculoskeletal structures requires advanced imaging. Ultrasound in particular is well suited for evaluation of peripheral/appendicular soft tissue pathology as it readily discriminates between types of soft tissues (tendon, ligament, muscle, vessel, connective tissue). The superficial nature of the peripheral limb soft tissues makes them readily accessible to ultrasound evaluation.

Despite its limited ability to evaluate soft tissues, radiography remains the mainstay of musculoskeletal imaging. For that reason, chapters on musculoskeletal radiography will focus on primarily on this modality. Advanced imaging with CT, MRI, and ultrasound is growing in use, and in some applications is preferred to radiography, so will be discussed where these modalities are most commonly used. The skull and spinal column are particularly complex structures, with intricate osseous anatomy (such as the vertebrae) surrounding soft tissue structures (such as the spinal cord), so the chapters on imaging of the head and spine will naturally include more MRI and CT images than in other areas of the body. As discussed above, the appendicular skeleton is more readily amenable to ultrasound imaging and so normal ultrasound anatomy of this area will be included in the relevant chapter.

This introductory chapter will outline the basic principles of musculoskeletal imaging, including choice of modality, patient positioning, and a review of normal anatomy (see also Appendix I). Clinically relevant anatomic variants are included and should not be misidentified as clinically significant pathology.

# Appendicular Skeleton

## Appendicular Skeleton: Basic Radiography Principles and Anatomy

As with other areas of the body, appendicular radiography requires a minimum of two orthogonal projections. Single radiographs can result in failure to recognize clinically significant abnormalities (Figure 6.1). The complexity of the skeleton dictates a wider variety of additional supplementary projections compared to the thorax or abdomen. Which projections constitute a "complete study" depends on the anatomic region,

clinician preference, and the clinical question to answer. As an example, the author considers four projections a minimum study for the carpus and tarsus, as two projections are frequently insufficient to fully characterize the complex anatomy of these areas. Table 6.1 lists body regions with recommended projections that constitute a "complete radiographic study" (and includes figure references). Optional projections and their indications are also listed.

As a reminder, radiographic projections are named for the direction of the x-ray beam; the region of entry and region of exit are listed in that order. If obliques are performed, the angle of obliquity relative to beam entry is listed. Table 6.1 lists projections with complete and colloquial names; a detailed description of radiographic naming conventions is available, though often shortened to a colloquial or abbreviated name for everyday use [1].

Proper positioning of musculoskeletal radiographs is critical. Even slight obliquity can hide clinically significant pathology (Figure 6.17). Poor positioning can give the false impression of pathology when none is present (Figure 6.18). Poor positioning also distorts normal anatomy (Figure 6.19).

## Appendicular Skeleton: Advanced Imaging

Ultrasound is increasingly used in appendicular imaging as a quick, relatively inexpensive test to diagnose and monitor a variety of soft tissue injuries. Peripheral tendon disease is

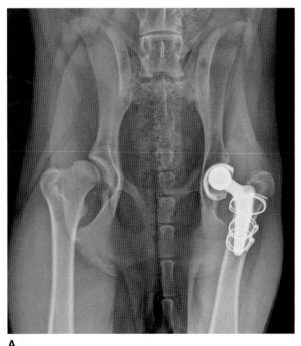
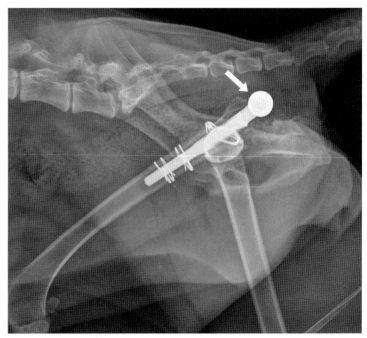

**A**  **B**

**FIGURE 6.1** Ventrodorsal (**A**) and lateral (**B**) projections of the pelvis demonstrating the importance of orthogonal projections. On the ventrodorsal projection, the ball of the left total hip replacement appears to be superimposed with the acetabulum, however on lateral projections it is dorsally luxated (arrow).

TABLE 6.1

**List of appendicular regions, with projections that constitute a complete baseline study and optional additional projections. Complete radiographic projections are included (and colloquial/abbreviated names for those projections are in parentheses).**

| Body part | Standard projections | Additional projections | Indication for projection |
|---|---|---|---|
| Carpus | Lateromedial (lateral; Figure 6.2a) | Extended lateromedial | Palmar instability |
| | Dorsopalmar (DP; Figure 6.2b) | Dorsopalmar with medial stress | Medial instability |
| | Dorsal 45° medial-palmarolateral oblique (45° medial oblique; Figure 6.4c) | Dorsopalmar with lateral stress | Lateral instability |
| | Dorsal 45° lateral-palmaromedial oblique (45° lateral oblique; Figure 6.3d) | | |
| Tarsus | Lateromedial (lateral; Figure 6.3a) | PD with medial stress (Chapter 8; Figure 8.32) | Medial instability |
| | Plantarodorsal (PD; Figure 6.3b) | PD with lateral stress | Lateral instability |
| | Dorsal 45° lateral-plantaromedial oblique (45° lateral oblique; Figure 6.3c) | | |
| | Dorsal 45° medial-plantarolateral oblique (45° medial oblique; Figure 6.4d). | | |
| Pes/manus | Lateromedial (lateral; Figure 6.4a) | Splay toe lateral (Figure 6.5) | Better identification of distal phalanx from a lateral perspective without superimposition of the other phalanges |
| | Dorsopalmar/plantar (DP; Figure 6.4b) | | |
| | Dorsal 45° lateral-palmaro-(plantaro-)medial oblique (45° lateral; Figure 6.4c) | | |
| | Dorsal 45 medial-palmaro-(plantaro-)lateral oblique (45° lateral; Figure 6.5d) | | |
| Elbow | Lateromedial (lateral; Figure 6.6a) | Flexed lateromedial (flexed lateral; Figure 6.7) | Better identify osteophytes on anconeal process, without superimposition of the humerus |
| | Craniocaudal (Figure 6.6b) | Cranial 15° medial-caudolateral oblique (15° oblique; Figure 6.8) | Better identification of the medial coronoid process and medial humeral condyle pathology |
| Shoulder | Lateromedial (lateral; Figure 6.9a) | Cranioproximal to craniodistal oblique (shoulder skyline; Figure 6.10) | Identify intertubercular pathology in cases with biceps tenosynovitis |
| | Craniocaudal (Figure 6.9b) | | |
| Pelvis | Ventrodorsal with hips extended (VD pelvis; Figure 6.11a) | Ventrodorsal with limbs abducted (frog-leg projection; Figure 6.12) | Better evaluates femoral neck pathology such as capital physeal fractures by allowing the femoral head and neck to malalign |
| | Lateromedial (lateral; Figure 6.11b) | Ventrodorsal with hip distraction (hip distraction view; Figure 6.13) | PennHip procedure used to screen for hip dysplasia (see Chapter 7) |
| | | Dorsal acetabular rim projection (DAR projection; Figure 6.14) | Identifies early osteophyte formation on the acetabular rim, an area usually obscured by superimposition with the femoral head |
| Scapula | Lateromedial (lateral; Figure 6.15a) | | |
| | Craniocaudal (Figure 6.15b) | | |

*(Continued)*

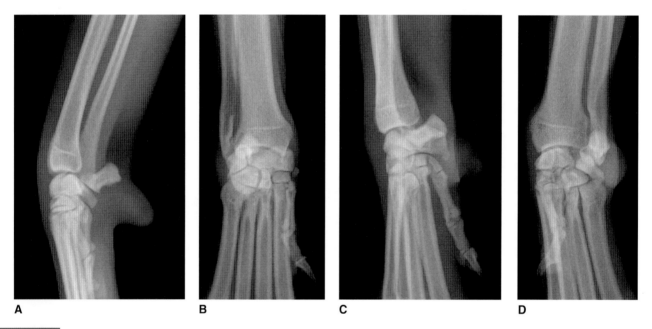

A   B   C   D

**FIGURE 6.2** Standard radiographs of the carpus consisting of lateromedial (**A**), dorsopalmar (**B**), dorsal 45 lateral-palmaromedial oblique (**C**), and dorsal 45 medial-palmarolateral oblique (**D**) images.

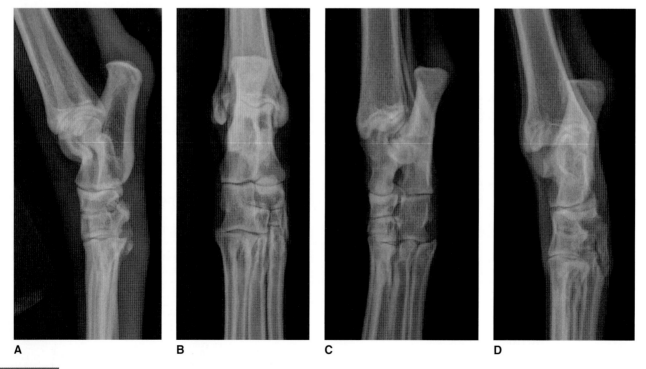

A   B   C   D

**FIGURE 6.3** Standard radiographs of the tarsus consisting of lateromedial (**A**), dorsoplantar (**B**), dorsal 45 lateral-plantaromedial oblique (**C**), and dorsal 45 medial-plantaromedial oblique (**D**) images.

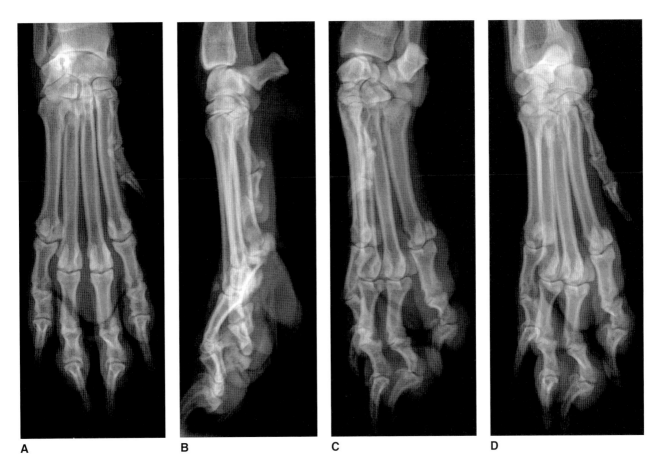

**FIGURE 6.4** Standard radiographs of the manus consisting of lateromedial (**A**), dorsopalmar (**B**), dorsal 45 lateral-palmaromedial oblique (**C**), and dorsal 45 medial-palmarolateral oblique (**D**) images. Notice that similar to carpus projections (Figure 6.2), the entire carpus is included on these projections, but unlike carpal projections the projection is not centered on the carpus and includes the entire digits.

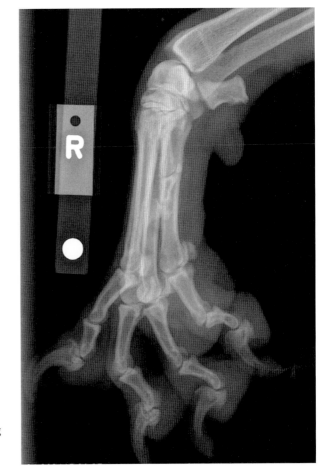

**FIGURE 6.5** Lateromedial splay toe projection of the manus, which allows evaluation of the digits within the superimposition present on a nonsplay toe lateromedial projection. This projection is acquired by placing gauze or tape around the nail of the first and fourth digits and displacing one dorsally and one palmarly.

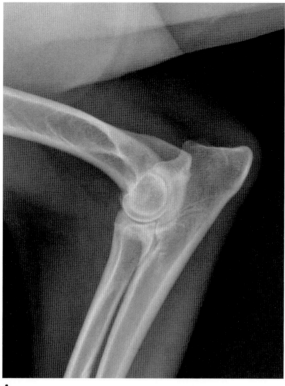

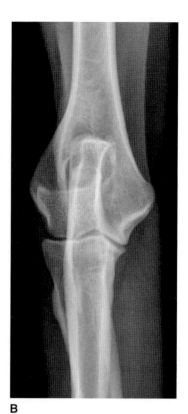

**A**

**B**

**FIGURE 6.6** Lateromedial (**A**) and craniocaudal (**B**) projections of the elbow.

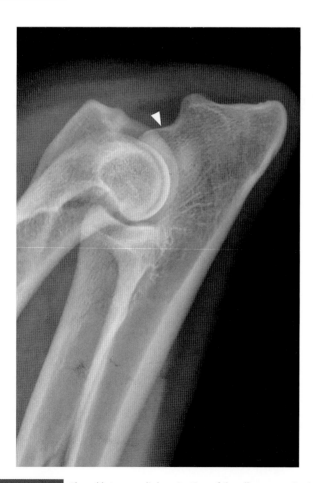

**FIGURE 6.7** Flexed lateromedial projection of the elbow, acquired when evaluation of the anconeal process (arrowhead) is necessary.

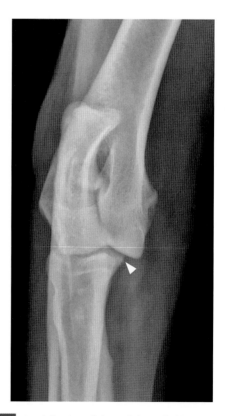

**FIGURE 6.8** Cranial 15° medial-caudolateral oblique projection of the elbow to better evaluate the medial coronoid process. By positioning the elbow in this manner, the medial coronoid process extends more medially without superimposition of the rest of the ulna, allowing visualization of more of it compared to the standard craniocaudal projection.

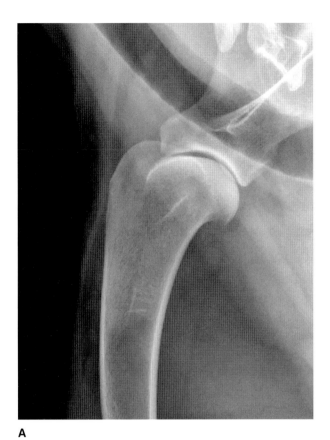

**A**

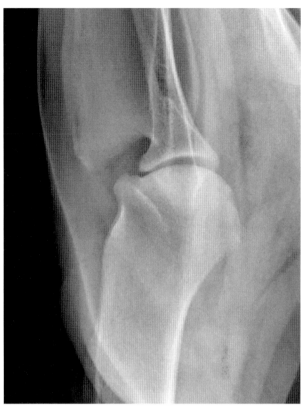

**B**

**FIGURE 6.9** Normal lateral (**A**) and craniocaudal (**B**) projections of the shoulder.

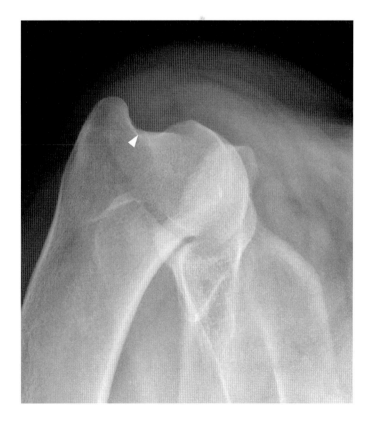

**FIGURE 6.10** Normal cranioproximal to craniodistal oblique of the shoulder, usually referred to as the shoulder skyline projection, used to see the greater tubercle and the intertubercular groove (arrowhead). Notice the smooth margins of the groove.

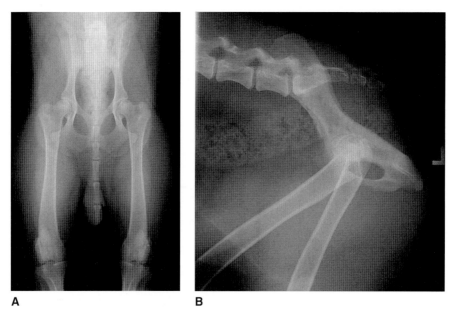

**FIGURE 6.11** Normal ventrodorsal (**A**) and lateral (**B**) projection of the pelvis. Note that the ventrodorsal projection includes the entire femurs.

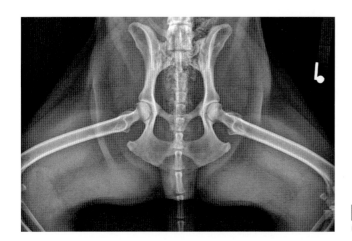

**FIGURE 6.12** Frog-leg ventrodorsal projection of the pelvis, used to better evaluate the femoral heads.

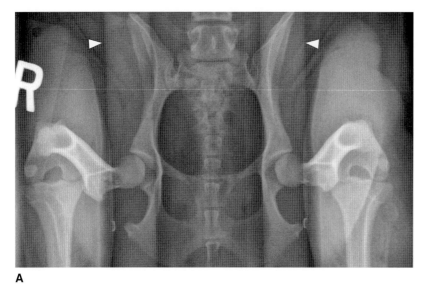

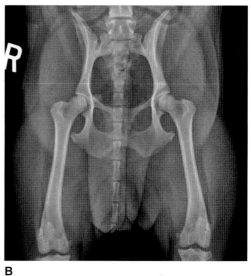

**FIGURE 6.13** Distraction view of the pelvis (**A**) compared to a standard ventrodorsal projection (**B**) in a normal dog. A PennHip distractor is used (margins of the distractor are indicated by arrowheads) to distract the hips. The coxofemoral joints are widened on the distracted view compared to the standard projection.

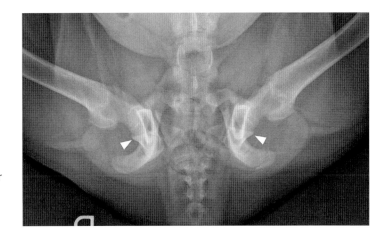

**FIGURE 6.14** Dorsal acetabular projection of the pelvis in a normal dog. This projection is used to evaluate the dorsal acetabulum margin (arrowheads) for osteophytes or fractures or other pathology. Normally the acetabular rim is superimposed with the femoral heads, preventing their evaluation on ventrodorsal projections.

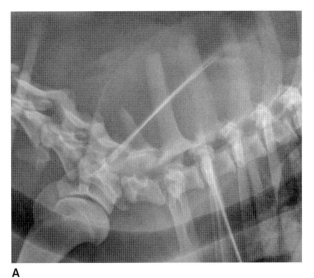

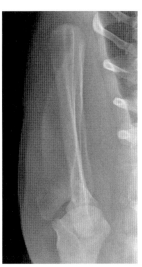

**FIGURE 6.15** Lateromedial and craniocaudal projection of the scapula in a normal dog. Note that on the lateral projection, there is superimposition of the scapula with the spine.

**A**

**B**

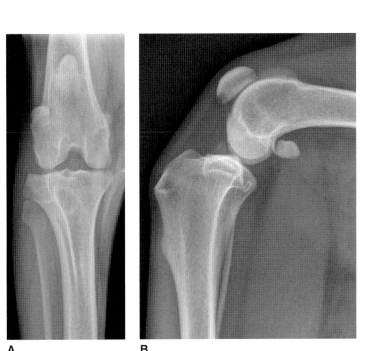

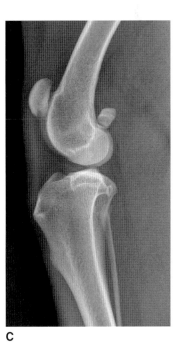

**A**

**B**

**C**

**FIGURE 6.16** Caudocranial (**A**), neutral lateral (**B**), and extended lateral (**C**) projections of the stifle in a normal dog. The neutral positioning (with the femur and tibia approximately 90° to one another) is the preferred position for radiographing the stifle prior to a TPLO procedure. In comparison, the stifle is extended when radiographs are performed prior to a TTA procedure. This positioning results in an angle closer to what a dog would have during normal standing (approximately 135° angle between the femur and tibia).

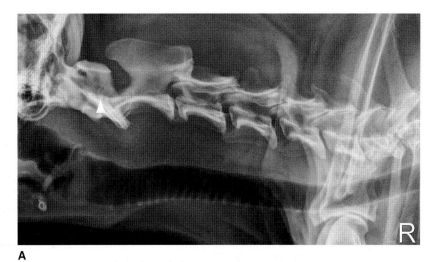

A

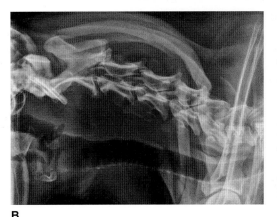

B

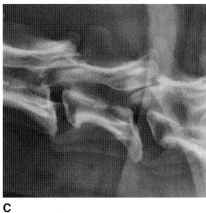

C

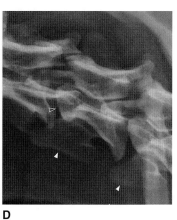

D

**FIGURE 6.17** Lateromedial projections of a well-positioned (**A**) and poorly positioned spine (**B**), with magnified C3–4 disc spaces of the well-positioned (**C**) and poorly positioned (**D**) images. On the well-positioned spine (**A,C**), intervertebral disc spaces are clearly identified without overlap of adjacent vertebral bodies. There is superimposition of the left and right transverse processes. On the poorly positioned spine (**B,D**), there is overlap of adjacent vertebral bodies (open arrowhead) and one set of transverse processes is more ventral than the others due to rotation along the long axis of the spine (closed arrowheads).

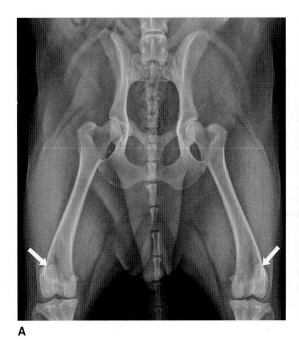

A

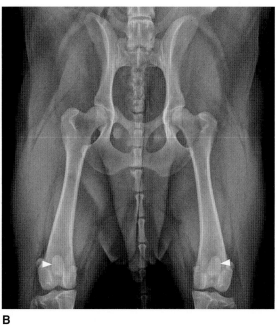

B

**FIGURE 6.18** Ventrodorsal projections of the pelvis with the legs slightly abducted compared to a properly positioned projection with the legs more adducted. Notice with proper positioning the patellas are superimposed with the distal femur (arrowheads) as opposed to the poorly positioned projection where they are laterally located (arrows). This poor positioning results in the false impression of lateral patellar luxation.

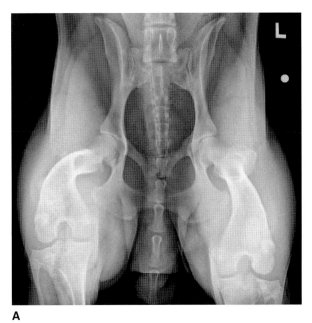

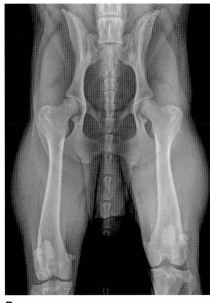

**A**                                        **B**

**FIGURE 6.19** Ventrodorsal projections with the legs incompletely extended (**A**), resulting in foreshortening compared to the better positioned pelvis with femurs more extended (**B**).

easily accessed with this modality, and new high-resolution linear transducers provide the detail necessary to identify the tendon ultrastructure for evidence of disruption. Biceps tenosynovitis and common calcaneal tendonitis or disruption are the most common diseases diagnosed with ultrasound, though it is suitable for examination of any soft tissues not surrounded by bone.

Computed tomography (CT) use in small animal appendicular imaging is more limited. Its primary use is evaluation of elbow dysplasia as radiographs may not be able to diagnose the subtle pathology present in early disease or may underrepresent the severity of disease even if changes are present. Given its ability to recreate complex three-dimensional structures, CT is useful for preoperative planning in patients with complex angular limb deformities. CT also sees use in evaluation of potentially aggressive peripheral bone lesions, as it is more sensitive to evidence of inflammation and bone neoplasia compared to radiographs.

Magnetic resonance imaging (MRI) evaluation of appendicular limb musculoskeletal pathology is rare. The high cost is prohibitive for many clients. Compared to humans, the small size of canine/feline joints, tendons, ligaments, and cartilage poses a challenge, as many MRI sequences cannot provide the high resolution necessary to image such small structures within a reasonable amount of time. Moreover, for most common canine and feline appendicular pathology, clinical examination paired with radiographs provides a definitive diagnosis without the need for an expensive imaging test. As an example, palpation of a cranial drawer sign in a patient with suspected cranial cruciate ligament pathology is diagnostic for that disease, and surgical stabilization methods do not depend on advanced preoperative imaging beyond radiographs.

# Appendicular Skeleton: Anatomic Variants or Easily Confused Anatomy

**Chondrodystrophy**  The tibia/fibula and radius/ulna are particularly affected in patients with chondrodystrophy (Figure 6.20). There is procurvatum and external rotation of the paws in these patients. No clinically significant elbow incongruity is expected. The femur in these breeds is typically short with larger peripheral features than other breeds. The humerus has a more curved proximal diaphysis, with a hook on the caudal aspect of the humeral head that is not an osteophyte.

**Sesamoid Bones**  Smaller sesamoid bones should not be confused with pathology (such as chip fragments). The supinator sesamoid bone is adjacent to the radial head, but is variable between patients, sometimes not seen at all, and in some patients seen unilaterally or bilaterally (Figure 6.21). The abductor pollicus longus sesamoid bone is consistent in dogs, seen medial to the carpus (Figure 6.22). The sesamoid bones palmar to the metacarpo/tarsophalangeal joints are always present (though the first digit only has one) and the dorsal sesamoid at these joints is also consistently identified. The popliteal sesamoid and fabellae (sesamoids of the gastrocnemius muscle) are common and well-understood sesamoid bones.

**Other Focal Mineralized Periarticular Bodies**  A focal, small mineralized body caudal to the glenoid cavity in a dog shoulder is an ossification variant and not associated with other degenerative change (Figure 6.23). Similarly,

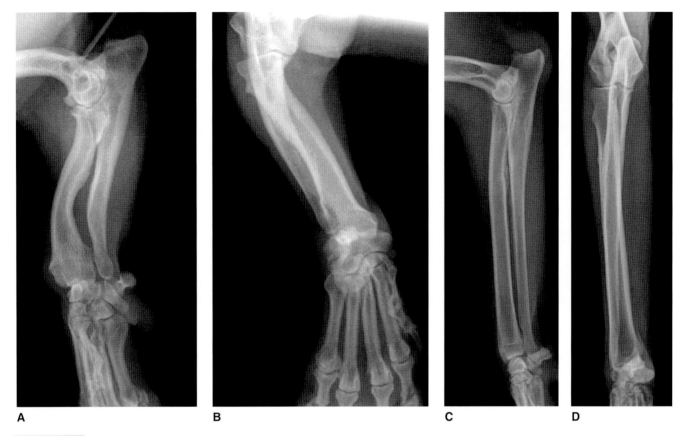

**FIGURE 6.20**  Lateromedial (**A**) and craniocaudal projection (**B**) of the thoracic limbs of a chondrodystrophic versus a nonchondrodystrophic dog (**C,D**). Notice in the chondrodystrophic dog there is cranial curvature of the middiaphysis of the radius (procurvatum) and ulna, with valgus and rotation of the manus centered at the carpus.

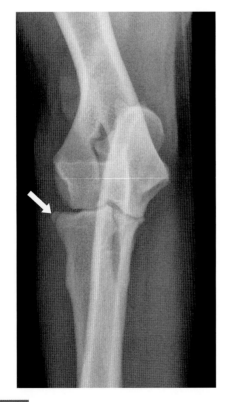

**FIGURE 6.21**  Normal-appearing supinator sesamoid bone adjacent to the radial head (arrow).

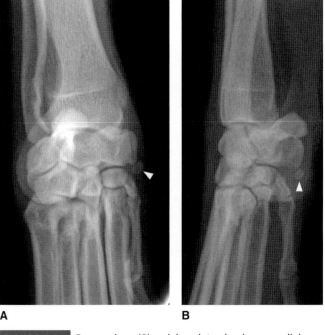

**FIGURE 6.22**  Dorsopalmar (**A**) and dorsolateral-palmaromedial oblique (**B**) radiographs of a normal-appearing abductor pollicis longus sesamoid bone medial to the carpus (arrowheads).

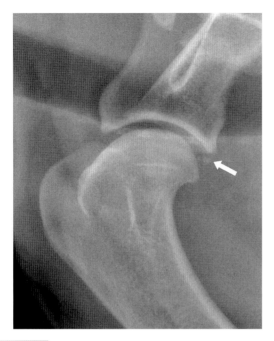

**FIGURE 6.23**   Lateromedial radiograph of the shoulder showing a small ossification center (arrow) caudal to the scapula.

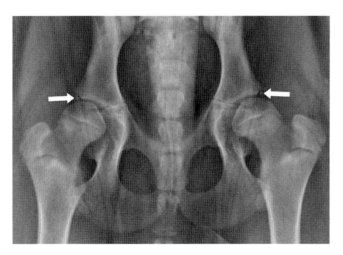

**FIGURE 6.24**   Ventrodorsal projection of the pelvis showing small secondary centers of ossification cranial to both acetabula (arrows).

a small secondary center of ossification of the cranial rim of the acetabulum in juvenile animals typically fuses by 1 year of age (Figure 6.24). A focal mineralized body may also be seen proximal to the greater trochanter, at the site of insertion of the gluteal musculature (Figure 6.25). This is not associated with clinical signs.

## Clavicles

Dog clavicles are small and inconsistently mineralized on radiographs, though some patients have large prominent clavicles (Figure 6.26). They may superimpose with the proximal humerus and should not be confused with bone fragments or mineralization in the area of the biceps tendon. Cat clavicles are relatively larger and less likely to be confused with pathology compared to dogs (Figure 6.27).

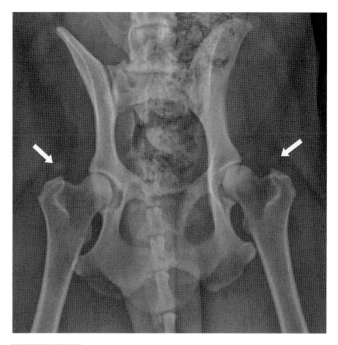

**FIGURE 6.25**   Ventrodorsal projection of the pelvis showing focal rounded mineralization proximal to both greater trochanters at the site of insertion of the gluteal musculature. This is not a clinically significant finding.

## Radial/Ulnar Interosseous Space

The opposed margins of the radius and ulna middiaphysis have a varied appearance. Undulation of the outer cortical margin is expected, as is increased opacity of the adjacent medullary cavity (Figure 6.28). Focal, geographic lysis near the nutrient foramen of these bones is also common, and has been termed "radial ulnar ischemic necrosis" (Figure 6.29). These interosseous changes do not cause lameness.

## Metaphyseal Cutback

In young, rapidly growing breeds (such as Great Danes), it is common to have peripheral irregularity of the distal ulnar metaphysis and to a lesser extent radial and other metaphyses (Figure 6.30). This is considered normal metaphyseal remodeling and sometimes termed "cutback." This peripheral irregularity should not be confused with hypertrophic osteodystrophy (see Chapter 7).

## Physes

Normal physes or separate centers of ossification may be confused with pathology without knowledge of normal closure times. As an example, the anconeal process maintains a separate center of ossification at its proximal tip; this should be fused to the remaining olecranon by 5 months of age. In some dogs, failure to close occurs, resulting in so-called ununited anconeal process which ultimately results in lameness and elbow degeneration (see Chapter 7).

Similarly, the medial and lateral humeral condyles should fuse by approximately 80 days after birth. Prior to that time,

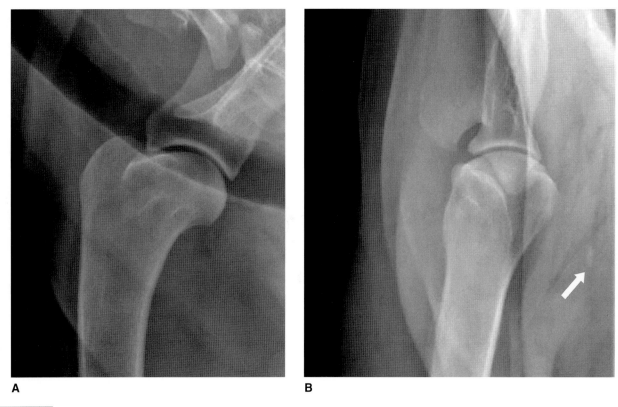

A   B

**FIGURE 6.26** Lateromedial (**A**) and craniocaudal (**B**) projections of the shoulders showing the normal canine clavicle (arrow). Note that the clavicle is not seen on lateral projection as it superimposes with the greater tubercle.

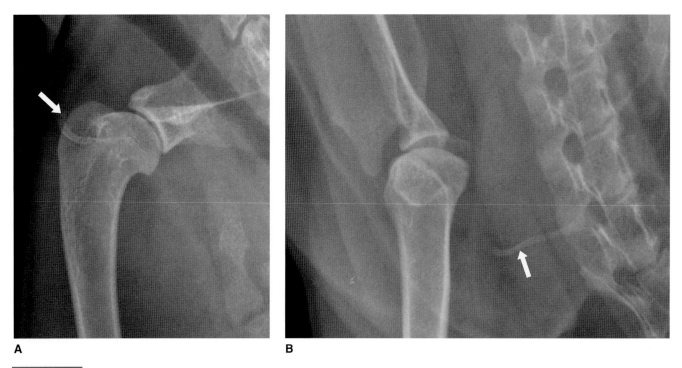

A   B

**FIGURE 6.27** Lateromedial (**A**) and craniocaudal (**B**) projections of the shoulders in a cat showing the large clavicle (arrow) when compared to the dog.

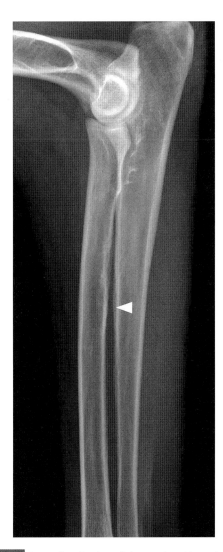

**FIGURE 6.28**  Lateral projection of the antebrachium showing irregularity of the opposed margins of the radius and ulna in the middiaphysis region (arrowhead).

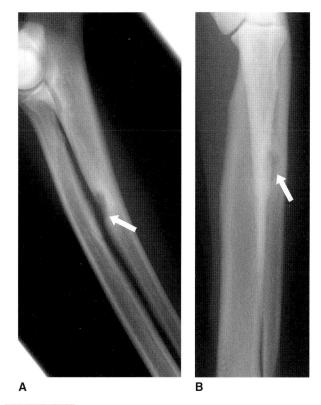

**A**  **B**

**FIGURE 6.29**  Craniocaudal and lateral projections of the antebrachium showing focal resorption of the ulna in the middiaphysis region (arrows), consistent with radial ulnar ischemic necrosis.

they are separated by a lucent line that extends to the articular margin of the distal humerus, and should not be misdiagnosed as a fracture. In some dogs, the medial and lateral condyles remain unfused, termed "incomplete ossification of the humeral condyle," which weakens the bone and can predispose to an articular fracture (see Chapter 7 for further details). Other physes and normal centers of ossification include the lesser trochanter (Figure 6.31) and accessory carpal bone (Figure 6.32).

Delayed closure of the physes has been described in male neutered cats, particularly affecting the distal femur, tibial tuberosity, greater trochanter, and possibly the capital physis [2]. Normal feline capital physeal closure time is approximately 9 months of age, though delayed closure as long as a year or more may occur in male cats, particularly those neutered at an early age (<4 months). The delayed capital physeal closure can predispose to nontraumatic fractures.

Some physes/apophyses may never close. An example is the crest of the ilium, where even mature dogs may have retained opened apophyses bilaterally (Figure 6.33).

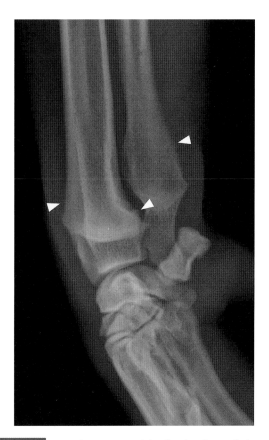

**FIGURE 6.30**  Lateral projection of the distal radius and ulna showing irregularity in the distal metaphyseal region (arrowheads), consistent with normal cutback zone.

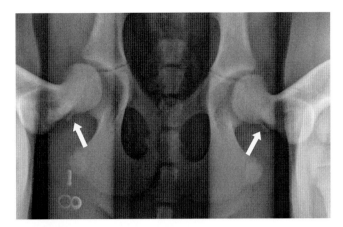

**FIGURE 6.31** Ventrodorsal PennHip projection in a young dog with secondary centers of ossification of the lesser trochanter (arrows), a normal finding.

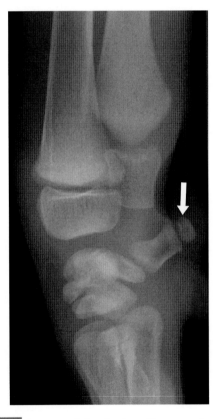

**FIGURE 6.32** Lateromedial projection of the carpus in a young dog showing the secondary center of ossification of the accessory carpal bone (arrow).

## Anal Sac Gas

Gas may normally reside within the anal sacs. This gas may superimpose with the ischium or caudal perineal soft tissues on the ventrodorsal (VD) projection and should not be confused with bone lysis or soft tissue abscessation (Figure 6.34).

## Coxofemoral Laxity

As a ball-in-socket joint, the coxofemoral joint allows a high degree of motion in all directions, including some degree of laxity. In a normal dog, the femoral head can distract slightly from the adjacent acetabulum. On

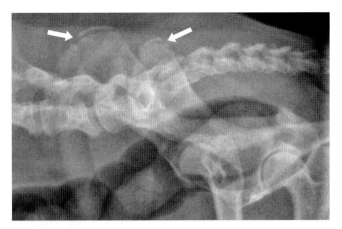

**FIGURE 6.33** Lateromedial projection of the pelvis in a geriatric Maltese showing the two ilial wings with residual secondary centers of ossification that have not closed (arrows). Note that the pelvis is intentionally oblique with one ilial wing cranial to the other.

the extended leg VD projection, normal laxity is characterized by slight medial widening of the joint and slight decreased coverage of the femoral head (Figure 6.35). The Orthopedic Foundation for Animals evaluates the coxofemoral joint on extended leg ventrodorsal projections and assigns grades for passing and dysplastic hips [3]. Passing classifications display excellent conformation (minimal joint space and a well-seated femoral head), good conformation (slight joint space widening but still a well-formed congruent hip), and fair conformation (even greater widening of the joint space and a shallow acetabulum) [3]. Hip dysplasia results in abnormal laxity, characterized by a more severe widening of the joint space and decreased femoral head coverage when compared to a normal dog. Evaluation of normal versus abnormal coxofemoral laxity on the extended leg VD projection is a subjective assessment, though is more likely abnormal if osteophytosis or other evidence of coxofemoral degeneration is present.

The PennHip distraction method provides a more objective measure of coxofemoral laxity (Figure 6.36). The femurs are placed in a neutral position, without caudal extension, relaxing the joint capsule when compared to the extended limb position. A distraction device is placed between the limbs and serves as a fulcrum allowing active coxofemoral distraction. A *distraction index* is calculated from the radiographs, quantifying the degree of coxofemoral laxity, and is compared against other dogs of the same breed in the PennHip database.

## Retained Cartilage Core in the Tibia

Dogs may have a small retained cartilage core in the area of the proximal tibial apophysis, which is particularly common in small/ toy breed dogs (Figure 6.37) [4]. This core does not cause clinical disease though it has been associated with medial patellar luxation. It should not be misdiagnosed as an area of bone lysis.

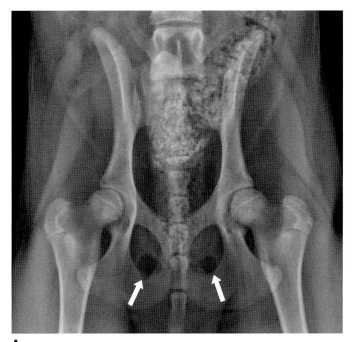
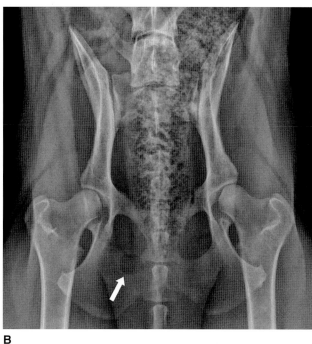

**A**   **B**

**FIGURE 6.34** Ventrodorsal projection of the pelvis showing bilateral (**A**) and unilateral (**B**) gas in the anal sacs. The gas may be more cranially located, as in the case with the bilateral gas, or more caudal and superimposed on the ischial table. This should not be confused for an osseous lytic lesion.

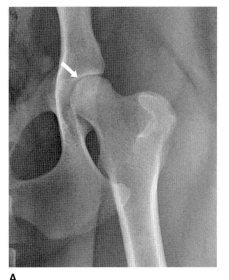
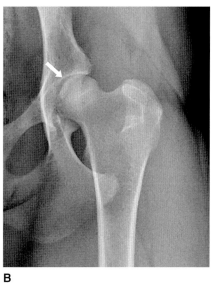
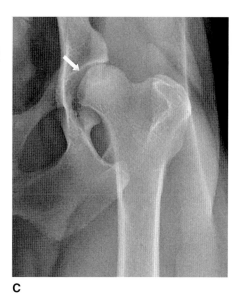

**A**   **B**   **C**

**FIGURE 6.35** Ventrodorsal projections of pelvis, showing a dog graded as excellent (**A**), good (**B**), and fair (**C**) conformation by the Orthopedic Foundation for Animals. Note that the joint space (arrow) is very thin/narrow on the excellent conformation but widens on the good and fair evaluations.

**Nutrient Foramina** All bones have nutrient foramina and while their location is generally similar between patients, in some patients they may occur in unusual locations or be more obvious in some patients compared to others. They are located in the distal diaphysis of some bones such as the humerus (Figure 6.38) and the proximal diaphysis of others, such as the

radius and ulna (Figure 6.39). The position tends to be consistent between patients.

**Digit Variations** Some breeds of dogs and cats have additional digits beyond the expected five. These digits may not have complete osseous connection to the carpus/tarsus,

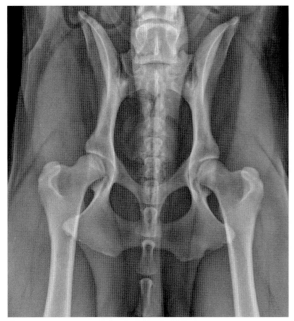
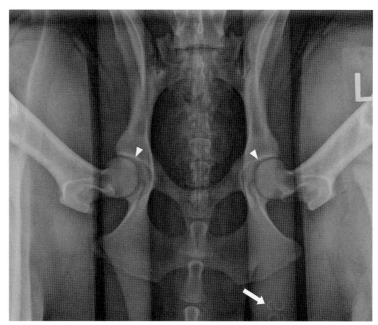

**A**

**B**

**FIGURE 6.36** Ventrodorsal projections of the pelvis in the traditional hip extended projection (**A**) as well as in the positioning used for the PennHip method (**B**). There is slight widening of the medial coxofemoral joint (arrowheads) in normal dogs. Each PennHip distractor has a unique embedded number (arrow) allowing its identification.

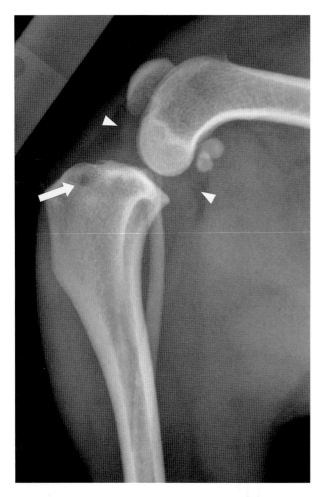

**FIGURE 6.37** Lateromedial projection of the stifle showing a focal lucency representing a retained tibial cartilage core (arrow). There is moderate effusion in the stifle joint causing cranial displacement of the infrapatellar fat pad and caudal distension of the joint capsule (arrowheads).

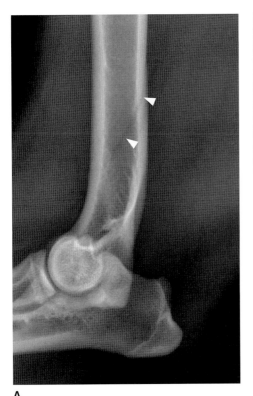
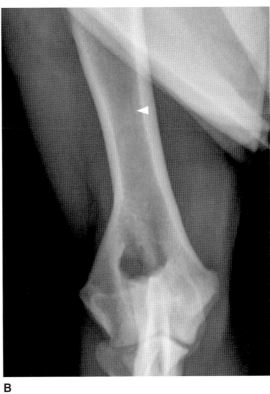

**A**    **B**

**FIGURE 6.38**    Lateromedial (**A**) and craniocaudal (**B**) projections of the distal humerus showing the position of a normal nutrient foramen (arrowheads). This should not be confused with a fissure fracture.

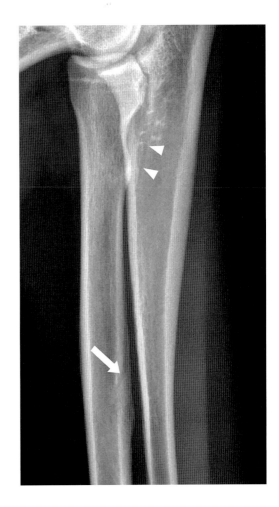

**FIGURE 6.39**    Lateral projection of the antebrachium showing the normal nutrient foramen of the radius (arrow) and ulna (arrowheads).

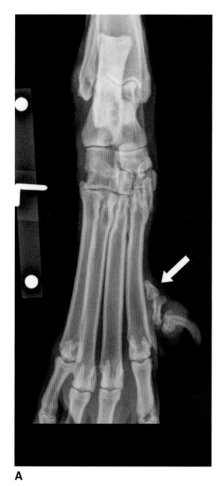

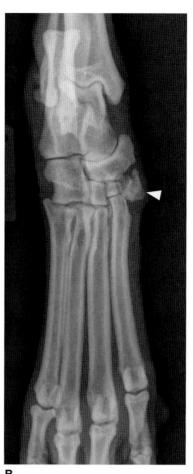

A                              B

**FIGURE 6.40**  Dorsoplantar projections of the hindlimb showing variations of the dew claw. They may be either large and defined externally as a separate digit (arrow) though may lack osseous connection to the underlying tarsus (**A**), or may be small remnants adjacent to the tarsus with little external digit seen (arrowhead, **B**).

and there can be separate bony thickening more proximally (Figure 6.40). These are usually intermittent anatomic variants, though are part of the breed standard expected in some types of dogs (such as Great Pyrenees or Icelandic sheepdogs). Polydactyly is intermittent in cats, and occurs most commonly in the thoracic limbs (Figure 6.41).

# Head

## Head: Basic Radiography Principles and Anatomy

The complex anatomy of the skull mandates careful positioning during radiography. The author finds the ventrodorsal projection of the skull often the most useful projection for the detection and characterization of many abnormalities on radiograph. Comparison between the left and right sides increases sensitivity of lesion detection, as pathology disrupts the expected left/right symmetry of the head.

Unfortunately, even slight obliquity of a ventrodorsal projection ruins left/right symmetry, preventing confident comparison between the left and right sides of the skull and decreasing diagnostic accuracy (Figure 6.42). Given the

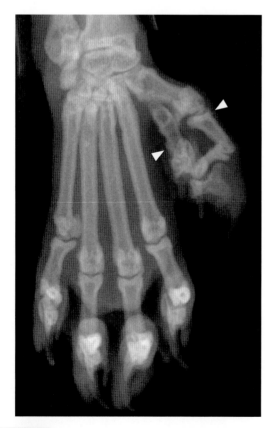

**FIGURE 6.41**  Dorsopalmar projection of the manus showing a cat with duplicated first digits (arrowheads), consistent with polydactyly.

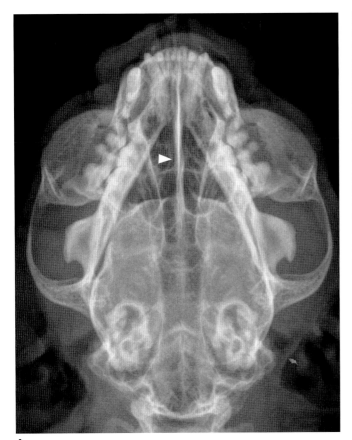

**A**

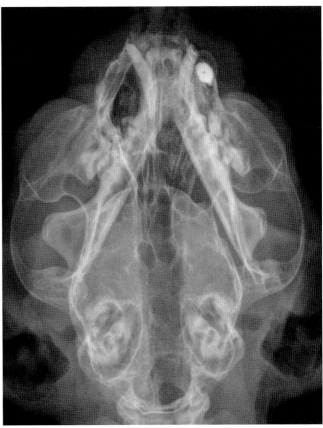

**B**

**FIGURE 6.42**   Ventrodorsal projections of the skull in a cat that are well positioned (**A**) and poorly positioned with obliquity (**B**). Notice that on well-positioned radiographs, the nasal septum (arrowhead) bisects the mandibular symphysis with symmetry between the left and right sides. On the poorly positioned radiographs, one mandible crosses the nasal cavity, creating asymmetry between the left and right sides of the skull.

importance of straight, well-positioned projections, successful skull radiography requires either very strong sedation or general anesthesia. If the latter is elected, the endotracheal tube is pulled laterally on VD projections to prevent superimposition with nasal structures or other anatomic structures of interest.

Many radiographic projections of the head are available, with projections performed depending on the area of interest and the clinical question to answer. Table 6.2 lists available projections of the skull, with figure references. At a minimum, a lateral and closed mouth VD projection are acquired.

Though the nasal cavity and osseous structures of the head are often a primary focus for radiography, radiographs also display abnormalities of the upper airway (nasopharynx, larynx, upper trachea). The nasopharynx is of particular interest given challenges of a direct airway examination in a patient, which usually otherwise requires retroflex endoscopy. Masses, strictures, and airway collapse can be identified on a lateral projection. As with the VD projection, careful positioning is necessary to achieve a straight lateral projection, as even slight obliquity can result in artifactual airway masses or collapse (Figure 6.51).

High-resolution dental radiography is a specialized imaging technique. Optimally, it requires use of a small field of view and high-resolution digital panels, designed to fit in the mouth and provide detailed images of a selected few teeth at a time. In reality, many practices do not have dedicated dental digital plates and rely on the larger, body/general digital plates to image the teeth. In that case, larger fields of view are achieved but with inferior resolution. More recently, cone beam CT units are available that provide high-detail cross-sectional imaging of the teeth. Dental imaging is the best use of this technology, as it otherwise displays poor contrast resolution/poor soft tissue anatomy and is negatively affected by motion.

Only basic dental anatomy will be included in this text (Figure 6.52), and advanced dental imaging and review of pathology is beyond the scope of the text.

A normal tooth has a crown (above the alveolar bone) and a root which is below the alveolar margin. There are three layers to a crown, including an inner pulp chamber, dentin, and the outer enamel layer. The pulp is radiolucent compared to the other two layers, and the enamel is very thin but the most opaque layer. The pulp chamber communicates with the root canal, which extends within the root. There is a thin layer of cementum that

**List of possible radiographic projections of the skull.**

| Projection name | Acquisition notes | Indication |
| --- | --- | --- |
| Lateromedial (lateral)[a] (Figure 6.43) | Patient placed in lateral recumbency | Evaluates overall morphology of skull |
| | | Best projection to evaluate gas in the nasopharynx, larynx, and upper trachea |
| Closed mouth ventrodorsal projection (VD)[a] (Figure 6.44) | Patient in dorsal recumbency with head extended. X-rays directed from ventral to dorsal with the mouth closed | Evaluates overall morphology of skull |
| | | Useful for evaluation of the temporomandibular joints |
| | | Useful for evaluation of the tympanic bullae |
| | | Limited use for evaluation of nasal cavity as the mandible superimposes it |
| [a]Dorsal 45 left-ventral right oblique (left 45 oblique) [a]Dorsal 45 right-ventral left oblique (right 45 oblique) (Figure 6.45) | Patient in lateral recumbency. Head is rotated 45° to achieve one oblique; the opposite oblique is then performed. Slightly opening the mouth allows better evaluation of the teeth | Useful for evaluation of tympanic bullae, maxilla, and mandible without superimposition of the contralateral side |
| Ventrodorsal projection of maxillary with open mouth (open mouth VD) (Figure 6.46) | Patient in dorsal recumbency Mandible retracted and x-rays directed from ventral to dorsal | Useful for intranasal pathology as the mandible does not superimpose the maxilla |
| | | Useful for evaluation of maxillary dental structures |
| Dorsoventral intraoral projection | Patient in sternal recumbency Digital plate placed within the mouth X-rays directed from dorsal to ventral through maxilla | Provides similar anatomy as the VD open mouth projection, but more limited in the caudal extent of anatomy that is visible as the digital plate may not fit entirely within the mouth |
| Ventrodorsal intraoral projection | Patient is placed in dorsal recumbency Digital plate is placed within the mouth X-rays directed from ventral to dorsal through the mandible | Useful for rostral mandibular pathology as the maxilla does not superimpose the mandible |
| Closed mouth rostrocaudal projection (frontal sinus skyline projection) (Figure 6.47) | Patient in dorsal recumbency, but head flexed Muzzle pointed toward x-ray tube X-rays directed from rostral to caudal to skyline the frontral sinuses | Frontal sinus evaluation |
| Open mouth rostrocaudal projection (open mouth bulla skyline) (Figure 6.48) | Similar to the closed mouth projection, but mouth is open X-rays directed from rostral to caudal through the oral cavity | Evaluation of the bullae |
| Rostral 10° ventral-caudal dorsal oblique (cat bulla skyline) (Figure 6.49) | The x-ray beam is directed ventral to the mandible, from rostral to caudal with the mouth closed | Alternative projection for bulla evaluation in the cat; does not require opening the mouth |
| Lateral 75° rostral-medial caudal oblique (TMJ oblique) (Figure 6.50) | Patient in lateral recumbency The nose is slightly elevated by 15° to highlight a temporomandibular joint. The opposite projection is then acquired | Temporomandibular joint evaluation from a lateral perspective, but without superimposition of the other skull anatomy |

[a] indicates this projection should be included as standard on all skull radiographic studies. Colloquial/abbreviated names for each projection are listed in parentheses.

coats the root, but is not seen radiographically as a separate layer. Typically, the alveolar bone should extend to within a millimeter or two of the cementoenamel junction; loss of alveolar bone can be recognized radiographically [5]. A normal root is surrounded by a thin lucent zone where the periodontal ligament is affixed to the tooth, and then a thin but dense layer of alveolar bone, termed the lamina dura, is seen. As a patient ages, the pulp chamber/root canal narrows, being much larger in a juvenile patient. Numeric tooth numbering via the Triadian system is preferred as a method to refer to each tooth.

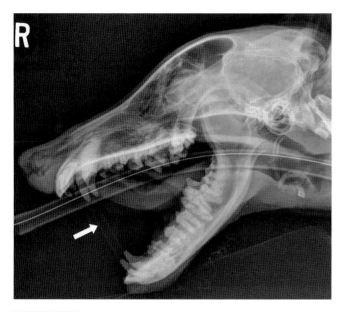

**FIGURE 6.43**  Lateral projection of the normal skull with the mouth opened, resulting in less than perfect position of mandibular and maxillary teeth. A small plastic tubular gag (arrow) spans between the maxillary and incisor canine teeth, separating the mandible from the maxilla.

## Head: Advanced Imaging

There are regions of the head that cannot be satisfactorially imaged with radiography. For the patient displaying central neurologic signs, an MRI is the preferred test to evaluate the brain and cranial nerves. CT can be used to image the brain, and is particularly useful for hemorrhage in the brain, but MRI remains the preferred imaging modality.

For other areas of pathology, particularly intranasal pathology, complex fractures, or soft tissue masses, CT is able to more exactly define the anatomy affected and refine differentials compared to radiography. Though MRI can be used to image pathology outside the brain/calvarium, the speed and lower cost of CT mean that modality is preferred for most other imaging indications, other than imaging the brain. Ultrasound is used more sparingly, typically in cases of cervical masses or ventral soft tissue masses of the head, when accessible structures such as the thyroid lobes, carotid body, larynx, or lymph nodes of the head are affected.

## Head: Anatomic Variants or Easily Confused Anatomy

**Superimposed Pinnae**   In some patients, particularly those with large pinnae, the pinnae may superimpose with anatomy of the skull/head. Because the pinna is surrounded by gas, it may appear strikingly opaque and can even mimic a mineralized structure or foreign object. Gas within the pinna will be prominent (Figure 6.53). When pinna superimposition occurs, reacquiring the radiograph with the pinna to the side can correct this artifact.

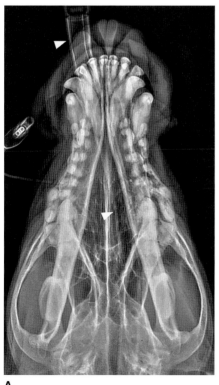

A

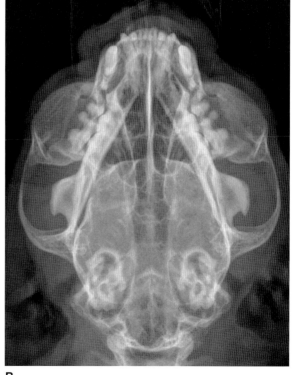

B

**FIGURE 6.44**  Closed mouth ventrodorsal projections in a dog (**A**) and cat (**B**), resulting in superimposition of the mandible with the rostral maxilla. An endotracheal tube (arrowheads) is present in the dog, and also superimposes the caudal nasal cavity. This should be retracted to the side when performing this projection to prevent superimposition.

---

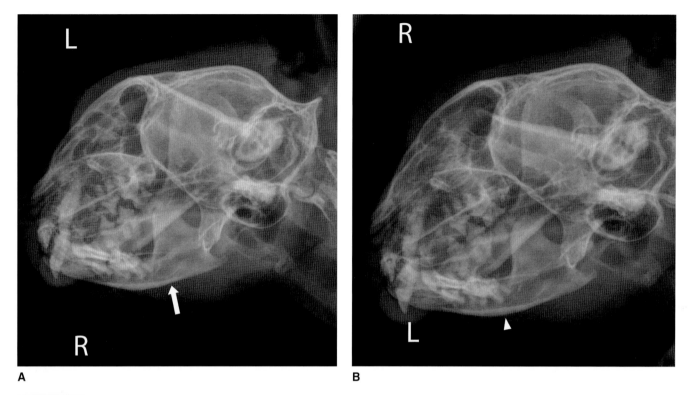

**FIGURE 6.45** Oblique projections of the maxilla and mandible from orthogonal directions. On (**A**), the left-sided anatomy is more dorsal and the right-sided anatomy more ventral. The arrow indicates the margin of the right mandible. On (**B**), the right-sided anatomy is more dorsal and the left-sided anatomy more ventral. The arrowhead indicates the margin of the left mandible. Double marking (using both R and L markers) radiographs is important to prevent confusion over sidedness.

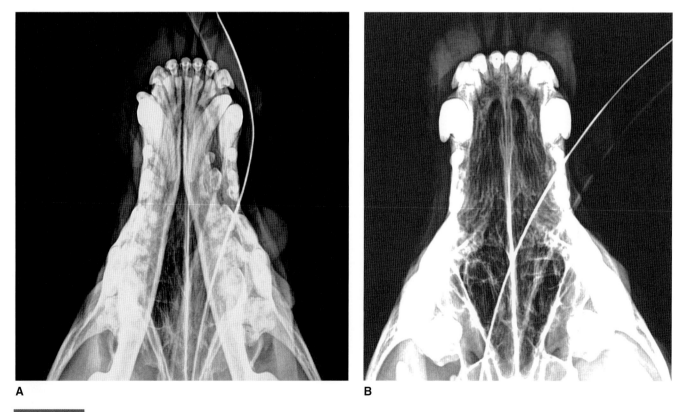

**FIGURE 6.46** Comparison of open mouth and closed mouth ventrodorsal projections. Notice when the mandible is closed (**A**), there is superimposition of the mandible with the rostral maxilla. With the mouth open (**B**), the maxillary turbinates of the rostral nasal cavity are clearly seen. The endotracheal tube has also been pulled to the side on the open mouth projection to limit superimposition with the rostral maxilla.

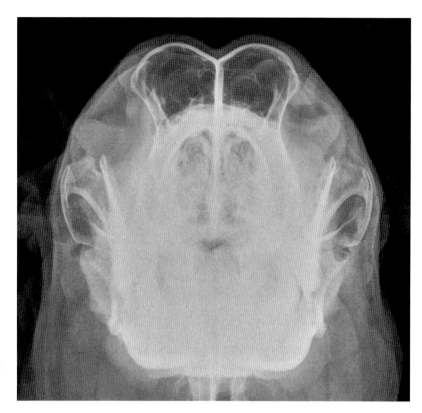

**FIGURE 6.47** Rostrocaudal closed mouth projection (frontal sinus skyline projection), demonstrating the normal gas-filled frontal sinuses.

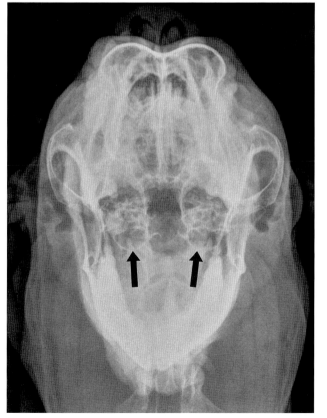

**A**

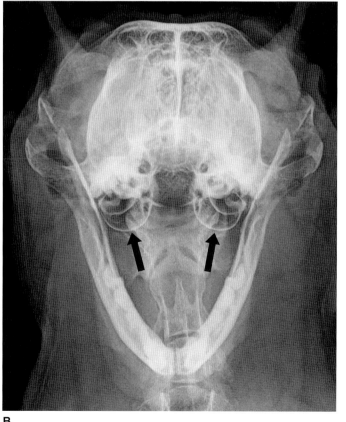

**B**

**FIGURE 6.48** Open mouth rostrocaudal projection in a dog (**A**) and cat (**B**) showing the bullae (arrows) which are normally gas filled.

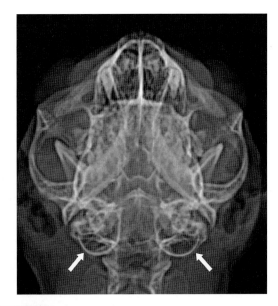

**FIGURE 6.49** Alternative projection to demonstrate the bulla in a cat. The mouth is closed and the x-ray beam angled proximally 10° rostral to caudal. This is technically easier and faster to perform than the open mouth rostrocaudal projection. The geometry of the skull does not allow this projection to be used in dogs, as the bulla superimposes the skull.

## Head Shape

Numerous anatomic variants are seen in brachycephalic dogs and cats related to their head conformation. Brachycephalic dogs typically have a hypoplastic or aplastic frontal sinus (Figure 6.54). A thick soft palate is often observed with radiography and CT. With advanced imaging, other more subtle abnormalities become apparent. This includes narrowing of the rostral choanae and caudal aberrant turbinates. Caudal aberrant turbinates from the nasal cavity into the rostral

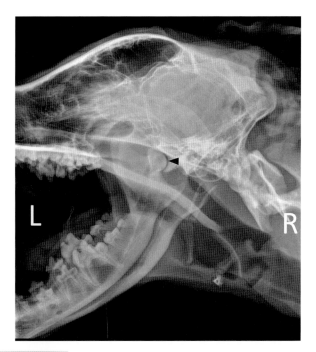

**FIGURE 6.50** Example of an oblique projection to demonstrate the temporomandibular joint (arrowhead). The nose is elevated from a lateral projection by approximately 15°; in this case the left temporomandibular joint is rostrally shifted and well seen. The right temporomandibular joint is not seen, so for complete evaluation the opposite oblique would also have to be performed. Notice that both R and L markers are used, to prevent confusion as to which joint is more cranial and which more caudal.

nasopharynx may contribute to the familiar stertor of brachycephalics as well as upper airway obstruction (Figure 6.55) [6]. There is typically prognathism of the mandible, with an elongated shape relative to the maxilla extending rostrally.

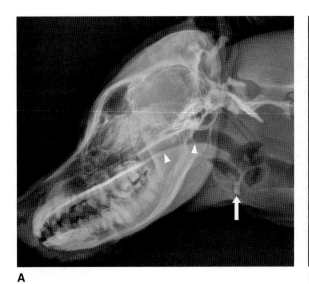

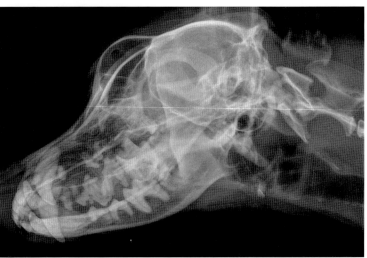

**A**  **B**

**FIGURE 6.51** Lateromedial projections of the skull in a dog that are well positioned (**A**) and poorly positioned (**B**) with obliquity. On the well-positioned radiographs, the air in the nasopharynx is readily apparent (arrowheads) but obscured on the oblique projection due to superimposed bone. When well positioned, the left and right sides of the hyoid apparatus superimpose (arrow).

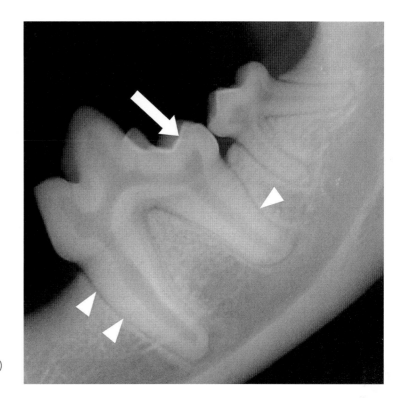

**FIGURE 6.52** Dental radiograph of a normal tooth. The pulp chamber is seen as a lucent central zone. Surrounding the tooth is the radiolucent periodontal space (arrowheads) with a thicker sclerotic lamina dura surrounding this space. Enamel is seen as an opaque layer of the outer crown (arrow) and dentin is seen as the thicker opacity under the enamel.

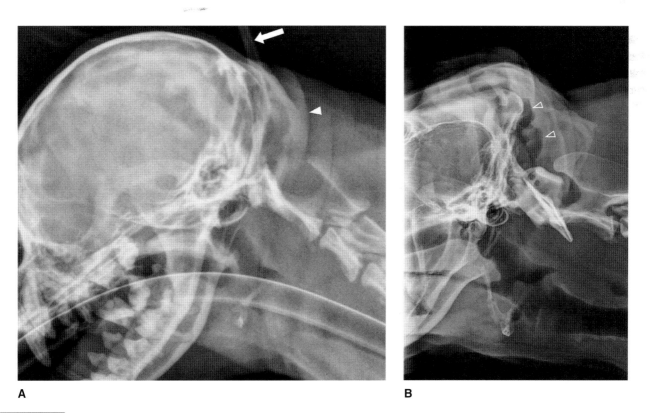

A

B

**FIGURE 6.53** Lateral radiographs of two dogs with superimposed pinna. The pinna can be seen outside the skull (arrow) but where it superimposes with the skull and neck it can appear more opaque than other tissues (closed arrowhead) and could mimic a foreign body or fracture. In some cases, the gas in the ear canal may be apparent and should not be confused with abnormal pathology (open arrowhead).

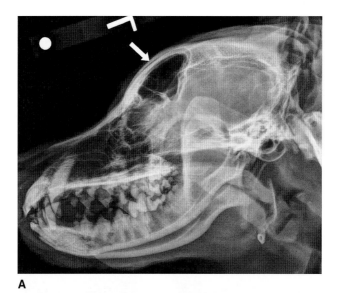

**A**

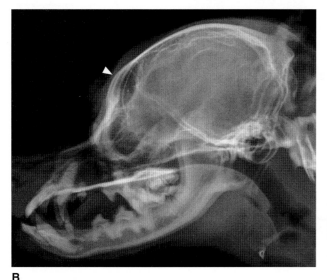

**B**

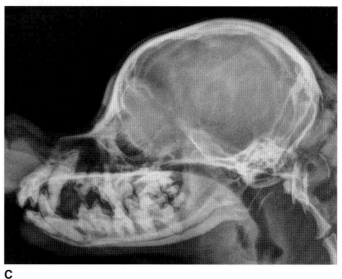

**C**

**FIGURE 6.54** Lateral projection of a Border collie (**A**), Maltese (**B**), and Chihuahua (**C**) showing normal breed variation in the frontal sinus. In the collie, the frontal sinus is large and gas filled (arrow). In the Maltese, it is reduced in size (arrowheads) and is absent in the Chihuahua.

Dolichocephalic dogs often have less pronounced anatomic abnormalities compared to brachycephalic dogs. Their skull is more narrow and elongated.

**Mandibular Salivary Gland** Intermittent medial location of the mandibular salivary gland occurs in dogs, resulting in it being located more rostral than normal and medial to the digastricus muscle (Figure 6.56). No clinical effects are seen in these patients [7].

**Foramen Magnum** In many small-breed dogs, the foramen magnum may have an abnormal shape. Rather than its

typical oval shape, it may be greatly elongated dorsally, appearing more keyhole-like (Figure 6.57). Where there should be bone, there may be a thin fibrous band appreciated on MRI, though on radiographs this may be seen on the rostrocaudal projection as an elongated lucent opening.

**Mandibular Symphysis** The mandibular symphysis normally has irregular margins where the left and right hemimandibles are opposed. The symphysis is wider in young patients and becomes more narrow with age, but may never completely close, and can be falsely interpreted as a fracture.

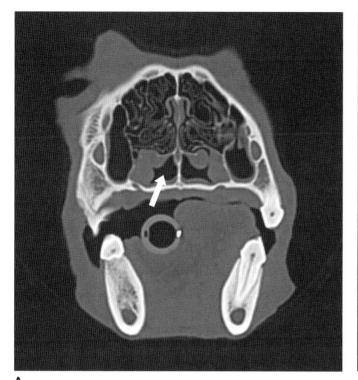

A

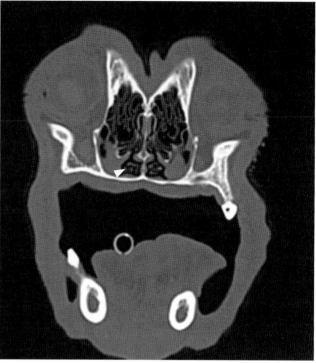

B

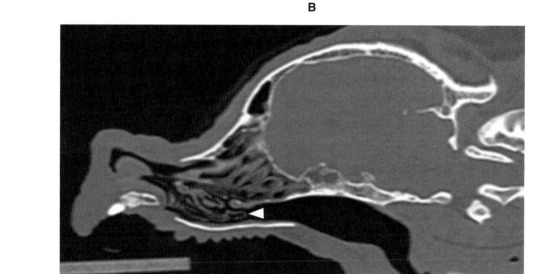

C

**FIGURE 6.55** Transverse CT image of a normal Labrador retriever without aberrant turbinates, showing an open nasopharyngeal meatus (arrow, **A**). In comparison, a bulldog is shown with caudal aberrant turbinates (arrowhead) extending through the nasopharyngeal meatus into the nasopharynx (**B**, transverse plane and **C**, parasagittal reconstruction image).

# Axial Skeleton

## Axial Skeleton: Basic Radiography Principles

Indications for spinal radiography are numerous. Pain on spinal palpation, nerve root signature displayed to a forelimb or hindlimb, and neurologic deficits to the limbs are reasons for spinal survey radiographs. In most patients, the length of the spine prevents inclusion of the entire cervical through lumbar spine on a single radiograph. For that reason, only a portion of the spine is radiographed in a given patient (using lateral and VD radiographs), with the area of interest selected based on physical examination findings, neurologic localization, and history.

Cervical radiographs include a lateral and VD projection, extending from the most caudal aspect of the skull through the third thoracic vertebral segment. Because the scapulae superimpose the caudal cervical spine, the author recommends two

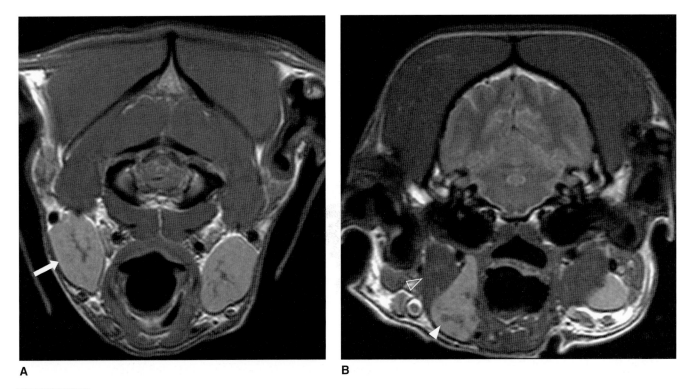

**A**

**B**

**FIGURE 6.56** Transverse PD image of a dog with normal mandibular salivary gland location (**A**, arrow) compared to a dog with a malpositioned mandibular salivary gland (**B**, closed arrowhead). In the dog with malpositioning, the salivary gland is more rostral than normal and medial to the digastricus muscle (open arrowhead).

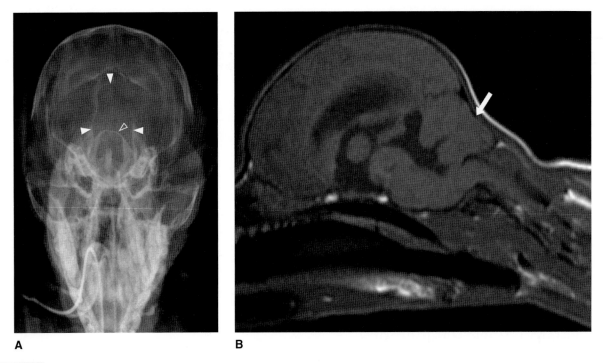

**A**

**B**

**FIGURE 6.57** Rostral 20° dorsal to caudal ventral oblique (**A**) acquired by directing the x-beam from rostral to caudal and slightly tipping the nose ventrally. This highlights the margin of the foramen magnum (closed arrowheads) which is greatly elongated dorsal to ventral. The dorsal lamina of C1 is superimposed with this area (open arrowhead). On the sagittal T1W MRI of this patient (**B**), the dorsal foramen magnum margin (arrow) is very dorsally located, allowing the cerebellum to extend caudally.

lateral radiographs of the cervical spine. One lateral radiograph is performed with the thoracic limbs cranially extended and then another lateral radiograph with the thoracic limbs caudally. Altering scapula position between radiographs moves the area of superimposition of the scapula with the cervical spine, allowing a more thorough evaluation of all vertebrae without superimposition (Figure 6.58). Often, if a lesion is neurologically localized to the T3–S3 location, separate radiographs of the thoracic region (lateral and VD) and lumbar region (lateral and VD) are performed, with the radiographs centered in the midthoracic and midlumbar spine respectively. Additional projections (lateral and VD) centered at the thoracolumbar junction are beneficial (for reasons discussed below). If lumbosacral clinical signs are present, than VD/lateral radiographs centered at this disc space are performed.

Intervertebral disc space narrowing occurs in patients with disc degeneration or herniation and in cases of discospondylitis. If the spine is rotated on lateral projections, disc narrowing will be less apparent (Figure 6.59).

Conversely, in a normal patient, rotation or obliquity of the spine results in the artifactual appearance of disc space narrowing as follows. When performing lateral radiographs of a normal patient, the spine should be parallel to the imaging plate. The disc spaces will then be parallel to the x-ray beam, resulting in a normal width on the resultant radiographs. If a portion of the spine is not well supported, there is resultant medial/lateral curvature of the spine (in other words, a portion of the spine will "sag" toward the table). Spinal curvature obliques the intervertebral disc space orientation relative to the x-ray beam, resulting in an artifactual impression of disc space narrowing on the resultant radiograph.

Even in a well-supported/positioned spine, disc spaces near the end of the lateral projection will appear narrowed. The x-ray beam at the edges of an exposed area normally

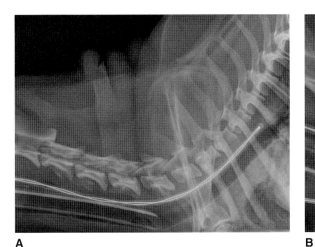
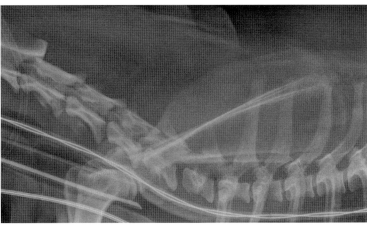

**FIGURE 6.58** Lateromedial radiographs of the cervical spine with the legs maximally caudally positioned (**A**) and cranially positioned (**B**). Notice that with the legs caudally positioned, the disc spaces of C5–6 and C6–7 are well seen but the scapula superimposes the more caudal disc spaces. When the legs are cranially positioned, those more caudal spaces are seen without superimposition of the scapula.

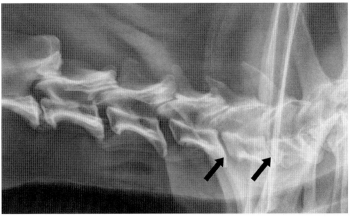
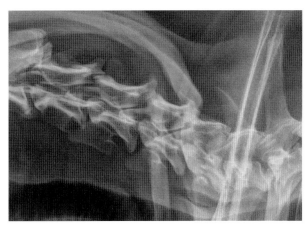

**FIGURE 6.59** Lateromedial radiographs of the cervical spine that are well positioned (**A**) and poorly positioned (**B**) due to rotation and obliquity of the disc spaces. On the well-positioned radiograph, caudal cervical disc narrowing (arrows) is readily seen, but is more difficult to see when the positioning is poor.

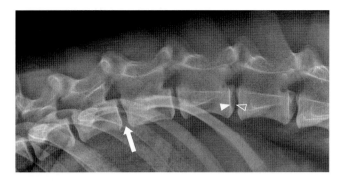

**FIGURE 6.60** Radiographs centered at the thoracolumbar junction. Notice that disc spaces at the center of the projection have well-defined margins without superposition of adjacent vertebral segments (arrow). Disc spaces at the edge of the projection, where the x-ray beam diverges from the intervertebral disc angle, result in normal superimposition of adjacent segments due to beam divergence. The closed arrowhead indicates one side of the caudal L1 endplate and the open arrowhead indicates the other side of the caudal L1 endplate. Notice that the margin of the endplate (open arrowhead) overlaps with cranial L2.

have a more oblique orientation relative to the patient. This normal x-ray beam divergence means that the x-rays are no longer parallel to the intervertebral disc space, artifactually causing an impression of disc space narrowing (Figure 6.60). For that reason, multiple projections centered over different areas of the spine allow evaluation of all intervertebral widths.

Though the spine is included as part of standard abdomen or thoracic radiography studies, abdominal or thoracic radiographs are no substitute for dedicated spinal radiographs. While spinal structures are included on thoracic and abdominal radiographs, optimal spinal positioning is rarely achieved when the area of the interest is the thorax or abdomen, as the focus of these studies is inclusion of thoracic or abdominal structures rather than spinal anatomy. Moreover, the spine is not in the center of the image for lateral thoracic and abdominal radiographs, resulting in oblique x-ray orientation relative to the spine.

Finally, radiographic technique (mAs/kVp) used for imaging the spine is different from that used for abdominal or thoracic radiographs. Optimal imaging of the spine requires higher mAs settings than typically used for thoracic or abdominal radiography, and while gross abnormalities may be apparent, subtle areas of bone loss or other pathology may not be seen when compared to centered, high-technique dedicated radiographs of the spine (Figure 6.61). Spinal radiographs also require tight collimation, excluding the thoracic or abdominal structures which otherwise would increase scatter and diminish radiographic contrast of the spine.

**Projections and Positioning**   As mentioned above, careful spinal positioning is necessary for adequate spinal radiography. In very thin patients, radiolucent pad placement under the lumbar or midcervical spine prevents "sagging"

of the spine toward the table, which can alter alignment of adjacent vertebral segments. Lateral projections should be inspected for superimposition of left/right-sided transverse and articular processes, which only occurs with true lateral projections. Obliquity results in ventral positioning of one transverse or articular process compared to the contralateral side.

Additional projections beyond lateral and VD spinal radiographs are rarely indicated, though exceptions exist. If dens hypoplasia or fracture is suspected, a lateral projection is acquired after intentionally rotating the head approximately 30° around its long axis. This displaces one wing of C1 more ventrally than the other, resolving superimposition of the dens that otherwise obscures its margins (Figure 6.62). Dorsoventral (DV) spinal projections are rarely performed, as the greater distance between the spine and the imaging plate allows more motion and magnification. Oblique spinal radiographs improve detection of subtle fractures or complex spinal pathology.

In rare cases, when instability is suspected between C1 and C2, lateral radiographs may be performed with gentle flexion of the spine. The dorsal lamina of C1 and spinous process of C2 should remain in close apposition due to the presence of the dorsal atlantoaxial ligament. Any widening of the space between these structures is evidence of atlantoaxial instability (Figure 6.62).

## Vertebral Development and Normal Anatomy

Vertebrae form from multiple different centers of ossification. C1 forms from three ossification centers: a pair of neural arches and intercentrum 1 (which forms the body). C2 arises from seven centers of ossification, with two of these fusing by approximately 100 days of age to form the dens. The remaining cervical, thoracic, and lumbar vertebrae form from a pair of neural arches and centrum, with cranial and caudal physes which remain radiographically visible until close to skeletal maturity (approximately 7–12 months of age).

The atlantoaxial junction has complex but important anatomy aimed at stabilizing this region. The atlantoaxial joint allows rotational movement around the dens, but has structures that prevent abnormal flexion, extension, or lateral movement. The dens is a short osseous protuberance on the cranial margin of C2 that is easily recognized on the ventrodorsal projection (Figure 6.62). Extending cranially from the dens are the short apical ligaments that insert on the foramen magnum margin and the occipital condyles. The alar ligaments extend at approximately a 45° angle from the dens and also anchor it to C1.

Finally, the transverse ligament extends dorsal to the dens, and prevents dorsal subluxation of C2 relative to C1 when the neck is flexed by holding the dens against the ventral arch of C1. Also preventing dorsal C2 subluxation is the dorsally positioned atlantoaxial ligament, which extends from the spinous process of C2 to the dorsal lamina of C1.

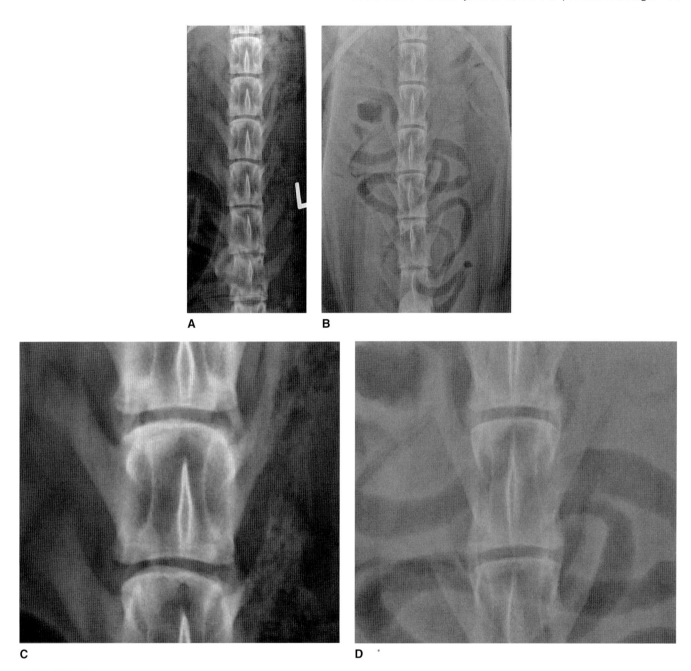

**A**   **B**

**C**   **D**

**FIGURE 6.61** Ventrodorsal projections of the lumbar spine acquired with dedicated spinal technique (**A**), using a high mAs/low KVP technique and collimation to the spine. This is compared to images of the spine included as part of this abdominal radiography series (**B**), using abdominal residence bound technique and wider collimation. Magnified images of the spinal technique (**C**) versus abdominal technique (**D**) are also included. Notice that the dedicated spinal radiographs have better detail and contrast of the vertebral segments compared to when the spine is included as part of the abdominal series.

## Axial Skeleton: Advanced Imaging

Radiography is a useful initial spinal imaging test, as it can screen for narrowed disc spaces, fractures, or evidence of bone loss. If radiographs are normal, CT better identifies subtle osseous pathology, such as fissure fractures or early aggressive lesions. Some anatomy such as endplate morphology and disc space width are best seen in other reformatted planes (Figure 6.63).

If spinal cord/soft tissue pathology is suspected, then MRI is the gold standard imaging test. Radiographs or CT may identify

some obvious changes, such as disc space narrowing or aggressive bone loss that suggests spinal cord compression could be present, but MRI is the best imaging test to directly characterize that soft tissue pathology (Figure 6.64). Radiographs can only identify gross soft tissue pathology, such as a large mass adjacent to the vertebral bodies and are not able to identify any soft tissues within the vertebral canal. CT can identify some soft tissue structures with more definition than radiographs, such as the musculature adjacent to the vertebral column, but is not as adept at identifying smaller soft tissue structures. Spinal

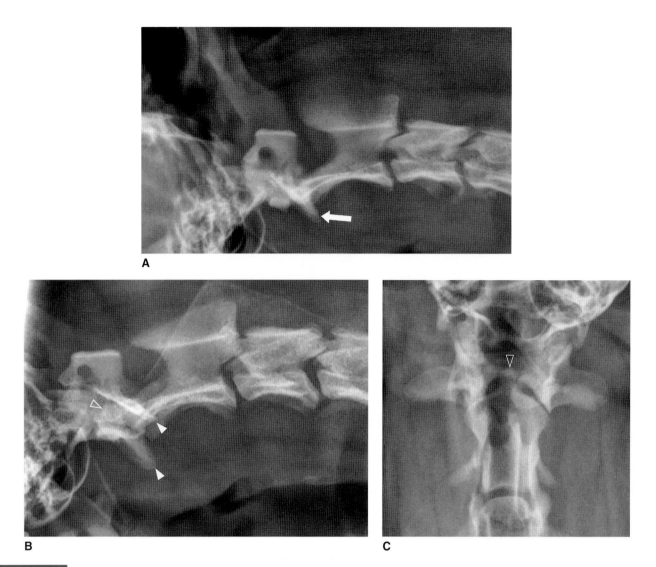

**FIGURE 6.62** Lateromedial (**A**), lateromedial with C1 wings obliqued (**B**), and ventrodorsal (**C**) projections of the cranial cervical region. When the wings of C1 are superimposed (arrow), the dens is not seen on the lateral projection. Obliquing the left and right wings of C1 (closed arrowhead) allows the dens to be seen (open arrowhead). The dens is well seen on the ventrodorsal projection (open arrowhead). Notice the lamina of C1 and spinous process of C2 are in close apposition on the lateral radiographs; this distance should not change with flexion of the spine.

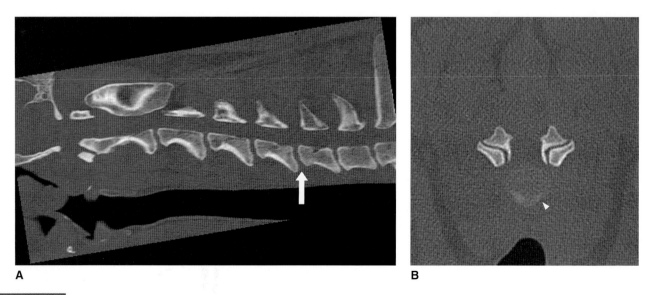

**FIGURE 6.63** Sagittal (**A**) and transverse (**B**) CT images of the cervical spine. The disc space width is appreciated on sagittal reformatted images (the arrow is at the C5–6 intervertebral disc). The transverse image (**B**) is at the level of C5–6. There is partial volume averaging resulting in the caudal aspect of C5 (arrowhead) being partially included in this image at the intervertebral disc.

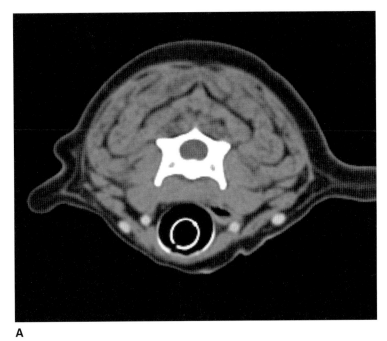

A

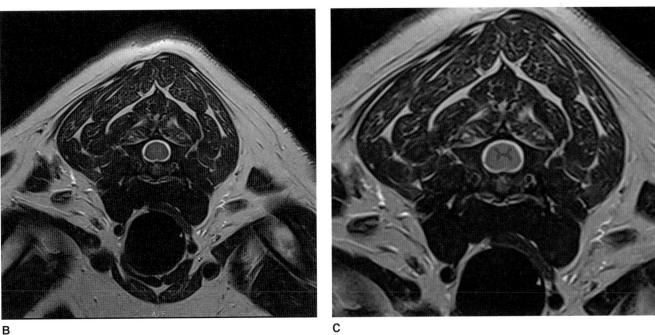

B                                    C

**FIGURE 6.64**   CT (**A**) and MRI (**B**) transverse images of the spine (same patient), with a magnified image (**C**) showing the spinal cord white matter in red, gray matter in blue, and the surrounding CSF/epidural tissues in yellow. Notice that the vertebrae are distinctly seen on CT images but have a hypointense appearance on MRI with less well-defined margins. In comparison, the distinction between fat and soft tissues of the superficial spinal cord is well seen on the MRI due to better differences in signal between fat and soft tissues. The internal spinal cord anatomy is discernible on MRI, but on CT is a homogeneous density.

nerves, for instance, are well defined on MRI, but either not seen at all on CT or only seen where they are grossly enlarged.

The difference between epidural fat and soft tissues allows visualization of the outer margin of the dura mater on CT imaging. The spinal cord itself is not seen, however, as the density differences between CSF and the spinal cord are too small to allow the spinal cord to be seen. In comparison, MRI readily separates signal from cerebrospinal fluid (CSF) and the spinal cord, allowing ready identification of spinal cord anatomy.

# Axial Skeleton: Anatomic Variants or Easily Confused Anatomy

**Congenital Vertebral Anomalies** Congenital vertebral anomalies are common in some breeds of dog, but rarely associated with any clinical signs (further discussed in Chapter 12). This may consist of hemivertebrae (malformed vertebral body development), block vertebrae (fusion of vertebral bodies) or aberrant ribs. Aberrant ribs are most common at T13, but C7 may have small aberrant vestigial ribs as well. In some dogs, these aberrant C7 vestigial ribs may contact or fuse with abnormally formed T1 ribs.

The caudal/tail vertebrae normally have numerous congenital abnormalities in certain breeds, such as bulldogs, resulting in a truncated, corkscrew shape.

Ventral to the cranial intervetebral spaces of the tail, there are small hemal arches (Figure 6.65). These are separate small osseous structures found in normal dogs, but there is some variation in their size and number between dogs. In most dogs, these are not seen caudal to the seventh caudal vertebral segment. These should not be confused for fracture fragments or spondylosis deformans.

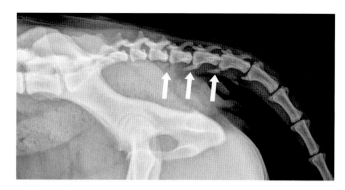

**FIGURE 6.65**  Lateral radiographs of the tail showing normal hemal arches (arrows).

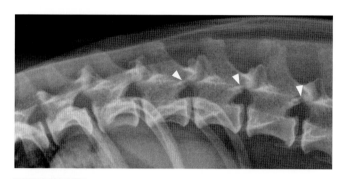

**FIGURE 6.66**  Lateral radiograph of the thoracolumbar junction showing accessory processes (arrowheads) superimposed with the dorsal intervertebral foramen. These cause the foramen to appear slightly smaller at this level but this is a normal feature in this region that should not be confused with superimposed disc material.

**C6 Transverse Processes** The transverse processes of C6 are larger than adjacent cervical transverse processes. As a result, they extend more ventrally and are more apparent on lateral projections. If the lateral projection is obliqued, one of the C6 transverse processes will extend significantly below the vertebral column and can be mistakenly confused with an esophageal mineralized foreign body.

**Accessory Process** The caudal thoracic vertebrae have larger accessary processes compared to those thoracic

vertebrae more cranially or lumbar vertebrae more caudally. These project caudally and dorsally from the pedicles of the caudal thoracic vertebrae, superimposing with the intervertebral foramen (Figure 6.66). These should not be confused for mineral material that has extruded dorsally from an abnormal, degenerative intervertebral disc.

# References

1.  Smallwood, J.E., Rendano, V.T., and Habel, R.E. (1985). A standardized nomenclature for radiographic projections used in veterinary medicine. *Vet. Radiol. Ultrasound* 26 (1): 2–9.

2.  Perry, K.L., Fordham, A., and Arthurs, G.I. (2014). Effect of neutering and breed on femoral and tibial physeal closure times in male and female domestic cats. *J. Feline Med. Surg.* 16 (2): 149–156.

3.  Orthopedic Foundation for Animals Website. What is canine hip dysplasia? www.ofa.org/diseases/hip-dysplasia#hipscreening

4.  Paek, M., Engiles, J.B., and Mai, W. (2013). Prevalence, association with stifle conditions, and histopathologic characteristics of tibial tuberosity radiolucencies in dogs. *Vet. Radiol. Ultrasound* 54 (5): 453–458.

5.  Bannon, K.M. (2013). Clinical canine dental radiography. *Vet. Clin. North Am. Small Anim. Pract.* 43 (3): 507–532.

6.  Vilaplana Grosso, F., Haar, G.T., and Boroffka, S.A. (2015). Gender, weight, and age effects on prevalence of caudal aberrant nasal turbinates in clinically healthy English bulldogs: a computed tomographic study and classification. *Vet. Radiol. Ultrasound* 56 (5): 486–493.

7.  Durand, A., Finck, M., Sullivan, M., and Hammond, G. (2016). Computed tomography and magnetic resonance diagnosis of variations in the anatomical location of the major salivary glands in 1680 dogs and 187 cats. *Vet. J.* 209: 156–162.

# CHAPTER 7

# Developmental Orthopedic Disease

Elizabeth Huynh

VCA West Coast Specialty and Emergency Animal Hospital, Fountain Valley, CA, USA

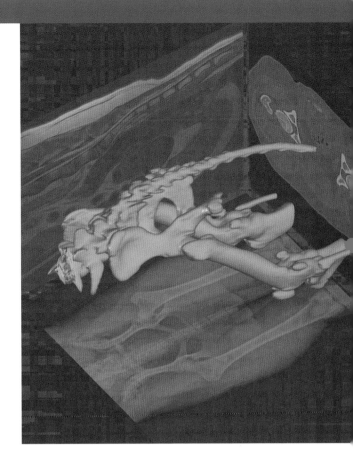

## Introduction

An understanding of normal radiographic anatomy and the pathogenesis of disease conditions is imperative when evaluating young dogs and cats for developmental orthopedic disease. There are unique factors that confound interpretation of orthopedic radiographs in juvenile patients. These include the presence of open physes, incomplete development of osseous structures, and variations of anatomy specific to species and breeds. A classic interpretation paradigm is not as helpful in developmental orthopedic disease, although specific diseases are associated with specific anatomic locations of the osseous structures.

One can develop a prioritized differential list based on some of the same questions asked of other orthopedic studies. These would include aggressive versus nonaggressive changes, position within the osseous structure (i.e., epiphysis, physis, metaphysis, diaphysis, joint centered, etc.), and number of bones involved (monostotic versus polyostotic).

Well-positioned orthogonal radiographs are critical for accurate interpretation. At times, comparison views of contralateral limbs (or other age-matched normal patients) provide a better understanding of normal developmental variations though some developmental orthopedic diseases may be bilateral. Unique radiographic views (i.e., oblique radiographs, etc.) will aid in interpretation for highlighting specific areas of the regional anatomy.

Finally, an awareness of the signalment and clinical signs associated with each developmental disease is imperative for the development of a prioritized differential list, as well as decisions around therapy (Table 7.1).

Developmental orthopedic disease can be broken down into three major categories.

- Dysplasia (abnormal cartilage and/or bone development) [1]
- Osteochondrosis (failure of normal endochondral ossification)

| TABLE 7.1 | Developmental orthopedic diseases with typical signalment, history, and imaging findings with recommended therapies. |

| Disease | Common breeds | Typical age of diagnosis | Clinical signs | Key radiographic changes | Therapy |
|---|---|---|---|---|---|
| Hip dysplasia | German shepherd, Labrador/ golden retriever | 24 mo | Hip pain, lameness | Coxal Incongruity, laxity, osteoarthritis | Weight loss, pain management, hip replacement |
| Fragmented medial coronoid process (FMCP) | Labrador/ golden retriever | 1 yr | Elbow pain | Flat or fragmented medial coronoid process, sclerosis of semilunar notch, osteoarthritis | Weight loss, pain management, surgical debridement |
| Ununited anco-neal process (UAP) | German shepherd | 5 mo | Elbow pain | Fissure between anconeal process and olecranon | Surgical removal |
| Osteochondritis dissecans (OCD) | Labrador/ golden retriever, German shepherd | 8–24 mo | Location specific | Flattening of humeral head, medial humeral condyle, medial or lateral femoral condyle, medial or lateral trochlear ridge of the talus | Surgical debridement |
| TMJ dysplasia | Basset hound, setter breeds, Cavalier King Charles spaniel | Any age | Asymptomatic, joint laxity, open mouth jaw locking, dental malocclusion | Flat mandibular fossa, misshapen condylar process, short retroarticular process, TMJ subluxation | Zygomatic arch ostectomy if jaw locking |
| Panosteitis | German shepherd | 5–12 mo | Shifting leg lameness, pain over diaphysis | Endosteal or subperiosteal new bone formation | Supportive, steroids, NSAIDs |
| Hypertrophic osteodystrophy (HOD) | Great Dane, Irish wolfhound, Rottweiler, Weimaraner | 3–5 mo | Shifting leg lameness, pain over metaphyses | Double physis sign, metaphyseal flare, metaphyseal periosteal response | Supportive, ± steroids, NSAIDs |
| Retained cartilage core | Large to giant breeds, Great Dane | 3–9 mo | Angular limb deformities; may be asymptomatic | Well-defined, triangular lucency of the distal ulnar metaphysis | Supportive |
| Incomplete ossification of the humeral condyle | Spaniel breeds | Any | Asymptomatic or lameness | Lucency of humeral intercondylar region, ± supracondylar fracture | Surgical stabilization |
| Avascular necrosis of the femoral head | Miniature to small-breed dogs | 5–8 mo | Lameness | Lucent, resorptive femoral head and neck, coxal osteoarthritis | Femoral head and neck ostectomy |
| Capital femoral physeal fracture (Cats) | Any | 7 mo to 2 yr | Traumatic or non-traumatic lameness | Salter Harris type I fracture of the femoral head, coxal osteoarthritis | Femoral head and neck ostectomy |
| Septic metaphysitis | Any | Young | Lameness | Soft tissue swelling, aggressive osseous proliferation and lysis | Antibiotics |
| Multiple cartilaginous exostoses | Great Danes, St Bernards, hounds | 6 wk to 11 yr | Lameness, firm masses | Single/multiple osseous masses, metaphyses of long bones, axial skeleton | Supportive |
| Multiple epiphyseal dysplasia | Beagles, miniature poodles, others | Young, adult | Disproportionate size, lameness | Shortened long bones, wide metaphysis, decreased epiphysis, vertebrae affected | Supportive |
| Craniomandibular osteopathy | West Highland white terriers | 3–7 mo | Difficult prehension | Thickened mandibular cortex, bulla with periosteal proliferation | Supportive, NSAIDs |
| Calvarial hyperostosis | Bull mastiffs | Any | Pain | Thickened external sagittal crest of the skull and frontal bone region | Supportive, NSAIDs |

NSAID, nonsteroidal antiinflammatory drug.

- Miscellaneous idiopathic diseases that are often polyostotic and involve specific anatomic regions of the long bones

# Dysplasia

Joint dysplasias are best defined as growth disorders resulting in joint incongruity, laxity, or other malformations. These disorders often have multifactorial etiologies; however, genetic predisposition plays a role. Joints commonly affected by dysplasia are the coxal (coxofemoral), cubital (elbow), and temporomandibular joints (TMJ).

Generalized osseous dysplasias include epiphyseal and metaphyseal dysplasias, abnormalities associated with congenital hormonal underdevelopment (i.e., congenital panhypopituitarism, congenital hypothyroidism), or secondary to an underlying osseous structural disorder (i.e., osteogenesis imperfecta, mucopolysaccharidosis, etc.). Metabolic disorders of nutrition and renal dysplasia result in generalized osteopenia, pathologic folding fractures, and fibrous dysplasia of the skull.

## Hip Dysplasia

**Etiology**  Hip dysplasia is a developmental abnormality associated with the soft tissues and osseous structures of the coxal joint. Hip dysplasia is primarily a developmental disorder of large-breed dogs but can affect small-breed dogs and cats. It is usually bilateral but can be unilateral and asymmetric when comparing the right and left sides. Hip dysplasia is heritable, with environmental, nutritional, and conformational factors affecting rate of progression of degenerative changes and degree of lameness in the dog or cat [2]. The phenotypic expression of dysplastic changes, particularly degenerative changes, is not apparent early but progresses with age. Clinical signs of pelvic limb lameness can develop as early as 4–6 months and typically are documented radiographically at 24 months of age. Common breeds affected include the German shepherd, Labrador retriever, golden retriever, and other large-breed dogs [1].

**Pathogenesis**  The underlying abnormality appears to be a laxity of the coxal joints resulting in incomplete development of the acetabular rim that leads to a shallow acetabulum and progressive coxal joint subluxation and resultant joint incongruity. This leads to secondary periarticular osteophyte formation associated with the acetabula and femoral heads. Enthesopathy will also develop over time in the region of the intertrochanteric fossa and femoral neck where a number of muscles and the coxal joint capsule insert. Other insertional abnormalities include lesser trochanter avulsion fractures associated with the iliopsoas muscle insertion and enthesopathy associated with the joint capsule. This is radiographically

characterized by an osseous fragment immediately adjacent to the lesser trochanter of the femur in the region of the iliopsoas muscle insertion.

**Radiographic Assessment and Indicators of Hip Dysplasia**  There are five radiographic views that evaluate the coxal joint (Figure 7.1): (i) lateral pelvis view (with the pelvic limbs scissored so that the dependent limb is cranial and the pelvic limb further away from the table is positioned caudally), (ii) extended limb ventrodorsal pelvis view, (iii) flexed limb ventrodorsal pelvis view, (iv) dorsal acetabular rim (DAR) view [3], and (v) PennHip evaluation view using a distraction device for determining degree of subluxation/laxity. The first two listed are obtained for routine evaluation of the pelvis. The other views may be obtained for evaluation of specific conditions as clinically warranted (Table 7.2).

Multiple radiographic abnormalities are seen with hip dysplasia (Figure 7.2). Coxal joint laxity is manifested as decreased coverage of the femoral head by the DAR resulting in incongruency of the femoral head and acetabular surfaces. Additionally, osseous proliferation is associated with the acetabulum, femoral head, and femoral neck. An early indicator of degenerative joint disease associated with osseous proliferation of the femoral neck has been termed the "Morgan line," which represents enthesophyte formation of the insertion of the coxal joint capsule.

## Elbow Dysplasia

Elbow dysplasia causes variable degrees of lameness in affected dogs and cats and is a multifactorial disease composed of one or more of the following developmental abnormalities: fragmented medial coronoid process (FMCP), ununited anconeal process (UAP), osteochondritis dissecans (OCD) of the medial humeral condyle, elbow joint incongruity, and secondary elbow joint osteoarthrosis [4]. FMCP and UAP can be related to asynchronous growth of the radius and ulna leading to joint incongruity, whereas osteochondrosis and osteoarthrosis can be primary disease conditions or secondary to elbow incongruity. To diagnose elbow dysplasia, knowledge of normal elbow anatomy is important (Figure 7.3).

### Fragmented Medial Coronoid Process of the Ulna

**Etiology**  Fragmented medial coronoid process is characterized by fragmentation or fissuring of the cartilage and bone over the craniolateral aspect of the medial coronoid process of the ulna. A recent change in terminology groups a number of related pathologies under the term "medial compartment syndrome": coronoid process sclerosis, coronoid eburnation and microfissuring, and coronoid fragmentation with or without

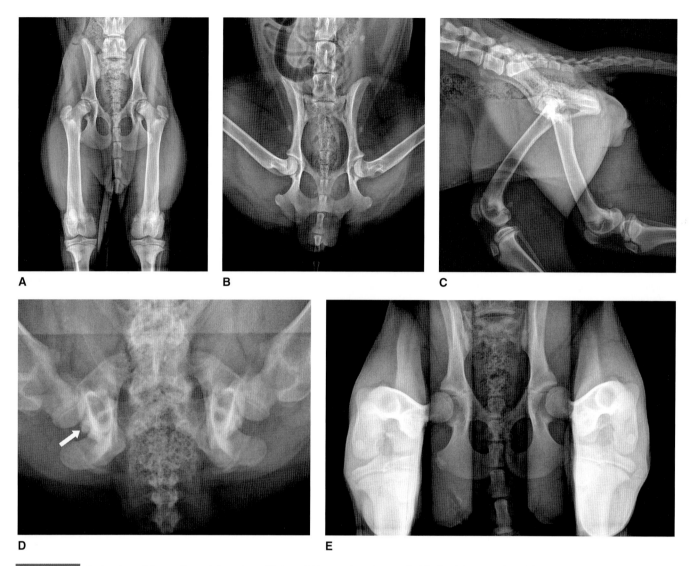

**FIGURE 7.1** Evaluation of the canine pelvis and coxal joints. (**A**) Ventrodorsal extended limbs, (**B**) ventrodorsal flexed limb, (**C**) lateral, (**D**) craniocaudal dorsal acetabular rim, and (**E**) PennHip radiographs. In (**D**), the dorsal acetabular rim (DAR) point is the lateral aspect of the dorsal acetabular rim that is seen in this radiograph (arrow).

documented incongruity. The frequency of disease and the commonality of breeds it affects have led to much investigation into this disease process and its underlying etiologies, including osteochondrosis, joint incongruities, and biomechanical force mismatch. Dog breeds commonly affected by FMCP include the Labrador retriever, golden retriever, Rottweiler, and Bernese mountain dog.

**Pathogenesis** Fragmented medial coronoid process is thought to represent a form of osteochondrosis, which has been histologically reported in one study [5] and more suggestive of an osteochondral fracture of the medial coronoid process in another study [6]. In the latter study, FMCP was determined to be more consistent with a fibrous nonunion, nonhealed osteochondral fracture. The medial coronoid process ossifies between 12 and 22 weeks and may be susceptible to osteochondrosis during this time.

The most recent research suggests that asynchronous growth of the radius and ulna leads to incongruity of the elbow joint and altered forces on the medial aspect of the elbow joint [7, 8]. The disease process begins as the radius and ulna are lengthening with onset of clinical signs between 6 and 9 months of age. A shortened radius, with respect to the ulna, subjects the medial coronoid process to increased weight-bearing load from the humeral condyle. This altered load causes microfractures of the medial coronoid, leading to alteration in bone density. Secondary subchondral bone sclerosis of the trochlear notch of the ulna develops.

Underdevelopment and the small size of the ulnar trochlear notch and relatively increased size of the proximal ulna could result in loading at the anconeal and medial coronoid processes of the ulna, which has also been proposed as the cause of elbow joint incongruity [7, 9]. Changes associated with the medial coronoid process, regardless of the underlying cause, cause

**TABLE 7.2**   **Radiographic views for evaluation of the canine and feline pelvis.**

| Radiographic view | Positioning | Comments | When used |
|---|---|---|---|
| Right (or left) lateral | Patient in right (left) lateral recumbency with the right (left) pelvic limb cranial and the left (right) pelvic limb caudal; coxal joints should be superimposed over each other for straight radiographic positioning; collimation is open to the stifle joints from the dorsal aspect of the pelvis | Useful for luxations of the coxal joints that are commonly cranial and dorsal (femoral head position relative to the acetabulum). Useful for evaluation of the lumbosacral joint and acute traumatic injuries | Routine view of the pelvis |
| Extended leg ventrodorsal radiograph of the pelvis | Dog/cat is in dorsal recumbency and the stifle joints and pelvic limbs are extended so that the stifle joints are internally rotated (patella in a central position and femoral condyles equal in size); pelvic limbs should be taped equidistant from the table | Useful for evaluation of the coxofemoral joints, coverage of the femoral heads, presence of degenerative changes of the coxal joint; joint space collapse; subluxation to luxation; presence of eburnation | Routine view of the pelvis |
| Flexed or neutral pelvic limb ventrodorsal radiograph of the pelvis | Dog/cat in dorsal recumbency with pelvic limbs flexed to the side; the pelvis should be straight; no tension on the coxofemoral joint compared with the extended leg view | Evaluation of the femoral head/physis and femoral neck for acute trauma or aggressive osteolytic changes | Follow-up image if acute trauma is suspected based on other views; however, fracture not confirmed |
| Dorsal acetabular rim (DAR) view | Dog in sternal recumbency with the pelvic limbs flexed under the pelvis and the x-ray collimation centered over the coxofemoral joints | Documents degree of development of the dorsal acetabular rim and coverage of the femoral heads | Fallen out of favor as triple pelvic osteotomies are not routinely performed any more |
| PennHip neutral, compression, traction views | Dog is in dorsal recumbency with the pelvic limbs in a neutral position (stifle joints pointing up toward the collimator) and the distraction device between the pelvic limbs | Allows for early detection of laxity and subluxation of the coxofemoral joints; can be done as early as 4 months for review and comparison with national/international database for a joint laxity score called the distraction index | Images are sent away for review and distraction index created and compared with database for interpretation |

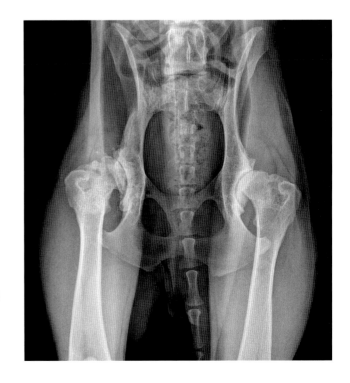

**FIGURE 7.2**   Canine hip dysplasia. Ventrodorsal radiograph of the pelvis of a 3-year-old German shepherd dog. There is severe osteophyte formation of the acetabular rims and femoral heads. The femoral heads are misshapen. There is severe enthesophyte formation of the femoral necks, causing marked femoral neck irregularity and thickening, representing joint capsule insertion osteoproliferation. There is marked subchondral sclerosis of the coxal joints, worse on the right. The acetabular rims are shallow, worse on the right. There is decreased acetabular coverage of the femoral heads, representing coxal joint subluxation. Within the soft tissues surrounding the right coxal joint, there are multifocal, well-defined, amorphous, mineral opaque structures, which may represent synovial osteochondromas or chronic avulsion fractures.

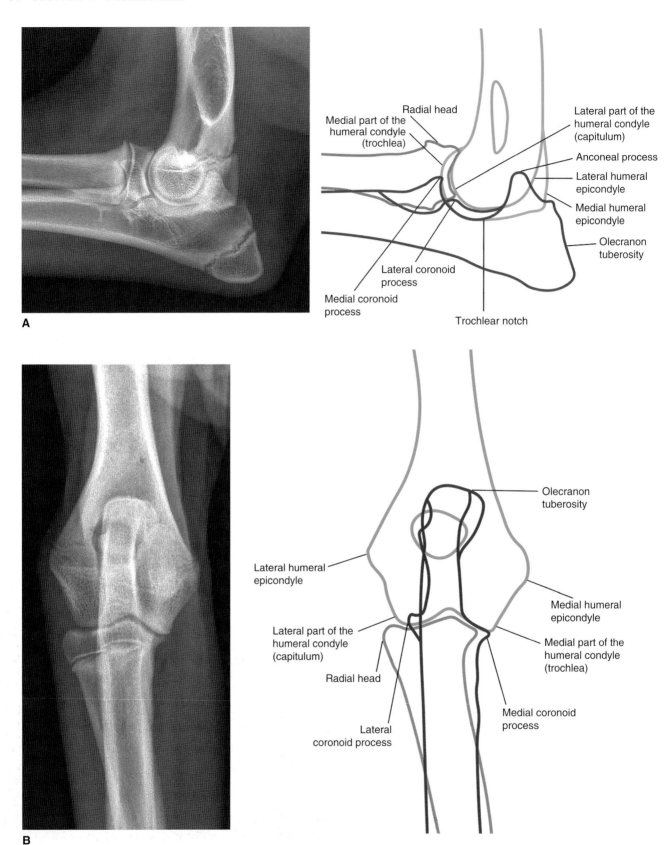

**FIGURE 7.3** Elbow radiographic anatomy. (**A**) Mediolateral radiograph of the elbow. (**B**) Caudocranial radiograph of the elbow.

secondary periarticular osseous proliferation associated with the radial head, anconeal process, and humeral epicondyles.

**Radiographic Assessment and Indicators** Radiographic diagnosis of FMCP is challenging. Secondary osseous proliferation of the elbow joint is commonly seen with or without radiographic changes associated with the medial coronoid process. Radiographically, the medial coronoid process is normally triangular shaped and well defined on both craniocaudal and mediolateral views. FMCP is characterized by indistinct or irregular margination of the medial coronoid process on mediolateral and craniocaudal views. Blunting of the cranial margin of the medial coronoid process on mediolateral views may also be present (Figure 7.4) [10]. Secondary FMCP changes include ulnar subtrochlear sclerosis and periarticular osseous proliferation associated with the radial head, anconeal process, and humeral epicondyles. Humeral condylar "kissing lesion" with subchondral sclerosis of the medial humeral condyle with or without associated articular margin lucency can also be seen.

At a minimum, standard orthogonal mediolateral and craniocaudal radiographic views are required for assessment of the elbow. The cranio15° lateral-caudomedial oblique view (Cr15L-CdMO) is the best radiographic view to completely evaluate the cranial margin of the medial coronoid process for the detection of FMCP [11]. Distomedial-proximolateral oblique views can also be helpful; however, the utility of oblique views is dependent on the viewer's familiarity with reading oblique projections which can be difficult to completely assess. A maximally flexed mediolateral projection identifies osteophytes on the proximal anconeal process without superimposition of the humerus.

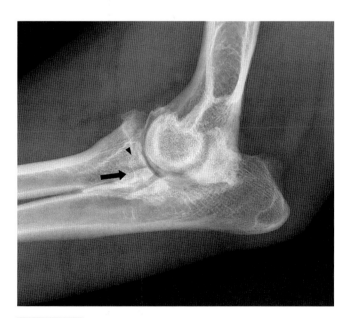

**FIGURE 7.4** Fragmented medial coronoid process of the ulna. Mediolateral radiograph of the elbow with flattening (arrow) and sclerosis of the medial coronoid process with a well-defined triangular shaped osseous fragment (arrowhead). There is also moderate cubital joint osteoarthrosis, further characterized by osteophyte formation of the humeral condyle, humeral epicondyle, anconeal process, and radial head.

## Ununited Anconeal Process of the Ulna

**Pathogenesis** Similar to FMCP, UAP has been described as a manifestation of osteochondrosis. Multiple theories of the pathogenesis of UAP are proposed, which include an inherited developmental anomaly, metabolic defect, nutritional deficiencies, trauma, and radioulnar mismatch and growth asynchrony secondary to radial lengthening. This causes increased proximal pressure on the humeral condyle, and subsequent excessive load on the anconeal process. The altered pressure causes proximal displacement of and lack of fusion of the anconeal process to the parent bone. The prompt healing of UAP reported after ulnar osteotomy further supports the hypothesis that asynchronous growth between the radius and ulna is the underlying cause of UAP. Lucency of the tip of the anconeal process representing a normal secondary center of ossification should not be confused with a pathologic UAP (Figure 7.5) [12]. As a location for separate center of ossification, the tip of the anconeal process should fuse to the parent bone by 150 days.

Breeds commonly affected by UAP include the German shepherd, St Bernard, Great Dane, Labrador retrievers, and others. The disease process is typically seen in dogs between 3 and 4 months of age, and is documented at 5 months of age, when the anconeal process secondary ossification center should have fused to the parent bone. Occasionally, UAP can be diagnosed in older dogs with an acute onset of lameness or considered incidental [13].

**Radiographic Assessment and Indicators** Radiographically, UAP is characterized by radioulnar incongruity with proximal displacement of the radial head with respect to the trochlear notch, a well-delineated lucency of the anconeal process and proximal displacement and lack of fusion of the anconeal process in relation to the parent bone (Figure 7.6).

The flexed mediolateral projection best evaluates for UAP, as there is no superimposition of the humerus with the anconeal process. Projections of both limbs are recommended as UAP is commonly bilateral.

## Osteochondrosis or Osteochondritis Dissecans of the Medial Humeral Condyle

**Pathogenesis** Osteochondrosis or osteochondritis dissecans (OC/OCD) is an erosive cartilage defect caused by disturbed endochondral ossification of the articular or epiphyseal cartilage which can be seen in conjunction with FMCP. OC/OCD of the medial humeral condyle may be categorized as primary or secondary. OC/OCD of the humeral condyle is of similar etiology to OC/OCD lesions in other anatomic regions: failure of endochondral ossification with thinning and flattening of the cartilage surface. More common is secondary erosion of the medial humeral condyle articular surface, as a result of altered forces such as incongruity between the ulnar trochlear notch and the humeral trochlea, leading to eburnation of the opposing cartilaginous surfaces. The resultant lesions are commonly known as "kissing

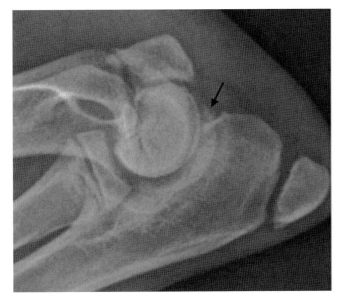 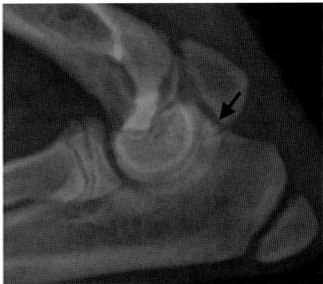

**FIGURE 7.5** Secondary center of ossification of the anconeal process. Note the small triangular-shaped secondary center of ossification of the anconeal process (arrow). The ossification center is small and poorly defined with an irregular line of separation from the ulnar diaphysis. Source: Jean K. Frazho DVM et al. [12] / with permission of John Wiley & Sons.

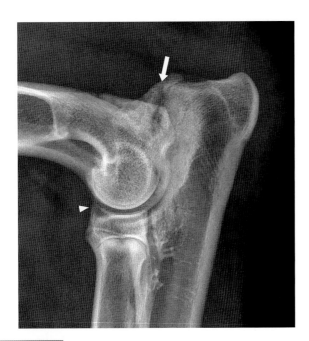

**FIGURE 7.6** Ununited anconeal process. Mediolateral radiograph of the elbow with a well-defined, irregular lucency (arrow) at the level of the anconeal process. There is also mild cubital joint osteoarthrosis, further characterized by osteophyte formation of the radial head (arrowhead).

lesions" and are better classified as a form of joint degeneration than osteochondrosis.

The most common dog breed affected by OC/OCD with a combination of FMCP is the Labrador retriever. Males are more commonly affected, which may be due to their quicker rate of overall growth or a sex-linked factor [14].

**Radiographic Assessment and Indicators** Radiographic changes associated with OC/OCD of the medial part of the humeral condyle include subchondral sclerosis of the medial humeral condyle with or without a concave articular margin lucency/defect (Figure 7.7). Small OC/OCD lesions may be difficult to evaluate radiographically. Diagnosing the concave articular margin defect is also dependent on the angle of the radiographic view. Severe joint erosion may result in secondary subchondral defects that can appear similar to OC/OCD on imaging.

OC/OCD of the medial part of the humeral condyle is most readily seen on the craniocaudal view. The best radiographic view includes the craniocaudal (CC) and Cr15L-CdMO (Figure 7.8) [15].

## Temporomandibular Joint Dysplasia

See also Chapter 12, Imaging of the Head.

**Etiology** Temporomandibular joint dysplasia is a congenital disease with an unclear underlying etiology; however, the underlying cause may be attributable to the rapid growth of chondrodystrophic breed dogs, prognathism, and laxity of the mandibular symphysis [16]. TMJ dysplasia is characterized by joint laxity, and commonly a flat and abnormally angled mandibular condyle with a shortened retroarticular process though the joint may also have an otherwise normal morphology. Joint laxity may result in open mouth locking of the jaw and dental malocclusion secondary to the coronoid process of the mandible translating lateral to the zygomatic arch. Not all dogs and cats with TMJ dysplasia result in dysfunction.

Common dog breeds affected include the basset hound, setter breeds, Cavalier King Charles spaniel, and others. It occurs less commonly in cats. It affects dogs and cats at any age of development as TMJ dysplasia is often asymptomatic and may be diagnosed incidentally.

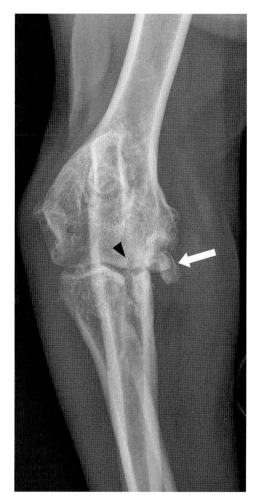

**FIGURE 7.7** Osteochondritis dissecans of the medial part of the humeral condyle and fragmented medial coronoid process of the ulna. Caudocranial radiograph of the cubital joint. Within the medial aspect of the cubital joint, there are two ovoid to rounded, smoothly marginated, osseous fragments, partially superimposed over one another (arrow). There is a large, irregularly marginated, concave defect of the medial humeral condyle with regional subchondral sclerosis (arrowhead). The adjacent soft tissues are markedly thickened, representing joint effusion and/or synovial proliferation.

## Radiographic Assessment and Indicators

Temporomandibular joint dysplasia is characterized by a flattened mandibular fossa, misshapen retroarticular process of the temporal bones, and a blunted retroarticular process with a shortened or absent lateral aspect, causing a distortion of the normal "C" shaped caudal aspect of the TMJ (Figure 7.9).

Positioning for skull radiographs to assess the TMJ can be difficult. Radiographs under heavy sedation or general anesthesia is the ideal method for obtaining diagnostic images. Standard radiographic images of the TMJs are needed (Figure 7.10) [17], which include the lateral-lateral (right to left lateral and left to right lateral) views, dorsoventral (DV) or ventrodorsal (VD) view, and latero-20°-rostral-laterocaudal oblique view [17–19].

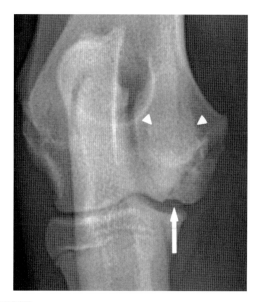

**FIGURE 7.8** Cranio15°lateral-caudomedial oblique (Cr15L-CdMO) radiograph for the detection of osteochondrosis or osteochondritis dissecans of the medial part of the humeral condyle. A mineralized fragment (arrow) is seen distal to the lucency. There is surrounding subchondral sclerosis of the medial part of the humeral condyle (arrowhead). Source: Cristi R. Cook DVM et al. [4] / with permission of John Wiley & Sons.

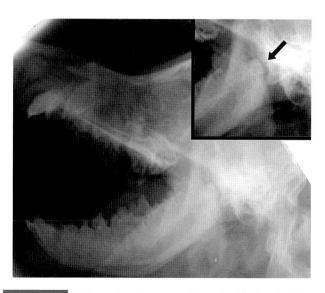

**FIGURE 7.9** TMJ dysplasia. Lateral radiograph of the head with a small magnification of the temporomandibular joint region. There is flattening of the mandibular fossa (arrow) and the misshapen condylar process of the mandible is evident and results in loss of parallelism and narrowing of the joint space. Source: Assaf Lerer et al. [16] / with permission of John Wiley & Sons.

# Osteochondrosis

## Etiology

Osteochondrosis (OC) is the general term used to describe a failure of endochondral ossification, the normal bone growth process by which the cartilarge model is replaced by bone. The

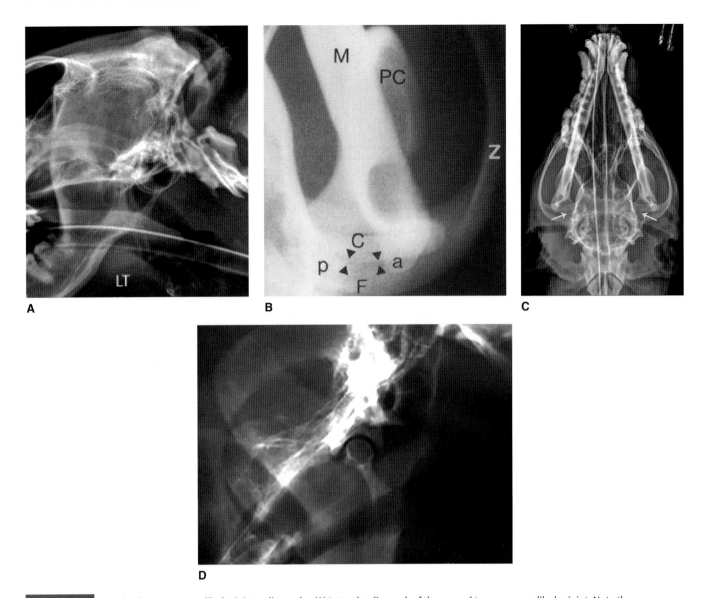

**FIGURE 7.10** Standard temporomandibular joint radiographs. (**A**) Lateral radiograph of the normal temporomandibular joint. Note the superimposed left and right temporomandibular joints. (**B**) Dorsoventral radiograph of the normal left temporomandibular joint in a dog. Note the zygomatic arch (Z), the mandibular fossa (F) and the retroarticular process (p) of the temporal bone, and the head of the condylar process (c), coronoid process (PC), and angular process a of the mandible (M) and the thin, lucent temporomandibular joint space (between arrowheads). Source: Courtesy of Tobias Schwarz MA et al. (2005), John Wiley & Sons. (**C**) Ventrodorsal radiograph of the skull. Note the normal, lucent temporomandibular joint (arrows) located between the head of the condylar process of the mandible and the retroarticular process. (**D**) Latero 20° rostral-laterocaudal oblique radiograph of the temporomandibular joint. LT, left. Source: Gawain Hammond et al. [19] / with permission of John Wiley & Sons.

disease process is further divided into subtypes: latens (lesion confined to the epiphyseal cartilage), manifesta (lesion accompanied by delay in endochondral ossification), and dissecans (cleft formation through the articular cartilage; OCD) [20]. Radiographically, OCD is diagnosed when a cartilage flap can be seen in conjunction with a cartilage margin defect; alternatively, osteochondrosis is diagnosed when only the cartilage defect is detectable. OC is considered to have multifactorial etiologies including rapid growth, hereditary, anatomic characteristics, trauma, and diet.

## Pathogenesis

Osteochondrosis may be related to disruption in the blood supply to the chondral and subchondral bone. The result is ischemic necrosis and retention of excessive cartilage at the site as transformation to bone stops and cartilage continues to grow. The end-result is abnormally thick regions of cartilage that are poorly resistant to mechanical stress [20]. The disease manifests as one of two common presentations: (i) chondral surface lesions and (ii) subchondral cyst-like lesions. In the chondral surface lesion type, a flap of cartilage may detach, becoming free within the joint. This often mineralizes following detachment, creating a free joint body. In the subchondral cyst-like lesion type, persistent necrosis may lead to the development of a cyst.

The most common sites affected are the caudal central aspect of the humeral head, the medial part of the humeral condyle, the medial and lateral femoral condyles, and the medial and lateral trochlear ridges of the talus. Lesions may develop in several locations in a single patient and are often bilateral.

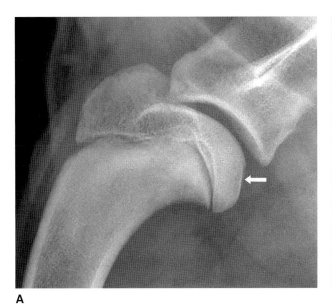

**A**

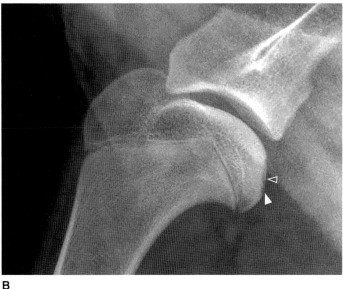

**B**

**FIGURE 7.11**   Osteochondrosis of the caudal humeral head. (**A**) Mediolateral radiograph of the scapulohumeral joint. There is flattening of the caudal humeral head (white arrow) with no overt evidence of an osseous fragment. (**B**) Mediolateral radiograph of the humeral joint of another patient. There is flattening of the caudal humeral head with a lucent curvilinear fissure (arrowhead), subchondral sclerosis, and thin osseous fragment (open arrowhead).

Medium- or large-breed dogs such as Labrador and golden retrievers, German shepherds, and Rottweilers, or breed specific depending on the location, may be affected. Males are afflicted more often than females. The age of affected dogs ranges between 6 and 24 months. Patients present with chronic intermittent to persistent lameness, attributable to the joint affected, that may worsen after periods of rest.

## Radiographic Assessment and Indicators

**Shoulder**   Osteochondrosis of the shoulder is typically associated with the caudal central aspect of the humeral head manifesting as humeral head flattening and irregularity on the lateral view (Figure 7.11). A flap of cartilage may be visualized if it becomes mineralized, and may remain attached, or detach, often migrating to the dependent aspect of the joint (Figure 7.12). If the cartilage defect is not readily seen on the lateral view, additional supinated mediolateral and pronated mediolateral views can be helpful [21].

**Elbow**   As discussed previously, osteochondrosis of the elbow most commonly affects the medial humeral condyle. The lesions appear as lucent chondral or subchondral defects, with some lesions causing an "osseous cyst-like lesion" in the humeral condyle on craniocaudal and cranial-15°-lateral-caudal medial oblique views [15] (Figure 7.7).

**Stifle**   Stifle OC most commonly affects the lateral condyle of the femur, though the medial condyle is also commonly

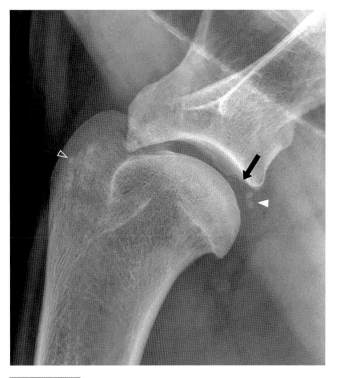

**FIGURE 7.12**   Osteochondritis dissecans of the caudal humeral head with fragment migration. Mediolateral radiograph of the scapulohumeral joint. There is flattening and irregular articular surface of the caudal aspect of the humeral head. Additionally, there is a large, well-defined, concave defect associated with the caudal aspect of the glenoid cavity (arrow), representing an osteochondral lesion of the glenoid cavity. Within the caudal aspect of the humeral joint, there are at least two round, irregularly marginated, osteochondral fragments (arrowhead). Superimposed over the bicipital tendon sheath, there are multifocal, faint, osteochondral fragments (open arrowhead).

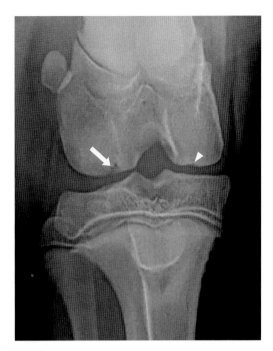

**FIGURE 7.13**  Osteochondrosis of the medial and lateral femoral condyles. Caudocranial radiograph of the stifle joint. There is a well-defined, lucent, irregularly marginated, concave defect of the subchondral bone with sclerosis of the lateral femoral condyle (arrow). There is also a smaller, well-defined, concave defect associated with the articular margin of the medial femoral condyle (arrowhead).

affected. Similar to humeral OC lesions, they appear as lucent chondral or subchondral defects, with some lesions causing an "osseous cyst-like lesion" in the femoral condyle or just subchondral sclerosis on craniocaudal views (Figure 7.13). Affected breeds include the German shepherd, bull mastiff, Samoyed, German wire-haired pointer, wolfhound, Labrador retriever, standard poodle, greyhound, Great Dane, St Bernard, boxer, chow chow, collie, giant schnauzer, Doberman pinscher, Border collie, and Staffordshire bull terrier.

**Tarsus**   Tarsal OC affects the medial and lateral ridges of the talus. Medial ridge lesions are more common in Rottweilers and Labrador retrievers, while lateral lesions are most common in golden retrievers. The disease manifests as flattening of the trochlear ridge on the lateral views and/or mineralized osseous fragments on the medial (Figure 7.14) or lateral (Figure 7.15) trochlear ridge of the talus on the plantarodorsal view.

# Miscellaneous Diseases

## Panosteitis

### Pathophysiology
Panosteitis is a spontaneously occurring, self-limiting disease of young (between 5 and 18 months of age), large-breed dogs, particularly German shepherd dogs [22],

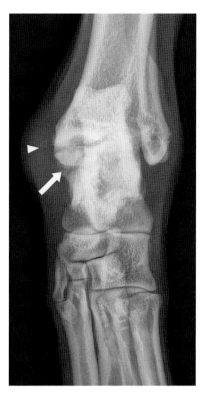

**FIGURE 7.14**  Osteochondritis dissecans of the medial trochlear ridge of the talus. Dorsoplantar radiograph of the tarsus. There is a large, osteochondral fragment (arrow) associated with the medial trochlear ridge of the talus. In the soft tissues adjacent to this region, there are multifocal, faint, mineral opaque fragments, likely representing additional osteochondral fragments (arrowhead). There is severe soft tissue swelling of the medial tarsocrural joint, representing joint effusion and/or synovial proliferation.

involving primarily the diaphysis of long bones. Occasionally, the metaphysis is involved.

Patients present with a shifting leg lameness and signs of systemic illness such as pyrexia, anorexia, and lethargy. On physical examination, pain can be elicited on deep palpation of the diaphysis of long bones. Radiographic imaging of the painful regions is recommended. Though all long bones may be affected, the proximal ulna is most commonly affected. Additionally, the distal humerus, middiaphysis of the femur, and proximal tibia are also regions that can be affected.

The etiology of panosteitis is poorly understood, though it may be related to protein or amino acid metabolism disorder [23, 24].

### Radiographic Assessment and Indicators
The predominant radiographic feature of panosteitis is poorly delineated regions of increased mineral opacity in the medullary cavity of long bones, particularly surrounding the nutrient foramen on the lateral views. Endosteal sclerosis and irregular periosteal osseous proliferation can also be seen in advanced cases (Figure 7.16).

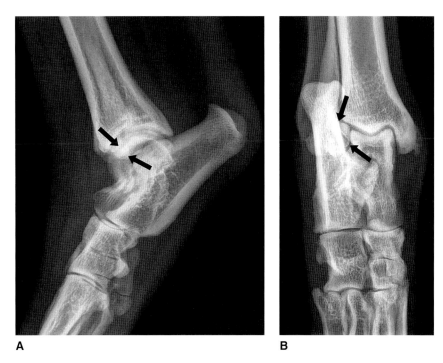

**A**        **B**

**FIGURE 7.15** Osteochondritis dissecans of the lateral trochlear ridge of the talus. Mediolateral (**A**) and plantarodorsal (**B**) radiographs of the tarsus of a golden retriever. There is a large, smooth, round, osseous fragment associated with the lateral trochlear ridge of the talus (arrows). There is mild to moderate osteophyte and enthesophyte formation of the tarsocrural joint and proximal intertarsal joint, representing secondary osteoarthrosis.

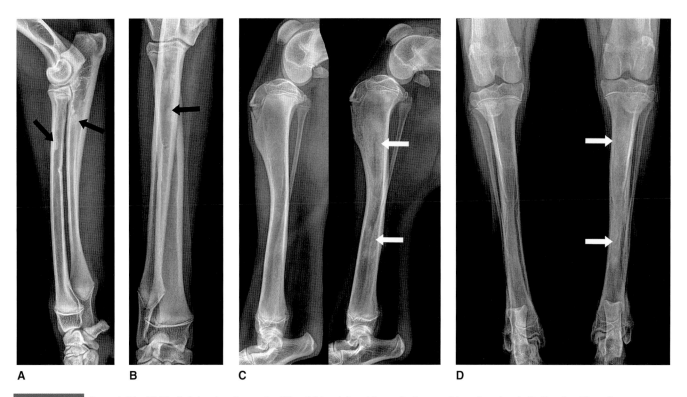

**A**        **B**        **C**        **D**

**FIGURE 7.16** Panosteitis. (**A**) Mediolateral radiograph of the right antebrachium of a 1-year-old neutered male Rottweiler. There is inhomogeneous increase in mineral opacity of the proximal radial and ulnar metaphyseal regions (black arrows). (**B**) Craniocaudal radiograph of the right antebrachium of the same Rottweiler. There is inhomogeneous increase in mineral opacity of the proximal aspect of the superimposed radius and ulna (black arrows). (**C**) Mediolateral radiograph of the affected left crus and normal right crus for comparison of an 8-month-old intact male German shepherd dog. There is inhomogeneous increase in mineral opacity of the entirety of the left tibial diaphysis (white arrows). (**D**) Craniocaudal radiograph of the affected left crus and normal right crus for comparison of the same German shepherd dog. Note the inhomogeneous increase in mineral opacity of the left tibial diaphysis (white arrows).

# Hypertrophic Osteodystrophy (Metaphyseal Dysplasia)

**Pathophysiology**  Hypertrophic osteodystrophy (HOD) is a spontaneously occurring, self-limiting disease of young, large-breed dogs involving the metaphyses of long bones. It affects dogs between the ages of 7 weeks and 8 months, and the highest incidence is reported between 3 and 4 months of age [25]. Common dog breeds affected include the Great Dane, boxer, German shepherd, Irish setters, Weimaraner, and other giant and large-breed dogs [26]. The underlying etiology is poorly understood. Numerous etiologies have been suggested including vitamin C deficiency, overnutrition, and infectious etiologies (i.e., canine distemper virus) [27].

Patients present with similar clinical signs to panosteitis, with shifting leg lameness. However, patients tend to be painful on palpation of the physes rather than the diaphyses. On physical examination, patients are often hyperthermic with pain and soft tissue swelling over the metaphyseal regions.

**Radiographic Assessment and Indicators**  Hypertrophic osteodystrophy usually causes bilateral "double physis" sign in the metaphysis of long bones, namely the distal radius,

ulna, and tibia. The vertebrae, ribs, mandible, scapulae, humeri, femurs, and optic foramina have been reported to be affected [27–29]. The "double physis" sign is further characterized by a radiolucent band parallel to and on the metaphyseal side of the physis (Figure 7.17). The epiphyses and physes proper are usually normal, though irregular widening of the growth plate may occur as the disease progresses. Subperiosteal or extraperiosteal new bone formation of the metaphyses may occur, which may progress to involve the entire diaphysis. Additionally, in advanced diseases, HOD may cause angular limb deformities.

# Retained Cartilage Core

**Pathophysiology**  Retained cartilage core is a failure of endochondral ossification that may occur at any physis (osteochondrosis manifesta), though most commonly it is bilateral and affects the distal ulnar physis. This should not be confused with hypertrophic osteodystrophy (i.e., double physeal sign) or metaphyseal osteomyelitis, where the lucent lesions are due to suppurative inflammation and necrosis of the metaphyseal regions. A core of cartilage extending into the metaphyseal bone and diaphysis fails to ossify with retention of the center of hypertrophied cartilage cells. The core may

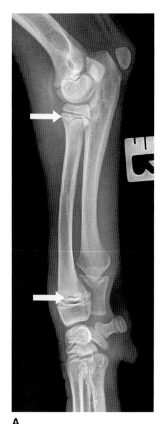
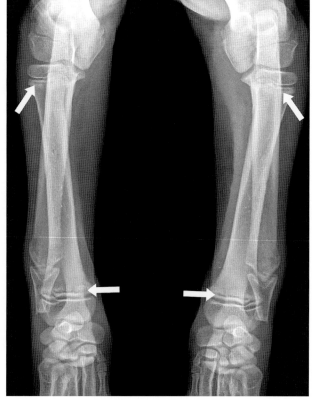

**A**    **B**

**FIGURE 7.17**  Hypertrophic osteodystrophy. Mediolateral radiograph (**A**) of the right antebrachium and (**B**) caudocranial radiograph of the right and left antebrachia of a young dog with hypertrophic osteodystrophy. There is a well-defined, irregularly marginated lucency affecting the proximal and distal radial metaphyses, distal ulnar metaphyses, distal metacarpal metaphyses with surrounding sclerosis, oriented parallel to the physes (arrows).

be asymptomatic, but may result in decreased growth from the distal ulnar physis. The degree of shortening determines the development of carpal valgus and radius procurvatum deformity of the limb [30].

Large- and giant-breed dogs, particularly Great Danes, have been reported to be affected. Retained cartilage core affects dogs during the developmental stages of ossification (between 3 and 9 months of age) with evident clinical signs if ulnar growth arrest occurs. On palpation of the affected regions, no pain can be elicited. The underlying cause of this disorder is undetermined, but genetic factors and diet have been proposed to have a role in its development [30–32].

**Radiographic Assessment and Indicators** The common characteristics of retained cartilage core are bilateral, well-circumscribed, triangular-shaped, smooth marginated, lucent regions of the distal ulnar metaphysis. Sclerotic margins immediately proximal to the lucent region can sometimes be seen [33] (Figure 7.18). Different radiographic variations of retained cartilage core have been reported: irregular shaped and irregularly marginated lucencies in the ulnar metaphyseal region, which could easily be mistaken for hypertrophic osteodystrophy or metaphyseal osteomyelitis [34].

# Angular Limb Deformities Secondary to Premature Closure of the Physis

**Pathophysiology** Angular limb deformities can affect the limb in the frontal, sagittal, and/or transverse planes. Orthogonal radiographs are used to assess affected limbs in these planes. A craniocaudal or caudocranial radiograph is used to assess angular limb deformities in the frontal plane, which includes valgus or varus deformities (lateral or medial angulation of the distal limb respectively). A lateromedial or mediolateral radiograph is used to assess angular limb deformities in the sagittal plane, which evaluates for procurvatum and recurvatum (cranial bowing and caudal bowing of the diaphysis, respectively). A transverse plane deformity can be assessed by obtaining an axially oriented x-ray beam radiograph to assess for torsional deformities. This is not commonly done. This plane is best assessed on computed tomography using transverse plane images. Some bones have deformities in more than one plane.

By convention, a deformity is described in terms of the relationship of the distal portion of the bone or point to the more proximal portion of the same structure.

Multiple etiologies of retardation or premature closure of growth plates have been reported, including physeal trauma, malunion, congenital malformation, nutritional imbalances, and radiation exposure [35, 36]. Premature closure of the physis of paired long bones, leading to asynchronous growth, may result in angular limb deformities. Antebrachial deformities are the most common limb malformations in dogs, particularly caused by premature closure of the distal ulnar

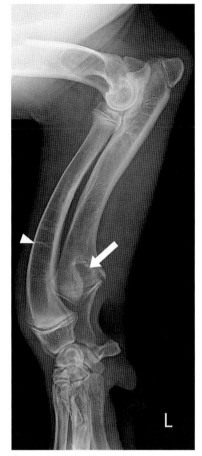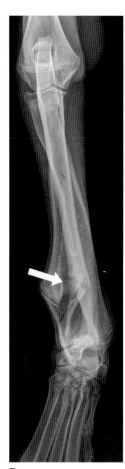

**A**           **B**

**FIGURE 7.18** Retained cartilage core. Mediolateral radiograph (**A**) and caudocranial radiograph (**B**) of the antebrachium. There is a well-defined, triangular to fusiform-shaped lucency extending from the distal ulnar physis into the distal ulnar metaphysis (arrow). There is mild sclerosis surrounding this lesion. There is cranial bowing of the distal radial metaphyseal region, representing radius procurvatum. The horizontally oriented mineral opaque bands in the middiaphysis of the radius represent incidental growth arrest lines (arrowheads). On the caudocranial radiograph (**B**), there is medial deviation of the manus in relation to the carpus, representing carpal valgus deformity.

physis [37, 38]. Premature closure of the distal ulnar physis results in carpal valgus deformity and radius procurvatum. In dogs, the growth plates of the radius and ulna grow at different rates. The distal ulnar growth plate is considered to grow at an equal rate to that of the proximal and distal radial growth plates combined. It is considered to contribute 85% of the total length of the ulna and all the length of the ulna distal to the humeroradial joint so is particularly at risk of insults which affect its growth [39].

Any breed can be affected at any age throughout the growth lengthening stages of long bone development. However, chondrodystrophic breeds such as the basset hound, English bulldog, and dachshund have a higher predisposition as they have been bred selectively for traits similar to disproportionate dwarfism.

**Radiographic Assessment and Indicators** Radiographic indicators of premature closure of the physis include increased mineral opacity of physis and the lack of visibility of a physeal lucency. Contralateral limb orthogonal radiographs should be done for comparison purposes. In patients chronically affected with a limb deformity, curvature of long bones toward side of closure with angulation of the affected joint can be seen (Figure 7.19). The radiocarpal joint is the joint most commonly affected. Concurrent joint incongruity can also be seen, most commonly affecting the cubital joint, which is further evidenced by increased width between the humeroulnar and radioulnar joint spaces with a step defect between the radioulnar joint.

## Physeal Fractures

See also Chapter 9, Fractures and Fracture Healing.

**Pathophysiology** Physeal fractures as a result of trauma are typically stratified according to Salter Harris classifications.

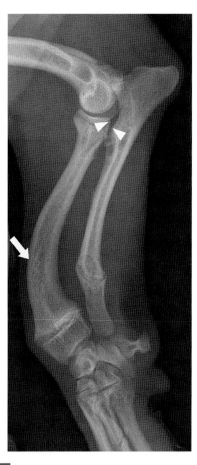

**FIGURE 7.19** Premature closure of distal ulnar physis. There is cranial bowing of the distal diaphysis of the radius (arrow) in relation to the ulna, representing radius procurvatum, with a step defect between the radioulnar joint (arrowheads) and resultant widening of the humeroulnar joint. The distal ulnar physis is subjectively decreased in conspicuity compared to the distal radial physis, representing the likely radiographic evidence of premature closure of the distal ulnar physis.

In veterinary medicine, Salter Harris fractures are divided into five types. Type I is a fracture along the physis. Type II is a fracture along the physis extending into the metaphysis. Type III is a fracture along the physis, extending through the epiphysis to the articular surface. Type IV is a fracture extending from the articular surface, across the physis, exiting through the metaphysis. Type V is a crushing injury to the physis often resulting in premature closure. Young dogs and cats of any breed with open physes can be affected.

**Radiographic Assessment and Indicators** Minimally displaced physeal fractures may be difficult to evaluate as the only radiographic sign is lucency and widening of the physis. Orthogonal (Figure 7.20) and/or contralateral limb radiographs may be helpful. Regional swelling can also indicate the presence of an otherwise occult fracture, and should prompt additional radiographs at different angles of obliquity. Soft tissue swelling is mostly dependent on the chronicity of the fracture. Soft tissue swelling is more evident in acute and subacute stages, whereas in peracute and chronic stages soft tissue swelling may not be as apparent.

## Incomplete Ossification of the Humeral Condyle and Humeral Condylar Fractures

**Pathophysiology** Incomplete ossification of the humeral condyle (IOHC) may be an incidental radiographic finding or may cause variable degrees of lameness, and can result in nontraumatic humeral condylar fractures. It is usually bilateral in distribution. The pathogenesis of IOHC is unclear. Several theories have been proposed including failure of fusion of the separate centers of ossification of the humeral condyle or normal physiologic loading on a weakened humeral condyle [40]. A fissure is seen extending from the articular margin of the condyle, through the physis, separating the medial and lateral portions. Spaniel breeds (i.e. springer spaniels and cocker spaniels) are overrepresented; a recessive mode of inheritance has been proposed [41]. Other affected breeds include Labrador retrievers and Rottweilers.

**Radiographic Assessment and Indicators** A linear sagittal lucency, representing humeral intercondylar fissure (HIF), of the humeral condyle may be partial or complete, extending from the articular margin of the humeral condyle through the supratrochlear foramen or extending partially to the supratrochlear foramen, between the trochlea and capitulum on the craniocaudal radiographic view. A lucent fissure may not be radiographically apparent unless the x-ray beam is oriented exactly parallel to the margins of the fissure (Figure 7.21). Multiple, variable angled, craniocaudal radiographic views may be needed to appreciate this subtle change. A cranio

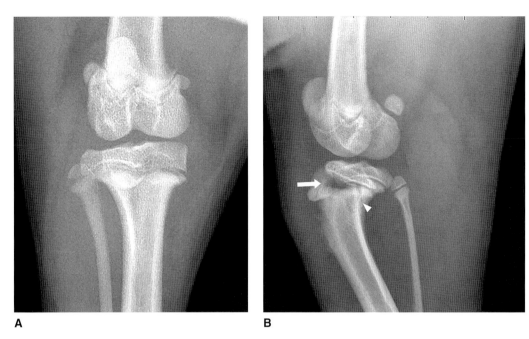

**FIGURE 7.20**   Benefits of orthogonal radiographs with mildly displaced physeal fractures. Caudocranial (**A**) and mediolateral (**B**) radiographs of the right crus including the stifle joint. Only seen on the mediolateral radiograph, the cranial aspect of the proximal tibial epiphysis is proximally and caudally displaced (arrow). There is an ill-defined lucent fissure extending from the caudal aspect of the proximal tibial metaphysis (arrowhead). There is mild to moderate irregular mineral opacity over the region of the tibial crest. The soft tissues of this region are thickened, representing edema and/or hemorrhage. The constellation of these findings is consistent with a Salter Harris type II fracture of the proximal tibia. Note the importance of orthogonal radiographs (mediolateral and caudocranial views) in diagnosing physeal fractures as they may not be evident on one of the two projections; in this case, the fracture is evidence on the mediolateral radiographic view.

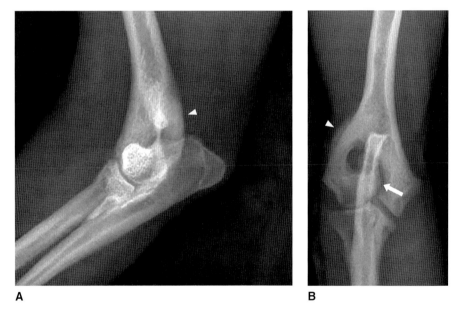

**FIGURE 7.21**   Incomplete ossification of the humeral condyle. Mediolateral (**A**) and caudocranial (**B**) radiographs of the elbow. There is a well-defined, linear lucent fissure associated with the distal humeral intercondylar region (arrow). There is mild to moderate, smoothly marginated, osseous proliferation associated with the lateral humeral epicondylar region (arrowheads), representing degenerative joint disease.

15°medial-caudolateral oblique radiographic view has been proposed as the projection that best demonstrates the fissure. If the intercondylar fissure is difficult to evaluate radiographically, computed tomography can be pursued. In conjunction with the intercondylar fissure, periosteal proliferation involving the lateral epicondyle, representing degenerative joint disease [42] (Figure 7.21) or a lateral epicondylar, medial epicondylar, Y-, or T-fracture may be seen (Figure 7.22) [40].

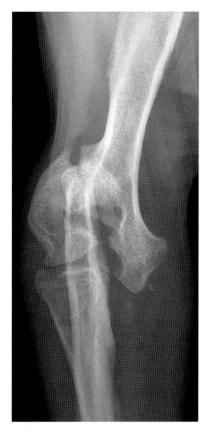

**FIGURE 7.22** Incomplete ossification of the humeral condyle with associated lateral humeral condylar fracture. Craniocaudal radiograph of the cubital joint of a 1-year-old cocker spaniel. The distal humeral intercondylar region is widened with smooth margins. There is a smoothly marginated, mildly displaced, lateral humeral condylar fracture with mild smooth periosteal proliferation.

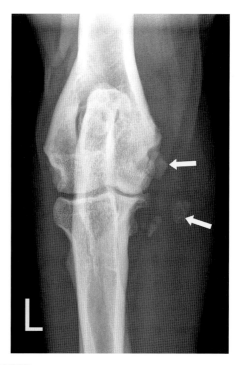

**FIGURE 7.23** Mineralization at the flexor tendon origin. Caudocranial radiograph of the cubital joint. There is a large, mineralized body at the level of the medial humeral epicondylar region with multifocal variably shaped osseous structures in the adjacent soft tissues (arrows). There is moderate to severe osteophyte formation of the medial coronoid process of the ulna. The regional soft tissues are moderate to markedly thickened.

## Ununited Medial Humeral Epicondyle

**Pathophysiology** Ununited medial humeral epicondyle has previously been thought to be a component of elbow dysplasia, but recent studies have demonstrated the absence of the failed fusion of the medial epicondyle to the parent bone [43]. Differential diagnoses of ununited medial humeral epicondyle include dystrophic calcification of the flexor tendon origin, traumatic avulsion of the medial humeral epicondyle, medial humeral condylar OCD, and development of a preformed ossification center (Figure 7.23). There is no breed predisposition but it has been reported in the German shepherd, Bernese mountain dog, Rottweiler, and Labrador retriever [44].

**Radiographic Assessment and Indicators** This condition is characterized by a small, well-defined, osseous structure superimposed over the soft tissues caudal and distal to the medial epicondyle on the mediolateral and craniocaudal radiographic views (Figure 7.24).

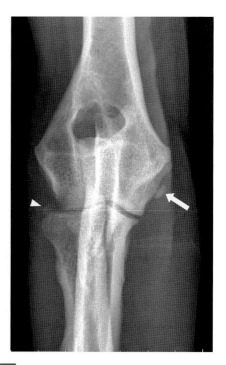

**FIGURE 7.24** Ununited medial humeral epicondyle. Craniocaudal radiograph of the cubital joints. Along the medial surface of the medial humeral epicondylar region, there is a well-defined, smoothly marginated, ovoid, mineral opaque structure (arrow). The supinator sesamoid is normal (arrowhead) and should not be confused with pathology.

## Avascular Necrosis of the Femoral Head

**Pathophysiology** Also referred to as aseptic necrosis of the femoral head and Legg–Calvé–Perthes disease, this disease causes ischemic necrosis of the femoral head which leads to trabecular bone collapse and ultimately to deformity of the subchondral bone, resulting in joint incongruency, joint instability, and predisposition to a pathologic fracture. This affects young (5–8 months of age), miniature and small-breed dogs (i.e. terriers, miniature pinscher, Pomeranian, miniature poodle, Chihuahua, pug, Lhasa apso, etc.) [45]. There is an inherited predisposition associated with the Manchester terrier. There is no sex predilection [45].

**Radiographic Assessment and Indicators** Marked lucency, resorptive lesions, and irregularity of the femoral head and neck are the radiographic indicators (Figure 7.25). Occasionally, pathologic fractures can be identified. Osteoarthritis develops with chronicity. Because affected patients are miniature or small-breed dogs, femoral head and neck ostectomy is the treatment of choice.

## Feline Femoral Neck Metaphyseal Osteopathy and Spontaneous Femoral Capital Physeal Fracture

**Pathophysiology** Metaphyseal osteopathy is a disease of young (between 7 months and 2 years of age), male neutered, obese cats. It has been reported that neutering causes a delay in growth plate closure of multiple physes, thereby predisposing

them to physeal fractures [46]. Histopathologically, the proximal femoral physes in cats with metaphyseal osteopathy almost double in size with irregular chondrocytes and evidence of necrosis [47]. This disease shares radiographic features with Legg–Calvé–Perthes disease in dogs. However, there is usually lucency and loss of cortical definition of the proximal femoral metaphysis with a pathologic capital (proximal) femoral physeal fracture. It is unclear whether metaphyseal osteopathy is the pathology in itself or a consequence of primary fracture and subsequent osseous remodeling.

**Radiographic Assessment and Indicators** Routine lateral and ventrodorsal radiographic views of the pelvis with extended pelvic limbs are recommended. An additional ventrodorsal view of the pelvis with flexed pelvic limbs ("frog-leg" view) can also be obtained in order to displace the fracture if present, as the ventrodorsal view with the pelvic limbs extended can reduce the proximal femoral physeal fracture [48].

Radiographically, metaphyseal osteopathy is characterized by lucency of the proximal femoral metaphysis. If a pathologic capital femoral physeal fracture is present, subtle or obvious changes can be seen, ranging from a step defect between the femoral epiphysis and metaphysis to widening and displacement of the femoral metaphysis in relation to the epiphysis (Figure 7.26).

## Septic Metaphysitis

**Pathophysiology** Septic metaphysitis is also known as metaphyseal bacterial osteomyelitis or bacterial metaphysitis. It is caused by bacteremia in young dogs and cats. Gram-positive bacteria such as *Staphylococcus* spp. are often isolated. Clinical examination findings of affected animals include fever, lameness,

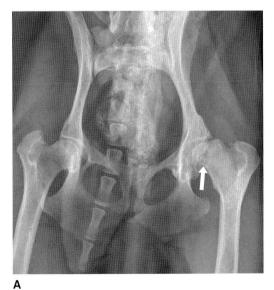
**A**

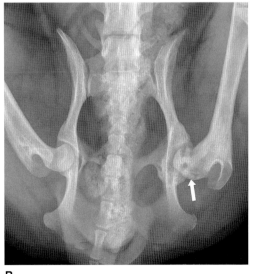
**B**

**FIGURE 7.25** Avascular necrosis of femoral head. (**A**) Ventrodorsal radiograph of the pelvis with the pelvic limbs extended. There is heterogeneous decrease in mineral opacity of the left femoral metaphyseal region (arrow). The left femoral head is irregular in shape with flattened margins. There is severe periarticular osteophyte formation of the acetabular rim. (**B**) Ventrodorsal radiograph of the pelvis with the pelvic limbs flexed or "frog-leg" view of the same patient. Similar radiographic changes of the left femoral neck (arrow) when compared to the ventrodorsal projection of the pelvis with the pelvic limbs extended are detected. No evidence of a pathologic fracture is detected.

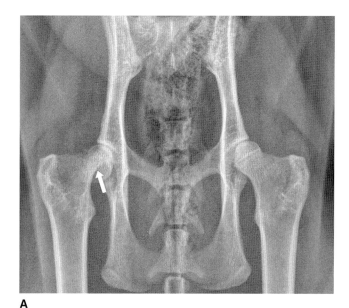 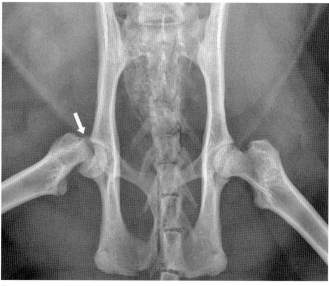

**A**                    **B**

**FIGURE 7.26** Capital femoral physeal fracture in a 2-year-old male neutered domestic shorthair cat. (**A**) Ventrodorsal radiograph of the pelvis with extended pelvic limbs. There is a right-sided capital femoral physeal fracture, characterized by discontinuity of the caudal aspect of the femoral metaphysis in relation to the epiphysis (arrow). (**B**) Ventrodorsal radiograph of the pelvis with flexed pelvic limbs or "frog-leg" view of the same patient. There is increased conspicuity of the right capital femoral physeal fracture (arrow).

and often bilaterally symmetric swelling of the metaphyses of long bones. A differential diagnosis for septic metaphysitis is hypertrophic osteodystrophy. Both diseases are radiographically similar in appearance. Radiographically, a lucent region of the metaphysis with periosteal proliferation is seen with septic metaphysitis, and a lucent band oriented parallel to the physis with sclerosis and periosteal proliferation is seen with hypertrophic osteodystrophy.

**Radiographic Assessment and Indicators** As radiography has limited sensitivity in detecting acute osteomyelitis, the only radiographic finding may be soft tissue swelling [49]. As the infection progresses, radiographic changes include aggressive periosteal proliferation, permeative or moth-eaten bone lysis, and increased mineral opacity (Figure 7.27).

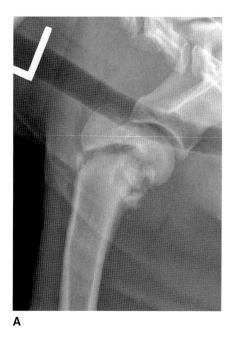 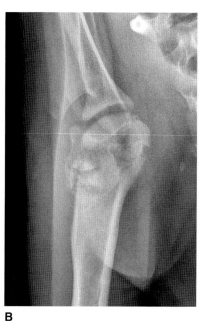

**A**                    **B**

**FIGURE 7.27** Septic metaphysitis. Mediolateral (**A**) and caudocranial (**B**) radiographs of the left shoulder. (**C**) The proximal humeral physis/metaphysis is markedly widened and lucent. There is moderate to marked, irregular osseous proliferation associated with the proximal humeral metaphysis. The surrounding soft tissues are moderate to markedly thickened. These findings are consistent with an aggressive process such as septic metaphysitis.

# Multiple Cartilaginous Exostosis

**Pathophysiology**  Multiple cartilaginous exostosis is also known as osteochondromatosis and multiple hereditary osteochondromata. It is considered a benign osseous disease of multiple, cartilage-capped bony nodules and masses that arise from the surface of any bone formed by endochondral ossification at the metaphyseal growth plate. The bones most frequently affected include the vertebrae, ribs, and other long bones. The cause of this disorder is unknown and it may affect both dogs and cats. Exostosis has been reported to undergo malignant transformation to chondrosarcoma or osteosarcoma in dogs and parosteal sarcoma in a cat [50, 51].

This disorder typically affects young dogs and cats but has been reported in a variety of ages ranging between 6 weeks to 11 years [50]. Both dogs and cats can be affected. There are no known breed or sex predilections, but Great Danes, St Bernards, and hounds appear to be overrepresented. In dogs, the disorder is inherited as an autosomal dominant trait, and is seen in young, growing dogs. Exostosis appears and enlarges before skeletal maturity. In cats, the disorder has been associated with feline leukemia virus. Exostosis occurs more commonly after skeletal maturity.

On physical examination, lameness can be noted depending on the affected anatomic structures. Additionally, the lesions can be palpated and pain may be elicited if it is associated with tendons, ligaments, vessels, or spinal cord compression.

**Radiographic Assessment and Indicators**  Single or multiple osseous masses, predominantly centered on the metaphyses of long bones, with thin cortices and medullary cavities that are confluent with the underlying bone with a foamy trabecular pattern can be identified (Figure 7.28). In dogs, growth of the exostoses should cease with closure of the adjacent growth plate. Collimated orthogonal radiographs of multiple regions of the body and limbs are recommended for complete evaluation.

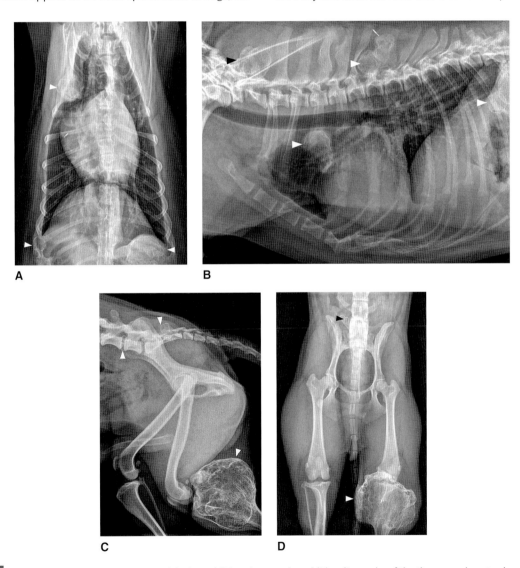

**A**    **B**    **C**    **D**

**FIGURE 7.28**  Multiple cartilaginous exostoses. Right lateral (**A**) and ventrodorsal (**B**) radiographs of the thorax, and ventrodorsal (**C**) and lateral (**D**) radiographs of the pelvis and proximal pelvic limbs. There are multifocal to coalescing, well-delineated, lobular, thin-walled, variable sized osseous nodules and masses, completely distorting the cortices and medullary bone (arrowheads). The masses associated with the body of the right 3rd rib, right 11th rib, and left 12th rib distort the lungs, causing an extrapleural sign.

# Multiple Epiphyseal Dysplasia

**Pathophysiology** Multiple epiphyseal dysplasia has been described in beagle puppies and miniature poodles. Punctate, stippled mineral opacities are seen in the epiphyses. There is failure of ossification at the epiphyseal centers. Affected puppies show a swaying hindlimb gait, sagging hocks, and forelimb lameness. Adult animals may show periodic lameness resulting from limb deformities or secondary degenerative joint disease.

Differentials for multiple epiphyseal dysplasia include mucopolysaccharidosis [52], hypervitaminosis A [53], congenital hypothyroidism [54], and osteochondrodysplasia of Scottish fold cats [55].

Mucopolysaccharidoses are a group of lysosomal disorders, each characterized by deficiency of one or multiple lysosomal enzymes needed to degrade glycosaminoglycans. Enzyme deficiency leads to an accumulation of glysoaminoglycan products in the lysosomes of multiple organs. This disease has been described in dogs and cats as well as humans and mice. Radiographically, patients exhibit epiphyseal dysplasia, generalized decreased mineral opacity of the skeletal structures, pectus excavatum, disproportionate body size, hyoid hypoplasia/aplasia, and hypoplasia and fragmentation or abnormal ossification of the dens of C2 [52].

Hypervitaminosis A affects animals restricted to a liveronly diet, which is rich in vitamin A. Hypervitaminosis A can be quickly excluded by noting the diet history. Affected animals display variable degrees of lameness depending on the bones affected, including thoracic limb lameness, stiffness, and reluctance to move. Radiographically, exostoses of the vertebral spine can be seen. Ankylosis of the elbows and shoulders and, less commonly, exostoses of the laryngeal region causing voice changes and regurgitation due to compression of the esophagus can be seen [53].

Congenital hypothyroidism has been reported in medium to large dog breeds such as the boxer and Great Dane. It results from aplasia or hypoplasia of the thyroid gland. Affected dogs and cats have thickened radial and ulnar cortices, bowing of the forelimbs, and short vertebral spines. Radiographically, there is delayed or reduced ossification of cartilage, particularly in the limbs and vertebrae. The skull may be foreshortened. Stunted and disproportionate growth with locomotor disability has been described associated with hypothyroidism in dogs and cats. Congenital hypothyroidism is rare and causes absence of or delayed appearance and development of epiphyseal growth centers. This results in a disproportionate dwarfism. Some cases are inherited [54]. If diagnosed early, abnormalities may regress with treatment.

Scottish fold cats are subject to a form of osteochondrodysplasia resulting in deformities of the metacarpus, metatarsus, and phalanges [55]. The bones are short and deformed. The caudal vertebral endplates are widened and the vertebrae foreshortened. Secondary changes occur in associated joints, causing severe locomotor problems. A similar condition has been described in Scottish deerhounds and bull terriers.

**Radiographic Assessment and Indicators** Radiographic findings include shortening of long bones and widening of the metaphysis. There is also decreased mineral opacity of the epiphyses, apophyses, and cuboidal bones of the appendicular skeleton and the epiphyses of the vertebrae. The mineral opacity of the metaphyses and diaphysis of the affected bones is normal [56]. Additionally, ossification of the affected cartilage can be seen (Figure 7.29).

# Cranial Mandibular Osteopathy and Calvarial Hyperostosis

See also Chapter 11, Imaging of the Head.

**Pathophysiology** Cranial mandibular osteopathy (CMO), also known as "lion jaw," is a proliferative, noninflammatory, nonneoplastic disorder of unknown etiology. Classically, the mandibles, occipital, and temporal bones are affected, further characterized by bilateral, irregular/palisading, osseous and periosteal proliferation. The parietal, frontal, and maxillary bones can also be affected. The tympanic bullae are often severely affected. No evidence of osteolysis is detected. CMO commonly affects West Highland white terriers. Other affected breeds include Scottish terriers, Labrador retrievers, Great Danes, Doberman pinschers, cairn terriers, German wire-haired pointers, Pyrenean mountain dogs, and less commonly the boxer, Boston terrier, and English bulldog. There is an autosomal recessive inheritance in West Highland white and Scottish terriers. CMO is usually diagnosed at around

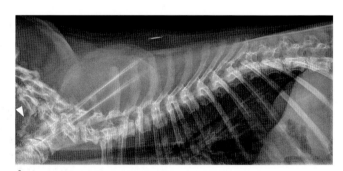

**A**

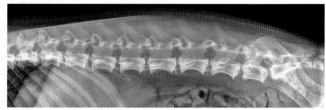

**B**

**FIGURE 7.29** Multiple epiphyseal dysplasia. Right lateral radiograph of the thoracic vertebral spine (**A**) and right lateral radiograph of the lumbar vertebral spine (**B**). The cranial and caudal physes of the caudal cervical, thoracic, and lumbar vertebral spine are markedly irregular with sclerotic endplates and irregularly shaped, thinned, heterogeneous endplates. There is marked, irregular osseous proliferation superimposed over the supraglenoid tubercles of the scapulae (arrowhead).

3–7 months of age. A common clinical complaint for CMO is difficult prehension. On physical examination, the osseous proliferation of the mandibles can be palpated and pain can be elicited by opening the mouth.

Calvarial hyperostosis resembles CMO and is characterized by progressive, often asymmetric, osseous proliferation of variable parts of the skull, with the dorsal calvarial area most commonly affected [57]. Calvarial hyperostosis affects young male and female bull mastiffs. Both CMO and calvarial hyperostosis are usually self-limiting. The osseous proliferation seen with both disorders usually ceases with skeletal maturity.

## Radiographic Assessment and Indicators

In dogs affected with CMO, the cortical bone of the mandibles, particularly the region of the mandibular angle, the tympanic bullae, and petrous part of the temporal bone are variably thickened with irregular/palisading periosteal, endosteal, and trabecular bone proliferation (Figure 7.30). The alveolar bone of the mandible is not usually affected. The regional soft tissues are variable in thickness. Dogs affected with calvarial hyperostosis exhibit variable degrees of smooth thickening of the external sagittal crest of the skull (Figure 7.31).

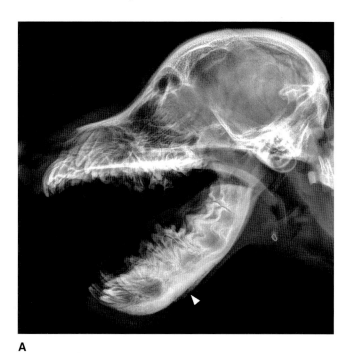

**A**

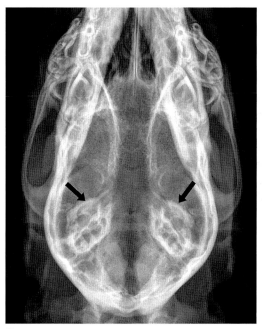

**B**

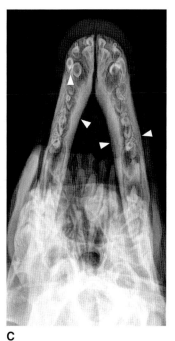

**C**

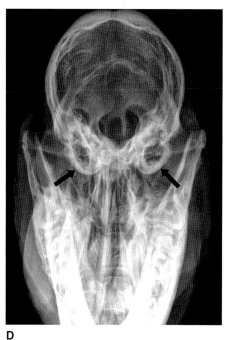

**D**

**FIGURE 7.30** Cranial mandibular osteopathy. Lateral (**A**), dorsoventral (**B**), open-mouth dorsoventral (**C**), and open-mouth rostrocaudal oblique (**D**) radiographs of the skull. There is irregular and smooth osseous proliferation of the left and right mandibles (arrowheads) and tympanic bullae walls (arrows). Incidental, multiple deciduous teeth are present. Note that the alveolar bone of the mandibles is unaffected.

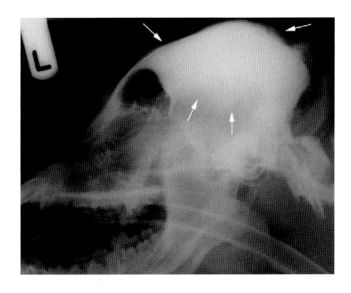

**FIGURE 7.31** Calvarial hyperostosis. Lateral radiograph of the skull of a dog. Note the focal thickening of the dorsal calvarium centered along the external sagittal crest (arrows). Source: J.F. McConnell et al. [57] / with permission of John Wiley & Sons.

# References

1. Schachner, E.R. and Lopez, M.J. (2015). Diagnosis, prevention, and management of canine hip dysplasia: a review. *Vet. Med.* 6: 181–192.
2. Fries, C.L. and Remedios, A.M. (1995). The pathogenesis and diagnosis of canine hip dysplasia: a review. *Can. Vet. J.* 36: 494–502.
3. Trumpatori, B.J., Mathews, K.G., Roe, S.R., and Robertson, I.D. (2003). Radiographic anatomy of the canine coxofemoral joint using the dorsal acetabular rim (DAR) view. *Vet. Radiol. Ultrasound* 44: 526–532.
4. Cook, C.R. and Cook, J.L. (2009). Diagnostic imaging of canine elbow dysplasia: a review. *Vet. Surg.* 38: 144–153.
5. Wolschrijn, C.F. and Weijs, W.A. (2005). Development of the subchondral bone layer of the medial coronoid process of the canine ulna. *Anat. Rec. A Discov. Mol. Cell. Evol. Biol.* 284: 439–445.
6. Guthrie, S., Plummer, J.M., and Vaughan, L.C. (1992). Aetiopathogenesis of canine elbow osteochondrosis: a study of loose fragments removed at arthrotomy. *Res. Vet. Sci.* 52: 284–291.
7. Gemmill, T.J. and Clements, D.N. (2007). Fragmented coronoid process in the dog: is there a role for incongruency? *J. Small Anim. Pract.* 48: 361–368.
8. Morgan, J.P., Wind, A., and Davidson, A.P. (2000). *Hereditary Bone and Joint Diseases in the Dog: Osteochondroses, Hip Dysplasia, Elbow Dysplasia.* Hannover: Schlütersche.
9. Wind, A. (1986). Elbow incongruity and developmental elbow disease in the dog: part 1. *J. Am. Anim. Hosp. Assoc.* 22: 711–724.
10. Lau, S.F., Theyse, L.F., Voorhout, G., and Hazewinkel, H.A. (2015). Radiographic, computed tomographic, and arthroscopic findings in labrador retrievers with medial coronoid disease. *Vet. Surg.* 44: 511–520.
11. Haudiquet, P.R., Marcellin-Little, D.J., and Stebbins, M.E. (2002). Use of the distomedial-proximolateral oblique radiographic view of the elbow joint for examination of the medial coronoid process in dogs. *Am. J. Vet. Res.* 63: 1000–1005.
12. Frazho, J.K., Graham, J., Peck, J.N., and De Haan, J.J. (2010). Radiographic evaluation of the anconeal process in skeletally immature dogs. *Vet. Surg.* 39: 829–832.
13. Sjöström, L. (1998). Ununited anconeal process in the dog. *Vet. Clin. North Am. Small Anim. Pract.* 28: 75–86.
14. Kirberger, R.M. and Fourie, S.L. (1998). Elbow dysplasia in the dog: pathophysiology, diagnosis and control. *J. S. Afr. Vet. Assoc.* 69: 43–54.
15. Chanoit, G., Singhani, N.N., Marcellin-Little, D.J., and Osborne, J.A. (2010). Comparison of five radiographic views for assessment of the medial aspect of the humeral condyle in dogs with osteochondritis dissecans. *Am. J. Vet. Res.* 71: 780–783.
16. Lerer, A., Chalmers, H.J., Moens, N.M. et al. (2014). Imaging diagnosis – temporomandibular joint dysplasia in a Basset Hound. *Vet. Radiol. Ultrasound* 55: 547–551.
17. Schwarz, T., Weller, R., Dickie, A.M. et al. (2002). Imaging of the canine and feline temporomandibular joint: a review. *Vet. Radiol. Ultrasound* 43: 85–97.
18. Wilson, M., Mauragis, D., and Berry, C. (2014). Radiography of the small animal skull: temporomandibular joints and tympanic bullae. *Today's Vet. Pract.* May/June: 53–58.
19. Hammond, G., King, A., and Lapaglia, J. (2012). Assessment of five oblique radiographic projections of the canine temporomandibular joint. *Vet. Radiol. Ultrasound* 53: 501–506.
20. Ytrehus, B., Carlson, C.S., and Ekman, S. (2007). Etiology and pathogenesis of osteochondrosis. *Vet. Pathol.* 44: 429–448.
21. Wall, C.R., Cook, C.R., and Cook, J.L. (2015). Diagnostic sensitivity of radiography, ultrasonography, and magnetic resonance imaging for detecting shoulder osteochondrosis/osteochondritis dissecans in dogs. *Vet. Radiol. Ultrasound* 56: 3–11.
22. Böhning, R.H., Suter, P.F., Hohn, R.B., and Marshall, J. (1970). Clinical and radiologic survey of canine panosteitis. *J. Am. Vet. Med. Assoc.* 156: 870–883.
23. Schawalder, P., Jutzi, K., Andres, H.U., and Blum, J. (2002). Canine panosteitis – an idiopathic bone disease investigated in the light of a new hypothesis concerning pathogenesis. Part two: biochemical aspects and investigations. *Schweiz. Arch. Tierheilkd.* 144: 163–173.

24. Schawalder, P., Andres, H.U., Jutzi, K. et al. (2002). Canine panosteitis: an idiopathic bone disease investigated in the light of a new hypothesis concerning pathogenesis. Part 1: clinical and diagnostic aspects. *Schweiz. Arch. Tierheilkd.* 144: 115–130.

25. Munjar, T., Austin, C., and Breur, G. (1998). Comparison of risk factors for hypertrophic osteodystrophy, craniomandibular osteopathy and canine distemper virus infection. *Vet. Comp. Orthop. Traumatol.* 1: 37–43.

26. LaFond, E., Breur, G.J., and Austin, C.C. (2002). Breed susceptibility for developmental orthopedic diseases in dogs. *J. Am. Anim. Hosp. Assoc.* 38: 467–477.

27. Watson, A. (1978). Hypertrophic osteodystrophy: vitamin C deficiency, overnutrition, or infection. *Aust. Vet. Pract.* 8: 107–108.

28. Meier, H., Clark, S., Schnelle, G., and Will, D. (1957). Hypertrophic osteodystrophy associated with disturbance of vitamin C synthesis in dogs. *J. Am. Vet. Med. Assoc.* 130: 483–491.

29. Franklin, M.A., Rochat, M.C., and Broaddus, K.D. (2008). Hypertrophic osteodystrophy of the proximal humerus in two dogs. *J. Am. Anim. Hosp. Assoc.* 44: 342–346.

30. Altunatmaz, K., Saroglu, M., and Guzel, O. (2005). Retained endochondral ossification of the distal ulnar growth plate in dogs. *Med. Weter.* 62: 40–42.

31. Richardson, D.C. and Zentek, J. (1998). Nutrition and osteochondrosis. *Vet. Clin. North Am. Small Anim. Pract.* 28: 115–135.

32. Trostel, C., McLaughlin, R., and Pool, R. (2002). Canine lameness caused by developmental diseases: osteochondrosis. *Compend. Contin. Ed. Pract.* 24: 836–854.

33. Johnson, K.A. (1981). Retardation of endochondral ossification at the distal ulnar growth plate in dogs. *Aust. Vet. J.* 57: 474–478.

34. Hickey, J. and Le Roux, A. (2016). What is your diagnosis? Variant of a bilateral distal ulnar retained cartilaginous core in a dog. *J. Am. Vet. Med. Assoc.* 249: 51–53.

35. Lau, R. (1977). Inherited premature closure of hte distal ulnar physis. *J. Am. Anim. Hosp. Assoc.* 13: 609–667.

36. Sande, R.D., Alexander, J.E., Spencer, G.R. et al. (1982). Dwarfism in Alaskan malamutes: a disease resembling metaphyseal dysplasia in human beings. *Am. J. Pathol.* 106: 224–236.

37. Johnson, J., Austin, C., and Breur, G. (1994). Incidence of canine appendicular musculoskeletal dirsorder in 16 veterinary teaching hospitals from 1980 to 1989. *Vet. Comp. Orthop. Traumatol.* 7: 56–69.

38. Ramadan, R.O. and Vaughan, L.C. (1978). Premature closure of the distal ulnar growth plate in dogs – a review of 58 cases. *J. Small Anim. Pract.* 19: 647–667.

39. Carrig, C. and Morgan, J. (1975). Asynchronous growth of the canine radius and ulna – early radiographic changes following experimental retardation of longitudinal growth of the ulna. *Vet. Radiol.* 16: 121–129.

40. Moores, A. (2006). Humeral condylar fractures and incomplete ossification of the humeral condyle in dogs. *In Pract.* 28: 391–397.

41. Marcellin-Little, D.L., Roe, S.C., and DeYoung, D.J. (1996). What is your diagnosis? Faint vertical condylar radiolucency, secondary to incomplete ossification of the humeral condyle. *J. Am. Vet. Med. Assoc.* 209: 727–728.

42. Marcellin-Little, D.J., DeYoung, D.J., Ferris, K.K., and Berry, C.M. (1994). Incomplete ossification of the humeral condyle in spaniels. *Vet. Surg.* 23: 475–487.

43. Walker, T.M. (1998). A redefined type of elbow dysplasia in the dog – 2 cases. *Can. Vet. J.* 39: 573–575.

44. de Bakker, E., Samoy, Y., Gielen, I., and Van Ryssen, B. (2011). Medial humeral epicondylar lesions in the canine elbow. A review of the literature. *Vet. Comp. Orthop. Traumatol.* 24: 9–17.

45. Cardoso, C.B., Rahal, S.C., Mamprim, M.J. et al. (2018). Avascular necrosis of the femoral head in dogs – retrospective study. *Acta Sci. Vet.* 46: 1537.

46. Stubbs, W.P., Bloomberg, M.S., Scruggs, S.L. et al. (1996). Effects of prepubertal gonadectomy on physical and behavioral development in cats. *J. Am. Vet. Med. Assoc.* 209: 1864–1871.

47. Craig, L.E. (2001). Physeal dysplasia with slipped capital femoral epiphysis in 13 cats. *Vet. Pathol.* 38: 92–97.

48. Lafuente, P. (2011). Young, male neutered, obese, lame? Non-traumatic fractures of the femoral head and neck. *J. Feline Med. Surg.* 13: 498–507.

49. Braden, T., Tvedten, H., Mostosky, U. et al. (1989). The sensitivity and specificity of radiology and histopathology in the diagnosis of posttraumatic osteomyelitis. *Vet. Comp. Orthop. Traumatol.* 2: 98–103.

50. Doige, C.E. (1987). Multiple cartilaginous exostoses in dogs. *Vet. Pathol.* 24: 276–278.

51. Pool, R. (1993). *Osteochondromatosis*. Philadelphia, PA: Lippincott Williams & Wilkins.

52. Konde, L., Thrall, M., Gasper, P. et al. (1987). Radiographically visualized skeletal changes associated with mucopolysaccharidosis VI in cats. *Vet. Radiol.* 28: 223–228.

53. Polizopoulou, Z.S., Kazakos, G., Patsikas, M.N., and Roubies, N. (2005). Hypervitaminosis A in the cat: a case report and review of the literature. *J. Feline Med. Surg.* 7: 363–368.

54. Saunders, H. and Jezyk, P. (1991). The radiographic appearance of canine congenital hypothyroidism: skeletal changes with delayed treatment. *Vet. Radiol.* 32: 171–177.

55. Malik, R., Allan, G.S., Howlett, C.R. et al. (1999). Osteochondrodysplasia in Scottish fold cats. *Aust. Vet. J.* 77: 85–92.

56. Rørvik, A.M., Teige, J., Ottesen, N., and Lingaas, F. (2008). Clinical, radiographic, and pathologic abnormalities in dogs with multiple epiphyseal dysplasia: 19 cases (1991–2005). *J. Am. Vet. Med. Assoc.* 233: 600–606.

57. McConnell, J.F., Hayes, A., Platt, S.R., and Smith, K.C. (2006). Calvarial hyperostosis syndrome in two bullmastiffs. *Vet. Radiol. Ultrasound* 47: 72–77.

# CHAPTER 8

# Imaging of Joint and Tendon Diseases

Nathan C. Nelson

Department of Molecular Biomedical Sciences, College of Veterinary Medicine, North Carolina State University, Raleigh, NC, USA

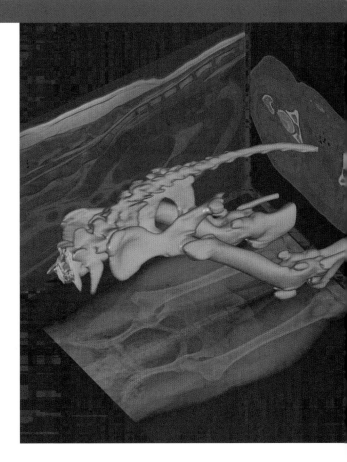

## Introduction

Joint diseases are broadly categorized as degenerative, inflammatory, or neoplastic in origin. Degenerative joint disease, also termed osteoarthritis or osteoarthrosis, is often seen in older patients as an incidental finding that does not cause clinical signs. While degenerative joint disease is typically less debilitating than other joint diseases, it is an ongoing process and can be quite painful when advanced. In comparison, neoplastic or inflammatory joint diseases are much more debilitating and rapidly progressive but less common. Imaging features for these types of joint disease are discussed below.

## Choice of Modality

Radiographs are the best initial imaging test when assessing joint disease, due to their low cost and widespread availability. Radiography readily allows assessment of overall joint alignment. Tendons and ligaments are not identifiable on radiographs, as their opacity is the same as regional soft tissues, resulting in effacement of tendon/ligament margins. Joint malalignment implies that the ligaments or tendons that support joints are abnormal. Similarly, articular cartilage is not seen on radiographs, being the same opacity as joint fluid. Subchondral bone is apparent on radiographs, and the presence of subchondral defects implies cartilage damage is present. Periarticular bone proliferation (termed *osteophytes*) is the cardinal sign of degenerative joint disease and identified on radiography even when small.

Ultrasound is most useful when evaluating periarticular structures such as tendons and ligaments, as their highly structured appearance is readily differentiated from surrounding soft tissues. Ultrasound has limited ability to image intraarticular structures as surrounding bones disrupt sound transmission into deeper soft tissues. Ultrasound may be used when an intraarticular or periarticular mass is suspected, to assess regional soft tissue involvement and guide tissue sampling.

While magnetic resonance imaging (MRI) is the gold standard for imaging joint and tendon/ligament diseases in people, its use is limited for musculoskeletal imaging in dogs and cats. MRI has more limited availability and the high cost deters some clients. The small size of veterinary patients requires higher image resolution, resulting in longer scan times and more image noise. Coils (MRI equipment that collects signal from the anatomic area of interest) are placed near the joint of interest, but are not specifically designed for veterinary patients, which can cause problems when positioning a patient or attempting to acquire high-resolution images.

Computed tomgraphy (CT) is rarely used in the assessment of musculoskeletal disease in veterinary patients. It is most effective when providing further imaging of equivocal or subtle osseous pathology identified on radiographs (such as suspected fissure fractures or areas of aggressive bone lysis). Evaluation of cartilage and other intraarticular structures requires intraarticular injection of iodinated contrast medium before the scan is performed. Contrast within soft tissues (such as muscle, ligaments, and tendons) is lower than MRI, so CT is rarely used for further evaluation of musculoskeletal soft tissue pathology.

# Degenerative Joint Disease

Degenerative joint disease is a slowly progressive degenerative disorder of synovial joints, which results in cartilage loss, synovial proliferation, and periarticular bony remodeling [1]. It has many names, including osteoarthrosis, osteoarthritis, and arthritis. The etiology is complex, but degenerative change to joint cartilage is the key underlying component.

Degeneration may be primary, as occurs with age, or due to underlying inherited cartilage defects (such as mucopolysaccharidosis). More commonly, degenerative joint disease is a secondary condition caused by conditions that alter joint stability, joint congruity, or acute injury, resulting in secondary damage to the cartilage and eventual cartilage degeneration [2]. Fractures that involve a joint, joint instability from trauma, hip dysplasia, viral infections, and immune-mediated diseases are some of the many causes of cartilage damage that eventually results in secondary degenerative joint disease [1].

Degenerative joint disease is very common in dogs and cats, and often is undiagnosed or diagnosed on radiography when imaging the patient for another reason.

# Radiographic Findings of Degenerative Joint Disease

## Swelling

Regardless of the underlying cause, joint diseases result in increased synovial fluid and synovial proliferation. Radiography cannot differentiate synovial fluid from

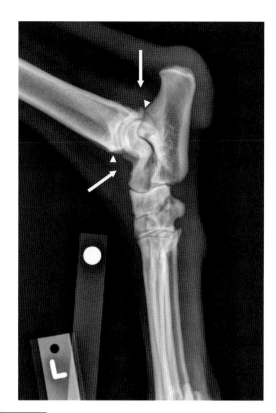

**FIGURE 8.1**   Lateral radiograph of mild tarsocrural osteoarthrosis. There is mild intracapsular swelling (arrows) seen dorsal and plantar to the tarsocrural joint and periarticular osteophytes (arrowheads).

synovial proliferation as both are similarly soft tissue opaque. Increased fluid/synovium causes soft tissue thickening which is concentrically centered on the affected joint. This appearance is termed *intracapsular swelling*. When mild, intracapsular swelling remains immediately adjacent to the joint margin on radiographs (Figure 8.1). As swelling progresses, the joint capsule distends and swelling may extend further along the margin of adjacent bones (Figure 8.2). Degenerative joint disease usually causes mild intracapsular swelling, whereas inflammatory and neoplastic joint diseases cause more severe swelling.

When structures outside the joint capsule (such as ligaments, subcutaneous structures, and muscles) are diseased, the soft tissue swelling tends to extend more proximally and distally on the limb, rather than being immediately at the level of the joint. This "extracapsular swelling" is usually eccentrically located, with the swelling being more severe in one area of the limb, centered on the most diseased tissue (Figure 8.3). Extracapsular swelling is rare in degenerative joint disease, and identification of significant extracapsular swelling should raise concern for some other soft tissue disease or concurrent injury to extracapsular structures.

## Osteophytes

Osteophytes are bony proliferations along the periarticular margins of synovial joints (Figures 8.1 and 8.2). They are

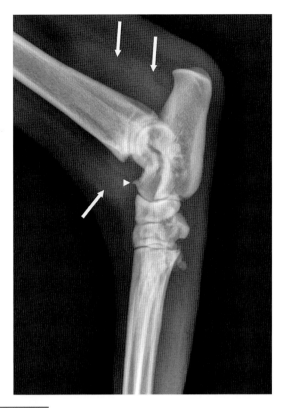

immediately adjacent to the joint margin, which distinguishes them from bony proliferation at the origin or insertion of tendons or ligaments (termed *enthesophytes*; see below). Osteophytes are the earliest radiographic evidence of degenerative joint disease, as direct visualization of articular cartilage is not possible on radiographs.

## Enthesophytes

An enthesophyte is a bony proliferation at the origin or insertion on bone of a tendon, ligament, or fascial plane. Enthesophytes may form as a consequence of degenerative joint disease, as the degenerative process of the joint may involve regional soft tissues. They are often a result of a previous traumatic episode to a soft tissue attachment (Figure 8.4), but tendons or ligaments undergoing primary degenerative processes may also form enthesophytes (Figure 8.5).

## Joint Collapse

There is partial or complete loss of the articular cartilage in cases of advanced degenerative joint disease. With weight bearing, cartilage loss allows narrowing of the joint space and if cartilage loss is complete, bone-on-bone contact occurs. In a nonweight-bearing patient, loss of downward pressure on the joint allows it to open to its normal width. For this reason, joint space narrowing is rarely recognized

**FIGURE 8.2** Lateral radiograph of severe tarsocrural effusion. There is severe intracapsular swelling (arrows) seen dorsal and plantar to the tarsocrural joint. An osteophyte is seen dorsal to the proximal intertarsal joint (arrowhead).

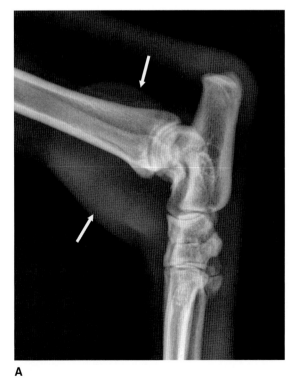

**A**

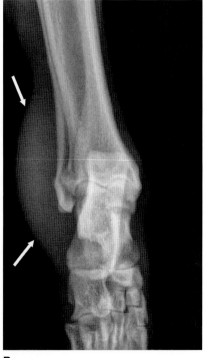

**B**

**FIGURE 8.3** Lateral (**A**) and DP (**B**) radiographs showing an extracapsular mass in the area of the tarsus (arrowheads). Notice the soft tissue swelling is not centered on the joint and is eccentric to the lateral aspect of the distal crus.

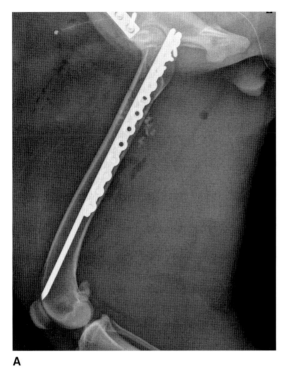
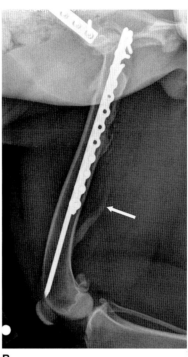

A

B

**FIGURE 8.4**   Immediate postoperative radiograph (**A**) of a femoral fracture, with recheck radiographs (**B**) 2 months later. There is a large enthesophyte that extends from the caudal margin of the femur (arrow), that was not present initially. Bony proliferation in this area is common after trauma, due to strain or avulsion of muscular attachments.

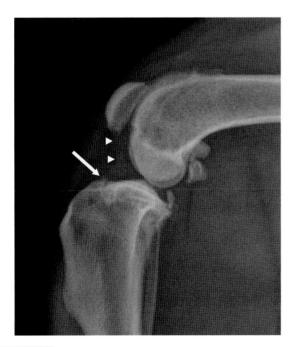

**FIGURE 8.5**   Lateral projection of the stifle showing moderate osteoarthrosis with an enthesophyte at the insertion of the cranial cruciate ligament (arrow). Increased fluid in the stifle joint is seen (arrowheads).

on radiography of dogs and cats even in severe joint degeneration, as most musculoskeletal radiographs are acquired in a nonweight-bearing position. More common is artifactual joint narrowing due to obliquity of the projection relative to the joint or flexion of a joint, allowing adjacent bones to summate (Figure 8.6).

## Subchondral Sclerosis

Loss of cartilage during the degenerative process results in decreased cartilage cushioning and increased forces on the adjacent subchondral bone. As a result, the subchondral bone remodels to become more opaque (Figure 8.7).

## Subchondral Resorption, Cysts

Resorption of subchondral bone occurs with more advanced degenerative joint disease and results in an irregular appearance to the articular margin of the subchondral bone. This resorption is uncommon, and when present is often very mild. If severe subchondral resorption is present or if this resorption occurs along the nonarticular peripheral margin of a joint, suspicion should be elevated for either septic arthritis or synovial neoplasia (see below).

Cyst-like lesions may occur as part of the degenerative process in a joint. This is particularly common in the intercondylar region of the stifle in patients with chronic cranial cruciate ligament ruptures, but other joints may be affected (Figure 8.8). As opposed to erosive lesions that tend to be poorly defined with an irregular shape, cyst-like lesions have well-defined margins and a more rounded shape.

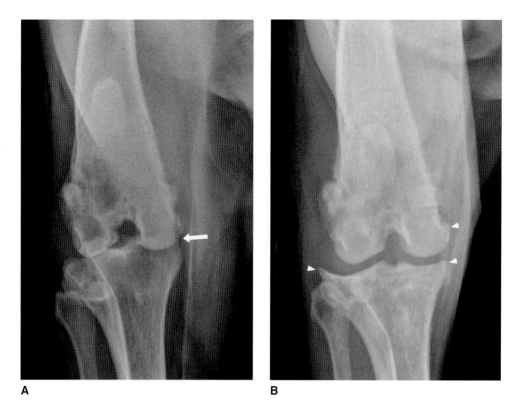

**A**　　　　　　　　　　　　**B**

**FIGURE 8.6** Craniocaudal projections of a stifle with flexion (**A**) and full extension (**B**). Notice when the stifle is flexed, there is overlap of the tibia and femur (arrow), resulting in artifactual joint narrowing. When appropriately extended, the joint space is normal and osteophytes are more apparent (arrowhead).

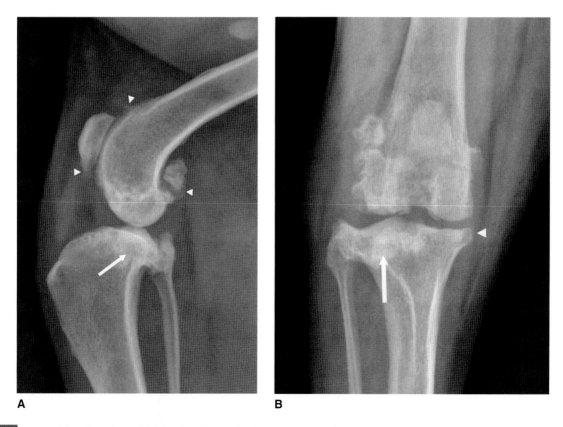

**A**　　　　　　　　　　　　**B**

**FIGURE 8.7** Lateral (**A**) and caudocranial (**B**) stifle radiographs showing severe stifle joint degeneration. There is subchondral sclerosis (arrow) and peripheral osteophytosis (arrowheads).

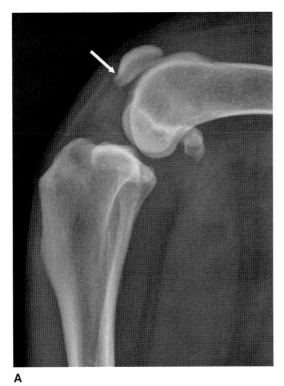
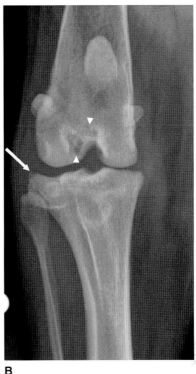

**A**

**B**

**FIGURE 8.8**   Lateral (**A**) and caudocranial (**B**) radiographs of mild stifle joint degeneration. Osteophytes (arrows) are present. There are also rounded cyst-like lesions within the intercondylar space (arrowheads).

# Degenerative Joint Disease of Specific Joints

## Coxofemoral Joint

The ventrodorsal, extended leg radiograph is best suited for evaluation of coxofemoral degeneration. Lateral pelvic radiographs rarely contribute significantly to screening for coxofemoral degeneration, but are useful in diagnosing dorsal femoral head luxation due to severe dysplasia.

In dogs with hip dysplasia (see Chapter 7), coxofemoral laxity eventually results in cartilage damage and degenerative joint disease. In younger dogs presenting with moderate to severe coxofemoral degenerative joint disease, the underlying cause of these changes is attributable to hip dysplasia. Subluxation of the joint is confirmatory of dysplasia, and is recognized by widening of the medial aspect of the joint relative to the lateral aspect of the joint (Figure 8.9).

One of the earliest signs of coxofemoral degeneration is a row of osteophytes on the femoral neck, sometimes termed a *Morgan's line* (Figures 8.9 and 8.10). This line may be subtle and seen in the absence of other degenerative changes, but is associated with progressive coxofemoral osteoarthritis [3].

Continued osteophyte formation causes progressive femoral neck thickening in the dysplastic patient (Figures 8.11

and 8.12). The acetabulum will become shallow due to osteophyte formation but also due to lack of femoral head contact, allowing acetabular remodeling to occur. The femoral head typically should have 50% or more coverage by the acetabulum, but is decreased in cases of dysplasia.

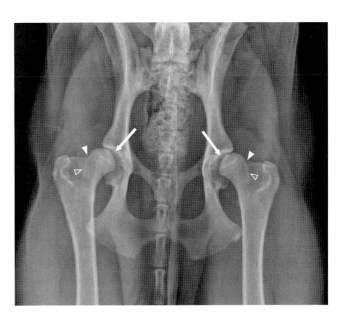

**FIGURE 8.9**   VD projection of the pelvis showing moderate subluxation of both femoral heads (arrows), osteophytes along the femoral neck resulting in thickening (arrowheads), and osteophytes at the area of joint capsule insertion.

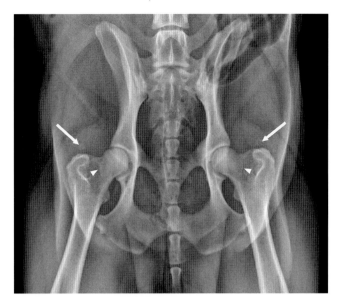

**FIGURE 8.10** VD projection of the pelvis showing mild coxofemoral osteoarthrosis, indicated by thin enthesophytes at the area of joint capsule insertion (arrowheads). There is also mineralization at the insertion of the gluteal musculature (arrows).

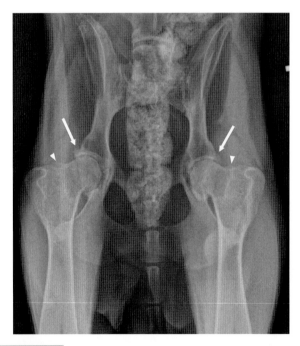

**FIGURE 8.11** Severe coxofemoral osteoarthrosis characterized by osteophyte formation on the acetabulum (arrows) and femoral necks (arrowheads).

## Elbow

Elbow osteoarthritis in dogs is often caused by elbow dysplasia (see Chapter 7), particularly if degeneration is recognized in a young dog. The anconeal process is the earliest site of osteophyte formation, recognized by proliferation on the proximal margin of the anconeal process on the flexed lateral elbow projection. Early osteophyte formation also occurs on the medial

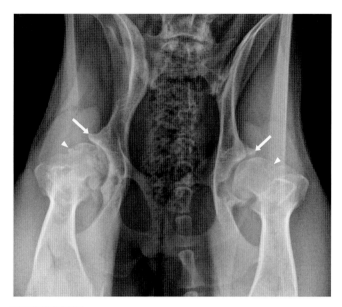

**FIGURE 8.12** Severe coxofemoral osteoarthrosis characterized by osteophyte formation on the acetabulum (arrows) and femoral necks (arrowheads). The acetabulae are shallow with decreased coverage of the femoral heads.

coronoid process, best seen on the craniocaudal projection. Enthesopathy of the medial and lateral humeral epicondyles, at the origin of the flexor and extensor muscles of the antebrachium, is often seen concurrently with elbow degenerative joint disease.

## Stifle

Most cases of stifle degenerative joint disease in dogs are attributable to degeneration of the cranial cruciate ligament. Enthesopathy of the cranial cruciate ligament insertion on the cranial intercondyloid region of the tibia is common (Figures 8.5 and 8.13). Osteophytosis is typically seen along the apex and base of the patella, proximal margin of the trochlear ridges, medial and lateral tibial condyles, and the fabella (Figure 8.14).

Mild joint effusion is easily recognized in the stifle because of the infrapatellar fat pad. In a normal stifle, this infrapatellar fat pad should extend caudally to the cranial margin of the tibial plateau (Figure 8.15). With mild increases in joint fluid, small strands of fluid extend more cranially in the joint and as synovial effusion becomes worse, the infrapatellar fat pad appears compressed cranially. Even mild amounts of joint effusion should alert the clinician to underlying joint disease.

Definitive clinical diagnosis of cranial cruciate rupture is through the detection of cranial drawer or positive tibial thrust on physical examination, but cranial displacement of the tibia relative to the femoral condyles may be seen radiographically in dogs with complete cranial cruciate rupture (Figure 8.16). When the stifle is positioned so that the diaphysis of the femur is perpendicular to the diaphysis of the tibia, the

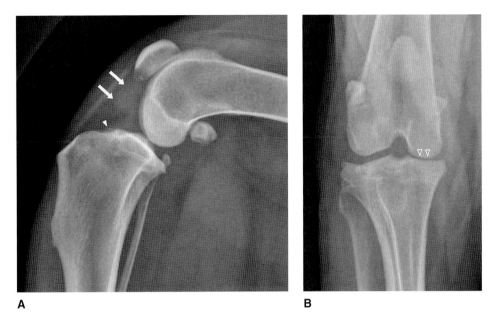

**FIGURE 8.13**   Lateral (**A**) and caudocranial (**B**) readiographs of mild stifle osteoarthrosis with increased fluid in the stifle joint (arrows) and an enthesophyte at the insertion of the cranial cruciate ligament (closed arrowhead). There is artifactual narrowing of the medial stifle joint (open arrowhead).

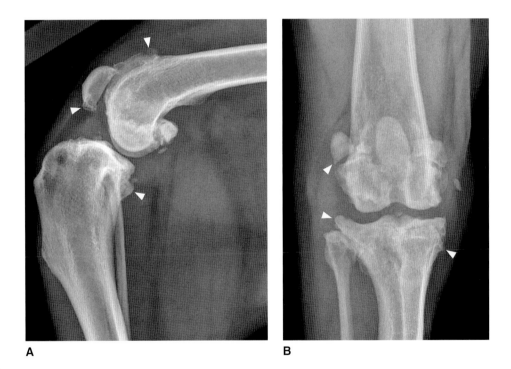

**FIGURE 8.14**   Lateral (**A**) and caudocranial (**B**) radiographs of severe stifle osteoarthritis due to cranial cruciate ligament rupture. There is severe osteophyte formation (arrowheads) along the margins of the stifle. The tibia is cranially subluxated relative to the femur due to the cranial cruciate rupture.

femoral condyles should align directly with the intercondylar eminences of the tibia. If cranial cruciate rupture is present, the intercondylar eminences are positioned more cranially. Dogs with partial cruciate rupture will maintain a normal orientation of the femur and tibia. Extension of the stifle masks the subluxation (Figure 8.17).

## Phalanges

Degenerative joint disease is common in the metacarpo/metatarsophalangeal and interphalangeal joints of dogs, and often seen concurrently with regional collateral ligament enthesopathy (Figure 8.18). These degenerative changes may

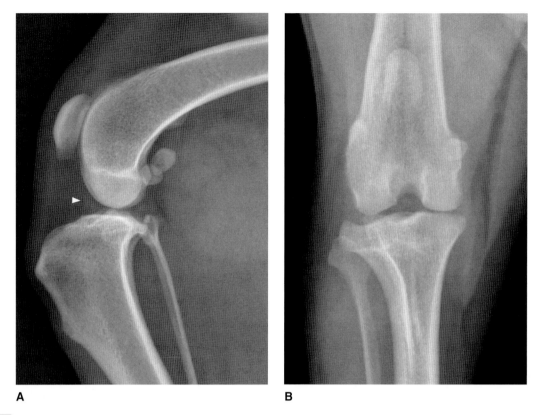

**A**                    **B**

Lateral (**A**) and caudocranial (**B**) projections of a normal stifle. The arrowhead indicates the normal soft tissue within the stifle.

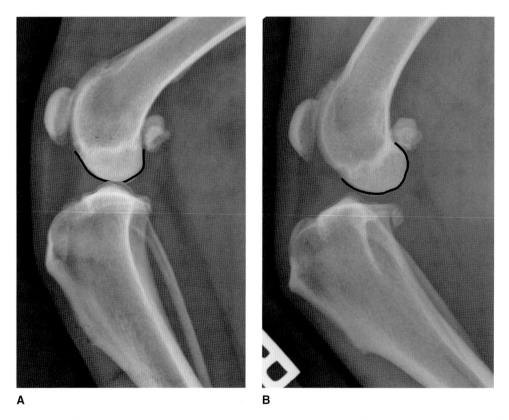

**A**                    **B**

**FIGURE 8.16** A normal stifle (**A**) compared to a stifle with cranial cruciate rupture and joint subluxation (**B**). In the normal stifle, the femoral condyle (black outline) is lined up with the tibial eminences (gray outline). In the patient with subluxation, the tibial eminences are cranially displaced relative to the femoral condyle.

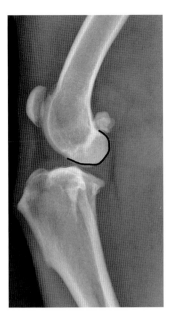

**FIGURE 8.17** Radiographs of a patient with cranial cruciate ligament rupture, but the stifle is more extended than in Figure 8.16. The tibial eminences (gray outline) are cranially displaced relative to the femoral condyle (black outline), but the subluxation is less severe due to the extended stifle positioning. The tibial eminences are smaller than the patient in Figure 8.16.

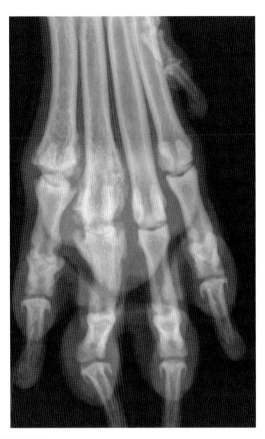

**FIGURE 8.19** Dorsopalmar projection of the manus showing severe osteoarthrosis of the fourth and fifth metacarpophalangeal joints. Osteophytes are seen at the joint margins. There is also proliferation further from joint margins, at the origin and insertion of the collateral ligaments. The patient was not lame and not painful on palpation of this area.

# Degenerative Changes to Nonsynovial Joints

Degenerative changes occur in other joint types besides synovial joints. The costochondral joint between the ribs and the costal arches is a type of hyaline cartilaginous (nonsynovial) joint. Mineralization of the costal arches is a normal consequence of aging in dogs and cats, and severe degenerative proliferation may occur at the costochondral junction. Though this may cause pain in humans, clinical signs associated with degeneration at the costochondral joints are not recognized in cats and dogs.

The intersternebral articulations are cartilaginous joints. Degenerative proliferation may occur at the intersternebral space and is characterized by rounded, smooth, mineralized proliferation, but does not cause clinical signs even when severe. Rarely, infection of the sternebrae or intersternebral spaces may occur, with a radiographic appearance similar to discospondylitis. There is erosion of opposing sternebral margins and active, irregular bony response. Degeneration of intervertebral discs (another cartilaginous joint) and

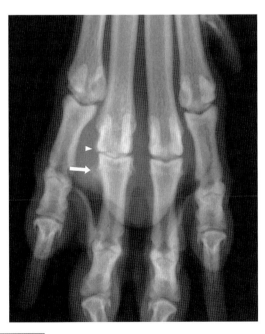

**FIGURE 8.18** Dorsopalmar projection of the manus showing mild osteoarthrosis of the fourth metacarpophalangeal joint. Osteophytes (arrowhead) are seen at periarticular margins. Enthesophytes are seen at the area of collateral ligament insertion (arrow).

be radiographically severe, but rarely result in clinically significant lameness (Figure 8.19). Degenerative changes to the manus/pes are rare in cats.

the synovial joints of the vertebral bodies is discussed in Chapter 12.

# Joint-Associated Neoplasia

Joint-associated neoplasms arise from the soft tissue structures of a joint, with histiocytic sarcomas and synovial cell tumors being the most common. Histiocytic sarcomas arise from either dendritic cell or macrophage lineage, and are particularly common in Bernese mountain dogs, Rottweilers, and retrievers [4, 5]. Joint-associated tumors are uncommon in smaller breed dogs, and rare in the cat. They may be localized to specific organs (such as spleen and skin) with secondary joint involvement, but may arise as a primary tumor surrounding a joint [4]. Synovial cell sarcoma has an identical radiographic appearance to histiocytic sarcoma, and requires special histopathologic staining to differentiate it from histiocytic sarcoma. Other joint tumors have been reported, such as fibrosarcoma, rhabdomyosarcoma, and hemangiosarcoma, but are uncommon [6].

Radiography of a joint affected by a neoplasm identifies a soft tissue mass effect circumferentially surrounding a joint. When the stifle is involved, the patella may be displaced cranially, which does not occur in diseases that merely cause an increase in joint fluid (such as degenerative joint disease; Figure 8.20). The soft tissue swelling is more severe, better defined, and more mass-like than that seen with degenerative or primary inflammatory joint diseases where the swelling tends to be mild and less well defined (Figure 8.21).

As the disease progresses, osseous changes occur primarily along the margins of a joint, near the sites of joint capsular attachment (Figure 8.20). Focal bone resorption results in small or larger coalescing areas of bone loss. In early cases, the bone loss may be geographic, mimicking the appearance of a bone cyst, but with time these areas will enlarge and assume a more aggressive appearance. There may be subchondral resorption of the joint articular surface, but this is less pronounced than bone loss at the peripheral margins of the joint. Periosteal reaction may occur along the margins of the joint, resulting in an irregular periarticular margin. This periosteal proliferation is differentiated from osteophytes due to its progressive nature and more irregular appearance. Bone reaction also extends further from the margin of the joint than expected for osteophytes.

Unlike a primary bone tumor, which is monostotic (affecting one bone), joint-associated neoplasms are locally polyostotic (affecting multiple bones in one area of the body).

# Septic Arthritis

Bacterial joint infection is uncommon in cats and dogs, but must be recognized early as articular cartilage damage occurs readily and leads to long-term joint degeneration and patient debilitation [7].

In most cases, septic arthritis results from direct inoculation such as during surgery or a penetrating wound, with cat bite wounds being the most common cause of feline septic arthritis. Secondary joint infection may occur from infected

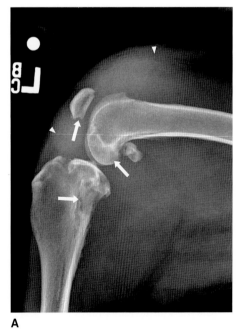
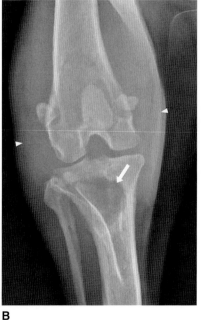

**A**    **B**

**FIGURE 8.20** Lateral (**A**) and caudocranial (**B**) projections of a stifle with joint-associated histiocytic sarcoma. There is severe lysis (arrows) at joint margins. There is also periosteal reaction extending at the margin of the adjacent joint (arrowheads). There is severe intracapsular soft tissue thickening cranially displacing the patella.

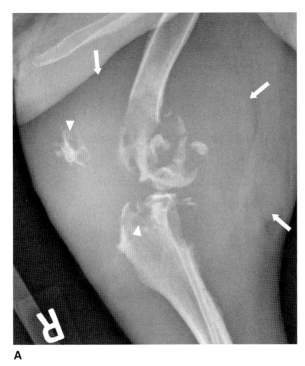
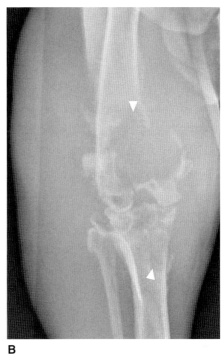

**A**                                                    **B**

**FIGURE 8.21**   Lateral (**A**) and caudocranial (**B**) projections of joint-associated histiocytic sarcoma. There is severe mass effect centered on the joint (arrows) with severe periarticular lysis (arrowheads).

adjacent superficial tissues or through hematogenous localization [8]. Hematogenous localization is more common in joints affected by degenerative joint disease, as the soft tissue proliferation and altered vascularization in a degenerative joint provide a suitable bed for initial bacterial colonization and growth. Animals with diabetes mellitus, urinary tract infections, and prosthetic joints are also predisposed to opportunistic hematogenous infection [7, 9].

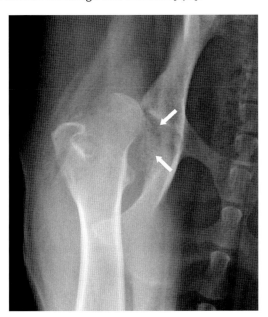

**FIGURE 8.22**   Ventrodorsal projection of a septic coxofemoral joint. There is a permeative lysis of the right acetabulum (arrows) and focally on the cranial femoral head. The femoral head is cranially subluxated.

Definitive diagnosis requires a positive culture of joint fluid or the synovial membrane, but high total protein and nucleated cell counts on synovial fluid analysis allow a presumptive diagnosis. Radiographs may also provide evidence of joint infection. Intracapsular soft tissue swelling is the initial radiographic finding, and the swelling tends to be more severe than that seen with joint degeneration. Additionally, with severe cases, extracapsular swelling may be present as the inflammation associated with the joint spreads to adjacent tissues. As infection continues, permeative or moth-eaten lysis develops along the periarticular and subchondral bone (Figure 8.22). Irregular periosteal reaction occurs along joint margins and there may be cellulitis in regional subcutaneous tissues (Figures 8.23 and 8.24). The lysis and periosteal reaction are often relatively subtle compared to the soft tissue swelling until later in the process (Figure 8.25).

Ultimately, the radiographic findings of septic arthritis overlap with the appearance of joint-associated neoplasia, though combining radiographic findings with other indicators of sepsis (pain, fever, leukocytosis) can raise the clinical suspicion of joint infection over neoplasia.

CT imaging of septic arthritis is rarely performed, but makes subtle areas of bone lysis or periosteal reaction more evident (Figure 8.24). CT guidance assists sampling of difficult-to-access joints (Figure 8.24). Ultrasound is occasionally used to image joint sepsis, as the synovial effusion and proliferation are readily apparent. Ultrasound cannot determine whether synovial proliferation is inflammatory or neoplastic in nature, so ultimate differentiation of tumor versus infection still relies on joint cytology or culture, though synovial biopsy may ultimately be necessary in some cases.

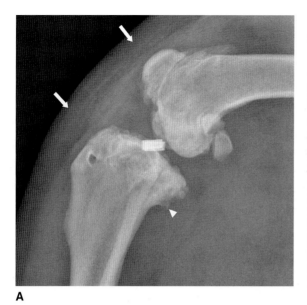
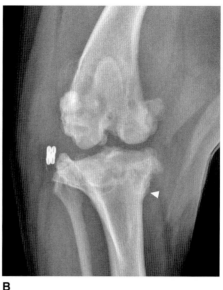

**A**

**B**

**FIGURE 8.23** Lateral (**A**) and caudocranial (**B**) projections of a septic stifle joint after extracapsular stabilization surgery. There is a metallic crimp lateral to the stifle from the surgery. There is thickening and soft tissue stranding in the subcutaneous tissues adjacent to the stifle (arrows). While osteophytes are present along joint margins from preexisting degenerative joint disease, there is also periosteal proliferation extending beyond the margin of the stifle joint, beyond where osteophytes would be expected (arrowheads).

# Immune-Mediated Arthritis

Immune-mediated joint disease is uncommon in dogs and rare in cats, but results in significant pain and lameness. These inflammatory diseases result in a polyarthropathy, with the distal limb joints typically most affected. They cause a type III hypersensitivity reaction where immune complexes accumulate in the joint space and cause joint inflammation [10]. These immune complexes are formed by antibodies combining with chronic antigenic stimuli (such as viral or bacterial infections or neoplasia) or as a result of antibodies being self-directed to certain immunoglobulins (rheumatoid factors) or nuclear elements normally found in the body [10]. Ultimately, immune complex deposition occurs in joints and results in pain and inflammation.

Due to the complex nature of these diseases, the diagnosis of multijoint inflammatory disease indicates the need for a thorough search for underlying infection, inflammation, or neoplasia, and involves imaging the abdomen and possibly head and neck for underlying sources of antigenic stimulation [11].

Radiographic abnormalities depend on the duration and type of immune-mediated joint disease. Polyarthropathies are divided into those that result in subchondral destruction on radiographs (erosive polyarthritis) and those that do not (nonerosive polyarthritis). Nonerosive polyarthritis does not result in any bone destruction, with inflammation localized to the soft tissues of the joints alone. Radiographically, this results in circumferential soft tissue swelling within multiple joints, particularly the carpus and tarsus. They are often idiopathic, but have been associated with vaccine- and drug-induced

versions, systemic lupus erythematosus, steroid-responsive meningitis-arteritis, and in some breeds (such as Akitas and familial shar pei fever) [10].

Erosive polyarthropathies are less common than nonerosive immune-mediated arthritis (less than 1% of cases) and result in bone destruction (Figure 8.26) [10]. Radiographically, this manifests as an irregular subchondral surface to the bone or resorptive lesions near the areas of joint capsular insertion. The subchondral erosion initially results in an apparent joint space widening, but joint collapse occurs as the disease progresses. On initial presentation, only soft tissue swelling may be present, as joint erosion requires weeks to months to appear. Rheumatoid arthritis (where antibodies in the body are self-directed to naturally occurring rheumatoid factors) is an example of an erosive polyarthritis, and typically affects middle-aged small-breed dogs. Erosive polyarthritis has also been described in greyhounds, and sporadically in other breeds. Though many causes are ultimately idiopathic, some viruses (notably distemper virus) are implicated in some cases.

Nonerosive immune-mediated polyarthritis in cats includes systemic lupus erythematosus and idiopathic/primary immune-mediated polyarthritis. There are two erosive forms of polyarthritis in cats: feline periosteal proliferative polyarthritis and feline rheumatoid-like arthritis. These erosive polyarthropathies are sporadic and not well characterized. In cats, infectious causes of polyarthritis are much more common than immune-mediated arthritis [8]. Most of the infectious causes of feline polyarthritis are nonerosive, and include feline infectious peritonitis virus, calicivirus, tick-borne rickettsial diseases, and fungal diseases.

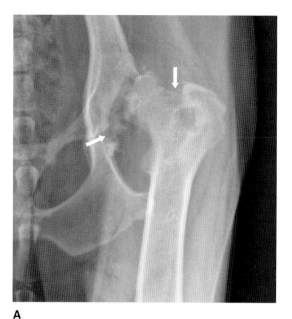

A

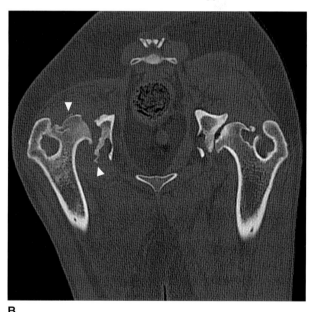

B

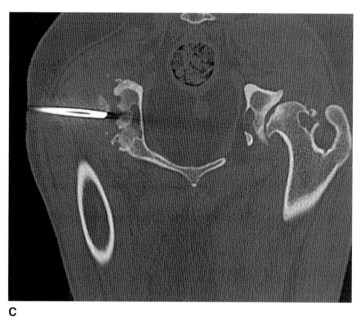

C

**FIGURE 8.24**   Radiograph (**A**) and CT image (**B**) of a septic coxofemoral joint. There is severe lysis of the acetabulum and femoral neck (arrow). Bony proliferation near the margins of the joint is more apparent on the CT image (closed arrowhead), and is more peripheral than expected for osteophytosis. CT was also performed to guide a biopsy instrument into regional soft tissues (**C**; open arrowhead) to rule out a joint neoplasm. Severe osteophytosis was seen on the contralateral coxofemoral joint.

# Luxations/Subluxations

A joint luxation is complete dissociation of two adjacent bones that normally share an articulation. Subluxation is a less severe dissociation of bones, so they maintain opposition but to a reduced degree compared to normal. Joint luxation/subluxation usually occurs due to trauma, and is recognized radiographically by malalignment of adjacent osseous structures.

Luxations/subluxations are inherently unstable, and the opposed bones may shift relative to one another. Depending on patient position, subluxation/luxations may reduce during radiography. In these cases, external pressure or altering patient position can result in distraction of the affected joint, allowing radiographic identification of subluxation/luxation. Coxofemoral subluxation is common in dogs with hip dysplasia, as the femoral head laterally displaces relative to the acetabulum, but in some dogs it is not apparent until hip distraction is performed (the so-called PennHip procedure; see Chapters 6 and 7). The cranial cruciate ligament in the stifle prevents cranial tibial subluxation relative to the femur. In a neutral position, the femur and tibia may properly align but when the stifle and tarsus are placed in a 90° angle, the tibia may subluxate cranially relative to the femur (so-called tibial thrust; Figure 8.16).

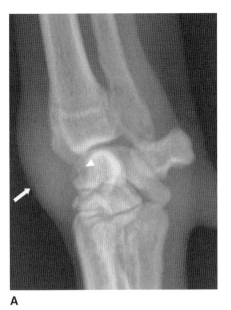
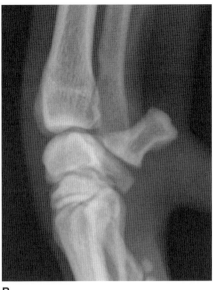

**A**    **B**

**FIGURE 8.25**   Lateral projection of a septic carpal joint (**A**) with a normal carpus for comparison (**B**). There is severe soft tissue swelling at the level of the affected carpal joint (arrow). There is also subtle lysis of the proximal carpal bones (arrowhead), most apparent when compared to the normal limb.

# Fractures Involving Joints

A fracture near a joint should alert the clinician to the possibility of extension through the subchondral bone. Joint involvement of a fracture carries a more guarded long-term prognosis, as fracture repair is more complex and degenerative joint disease is expected as a long-term sequela. Gross joint involvement may be readily identified on radiographs, but thin fissures or minimally displaced fractures may require additional oblique radiographs to identify (Figure 8.27). Carpal, tarsal, and pes/manus fractures in particular often have complex morphology, with oblique radiographs often demonstrating additional fractures or fragments not seen on lateral and dorospalmar radiographs alone (Figure 8.28). A distal humeral condylar fracture in a young dog should prompt radiographic evaluation of the contralateral elbow to rule out incomplete humeral ossification as a predisposing factor (see Chapter 7).

# Sesamoid Diseases

Sesamoid bones are small round bones adjacent to joints and typically embedded within tendons. Knowledge of normal sesamoid anatomy prevents misinterpretation as fracture fragments, but variation in their frequency and normal position exists. The supinator sesamoid is lateral to the head of the radius, and variably mineralized in dogs and cats (identified radiographically in 31% of dogs and 40% of cats) [12, 13]. The supinator sesamoid is typically symmetric between left and right limbs, but may only be radiographically apparent on one limb. In some smaller dogs, the medial fabella may not be mineralized.

Displacement of sesamoid bones can indicate the presence of regional soft tissue pathology. Distal displacement of the popliteal sesamoid may be seen with cranial cruciate rupture in the dog (Figure 8.29) [14]. Some dogs, particularly West Highland white terriers and other smaller dogs, may normally have a more distally positioned medial fabella, without evidence of other pathology (Figure 8.30) [15]. Acute distal displacement of a febella indicates rupture of the tendon of origin of the gastrocnemius muscle. Traumatic luxation of palmar/plantar sesamoid bones can also occur with disruption of regional supporting soft tissues (Figure 8.31).

Sesamoid bones may fracture, with the palmar/plantar sesmoid bones of the metacarpo/tarsophalangeal joints most affected. This condition is most common in racing greyhounds [16]. Sesamoids may be congenitally multipartite, where there are multiple small mineralized areas which mimic a fracture. Sesamoid pathology should be correlated with physical examination findings of lameness and pain on direct palpation, as fragmentation or fractures may be seen without causing any clinical signs.

# Other Joint Diseases

## Synovial Osteochondromatosis

Primary synovial chondromatosis is a rare disease affecting a single joint (or sometimes tendon sheath or bursa). There is intraarticular production of cartilage nodules which may ossify, resulting in the term *osteochondromatosis* [17]. Secondary synovial osteochondromatosis is much more common and due to underlying joint abnormalities such as osteoarthritis that result in mineralized chondral bodies associated with a joint [17].

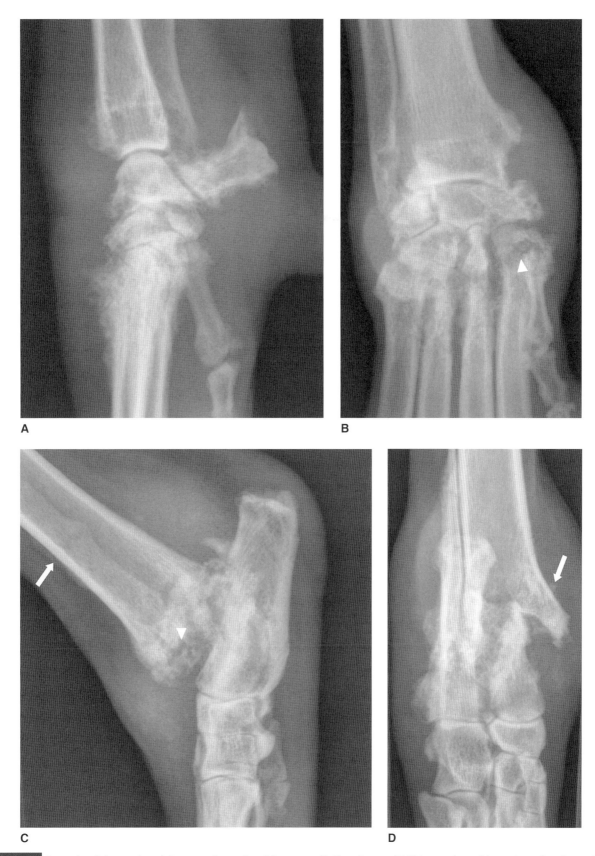

**FIGURE 8.26** Lateral and dorsopalmar/plantar radiographs of the carpus (**A,B**) and tarsus (**C,D**) in a patient with erosive polyarthropathy. There is severe soft tissue swelling surrounding the carpus and tarsus. There is multifocal regional lysis (arrowheads) and periosteal reaction (arrows). The tarsus is also subluxated.

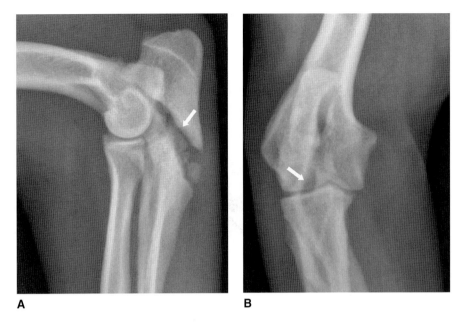

**FIGURE 8.27** Lateral (**A**) and craniocaudal (**B**) radiographs of an articular ulnar fracture (arrows). Fracture margins are less distinct on the craniocaudal projection and articular involvement cannot be seen on that projection.

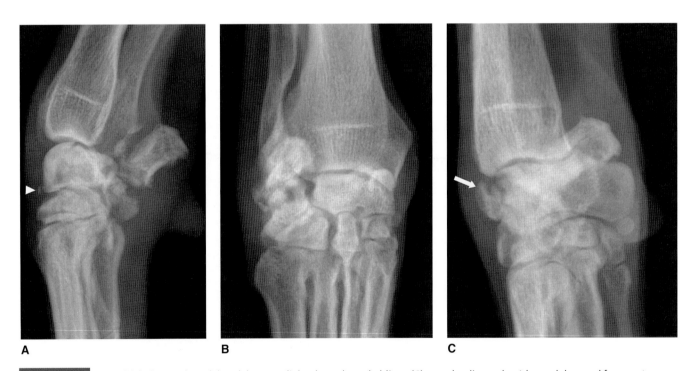

**FIGURE 8.28** Lateral (**A**), dorsopalmar (**B**) and dorsomedial-palmarolateral oblique (**C**) carpal radiographs. A large slab carpal fragment (arrow) from the intermedioradial carpal bone is only apparent on the oblique image. A small chip fragment (arrowhead) is seen on the lateral projection.

# Imaging of Tendons/Ligaments

Tendons and ligaments are not directly visible on radiographs, as surrounding soft tissue structures efface their margins. Despite this limitation, radiographs do have value in imaging of tendon/ligament ruptures as described below,

as positional radiography is more easily achieved than with ultrasound, CT, or MRI.

## Strains/Sprains

Although incorrectly used interchangeably, *sprain* refers to injury of a ligament and *strain* refers to injury of a musculotendinous unit [18]. Ligamentous sprains range from mild, where there are

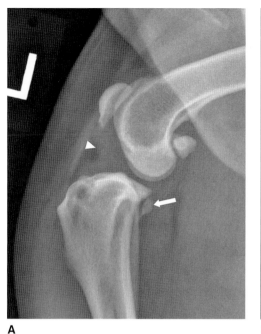
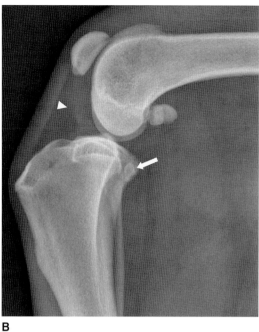

**A**                                    **B**

**FIGURE 8.29** Lateral projections of patients with cranial cruciate rupture with (**A**) and without (**B**) cranial tibial subluxation. There is distal displacement of the popliteal sesamoid (arrow) on the patient with tibial subluxation, most apparent when compared to the popliteal sesamoid location in the other patient. Both patients have increased fluid within the stifle joint (arrowheads).

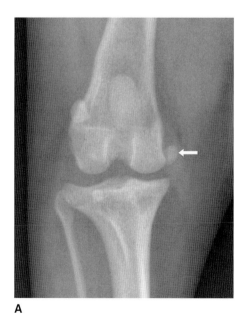
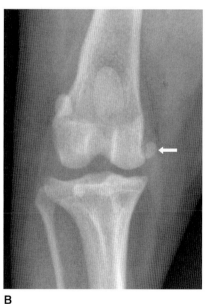

**A**                                    **B**

**FIGURE 8.30** Caudocranial projections of the right (**A**) and left (**B**) stifles in a patient. There is bilateral distal location of the medial fabella (arrow) compared to the normally positioned lateral fabella. This patient is not lame. The distal location of the medial fabella is a normal variant.

no collagen fiber ruptures and the adjacent joint remains stable, to severe where there is partial or complete rupture of a ligament or avulsion of the ligament from its bony attachment.

Radiographically, ligament damage is only recognized with stress radiography when a joint is abnormally positioned (implying the supporting ligament is severely disrupted). With mild and moderate sprains (when collagen fibers are not completely disrupted), there may not be joint instability, and only

mild regional soft tissue swelling is seen on radiography. When performing stress radiography, forces in different directions are applied to a joint and radiographs performed. For suspected collateral ligament disruption, the lateral collateral ligament is first stressed by pulling the distal limb medially relative to the proximal limb, and a radiograph performed. The process is repeated by pulling the distal limb laterally, stressing the medial collateral ligament. If a collateral ligament is disrupted,

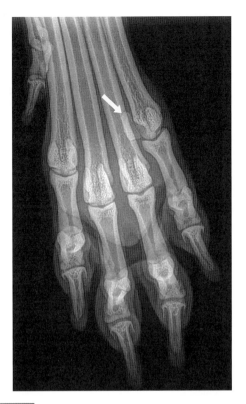

**FIGURE 8.31** Dorsopalmar projection of an axial subluxation of a palmar sesamoid bones of the fifth metacarpophalangeal joint (arrow).

there will be abnormal ipsilateral widening of the affected joint. Use of a fulcrum (such as a paddle) applied at the level of the affected joint is helpful when applying stress. Comparison to the contralateral, unaffected limb is also useful to determine the expected degree of joint laxity (Figure 8.32).

Imaging of pathologic change to specific tendons and ligaments is discussed below.

## Biceps Tendon and Supraspinatus Tendon

The biceps tendon arises on the supraglenoid tubercle of the scapula and inserts on the proximal ulna and radius at a small biceps tubercle on each respective bone. While traumatic tearing of the muscle belly or tendons of insertion may occur, most pathology is of the tendon near its origin. The biceps tendon sheath is confluent with the glenohumeral joint, so pathology in the tendon may affect the joint and vice versa. Bicipital tenosynovitis is a common cause of shoulder pain in dogs and recognized clinically by pain while flexing the shoulder.

While radiography cannot directly visualize the tendon, enthesophyte formation within the intertubercular groove is seen in nearly all dogs with chronic bicipital tenosynovitis and is recognized most readily through a skyline projection of the shoulder region (Figure 8.33) [19].

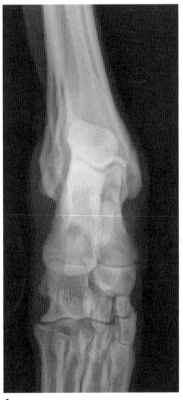
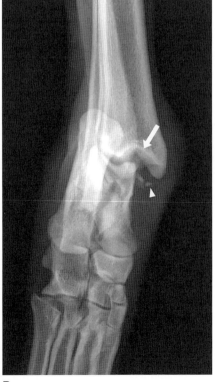

A                               B

**FIGURE 8.32** Plantarodorsal projections of a patient with medial collateral ligament rupture, without (**A**) and with (**B**) stress. Note that when stress is applied to the joint (by pulling the pes laterally), there is widening of the medial aspect of the tarsocrural joint (arrow). Small avulsion fragments also become apparent (arrowhead).

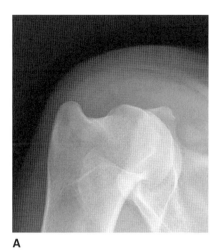
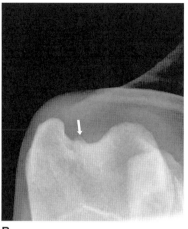
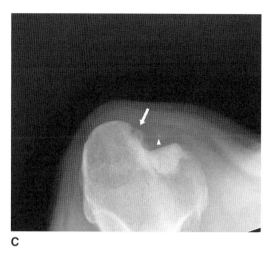

**A**  **B**  **C**

**FIGURE 8.33**  Proximal to distal skyline shoulder projection of a normal patient (**A**) and two patients with bicipital tenosynovitis (**B,C**). In the normal patient (**A**), the intertubercular groove has smooth margins. With bicipital tenosynovitis, there may be focal enthesophyte formation in the groove (arrow) or soft tissue mineralization (arrowhead).

Ultrasound is often the first advanced imaging modality used to confirm a diagnosis of biceps tenosynovitis. The biceps tendon is readily imaged with ultrasound given its superficial location and recognizable regional landmarks. The curved shape of this tendon poses difficulties when performing the ultrasound examination, due to an artifact termed *anisotropy*. When the direction of tendon or ligament fibers is perpendicular to the direction of the ultrasound beam, they are highly reflective to the sound beam, resulting in a recognizable linear appearance (Figure 8.34). When the ultrasound beam is not perpendicular to the fibers, the fibers direct the ultrasound reflections away from the transducer, resulting in a very hypoechoic appearance and loss of normal fiber pattern (Figure 8.34). The curved course of the biceps tendon means the sonographer must constantly adjust the angle of the ultrasound transducer relative to the biceps tendon.

A linear ultrasound transducer is best suited for biceps imaging. Biceps tendonitis is recognized by increased fluid within the biceps tendon sheath, typically greater than 2 mm thick, with a tendon that may be heterogeneous in its echogenicity (Figure 8.35). Enthesophytes may be seen in the intertubercular groove [20]. Complete biceps tendon rupture causes complete disruption of the normal tendon fiber pattern, and partial rupture recognized by asymmetric loss of fiber pattern of the biceps tendon.

MRI is a useful imaging test for shoulder pathology, but less seldom pursued compared to ultrasound given the greater expense, limited availability, and requirement for anesthesia. There is limited information on CT imaging of biceps and supraspinatus disease. In general, CT arthrography is more sensitive for diagnosis of biceps disease than noncontrast CT examinations, but provides less information on regional soft tissues compared to MRI [21].

Injury of the supraspinatus tendon is less common than biceps disease, but can result in significant lameness. Mineralization of the supraspinatus insertion is common in dogs, and frequently seen in dogs that do not demonstrate lameness, but can also indicate underlying pathology that results in lameness [22, 23]. This mineralization is proximal to the greater tubercle on lateral projections and along the lateral margin of the intertubercular groove on skyline projections (Figure 8.36).

Ultrasound and MRI of the supraspinatus are challenging, as the supraspinatus tendon has a central greater collagen content than other tendons, resulting in a less distinct linear fiber pattern compared to those typically expected elsewhere. With severe disease, the supraspinatus tendon may become swollen and extend into the intertubercular groove, resulting in impingement or medial displacement of the biceps tendon [24]. Mineralization is recognized by discrete, hyperechoic shadowing regions in the tendon [25].

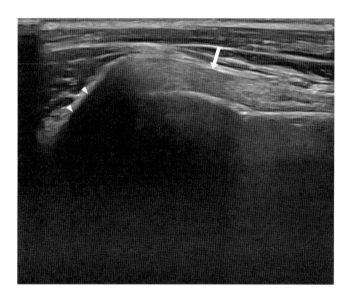

**FIGURE 8.34**  Ultrasound longitudinal image of a normal biceps tendon. Notice the linear fiber pattern of a normal tendon in long axis (arrow). When the tendon curves around the point of the shoulder, the tendon becomes dark due to the central beam anisotropy (arrowheads).

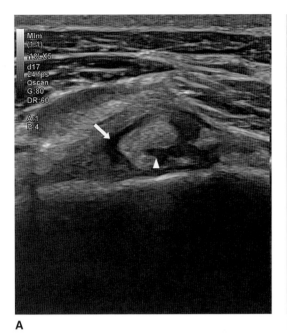

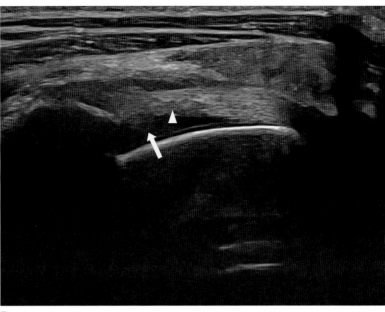

A B

**FIGURE 8.35** Transverse (**A**) and longitudinal (**B**) ultrasound images of a patient with bicipital tenosynovitis. There is fluid surrounding the biceps tendon on transverse images (arrows). There is also altered echogenicity within the biceps tendon (arrowheads).

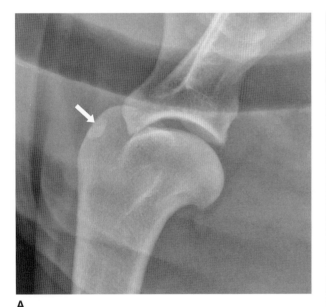

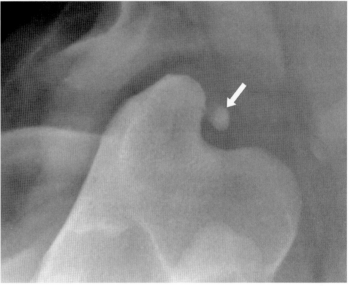

A B

**FIGURE 8.36** Lateral (**A**) and proximal to distal skyline (**B**) projections of mineralizing supraspinatus tendinopathy. There is focal mineralization just medial to the supraglenoid tubercle, best seen on the skyline projection (arrows), and is superimposed with the greater tubercle on the lateral projection.

## Iliopsoas Tendon

The iliopsoas muscle arises from the transverse processes and vertebral bodies of the mid/caudal lumbar spine. The tendon inserts on the lesser trochanter. Acute injury of this tendon is common in patients that splay their legs during trauma, and can result in an acute avulsion fragment. Mineralization of the insertional tendon may occur from repetitive stress during work/training [26]. On radiographs, mineralization or a fragment is seen immediately proximal to the lesser trochanter, the site of insertion of the iliopsoas tendon (Figure 8.37). On ultrasound, thickening and altered echogenicity of the insertional tendon can be seen (Figure 8.38).

## Calcaneal (Achilles) Tendon

The calcaneal tendon inserts on the calcaneal tuber of the tarsus and has three closely apposed components (gastrocnemius tendon, superficial digital flexor tendon, and conjoined tendon of the biceps femoris, semitendinosus, and gracilis). Trauma

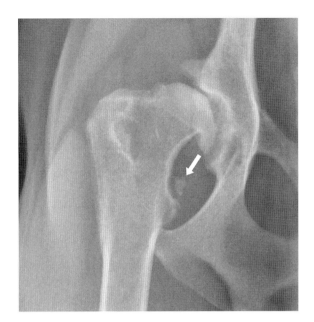

**FIGURE 8.37** Craniocaudal projection of the proximal femur showing a focal mineral body proximal to the lesser trochanter of the femur (arrow). There is also severe degeneration of the adjacent coxofemoral joint.

can result in partial or complete rupture of the tendon. Primary calcaneal degeneration occurs, resulting in secondary tendon laxity. Radiographically, calcaneal tendinopathy is recognized by soft tissue swelling at its insertion. With chronicity, mineralization and enthesopathy of the calcaneal tuber may be present (Figure 8.39).

Ultrasound is ideally suited to evaluate the tendon as the three major anatomic components are readily seen, and have the expected linear appearance in long axis images [27] (Figure 8.40). Partial or complete tendon ruptures are readily apparent as a loss of those linear echoes within the tendon and inflammation or degeneration identified through a decrease in echogenicity. Avulsion fragments or tendon mineralization

are identified by characteristic distal acoustic shadow artifacts (Figure 8.41).

## Carpal Palmar Fibrocartilage

The carpal palmar fibrocartilage is strong, thick connective tissue which provides support to the palmar aspect of the carpus and prevents its hyperextension. With hyperextension injuries (such as falling from a great height), this tissue may be disrupted, along with excessive extension of the carpus appreciated on stress radiography (Figure 8.42).

## Collateral Ligaments

As mentioned above, collateral ligament disruption results in abnormal medial/lateral instability of a joint. While instability is palpable clinically, radiography can confirm this instability through use of medial/lateral stressed projections, with the side of the joint with the ruptured collateral ligament becoming abnormally widened. An exception is the shoulder joint, which has a high degree of medial and lateral mobility. Medial or lateral angulation of the limb in a normal patient results in a high degree of joint widening, which should not be misdiagnosed as joint luxation (Figure 8.43).

## Patellar Ligament

Patellar ligament desmitis is common after tibial plateau leveling osteotomy (TPLO) surgery, when thickening may be appreciated on postoperative and recheck radiographs. This is not always associated with lameness (Figure 8.44). Rarely, an enthesophyte may be seen at the insertion of the patellar ligament, typically incidental and not associated with lameness (Figure 8.45).

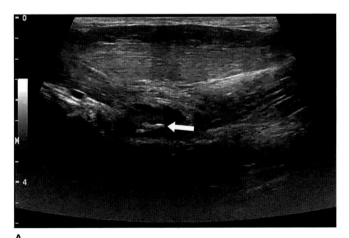
**A**

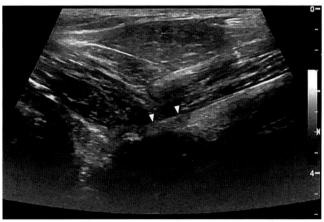
**B**

**FIGURE 8.38** Transverse (**A**) and longitudinal (**B**) ultrasound images of iliopsoas tendonitis and insertional mineralization. There is mineralization at its insertion characterized by a focal hyperechogenic (arrow) and slight decreased echogenicity of the adjacent iliopsoas tendon of insertion (arrowhead).

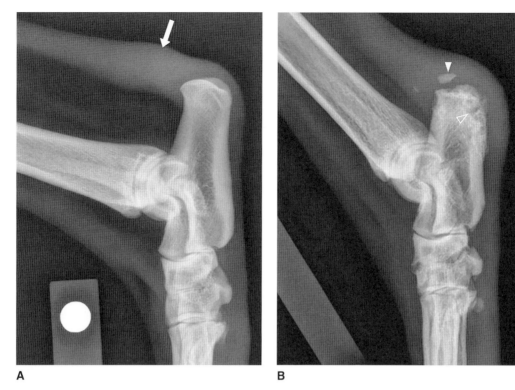

**FIGURE 8.39** Lateral projections of a patient with mild (**A**) and severe (**B**) calcaneal tendinopathy. On a more mildly affected patient, soft tissue swelling may be apparent at the calcaneal tendon insertion (arrow). With more severe chronic disease, soft tissue swelling may be worse, and there may be mineralization of the adjacent soft tissues (arrowhead) and bony resorption (open arrowhead).

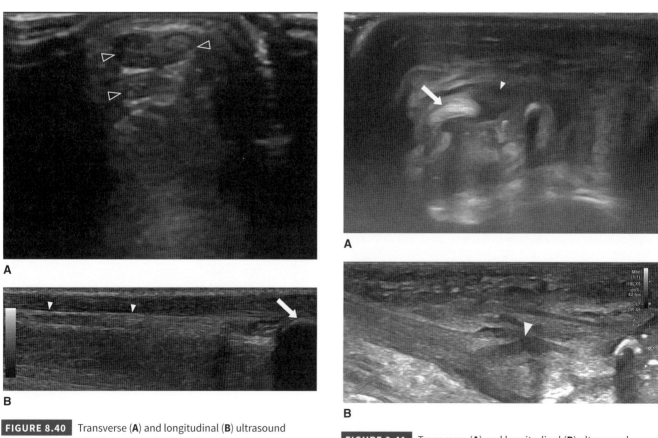

**FIGURE 8.40** Transverse (**A**) and longitudinal (**B**) ultrasound images of a normal calcaneal tendon insertion. The calcaneus causes distal shadowing and has a smooth margin (arrow). The linear pattern of the tendon is apparent on longitudinal images (arrowheads). In transverse images, the three components of the tendon are apparent as separate bundles (open arrowheads).

**FIGURE 8.41** Transverse (**A**) and longitudinal (**B**) ultrasound images of a ruptured calcaneal tendon. There are some residual tendon fibers seen (arrow) but in general the regional tissues are hypoechoic without apparent tendon fibers (arrowheads).

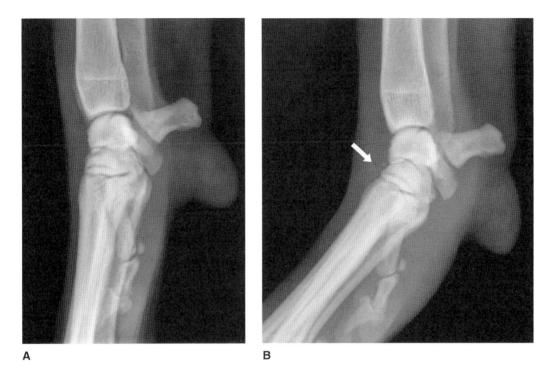

A                                               B

**FIGURE 8.42**   Lateral projections of the normal carpus (**A**) and one with hyperextension injury (**B**). Both projections were acquired under pressure to cause extension. Notice that in the patient with hyperextension injury, there are dorsal chip fragments (arrow) and an increased angle between the metacarpal bones and the antebrachium. There is also mild dorsal soft tissue swelling.

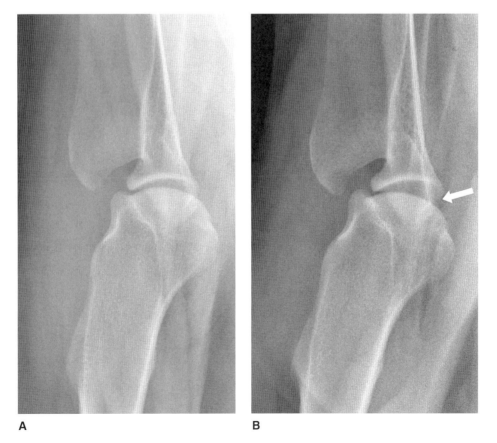

A                                               B

**FIGURE 8.43**   Craniocaudal projections of a normal shoulder in neutral position (**A**) and slightly abducted (**B**). With abduction, the medial aspect of the shoulder joint widens (arrow).

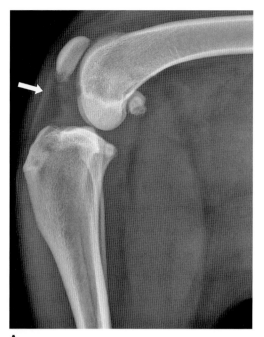

**A**

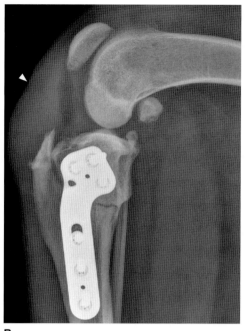

**B**

**FIGURE 8.44**   Lateral preoperative (**A**) and postoperative TPLO (**B**) radiographs of the stifle. On preoperative images in a patient with cranial cruciate ligament rupture, the patellar ligament has a normal thickness (arrow). Postoperatively, after tibial surgery, the patella ligament is severely thickened (arrowhead). Increased soft tissue opacity is seen within both stifles.

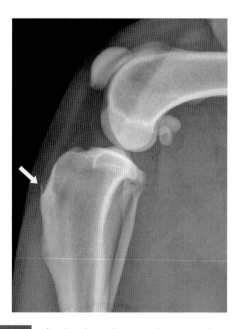

**FIGURE 8.45**   A focal enthesophyte may be seen at the patellar ligament insertion in clinically normal dogs (arrow).

## Abductor Pollicis Longus

The abductor pollicis longus is a muscle on the medial aspect of the distal antebrachium which arises from the radius and ulna. It has a strong tendon which extends along the medial sulcus of the radius to insert on the first digit, passing through a small tendon sheath medially [28]. Stenosing tenosynovitis has been recently described, where inflammation of this tendon sheath causes regional bony proliferation and stenosis, resulting in pain and lameness [28]. This is recognized radiographically by proliferation along the distal radial sulcus and soft tissue swelling (Figure 8.46). Ultrasound may confirm these lesions, though the radiographic appearance is distinct and often diagnosis may be made from radiographs alone.

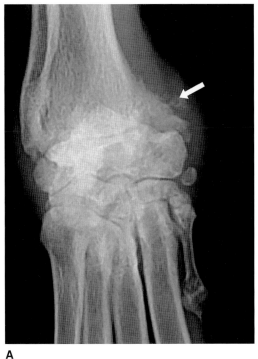

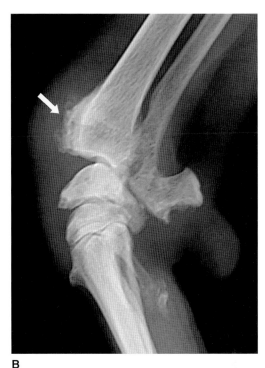

**A**                    **B**

**FIGURE 8.46** Dorsopalmar (**A**) and lateral (**B**) projections of a patient with abductor pollicis longus stenosing tendinopathy. Notice there is bony proliferation on the craniomedial aspect of the distal radius (arrow). There is adjacent soft tissue swelling.

# References

1. Allan, G.S. (2000). Radiographic features of feline joint diseases. *Vet. Clin. North Am. Small Anim. Pract.* 30 (2): 281–302, vi.

2. Rychel, J.K. (2010). Diagnosis and treatment of osteoarthritis. *Top. Companion Anim. Med.* 25 (1): 20–25.

3. Szabo, S.D., Biery, D.N., Lawler, D.F. et al. (2007). Evaluation of a circumferential femoral head osteophyte as an early indicator of osteoarthritis characteristic of canine hip dysplasia in dogs. *J. Am. Vet. Med. Assoc.* 231 (6): 889–892.

4. Moore, P.F. (2014). A review of histiocytic diseases of dogs and cats. *Vet. Pathol.* 51 (1): 167–184.

5. van Kuijk, L., van Ginkel, K., de Vos, J.P. et al. (2013). Peri-articular histiocytic sarcoma and previous joint disease in Bernese mountain dogs. *J. Vet. Intern. Med.* 27 (2): 293–299.

6. Craig, L.E., Julian, M.E., and Ferracone, J.D. (2002). The diagnosis and prognosis of synovial tumors in dogs: 35 cases. *Vet. Pathol.* 39 (1): 66–73.

7. Mielke, B., Comerford, E., English, K., and Meeson, R. (2018). Spontaneous septic arthritis of canine elbows: twenty-one cases. *Vet. Comp. Orthop. Traumatol.* 31 (6): 488–493.

8. Lemetayer, J. and Taylor, S. (2014). Inflammatory joint disease in cats: diagnostic approach and treatment. *J. Feline Med. Surg.* 16 (7): 547–562.

9. Benzioni, H., Shahar, R., Yudelevitch, S., and Milgram, J. (2008). Bacterial infective arthritis of the coxofemoral joint in dogs with hip dysplasia. *Vet. Comp. Orthop. Traumatol.* 21 (3): 262–266.

10. Johnson, K.C. and Mackin, A. (2012). Canine immune-mediated polyarthritis: part 1: pathophysiology. *J. Am. Anim. Hosp. Assoc.* 48 (1): 12–17.

11. Johnson, K.C. and Mackin, A. (2012). Canine immune-mediated polyarthritis: part 2: diagnosis and treatment. *J. Am. Anim. Hosp. Assoc.* 48 (2): 71–82.

12. Wood, A.K., McCarthy, P.H., and Martin, I.C. (1995). Anatomic and radiographic appearance of a sesamoid bone in the tendon of origin of the supinator muscle of the cat. *Am. J. Vet. Res.* 56 (6): 736–738.

13. Wood, A.K., McCarthy, P.H., and Howlett, C.R. (1985). Anatomic and radiographic appearance of a sesamoid bone in the tendon of origin of the supinator muscle of dogs. *Am. J. Vet. Res.* 46 (10): 2043–2047.

14. de Rooster, H. and van Bree, H. (1999). Popliteal sesamoid displacement associated with cruciate rupture in the dog. *J. Small Anim. Pract.* 40 (7): 316–318.

15. Stork, C.K., Petite, A.F., Norrie, R.A. et al. (2009). Variation in position of the medial fabella in West Highland white terriers and other dogs. *J. Small Anim. Pract.* 50 (5): 236–240.

16. Harasen, G. (2009). Sesamoid disease. *Can. Vet. J.* 50 (10): 1095.

17. Aeffner, F., Weeren, R., Morrison, S. et al. (2012). Synovial osteochondromatosis with malignant transformation to chondrosarcoma in a dog. *Vet. Pathol.* 49 (6): 1036–1039.

18. DeCamp, C., Johnston, S., Dejardin, L. et al. (2006). Principles of joint surgery. In: *Brinker, Piermattei, and Flo's Handbook of Small*

*Animal Orthopedics and Fracture Repair*, 4e (ed. D. Piermattei, G.L. Flo and C. DeCamp), 216–232. St Louis: Saunders Elsevier.

19. Stobie, D., Wallace, L.J., Lipowitz, A.J. et al. (1995). Chronic bicipital tenosynovitis in dogs: 29 cases (1985–1992). *J. Am. Vet. Med. Assoc.* 207 (2): 201–207.

20. Kramer, M., Gerwing, M., Sheppard, C., and Schimke, E. (2001). Ultrasonography for the diagnosis of diseases of the tendon and tendon sheath of the biceps brachii muscle. *Vet. Surg.* 30 (1): 64–71.

21. Eivers, C.R., Corzo-Menendez, N., Austwick, S.H. et al. (2018). Computed tomographic arthrography is a useful adjunct to survey computed tomography and arthroscopic evaluation of the canine shoulder joint. *Vet. Radiol. Ultrasound* 59 (5): 535–544.

22. Laitinen, O.M. and Flo, G.L. (2000). Mineralization of the supraspinatus tendon in dogs: a long-term follow-up. *J. Am. Anim. Hosp. Assoc.* 36 (3): 262–267.

23. Spall, B.F., Fransson, B.A., Martinez, S.A., and Wilkinson, T.E. (2016). Tendon volume determination on magnetic resonance imaging of supraspinatus tendinopathy. *Vet. Surg.* 45 (3): 386–391.

24. Fransson, B.A., Gavin, P.R., and Lahmers, K.K. (2005). Supraspinatus tendinosis associated with biceps brachii tendon displacement in a dog. *J. Am. Vet. Med. Assoc.* 227 (9): 1429–1433.

25. Mistieri, M.L., Wigger, A., Canola, J.C. et al. (2012). Ultrasonographic evaluation of canine supraspinatus calcifying tendinosis. *J. Am. Anim. Hosp. Assoc.* 48 (6): 405–410.

26. Cook, C.R. (2016). Ultrasound imaging of the musculoskeletal system. *Vet. Clin. North Am. Small Anim. Pract.* 46 (3): 355–371.

27. Lamb, C.R. and Duvernois, A. (2005). Ultrasonographic anatomy of the normal canine calcaneal tendon. *Vet. Radiol. Ultrasound* 46 (4): 326–330.

28. Hittmair, K.M., Groessl, V., and Mayrhofer, E. (2012). Radiographic and ultrasonographic diagnosis of stenosing tenosynovitis of the abductor pollicis longus muscle in dogs. *Vet. Radiol. Ultrasound* 53 (2): 135–141.

# CHAPTER 9

# Fractures and Fracture Healing

**Nathan C. Nelson**

Department of Molecular Biomedical Sciences, College of Veterinary Medicine, North Carolina State University, Raleigh, NC, USA

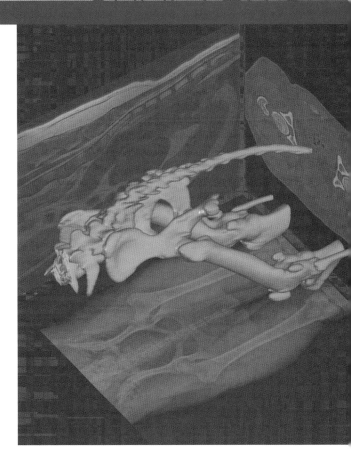

## Introduction

Radiography plays a key role in the diagnosis and classification of orthopedic fractures and monitoring of bone healing after stabilization. Diligent monitoring with radiography is necessary for early diagnosis and avoidance of complications to healing such as nonunion or bone infection. This chapter will describe proper radiographic technique to diagnose fractures, description of fracture location, normal appearance of healing, and potential complications of fracture healing.

## Radiographic Examination of Fractures

Complete evaluation of a fractured bone requires a minimum of two orthogonal radiographs, as single radiographs are insufficient to display the complex geometry of most fractures (Figure 9.1). Acquiring multiple radiographs of a fractured leg can be challenging, depending on the site of fracture as well as the degree of patient pain, so high-quality, well-positioned radiographs require strong sedation or anesthesia. Radiographs are usually the only imaging performed to plan for surgical repair. Errors in positioning (such as obliquity of the limb) result in incorrect bone geometry on the radiograph, by distorting the bone. This complicates eventual repair by obscuring parts of the fracture or artifactually altering bone measurements.

Some fractures require additional projections to identify or categorize the fracture. Fissure fractures, where there is no displacement of adjacent bone margins, can be particularly difficult to identify as the x-ray beam must be tangential with the fracture to appear on radiographs (Figure 9.2). This type of fracture is common in juvenile dogs as immature cortical bone tolerates more strain and elastic deformation than mature bone, allowing a fracture to occur through only one cortical edge, rather than completely through the bone (so-called greenstick fractures) [1]. If clinical suspicion for a fissure fracture is high,

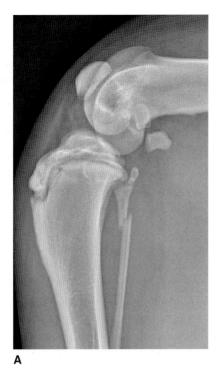
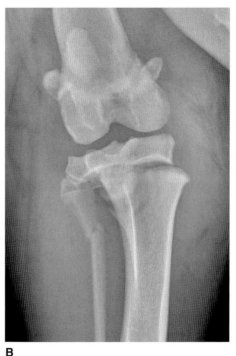

**A**    **B**

**FIGURE 9.1** Lateral (**A**) and craniocaudal (**B**) projections of a proximal tibia demonstrating the importance of orthogonal projections. On the lateral projection, no fracture of the tibia is seen (though an oblique fibular fracture is identified). On the craniocaudal projection, a Salter Harris type II fracture of the proximal tibial physis is seen.

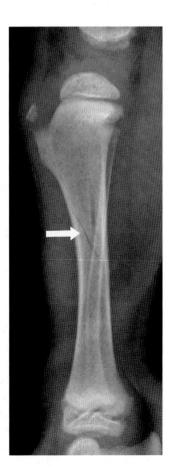

**FIGURE 9.2** Lateral radiograph of a tibia showing a nondisplaced fissure (arrow). Notice the cortices of this bone remain well aligned, without displacement.

additional oblique projections at 10–20° intervals can make them more apparent.

Fracture of the small bones in the carpus, tarsus, and digits can be particularly difficult to identify; studies in this region should include not only lateral and dorsopalmar(plantar) projections, but oblique projections as well (Figure 9.3). Fractures of the femoral neck may not align tangentially with the x-ray beam on lateral projections. Additionally, extension of the hips for traditional positioning of the ventrodorsal (VD) pelvic projection can result in artifactual alignment of the fracture margins, making them difficult to identify. A "frog-leg" position radiograph in such cases makes diagnosis easier, by relaxing the coxofemoral joint and allowing adjacent fracture margins to malalign (Figure 9.4). While the frog-leg position is more comfortable for the patient, the extended VD projection of the pelvis should also be performed in such cases as it provides a more complete understanding of fracture geometry, and positions the femur in a craniocaudal projection, allowing better surgical planning.

Spinal radiographs have only moderate sensitivity in detecting spinal fractures and subluxations compared to computed tomography (CT), and are particularly poor in diagnosing fracture fragments within the vertebral canal [2]. Manipulation should be kept to a minimum in patients with suspected spinal fractures, particularly when sedation or anesthesia is used, as this limits the protective bracing of the paraspinal musculature compared to an awake patient, and may predispose to further injury with manipulation [2]. Lateral radiographs are readily achieved in the recumbent trauma patient, but patient safety may dictate

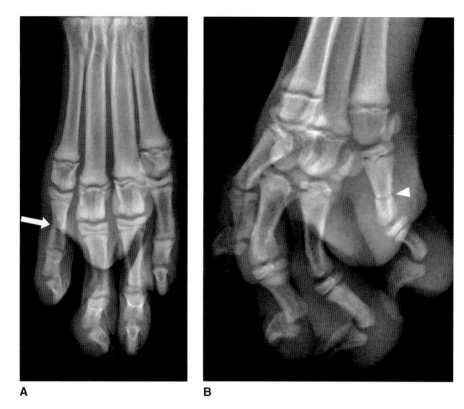

**FIGURE 9.3** Dorsopalmar (**A**) and dorsolateral-palmaromedial oblique (**B**) radiographs of a fracture of the proximal phalanx of the fifth digit. Note that on the dorsopalmar projection (**A**), the transverse fracture (arrow) is not readily apparent as it superimposes with external soft tissue margins. This fracture is more apparent on the oblique projection (arrowhead), as this oblique projection shows a fracture in a different orientation.

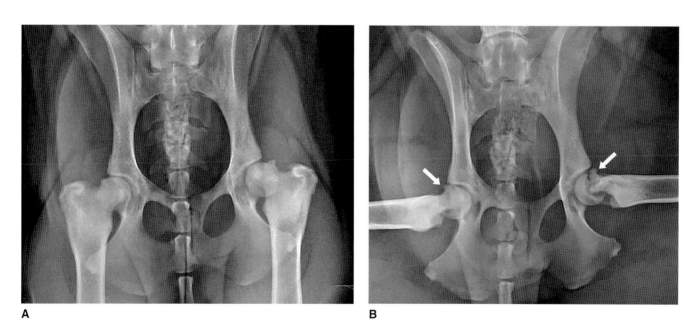

**FIGURE 9.4** Ventrodorsal extended leg projection (**A**) and frog-leg position (**B**) of a dog with bilateral capital physeal fractures. Note that on (**A**) with the pelvic limbs caudally positioned, capital physeal fractures are not readily apparent. On (**B**), with the legs in a more neutral frog-leg position, displacement of the femoral heads from the femoral necks (arrows) is apparent and the fracture lines are seen.

that orthogonal spinal radiographs employ a horizontal beam to prevent rolling the patient, which may result in some image compromise or less than ideal patient position (Figure 9.5).

Ultimately, if radiographs are deemed insufficient to diagnose or fully characterize a fracture, CT imaging of the fracture site should be pursued.

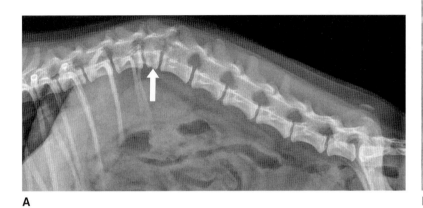
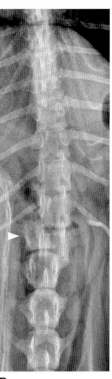

**A**

**B**

**FIGURE 9.5** Lateral (**A**) and horizontal beam ventrodorsal (**B**) projections of a patient with a traumatic fracture of L1. On the lateral projection, shortening of the first vertebral segment is appreciated (arrow). On the orthogonal horizontal beam projection, a significant rightward displacement of the fracture is identified (arrowhead).

# Fracture Description and Classification

A complete radiographic description of a fracture should convey all pertinent features and allow a second party (such as a radiologist or orthopedic surgeon) to mentally reconstruct the image of the fracture and its effect on adjacent tissues without actually seeing the radiographs in question [3].

The description begins with the bone(s) involved and the location of the fracture [3]. The fracture may involve the diaphyseal, epiphyseal, or metaphyseal region of the bone. Displacement and the severity of displacement are described by the orientation of the distal fracture fragment relative to the more proximal fragment (Figure 9.6). The term *overriding* or *proximal displacement* describes proximal translation of a distal fracture fragment. *Distraction* occurs when two fracture margins separate from each other, resulting in a wide fracture gap. Numerous other descriptive terms may apply. Fractures are *complete* when the fracture completely traverses the width of bone, or *incomplete* when only a portion of the cortical margin is affected (greenstick fractures are examples of incomplete fractures).

As previously mentioned, fractures may be described as *fissures* when no displacement of the fracture margins is present and the fracture is incomplete (Figure 9.7). Fissures often occur in conjunction with complete fractures, where a thin fissure line may extend for a significant distance from the major

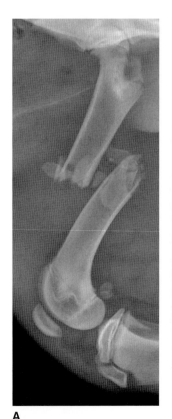
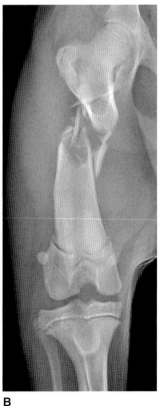

**A**

**B**

**FIGURE 9.6** Lateral (**A**) and caudocranial (**B**) radiographs of a comminuted, caudolaterally displaced fracture of the femoral middiaphysis. There is mild overriding of the fracture.

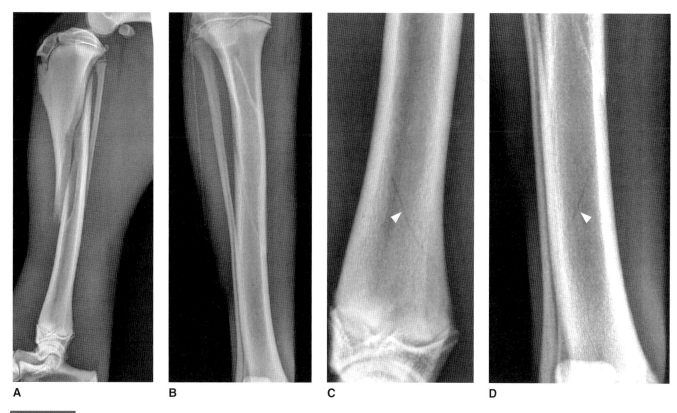

A          B          C          D

**FIGURE 9.7** Lateral (**A**) and caudocranial (**B**) and magnified projections (**C,D**) images of a fissure fracture (arrowhead) extending distally from a more proximal complete displaced fracture.

fracture line, and are important to recognize if surgical stabilization is attempted (Figure 9.7).

A *segmental* or *multiple* fracture is one in which there are two complete fractures on either side of a portion of bone, resulting in a separate osseous fragment.

A fracture is *open* if there is clear extension of bone beyond soft tissue margins. Any gas adjacent to an acute fracture indicates that skin margins were disrupted, and the fracture is assumed open. Lack of gas in the surrounding tissues does not mean a fracture is not open; confirming a fracture to be closed requires visual inspection during physical examination to ensure lack of skin disruption. A fracture is *closed* if the surrounding skin surface is intact.

A *comminuted* fracture contains adjacent fracture fragments (but not a complete osseous segmental fracture) which may be large or small (Figure 9.6).

A *folding* fracture occurs when an underlying osseous disease results in loss of mineralization, so that only soft matrix remains, increasing bone compliance (Figure 9.8). When an affected patient bears weight, the bone distorts but does not disrupt cortical margins, resulting in the impression of bone folding. This type of fracture is rare and only occurs in endocrinopathies such as renal secondary hyperparathyroidism or inherited dysplasias such as osteogenesis imperfecta.

Complete fractures are described based on the orientation of the fracture line. A *transverse* fracture occurs perpendicular to the long axis of a bone. A *short oblique* fracture is angled between a transverse fracture and 45° from the long axis of

the bone. A *long oblique* fracture has an angle greater than 45° from the long axis of a bone (Figure 9.9). A *spiral* fracture wraps around the long axis of its bone, changing its orientation at different locations along the length of the bone.

If the fracture line extends to the surface of a joint, the fracture is *articular* (Figure 9.10). The terms "T" or "Y" fracture describe fractures that extend from an articular surface to the condylar or supracondylar region along both margins of a bone, resulting in a T or Y shape (Figure 9.10). These are most common in the distal humerus.

*Avulsion* fractures occur at sites of soft tissue attachments on bone, such as the origin or insertion of tendons or ligaments (Figure 9.11). When a traumatic insult increases strain on those soft tissue structures, a segment of bone may pull from the underlying bone, resulting in a separate fragment.

*Compression* fractures are common in the spine, and occur when forces are applied along the long axis of a bone, resulting in the two fracture margins being driven into each other and an overall shortening of the bony segment. This type of fracture may be difficult to identify, and should be suspected when there are differences in vertebral length between adjacent segments (Figure 9.12).

A *pathologic* fracture occurs at a site of underlying bone disease, such as neoplastic or inflammatory lesions. Pathologic fractures are suspected when there is no history of trauma or only mild trauma is reported. Pathologic fractures occur most commonly when there is underlying osseous neoplasia, which weakens the bone, predisposing to fracture.

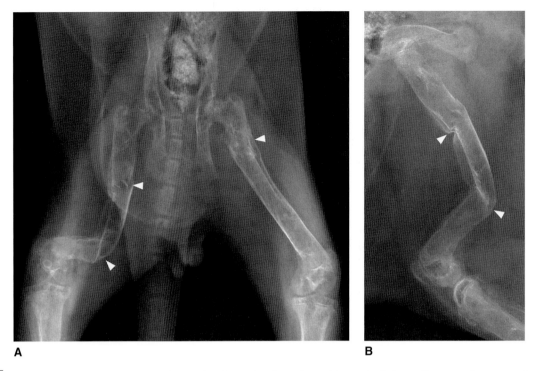

**A**　　　　　　　　　　　　　　　　　**B**

**FIGURE 9.8** Ventrodorsal pelvic (**A**) and lateral femur (**B**) radiographs of a patient with metabolic bone disease and numerous folding fractures. Notice the diffuse decreased opacity of the bones and the thin cortices. Multiple folding fractures are present (arrowhead).

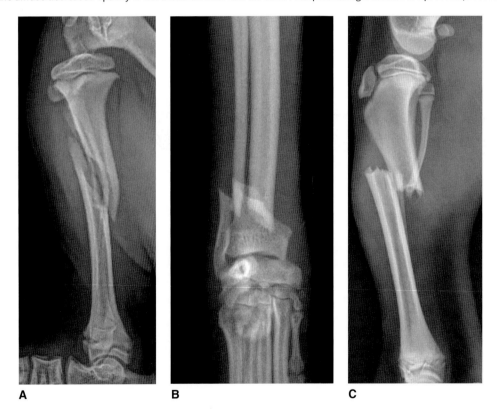

**A**　　　　　　　　　**B**　　　　　　　　　**C**

**FIGURE 9.9** Radiographs of fractures with multiple different orientations. Long oblique fractures are identified on (**A**). Short oblique fractures of the distal radius and ulna are identified on (**B**), and transverse fractures of the tibia and fibula are identified on (**C**).

The fracture may distort the osseous anatomy, obscuring the underlying pathology, but the bone fragments should be carefully scrutinized for any underlying bone loss or periosteal proliferation. Underlying bone distortion (collapse, displacement, etc.) also signals that the fracture could be pathologic in origin (Figure 9.13). CT is more sensitive to the lysis or altered medullary architecture that more definitively indicates a fracture as pathologic in nature. For that reason, when radiographs are indeterminate for underlying pathology at a fracture site, CT should be considered as the next imaging procedure.

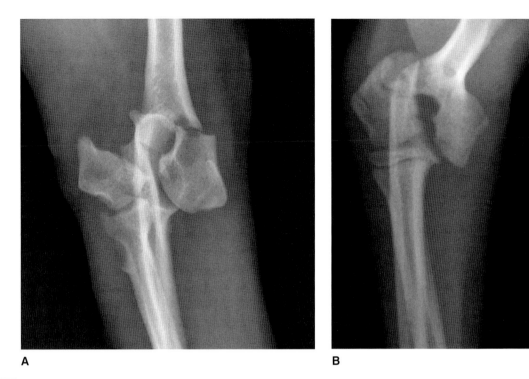

**A**                                                                **B**

**FIGURE 9.10**   Craniocaudal projections of the distal humerus in two dogs. Notice on (**A**) the fracture extends from the articular surface of the distal humerus through the medial and lateral supracondylar region; this is a T type fracture configuration. In comparison, on (**B**), the fracture extends from the articular surface to the lateral supracondylar region only, with the medial supracondylar region being normal.

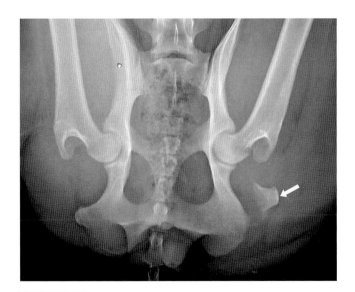

**FIGURE 9.11**   Ventrodorsal projection of the pelvis with an avulsion fragment of the left tibial tuberosity (arrow).

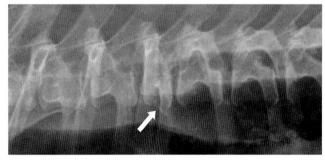

**FIGURE 9.12**   Lateral projection of the thoracic spine showing a compression type fracture of a midthoracic vertebral segment (arrow), occurring after the dog fell from a great height. The dog was painful on palpation of the midthoracic spine. Notice the decreased craniocaudal length of the segment as well, with mild ventral bony irregularity (arrow) which helps discriminate this from a congenital malformation.

The Salter Harris classification scheme describes fractures involving the physis, and only applies to juvenile animals prior to physeal closure [4, 5]. A Salter Harris type I fracture occurs transversely through the physis, and is an uncommon fracture conformation. Type II fractures extend through the physis and metaphysis, without involvement of the epiphysis (Figure 9.1). These most commonly occur in the distal femur [4]. Type III fractures extend through the physis and epiphysis, sparing the metaphysis, and are typically articular fractures that extend to the joint surface (Figure 9.14).

This is an uncommon fracture conformation [6]. Type IV fractures occur through the physis, epiphysis, and metaphysis and are most common in the distal humerus (Figure 9.15) [4]. Type IV fractures are also articular in nature. Type V fractures are compression fractures of the physis, and may be difficult to recognize as they only result in a decreased width of the physis, and may require images of the contralateral limb to recognize. Type VI Salter Harris fractures are fractures through only a portion of a physis. Because there is no displacement of bone margins, these may only be detected late in the healing process when the affected portion of the physis is closed or peripherally bridged by bone.

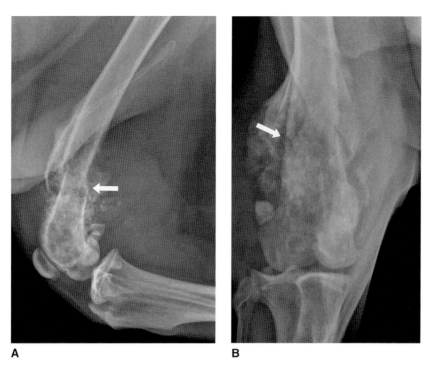

A          B

**FIGURE 9.13** Lateral (**A**) and caudocranial (**B**) projections of a pathologic fracture of the distal femur through a primary bone tumor. The fracture margin is difficult to identify given the regional bony reaction, but there is caudal displacement of the distal femoral segment relative to the proximal (at level of arrow).

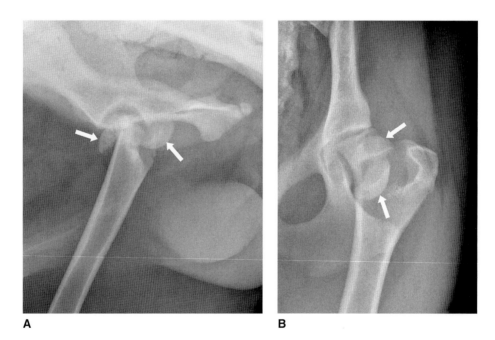

A          B

**FIGURE 9.14** Lateral (**A**) and caudocranial (**B**) radiographs of the proximal femur. There is a type III Salter Harris fracture of the proximal femur. The fracture extends through the capital physis and then through the femoral head, resulting in the femoral head having two displaced portions (arrows indicate the two fragments of the femoral head).

# Unique Fractures

Certain bones are predisposed to specific fracture types. For instance, racing greyhounds are predisposed to right central tarsal bone fractures, presumably due to repeated stress from racing at high speed in a counter-clockwise direction, resulting in adaptive modeling and eventually microdamage and fatigue fracture of the bones [7, 8]. These fractures have repeatable conformations and may be combined with fractures elsewhere in the tarsus; they are described based

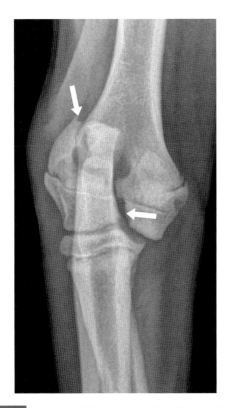

**FIGURE 9.15**   Craniocaudal projection of the elbow with a Salter Harris type IV fracture (arrow) extending from the articular surface of the humerus through the lateral supracondylar region.

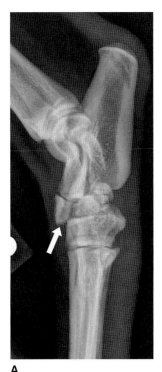 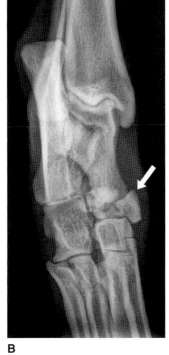

A                                   B

**FIGURE 9.16**   Lateral (**A**) and dorsolateral-plantaromedial oblique (**B**) radiographs of a racing greyhound with a central tarsal bone fracture. This results in displacement of a large fragment dorsally and medially (arrows indicate fracture fragments).

on the orientation and number of fracture fragments (Figure 9.16) [7, 9].

The humeral condyle is another site predisposed to a unique fracture conformation, related to incomplete humeral ossification during development. The medial and lateral centers of ossification of the humeral condyle should fuse by 10 weeks of age. In some dogs, these ossification centers fail to fuse, resulting in a radiolucent line that extends to the articular surface, and predisposes to fracture through this area of weakened bone (Figure 9.17) [10–12]. The fracture extends to the central articular portion of the humeral condyle, and extends proximally to the supracondylar region. This condition can occur in any breed but is more common in the cocker spaniel and English springer spaniel [11, 12]. Affected dogs present with spontaneous humeral condylar fractures that occur after no or minimal trauma, though prodromal lameness may occur [13]. The incomplete condylar ossification is typically bilateral. Therefore, in dogs with a compatible history, radiographs of the contralateral (nonfractured) limb are performed to identify the incomplete ossification. Superimposition of the ulna may obscure the area of incomplete ossification, so diagnosis may require oblique radiographs or CT examination of the elbow.

The feline femoral neck has several conditions that may result in a fracture, and recognition of these fractures may be difficult without proper radiographic positioning. Slipped capital femoral epiphysiolysis occurs when displacement of the femoral head from the neck occurs at the physis, and is often bilateral [12, 14]. It is associated with prepubertal gonadectomy, and the degree of femoral head/neck malalignment may be subtle. Cats are usually 5–24 months old with a history of chronic lameness, with the majority being male and neutered between 4 and 8 months of age [12, 14]. Radiographic diagnosis requires femoral head/neck malalignment, which may be obscured when a VD projection is performed with legs in the extended position. A frog-leg VD projection facilitates diagnosis by displacing the femoral head relative to the femoral neck (Figure 9.18).

Feline femoral neck metaphyseal osteopathy has also been described. Unlike slipped femoral capital physis, metaphyseal osteopathy results in significant necrosis of the femoral neck and an "apple core" appearance that may inhibit healing. Eventually, a pathologic fracture will occur, at which point the cat typically shows more severe clinical signs and will present for examination. This may represent a form of chronic slipped capital physeal fracture, though other etiologies are proposed [12, 15].

Finally, certain types of fractures are more common in cases of animal abuse, with characteristics similar to human abuse victims [16]. Transverse fractures are more common in cases of nonaccidental injury compared to dogs undergoing accidental trauma. Multiple fractures in multiple regions of the body (forelimb, hindlimb, axial) should also alert the clinician to the possibility of abuse. Multiple fractures in different stages of healing, or fractures presenting already in a delayed state of healing, also suggest a pattern of abuse [16]. Fractures of the pelvis are more commonly associated with motor vehicle

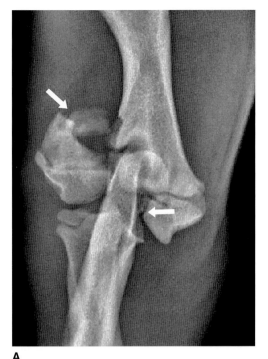 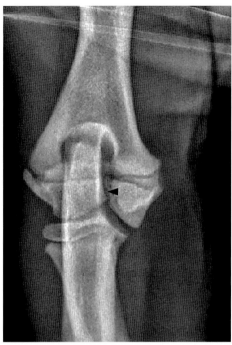 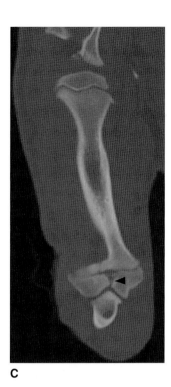

**A**                                    **B**                                    **C**

**FIGURE 9.17**  Craniocaudal projection of the left (**A**) and right (**B**) elbows of a patient, and dorsal reformatted CT image of the right elbow (**C**) in the same patient. There is incomplete ossification of the right elbow (arrowheads), better appreciated on the CT image as an area of decreased ossification between the medial and lateral condylar regions. This was also present on the left resulting in fracture (arrow) extending through the lateral supracondylar region. On the contralateral limb (**B**), a lucent line can be seen extending from the articular surface of the humerus to the distal humeral physis secondary to incomplete ossification.

accidents, while injuries of the skull and teeth, or areas clustered on the cranial aspect of the body, are more often associated with nonaccidental blunt force trauma [17, 18]. Rib fractures from motor vehicle accidents typically cluster on one side of the body in the cranial ribs, whereas those from abuse are more likely to be bilateral and may be anywhere along the thoracic cavity [17]. Young male dogs and cats, and those of certain breeds (such as the Staffordshire bull terrier) are particularly at risk for these sort of injuries [18].

# Normal Fracture Healing and Expected Radiographic Changes

Understanding the normal radiographic appearance of healing bone requires a basic knowledge of bone cellular structure and the physiology of fracture repair. This is an extremely complicated process, but can be broken into three overlapping phases of bone healing, each with a typical radiographic appearance.

The *inflammatory phase* persists for several weeks after the initial injury [19]. There is inflammation of the surrounding soft tissues and the periosteal envelope of bone, with resorption of the organic matrix of bone. With time, osteoclasts are stimulated and begin the process of resorbing and removing dead bone. During this phase, radiographic swelling of surrounding soft tissues is seen. Callous tissues are fibrous in nature and not identified radiographically, as they have the same opacity as the surrounding soft tissue swelling [20]. Within the first 2 weeks, the fracture fragments may have more indistinct margins and there may be a widening of the fracture margins by this demineralization. Healing biologic processes and the secondary radiographic appearance occur much more rapidly in the immature patient.

During the *repair phase*, the hematoma surrounding the fracture becomes organized and osteoprogenitor cells migrate to the fracture site [19]. As blood supply is reestablished, a periosteal callus begins to form (Figure 9.19). The osteoprogenitor cells differentiate into the cellular components necessary to produce bone. Collagen and calcium hydroxyapatite are deposited, resulting in a radiographic appearance of a mineralized callous at the fracture site which will become more opaque with time. Radiographic mineralization of callus is typically expected at least 14 days after the fracture occurs in an adult animal (earlier in a juvenile animal). This mineralized callus is disorganized and does not have the typical structure of uninjured lamellar bone. It extends along a greater length of adjacent bone than the more mature callus seen later, and has an irregular and feathery boundary without well-defined limits [20]. The mineralized

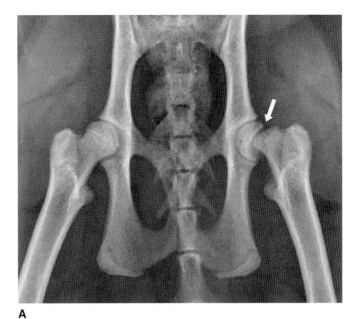

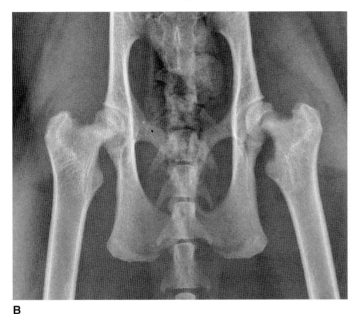

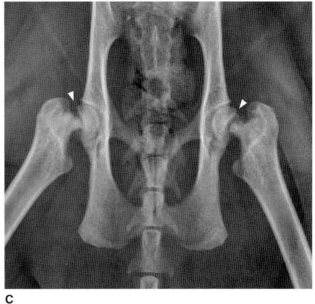

**FIGURE 9.18** Ventrodorsal radiographs of two cats with capital physeal fractures. On (**A**), the capital physeal fracture on the left is apparent when the limbs are caudally extended. In comparison, on (**B**) the capital physis of fracture is not well seen until the limbs are placed in a more frog-leg position (**C**), in which case bilateral fractures are seen.

callus crossing the fracture gap is not as solid a bridge as more mature callus that occurs after bone remodeling [20]. At this point (>14 days after fracture stabilization), the fracture line will also become smaller and less distinct as endosteal callus forms (Figure 9.20).

The *remodeling phase* begins when the fracture is bridged by callus and the mineralized cartilage remodels to woven, then lamellar bone, with an underlying structure similar to that seen in adjacent uninjured bone [19]. This phase may last for a very long time (potentially even years) after the initial injury. Radiographically, the callus remodels by smoothing and decreasing in size and with time assumes the typical appearance of cortical and medullary bone (Figure 9.21). There will be

no irregular borders, and the callus should connect adjacent fragments [20]. This process takes a longer period to begin, typically occurring 30 or more days after fracture reduction and stabilization.

The process described above is referred to as *secondary* or *indirect* bone healing, where a fibrocartilagenous callus remodels to a final bony callus. This type of repair is common in many types of fracture stabilzation where micromotion or a large fracture gap is present. In some types of rigid fixation with small fracture gaps (<1 mm), primary or direct bone healing may occur where there is direct deposition of lamellar bone without the initial fibrocartilagenous callus [19]. Radiographically, this would result in a loss of the normal fracture

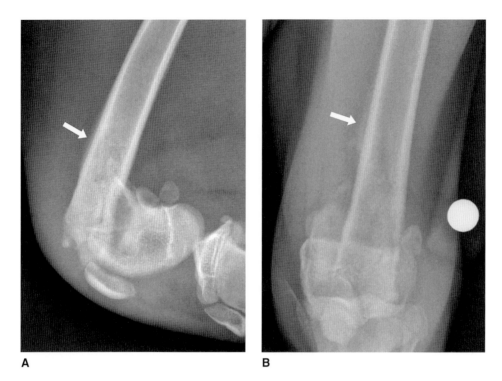

**FIGURE 9.19** Lateral (**A**) and caudocranial (**B**) radiographs of a distal femoral fracture, 18 days after initial trauma. There is very mild periosteal proliferation on the distal femur (arrow).

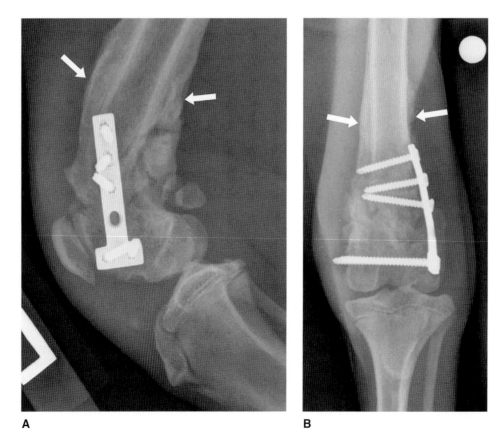

**FIGURE 9.20** Lateral (**A**) and caudocranial (**B**) radiographs of the same patient as illustrated in Figure 9.19. These radiographs are 2 months postoperative fracture stabilization. There is progressive smooth bony proliferation extending proximal and distal to the fracture site, causing bony bridging.

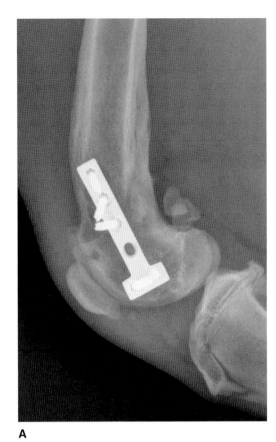 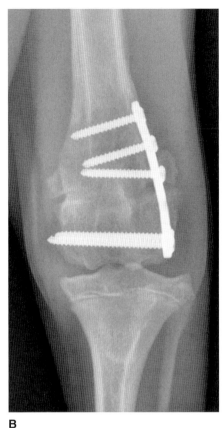

**A**      **B**

**FIGURE 9.21** Lateral (**A**) and caudocranial (**B**) radiographs of the same patient as Figures 9.19 and 9.20, 6 months postoperatively. There is remodeling and decreased size of the regional periosteal response. The fracture is no longer identified.

line with no or minimal callus appreciated, and the fracture line will gradually become more opaque with time. Primary bone healing is most common when rigid fixation devices (like bone plates) are used to closely reduce simple fractures or surgical osteotomy sites, so that the bony margins are in close, tight apposition [20].

# Radiographic Assessment of Orthopedic Implants and Bone Healing

Ideally, fracture fixation provides a biomechanically stable environment that facilitates bone healing, with proper anatomic reduction and alignment [1]. Many methods of fracture stabilization are used, including casting and splinting (referred to as external coaptation) which provide less rigidity and allow more motion than other methods, meaning the radiologist should be alert for potential fracture complications (see below). Internal and external fixation use internal or external implants respectively that rigidly stabilize the fracture site [1]. Bony callus formation tends to be larger and

more exuberant in poorly stabilized fractures, as the bone responds to continued instability with further proliferation, so the amount of callus is indirectly proportional to fracture stability [20].

Bony union is defined as the stage where the marrow cavity and cortices are continuous from one fracture margin to the other, and means that a bone has healed [20, 21]. Clinical questions often arise as to when an implant may be removed prior to complete bony union. The term "clinical union" is defined as the stage of the healing process where fixation devices may be removed and the bone will remain in the same alignment as before removal [20]. The bone may still be undergoing the healing, remodeling process, but maintain enough strength to allow continued stability. Radiographic assessment is key to this determination, though the exact qualifications that define "clinical union" are not uniform. Mature callus described above is nearly as strong as mature bone and occurs during clinical union [20].

Thorough evaluation of postoperative radiographs includes assessment of the stabilization apparatus. There are numerous methods and fixation devices used to stabilize fractures and a review of all the different orthopedic implants is beyond the scope of this chapter. When viewing postoperative radiographs, the mnemonic AAAAA ensures a complete radiographic evaluation. This stands for apposition, alignment, angulation, apparatus, and activity and refers to assessed radiographic features of healing.

With regard to fracture *apposition*, ideally the fractured bone margins will be in close contact to stimulate as much primary bone healing as possible. For *alignment* and *angulation*, the bones should be in a normal anatomic position, with the proximal and distal fracture margins well aligned with each other, and without malangulation of the long axes of the proximal and distal fracture segments. This assessment can be complex, making two high-quality orthogonal radiographs absolutely mandatory. *Apparatus* indicates that assessment of the fixation device is required, which includes estimation of appropriateness of length, size, and implant positioning, noting particularly whether implants have violated the joint or if there is any evidence of implant-associated infection. Finally, *activity* requires an assessment of the degree of bony healing on follow-up radiographs, determining if there are any issues with healing or if delayed or nonunion is developing.

# Complications of Fracture Healing

There are many potential complications that can occur during fracture healing. Bone infection may occur as a complication of surgical repair or as a result of an open fracture that occurred during the initial trauma. Sequestrum formation is an uncommon complication of fracture healing and is discussed more completely in Chapter 10. Ischemia of bone from trauma or disruption of blood supply from surgical repair can delay or completely prevent fracture healing and lead to avascular necrosis. This is particularly common in repair of femoral neck fractures (Figures 9.22 and 9.23). Joint involvement will eventually lead to osteoarthritis, and the presence of synovial fluid along the fracture margin may inhibit healing. Unstable fixation devices or unstable immobilization (especially a problem with external coaptation) result in too much bone movement and limit bone healing. In some instances, fractures may achieve bony union but have an inappropriate orientation of the two previous fracture fragments, resulting in an alignment that is not anatomic. Radiographically, such healed fractures are referred to as *malunions* (Figures 9.24 and 9.25).

Ultimately, if healing is inhibited, bone formation may not progress appropriately and a nonunion or delayed union will occur. Delayed union is a vague term, but indicates a fracture where the healing time exceeds the expected time of healing, and often occurs where there is excessive soft tissue damage or blood supply disruption [19, 21]. Twice the normal time or longer is often used for this determination, though this rule is applied loosely given the natural variation in bone healing between fracture locations, patient age, and so on [20, 21]. With enough time, a delayed union fracture would be expected to heal completely. Determination of delayed union is not possible from radiographs alone, but requires additional clinical

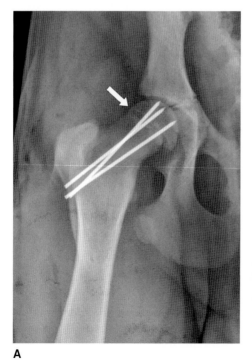 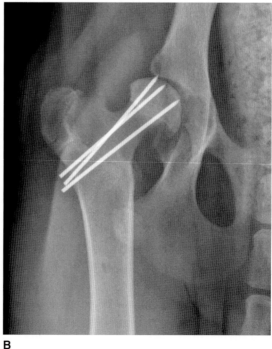

A         B

**FIGURE 9.22**  Immediate postoperative (**A**) and 8 weeks postoperative (**B**) images of a right proximal femoral fracture (arrow). Notice on recheck radiographs, the femoral neck is thinner than the prior radiograph, secondary to bony resorption; however, complete healing of the fracture has occurred.

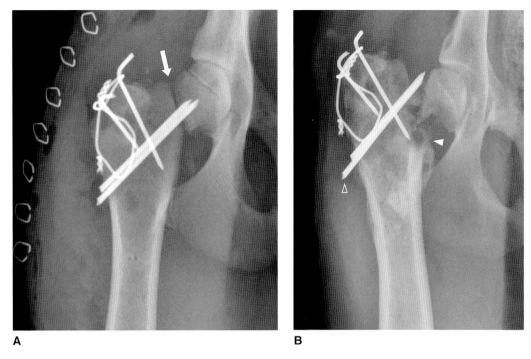

A                                        B

**FIGURE 9.23**   Immediate postoperative (**A**) and 8 weeks postoperative (**B**) images of a patient with a proximal femoral neck fracture (arrow). Notice that there has been severe resorption of the femoral neck (closed arrowheads) without evidence of bony bridging. One of the pins has retracted laterally (open arrowhead).

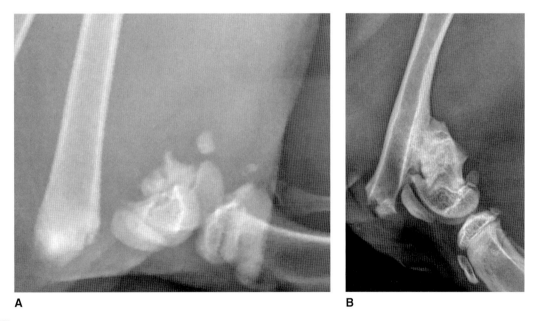

A                                        B

**FIGURE 9.24**   Distal femoral physeal fracture immediately after trauma (**A**) and 10 weeks later (**B**). A malunion has occurred with the distal femoral epiphysis healed to the distal diaphysis.

information such as time from the fracture, patient age, and other comorbidities [3].

Nonunion fractures are those where fibrous tissue separates the two fracture fragments, and demonstrable healing processes have ceased with subsequent recheck radiographs. Adjacent bone fragments will not unite without intervention [21, 22]. This occurs for many reasons, particularly if

fixation is inadequate, which leads to excessive motion and disruption of blood supply to the fracture, though it will also occur with ischemia from trauma, severe regional soft tissue trauma, loss of bone fragments from trauma, too early weight bearing, or infection [19, 21]. Nonunion fractures are identified after a long period of time, where subsequent radiographs demonstrate no progressive evidence of healing, and there is

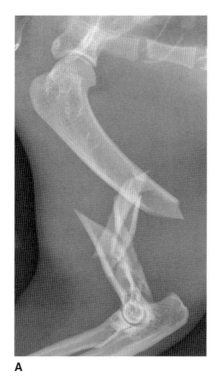 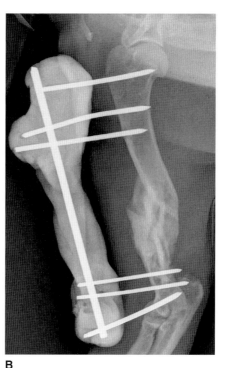

**A**                                           **B**

**FIGURE 9.25**    Preoperative (**A**) and 8 weeks postoperative external fixator placement (**B**) of a humeral fracture. A malunion has formed with cranial displacement of the distal humerus relative to the proximal.

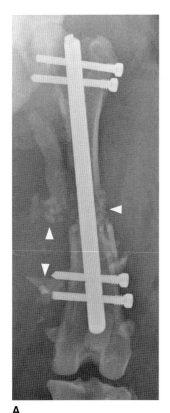 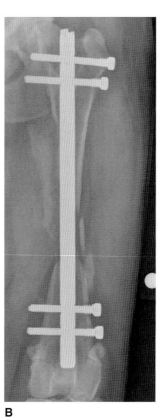

**A**                                  **B**

**FIGURE 9.26**    Immediate postoperative (**A**) and 8 weeks postoperative (**B**) radiographs of a patient with a femoral fracture stabilized by an intramedullary nail. There has been severe resorption of mineralized graft material (arrowheads) at the fracture repair as well as thinning and tapering of numerous cortical margins, consistent with bone atrophy.

lack of progressive periosteal or endosteal response, and no progressive fracture margin resorption (Figure 9.26). *Pseudarthrosis* is a nonunion where there is continued motion at the fracture site, resulting in the radiographic impression of a false joint in that area [21].

There are two classes of nonunion fractures as defined by their radiographic morphology and callus formation: *viable* and *nonviable.* Viable nonunions are fractures that are not bridging but have radiographic evidence of continued attempts to heal and are assumed to retain blood flow. There are three subclasses of viable nonunion fractures. *Hypertrophic nonunion* fractures have abundant callus with an "elephant foot" conformation, though none of the callus bridges the fracture margins. *Slightly hypertrophic nonunion* fractures have a moderate amount of nonbridging callus (Figure 9.27). *Oligotrophic nonunion fractures* have little or no callus, though still retain the potential for bone activity at their margins.

*Nonviable nonunion fractures* may appear similar to oligotrophic nonunion fractures, except they do not retain the blood supply to support further bone healing. The most common of these fractures are referred to as *atrophic nonunion.* These are recognized by resorption and rounding of fracture ends which decrease in opacity (Figure 9.28).

Some anatomic sites are predisposed to delayed or nonunion. Distal radial and ulnar fractures in small- and toy-breed dogs are particularly prone to nonviable nonunion fractures (particularly atrophic nonunions) due to poor vascular density and subsequent poor callus formation. The metacarpal and

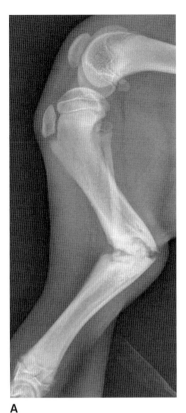
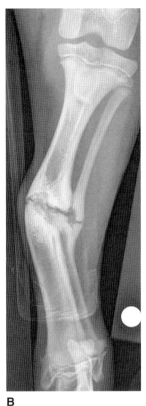

**A**    **B**

**FIGURE 9.27** Lateral (**A**) and craniocaudal (**B**) radiographs of a patient with a slightly hypertrophic nonunion fracture. Notice there is moderate bony proliferation along the proximal and distal fracture margins but no bridging of the fracture has occurred.

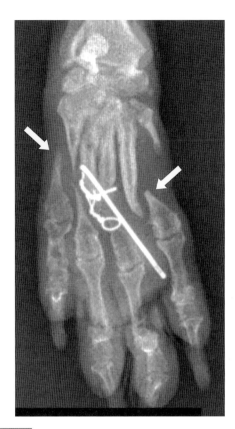

**FIGURE 9.29** Atrophic nonunion of chronic metacarpal fractures with unstable fixation (arrows). The fracture margins are atrophic, with a thinned pointed appearance.

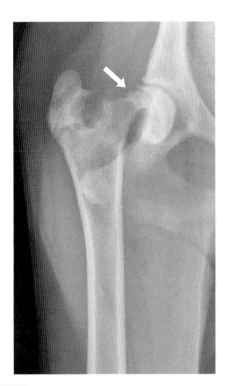

**FIGURE 9.28** Atrophic nonunion of a chronic capital physeal fracture, with persistent cranial displacement of the femoral neck (arrow) compared to the femoral head. The femoral neck is thin, consistent with resorption.

metatarsal bones are also prone to this type of nonunion (Figure 9.29) [19].

Bacterial infection of fracture sites is common with open fractures or as a complication of orthopedic stabilization, even if the fracture was initially closed. Radiographic evidence of infection may be difficult to distinguish from the normal periosteal response expected as part of a healing process. Infection of a fracture site or infection of an orthopedic apparatus is suspected in part based on clinical history. If the patient remains lame longer than suspected, displays more pain than expected during palpation of a fracture site, or has persistent swelling or drainage from a fracture site, clinical suspicion for bacterial infection exists. Radiographically, infection is suspected if there is soft tissue swelling over the plate and resorption surrounding the implants (Figure 9.30). There may also be infection if the periosteal reaction extends a significant distance from a fracture site, and if it does not change appearance over time to more mature bone.

Superimposition of orthopedic implants may obscure radiographic evidence of infection, meaning that orthogonal radiographs are required at a minimum, and oblique radiographs should be pursued if there is suspicion of infection but no initial radiographic evidence.

Recognition of orthopedic implant infection and complications of osteomyelitis is discussed in greater depth in Chapter 10.

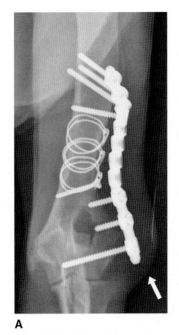
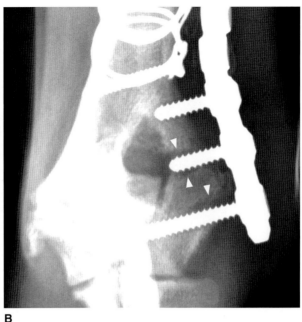

A                                 B

**FIGURE 9.30** Craniocaudal radiograph (**A**) and magnified image (**B**) showing implant-associated infection. There is regional soft tissue swelling (arrow). On the magnified image, the contrast is been adjusted to demonstrate subtle bony resorption (arrowheads) surrounding multiple screws.

# References

1. Radasch, R.M. (1999). Biomechanics of bone and fractures. *Vet. Clin. North Am. Small Anim. Pract.* 29 (1045–1082): v–vi.
2. Kinns, J., Mai, W., Seiler, G. et al. (2006). Radiographic sensitivity and negative predictive value for acute canine spinal trauma. *Vet. Radiol. Ultrasound* 47: 563–570.
3. Sande, R. (1999). Radiography of orthopedic trauma and fracture repair. *Vet. Clin. North Am. Small Anim. Pract.* 29: 1247–1260.
4. Marretta, S.M. and Schrader, S.C. (1983). Physeal injuries in the dog: a review of 135 cases. *J. Am. Vet. Med. Assoc.* 182: 708–710.
5. Salter, R.B. and Harris, W.R. (1963). Injuries involving the epiphyseal plate. *J. Bone Joint Surg.* 45: 587–622.
6. Hayes, G.M., Radke, H., and Langley-Hobbs, S.J. (2011). Salter-Harris type III fractures of the distal humerus in two dogs. *Vet. Comp. Orthop. Traumatol.* 24: 478–482.
7. Boudrieau, R.J., Dee, J.F., and Dee, L.G. (1984). Central tarsal bone fractures in the racing greyhound: a review of 114 cases. *J. Am. Vet. Med. Assoc.* 184: 1486–1491.
8. Johnson, K.A., Muir, P., Nicoll, R.G. et al. (2000). Asymmetric adaptive modeling of central tarsal bones in racing greyhounds. *Bone* 27: 257–263.
9. Guilliard, M.J. (2010). Third tarsal bone fractures in the greyhound. *J. Small Anim. Pract.* 51: 635–641.
10. Moores, A.P. and Moores, A.L. (2017). The natural history of humeral intracondylar fissure: an observational study of 30 dogs. *J. Small Anim. Pract.* 58: 337–341.
11. Butterworth, S.J. and Innes, J.F. (2001). Incomplete humeral condylar fractures in the dog. *J. Small Anim. Pract.* 42: 394–398.
12. von Pfeil, D.J., DeCamp, C.E., and Abood, S.K. (2009). The epiphyseal plate: nutritional and hormonal influences; hereditary and other disorders. *Compend. Contin. Educ. Vet.* 31: E1–E13. quiz E14.
13. Macias, C. and Marcellin-Little, D.J. (2002). Incomplete humeral condylar fractures in the dog. *J. Small Anim. Pract.* 43: 93.
14. McNicholas, W.T. Jr., Wilkens, B.E., Blevins, W.E. et al. (2002). Spontaneous femoral capital physeal fractures in adult cats: 26 cases (1996–2001). *J. Am. Vet. Med. Assoc.* 221: 1731–1736.
15. Queen, J., Bennett, D., Carmichael, S. et al. (1998). Femoral neck metaphyseal osteopathy in the cat. *Vet. Rec.* 142: 159–162.
16. Tong, L.J. (2014). Fracture characteristics to distinguish between accidental injury and non-accidental injury in dogs. *Vet. J.* 199: 392–398.
17. Intarapanich, N.P., McCobb, E.C., Reisman, R.W. et al. (2016). Characterization and comparison of injuries caused by accidental and non-accidental blunt force trauma in dogs and cats. *J. Forensic Sci.* 61: 993–999.
18. Munro, H.M. and Thrusfield, M.V. (2001). 'Battered pets': non-accidental physical injuries found in dogs and cats. *J. Small Anim. Pract.* 42: 279–290.
19. Remedios, A. (1999). Bone and bone healing. *Vet. Clin. North Am. Small Anim. Pract.* 29: 1029–1044, v.
20. Braden, T.D. and Brinker, W.O. (1976). Radiologic and gross anatomic evaluation of bone healing in the dog. *J. Am. Vet. Med. Assoc.* 169: 1318–1323.
21. Sumner-Smith, G. (1991). Delayed unions and nonunions. Diagnosis, pathophysiology, and treatment. *Vet. Clin. North Am. Small Anim. Pract.* 21: 745–760.
22. Nolte, D.M., Fusco, J.V., and Peterson, M.E. (2005). Incidence of and predisposing factors for nonunion of fractures involving the appendicular skeleton in cats: 18 cases (1998–2002). *J. Am. Vet. Med. Assoc.* 226: 77–82.

# CHAPTER 10

# Aggressive Bone Disease

**Erin Porter[1] and Nathan C. Nelson[2]**

[1] Department of Small Animal Clinical Sciences, College of Veterinary Medicine, University of Florida, Gainesville, FL, USA
[2] Department of Molecular Biomedical Sciences, College of Veterinary Medicine, North Carolina State University, Raleigh, NC, USA

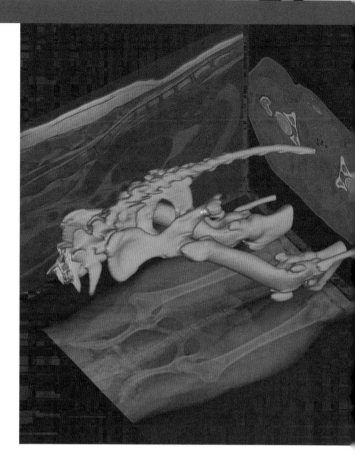

## Introduction

Radiographs are often the first diagnostic step when evaluating dogs and cats presenting with orthopedic pain, swelling, and/or lameness. Although not definitive, radiographic findings are supportive of a likely diagnosis when attempting to differentiate neoplastic, inflammatory, and benign bone diseases. The former two types of bone disease (neoplastic and inflammatory disease) tend to cause an *aggressive* radiographic appearance, whereas benign bone diseases cause a *nonaggressive (or benign)* radiographic appearance. This chapter will describe radiographic features that define an aggressive versus nonaggressive process.

The patient's signalment, history, clinical signs, and physical exam findings combined with the radiographic appearance allow creation of a prioritized differential list and formulation of an appropriate diagnostic plan. In addition to the initial radiographic study, it is important to evaluate for changes in the lesion or lesions over time to assess rate of disease progression or healing. Aggressive bone diseases tend to progress rapidly, whereas nonaggressive (benign) diseases remain static or regress (Figure 10.1). Screening of other organs, such as the lungs and draining lymph nodes, is also critical in determination of concurrent sites and/or staging if aggressive disease is suspected. Serologic and PCR analyses can evaluate for fungal and other types of infectious processes. Though history/signalment and radiographic appearance allow prioritization of differential diagnoses, in most cases a definitive diagnosis requires histopathologic evaluation of bone samples and culture if necessary.

## Radiographic Features of Bone Disease

Bone is composed of metabolically active tissue, which continually remodels throughout life. Cells called osteoblasts make osteoid, a matrix that mineralizes over time to become bone. Osteoblasts are embedded in the osteoid matrix and become

*Atlas of Small Animal Diagnostic Imaging*, First Edition. Edited by Clifford R. Berry, Nathan C. Nelson, and Matthew D. Winter.
© 2023 John Wiley & Sons, Inc. Published 2023 by John Wiley & Sons, Inc.
Companion website: www.wiley.com/go/berry/atlas

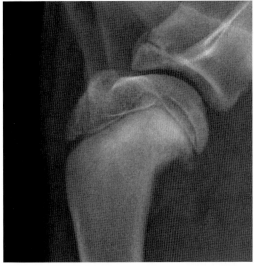

**A**

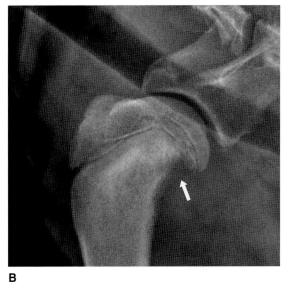

**B**

**FIGURE 10.1** Initial lateral projection (**A**) and recheck lateral projection 4 days later (**B**) of the proximal humerus in a 9-month-old boxer with acute left limb lameness due to clostridial osteomyelitis. There is lysis seen on the later image (arrow) not identified on initial radiographs. This rapid change over a short period is characteristic of aggressive bone disease.

osteocytes, which maintain the bone matrix. Osteoclasts break down and resorb bone via enzymatic activity. A fine balance between osteoclastic and osteoblastic activity occurs constantly, on a microscopic level, to maintain the normal homeostasis of bone, and allows bone to remodel and adapt to stress. Osteoclastic and osteoblastic activity, if severe enough, will result in radiographically apparent osteolytic or proliferative change respectively.

Aggressive bone diseases (neoplasia and osteomyelitis) rapidly disrupt the homeostasis of bone. These diseases can range from almost exclusively osteolytic to almost exclusively osteoproliferative; however, the most common radiographic appearance consists of a combination of both. The extent of osseous proliferation or osteolysis cannot differentiate neoplastic or inflammatory bone disease, as their appearance overlaps. Nonaggressive (benign) bone diseases (such as panosteitis, cysts, osteophytes) tend to remodel more slowly and consist entirely of bone proliferation or bone resorption.

As with all radiographic findings, aggressive and nonaggressive bone diseases are characterized using a Roentgen approach: number, location, size, shape, margination, and opacity. When evaluating a lesion, the reviewer should ask the following questions:

- *Number*: how many lesions are there? Is a single bone (monostotic) or are multiple bones (polyostotic) affected?
- *Location*: is the axial or appendicular skeleton affected? If appendicular, which portion of the bone is affected (diaphysis, metaphysis, epiphysis)? Does the lesion cross a joint space?
- *Size/shape*: how extensive is the lesion? Are multiple portions of a long bone affected? Is there a sharply demarcated

or poorly demarcated zone of transition between the lesion and adjacent, normal-appearing bone?
- *Margination*: are the margins of the lysis or proliferation smooth and well defined, or irregular and poorly defined? Are the margins continuous or interrupted?
- *Opacity*: is there increased or decreased mineral opacity, or a combination of both? If opacity is decreased, what type of lysis is present?

Evaluation of margins, opacity, shape, and size is central to determining if a lesion is likely to be aggressive. Aggressive bone lesions most often have some combination of increased and decreased mineral opacity, with ill-defined, irregular margins and a long zone of transition between the lesion and normal bone. The number and location of the lesion(s) are helpful for developing a differential diagnosis list once the lesion is characterized as aggressive or nonaggressive.

# Zone of Transition

The zone of transition between an osseous lesion and adjacent, normal bone can help to differentiate aggressive from nonaggressive disease processes. Lesions that are sharply demarcated from adjacent, normal-appearing bone are described as having a "short" zone of transition, and tend to be benign in nature. Examples would be a healing fracture, bone cyst, or cyst-like lesion at the margin of a joint (see Chapter 8, Figure 8.8). Conversely, aggressive lesions tend to have a poorly demarcated or "long" zone of transition between diseased and normal bone (Figure 10.2).

Determining the complete extent of pathology in a bone can be clinically imperative, particularly for planning surgical procedures, such as limb-sparing or complete or partial limb

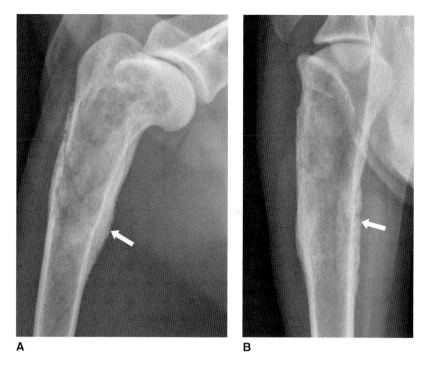

A                                             B

**FIGURE 10.2**   Lateral (**A**) and craniocaudal (**B**) radiographs of a dog with proximal humeral osteosarcoma. A long zone of transition is identified at the distal aspect of the lesion; the periosteal reaction (arrows) tapers distally, becoming less severe. Similarly, medullary lysis becomes less severe at the distal aspect of the lesion.

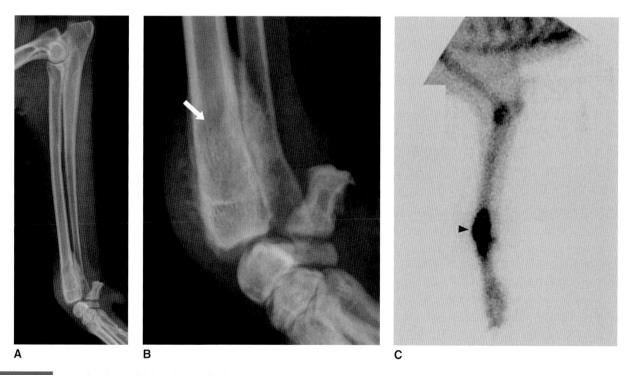

A                      B                                     C

**FIGURE 10.3**   Lateral radiograph (**A**) and magnified image of the distal radius (**B**) in a dog with osteosarcoma. A bone scan (**C**) was also performed. There is moth-eaten lysis (arrow) and irregular bony proliferation. On bone scan of the same patient, there is intense distal radial uptake (closed arrowhead) which extends more proximally than is apparent on radiographs due to greater sensitivity of bone scan for early/mild bone turnover.

amputations. When planning such surgical procedures, other imaging modalities such as nuclear scintigraphy, computed tomography (CT) and magnetic resonance imaging (MRI) may be useful to more accurately demarcate the lesion margins (Figure 10.3). For estimating the extent of intramedullary osteosarcoma, MRI has been shown to be more accurate than both CT and radiographs, which largely overestimate the extent of osseous neoplasia in dogs [1].

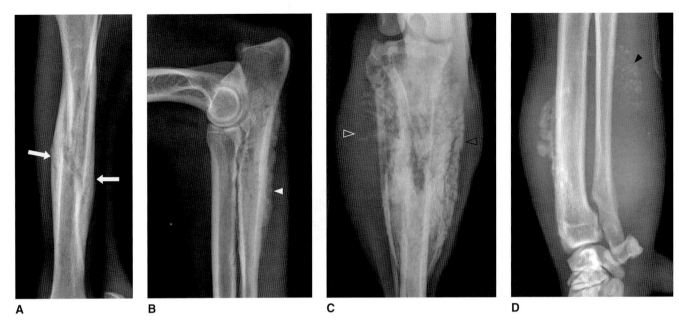

**A**           **B**           **C**           **D**

**FIGURE 10.4** Examples of periosteal reaction, from most benign to most aggressive. Lateral projection of the tibia (**A**) showing a healing fracture with smooth periosteal reaction (arrows). Lateral radiograph of the elbow (**B**) showing irregular periosteal proliferation (white closed arrowhead). Craniocaudal radiograph of the tibia (**C**) showing a laminated periosteal reaction (black open arrowhead) and sunburst periosteal reaction (white open arrowhead). Lateral radiograph of the antebrachium (**D**) showing amorphous periosteal reaction (black closed arrowhead).

# Increased Mineral Opacity and Periosteal Proliferation

Increased mineral opacity can be due to medullary sclerosis, superimposed periosteal proliferation, or a combination of both. Medullary sclerosis does occur with nonaggressive etiologies, such as panosteitis and bone infarction, but is common with osteomyelitis and neoplasia. When periosteal proliferation is present, it can be difficult to determine whether the increased mineral opacity is due to medullary sclerosis or superimposition of the overlying periosteal proliferation. Orthogonal radiographic projections can help to make this differentiation.

The periosteum can be stimulated to react by many causes, including trauma or strain at the attachment of soft tissue structures (e.g., ligaments and joint capsules), invasion by neoplastic cells, infection, and vascular etiologies. In general, the appearance of the periosteal proliferation depends on the intensity and duration of the insult. High-intensity, rapidly progressing processes result in a more aggressive appearance and less intense, more slowly progressing processes have a less aggressive appearance [2]. Some of the described types of periosteal proliferation, listed from least to most aggressive in appearance, include thin, solid, thick, irregular, septated, laminated or onionskin, sunburst, hair-on-end, and disorganized/amorphous (Figure 10.4).

Another type of periosteal proliferation, a *Codman triangle*, is formed when the periosteum is elevated and separated from the underlying cortex by subperiosteal bone formation, creating a triangular shape at the margin of the periosteal elevation (Figure 10.5). A Codman triangle is most

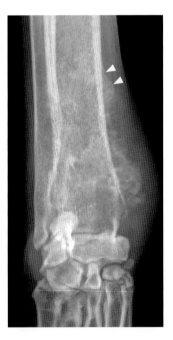

**FIGURE 10.5** Craniocaudal projection of a distal radial osteosarcoma showing the Codman triangle (arrowheads) where the periosteal reaction smooths toward normal cortical bone.

often associated with aggressive bone diseases; however, it is not pathognomonic, and may be seen with nonaggressive diseases as well.

Attempting to categorize the type of periosteal proliferation using specific terminology for every lesion can be confusing, and much overlap exists between nonaggressive and aggressive types of proliferation. However, the type of periosteal proliferation can be suggestive of certain diseases.

When evaluating periosteal proliferation, it is most important to first identify its presence and, secondly, recognize that in general, smooth, continuous, well-defined proliferation tends to result from less aggressive/benign etiologies, while irregular, poorly defined, interrupted periosteal proliferation tends to be formed by more aggressive etiologies.

## Osteolysis

Osteolysis is the resorption of bone by osteoclasts, a normal part of bone formation and remodeling. Excessive osteolysis can occur with both benign and aggressive bone diseases. Regardless of the etiology, approximately 50% of the mineral content of bone has to be lost before lysis becomes radiographically apparent [3]. Radiographically, the margins, extent, and zone of transition of any region of lysis should be carefully evaluated. Similar to periosteal proliferation, well-defined lysis tends to be less aggressive, while poorly defined lytic lesions indicate more aggressive processes.

Three basic patterns of osteolysis have been described and, in order of least to most aggressive, include the following: geographic, moth-eaten, and permeative lysis. As with periosteal proliferation, there is overlap between the different types of lysis and they do not definitively indicate one disease process over another, but the nature of the lysis may help to form a list of prioritized differential diagnoses (Figure 10.6).

- *Geographic lysis* is characterized by well-defined regions of decreased mineral opacity that do not usually involve the cortex. Geographic lysis is commonly caused by nonaggressive pathology such as bone cysts or cyst-like lesions, and synovial hyperplasia.
- *Moth-eaten lysis* is characterized by multifocal, small regions of decreased mineral opacity that become confluent with each other and have indistinct margins and a long zone of transition. Aggressive disease processes, such as neoplasia and osteomyelitis, typically cause moth-eaten lysis.
- *Permeative lysis* is characterized by a conglomeration of pinpoint regions of decreased mineral opacity, which are indistinguishable from one another, with indistinct margins and a long zone of transition. Permeative lysis is almost always seen with aggressive disease processes.

Osteolysis may involve the trabecular, endosteal, and/or cortical bone. Endosteal lysis can result in cortical deformation, which can cause compensatory bone to form on the periosteal surface, resulting in expansion of the affected portion of bone. This can occur with both malignant and nonmalignant diseases such as bone cysts, fibrous dysplasia, retained cartilage, and neoplasia [4].

When lysis weakens the cortex of diseased bones, pathologic fractures may develop (Figure 10.7). Therefore, on radiographic examinations, the cortices in the region of any osseous abnormality should be carefully evaluated for any areas of thinning or discontinuity. Pathologic fractures can be extremely subtle radiographically. Abnormalities, such as bone edema, a nonspecific finding, can indicate microfractures and early bone trauma, and may be seen earlier on MR images than radiographs [2].

On occasion, pathologic fractures are the reason for initial presentation, with no clinical history of prior disease. When a

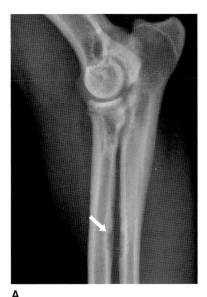
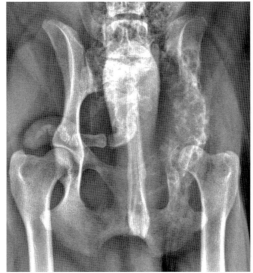
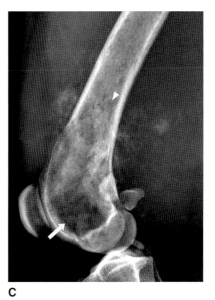

**A**    **B**    **C**

**FIGURE 10.6**  Lateral projection of the radius/ulna (**A**) showing an area of geographic lysis of the radius (arrow). This has a benign appearance. Ventrodorsal projection of the pelvis (**B**) showing diffuse moth-eaten lysis of the left pelvis due to osteosarcoma; there are large areas of lysis throughout this area. Lateral projection of the femur (**C**) showing areas of permeative lysis (arrowhead) above a larger area of moth-eaten lysis (arrow), due to osteosarcoma.

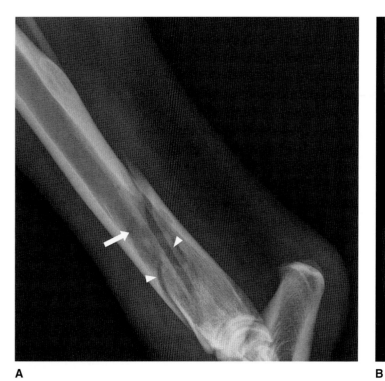

**A**

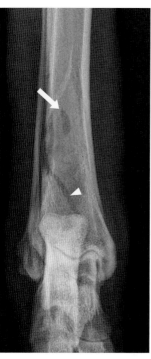

**B**

FIGURE 10.7    Lateral (**A**) and craniocaudal (**B**) radiographs of a distal tibial osteosarcoma with pathologic fracture (arrowheads). No periosteal reaction is seen, but this aggressive lesion is characterized by moth-eaten lysis (arrows).

patient presents with an acute fracture and history of minimal/no trauma, or a history of trauma that seems disproportionate in severity to the clinical presentation, radiographs should be highly scrutinized for evidence of an underlying aggressive lesion at the fracture site. The examiner should be aware that the radiographic findings can be as subtle as mildly ill-defined fracture margins or faint periosteal proliferation near the fracture site.

In some cases, the degree of bone lysis or periosteal proliferation is insufficient to allow a confident diagnosis of an underlying aggressive lesion in a fractured bone. In these cases, CT of the affected limb should be considered. CT is more sensitive in detecting underlying bone loss and subtle periosteal reaction than radiographs. For that reason, it will often allow a more confident diagnosis of an aggressive, pathologic fracture if screening radiographs are equivocal.

# Differentials for Aggressive Bone Disease

Neoplasia and bone infection (osteomyelitis) are the two primary differentials for aggressive bone disease, and cannot be differentiated from each other based on radiographic characteristics alone. Additionally, both neoplastic and infectious bone disease may present with similar clinical signs, such as

pain, lameness, local swelling, and/or neurologic signs ranging from ataxia to paralysis.

When differentiating between osseous neoplasia and osteomyelitis, the patient's signalment and history should be considered. Lesion number and location, including whether it is polyostotic or monostotic, axial or appendicular skeletal location, and whether the epiphyseal, metaphyseal, or diaphyseal portion of any long bone is affected, should also be taken into consideration. For example, primary osseous neoplasia, such as osteosarcoma, tends to be monostotic and affect the metaphyseal region of long bones in older dogs, while metastatic neoplasia is more likely to be middiaphyseal and polyostotic (Figure 10.8). Fungal osteomyelitis typically has a polyostotic distribution in the axial or appendicular skeleton with a history of travel to endemic regions.

When an aggressive lesion is identified, other organs should be screened for disease. Screening may include cytologic or histologic evaluation of draining lymph nodes, thoracic radiographs (including right and left lateral as well as orthogonal projections), and evaluation for other sites of osseous involvement. Nuclear scintigraphy, an imaging modality which utilizes a radiopharmaceutical (phosphate analog labeled with radioactive technetium-99m) to indicate areas of rapid bone turnover, is more sensitive than radiographs for early detection of skeletal lesions and can be used to detect osseous metastasis [5]. Finally, other diagnostics such as serologic and PCR analysis for fungal and other infectious agents, and histopathology and culture of samples of the affected bone should be performed to confirm the suspected diagnosis.

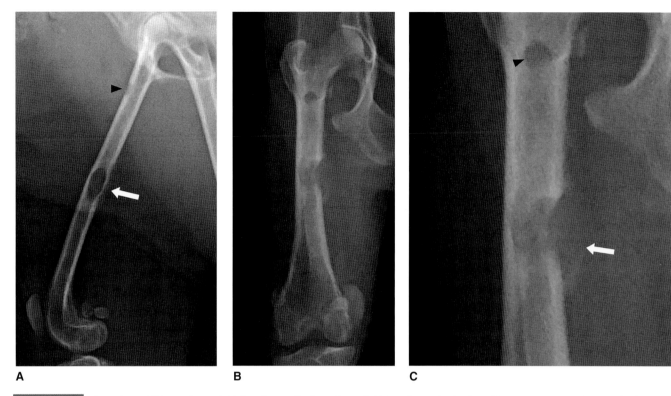

**A**          **B**          **C**

**FIGURE 10.8**   Figure lateral (**A**), craniocaudal (**B**) and magnified craniocaudal (**C**) radiograph of a dog with metastatic neoplasia to the femur. There are aggressive lesions in the middiaphysis (arrow) and proximal diaphysis (arrowhead) in the area of the nutrient foramen. There is a long zone of transition and irregular periosteal response. This location is more consistent with spread of an aggressive lesion (in this case neoplasia) to the femur rather than a primary osseous neoplasm.

# Primary Osseous Neoplasia

Osteosarcoma is responsible for up to 85% of skeletal malignancies, and is the most common primary bone neoplasia dogs and cats. It most commonly affects large- and giant-breed dogs, and has a bimodal distribution, with a small peak in 18–24-month-old dogs, but the majority of affected animals are middle aged and older. The most commonly affected locations include the proximal humeral and distal radial metaphyses in the thoracic limb, and the distal femoral and proximal tibial metaphyses in the pelvic limb, leading to the expression "away from the elbow, toward the knee (stifle)." However, the distal tibial metaphysis is also commonly affected.

The anatomic distribution of osteosarcoma is different in small-breed dogs and cats compared to large-breed dogs. In small dogs, osteosarcoma more frequently affects the axial skeleton [6, 7], and in cats it tends to be equally distributed between the axial and appendicular skeleton, with appendicular lesions more commonly affecting the thoracic limbs in dogs and pelvic limbs in cats [8, 9]. In both dogs and cats, osteosarcoma is extremely locally invasive and aggressive; however, while it is highly metastatic, often resulting in death within months of the initial diagnosis in dogs, it is slower to metastasize in cats. Osteosarcoma does not typically cross the joint, but can extend into the adjacent soft tissues and may affect adjacent bones. Less common, aggressive primary

bone tumors in dogs include chondrosarcoma (10%), fibrosarcoma (less than 5%), and hemangiosarcoma (less than 5%) [10–12].

# Neoplasia of the Axial Skeleton

Although primary bone neoplasia most commonly affects the appendicular skeleton, it can also affect the axial skeleton, with osteosarcoma being the most common primary vertebral tumor [13]. Further, some types of neoplasia, such as mammary carcinoma, have an affinity for metastasis to the axial skeleton, and a small subset of neoplasia has a predilection for the axial skeleton. Examples of these include multilobular tumor of bone and plasma cell tumors such as multiple myeloma, and solitary osseous plasmacytoma.

Multilobular osteochondrosarcoma (MLO) (also known as multilobular tumor of bone, multilobular osteoma, and chondroma rodens) is an uncommon, primary osseous neoplasm of dogs and cats that usually arises from the skull (see also Chapter 11) [12]. These tumors are usually slowly growing and locally invasive. They may occur after incomplete excision and may metastasize. Radiographically, these tumors have a characteristic "popcorn ball" appearance, with a granular mineral opacity, well-defined margins, and limited osteolysis. Computed tomography may be helpful to more thoroughly evaluate for tumor ossification and to determine the extent of cortical and soft tissue involvement.

The MR imaging features of MLO have also been described [14]. On T1-weighted images, the tumors have low signal intensity relative to the brain but not cerebrospinal fluid (CSF), and large areas of contrast enhancement. On proton density and T2-weighted images, the tumors also have low signal intensity relative to the brain with regions of centrally located hyperintensity. In general, MRI is highly useful when evaluating skull tumors, and can help to determine the presence and extent of brain involvement and/or compression, as well as adjacent soft tissue extension. When an ostectomy is elected as treatment for MLO, both CT and MR imaging can assist in surgical planning [14].

Multiple myeloma and plasmacytoma are neoplasms arising from the B-lymphocyte plasma cell lineage (see also Chapter 12). Solitary osseous plasmacytomas represent a small population of osseous neoplasia in dogs. They tend to occur in the axial skeleton and carry a better prognosis than multiple myeloma [15]. Multiple myeloma is the more prevalent plasma cell tumor in small animals. In 25–50% of dogs affected with multiple myeloma, multifocal, small osseous lesions are present, having a characteristic appearance of well-defined "punched-out" lysis without surrounding sclerosis [16–18]. The bones most commonly involved include the vertebrae, pelvic bones, ribs, and bones of the proximal extremities. Although the lytic lesions tend to look small, pathologic fractures can occur [19]. In addition to osteolysis, affected patients may have bone marrow plasmacytosis, serum or urine monoclonal gammopathy, hypercalcemia, and Bence Jones proteinuria. Multiple myeloma-related osteolysis is less common in cats than in dogs.

Clinical signs of neoplasia affecting the axial skeleton depend on the site(s) and severity of the lesion. For example, a dog with a multilobular tumor of bone near the temporomandibular joint may present with pain or difficulty upon opening the mouth, while a cat with multiple myeloma is more likely to present with nonspecific signs such as lethargy, weakness, and anorexia. Tumors of the axial skeleton can extend into the vertebral canal and compress the spinal cord and/or nerve roots. In these patients, the presenting sign may be progressive ataxia, paresis or even paralysis. When spinal cord or nerve root compression is suspected, spinal radiographs should be obtained to evaluate for aggressive lesions of the vertebral column; however, advanced imaging methods such as MRI, or radiographic or CT myelography are more sensitive for identifying the site of compressive myelopathy/radiculopathy.

# Periarticular Neoplasia

When an aggressive lesion affects the subchondral and/or adjacent cortical or trabecular bone on either side of a joint, diagnostic differentials should include septic or erosive arthritis as well as periarticular neoplasia (see also Chapter 8).

Histiocytic sarcoma and synovial cell sarcoma are the most common malignant periarticular tumors in small animals, although other types of joint-centric sarcomas have also been reported [20]. Localized histiocytic sarcoma arising near an appendicular joint has been suggested to represent a subtype of the disease [21]. Both synovial cell sarcoma and periarticular histiocytic sarcoma more commonly occur in large-breed dogs, with Rottweilers being overrepresented for periarticular histiocytic sarcoma [20]. There is a predilection for larger joints, such as the shoulder, elbow, and stifle, to be affected. Synovial cell sarcoma occurs uncommonly in cats. Both synovial cell and histiocytic sarcoma may develop from the synoviocytes of joint capsule and tendon sheaths and may invade adjacent bones.

Radiographic features include soft tissue thickening surrounding a joint and possibly aggressive bone lesions such as moth-eaten or permeative osteolysis and irregular osseous proliferation (Figure 10.9). Regional lymphadenopathy may also occur so fine needle aspirates should be obtained from palpable, regional lymph nodes for cytologic evaluation.

# Metastatic and Multicentric Neoplasia Involving Bone

Bone metastasis occurs primarily via the hematogenous route, but may also spread by contiguous extension [22]. Bone marrow has a rich blood supply and contains fenestrations between the endothelial cells and no basement membrane of the medullary sinusoids, which increases vessel permeability and allows circulating neoplastic cells to enter the bone marrow [22, 23]. Bone metastasis occurs less commonly than primary bone tumors in dogs, and more commonly affects the axial skeleton [24]. The most common sites for metastatic neoplasia overall include the vertebrae, humerus, ribs, and pelvis (Figure 10.10) [12, 24], although osseous metastasis tends to be polyostotic, and the patient is often not symptomatic for all sites of metastasis. Metastatic lesions in long bones tend to occur in the middiaphyseal region; however, metaphyseal sites of metastasis do occur.

Mammary, musculoskeletal, and pulmonary tumors were the most prevalent source of osseous metastasis in one study [24], although urogenital tumors of the prostate and urinary bladder also have a predilection for osseous metastasis [7, 12]. Some urogenital tumors, such as prostatic adenocarcinoma, have a tendency to metastasize to adjacent bones such as the sacrum, lumbar vertebrae, and iliac wings. Therefore, regional osseous structures should be carefully evaluated when urogenital neoplasia is suspected. Osseous involvement can also occur with different types of multicentric neoplasia, including histiocytic sarcoma and lymphoma, and lesions may be polyostotic with an aggressive radiographic appearance.

Nuclear bone scintigraphy is recommended to identify more subtle or subclinical osseous lesions due to metastatic or multicentric neoplasia.

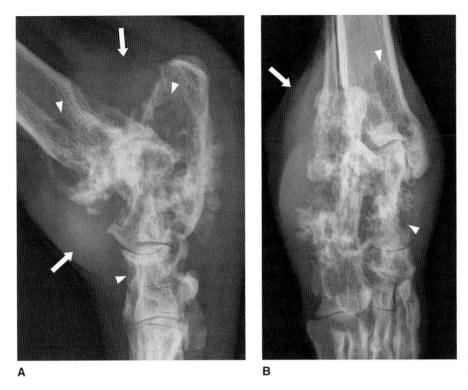

**FIGURE 10.9**   Lateral (**A**) and dorsopalmar (**B**) radiographs of a tarsus with joint-associated histiocytic sarcoma. There is severe regional soft tissue swelling centered at the joint (arrows) and multifocal lysis of the adjacent bones (arrowheads) representing locally polyostotic aggressive change.

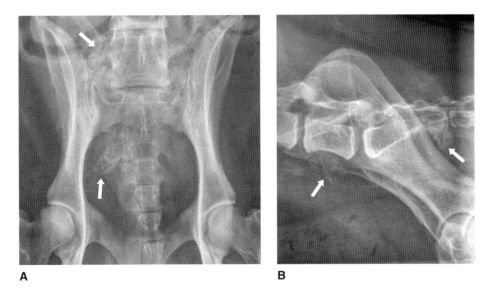

**FIGURE 10.10**   Ventrodorsal (**A**) and lateral (**B**) radiographs of the pelvic region showing a metastatic carcinoma to the sacrum and seventh lumbar vertebral body. There is irregular periosteal proliferation (arrows). Lysis is not well appreciated, as radiographs are relatively insensitive in detecting lysis when less than 50% of bone density has been lost.

# Benign Bone Tumors

Benign bone tumors such as osteomas, osteochondromas or multiple cartilaginous exostoses (MCE) and bone cysts occur uncommonly. Osteomas are histologically similar to reactive bone, are usually nonpainful on presentation and most often

affect the facial bones in small animals [25]. Radiographically, osteomas appear as smoothly margined, well-defined regions of osseous proliferation. Surgical excision is usually curative.

Osteochondromas (called MCE when more than one lesion is present; see also Chapter 7) are proliferations of bone and cartilage that result from aberrant growth of displaced chondrocytes from the growth plates [25]. Presentations of osteochondromas and MCE differ between dogs and cats. In dogs, these lesions most often affect the metaphyseal region of long bones, and occur in skeletally immature dogs [25]. Conversely, in cats, the flat bones are most commonly affected and lesions tend to appear after skeletal maturity, and a link between feline leukemia virus and MCE has been reported [25, 26]. Radiographically, these appear as smooth, well-defined regions of osseous proliferation. If the vertebrae are affected, spinal pain, paresis, or paralysis may result. Malignant transformation of these lesions is possible as the animal ages [27, 28].

True intraosseous bone cysts, consisting of a fluid-filled space with an epithelial lining, rarely occur. They most commonly occur in the metaphysis of long bones, and may communicate with the articular surface. Radiographically, they may appear as singular (simple), or multilocular, well-defined regions of geographic osteolysis, and may result in cortical thinning. In severe cases, pathologic fractures can occur secondary to bone cysts [29]. Aneurysmal bone cysts are multiloculated intraosseous regions that are filled with blood. Affected patients may present with lameness, pain, and swelling. The exact etiology is not known but they may result from any condition disrupting blood flow through the bone marrow, such as trauma, and a hereditary predisposition has been reported in Doberman pinschers [30–32]. The typical radiographic appearance is a well-defined, expansile lesion containing thin, mineral opaque septae and they often result in cortical thinning. Aneurysmal bone cysts most commonly occur in the metaphysis of long bones and can extend into the diaphyseal region. Although they are benign in nature, recurrence of these lesions after treatment and malignant transformation have been described [30, 31].

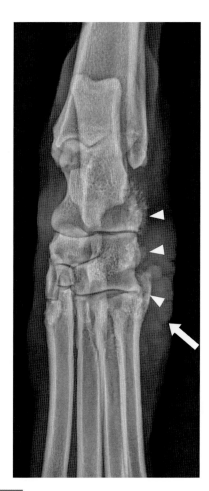

**FIGURE 10.11**  Dorsoplantar radiograph of an 8-year-old intact male mixed-breed dog with 2-year history of frequent tarsal licking. There is an irregular periosteal response (arrowheads) and adjacent lobular soft tissue thickening (arrow) confirmed as an acral lick granuloma with adjacent periostitis.

# Osteomyelitis

In addition to neoplasia, osteomyelitis, an infection of the bone or bone marrow, should be considered as a differential diagnosis when aggressive bone changes such as ill-defined lysis and irregular osseous proliferation are seen radiographically. Rarely, reaction of the periosteum alone (termed *periostitis*) may be present with primary soft tissue inflammation adjacent to osseous structures in the absence of an infectious agent (Figure 10.11).

Bacterial, fungal, and protozoal causes of osteomyelitis have been reported, with bacterial infections being most common. Bacterial infections tend to form focally from traumatic or iatrogenic causes; however, hematogenous spread can also occur (Figure 10.12). More than one bone in a particular area may be affected, a useful radiographic feature which differentiates osteomyelitis from primary bone neoplasms (Figure 10.13). Fungal infections are less common than bacterial osteomyelitis, and tend to follow a hematogenous route. The source of the infection (i.e., focal or hematogenous) and pathogen type will affect the anatomic distribution of osteomyelitis.

Clinically, osteomyelitis often results in local swelling, severe pain, lameness, and often pyrexia and lethargy. Non-healing wounds or recurrent draining tracts also raise concern for underlying osteomyelitis.

## Bacterial Osteomyelitis

Bacterial infections are responsible for the majority of cases of osteomyelitis in small animals, with *Staphylococcus* spp. being the most common [33]. The infections most often develop focally, secondary to penetrating trauma, extension of adjacent soft tissue infections, iatrogenic causes, and even migrating foreign bodies, such as plant material. Because of the local source of infection, bacterial osteomyelitis tends to involve only one limb, although multiple bones within the affected region/limb may be affected.

Hematogenous forms of bacterial osteomyelitis are less common, and rarely affect long bones of immunocompetent, skeletally mature, small animals because of the natural protective barriers in place. When hematogenous cases of bacterial osteomyelitis occur, a polyostotic, metaphyseal distribution is more likely.

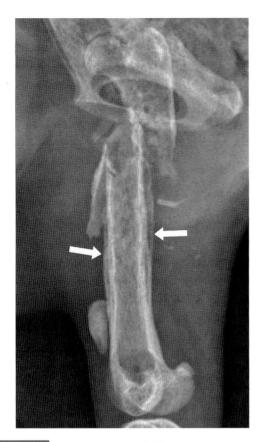

**FIGURE 10.12** Lateral projection of a femur showing severe permeative lysis and smooth periosteal reaction (arrows), with a pathologic fracture in a 3-year-old Persian cat. The cat had previous aortic thromboembolus due to aortic valve endocarditis. There was hematogenous bacterial spread to the femur.

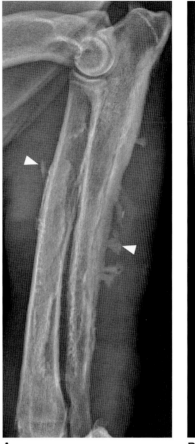
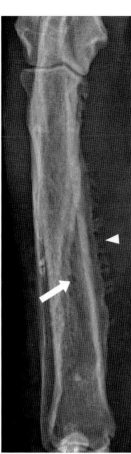

A                                                              B

**FIGURE 10.13** Lateral (**A**) and craniocaudal (**B**) radiographs of a 5-year-old pit bull presented for swollen limb and bacterial osteomyelitis. Active periosteal response is seen on the radius and ulna (arrowheads) with other areas of lysis (arrow). *Actinomyces canis* was cultured.

In adult dogs, discospondylitis is one of the more commonly seen forms of hematogenous osteomyelitis (Figure 10.14; see also Chapter 12). Discospondylitis is an intervertebral disc infection with concurrent osteomyelitis of the adjacent vertebral endplates. Clinically affected dogs present with back pain and signs of systemic infection. The infection can be bacterial or fungal in origin. Common sources of infection include the urogenital tract, skin, dental disease, or endocarditis [34]. Radiographic findings may include intervertebral disc space narrowing or collapse, irregular lysis and sclerosis of the adjacent vertebral endplates and ill-defined, irregular osseous proliferation surrounding the disc space. Multiple intervertebral disc spaces are often concurrently affected, and there may be associated spinal cord compression. Magnetic resonance findings of discospondylitis are well described and MR imaging is extremely helpful in determining presence or severity of associated spinal cord compression [35, 36]. Discospondylitis rarely occurs in cats.

Pododermatitis can spread to the underlying bones of the digit and result in osteomyelitis in severe cases (Figure 10.15). Subungual tumors, such as squamous cell carcinoma and melanoma, are not uncommon in the digits of the dog, and may be impossible to differentiate radiographically from pododermatitis with underlying osteomyelitis. Neoplasia

and inflammatory lesions can occur in the manus and pes with equal frequency, and both can result in moderate to severe soft tissue thickening and aggressive, osseous changes, including ill-defined lysis and/or osseous proliferation of the affected digit [37]. However, lesions characterized primarily by lysis rather than proliferation are more likely to be neoplastic than infectious [37].

Pododermatitis is less common in cats, and when aggressive lesions of one or multiple digits are identified, neoplasia should be considered a top differential diagnosis and can only be ruled out with cytology or histologic evaluation. In cats, primary lung tumors, such as bronchial and bronchioalveolar carcinoma, may metastasize to the digits. This unusual pattern of metastasis is termed lung–digit syndrome [38]. In these patients, extensive, ill-defined lysis and, sometimes, irregular osseous proliferation are seen affecting the distal phalanges of the weight-bearing digits. The lesions tend to be polyostotic, affecting the distal phalanges of limbs. If polyostotic, aggressive lesions are identified affecting the digits in a cat, thoracic imaging is indicated, as these lesions may be the presenting complaint in a cat with primary lung neoplasia (Figure 10.16).

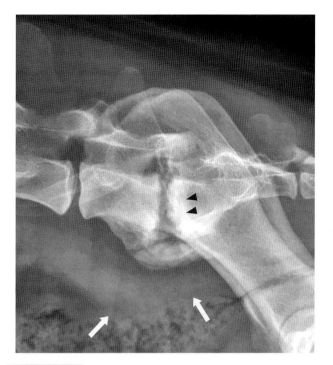

**FIGURE 10.14** Lateral radiograph of the lumbosacral junction in a dog with discospondylitis. There is irregularity of the L7–S1 endplates, particularly in comparison to the normal appearance of the L6–7 endplates. There is sclerosis of the adjacent vertebra (arrowheads) and ventral soft tissue swelling (arrows).

## Implant-Associated Infections

The presence of an orthopedic implant predisposes bone to bacterial colonization and the development of osteomyelitis, particularly if trauma or necrosis occurs during implant placement.

Radiographic signs depend on the duration of implant infection. A lucent halo surrounding the implant is an early indicator of potential infection, particularly if periosteal reaction is present (Figure 10.17). The presence of this lucent halo is not definitive for infection, as sterile loosening results in a similar appearance. Additionally, digital radiographic units employ edge enhancement algorithms that can also result in an artifactual lucent halo surrounding orthopedic implants, termed an "Uberschwinger" artifact. Improvement in digital algorithms has reduced this artifact with newer systems, but it should not be confused with implant infection. This artifact may be differentiated from true implant infection by comparing immediate postoperative radiographs with later radiographs, as the Uberschwinger artifact will be present immediately after implant placement and will not change over time, whereas infection-associated lucency will become more severe. Periosteal response will develop and may be smooth if subperiosteal infection is established or more irregular and active in appearance (Figure 10.18).

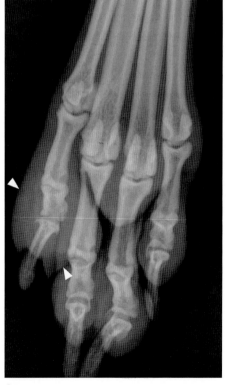

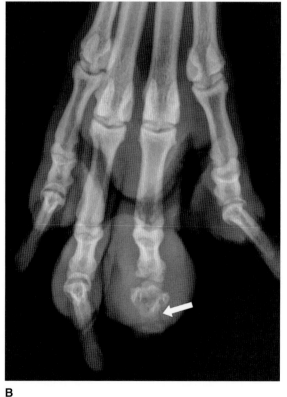

A                                         B

**FIGURE 10.15** Dorsopalmar radiographs of a dog with pododermatitis (**A**) compared to a dog with digital squamous cell carcinoma (**B**). In the dog with pododermatitis, swelling is present (arrowhead) but no lysis is seen. In the dog with carcinoma, there is swelling but also lysis of the distal phalanx (arrow). Unfortunately, the radiographic appearances of these diseases overlap, so final diagnosis in these patients was reliant on cytology of the swollen area and not radiographic appearance.

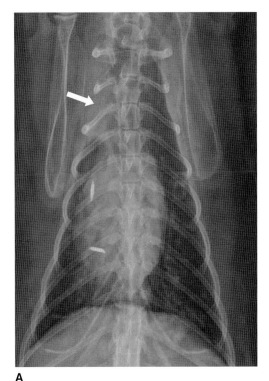
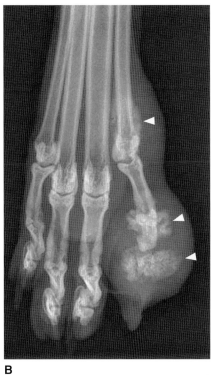

A                    B

**FIGURE 10.16** Ventrodorsal thoracic radiograph (**A**) and dorsopalmar radiograph (**B**) of the pes. A mass is seen in the right cranial lung lobe (arrow) diagnosed as pulmonary carcinoma. The second digit of the manus has multiple metastases (arrowheads) causing irregular bony proliferation (so-called "lung–digit syndrome").

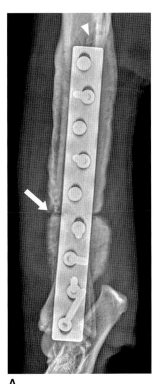
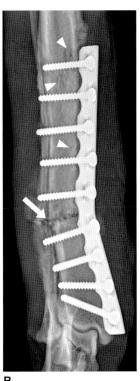

A                    B

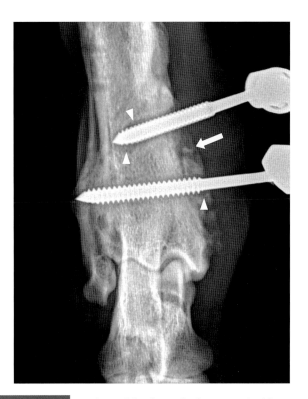

**FIGURE 10.17** Lateral (**A**) and craniocaudal (**B**) radiographs of a 6-year-old Newfoundland. A tibial osteotomy was performed for an angular limb deformity, but there was a more recent swollen limb and increased drainage from incision. Osteomyelitis is present and can be recognized by areas of lysis (arrowheads) and extensive periosteal reaction far from the osteotomy site (arrowhead) that has an active appearance at the osteotomy margins.

**FIGURE 10.18** Craniocaudal radiograph of a 12-month-old Chesapeake Bay retriever. An external fixator was placed to fix a tibial fracture (fracture not included in the image). The patient had drainage from the pin tracts. There is severe periosteal response (arrow) adjacent to the pins and subtle lucency (arrowheads) around the pins, consistent with pin infection. *Staphylococcus pseudintermedius* was cultured.

Soft tissue swelling focused over the implant is another expected, early sign of implant infection. With chronic infections, other signs of aggressive bone disease, such as an active periosteal response or widespread aggressive lysis, will eventually develop. Unfortunately, radiographic remodeling from bone healing may preclude determination of the presence of low-grade osteomyelitis [4].

## Sequestrum Formation

Sequestrum formation is an uncommon complication of osteomyelitis that occurs when a portion of infected bone loses its vascular supply and becomes necrotic. The devascularized segment of bone, termed the *sequestrum*, becomes completely surrounded by an infectious envelope which prevents revascularization and resorption of the bone (Figure 10.19). As a result, the segment of devitalized bone appears radiographically as a well-defined mineralized structure surrounded by a thick lucent zone where the infectious debris is concentrated. This may be difficult to identify if the sequestrum occurs with a concurrent

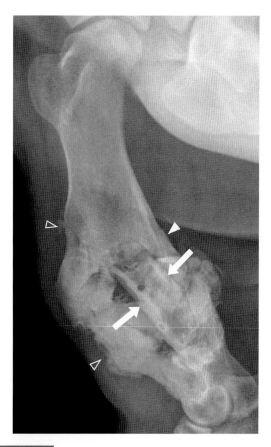

**FIGURE 10.19** Lateral radiograph of a 10-month-old Labrador retriever. The dog was hit by a car 3 months prior, with open fracture of the humerus managed by external fixation. Drainage from the pin tracts was noted and the dog became more lame 1 month after surgery. A large sequestrum is identified by its well-defined margins (arrows) and surrounded by a large lucent zone. There is some smooth periosteal response (closed arrowhead) characteristic of a healing fracture, but more active response (open arrowhead) due to underlying infection.

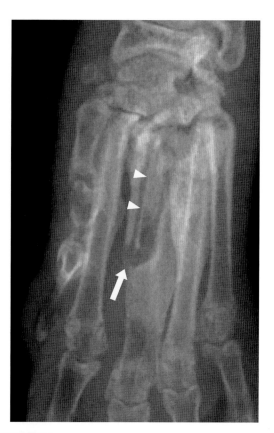

**FIGURE 10.20** Dorsopalmar radiograph of the manus of a 6-month-old mixed-breed cat. There were multiple fractures of the metacarpal bones 2 months prior, and now draining tract and swelling at the site of fracture. A sequestrum is present within the third metacarpal bone (arrowheads). The cloaca is identified more distally (arrow). There is thickening of the surrounding third metacarpal bone, with more mild thickening of the second and fourth metacarpal bone representing healed fractures.

fracture or if the surrounding viable bone, termed the *involucrum*, has exuberant reactive tissue and increased opacity (Figure 10.20). Soft tissue swelling and a possible draining tract (termed the *cloaca*) that connects to the lucent area around the sequestrum may be identified radiographically and can assist diagnosis (Figure 10.21).

## Fungal Osteomyelitis

Fungal osteomyelitis is less common than bacterial osteomyelitis in dogs and is rarely seen in cats. Contrary to bacterial causes, fungal causes of osteomyelitis are more commonly hematogenous in origin, and are therefore often polyostotic, with the metaphases of long bones being preferentially affected [39, 40]. The predilection for metaphyseal involvement has been explained by various hypotheses and is likely multifactorial. The rich vascular network connecting metaphyseal capillaries and venules may result in sluggish blood flow in the metaphysis. Additionally, the capillary endothelium in the physeal region lacks a basement membrane, allowing for extravasation of blood and associated infectious agents in the metaphyseal region [39]. Transphyseal blood vessels do not

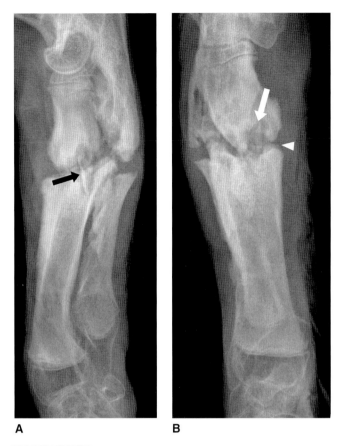

**A**                    **B**

**FIGURE 10.21** Lateral (**A**) and craniocaudal (**B**) radiographs of a 5-month-old German shepherd dog, with open fractures of the radius and ulna managed by intramedullary pinning (pins removed). The fractures are not healed, with a well-defined sequestrum (arrows) seen within the fracture segment. The cloaca (arrowhead) is seen adjacent to the sequestrum.

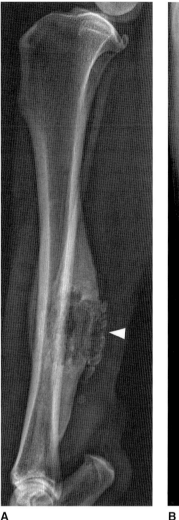
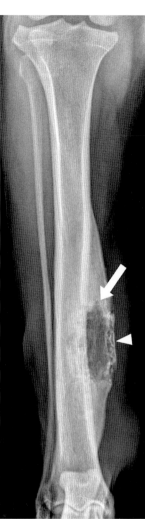

**A**                    **B**

**FIGURE 10.22** Lateral (**A**) and craniocaudal (**B**) radiographs of a 1-year-old Alaskan Malamute. There is mixed moth-eaten and permeative lysis (arrows) and severe periosteal reaction which is irregular at the level of the lucent lesion (arrowheads). Blastomycosis was identified on cytologic examination.

exist at birth in dogs and cats, so infections are usually isolated to the metaphyseal side of the bone prior to physeal closure. Nonetheless, hematogenous fungal osteomyelitis can have a diaphyseal distribution in long bones, with infectious seeding likely occurring via the nutrient artery.

Fungal osteomyelitis in the United States occurs most often in geographic regions where the fungal agents are endemic, often the southeast and southwest. The most common fungal isolates from bone in the United States are *Blastomyces*, *Coccidioides*, *Histoplasma*, and *Cryptococcus* [34]. Additionally, young German shepherd dogs have a genetic predisposition for disseminated aspergillosis, due to *Aspergillus terreus* [4, 34, 41].

Fungal infections are commonly transmitted via inhalation, with dissemination to other organ systems occurring later in the disease process. Patients often present with nonspecific signs of systemic infection including fever, anorexia, weight loss, depression, weakness, and peripheral lymphadenopathy. In addition, affected patients may show signs of more specific disease such as pneumonia, cutaneous infections, ocular disease such as keratitis, uveitis or acute blindness, ataxia, seizures or behavioral changes and gastrointestinal signs, depending on the fungal organism and organ system involved.

Whenever a polyostotic, aggressive lesion is identified, fungal osteomyelitis should be considered as a differential diagnosis. The radiographic appearance can appear similar to osseous neoplasia (Figure 10.22). In these cases, careful consideration should be given to the patient's travel history and thoracic imaging should be performed to evaluate for tracheobronchial lymphadenopathy and lung pathology. More definitive diagnosis can be obtained via serology, evaluation of urine for fungal hyphae, and bone biopsy for cytologic evaluation and culture.

## Protozoal Osteomyelitis

Protozoan and other causes of osteomyelitis are rare. Canine hepatozoonosis is a tick-borne protozoal disease, carried primarily by the brown dog tick, *Rhipicephalus sanguineus*, and is seen in the southern United States and throughout the world. Dogs affected with *Hepatozoon americanum* are systemically ill, with pyrexia, mucopurulent ocular discharge, muscle atrophy, weight loss, and generalized muscle and bone pain [4, 42]. Typically, a polyostotic pattern of smooth or irregular periosteal proliferation is seen at the muscle attachment sites on long bones, vertebrae, and pelvic and skull bones, which is thought to be due to myositis at skeletal muscle attachment sites [4, 42, 43]. The polyostotic distribution and lack of cortical disruption make it radiographically difficult to differentiate from hypertrophic osteopathy. Early osseous lesions from canine hepatozoonosis often occur proximal to the carpus or tarsus and on the axial skeleton are associated with high-intensity, diffuse, symmetric radiopharmaceutical uptake on bone scintigraphy [43].

## Differentiating Neoplasia from Osteomyelitis

Both neoplasia and osteomyelitis may present with similar clinical signs, including soft tissue swelling, pain, lameness, and lethargy. Radiographically, both display aggressive characteristics including some combination of ill-defined osseous proliferation and osteolysis (usually moth-eaten or permeative) with a long zone of transition, and in more severe cases, cortical thinning and pathologic fractures may develop. In general, osteomyelitis tends to progress more slowly than osseous neoplasia, so serial radiography can be helpful, but this is variable and cannot be depended upon for definitive differentiation of infection from neoplasia.

When attempting to differentiate neoplasia from osteomyelitis, many factors should be considered, including the patient's signalment, history and clinical signs, as well as the anatomic distribution of the lesion. Typically, primary bone tumors are monostotic with a metaphyseal location in long bones, while metastatic bone tumors are more likely to be polyostotic and diaphyseal in location, and are more likely to affect the axial skeleton.

Bacterial osteomyelitis tends to be localized to one region and affected patients often present with a history of trauma, local infection or a recent, invasive medical procedure. Fungal osteomyelitis tends to have a polyostotic, metaphyseal distribution, and affected patients may have a history of travel to endemic regions. Additionally, patients with fungal osteomyelitis are more likely to be systemically ill, with clinical signs such as anorexia, depression, fever, respiratory signs, or lymphadenopathy.

# References

1. Wallack, S.T., Wisner, E.R., Werner, J.A. et al. (2002). Accuracy of magnetic resonance imaging for estimating intramedullary osteosarcoma extent in pre-operative planning of canine limb-salvage procedures. *Vet. Radiol. Ultrasound* 43 (5): 432–441.

2. Rana, R.S., Wu, J.S., and Eisenberg, R.L. (2009). Periosteal reaction. *Am. J. Roentgenol.* 193 (4): W259–W272.

3. Kealy, J. (1987). *Diagnostic Radiology of the Dog and Cat.* Philadelphia, PA: WB Saunders.

4. Robert, H.W. (2000). Malignant versus nonmalignant bone disease. *Vet. Clin. North Am. Small Anim. Pract.* 30 (2): 315–347.

5. Forrest, L.J. and Thrall, D.E. (1994). Bone scintigraphy for metastasis detection in canine osteosarcoma. *Vet. Radiol. Ultrasound* 35 (2): 124–130.

6. Amsellem, P.M., Selmic, L.E., Wypij, J.M. et al. (2014). Appendicular osteosarcoma in small-breed dogs: 51 cases (1986–2011). *J. Am. Vet. Med. Assoc.* 245 (2): 203–210.

7. Cooley, D.M. and Waters, D.J. (1997). Skeletal neoplasms of small dogs: a retrospective study and literature review. *J. Am. Anim. Hosp. Assoc.* 33 (1): 11–23.

8. Quigley, P.J. and Leedale, A.H. (1983). Tumors involving bone in the domestic cat: a review of fifty-eight cases. *Vet. Pathol. Online* 20 (6): 670–686.

9. Heldmann, E., Anderson, M., and Wagner-Mann, C. (2000). Feline osteosarcoma: 145 cases (1990–1995). *J. Am. Anim. Hosp. Assoc.* 36 (6): 518–521.

10. Farese, J.P., Kirpensteijn, J., Kik, M. et al. (2009). Biologic behavior and clinical outcome of 25 dogs with canine appendicular chondrosarcoma treated by amputation: a Veterinary Society of Surgical Oncology Retrospective Study. *Vet. Surg.* 38 (8): 914–919.

11. Waltman, S.S., Seguin, B., Cooper, B.J., and Kent, M. (2007). Clinical outcome of nonnasal chondrosarcoma in dogs: thirty-one cases (1986–2003). *Vet. Surg.* 36 (3): 266–271.

12. Withrow, S.J. and Vail, D.M. (2006). *Withrow and MacEwen's Small Animal Clinical Oncology,* 4e, 540–582. Philadelphia, PA: Saunders.

13. Morgan, J.P., Med, V., Ackerman, N. et al. (1980). Vertebral tumors in the dog: a clinical radiologic, and pathologic study of 61 primary and secondary lesions. *Vet. Radiol.* 21 (5): 197–212.

14. Lipsitz, D., Levitski, R.E., and Berry, W.L. (2001). Magnetic resonance imaging features of multilobular osteochondrosarcoma in 3 dogs. *Vet. Radiol. Ultrasound* 42 (1): 14–19.

15. Rusbridge, C., Wheeler, S.J., Lamb, C.R. et al. (1999). Vertebral plasma cell tumors in 8 dogs. *J. Vet. Intern. Med.* 13 (2): 126–133.

16. Matus, R.E., Leifer, C.E., MacEwen, E.G., and Hurvitz, A.I. (1986). Prognostic factors for multiple myeloma in the dog. *J. Am. Vet. Med. Assoc.* 188 (11): 1288–1292.

17. Osborne, C.A., Perman, V., Sautter, J.H. et al. (1968). Multiple myeloma in the dog. *J. Am. Vet. Med. Assoc.* 153 (10): 1300–1319.

18. MacEwen, E.G. and Hurvitz, A.I. (1977). Diagnosis and management of monoclonal gammopathies. *Vet. Clin. North Am.* 7 (1): 119–132.

19. Bartels, J.E., Cawley, A.J., McSherry, B.J., and Percy, D.H. (1972). Multiple myeloma (Plasmacytoma) in a dog. *Vet. Radiol.* 13: 36–42.

20. Craig, L.E., Julian, M.E., and Ferracone, J.D. (2002). The diagnosis and prognosis of synovial tumors in dogs: 35 cases. *Vet. Pathol.* 39 (1): 66–73.

21. Klahn, S.L., Kitchell, B.E., and Dervisis, N.G. (2011). Evaluation and comparison of outcomes in dogs with periarticular and non-periarticular histiocytic sarcoma. *J. Am. Vet. Med. Assoc.* 239 (1): 90–96.

22. Berrettoni, B.A. and Carter, J.R. (1986). Mechanisms of cancer metastasis to bone. *J. Bone Joint Surg. Am.* 68 (2): 308–312.

23. Nguyen, D.X., Bos, P.D., and Massagué, J. (2009). Metastasis: from dissemination to organ-specific colonization. *Nat. Rev. Cancer* 9 (4): 274–284.

24. Trost, M.E., Inkelmann, M.A., Galiza, G.J.N. et al. (2014). Occurrence of tumours metastatic to bones and multicentric tumours with skeletal involvement in dogs. *J. Comp. Pathol.* 150 (1): 8–17.

25. Vanel, M., Blond, L., and Vanel, D. (2013). Imaging of primary bone tumors in veterinary medicine: which differences? *Eur. J. Radiol.* 82 (12): 2129–2139.

26. Turrel, J.M. and Pool, R.R. (1982). Primary bone tumors in the cat. *Vet. Radiol.* 23 (4): 152–166.

27. Owen, L.N. and Bostock, D.E. (1971). Multiple cartilaginous exostoses with development of a metastasizing osteosarcoma in a Shetland sheepdog. *J. Small Anim. Pract.* 12 (9): 507–512.

28. Green, E.M., Adams, W.M., and Steinberg, H. (1999). Malignant transformation of solitary spinal osteochondroma in two mature dogs. *Vet. Radiol. Ultrasound* 40 (6): 634–637.

29. Choate, C.J. and Arnold, G.A. (2011). Elbow arthrodesis following a pathological fracture in a dog with bilateral humeral bone cysts. *Vet. Comp. Orthop. Traumatol.* 24 (5): 398–401.

30. Vignoli, M., Stehlik, L., Terragni, R. et al. (2015). Computed tomography-guided cementoplasty combined with radiation therapy for an aneurysmal bone cyst in a dog: a case report. *Vet. Med.* 60 (2): 109–114.

31. Shimada, A., Yanagida, M., Umemura, T., and Tsukamoto, S. (1996). Aneurysmal bone cyst in a dog. *J. Vet. Med. Sci.* 58 (10): 1037–1038.

32. Sarierler, M., Cullu, E., Yurekli, Y., and Birincioglu, S. (2004). Bone cement treatment for aneurysmal bone cyst in a dog. *J. Vet. Med. Sci.* 66 (9): 1137–1142.

33. Siqueira, E.G.M., Rahal, S.C., Ribeiro, M.G. et al. (2014). Exogenous bacterial osteomyelitis in 52 dogs: a retrospective study of etiology and in vitro antimicrobial susceptibility profile (2000–2013). *Vet. Q.* 34 (4): 201–204.

34. Greene, C.E. and Budsberg, S.C. (2006). *Musculoskeletal Infections. Infectious Diseases of the Dog and Cat*, 3e, 823–841. St Louis, MO: Saunders Elsevier.

35. Carrera, I., Sullivan, M., McConnell, F., and Gonçalves, R. (2011). Magnetic resonance imaging features of discospondylitis in dogs. *Vet. Radiol. Ultrasound* 52 (2): 125–131.

36. Gendron, K., Doherr, M.G., Gavin, P., and Lang, J. (2012). Magnetic resonance imaging characterization of vertebral endplate changes in the dog. *Vet. Radiol. Ultrasound* 53 (1): 50–56.

37. Voges, A.K., Neuwirth, L., Thompson, J.P., and Ackerman, N. (1996). Radiographic changes associated with digital, metacarpal and metatarsal tumors, and pododermatitis in the dog. *Vet. Radiol. Ultrasound* 37 (5): 327–335.

38. Goldfinch, N. and Argyle, D.J. (2012). Feline lung-digit syndrome: unusual metastatic patterns of primary lung tumours in cats. *J. Feline Med. Surg.* 14 (3): 202–208.

39. Rabillard, M., Souchu, L., Niebauer, G.W., and Gauthier, O. (2011). Haematogenous osteomyelitis: clinical presentation and outcome in three dogs. *Vet. Comp. Orthop. Traumatol.* 24 (2): 146–150.

40. Whalen, J.L., Fitzgerald, R.H., and Morrissy, R.T. (1988). A histological study of acute hematogenous osteomyelitis following physeal injuries in rabbits. *J. Bone Joint Surg.* 70 (9): 1383–1392.

41. Berry, W.L. and Leisewitz, A.L. (1996). Multifocal aspergillus terreus discospondylitis in two German shepherd dogs. *J. S. Afr. Vet. Assoc.* 67 (4): 222–228.

42. Potter, T.M. and Macintire, D.K. (2010). Hepatozoon americanum: an emerging disease in the south-central/southeastern United States. *J. Vet. Emerg. Crit. Care* 20 (1): 70–76.

43. Drost, W.M., Cummings, C.A., Mathew, J.S. et al. (2003). Determination of time of onset and location of early skeletal lesions in young dogs experimentally infected with *Hepatozoon americanum* using bone scintigraphy. *Vet. Radiol. Ultrasound* 44 (1): 86–91.

# CHAPTER 11

# Imaging of the Head

Nathan C. Nelson

Department of Molecular Biomedical Sciences, College of Veterinary Medicine, North Carolina State University, Raleigh, NC, USA

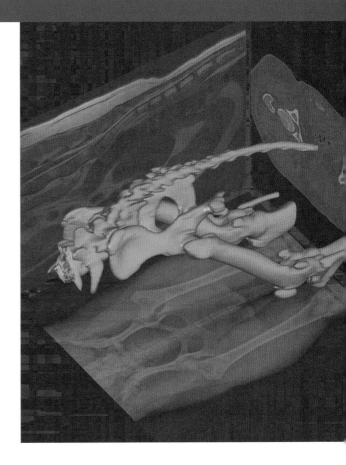

## Choice of Modality

More than any other body region, when contemplating an imaging study of the head, the clinician should ask, "What question needs to be answered?" The choice of imaging modality depends on whether the suspected disease process involves osseous or soft tissue structures, the location of the affected structures in the head, and the availability and cost of different imaging modalities.

Radiographs are a useful initial diagnostic test for suspected osseous pathology, as radiography is more widely available in general veterinary practice and has a lower financial cost. Radiographs provide a rapid global survey of the skull in cases of head trauma and identify major fractures or dislocations. They can serve as an initial imaging test for intranasal pathology, but superimposition of the osseous structures of the nasal cavity complicates interpretation. Skull morphology is complex, and requires careful positioning for radiographs,

as even slight obliquity of the patient will significantly limit diagnostic interpretation of osseous structures.

In comparison, computed tomography (CT) and magnetic resonance imaging (MRI) are more sensitive and specific tests for imaging of the head. Generally, CT is the preferred imaging test for intranasal pathology, as it is rapid and provides good contrast resolution between gas, osseous structures, and soft tissue pathology. MRI is the preferred test for intracalvarial disease and disease affecting neurologic structures, as it has superior soft tissue contrast resolution compared to CT. The continued increase in availability of CT and MRI, along with their superior imaging abilities, explains the decrease in skull radiography in recent years at major referral centers though radiography of the head remains common in general practice.

Ultrasound is the preferred first-line imaging test for superficial soft tissue pathology in the head. The eye and structures in the ventral neck (such as the thyroid lobes, lymph nodes, and salivary glands) are readily accessible to ultrasound imaging. Additionally, only mild sedation or manual restraint alone is typically sufficient to complete an ultrasound examination of these areas, providing a more reasonable cost to the client compared to CT or MRI. Surrounding osseous anatomy prevents ultrasound evaluation of intranasal or intra-calvarial soft tissue diseases.

Dental imaging requires high resolution given the small size of teeth in canine/feline patients. Dental pathology may be relatively subtle and affects small anatomic structures. Standard digital radiography detectors, such as the type used for abdominal/thoracic radiographs, may not provide the high-resolution imaging necessary to detect subtle dental disease. Additionally, the large size of standard digital radiography detectors limits detector positioning around the head. Ideally, dental radiography is performed with dedicated dental digital imaging plates, which are much smaller than standard digital

plates, allowing intraoral positioning of the plate. Additionally, dental digital plates are also higher resolution than standard digital imaging systems, allowing optimal diagnostic ability of dental pathology.

Cone beam CT units are becoming more common in veterinary practice. Cone beam CT units produce cross-sectional images similar to standard CT units, but have higher spatial resolution, making them ideal for dental imaging (Figure 11.1). Cone beam CT units have limited contrast resolution, providing inadequate imaging of soft tissue structures of the head. They scan more slowly than traditional CT scanners, making them especially sensitive to patient motion artifacts (Figure 11.2). For these reasons, their use should be limited to evaluating dental or other osseous structure of the head and not for evaluation of soft tissue pathology.

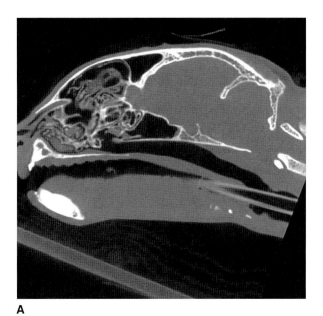

**A**

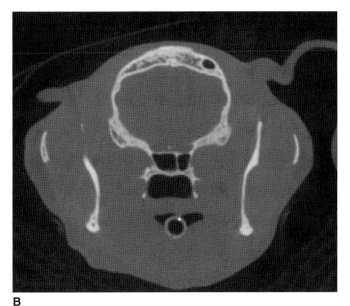

**B**

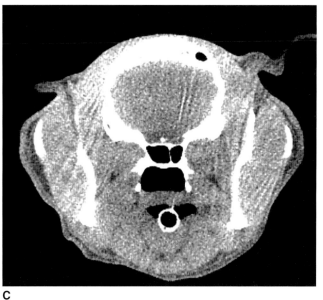

**C**

**FIGURE 11.1**   Cone beam CT images in a cat in a sagittal bone window (**A**), transverse bone window (**B**) and soft tissue window (**C**). Note the fine osseous detail on the bone window/level images, but poor soft tissue contrast.

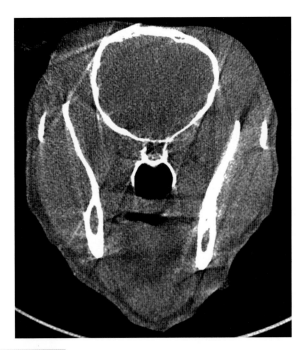

**FIGURE 11.2**   Cone beam CT image showing numerous streak artifacts related to mild patient motion.

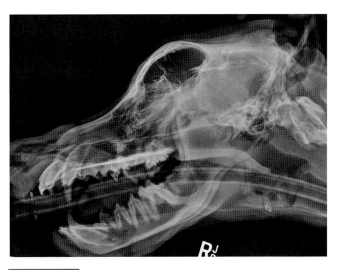

**FIGURE 11.3**   Well-positioned normal lateral skull. Note the near complete superimposition of the right and left maxilla, mandible, and bullae. An endotracheal tube is present as the patient is anesthetized; this greatly facilitates patient positioning.

# Imaging Protocols

## Radiography

High-quality, diagnostic radiographs of the head require careful patient positioning. Ventrodorsal projections are particularly important for intranasal pathology. Comparison between the left and right nasal cavities on the VD projection facilitates identification of subtle, unilateral abnormalities which disrupt left/right nasal symmetry. Left/right comparison is only possible when the patient is straight and the left/right nasal cavities are symmetrically positioned, which can be challenging or impossible in the awake patient.

Some areas of the skull require specialized oblique projections for complete evaluation (as discussed below), and may result in the patient discomfort if performed when the patient is awake. Strong sedation or anesthesia allows careful patient positioning, prevents patient discomfort, and is required for skull radiographic procedures.

Due to the complex skull anatomy, there are many potential radiographic projections that may be employed to "pick off" or accentuate a particular area of interest. A standard skull examination may include some or all of these projections. The following skull projections are available.

### Lateral Projection
The patient is placed in either a right or left lateral recumbent position, and x-rays traverse the patient lateromedially. This projection shows alignment of the maxilla and mandible, and generally provides an overview of skull morphology (Figure 11.3).

### Closed Mouth Ventrodorsal Projection
The patient is placed in dorsal recumbency and x-rays transverse the patient from ventral to dorsal. This projection is useful to display left/right alignment of the mandible with the skull and for evaluating congruency of the temporomandibular joints (TMJs) (Figure 11.4). Superimposition of the mandible with the nasal cavity limits the ability to interpret intranasal pathology on this projection.

### Open Mouth Ventrodorsal Projection
This projection is performed with the patient in dorsal recumbency. The mandible is maximally retracted (often using gauze or other material) and the x-ray beam is directed through the nasal cavity without superimposition of the mandible. This projection is the most useful to diagnose pathology in the nasal passage (Figure 11.4). If the patient is anesthetized, the endotracheal tube should be distracted to the side to prevent superimposition with the nasal cavity.

### Frontal Sinus Skyline Projection
The patient is placed in dorsal recumbency. The neck is flexed, so that the rostral tip of the nose is directed toward the x-ray tube, with x-rays directed in a rostral to caudal direction. This projection is useful for showing pathology within the frontal sinus (Figure 11.5).

### Left 45° Ventral-Right Dorsal Oblique and Right 45° Ventral-Left Dorsal Oblique
These are often referred to as "45° oblique projections." With the patient in a laterally recumbent position, the head is rotated in one direction along its axis. The x-ray beam is then directed at an approximately 45° angle relative to the nasal cavity from left ventral to right dorsal and vice versa (Figure 11.6). The orthogonal (opposite 45°) projection is then acquired by rotation of the head in the other direction

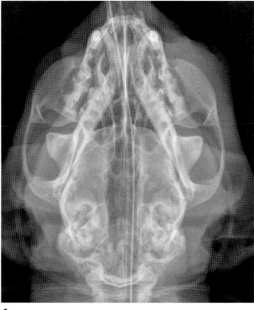 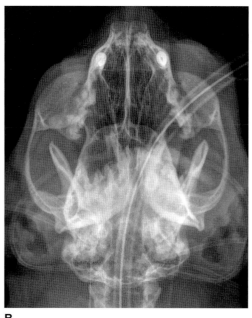

**A**   **B**

**FIGURE 11.4**  Closed mouth (**A**) and open mouth (**B**) ventrodorsal projections of the skull. Note the turbinates are seen in (**B**) but not (**A**) due to superimposition of the mandible. The endotracheal tube is also pulled to the side in (**B**).

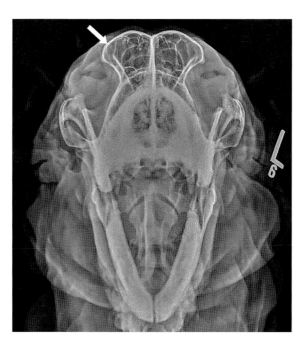

**FIGURE 11.5**  Normal frontal sinus skyline projection showing the gas-filled frontal sinuses (the right frontal sinus is indicated by an arrow).

along its long axis. These projections are useful for overall survey of the maxilla, but also useful when evaluating the bullae as one will be more ventrally located on each oblique, allowing evaluation without other osseous superimposition.

## Left 10° Rostral-Right Caudal Oblique and Right 10° Rostral-Left Caudal Oblique [1]

These are often referred to as the "TMJ oblique projections." They

show the TMJs in a lateral-type position, without superimposition of the contralateral side. Starting with the patient in a lateral recumbent position, the nose is slightly elevated (approximately 10°) from the radiographic table (Figure 11.7). This places one TMJ rostral to the other. The patient is then placed in the opposite recumbency and the same procedure followed to provide a projection of the contralateral TMJ.

## Bulla Projections

Though the 45° oblique projections and ventrodorsal projections allow evaluation of the bullae, additional projections may be performed when middle or inner ear disease is suspected. In both dogs and cats, the patient is placed in dorsal recumbency. The neck is flexed, and the mouth opened; the x-ray beam is then directed in a rostral to caudal direction through the mouth, highlighting the bullae. In the cat, an alternative projection is available. Rather than opening the mouth, the neck may be slightly less flexed, resulting in an approximately 10° ventral angulation of the x-ray beam relative to the nasal planum (Figure 11.8).

As the head is symmetric, images must be labeled with indicators for sidedness. On ventrodorsal and rostrocaudal projections, a single L or R indicator is sufficient to unambiguously label the side of the head. On oblique images, double simultaneous marking with both L and R indicators leaves no question as to which is left and which is right anatomy (Figure 11.6).

Typically, closed mouth ventrodorsal and lateral projections are the minimum requirements for a study of the skull, but additional projections are recommended depending on the clinical question to answer (Figure 11.9). Below are recommended imaging protocols for each area of interest.

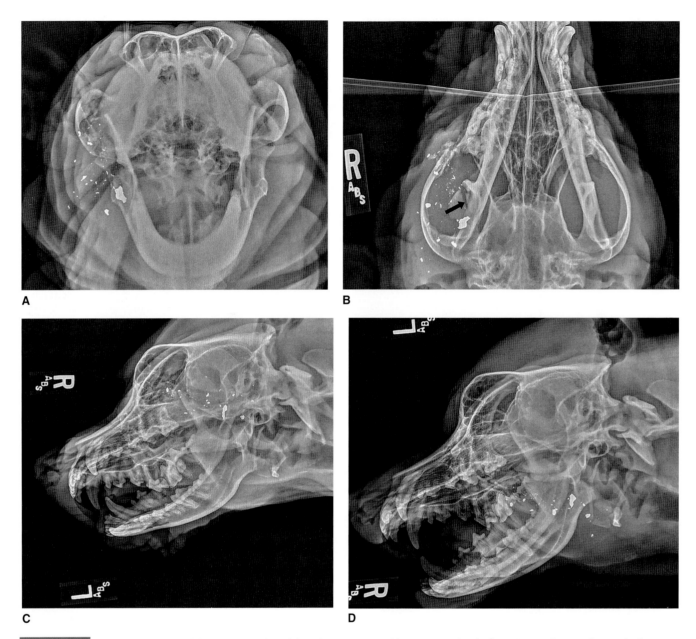

**FIGURE 11.6** Frontal sinus skyline (**A**), closed mouth VD (**B**), and opposite 45° oblique images (**C,D**) of a patient with a gunshot to the face. Note that the mandibular ramus fracture is only readily visible on the VD projection (arrow). Note also that on oblique images, both L and R markers are included so there is no ambiguity as to what is right- versus left-sided anatomy. Numerous metallic remnants from a ballistic projectile remain within the tissues of the right side of the head.

**Nasal Disease** Closed mouth ventrodorsal projection, open mouth ventrodorsal projection, lateral projection, orthogonal 45° projections, frontal sinus skyline projection.

**Middle Ear Disease** Closed mouth ventrodorsal projection, lateral projection, left/right 45° orthogonal projections, rostrocaudal bulla projection.

**TMJs** Lateral projection, closed mouth ventrodorsal projection, left/right temporomandibular oblique projections.

**Routine Trauma Survey** Lateral, closed mouth ventrodorsal projection, orthogonal 45° projections.

## Computed Tomography

Where available, CT has largely replaced skull radiography as the preferred modality for imaging the skull or nasal cavity. Indications for head CT are broad, with scanning commonly performed in patients with epistaxis or chronic/recurrent intranasal symptoms, masses anywhere in the head (outside the brain), oral tumors, swelling in the laryngeal/pharyngeal reason, or retrobulbar disease.

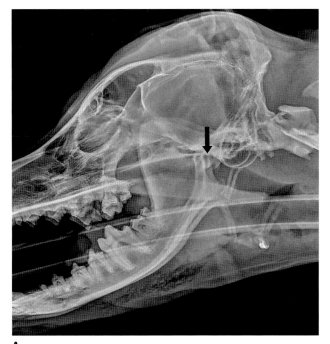

**A**

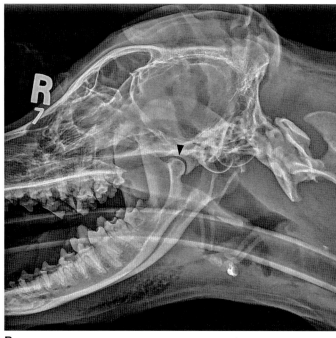

**B**

**FIGURE 11.7**   Lateral (**A**) and (**B**) 10° rostral TMJ oblique projection of the temporomandibular joint. Note the TMJs are superimposed on the lateral image (arrow), but one is projected rostrally and well seen on the oblique image (arrowhead).

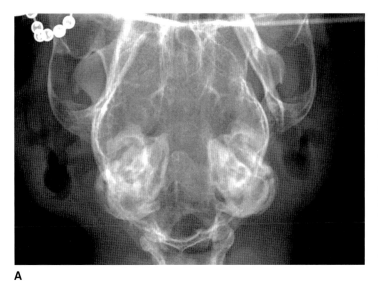

**A**

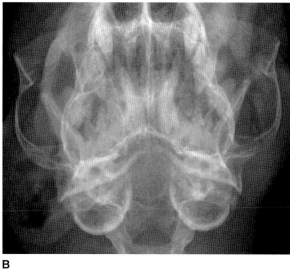

**B**

**FIGURE 11.8**   Ventrodorsal projection (**A**) and 10° ventral bulla oblique (**B**) projections in a cat. Not that the oblique image displays the bullae with less superimposition of the skull. The bullae are bilaterally thickened and contain fluid (are less gas filled than normal).

Imaging before and after the administration of intravenous iodinated contrast is standard, except in cases of trauma when surveying for osseous abnormalities. Scanning after the administration of intravenous contrast improves the visibility of most soft tissue pathology, and is particularly important when evaluating intracranial lesions if MRI is not available. When scanning for disease within the oral cavity or pharyngeal region, the mouth should be opened, which helps separate soft tissues of the oral and laryngeal regions. Compression on the ventral head/neck should be avoided, as it can distort regional anatomy.

## Magnetic Resonance Imaging

Magnetic resonance imaging provides superior contrast resolution of soft tissue structures, and is preferred over CT when imaging the brain. Though MRI can image other structures of the head, such as the nasal or oral cavity, the increased time and cost of MRI compared to CT mean that it is rarely used for other purposes (Figure 11.10). Additionally, MRI artifacts at gas–soft tissue interfaces interfere with evaluation of structures in the nasal cavity and airway.

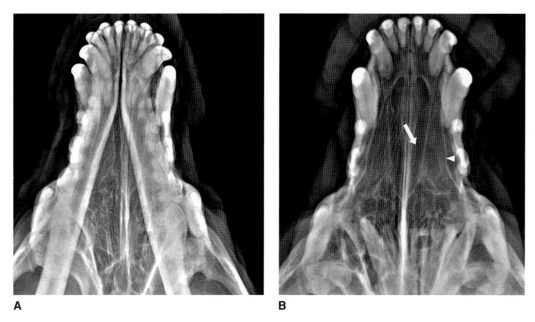

**A**    **B**

**FIGURE 11.9**    Closed mouth VD (**A**) and open mouth VD (**B**) projections of the maxillary region in a dog with unilateral *Aspergillus* rhinitis. Note that there is mild turbinate loss (arrow) and soft tissue thickening (arrowhead) on the left nasal cavity not seen when the mandible is closed. Inclusion of the open mouth VD projection is critical to diagnosis. The closed mouth VD projection is also slightly oblique (note the mandibular symphysis is not aligned with the nasal septum). This further superimposes the left mandible with the left nasal cavity, further hindering diagnosis.

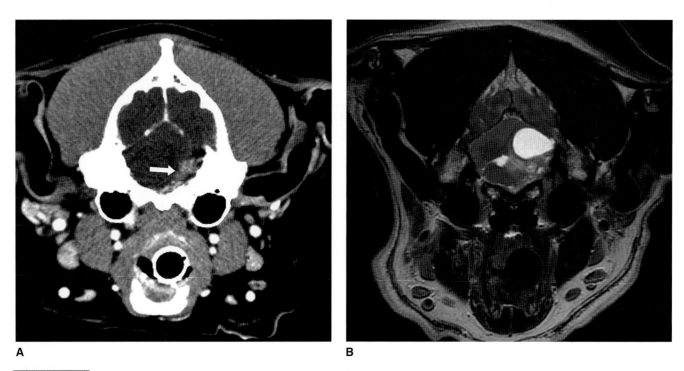

**A**    **B**

**FIGURE 11.10**    Transverse CT (**A**) and MRI (**B**) images of a cystic meningioma within the caudal skull. There is mild contrast enhancement of the mass on the CT images (arrow), but the cystic nature of the mass is much more apparent on the MRI and it is much larger than appreciated on the CT images.

## Ultrasound

Ultrasound is infrequently used in head imaging compared to other modalities, and is primarily used to investigate the ventral soft tissues of the head or in cases of ocular pathology.

The osseous structures of the skull block ultrasound beam transmission, so it can only be used for intracranial evaluation in neonatal patients (where the open sutures are used as acoustic windows) or in patients with persistent open fontanelles (Figure 11.11).

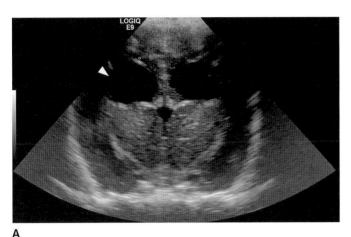

**A**

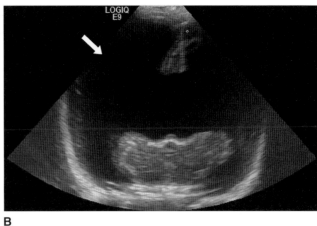

**B**

**FIGURE 11.11**   Ultrasound images of a normal brain (**A**) and brain with hydrocephalus (**B**). Note the distended lateral ventricles in the patient with hydrocephalus (arrow) compared to their normal size in (**A**) (arrowhead).

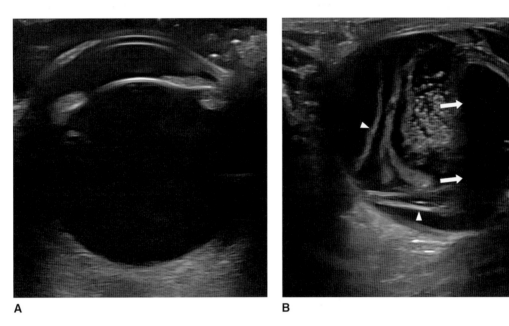

**FIGURE 11.12**   Ultrasound images of a normal eye (**A**) and dog with cataracts and retinal detachment (**B**). In the patient with cataracts, the affected lens causes distal acoustic shadowing (arrows) due to mineralization in the lens. The detached retina (arrowhead) attaches at the posterior aspect of the globe.

Ultrasound is ideally suited for imaging of the eye and readily identifies structures such as the cornea, lens, iris, and posterior chamber. The cornea is anesthetized through topical medications. The ultrasound transducer is placed directly on the cornea (coupled with sterile ultrasound gel) or on the closed eyelids. Light sedation limits patient movement, though many patients will allow imaging without sedation and only manual restraint.

Indications for ocular ultrasound are many. Patients with cataracts are imaged to ensure lack of retinal separation prior to phacoemulsification (Figure 11.12). Ocular trauma or acute onset of hyphema are indications for ultrasound to evaluate for ocular damage, lens luxation, or masses that are otherwise obscured from direct examination by the presence of intra-ocular blood (Figure 11.13). Intraocular tumors are readily

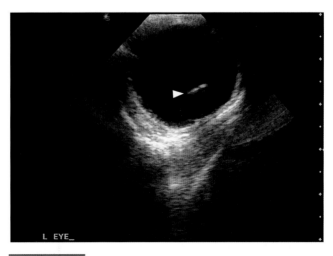

**FIGURE 11.13**   Ultrasound image of a lens luxation. The lens (arrowhead) is displaced to the posterior aspect of the globe.

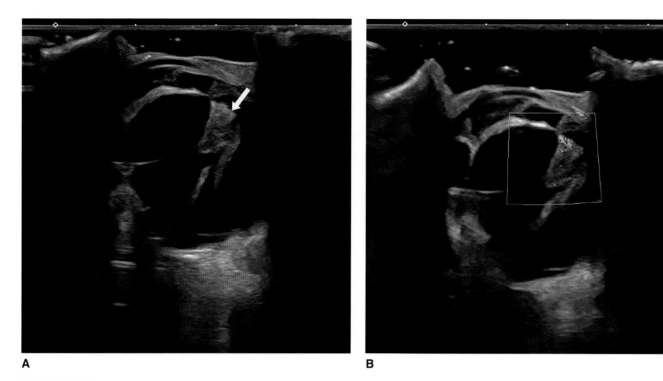

A

B

**FIGURE 11.14**  Ultrasound images of a uveal neoplasm without (**A**) and with (**B**) Doppler ultrasound. There is thickening of the iris and ciliary body (arrow). The blue indicates blood flow in the mass on the Doppler image.

identified on ocular ultrasound and the tissue of origin may be identified (Figure 11.14).

Retrobulbar ultrasound is performed in cases of exoph-thalmos or when a retrobulbar mass or inflammation is suspected. The globe may be used as an acoustic window to investigate the retrobulbar space, though approaches dorsal or ventral to the zygomatic arch allow imaging posterior to the globe as well.

Other areas of the head and neck, primarily around the pharyngeal/laryngeal region, are accessible to ultrasound imaging. When examining this region, a routine methodology is followed to identify the following structures: medial retropha-ryngeal and mandibular lymph nodes, carotid artery, thyroid lobes, mandibular salivary glands, esophagus, trachea, laryn-geal tissues.

# Specific Diseases of the Head/Skull

## Nasal Diseases

The goal of imaging with radiographs, CT, or MRI is to determine whether nasal disease is more likely to be inflammatory (some form of rhinitis) or neoplastic in origin, and the extent of disease [2]. While radiographs may provide this information, CT or MRI better define the boundary of nasal pathology, and allow a more definitive or specific prioritized differential diagnosis list.

**Rhinitis**  There are many causes of nasal inflammation, including infectious rhinitis, immune-mediated rhinitis, and for-eign body rhinitis, though many cases are idiopathic in nature. Rhinitis typically results in bilateral increase in soft tissue within the nasal cavity, without destruction of the turbinates or surrounding bones. Fine turbinate detail is retained but with chronic rhinitis, mild turbinate atrophy may occur. Concurrent sinusitis causes mild fluid accumulation within the sinuses and/or thin soft tissue thickening along the luminal margin of the sinus due to inflamed or hyperplastic sinus mucosa.

The appearance of *Aspergillus* rhinitis in dogs is unique, and does not conform to the description of other causes of rhi-nitis described above. While *Aspergillus* does cause increased opacity in the nasal cavity, it also causes extensive turbinate lysis (Figure 11.15) and tends to be unilateral. Unlike neo-plasia (which also causes turbinate lysis), the turbinate loss due to *Aspergillus* is more multifocal, resulting in larger gas-filled voids throughout the nasal cavity. A solitary, large mass is not present but instead, the soft tissue thickening is more peripheral among the margins of the nasal cavity and along the residual turbinates. Fungal plaques in the frontal sinuses are common, and appear as heterogeneous mixed gas and fluid (unlike other causes of sinusitis where the thickening is homo-geneous). The frontal sinus skyline projection in particular is useful to identify these changes. Other less common fungal agents may also cause rhinitis, and can appear mass-like or more diffuse [3].

Fungal rhinitis in cats is rare, but *Aspergillus* and *Cryp-tococcus* are most common and appear as a solitary mass or more diffuse disease (Figure 11.16) [4].

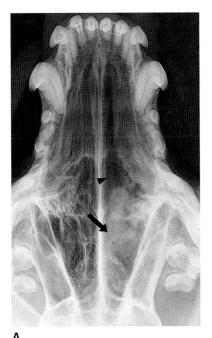
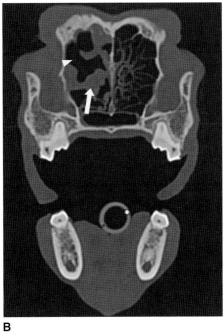
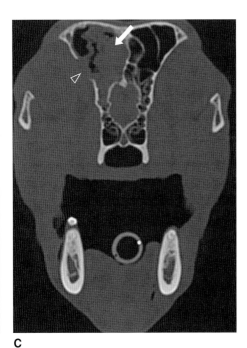

**A**                    **B**                    **C**

**FIGURE 11.15**  Open mouth ventrodorsal radiograph (**A**), transverse midnasal CT image (**B**), and transverse caudal nasal CT image (**C**) of a dog with *Aspergillus* rhinitis. There is soft tissue in the caudal nasal cavity on radiographs and CT (arrow), with large gas-filled areas of turbinate loss (closed arrowhead). There is peripheral bone loss not seen on radiographs (open arrowhead).

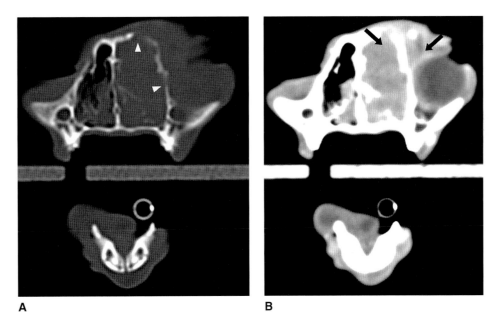

**A**                    **B**

**FIGURE 11.16**  Transverse CT images of a cat with cryptococcus fungal disease within the left nasal cavity in a bone window/level (**A**) and soft tissue window/level (**B**). There is a large contrast-enhancing mass (arrows) extending into the retrobulbar space, causing lysis of the adjacent maxillary bone (arrowhead).

**Nasal Foreign Bodies**  Foreign body rhinitis typically localizes around the foreign body, resulting in a more focal and unilateral abnormality compared to other causes of rhinitis (Figure 11.17). The rostral nasal cavity is typically affected, as the nasal aperture is the point of entry for most foreign bodies (Figure 11.18). The foreign body establishes conditions ideal for secondary *Aspergillus* infection, which can result in more extensive turbinate lysis in the area of the foreign body. Unless

mineral or metallic, the foreign body is not often easily identified, particularly for small foreign bodies such as plant material (grass) or other soft tissue material (such as nasal parasites) (Figure 11.19).

**Nasal Neoplasia**  Neoplasms arise from the soft tissues or osseous structures of the nasal cavity. There is a wide variety of tumor types reported, with epithelial origin (carcinoma)

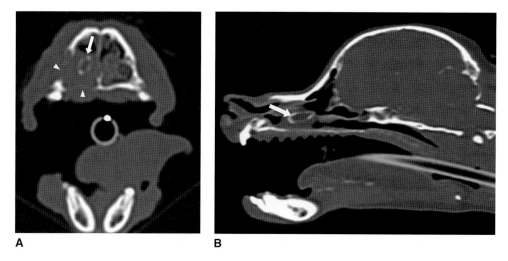

**FIGURE 11.17** Transverse (**A**) and sagittal (**B**) CT images of a patient with a nasal foreign body (a plant seed). Note the nasal foreign body is mineral attenuating (arrow) and has surrounding soft tissue thickening and lysis of the palate and maxillary bones (arrowhead).

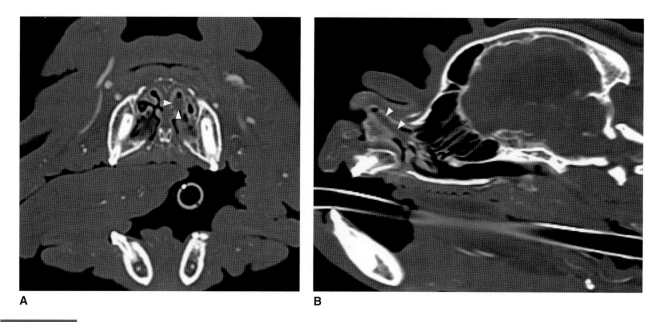

**FIGURE 11.18** Transverse (**A**) and sagittal (**B**) CT postcontrast images showing a subtle stick nasal foreign body. A thin linear soft tissue attenuating structure (arrowheads) extends caudally into the nasal cavity. This was more obvious on postcontrast images.

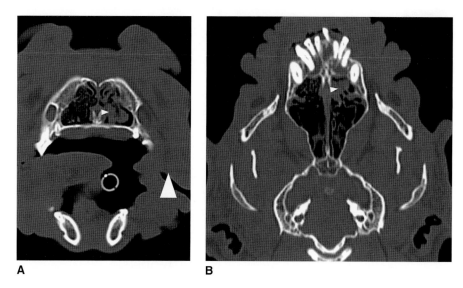

**FIGURE 11.19** Transverse (**A**) and sagittal (**B**) CT images of a patient with a foreign body (piece of grass) where there is regional soft tissue thickening (arrowheads) but the foreign body itself is not identified.

being the most common tumor type in dogs (up to 75% of cases), but tumors arising from connective tissue (sarcomas) are also common. Lymphoma, osseous tumors, and other uncommon tumor types (such as leiomyoma and transmissible veneral tumor) also occur [5–7].

Most nasal neoplasms result in a solid, solitary mass that causes local turbinate destruction (Figures 11.20 and 11.9). If the mass become very large, it causes lysis of the larger osseous structures surrounding the nasal cavity, such as the nasal or maxillary bones, but this tends to be reserved for only the largest, most advanced masses. Commonly, there will be a large amount of fluid among the remaining turbinates due to secondary hemorrhage or rhinitis. Large masses trap fluid caudally in the nasal cavity or frontal sinus due to obstruction of nasal drainage.

Most nasal tumors (carcinomas, sarcomas) do not have unique features that allow further differentiation of tumor type,

though some have unique characteristics that can be identified on CT. For instance, nasal chondrosarcoma typically has patchy mineral regions within it, a feature not expected in carcinomas [8]. Nasal lymphoma may be a solitary mass but tends to be more widespread than other nasal tumors and can cause mild diffuse thickening that mimics rhinitis (Figure 11.21). Tumors (e.g., osteosarcoma) arising from the larger bones surrounding the nasal cavity are centered on the osseous structures rather than within the nasal cavity. Olfactory neuroblastomas are uncommon tumors that arise from the sensory neuroendocrine olfactory cells in the upper part of the nasal cavity. These center on the cribriform plate with invasion into the cranial vault and caudal nasal cavity (Figure 11.22) [9]. Most of these features are not distinguishable on radiography, but readily are identified on CT, allowing more specific prioritization of neoplastic differential diagnoses [10].

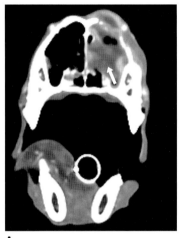
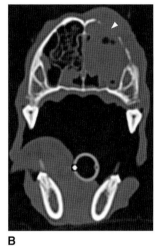
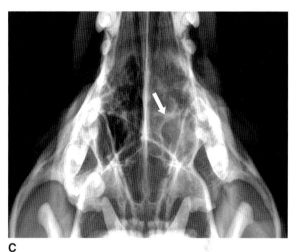

**A**    **B**    **C**

**FIGURE 11.20**  Transverse soft tissue window/level (**A**) CT image, bone window/level (**B**) CT image, and open mouth VD projection (**C**) of a dog with nasal adenocarcinoma. There is a soft tissue mass causing regional turbinate lysis (arrow). The soft tissue thickening and bone loss are more apparent on the CT than the radiographs. The maxillary bone loss (arrowhead) was only visible on CT images.

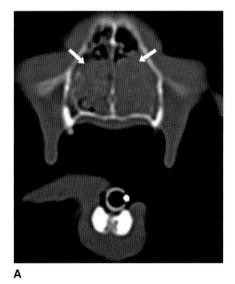
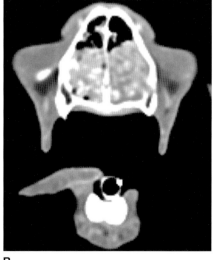

**A**    **B**

**FIGURE 11.21**  Transverse bone window/level (**A**) and soft tissue window/level (**B**) CT of a cat with diffuse nasal lymphoma. There is diffuse soft tissue thickening (arrows) through the left and right nasal cavity, but no turbinate lysis. This appearance mimics rhinitis.

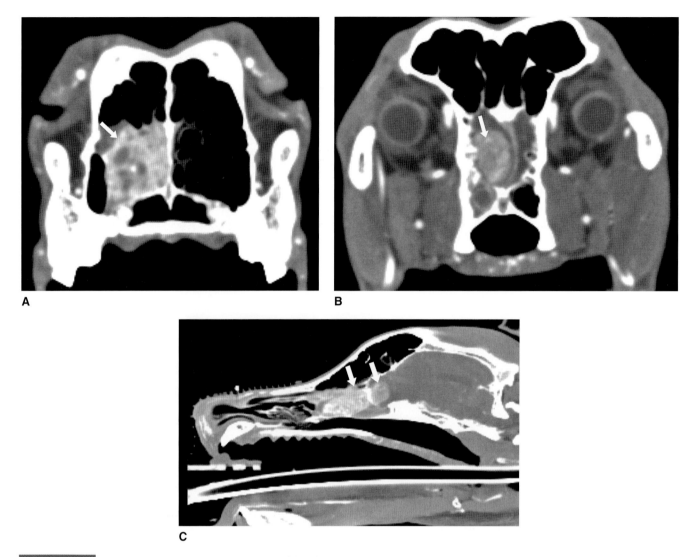

**A**

**B**

**C**

**FIGURE 11.22** Transverse CT images at the nasal cavity (**A**) and rostral brain (**B**) with a sagittal image (**C**) in a patient with a neuroblastoma centered on the cribriform plate. Note that the mass (arrows) extends into the nasal cavity as well as into the olfactory region of the brain.

CT allows assessment of draining lymph nodes in cases with nasal neoplasia, which can guide the decision on whether to sample them for complete staging purposes. CT lacks specificity to distinguish inflammatory/reactive lymph nodes from neoplastic lymph nodes, so ultimately image-guided aspiration and cytologic/histopathologic evaluation may be necessary to make the final determination [11].

Though MRI can be used to image nasal neoplastic disease, it is less commonly employed compared to CT, due to the necessity of general anesthesia, greater cost, and longer scan times. MRI provides additional information about structures that are difficult to assess on CT, such as reactive meningeal changes surrounding a tumor or bone marrow involvement of the calvarium [12] (Figure 11.23).

### Intranasal Epidermoid Cysts

Intranasal epidermoid cysts are rare causes of mass effects within the nasal cavity of brachycephalic dogs. They have a characteristic appearance on CT and MRI, being entirely fluid attenuating on CT or

homogenously fluid hyperintense on MRI (Figure 11.24). They cause resorption of adjacent osseous structures via pressure necrosis [13].

## Retrobulbar Diseases

Patients with retrobulbar disease often present with a complaint of exophthalmos or loss of vision. Ultrasound is a useful first-line imaging test in these patients given its accessibility, speed, and ease of use. Because deeper tissues are imaged, a microconvex transducer is more useful than a linear transducer. Multiple imaging approaches are available to examine the retrobulbar tissues. The globe can be used as a standoff, imaging the deeper retrobulbar tissues through the globe. Approaches dorsal to the globe (just above the upper eyelid) or just dorsal or ventral to the zygomatic arch provide a more complete retrobulbar examination. The osseous orbit limits ultrasound examination by preventing evaluation of the most medial aspect of the retrobulbar space, so

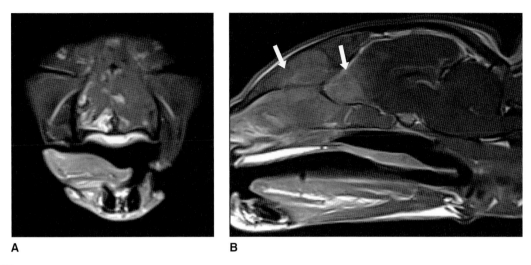

**FIGURE 11.23**   Transverse (**A**) and sagittal (**B**) postcontrast T1-weighted MRI image of a cat with nasal lymphoma extending into the calvarium. This causes diffuse soft tissue thickening in the left and right nasal cavities and also extends into the brain (arrow).

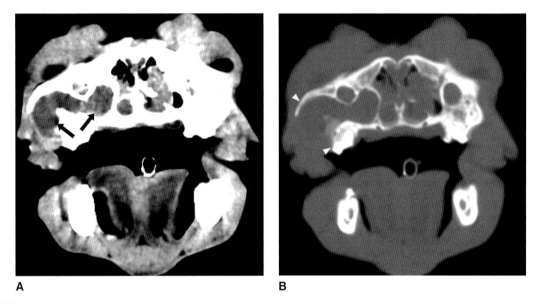

**FIGURE 11.24**   Transverse soft/tissue window (**A**) and bone window/level (**B**) CT image of a patient with an epidermoid cyst. There is a cyst-like lesion (arrow) within the right maxillary bone causing regional bony expansion and thinning (between arrowheads).

ultimately CT or MRI may be necessary for further examination if ultrasound is unsuccessful in identifying the cause of clinical signs.

External puncture wounds or wounds extending from the oral cavity into the retrobulbar region from oral or external foreign body puncture cause retrobulbar abscesses (Figure 11.25). Foreign material often causes distal acoustic shadowing on ultrasound, though very small or nondense/nonattenuating material (such as chronic, water-logged plant material) lacks a shadow. Regional fat appears reactive, being hyperechoic/hyperattenuating on ultrasound and causing stranding within retrobulbar fat on CT. Distinct fluid pockets may be seen. Regional contrast enhancement is expected on CT and MRI (Figure 11.26).

Retrobulbar neoplasia may arise from the osseous structures of the skull or the retrobulbar soft tissues (Figure 11.27). CT and MRI are more useful than ultrasound to determine tissue of origin, particularly if the tumor is deep in the retrobulbar space where shadowing from osseous structures prevents definitive determination with sonography [14]. Myxosarcomas often extend into the retrobulbar space [15]. Uncommonly, retrobulbar lipomas and rhabdomyosarcomas occur [14, 16]. Primary bone tumors such as osteosarcoma, chondrosarcoma, or multilobular tumor of bone may become large enough to extend into the retrobulbar space; osseous involvement makes neoplasia much more likely than inflammatory causes of retrobulbar disease [14].

Zygomatic sialadenitis is a rare cause of retrobulbar mass effect and is discussed below.

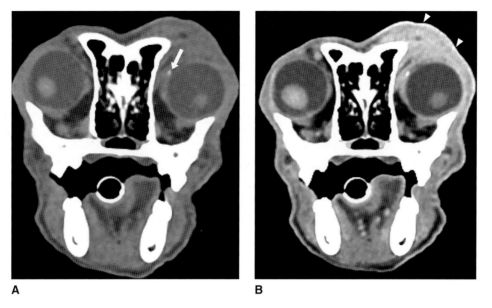

**FIGURE 11.25** Transverse precontrast (**A**) and postcontrast (**B**) CT images showing a grass awn (arrow) medial to the globe. There is regional soft tissue thickening that enhances, representing cellulitis (arrowhead).

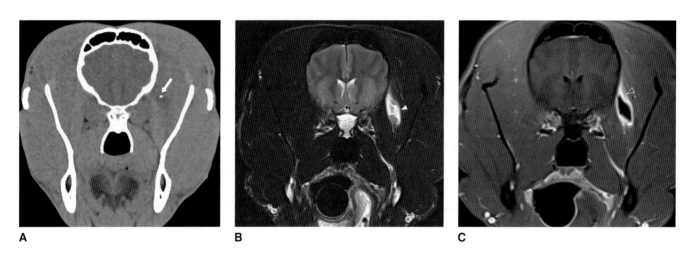

**FIGURE 11.26** Transverse CT image (**A**), transverse T2W MRI image (**B**) and transverse postcontrast MRI image (**C**) of a patient with a retrobulbar plastic foreign body. On the CT image, the foreign body is identified (arrow) but the regional abscessation is not well seen. On the MRI sequences, the foreign body is not seen, but the hyperintense abscess (closed arrowhead) and regional enhancement (open arrowhead) are well seen.

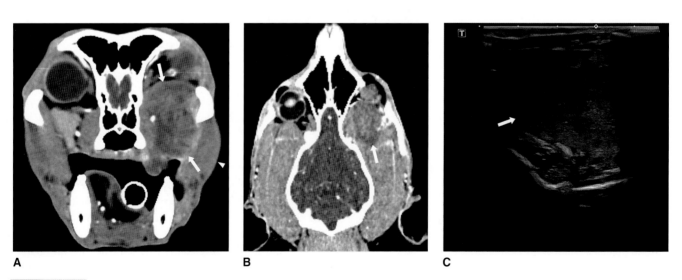

**FIGURE 11.27** Transverse (**A**) and dorsal (**B**) postcontrast CT images and ultrasound image (**C**) of a patient with a retrobulbar sarcoma. There is a large mass seen on all images, but only a portion of the mass is accessible for ultrasound imaging. The arrowhead indicates the location of placement for the ultrasound transducer, to produce the image in (**C**).

# Trauma

Traumatic injuries unpredictably damage osseous and soft tissue structures of the head. Survey radiography provides a broad overview of affected structures, but is insensitive to fissures and small fractures in some areas. Fractures of the mandibular ramus are difficult to identify as they superimpose with the zygomatic arch. In comparison, mandibular fractures are readily identified. Calvarial or maxillary fractures may require multiple oblique projections as the fractures are seen only in a tangential plane.

CT is preferred over radiography when surveying for head trauma due to improved performance in identifying small fractures and areas of soft tissue pathology. Intravenous contrast is typically not necessary, but improves the ability to screen for some types of soft tissue pathology or intranasal

trauma (Figure 11.28). If acute brain trauma is suspected, then MRI is preferred as it better identifies brain contusions or direct brain injury, though CT is relatively sensitive for acute hemorrhage so may be a useful screening test in patients with subdural or subarachnoid hemorrhage (Figure 11.29) [17].

## Temporomandibular Joint Disorders

Temporomandibular joint degeneration is characterized by peripheral osteophytosis (especially medially), subchondral sclerosis, and/or small cyst-like lesions but clinical symptoms are rare unless the disease is severe or accompanied by other concurrent malformation of the joint [18].

Temporomandibular dysplasia is a rare disease in which the TMJ displays increased laxity, allowing the mandibular process to impinge on the zygomatic arch. This results in locking

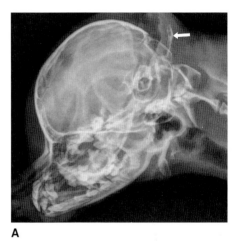
**A**

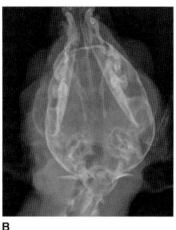
**B**

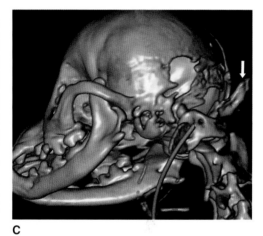
**C**

**FIGURE 11.28**   Poorly positioned oblique (**A**) and ventrodorsal projection (**B**) of the skull in a patient with head trauma. A fragment can be seen displaced caudally from the occipital region of the skull on the radiographs (arrow), but the more extensive fracturing of the caudal skull is not apparent, being more easily seen on the three-dimensional reformatted images from the CT examination (**C**).

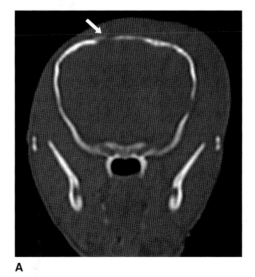
**A**

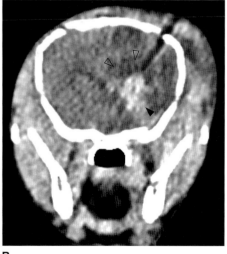
**B**

**FIGURE 11.29**   Transverse CT images in a bone window/level (**A**) and soft tissue window/level (**B**) in a patient with head trauma. Focal fractures are seen (arrow). There is a focal hyperattenuating area in the brain consistent with hemorrhage (closed arrowhead). This is surrounded by poorly defined edema, characterized by a thick hypoattenuating zone (open arrowheads).

of the jaw in an open position [19]. Radiographs of the skull with the jaw locked in an open position display the lateral shifting of the mandible characteristic of the disease (Figure 11.30). This disease predominates in bassett hounds, Irish setters, and cocker setter breeds [20, 21].

Temporomandibular fractures can be difficult to identify on survey radiographs, as disruption of the retroarticular process may be subtle and special projections may be necessary to fully see the mandibular condyle without other osseous superimposition (Figure 11.31). A well-positioned closed mouth VD projection is often the most useful projection to screen for TMJ trauma, as careful comparison between the left and right sides makes subtle lesions more apparent. Ultimately, CT provides a more accurate and complete assessment of TMJ traumatic lesions (Figure 11.32).

Joint-associated neoplasia of the TMJ is uncommon, though osteosarcoma and multilobular tumor of bone have been reported [18]. Myxosarcoma has a unique, expansile, cyst-like appearance on imaging [15]. The mass frequently extends into the retrobulbar space and usually results in resorption of the articular margins of the TMJ (Figure 11.33). On CT, the mass is predominantly hypoattenuating fluid pockets surrounded by thin soft tissue of variable contrast enhancement. On MRI, the mass is strongly hyperintense/fluid intense and on ultrasound will appear mostly anechoic (Figure 11.34). Radiographs are frequently unrewarding.

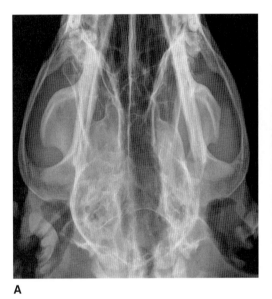
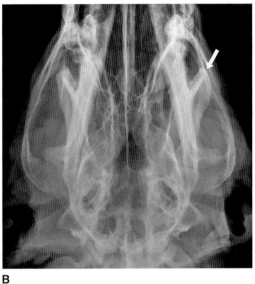

A    B

**FIGURE 11.30**  Ventrodorsal closed mouth (**A**) and open mouth (**B**) images of a patient with TMJ dysplasia. No abnormalities are seen on the closed mouth projection but when the mouth is opened, the mandible displaces to the left with the left zygomatic arch impinged by the left ramus (arrow).

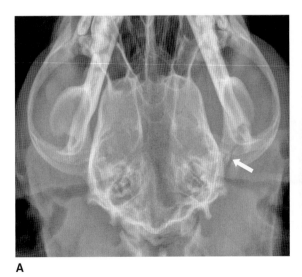
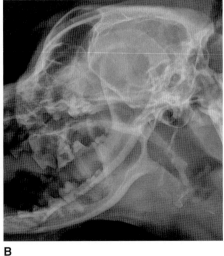

A    B

**FIGURE 11.31**  Ventrodorsal (**A**) and oblique (**B**) images in a patient with a traumatic fracture of the retroarticular process of the TMJ (white arrow). Note that the fracture is only seen on the ventrodorsal image and not apparent on the oblique projection.

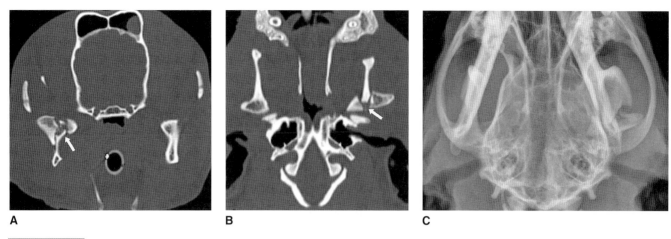

**FIGURE 11.32**   Transverse (**A**) and dorsal (**B**) CT images and ventrodorsal radiograph (**C**) of a patient with a mandibular condylar fracture (arrows). The fracture is more extensive as identified on CT when compared to radiographs.

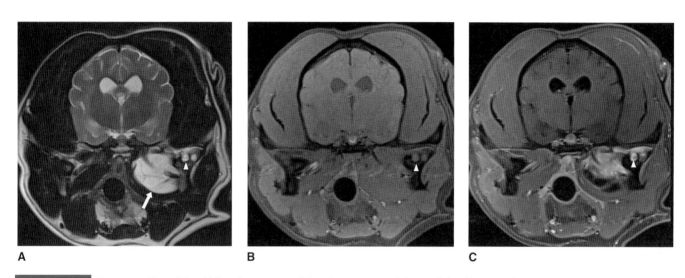

**FIGURE 11.33**   Transverse T2-weighted (**A**) and precontrast (**B**) and postcontrast (**C**) T1-weighted images of a patient with a myxosarcoma affecting the TMJ. Note the large fluid-intense region medial to the left TMJ (arrow), that contrast enhances, as well as the cyst-like areas of bony resorption affecting the mandibular condyle (arrowheads).

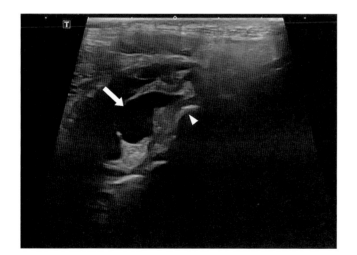

**FIGURE 11.34**   Ultrasound image of a myxosarcoma affecting the left temporomandibular joint. There are large fluid-filled regions (arrow) as well as some regional soft tissue thickening adjacent to the bone. The margin of bone is indicated by arrowheads.

## Pharyngeal/Laryngeal Diseases

Due to its ready inspection during a sedated examination, direct visualization is the best first diagnostic step when a structural abnormality of the pharynx/larynx is suspected. Plain radiographs are rarely helpful given the limited ability to discriminate specific soft tissues around pharynx/larynx. CT is reserved when deeper or more complex soft tissue abnormalities are present. Fluoroscopy, a real-time x-ray modality, is useful in the evaluation of dynamic processes such as pharyngeal or tracheal collapse.

## Nasopharyngeal Polyps

Nasopharyngeal polyps are usually identified on visual oropharyngeal or external ear evaluation, but imaging can better define involvement of the nasopharynx or middle ear. When performing radiographs, it is crucial that lateral radiographs

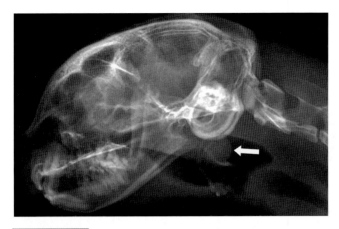

**FIGURE 11.35** Lateral radiograph of a patient with a nasopharyngeal polyp. There is a large mass effect with a rounded caudal margin within the nasopharynx (arrow). The bullae are bilaterally thickened but superimposed with one another, indicating this is a well-positioned lateral radiograph.

are well positioned, as obliquity hides the normally gas-filled nasopharynx (Figure 11.35). For cats with concurrent vestibular signs, CT or MRI are better able to define potential middle or inner ear involvement (Figure 11.36). Polyps display a characteristic rim enhancement pattern, though otitis media alone may also have this appearance.

## Pharyngeal/Laryngeal Neoplasia

Carcinomas are the most common pharyngeal/laryngeal tumor in dogs and lymphoma is most common in cats [22]. Ectopic thyroid carcinoma often disrupts the bones of the hyoid apparatus (especially the basihyoid bone) [23]. Radiographs may demonstrate a mass effect which disrupts the normally gas-filled pharynx or larynx, but rarely gives additional information about regional infiltration or lymph node involvement (Figure 11.37). Pharyngeal masses outside the

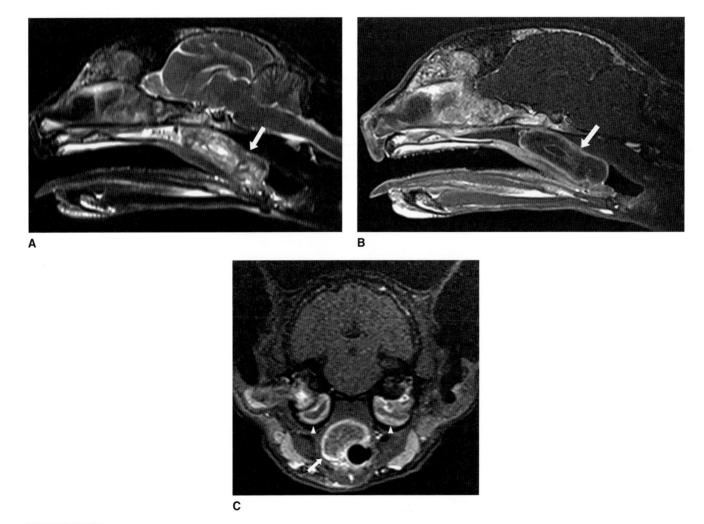

A

B

C

**FIGURE 11.36** Sagittal T2-weighted (**A**), sagittal (**B**) and transverse (**C**) postcontrast T1-weighted images of a patient with a nasopharyngeal polyp. Notice the rim-enhancing, T2 hyperintense mass within the nasopharynx on sagittal images (arrows). Both bullae are filled with fluid and peripheral contrast enhancement (arrowheads), consistent with otitis media.

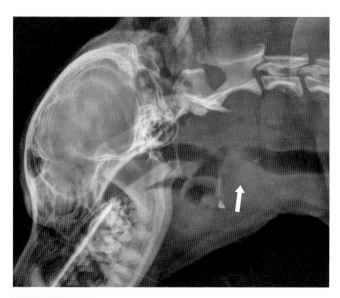

**FIGURE 11.37**   Lateral radiograph of a patient with laryngeal neoplasia. Note the large mass effect narrowing the airway, caudal to the hyoid apparatus (white arrow).

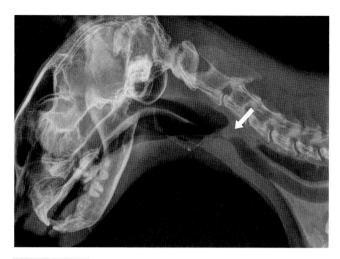

**FIGURE 11.39**   Lateral radiograph of a patient with laryngeal lymphoma. There is caudal displacement of the larynx and overdistension of the pharyngeal structures, common in patients with upper airway obstruction at the level of the larynx. The soft tissues of the larynx are diffuse and thick with severe airway narrowing at the level of the neoplasm (arrow).

airway result in minimal effect on the airway (Figure 11.38). If the mass is resulting in significant airway obstruction at the level of the larynx, the more rostral airway (pharynx) may be excessively gas dilated and the larynx caudally displaced (Figure 11.39). Ultrasound may identify involvement of other regional structures, but gas in the larynx/trachea interferes with the examination. CT more clearly identifies tissue of origin, regionally invaded structures, and evidence of lymph node metastasis. Rarely, benign soft tissue growths may be encountered, including laryngeal cysts, inflammatory polyps or other inflammatory diseases [24].

## Pharyngeal/Laryngeal Foreign Bodies

Foreign material such as sticks or bones may penetrate the tissues of the pharynx while chewing or during a swallowing attempt, and can migrate dorsally into the retrobulbar space or more caudally in the cervical region. Radiographs are insensitive in detecting "soft tissue" plant foreign material (such as grass awns and sticks), but more readily identify mineral or metallic objects. CT and MRI are also limited in identifying plant foreign material as regional inflammation has similar imaging characteristics as the material, obscuring the foreign body margins (Figure 11.40). Ultrasound more readily detects foreign material (including plant material) as most foreign material causes beam attenuation and shadowing, regardless of its consistency. Gas may track along the path of the foreign material.

Ultimately, surgical exploration of the affected area may be necessary in a patient with a compatible clinical history and evidence of regional inflammation, fluid pocketing or gas tracking, even if foreign material itself is not identified on imaging.

## Nasopharyngeal Stenosis

Nasopharyngeal stenosis occurs at the level of the hard or soft palate. It is typically a sequela of chronic inflammatory disease (rhinitis, aspiration, trauma) though congenital forms exist. Both dogs and cats are affected [25]. Evidence of rhinitis is expected and there may be adjacent bony reaction. Diagnosis is often made during retroflex rhinoscopy of the nasopharynx, but may be identified on CT (though fluid adjacent to the stenosis may mask its presence; Figure 11.41). Survey radiographs may identify increased opacity within the nasopharynx.

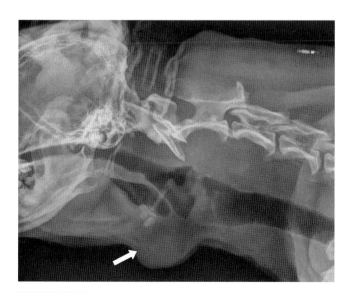

**FIGURE 11.38**   Lateral radiograph of a patient with ectopic thyroid carcinoma causing a large mass effect protruding ventrally from the ventral laryngeal region (arrow).

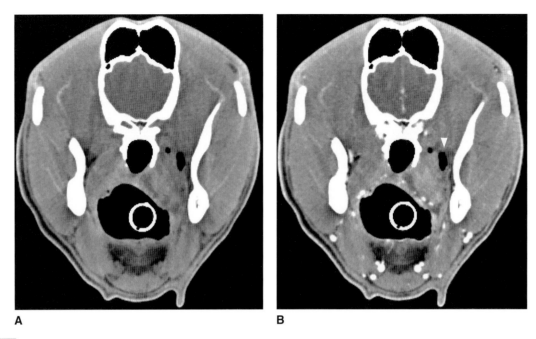

**A**　　　　　　　　　　　　**B**

**FIGURE 11.40** Transverse precontrast (**A**) and postcontrast (**B**) CT images of a patient with a retropharyngeal foreign body, which penetrated from the oral cavity. There is gas within the foreign body (arrowhead) and regional soft tissue thickening and fluid.

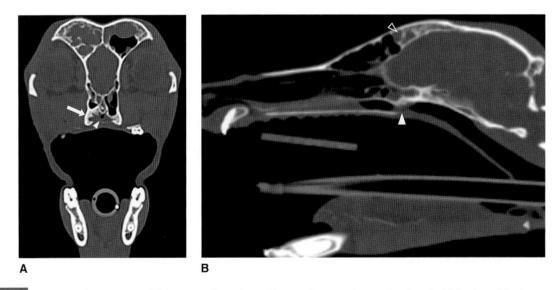

**A**　　　　　　　　　　　　**B**

**FIGURE 11.41** Transverse (**A**) and sagittal (**B**) images of a patient with nasopharyngeal stenosis. There is thickening of the bone surrounding the nasopharynx (arrow) with soft tissue proliferation causing narrowing of the airway (closed arrowhead). There is also evidence of bilateral frontal sinusitis (open arrowhead).

## Pharyngeal Collapse

Dynamic pharyngeal collapse is most common in dogs with brachycephalic airway syndrome, but also occurs in patients with other airway diseases including tracheal and mainstem bronchial collapse [26]. Dorsal displacement of the soft palate and/or ventral deviation of the dorsal pharyngeal wall causes complete or partial collapse of the pharynx [26, 27]. While CT or endoscopy may diagnose this condition, it is most commonly identified on dynamic fluoroscopic examination of the upper airway where the pharyngeal lumen is narrowed on inspiration by collapse of adjacent structures (particularly the dorsal pharyngeal wall) (Figure 11.42).

## Epiglottic Retroversion

While rare, epiglottic retroversion causes dyspnea/upper airway obstruction in dogs by obstructing the rima glottidis [28, 29]. On fluoroscopy, paradoxical caudal retroflexion of the epiglottis occurs during inspiration (Figure 11.43).

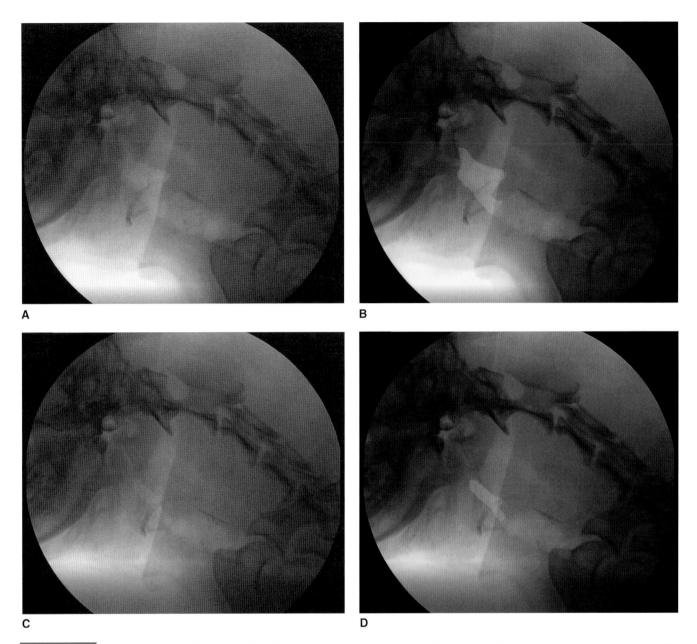

A

B

C

D

**FIGURE 11.42**   Expiratory (**A**,**B**) and inspiratory (**C**,**D**) fluoroscopic images of a patient with collapse of the nasopharynx on inspiration. On (**B**) and (**D**), the airway lumen is indicated with a color overlay, and is collapsed on inspiration.

## Laryngeal Paralysis

Laryngeal paralysis is typically a unilateral or bilateral disorder in older large-breed dogs. This condition most commonly affects the Labrador retriever, though cats and other dog breeds are also affected. Laryngeal paralysis is usually idiopathic, but can be caused by a variety of poly-neuropathies, trauma, and masses [24]. Laryngeal exami-nation under sedation provides definitive diagnosis when there is failure of arytenoid abduction during inspiration, but ultrasound examination using a ventral approach can identify abnormal movement of the arytenoid or cuneiform processes [30].

# Dental and Oral Disorders

## Neoplasia

Oral soft tissue neoplasms, such as melanoma and squamous cell carcinoma, are usually first recognized on direct oral examination. Imaging identifies secondary regional osseous destruction that may be apparent and screens for metasta-sis [31]. Radiographs are less sensitive than CT or MRI for osse-ous involvement [10].

Primary bone tumors of the mandible and maxillary have an aggressive appearance similar to malignant osseous tumors

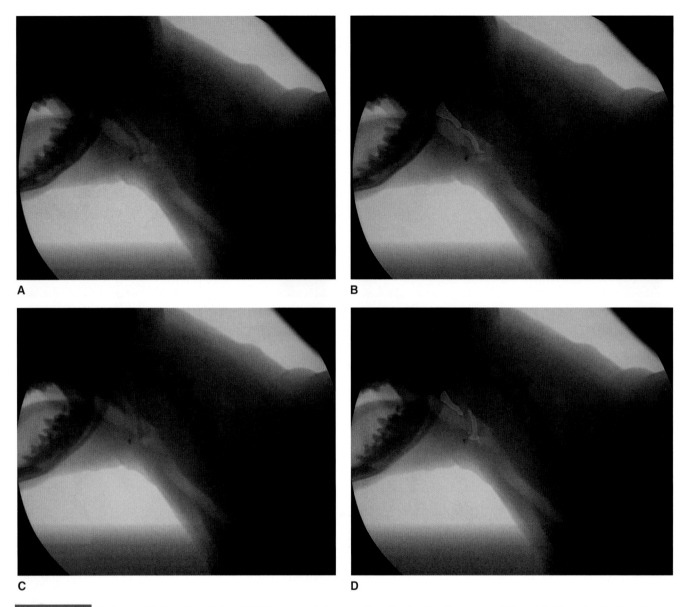

A

B

C

D

**FIGURE 11.43** Expiratory (**A,B**) and inspiratory (**C,D**) fluoroscopic images of a patient with retroversion of the epiglottis on inspiration. On inspiration, the epiglottis (red overlay) moves caudally away from the soft palate (yellow overlay) to contact the dorsal nasopharyngeal wall.

elsewhere in the body. Fibrosarcoma and chondrosarcoma are more common than in the appendicular skeleton [32].

Odontogenic neoplasms derive from the tooth-forming apparatus and are the most common oral masses in dogs [33]. There are numerous types of odontogenic neoplasms and all cause osseous destruction centered on the affected tooth roots, but some distinguishing characteristics exist. Fibromatous epulides of periodontal ligament origin often have a large contrast-enhancing extraosseous component. Acanthomatous ameloblastomas often have more pronounced aggressive characteristics compared to other odontogenic tumor types (Figure 11.44) [33].

Tonsillar neoplasia in dogs can have a unique appearance as identified on CT. The primary tonsillar tumor (usually squamous cell carcinoma) may be relatively small but the metastatic medial retropharyngeal lymph nodes can be disproportionally large (Figure 11.45) [34].

## Periodontal/Endodontal Disease

Dental disease is very common in companion animals, with dental abnormalities present in 27.8% of dogs with visibly normal teeth [35]. A full review of dental imaging is beyond the purview of this chapter, though the high prevalence of dental disease warrants familiarity with the imaging appearance of the most common changes. Dental digital radiography plates have a smaller footprint that facilitates intraoral use. These units also acquire higher resolution images than standard digital radiography plates, necessary to detect the subtle radiographic findings of early dental disease. CT and cone beam CT for dental disease are becoming more common, but are still typically reserved for the more complex cases given the increased cost of these modalities.

Periodontal disease is the most common oral disease encountered on imaging [35]. Periodontal disease results in widening of the periodontal ligament space, sometimes

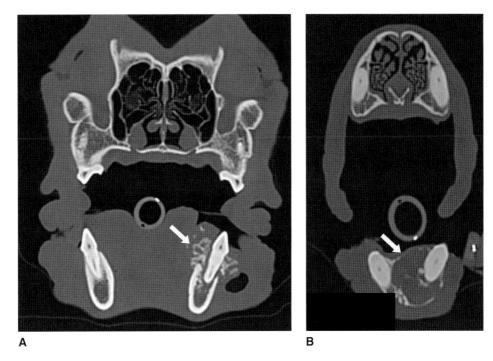

**A**    **B**

**FIGURE 11.44**   Transverse CT images of two patients with amyloid-producing odontogenic tumors. The patient in (**A**) has a more irregular bony response compared to the one in (**B**) where there is a more soft tissue expansile appearance.

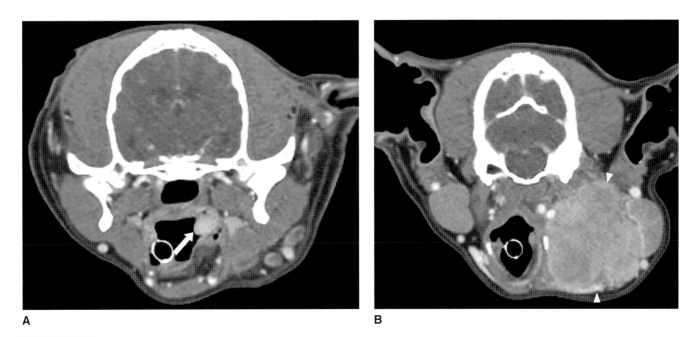

**A**    **B**

**FIGURE 11.45**   Transverse postcontrast CT images at the level of the caudal oral cavity (**A**) and larynx (**B**). The left tonsil (arrow) is enlarged. The left medial retropharyngeal lymph node (arrowhead) is severely enlarged due to metastatic carcinoma, with the enlargement of the lymph node proportionally much greater than the degree of tonsillar enlargement.

termed vertical bone loss, and loss of alveolar bone between teeth, referred to as horizontal bone loss (Figure 11.46).

Endodontic disease causes inflammation at the apex of the tooth [35]. This results in resorption of the root tip of the affected tooth, regional loss of lamina dura, or circular lesions at the root tip (Figure 11.47). The pulp canal may become abnormally wide (seen with pulp necrosis) or abnormally small if chronic pulp irritation is seen. Increased width of the periodontal

ligament space is also typically present. Both periodontal and endodontic disease may be concurrently present.

## Trauma

Traumatic injury to the rostral osseous and soft tissues of the head is common. While physical examination/oral examination is important to identify obvious pathology in this region,

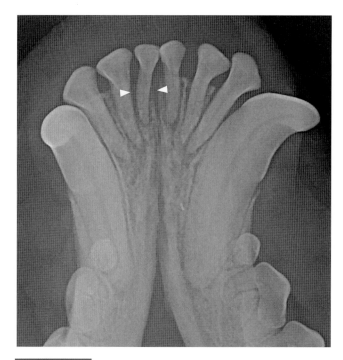

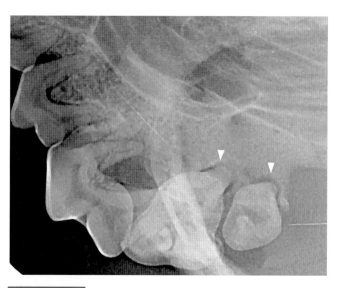

**FIGURE 11.47** Radiograph of the caudal maxillary molars using a dental digital radiography unit, showing periapical halos (arrowheads) of two teeth.

**FIGURE 11.46** Ventrodorsal projection of the mandible using a dental digital radiography unit, showing bone loss (arrowhead) along the periodontal margin of a mandibular incisor tooth.

radiographs and CT more fully identify the extent of disease. CT in particular is helpful to evaluate for possible dental or TMJ involvement of any fractures.

## Salivary Diseases

### Sialadenitis
Sialadenitis is inflammation of the salivary glands, and is periodically reported in dogs [22]. The cause is often unknown, though may be due to trauma, ascending infection, or immune-mediated causes. On CT, MRI, or ultrasound, it causes enlargement of the salivary gland and disruption of the normal homogeneous gland architecture by areas of increased fluid or inflammation (Figure 11.48). The mandibular and parotid salivary glands are most readily approached with ultrasound, though a supra- or subzygomatic approach may be used with ultrasound to image the zygomatic salivary gland (Figure 11.49).

### Sialocele/Salivary Mucocele
Sialoceles (also referred to as salivary mucocele) are the most common salivary disorder in dogs, and especially affect the sublingual salivary glands or ducts (referred to as a ranula) [36, 37]. Sialoceles result in fluid distension of the affected salivary

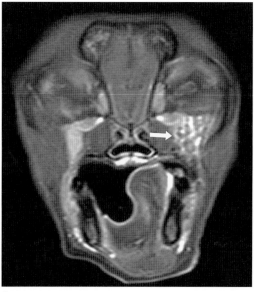

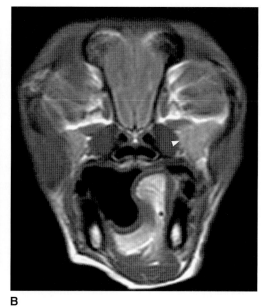

A                                                    B

**FIGURE 11.48** Transverse T1-weighted postcontrast (**A**) and T2-weighted images (**B**) in a patient with left zygomatic sialoadenitis. The zygomatic salivary gland is enlarged (arrowhead) and increased in enhancement (arrow) compared to the right.

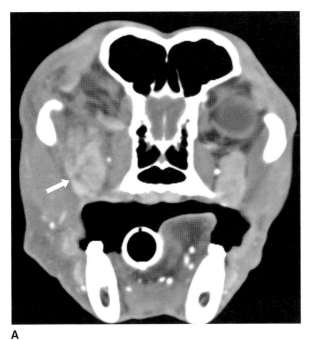
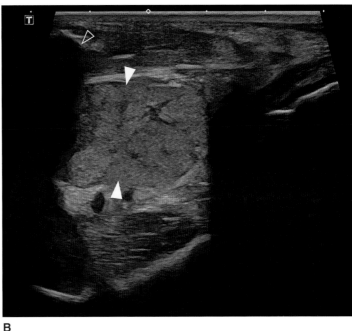

**A**                                                                                                          **B**

**FIGURE 11.49**   CT image (**A**) and ultrasound image (**B**) of a patient with zygomatic sialadenitis. The CT demonstrates enlargement of the right zygomatic salivary gland (arrow) compared to the left. On ultrasound, the zygomatic salivary gland (between closed arrowheads) has internal hypoechoic septations. The zygomatic arch (open arrowhead) causes distal shadowing.

gland or salivary duct. These are recognized on CT, MRI, or ultrasound as a fluid-filled rounded structure with a thin wall and may be unilateral (Figure 11.50) or bilateral (Figure 11.51). The appearance of ranula is characteristic and diagnosed on physical examination by an elliptical fluid fluctuant mass in a sublingual location. Advanced imaging modalities differentiate sialoceles from other causes of more caudal neck/pharyngeal region masses. When the zygomatic salivary gland is involved, a retrobulbar mass effect may result in exophthalmos [38].

## Sialolithiasis

Sialoliths are mineral concretions within the salivary glands or ducts, typically composed of calcium carbonate or phosphate. The cause is unknown. Sialoliths may accumulate within any salivary tissue, though only cause

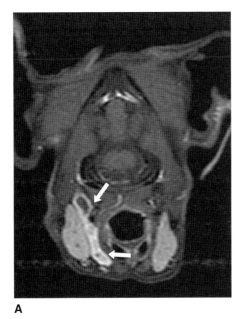
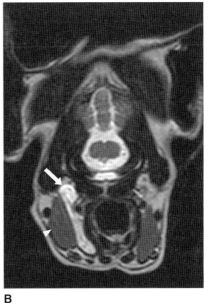

**A**                                                          **B**

**FIGURE 11.50**   Postcontrast T1-weighted (**A**) and T2-weighted (**B**) images of a patient with a unilateral mandibular sialocele. Notice the contrast rim enhancement of the sialocele (arrow) and its location just medial to the mandibular salivary gland (salivary gland indicated by arrowhead).

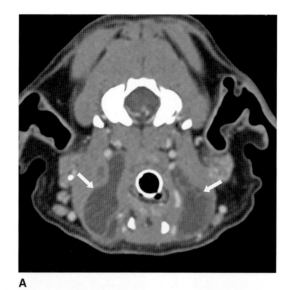

**A**

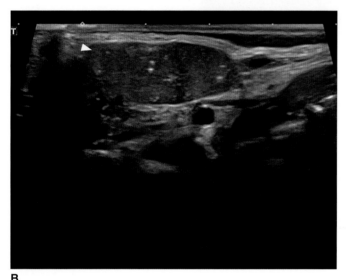

**B**

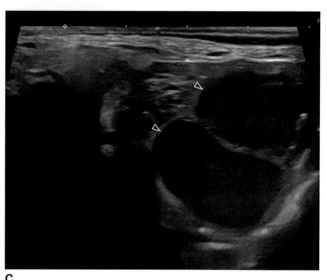

**C**

**FIGURE 11.51** Postcontrast CT (**A**) and ultrasound images (**B,C**) of a patient with bilateral mandibular sialoceles. On CT, the sialoceles cause a fluid-attenuating pocket (arrows) medial to the mandibular salivary glands. The mandibular salivary glands appear normal on ultrasound (closed arrowhead) but a fluid pocket is clearly seen extending from them medially (open arrowhead).

signs when lodged in the salivary duct, causing dilation and regional inflammation [39, 40]. They are often obscured on radiographs by superimposed osseous anatomy, and are more readily identified on CT (Figure 11.52). They may be challenging to identify on MRI given the inherent low signal of mineralized structures on MRI. CT sialography can definitively identify the duct involved, though is rarely necessary as the affected duct may be deduced by the anatomic location of the sialolith [41].

### Salivary Gland Neoplasia
Salivary gland neoplasia is rarely reported in dogs and cats. Adenocarcinoma is most common but adenomas, carcinomas, myxosarcomas, and others have been reported [42]. The neoplastic mass distorts

regional soft tissue anatomy (Figure 11.53). Rarely, salivary melanosis has been reported, which results in unusual signal characteristics on MRI (being T2 hypointense due to the presence of melanin, as opposed to most neoplastic masses which are T2 hyperintense) [43]. If fluid filled, salivary gland neoplasia can be difficult to distinguish from salivary mucoceles, but the presence of soft tissue thickening or adjacent bony lysis makes neoplasia more likely [38].

### Sialadenosis
This idiopathic painless, bilateral, noninflammatory enlargement of the salivary glands is a rare condition in dogs (Figure 11.54). It is responsive to phenobarbital and is diagnosed using imaging and exclusion of other causes of salivary gland enlargement described above [44].

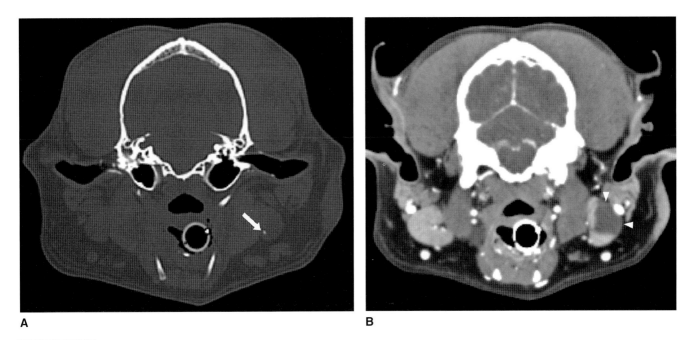

**FIGURE 11.52** Transverse CT images in bone window/level (**A**) and postcontrast soft tissue window/level (**B**) images showing a sialolith within the left mandibular salivary gland. The sialolith is a focal mineralization (arrow) and is obstructing the salivary duct, resulting in a large accumulation of fluid in the salivary gland (arrowhead).

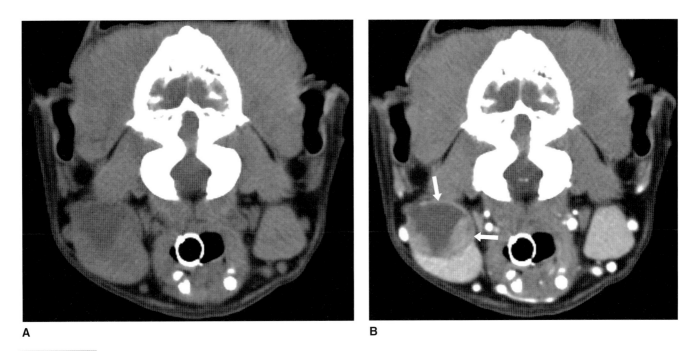

**FIGURE 11.53** Transverse precontrast (**A**) and postcontrast (**B**) images of a patient with a salivary carcinoma. Notice the mass (arrows) in the dorsal right mandibular salivary gland. This mass contains a large region of fluid within its center.

## Thyroid Disorders

**Neoplasia** Up to 88% of canine thyroid masses are malignant carcinoma, with the remainder representing benign adenoma formation (the latter usually only found incidentally as they tend to remain very small and noninvasive) [45].

Thyroid carcinoma, though slow growing, can become quite large. Thyroid carcinoma is highly vascular, characterized by strong contrast enhancement on MRI and CT imaging (Figure 11.55) and increased Doppler signal on ultrasound investigation (Figure 11.56). Nearly a third of canine thyroid carcinoma may be bilateral. Radiographs are less definitive in confirming thyroid origin, with a nonspecific increased soft

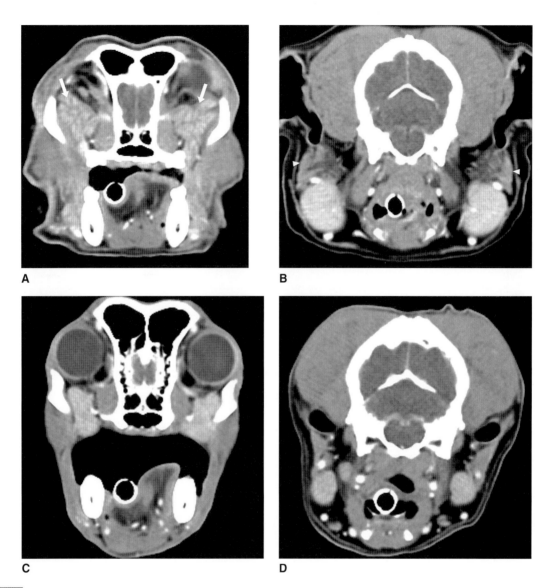

**FIGURE 11.54** Transverse postcontrast weighted images of a patient with phenobarbital-responsive sialoadenosis (**A,B**) compared to a normal patient (**C,D**). The zygomatic salivary glands (arrows) and parotid salivary glands (arrowheads) in the affected patient are enlarged and have a striated appearance compared to the normal patient.

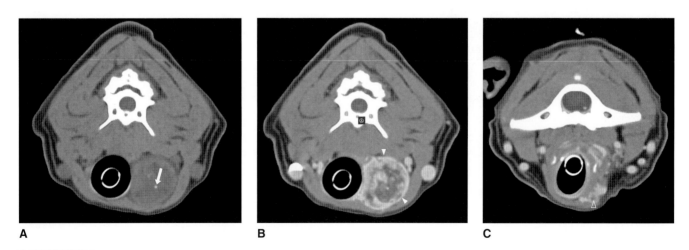

**FIGURE 11.55** Transverse precontrast (**A**) and postcontrast (**B,C**) CT images of a patient with thyroid carcinoma. The thyroid carcinoma has internal areas of mineralization (arrow) and is strongly contrast enhancing (**B**, closed arrowheads), though it has internal areas which are less enhancing and are consistent with either fluid or necrosis. There is vascular invasion seen caudal to the mass, characterized by a filling defect (open arrowhead) in a vessel.

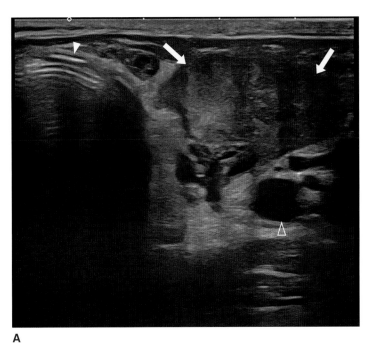

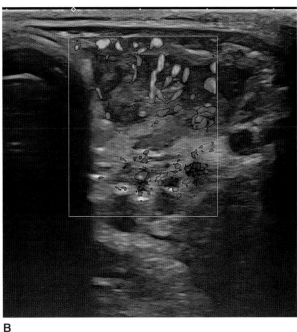

**A**                                          **B**

**FIGURE 11.56**  Transverse (**A**) and Doppler (**B**) ultrasound images of a thyroid carcinoma. The mass (arrows) is located between the trachea (closed arrowheads) and the carotid artery (open arrowheads) and has a high level of vascularity on Doppler imaging.

tissue opacity that causes ventral or dorsal displacement of the trachea (Figure 11.57). CT better assesses resectability of the mass, and plays an important role in staging and screening for metastasis to regional lymph nodes or the lungs. Both benign and malignant thyroid masses are prone to fluid-filled areas representing colloid accumulation or necrosis (Figure 11.58).

Approximately 50% of dogs have ectopic thyroid tissue on necropsy, and neoplastic transformation of this tissue may occur [46]. This tissue may be seen anywhere between the base of the tongue and base of the heart. When it occurs at the base of the tongue, it results in a large, contrast-enhancing mass that causes lysis of the basihyoid bone [47] (Figure 11.59).

Malignant thyroid tumors are uncommon in cats, as benign nodules and masses predominate [48]. A large or fixed thyroid mass should raise suspicion of malignancy, and they tend to be highly metastatic in cats [48]. Adenomatous nodules in cats typically autonomously secrete thyroid hormone, resulting in hyperthyroidism. They are identified on ultrasound

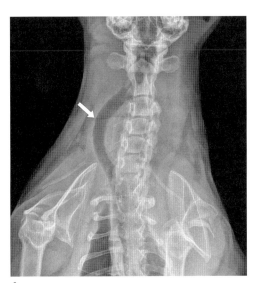

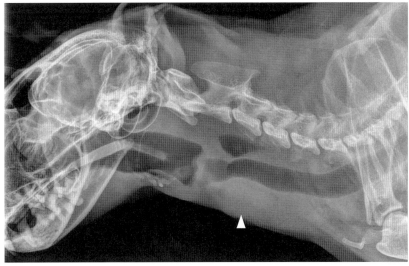

**A**                                          **B**

**FIGURE 11.57**  Ventrodorsal (**A**) and lateral (**B**) radiographs of a patient with thyroid carcinoma. Notice the severe rightward deviation of the trachea (arrow) on the ventrodorsal projection. On the lateral projection there is increased soft tissue mass adjacent and ventral to the cranial cervical trachea (arrowhead), causing dorsal displacement.

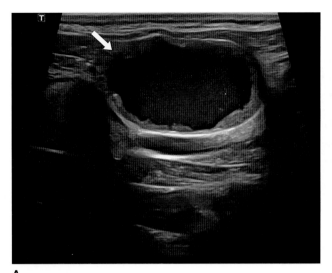

**A**

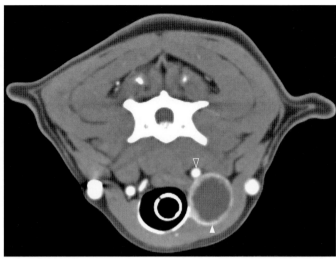

**B**

**FIGURE 11.58** Ultrasound (transverse) (**A**) and postcontrast CT (**B**) images of a thyroid carcinoma. On ultrasound, the fluid-filled region is hypoechoic with a thick rim (arrow). The wall of this fluid-filled region is strongly enhancing on the CT image (closed arrowhead). Notice that the thyroid carcinoma is displacing the carotid artery dorsally and medially (open arrowhead), rather than laterally as more typically seen.

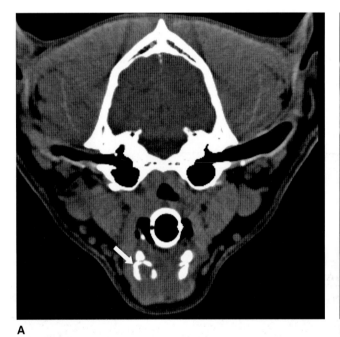

**A**

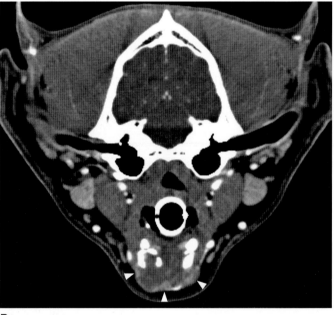

**B**

**FIGURE 11.59** Precontrast (**A**) and postcontrast (**B**) images of a patient with ectopic thyroid carcinoma. This is causing lysis of the basihyoid bone (arrow). The mass has peripheral contrast enhancement (arrowhead).

or CT imaging as well-defined, unilateral or bilateral nodules. The remaining normal thyroid parenchyma may be reduced in size due to suppression by the hypersecretory nodules. When a hyperactive nodule is present, the normal thyroid tissue may become less attenuating, and the affected lobe becomes heterogeneous in its pattern on CT [49].

**Hypothyroidism** Hypothyroidism is definitively diagnosed through identification of low circulating thyroid hormone levels. Structural thyroid gland changes are seen on imaging of the hypothyroid patient, and should prompt measurement of thyroid hormone levels if not already performed.

On ultrasound, a normal thyroid lobe should be more echogenic than surrounding musculature. It should have a prominent fusiform shape on longitudinal images and triangular shape on transverse images. With the hypothyroid state, the thyroid lobes become small, more hypoechoic, and more rounded, making them more difficult to identify [50, 51] (Figure 11.60). While not typically a

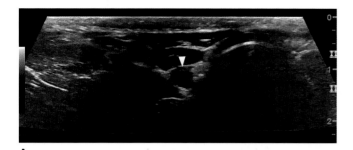

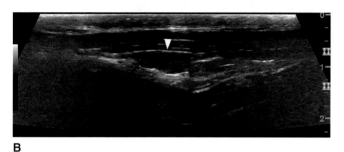

**B**

**FIGURE 11.60** Transverse (**A**) and sagittal (**B**) ultrasound images of a patient with hypothyroidism. Note that the thyroid lobe (arrowhead) in this image is more hypoechoic than expected and has rounded margins, also being smaller than typically seen.

diagnostic test for the disease, ultrasound can be used to discriminate between euthyroid sick and hypothyroid dogs [52].

On CT, a normal thyroid lobe is hyperattenuating to adjacent tissues on preintravenous contrast images, due to the inherently high iodine present in the normal thyroid gland (Figure 11.61) [53]. With hypothyroidism, the lobes become small and reduced in attenuation, being similar to adjacent soft tissue structures (Figure 11.61).

## Parathyroid Disorders

While normal parathyroid glands are readily seen with ultrasound, they are not typically identified on CT imaging unless abnormal [54, 55]. On ultrasound, parathyroid glands are round or ellipsoid hypoechoic structures, less than 2 mm diameter, typically along the cranial and midmargin portions of the thyroid gland. The thyroid gland may contain other small round hypoechoic structures that appear similar to normal parathyroid glands, but represent thyroid lobules (Figure 11.62) [55].

The degree of parathyroid enlargement and the number of enlarged parathyroid glands determine differential diagnoses for parathyroid enlargement. Secondary hyperparathyroidism, as seen with chronic renal disease or nutritional imbalance, results in mild to moderate enlargement of all parathyroid glands (typically between 2 and 6 mm in diameter). Patients with acute renal failure may be differentiated from those with chronic renal failure, as the former will not demonstrate parathyroid enlargement [56]. A hyperactive parathyroid adenoma or adenocarcinoma results in a solitary, moderately to severely enlarged parathyroid gland (Figure 11.63). Parathyroid tumors typically result in more enlargement of the affected gland than seen in cases of secondary hyperparathyroidism (often more than 6 mm diameter). If large enough, parathyroid tumors may be recognized on CT (Figure 11.64), though there is overlap in the appearance of parathyroid adenoma, parathyroid carcinoma, and thyroid carcinoma (Figure 11.65).

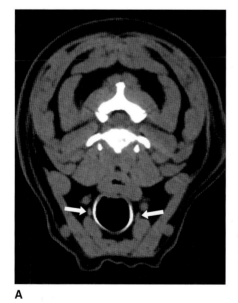

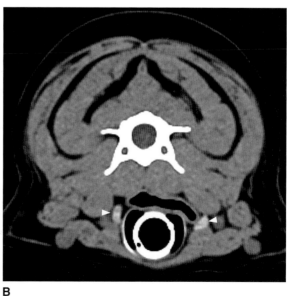

**A**                    **B**

**FIGURE 11.61** Transverse precontrast CT images in a patient with hypothyroidism (**A**) compared to a normal patient (**B**). Notice that in the hypothyroid patient, the thyroid lobes (arrows) are very small and decreased in attenuation due to low iodine content, compared to the normal patient with thyroid lobes (arrowheads) which are normally hyperattenuating to adjacent musculature in the precontrast images.

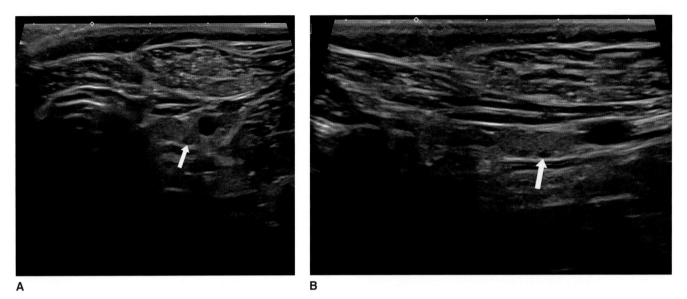

**FIGURE 11.62** Transverse (**A**) and sagittal (**B**) ultrasound images of normal parathyroid glands (arrows). The adjacent thyroid parenchyma is normal.

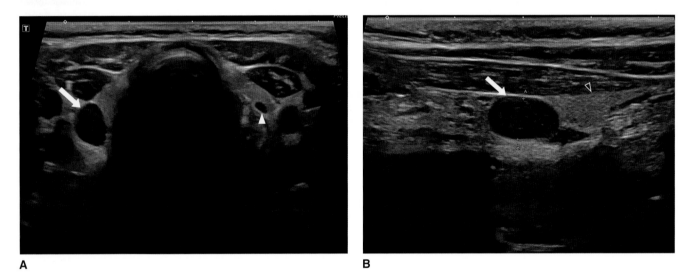

**FIGURE 11.63** Transverse (**A**) and sagittal (**B**) ultrasound images of the right thyroid lobe with a large parathyroid adenoma (arrows). The left thyroid lobe had a smaller hypoechoic nodule (closed arrowhead). This smaller nodule is nonspecific and in this case was a thyroid follicle; however, a thyroid cyst or normal parathyroid gland could also have this appearance. Adjacent thyroid tissue is normal (open arrowhead).

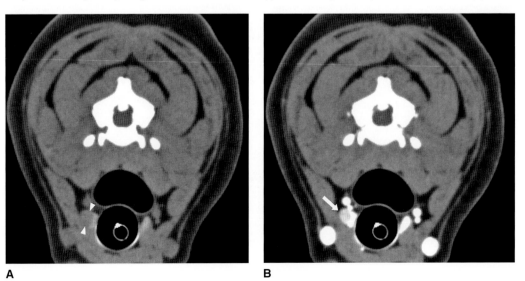

**FIGURE 11.64** Precontrast (**A**) and postcontrast (**B**) CT images of a patient with a primary right parathyroid adenoma. On precontrast images, the nodule (arrowheads) is less attenuating than adjacent thyroid parenchyma. It enhances less than thyroid parenchyma on postcontrast images (arrow).

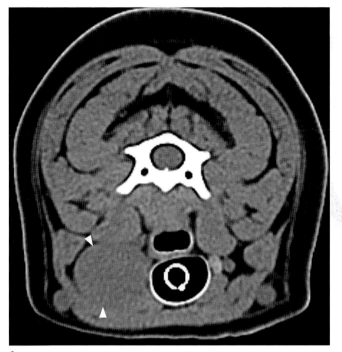
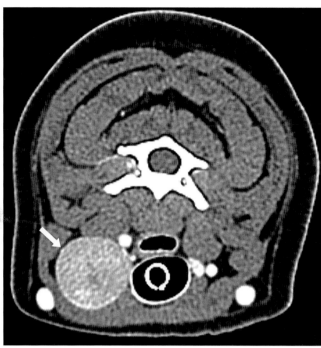

**A**  **B**

**FIGURE 11.65** Precontrast (**A**) and postcontrast (**B**) CT images of the patient with parathyroid carcinoma. On precontrast images, the mass (arrowhead) displaces regional anatomy but is more apparent on postcontrast images (arrow).

# External/Middle/Inner Ear Disease

Otitis externa is best diagnosed through careful aural examination, but when chronic will result in mineralization and thickening of the ear canal wall and luminal narrowing on radiographs, CT or MRI [57]. Imaging studies are more useful in the diagnosis and management of otitis media. Affected bullae will have variable degrees of fluid filling, bulla thickening, and increased contrast enhancement (Figure 11.66). While radiographs may identify the changes seen on otitis media, it is less sensitive than CT or MRI for mildly affected cases. If chronic, the bullae may become mildly, diffusely thickened (Figures 11.67 and 11.68).

Primary secretory otitis media is common in Cavalier King Charles spaniels, and often seen incidentally in imaging studies performed for reasons unrelated to the middle ear

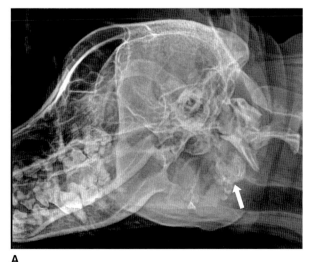
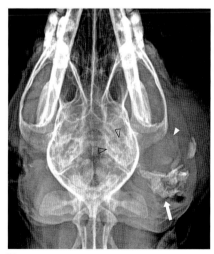

**A**  **B**

**FIGURE 11.66** Oblique (**A**) and ventrodorsal (**B**) projections of a patient with an external ear canal abscess (closed arrowhead) and extensive ear canal mineralization (arrow). The abscess displaces the ear canal and occludes the lumen. There is also increased opacity of the left middle ear (open arrowheads), consistent with otitis media.

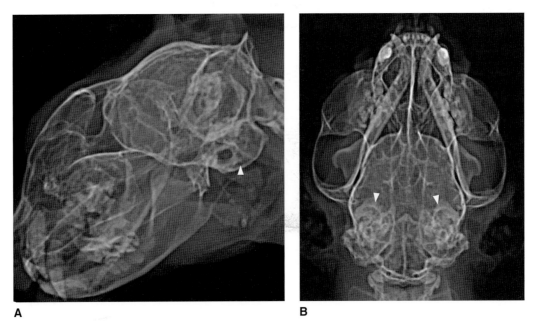

A          B

**FIGURE 11.67** Oblique (**A**) and ventrodorsal (**B**) projections of a patient with bilateral otitis media. There is diffuse increased opacity of the lumen of the tympanic bullae (arrowheads).

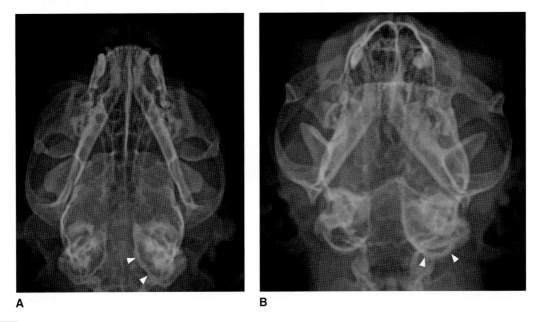

A          B

**FIGURE 11.68** Ventrodorsal (**A**) and rostrocaudal oblique (**B**) images of a patient with unilateral chronic otitis media. The left tympanic bulla wall is thickened (arrowhead) and the lumen of the bulla is increased in opacity.

(Figure 11.69) [58]. It causes partial or complete fluid filling of the bullae (often bilaterally) without significant regional contrast enhancement [58, 59].

Otitis interna cannot be diagnosed on radiographs. T2-weighted and FLAIR sequences on MRI are sensitive to loss of the normally fluid-filled inner ear structures as occurs with otitis interna. On postcontrast, T1-weighted images, inner ears affected with otitis interna display abnormal, increased contrast enhancement compared to the contralateral side (Figure 11.70) [60]. If severe enough, inflammation will spread from the inner ear to adjacent meninges and brain parenchyma, resulting in regional meningeal and neuroparenchymal contrast enhancement and increased T2 signal (Figure 11.71).

Cholesteatoma is an epidermoid cyst that contains keratin and is frequently associated with chronic otitis media. It is infrequently diagnosed in dogs, and has features that distinguish it from typical otitis media or neoplasia. Growth is slowly progressive, resulting in expansion of the tympanic cavity with thickening and concurrent osteolysis of the bulla (Figure 11.72) [61, 62]. If severe, it may cause resorption of the petrosal part of the temporal bone. This appearance can help differentiate it from otitis media (which lacks bulla expansion and adjacent osseous resorption) [61].

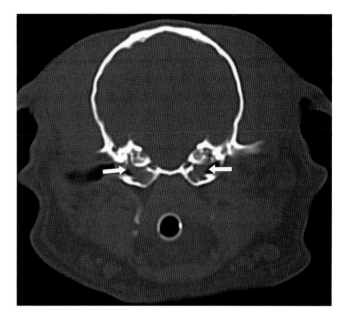

**FIGURE 11.69** Transverse CT images of a Cavalier King Charles spaniel with primary secretory otitis media. There is soft tissue attenuating fluid within tympanic bullae (arrows) but otherwise no evidence of osseous reaction.

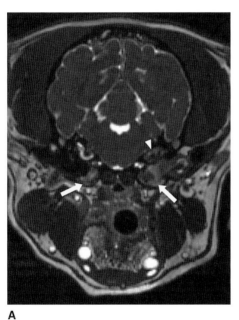

**A**

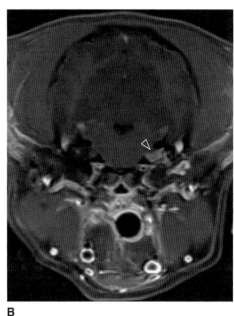

**B**

**FIGURE 11.70** Transverse T2-weighted (**A**) and postcontrast T1-weighted (**B**) images of a patient with otitis media bilaterally and left otitis interna. Both tympanic bullae are filled with T2 hyperintense and mildly contrast-enhancing material (arrows). The left inner ear structures are decreased in signal in T2-weighted images (closed arrowhead) and have increased enhancement on T1-weighted images (open arrowhead).

# Brain Imaging

Intracranial neoplasms may be described as either intraaxial or extraaxial based on their imaging features. Intraaxial tumors include most primary brain tumors such as glioma (Figure 11.73). The brain parenchyma completely surrounds intraaxial tumors. Contrast enhancement is variable, with many gliomas demonstrating poor enhancement. In comparison, extraaxial tumors arise outside the neuroparenchyma and include meningiomas, round cell neoplasia of the meninges, chroid plexus tumors, and pituitary tumors (Figure 11.74). These typically enhance more strongly than intraaxial tumors. Meningiomas and pituitary

tumors may have internal cystic or mineralized regions. Extraaxial tumors originate peripherally in the brain, with a broad base of contact with the adjacent calvarium, falx cerebri, or ventricular system. A dural tail is a thick area of contrast enhancement that extends away from the base of a meningioma into the adjacent meninges. While common in meningiomas, dural tail may occur with other neoplastic or inflammatory diseases that affect the meninges. Extraaxial tumors may also arise from adjacent osseous structures or within the caudal nasal cavity and secondarily affect the neuroparenchyma.

Ischemic and hemorrhagic cerebrovascular accidents (CVAs; also called strokes) have some unique features on MRI, though there is overlap in the appearance with neoplastic and

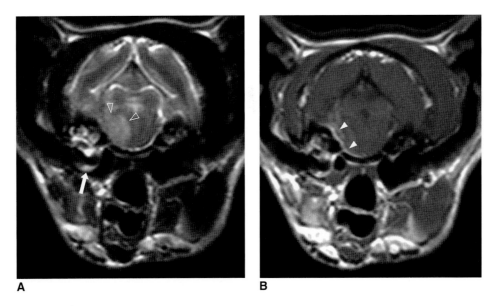

**FIGURE 11.71** Transverse T2-weighted (**A**) and postcontrast T1-weighted (**B**) images of a patient with right-sided otitis media and interna with extension of infection into the brain. The right tympanic bulla contains contrast-enhancing, T2 hyperintense material (arrows) representing otitis media. There is also increased enhancement of the right inner ear structures. The meninges adjacent to the right inner ear are contrast enhancing (closed arrowhead) and there is T2 hyperintensity within the brainstem representing adjacent inflammation and edema (open arrowhead).

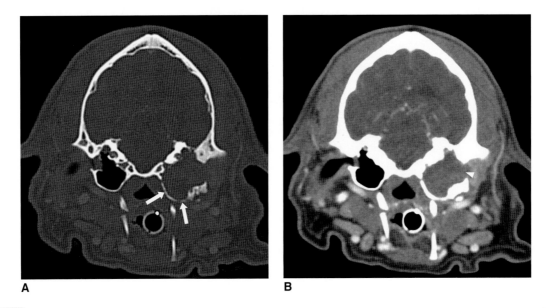

**FIGURE 11.72** Transverse precontrast (**A**) and postcontrast (**B**) images of a patient with a left-sided cholesteatoma. This causes thinning and multifocal lysis of the left tympanic bulla (arrows). The left bulla is also expansile and filled with fluid attenuating material (arrowhead).

inflammatory diseases. The location of the CVA depends on the affected vessel, and the cerebrum, cerebellum, and deeper white and gray matter may be affected. Acute ischemic strokes result in a well-marginated T2 hyperintense focus. Contrast enhancement is absent initially, but is expected with chronicity as revascularization occurs (Figure 11.75). Hemorrhagic strokes occur with vessel rupture, and can occur secondary to ischemic strokes. Extravasation of blood results in mixed signal on T2- and T1-weighted images and variable enhancement depending on

chronicity. The appearance of hemorrhage also changes rapidly after the initial hemorrhage occurs, being either T2/T1 hyper- or hypointense, or some combination of mixed intensities.

Inflammatory brain diseases tend to be more widespread and multifocal than neoplastic or vascular brain disease [63]. Immune-mediated causes of inflammation (such as meningo-encephalitis of unknown origin) and infectious causes of brain inflammation (such as toxoplasmosis, *Neospora*, fungal disease, viral diseases) have overlapping imaging characteristics

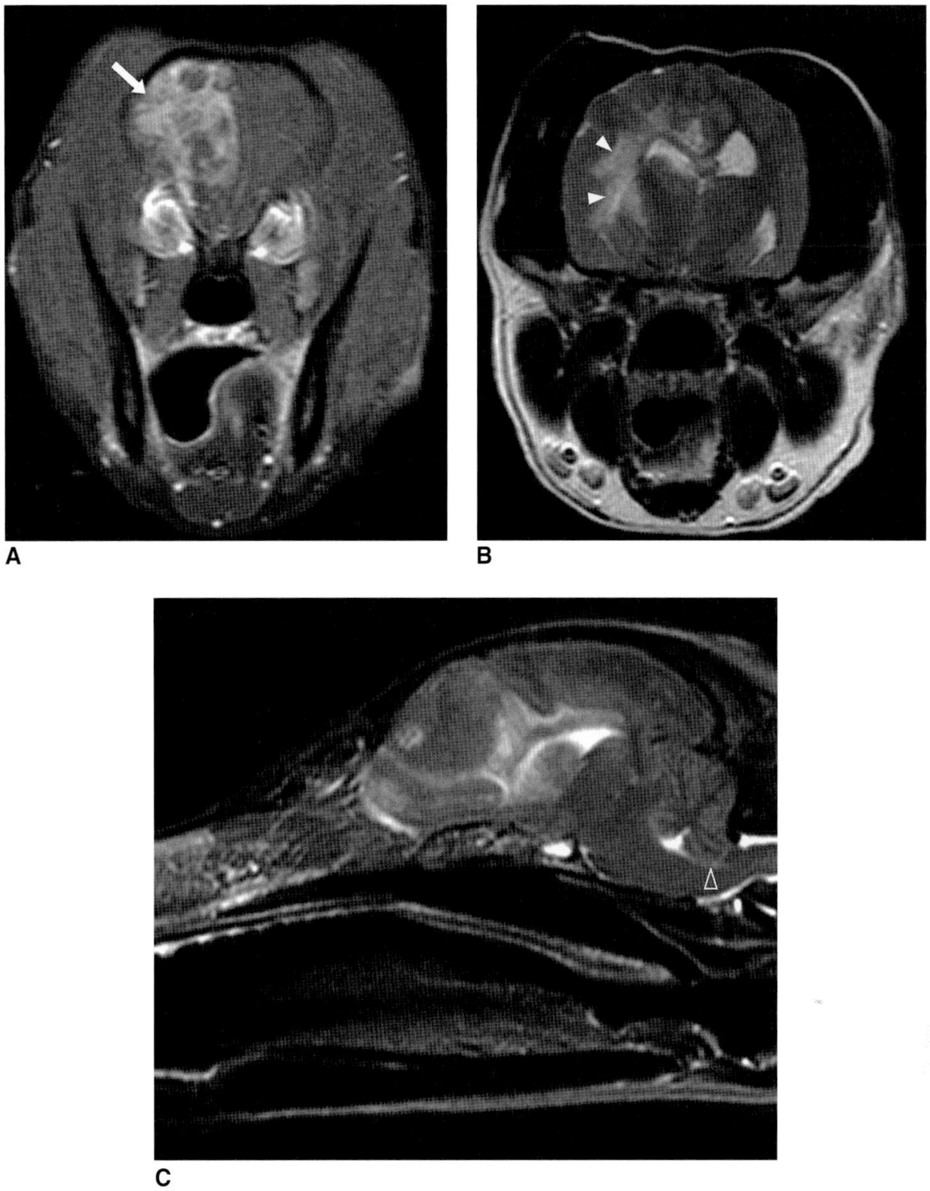

**FIGURE 11.73**  Transverse postcontrast T1-weighted (**A**), transverse T2-weighted (**B**) and sagittal T2-weighted (**C**) images of a patient with a glioma. There is a contrast-enhancing mass (arrow) in the right frontal lobe region. Caudal to this, there is edema in the internal capsule, characterized by high T2 signal (closed arrowhead). There is also herniation of the cerebellum at the foramen magnum (open arrowhead).

on MRI. Multifocal T2 hyperintensities with contrast enhancement are typical (Figure 11.76). Meningeal thickening and contrast enhancement are often present and diffuse.

Metabolic, nutritional, toxic, and degenerative encephalopathies are uncommon causes of structural brain disease. These diseases tend to cause bilaterally symmetric change on MRI. The area of the brain affected depends on the underlying cause. As an example, thiamine deficiency in cats results in symmetric multifocal T2/postcontrast T1 hyperintensities in the brainstem (affecting specific structures such as the red nucleus and caudal colliculus; Figure 11.77). Hepatic encephalopathy results in diffuse brain atrophy and hyperintensity in the lentiform nuclei. There are a large number of inherited

mitochondrial encephalopathies and lysosomal storage diseases intermittently reported in cats and dogs with similar findings [64].

Tumors, infarcts, and inflammatory disease result in regional vasogenic edema, caused by increased permeability of the blood–brain barrier and extravasation of fluid and protein into the brain parenchyma. On MRI, this causes increased T2 signal that does not contrast enhance surrounding the area of pathology. White matter is most affected (Figure 11.73). A mass effect or regional edema may obstruct the ventricular system resulting in hydrocephalus, recognized by ventricular dilation (Figure 11.73). Regardless of cause, when intracranial pressure becomes elevated, herniation of the brain parenchyma under

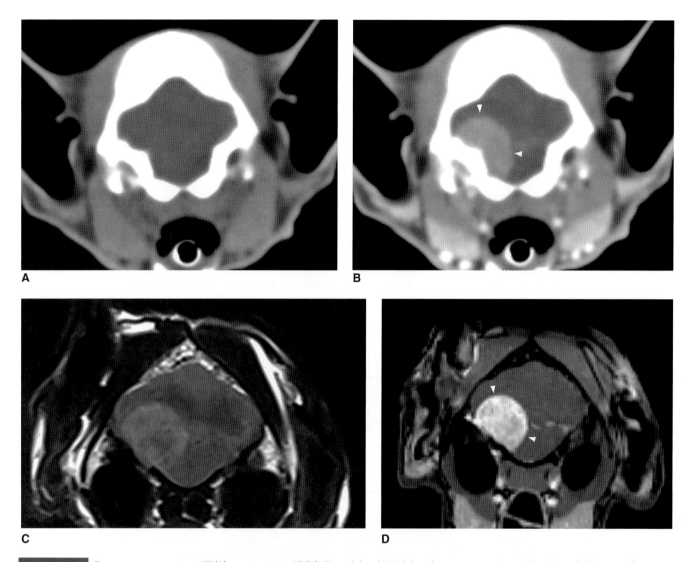

**FIGURE 11.74** Transverse precontrast CT (**A**), postcontrast CT (**B**), T2-weighted MRI (**C**) and postcontrast T1-weighted MRI (**D**) images of a meningioma. The mass strongly enhances on CT and MRI (arrowheads) and is only mildly T2 hyperintense.

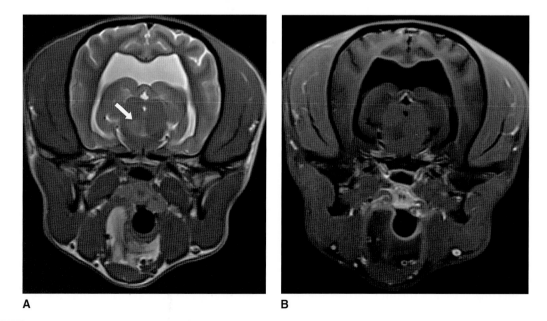

**FIGURE 11.75** Transverse T2 weighted (**A**) and postcontrast T1-weighted (**B**) MRI images of a patient with an acute arterial infarction. The infarct is T2 hyperintense (arrow) and there is no enhancement.

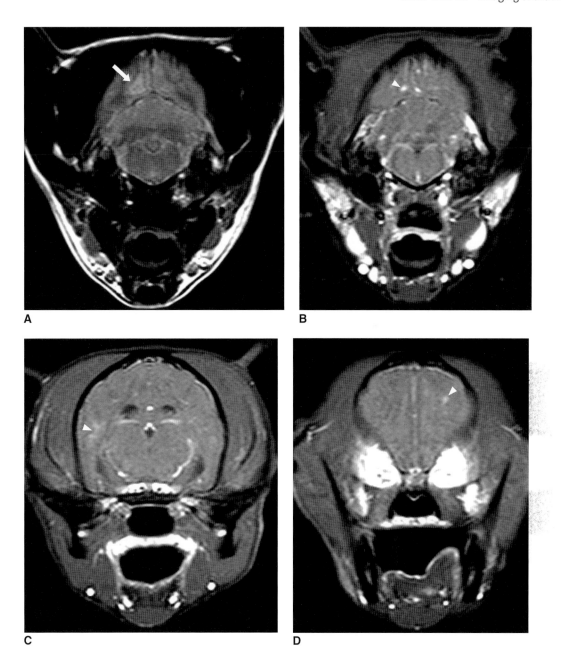

**FIGURE 11.76** Transverse FLAIR (**A**) and postcontrast T1-weighted (**B,C,D**) images of a patient with granulomatous meningoencephalitis. Multiple contrast-enhancing areas are seen in the brain (arrowheads) but only have a small amount of regional T2 change representing either edema or inflammation (arrow).

the tentorium cerebelli or through the foramen magnum occurs (referred to as transtentorial or cerebellar herniation respectively; Figure 11.73).

## Other Tumors of the Head

### Multilobular Osteochondrosarcoma

Multilobular osteochondrosarcoma (MLO), also referred to as multilobular tumor of bone, is an osseous tumor arising from the flat bones of the skull. It may affect the mandible, maxilla, cranium, zygoma, and tympanic bullae, and is usually limited to medium- and large-breed dogs [65, 66]. On imaging, it has a high degree of internal mineralization resulting in a unique mineralized "popcorn ball" appearance [67] (Figure 11.78). On MRI, the signal intensity varies, having a heterogeneous appearance, but tends to contrast enhance [68] (Figure 11.79).

### Carotid Body Tumor/Paraganglioma

Carotid body tumors arise from the carotid body at the base of the internal carotid artery, and are sometimes

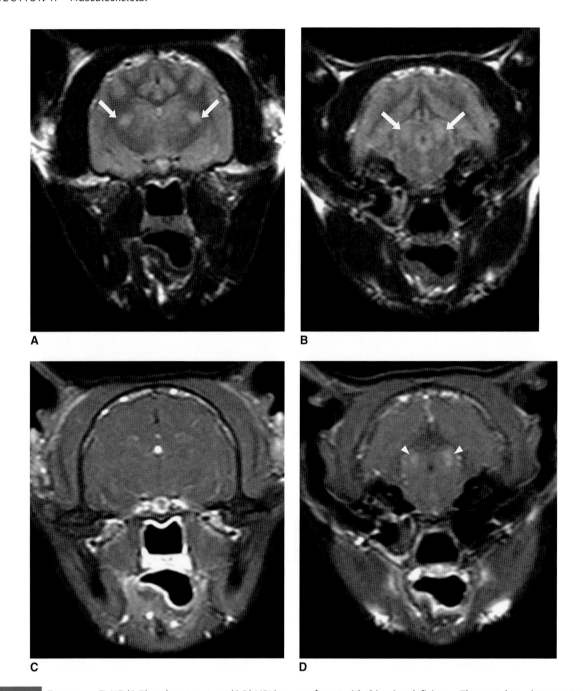

**FIGURE 11.77** Transverse FLAIR (**A,B**) and postcontrast (**C,D**) MRI images of a cat with thiamine deficiency. There are hyperintense structures on FLAIR that are symmetric between the left and right sides (arrows). There is some enhancement of the more caudal foci (arrowheads).

referred to as paraganglioma or chemodectoma. They are recognized on US, CT or MRI due to this characteristic location, and usually displace the common carotid artery ventrally (Figures 11.80 and 11.81) [69]. They strongly contrast enhance on CT and MRI, and may be well defined or creep along the carotid artery into the basilar region of the skull. They are differentiated from thyroid carcinoma due to their more rostral location and characteristic deviation of the common carotid artery.

# Other Miscellaneous Disorders

## Masticatory Muscle Myositis

Masticatory muscle myositis is an immune-mediated inflammatory disease where the immune system causes inflammation directed at the 2M masticatory muscle fibers. Dogs typically present at a young age, and are usually large-breed

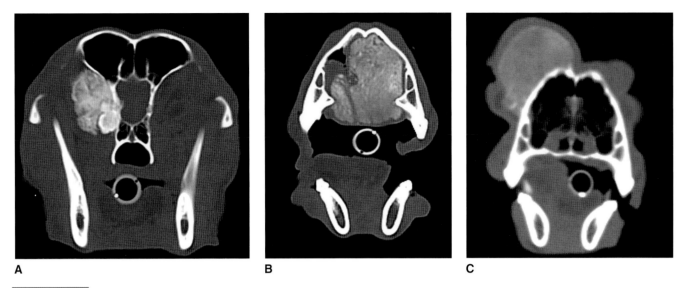

**FIGURE 11.78** (**A,B,C**) Transverse bone/window level images of multiple patients with multilobular osteochondrosarcoma. Notice the characteristic highly attenuating mineralization within each of these masses.

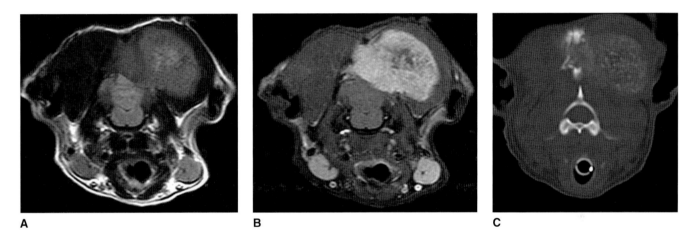

**FIGURE 11.79** Transverse T2-weighted (**A**) and postcontrast T1-weighted (**B**) MRI images and a CT image (**C**) of a dog with multilobular osteochondrosarcoma. The mass is intermediate in signal on T2-weighted images and strongly contrast enhancing. On the CT image, it has the characteristic mineralized appearance.

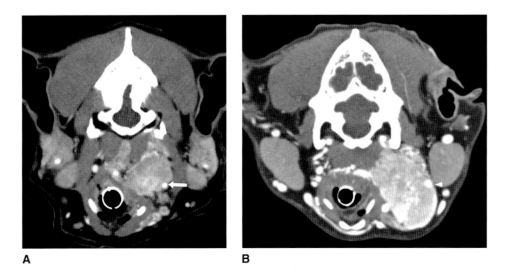

**FIGURE 11.80** Transverse postcontrast CT images (**A,B**) of two dogs with carotid body tumors. Both masses are strongly contrast enhancing and displacing the common carotid artery (arrowhead) lateral and ventrally.

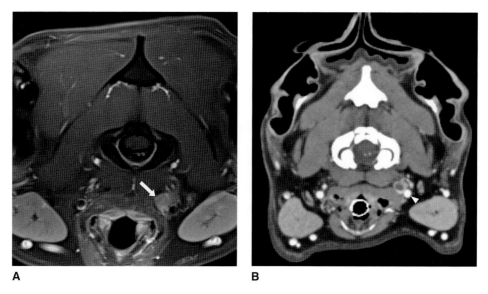

**A**                                              **B**

Transverse postcontrast T1-weighted MRI (**A**) and postcontrast CT (**B**) images of a small left carotid body tumor (arrow). The mass is dorsal medial to the left carotid artery (arrowhead).

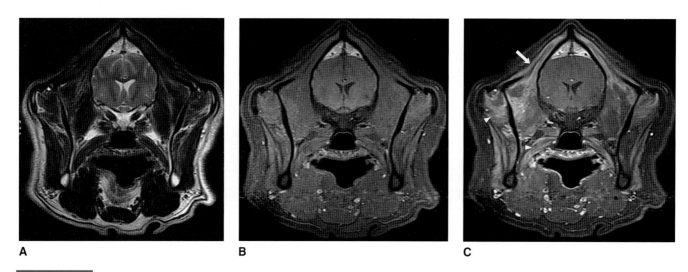

**A**                              **B**                              **C**

Transverse T2-weighted (**A**), precontrast (**B**) and postcontrast (**C**) T1-weighted images of a patient with immune-mediated masticatory myositis. The temporalis muscle (arrows) is decreased in size and contrast enhancing, being also more T2 hyperintense than expected. Other regional masticatory muscles also abnormally contrast enhance (arrowheads).

dogs such as golden retrievers and German shepherds, though Cavalier King Charles spaniels are also overrepresented (cats are rarely reported) [70]. The dogs have painful muscles on palpation and inability to open the mouth or eat.

The definitive test for masticatory myositis in dogs is identification of 2M antibodies (antibodies to the 2M muscle fiber types in masticatory muscles), but CT or MRI imaging is often performed on dogs with signs of masticatory myositis to rule out other potential causes of pain, such as foreign bodies or tumors [71]. On MRI, dogs develop bilateral increased T2 signal and contrast enhancement of the temporalis, masseter, and pterygoid muscles (the digastricus tends to be spared; Figure 11.82). On CT, muscles may demonstrate increased contrast enhancement (Figure 11.83). While changes are typically bilateral, one side may be more affected than the other.

With chronicity, masticatory muscles may become atrophic. Regional lymph nodes are often enlarged.

## Craniomandibular Osteopathy

See also Chapter 7.

The etiology of this disease is unknown, but it results in pain and swelling of the mandibular region in young dogs (usually 3–8 months of age) and is most common in young terrier breeds. It results in irregular bony proliferation of the mandible, which may extend to the tympanic bullae in severe cases (Figure 11.84). The proliferation is typically bilateral, but may be asymmetric with one mandible more affected than the other and may impede mastication (Figure 11.85).

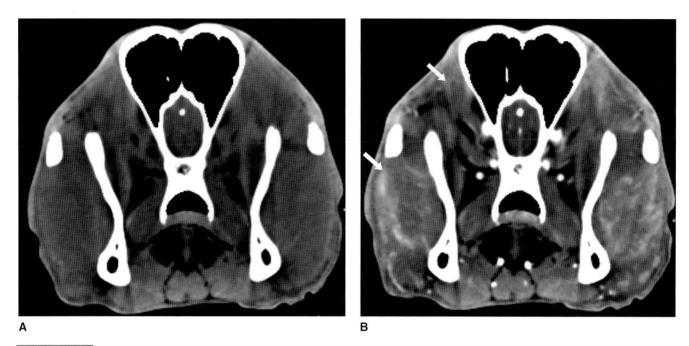

**FIGURE 11.83** Transverse precontrast (**A**) and postcontrast (**B**) CT images of a patient with masticatory myositis. The affected muscles are increased in size and have patchy internal contrast enhancement (arrows).

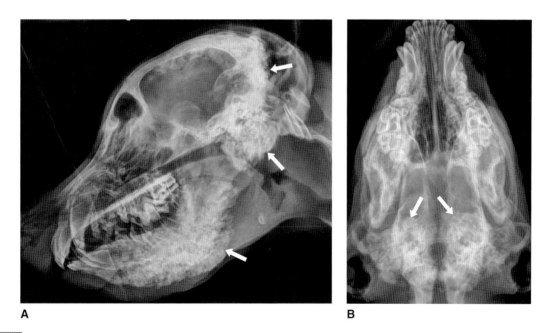

**FIGURE 11.84** Lateral (**A**) and ventrodorsal (**B**) projections of a patient with craniomandibular osteopathy. There is severe irregular bony proliferation (arrows) along both mandibular bodies and in the area of the tympanic bullae and caudal occiput.

## Calvarial Hyperostosis

See also Chapter 7.

The etiology of this disease is also unknown, but it results in pain of the skull accompanied by hyperostosis of the frontal and parietal bones (Figure 11.86). It typically affects bull mastiffs around 6 months of age. The mandible is unaffected.

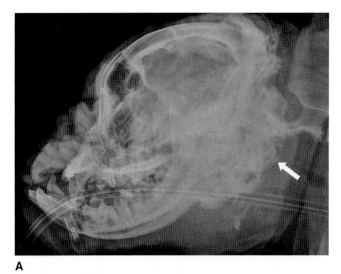

**A**

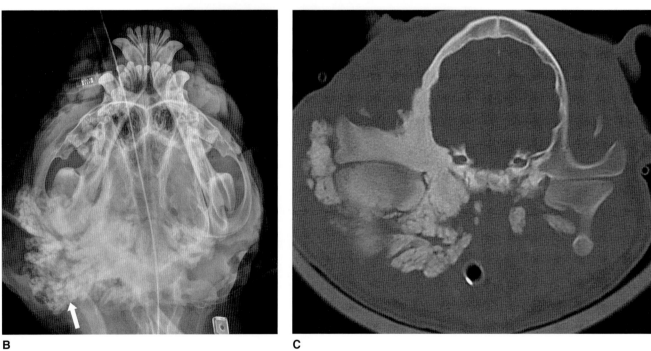

**B**

**C**

**FIGURE 11.85**   Lateral (**A**) and ventrodorsal (**B**) radiographs and transverse CT image (**C**) of a patient with craniomandibular osteopathy. There is severe bony reaction surrounding the right caudal mandible and tympanic bullae (arrows). The asymmetric dissipation of right versus left is unusual for this disease process, as the changes are typically more bilaterally symmetric and affect the rostral mandible.

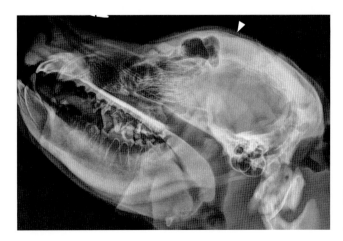

**FIGURE 11.86**   Lateral radiograph of a bull mastiff with calvarial hyperostosis. There is severe thickening of the dorsal calvarial osseous structures (arrowhead).

# References

1. Schwarz, T., Weller, R., Dickie, A.M. et al. (2002). Imaging of the canine and feline temporomandibular joint: a review. *Vet. Radiol. Ultrasound* 43 (2): 85–197.

2. Lefebvre, J., Kuehn, N.F., and Wortinger, A. (2005). Computed tomography as an aid in the diagnosis of chronic nasal disease in dogs. *J. Small Anim. Pract.* 46 (6): 280–285.

3. Ostrzeszewicz, M. and Sapierzynski, R. (2015). Fungal rhinitis in dogs. *Pol. J. Vet. Sci.* 18 (4): 683–688.

4. Karnik, K., Reichle, J.K., Fischetti, A.J., and Goggin, J.M. (2009). Computed tomographic findings of fungal rhinitis and sinusitis in cats. *Vet. Radiol. Ultrasound* 50 (1): 65–68.

5. Hamon, M., Dequeant, B., Decambron, A. et al. (2019). Leiomyoma in the nasal cavity of a dog. *J. Small Anim. Pract.* 60 (5): 319–322.

6. Ojeda, J., Mieres, M., Soto, F. et al. (2018). Computer tomographic imaging in 4 dogs with primary nasal canine transmissible venereal tumor and differing cellular phenotype. *J. Vet. Intern. Med.* 32 (3): 1172–1177.

7. Avner, A., Dobson, J.M., Sales, J.I., and Herrtage, M.E. (2008). Retrospective review of 50 canine nasal tumours evaluated by low-field magnetic resonance imaging. *J. Small Anim. Pract.* 49 (5): 233–239.

8. Jania, R., Boudreaux, B., Langohr, I. et al. (2019). Computed tomography imaging characteristics of canine nasal chondrosarcoma. *J. Small Anim. Pract.* 60 (11): 678–682.

9. Gumpel, E., Moore, A.S., Simpson, D.J. et al. (2017). Long-term control of olfactory neuroblastoma in a dog treated with surgery and radiation therapy. *Aust. Vet. J.* 95 (7): 227–231.

10. Ghirelli, C.O., Villamizar, L.A., and Pinto, A.C. (2013). Comparison of standard radiography and computed tomography in 21 dogs with maxillary masses. *J. Vet. Dent.* 30 (2): 72–76.

11. Skinner, O.T., Boston, S.E., Giglio, R.F. et al. (2018). Diagnostic accuracy of contrast-enhanced computed tomography for assessment of mandibular and medial retropharyngeal lymph node metastasis in dogs with oral and nasal cancer. *Vet. Comp. Oncol.* 16 (4): 562–570.

12. Lux, C.N., Culp, W.T.N., Johnson, L.R. et al. (2017). Prospective comparison of tumor staging using computed tomography versus magnetic resonance imaging findings in dogs with nasal neoplasia: a pilot study. *Vet. Radiol. Ultrasound* 58 (3): 315–325.

13. Murgia, D., Pivetta, M., Bowlt, K. et al. (2014). Intranasal epidermoid cyst causing upper airway obstruction in three brachycephalic dogs. *J. Small Anim. Pract.* 55 (8): 431–435.

14. Winer, J.N., Verstraete, F.J.M., Cissell, D.D. et al. (2018). Clinical features and computed tomography findings are utilized to characterize retrobulbar disease in dogs. *Front. Vet. Sci.* 5: 186.

15. Dennis, R. (2008). Imaging features of orbital myxosarcoma in dogs. *Vet. Radiol. Ultrasound* 49 (3): 256–263.

16. Charnock, L., Doran, B., Milley, E., and Preston, T. (2020). Canine retrobulbar lipoma excision through a ventral transpalpebral anterior orbitotomy. *Can. Vet. J.* 61 (3): 257–262.

17. Chai, O., Peery, D., Bdolah-Abram, T. et al. (2017). Computed tomographic findings in dogs with head trauma and development of a novel prognostic computed tomography-based scoring system. *Am. J. Vet. Res.* 78 (9): 1085–1090.

18. Arzi, B., Cissell, D.D., Verstraete, F.J. et al. (2013). Computed tomographic findings in dogs and cats with temporomandibular joint disorders: 58 cases (2006–2011). *J. Am. Vet. Med. Assoc.* 242 (1): 69–75.

19. Gatineau, M., El-Warrak, A.O., Marretta, S.M. et al. (2008). Locked jaw syndrome in dogs and cats: 37 cases (1998–2005). *J. Vet. Dent.* 25 (1): 16–22.

20. Hoppe, F. and Svalastoga, E. (1980). Temporomandibular dysplasia in American Cocker Spaniels. *J. Small Anim. Pract.* 21 (12): 675–678.

21. Lerer, A., Chalmers, H.J., Moens, N.M. et al. (2014). Imaging diagnosis – temporomandibular joint dysplasia in a Basset Hound. *Vet. Radiol. Ultrasound* 55 (5): 547–551.

22. Cannon, M.S., Paglia, D., Zwingenberger, A.L. et al. (2011). Clinical and diagnostic imaging findings in dogs with zygomatic sialadenitis: 11 cases (1990–2009). *J. Am. Vet. Med. Assoc.* 239 (9): 1211–1218.

23. Ramirez, G.A., Altimira, J., and Vilafranca, M. (2015). Cartilaginous tumors of the larynx and trachea in the dog: literature review and 10 additional cases (1995–2014). *Vet. Pathol.* 52 (6): 1019–1026.

24. MacPhail, C.M. (2020). Laryngeal disease in dogs and cats: an update. *Vet. Clin. North Am. Small Anim. Pract.* 50 (2): 295–310.

25. Berent, A.C. (2016). Diagnosis and management of nasopharyngeal stenosis. *Vet. Clin. North Am. Small Anim. Pract.* 46 (4): 677–689.

26. Rubin, J.A., Holt, D.E., Reetz, J.A., and Clarke, D.L. (2015). Signalment, clinical presentation, concurrent diseases, and diagnostic findings in 28 dogs with dynamic pharyngeal collapse (2008–2013). *J. Vet. Intern. Med.* 29 (3): 815–821.

27. Pollard, R.E., Johnson, L.R., and Marks, S.L. (2018). The prevalence of dynamic pharyngeal collapse is high in brachycephalic dogs undergoing videofluoroscopy. *Vet. Radiol. Ultrasound* 59 (5): 529–534.

28. Skerrett, S.C., McClaran, J.K., Fox, P.R., and Palma, D. (2015). Clinical features and outcome of dogs with epiglottic retroversion with or without surgical treatment: 24 cases. *J. Vet. Intern. Med.* 29 (6): 1611–1618.

29. Flanders, J.A. and Thompson, M.S. (2009). Dyspnea caused by epiglottic retroversion in two dogs. *J. Am. Vet. Med. Assoc.* 235 (11): 1330–1335.

30. Rudorf, H., Barr, F.J., and Lane, J.G. (2001). The role of ultrasound in the assessment of laryngeal paralysis in the dog. *Vet. Radiol. Ultrasound* 42 (4): 338–343.

31. Soukup, J.W., Snyder, C.J., Simmons, B.T. et al. (2013). Clinical, histologic, and computed tomographic features of oral papillary squamous cell carcinoma in dogs: 9 cases (2008–2011). *J. Vet. Dent.* 30 (1): 18–24.

32. Gardner, H., Fidel, J., Haldorson, G. et al. (2015). Canine oral fibrosarcomas: a retrospective analysis of 65 cases (1998–2010). *Vet. Comp. Oncol.* 13 (1): 40–47.

33. Amory, J.T., Reetz, J.A., Sanchez, M.D. et al. (2014). Computed tomographic characteristics of odontogenic neoplasms in dogs. *Vet. Radiol. Ultrasound* 55 (2): 147–158.

34. Thierry, F., Longo, M., Pecceu, E. et al. (2018). Computed tomographic appearance of canine tonsillar neoplasia: 14 cases. *Vet. Radiol. Ultrasound* 59 (1): 54–63.

35. Bannon, K.M. (2013). Clinical canine dental radiography. *Vet. Clin. North Am. Small Anim. Pract.* 43 (3): 507–532.

36. McGill, S., Lester, N., McLachlan, A., and Mansfield, C. (2009). Concurrent sialocoele and necrotising sialadenitis in a dog. *J. Small Anim. Pract.* 50 (3): 151–156.

37. Karbe, E. and Nielsen, S.W. (1966). Canine ranulas, salivary mucoceles and branchial cysts. *J. Small Anim. Pract.* 7 (10): 625–630.

38. Atkins, R.M., Hecht, S., Westermeyer, H.D., and McLean, N.J. (2010). What is your diagnosis? A zygomatic salivary gland mucocele. *J. Am. Vet. Med. Assoc.* 237 (12): 1375–1376.

39. Han, H., Mann, F.A., and Park, J.Y. (2016). Canine sialolithiasis: two case reports with breed, gender, and age distribution of 29 cases (1964–2010). *J. Am. Anim. Hosp. Assoc.* 52 (1): 22–26.

40. Coutin, J.V., Reese, S.L., Thieman-Mankin, K., and Ellison, G.W. (2014). What is your diagnosis? Mandibular sialolithiasis. *J. Am. Vet. Med. Assoc.* 244 (5): 535–537.

41. Kneissl, S., Weidner, S., and Probst, A. (2011). CT sialography in the dog – a cadaver study. *Anat. Histol. Embryol.* 40 (6): 397–401.

42. Hammer, A., Getzy, D., Ogilvie, G. et al. (2001). Salivary gland neoplasia in the dog and cat: survival times and prognostic factors. *J. Am. Anim. Hosp. Assoc.* 37 (5): 478–482.

43. Pownder, S., Fidel, J.L., Saveraid, T.C. et al. (2006). What is your diagnosis? Incidental melanosis of a salivary gland lesion. *J. Am. Vet. Med. Assoc.* 229 (2): 209–210.

44. Alcoverro, E., Tabar, M.D., Lloret, A. et al. (2014). Phenobarbital-responsive sialadenosis in dogs: case series. *Top Compan. Anim. Med.* 29 (4): 109–112.

45. Liptak, J.M. (2007). Canine thyroid carcinoma. *Clin. Tech. Small Anim. Pract.* 22 (2): 75–81.

46. Broome, M.R., Peterson, M.E., and Walker, J.R. (2014). Clinical features and treatment outcomes of 41 dogs with sublingual ectopic thyroid neoplasia. *J. Vet. Intern. Med.* 28 (5): 1560–1568.

47. Rossi, F., Caleri, E., Bacci, B. et al. (2013). Computed tomographic features of basihyoid ectopic thyroid carcinoma in dogs. *Vet. Radiol. Ultrasound* 54 (6): 575–581.

48. Barber, L.G. (2007). Thyroid tumors in dogs and cats. *Vet. Clin. North Am. Small Anim. Pract.* 37 (4): 755–773, vii.

49. Lautenschlaeger, I.E., Hartmann, A., Sicken, J. et al. (2013). Comparison between computed tomography and (99m)TC-pertechnetate scintigraphy characteristics of the thyroid gland in cats with hyperthyroidism. *Vet. Radiol. Ultrasound* 54 (6): 666–673.

50. Bromel, C., Pollard, R.E., Kass, P.H. et al. (2005). Ultrasonographic evaluation of the thyroid gland in healthy, hypothyroid, and euthyroid Golden Retrievers with nonthyroidal illness. *J. Vet. Intern. Med.* 19 (4): 499–506.

51. Taeymans, O., Daminet, S., Duchateau, L., and Saunders, J.H. (2007). Pre- and post-treatment ultrasonography in hypothyroid dogs. *Vet. Radiol. Ultrasound* 48 (3): 262–269.

52. Reese, S., Breyer, U., Deeg, C. et al. (2005). Thyroid sonography as an effective tool to discriminate between euthyroid sick and hypothyroid dogs. *J. Vet. Intern. Med.* 19 (4): 491–498.

53. Drost, W.T., Mattoon, J.S., Samii, V.F. et al. (2004). Computed tomographic densitometry of normal feline thyroid glands. *Vet. Radiol. Ultrasound* 45 (2): 112–116.

54. Lautscham, E., von Klopmann, C., Schaub, S. et al. (2020). CT imaging features of the normal parathyroid gland in the dog. *Tierarztl Prax Ausg K Kleintiere Heimtiere* 48 (5): 313–320.

55. Liles, S.R., Linder, K.E., Cain, B., and Pease, A.P. (2010). Ultrasonography of histologically normal parathyroid glands and thyroid lobules in normocalcemic dogs. *Vet. Radiol. Ultrasound* 51 (4): 447–452.

56. Reusch, C.E., Tomsa, K., Zimmer, C. et al. (2000). Ultrasonography of the parathyroid glands as an aid in differentiation of acute and chronic renal failure in dogs. *J. Am. Vet. Med. Assoc.* 217 (12): 1849–1852.

57. Lorek, A., Dennis, R., van Dijk, J., and Bannoehr, J. (2020). Occult otitis media in dogs with chronic otitis externa – magnetic resonance imaging and association with otoscopic and cytological findings. *Vet. Dermatol.* 31 (2): 146–153.

58. Cole, L.K., Samii, V.F., Wagner, S.O., and Rajala-Schultz, P.J. (2015). Diagnosis of primary secretory otitis media in the cavalier King Charles spaniel. *Vet. Dermatol.* 26 (6): 459–466.

59. Belmudes, A., Pressanti, C., Barthez, P.Y. et al. (2018). Computed tomographic findings in 205 dogs with clinical signs compatible with middle ear disease: a retrospective study. *Vet. Dermatol.* 29 (1): 45-e20.

60. Castillo, G., Parmentier, T., Monteith, G., and Gaitero, L. (2020). Inner ear fluid-attenuated inversion recovery MRI signal intensity in dogs with vestibular disease. *Vet. Radiol. Ultrasound* 61 (5): 531–539.

61. Travetti, O., Giudice, C., Greci, V. et al. (2010). Computed tomography features of middle ear cholesteatoma in dogs. *Vet. Radiol. Ultrasound* 51 (4): 374–379.

62. Hardie, E.M., Linder, K.E., and Pease, A.P. (2008). Aural cholesteatoma in twenty dogs. *Vet. Surg.* 37 (8): 763–770.

63. Wolff, C.A., Holmes, S.P., Young, B.D. et al. (2012). Magnetic resonance imaging for the differentiation of neoplastic, inflammatory, and cerebrovascular brain disease in dogs. *J. Vet. Intern. Med.* 26 (3): 589–597.

64. Hecht, S. and Adams, W.H. (2010). MRI of brain disease in veterinary patients part 2: acquired brain disorders. *Vet. Clin. North Am. Small Anim. Pract.* 40 (1): 39–63.

65. Straw, R.C., LeCouteur, R.A., Powers, B.E., and Withrow, S.J. (1989). Multilobular osteochondrosarcoma of the canine skull: 16 cases (1978–1988). *J. Am. Vet. Med. Assoc.* 195 (12): 1764–1769.

66. Dernell, W.S., Straw, R.C., Cooper, M.F. et al. (1998). Multilobular osteochondrosarcoma in 39 dogs: 1979–1993. *J. Am. Anim. Hosp. Assoc.* 34 (1): 11–18.

67. Hathcock, J.T. and Newton, J.C. (2000). Computed tomographic characteristics of multilobular tumor of bone involving the cranium in 7 dogs and zygomatic arch in 2 dogs. *Vet. Radiol. Ultrasound* 41 (3): 214–217.

68. Lipsitz, D., Levitski, R.E., and Berry, W.L. (2001). Magnetic resonance imaging features of multilobular osteochondrosarcoma in 3 dogs. *Vet. Radiol. Ultrasound* 42 (1): 14–19.

69. Mai, W., Seiler, G.S., Lindl-Bylicki, B.J., and Zwingenberger, A.L. (2015). CT and MRI features of carotid body paragangliomas in 16 dogs. *Vet. Radiol. Ultrasound* 56 (4): 374–383.

70. Blazejewski, S.W. and Shelton, G.D. (2018). Trismus, masticatory myositis and antibodies against type 2M fibers in a mixed breed cat. *JFMS Open Rep.* 4 (1): 2055116918764993.

71. Reiter, A.M. and Schwarz, T. (2007). Computed tomographic appearance of masticatory myositis in dogs: 7 cases (1999–2006). *J. Am. Vet. Med. Assoc.* 231 (6): 924–930.

# CHAPTER 12

# Imaging of the Spine

Nathan C. Nelson

Department of Molecular Biomedical Sciences, College of Veterinary Medicine, North Carolina State University, Raleigh, NC, USA

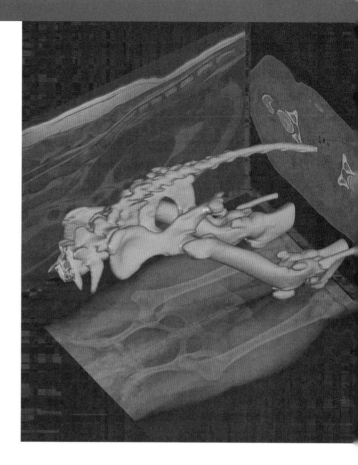

## Introduction

Indications for spinal imaging are numerous. Radiographs screen for occult spinal fractures in patients recently subjected to a traumatic event (hit by car, dog bite, etc.). Spinal imaging, particularly magnetic resonance imaging (MRI), is indicated in patients that are acutely paraplegic or display significant spinal pain. Patients with chronic limb neurologic deficits also warrant imaging, and MRI is the modality most likely to give a definitive diagnosis. Many patients with thoracic or hindlimb "lameness" in reality display nerve root signatures that localize to the spine, and rather than imaging the limbs, imaging tests should be directed toward the spine. Acquiring a thorough anamnesis and performing a careful orthopedic and neurologic examination are essential when determining the body part to image and imaging test (or tests) most likely to provide a diagnosis.

As indications to image the spine are broad, availability, client cost, and the clinical question dictate the choice of modality. As an example, in a patient with a history of recent vehicular trauma displaying neurologic symptoms, radiographs are a quick and cost-effective test to answer the question "Are there obvious fractures that could explain the clinical signs and would immediately alter the course of treatment?" If the answer is "no," then the decision to either medically manage the patient or pursue advanced imaging with computed tomography (CT) or MRI must be made (keeping in mind the limitations of radiography in detecting subtle bone or soft tissue pathology). In comparison, a patient with more chronic neurologic symptoms localized to the nerve roots is less likely to benefit from spinal radiographs as soft tissue lesions would not be detected. CT is more widely available and less expensive than MRI, and displays greater sensitivity than radiography for many soft tissue lesions of the spine. For those reason, CT might be the best imaging test available for a client, even if MRI might ultimately be more the more sensitive test for some conditions.

# Modalities for Imaging the Spine

## Radiography

Despite the development of advanced cross-sectional techniques, radiography remains the most common first-line imaging test when evaluating patients with pain or neurologic symptoms localized to a spinal segment. Two orthogonal projections are acquired, albeit with caveats. Patients that have undergone trauma should initially have lateral radiographs performed, followed by ventrodorsal projections when there is confirmation that no gross spinal instability or fracture is present. In this situation, when orthogonal projections are required, cross-table horizontal beam projections are a consideration as the patient does not need to be rolled into dorsal recumbency (as would otherwise be the case for ventrodorsal radiographs). Radiographs also allow careful stress radiography (with the vertebrae in flexion or extension), which is much more challenging with CT or MRI. Positional radiography can evaluate for spinal instability, such as with atlantoaxial instability.

## Myelography

Radiographs readily identify the vertebral canal margins but the actual spinal cord is not seen due to effacement with surrounding soft tissues. Myelography involves injection of nonionic iodinated contrast medium into the subarachnoid space around the spinal cord, delineating its margins. Pathology that compresses or expands the spinal cord will be apparent. The subarachnoid space should remain a thin "column" that parallels the margin of the spinal cord. Spinal cord compression is recognized by distortion or narrowing of the subarachnoid space, with different patterns depending on whether the pathology is outside the dura mater (extradural pathology), within the spinal cord (intramedullary pathology), or between the dura mater and spinal cord (intradural-extramedullary) (Figure 12.1).

## Computed Tomography

Computed tomography provides better three-dimensional anatomy of the spine and better soft tissue contrast than radiography, allowing earlier diagnosis of many spinal diseases compared to radiography. CT has advantages over MRI in that it is more accessible, cheaper, and faster. A typical CT examination of the spine lasts approximately 10 minutes from start to finish whereas an MRI examination is typically a minimum of 30 minutes. Unlike MRI, CT cannot distinguish the spinal cord as separate from the surrounding cerebrospinal fluid (CSF) or meninges. While it does allow visualization of the epidural space and other spinal structures, the soft tissue detail is inferior to MRI. CT may be combined with myelography, allowing better diagnosis by direct visualization of the spinal cord, more similar to MRI, but still provides limited internal detail of the spinal cord.

## Magnetic Resonance Imaging

Magnetic resonance imaging is the gold standard for imaging the spinal cord and paraspinal soft tissues. By separating the signal of CSF, spinal tissue, and epidural fat, spinal

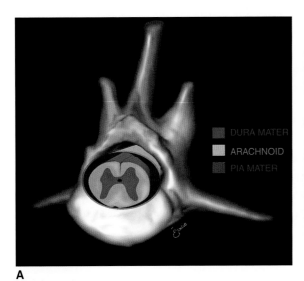

**A**

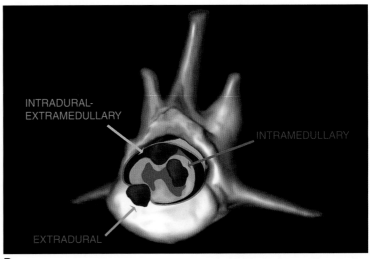

**B**

**FIGURE 12.1**   Relevant spinal anatomy, including dura mater, arachnoid membrane, and pia mater (**A**). Lesions in this area arise from the spinal cord (intramedullary), outside the dura mater (extradural) or within the dura but outside the spinal cord (intradural extramedullary) (**B**). Imaging tests attempt to determine whether pathology is located within one of these three areas, as that ultimately determines the most likely differential diagnosis present.

pathology is directly imaged without the need for intrathecal contrast agent. The downsides of MRI are the longer acquisition time, requirement of anesthesia, and greater expense of an examination.

Typical MRI protocols include T2-weighted and T1-weighted images, pre- and post-IV contrast. IV contrast is not necessary for all spinal examinations, particularly those where intervertebral disc extrusion is the most likely clinical diagnosis based on presentation and history. Withholding IV contrast saves time (as postcontrast images are unnecessary) and expense if the diagnosis is made on precontrast images.

# Congenital Vertebral Disorders

Numerous congenital anomalies affect osseous and soft tissue structures of the spine. Some of these have no clinical effect on the patient and do not result in clinical signs. Others present when the patient is young, as the malformation may result in early spinal cord compression. Some may not initially affect the patient, but may predispose to instability and present with clinical signs when older and instability becomes more pronounced.

## Atlantoaxial Subluxation

Atlantoaxial instability is a common disorder in small- and toy-breed dogs. The etiology is complex, but typically involves both soft tissue and orthopedic malformations. Clinical signs are chronic and insidious, affecting all four limbs, though sometimes an acute exacerbation may be present. Though atlantoaxial subluxation may occur due to trauma, it typically is due to incomplete development of the soft tissues and osseous structures in this region. Specifically, ligaments that stabilize this joint are incompletely developed. Moreover, the dens may be shortened and hypoplastic, further leading to instability (Figure 12.2). The result is increased mobility at this joint, resulting in soft tissue inflammation, hypertrophy, and eventual spinal cord compression.

Classically, diagnosis of atlantoaxial instability was achieved through a standard lateral radiograph performed in neutral position compared to a radiograph acquired during gentle neck flexion. Neck flexion results in separation of the lamina of C1 and the spinous process of C2, with dorsal displacement of C2 relative to C1, a motion prevented in normal dogs by the strong, thick atlantoaxial dorsal ligament. On the lateral projection, the normal alignment of C2 relative to C1 is altered, so that the angle of flexion between these vertebrae increases. Risk of spinal flexion in a dog with atlantoaxial instability is obvious, as flexion in a dog with instability can result in significant spinal cord compression as C2 subluxates dorsally and a worsening of clinical signs or even death.

In recent years, other lesions associated with this instability have been recognized with the increased use of CT and MRI imaging. Specifically, atlantoaxial instability may be seen in concert with atlantooccipital overlapping, where the dorsal lamina of C1 protrudes into the caudal fossa of the skull and can result in cerebellar compression (Figure 12.3). This is only possible if there is concurrent malformation and incomplete

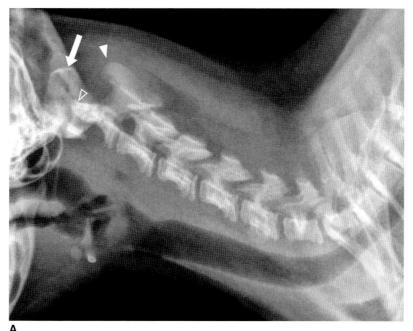

A

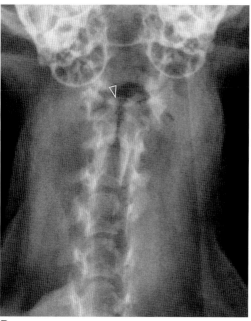

B

**FIGURE 12.2**    Lateral (**A**) and VD (**B**) projections of a dog with dens hypoplasia (arrow) and C1–2 subluxation. Note the increased distance between the lamina of C1 (arrow) and spinous process of C2 (closed arrowhead). C2 is displaced dorsally relative to C1 and the dens is blunted (open arrowhead).

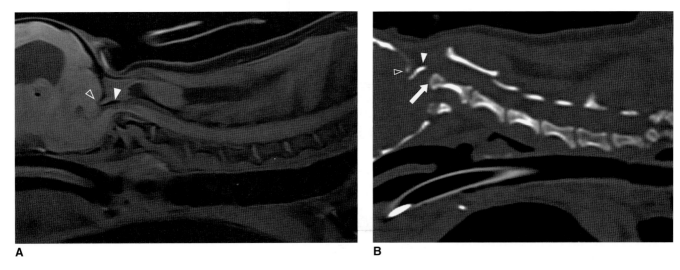

A                                                    B

**FIGURE 12.3** Sagittal T1-weighted MR (**A**) and sagittal CT (**B**) images of a dog with dens hypoplasia, C1–2 subluxation, and cranial displacement of C1 into the caudal fossa. The dens is blunted (arrow). The C1 lamina (closed arrowhead) is displaced cranially, being ventral to the dorsal margin of the foramen magnum (open arrowhead). The spinal cord is severely compressed at this level, but this is only appreciated on the MRI image as the spinal cord is not distinctly seen on the CT.

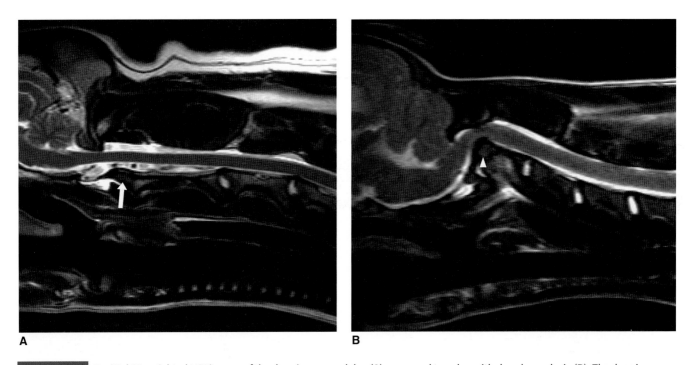

A                                                    B

**FIGURE 12.4** Sagittal T2-weighted MRI images of the dens in a normal dog (**A**) compared to a dog with dens hypoplasia (**B**). The dens in the normal dog (arrow) is much larger than the small one in the affected dog (arrowhead). There is also subluxation of C1–2 and spinal cord compression (arrowhead).

ossification of the foramen magnum, resulting in a keyhole shape that allows C1 to protrude into the skull (often termed occipital dysplasia). This is difficult to recognize radiographically and requires either CT or MRI to definitively diagnose.

Dens hypoplasia is commonly present in dogs with atlantoaxial instability (Figures 12.2 and 12.4). This is difficult to identify on a straight lateral projection of the spine as the large superimposed wings of C1 overlap the dens of C2, making identification of the dens difficult in all dogs. Slight, intentional obliquity of the head rotates the wings of C1 in a way

that the dens may be appreciated (see Chapter 6). The ventro-dorsal projection also highlights the dens and is another way to assess potential hypoplasia, though the risks of positioning a dog with suspected subluxation should be weighed against the information provided by a VD projection. Moreover, some dogs that are clinically normal may have undeveloped dens, so identification of this anomaly alone cannot diagnose instability without the dynamic positioning.

Both MRI and CT are able to recognize morphologic abnormalities of C2 and C1, and can help confirm spinal cord compression, but dynamic imaging of the spine to confirm atlantoaxial subluxation is typically still reserved to radiography given the dangers with prolonged flexion required by MRI and CT to diagnose this instability.

## Transitional Vertebrae

Transitional vertebrae have characteristics of two different vertebral types, and may be symmetric or asymmetric between their left and right halves. These anomalies typically are of the vertebral arch rather than the vertebral body. For instance, a thoracolumbar vertebral segment will have one lateral half that appears to be a thoracic vertebral body with a small adjacent rib, whereas the other lateral half will appear similar to a lumbar segment and have a broad transverse process (Figure 12.5). The most caudal ribs may be hypoplastic or aplastic bilaterally. Similarly, a lumbosacral transitional segment may have one lumbarized half and one sacralized half or both may be lumbarized. This may be seen involving only one vertebral segment (Figure 12.6) or multiple segments (Figure 12.7).

Transitional segments are most common at the thoracolumbar and lumbosacral junctions, but cervicothoracic transitional segments do occur, most commonly characterized by small vestigial ribs on C7. Those at the cervicothoracic and thoracolumbar junctions are typically incidental and do not result in clinical signs, though thoracolumbar transitional segments may complicate vertebral counting prior to spinal surgery and cause crowding of regional anatomy (Figure 12.8). Transitional segments at the lumbosacral junction increase the risk of intervertebral disc degeneration and instability, which can result in nerve impingement and cauda equina

syndrome (Figure 12.9). Lumbosacral transitional segments may also affect normal hip development [1, 2]. Sacral congenital abnormalities are expected in some breeds (such as English bulldogs) and typically do not result in clinical signs (Figure 12.10).

## Hemivertebrae

Hemivertebrae are congenital vertebral body malformations that represent a defect that occurred during vertebral body formation [3]. They are the most common malformation seen in the spine, and are most common in brachycephalic breeds such as the pug and English bulldog. They are most common in the midthoracic region, but occur as far caudal as the thoracolumbar junction, and are rare in the cervical or lumbar area (Figure 12.5). They may result in deviation of the long axis of the spine, directing it dorsally (kyphosis), ventrally (lordosis), or to the side (scoliosis). This degree of deviation is typically mild, but hemivertebrae result in vertebral canal stenosis and spinal cord compression if severe (Figure 12.11).

Though most dogs with hemivertebrae are neurologically normal, kyphosis in particular is a risk factor for development of clinical signs from spinal cord compression [3, 4].

Classification schemes for the different shapes of hemivertebrae are based on which portions of the vertebral body are incompletely formed and to what degree [3, 5]. In general, hemivertebrae have a wedge type of shape, with some degree of ventral and/or lateral vertebral body hypoplasia or aplasia [3, 5]. Hemivertebrae are not always wedge shaped, however, and median aplasia, where there is incomplete or absence of the central region of the vertebrae, results in a "butterfly

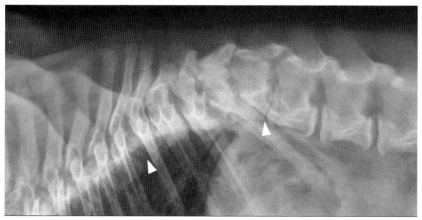

**A**

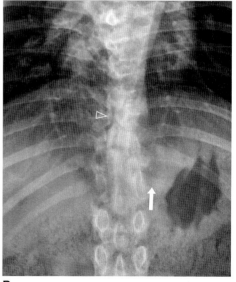

**B**

**FIGURE 12.5**   Lateral (**A**) and VD (**B**) projections of a dog with congenital malformations at the thoracolumbar junction. The left 13th rib is aplastic and instead the left side of T13 appears similar to lumbar vertebrae (arrow). Multiple hemivertebrae are present which result in kyphosis (closed arrowhead). T10 is a butterfly vertebrae, as seen on the VD projection (open arrowhead).

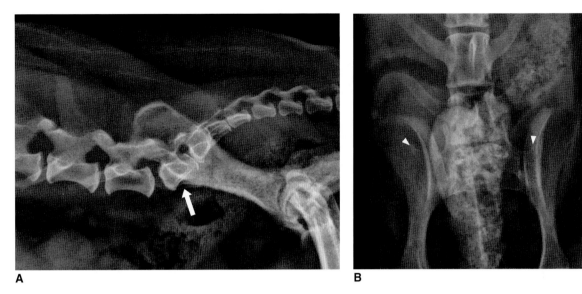

**FIGURE 12.6** Lateral (**A**) and VD (**B**) projections of a lumbosacral transitional segment. S1 is separate from the other two sacral segments (arrow) and has two small lumbar-like transverse processes (arrowheads).

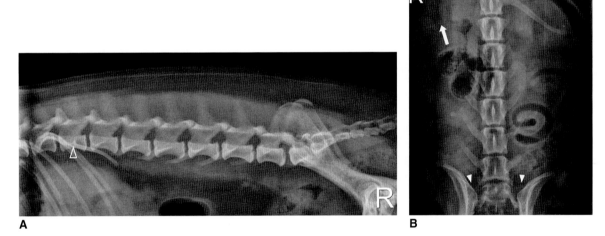

**FIGURE 12.7** Lateral (**A**) and VD (**B**) projections of the lumbar spine in a dog with congenital malformations. The right 13th rib is hypoplastic with only a small remnant present (arrow), and the left 13th rib is broad and lumbarized (open arrowhead). L7 has broad transverse processes (closed arrowheads). Three fused sacral segments are present, best appreciated on the lateral projection.

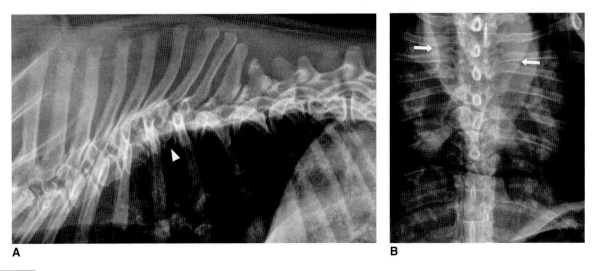

**FIGURE 12.8** Lateral (**A**) and VD (**B**) projections of a dog with congenital malformations in the midthoracic region. T5–7 hemivertebrae have a wedge-shaped vertebral body (arrowheads) and result in kyphosis. There is crowding of the ribs on the VD projection (arrows).

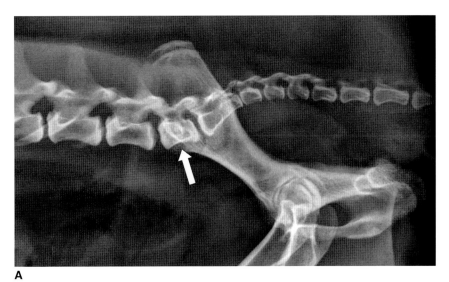
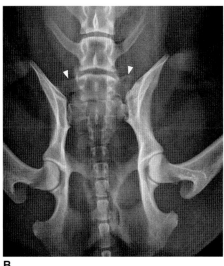

**A**  **B**

**FIGURE 12.9**  Lateral (**A**) and VD (**B**) projections of a dog with a transitional first sacral segment. On the lateral projection, the first sacral segment (arrow) is unfused to the other two, and has an angulation between the lumbar and other sacral segments. On the VD, this vertebrae has short left and right margins which appear similar to lumbar transverse processes (arrowheads). This patient had cauda equina syndrome.

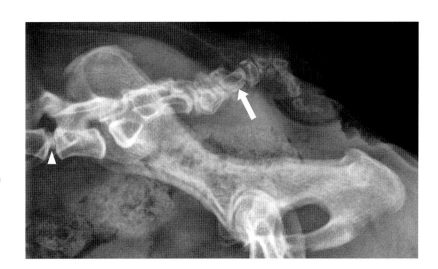

**FIGURE 12.10**  Lateral projection of a bulldog with congenital malformations of the sacrum and caudal vertebrae, typical of the breed. The sacrum has a convex shape on the lateral projection, and multiple malformed caudal vertebrae are seen (arrow). The L6–7 disc is mineralized in situ (arrowhead).

vertebrae" recognized by the resemblance to a butterfly when evaluated on the ventrodorsal projection (Figure 12.5). In some dogs, there may be symmetric and incomplete development of a vertebral body (termed symmetric hypoplasia), resulting in a diffusely shortened vertebral body but this does not cause any spinal malalignment.

## Block Vertebra

Block vertebrae are congenital defects in segmentation, where adjacent vertebral developmental bodies do not separate into two different vertebrae. The result is one long vertebral segment with adjacent fusion of the vertebral bodies and possibly the vertebral arches (Figure 12.12). These are usually not clinically relevant and do not cause symptoms, but can predispose to intervertebral disc degeneration (Figure 12.13) and

herniation (Figure 12.14) in the adjacent discs due to increased loading from a fulcrum effect [6].

## Facet Dysplasia

Incomplete development of the caudal articular processes of the vertebrae at the thoracolumbar junction has been described in brachycephalic dogs. These articular processes may be either hypoplastic or completely aplastic, resulting in decreased vertebral column stability (Figure 12.15). Pugs are particularly affected. This malformation is associated with progressive neurologic symptoms from chronic cord disease from chronic instability. This may be recognized on survey radiographs by incompletely formed or absent articular processes, but is most easily recognized when cross-sectional imaging is performed in these patients (Figure 12.16) [7].

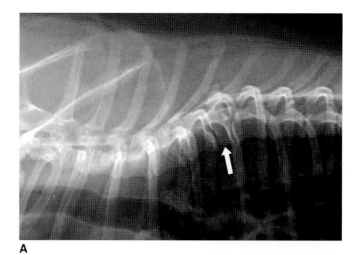

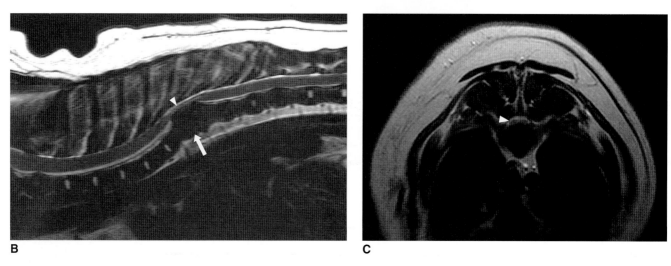

**FIGURE 12.11** Lateral radiograph (**A**), sagittal T2W image (**B**) and transverse T2W image (**C**) of a dog with a T7 hemivertebrae (arrow) resulting in kyphosis. There is spinal cord compression (arrowheads) as seen on the MRI images due to this malformation and presumably intervertebral disc herniation.

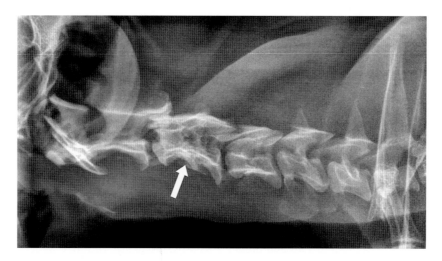

**FIGURE 12.12** Lateral radiograph of a dog with a C3–4 block vertebrae (arrow). The dog had no clinical symptoms.

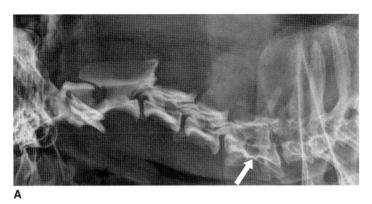
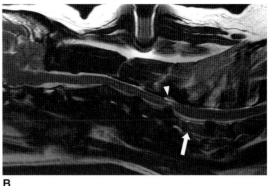

**A**   **B**

**FIGURE 12.13**   Lateral radiograph (**A**) and sagittal T2-weighted MRI (**B**) of a dog with C5–6 block vertebrae (arrow) and disc compression of the spinal cord at C4–5 (arrowhead). The spinal cord has an hour-glass shape and increased T2 signal consistent with atrophy and gliosis from chronic compression.

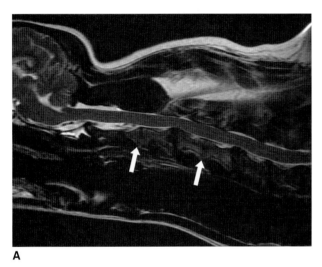
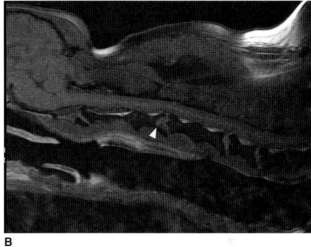

**A**   **B**

**FIGURE 12.14**   Sagittal T2W image (**A**) and sagittal T1W image (**B**) of a dog with C2–3 and C4–5 block vertebrae (arrows). The spinal cord is not significantly compressed. There is also concavity of the caudal C3 endplate, consistent with disc herniation into the vertebrae (arrowhead) sometimes termed a "Schmorl's node."

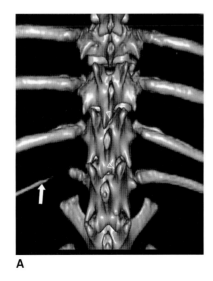
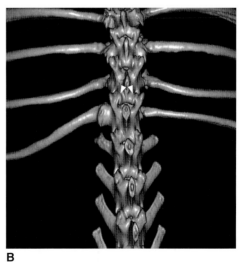

**A**   **B**

**FIGURE 12.15**   3D image of a pug with facet hypoplasia (**A**) and a pug without facet hypoplasia (**B**). In the affected dog, multiple caudal articular facts are absent or hypoplastic (open arrowheads) when compared to the nonaffected dog where the caudal articular facets are normal (closed arrowheads). Note that in (**A**) there is hypoplasia of the right 13th rib (arrow) and in (**B**) there is a lumbarized transitional right 13th rib.

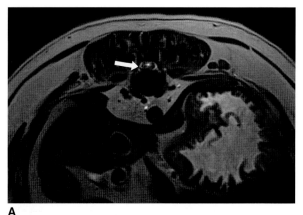
**A**
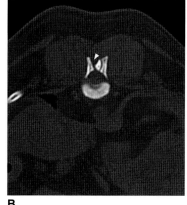
**B**
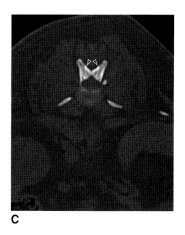
**C**

**FIGURE 12.16** Transverse T2W image (**A**) and transverse CT image (**B**) of a dog with facet hypoplasia, compared to CT images of a normal dog (**C**). These are the same dogs as in Figure 12.15. On MRI images, there is a herniated disc causing spinal cord compression (arrowhead) at T12–13. A transverse process is unilaterally absent (closed arrowhead) in the affected dog (closed arrowhead) but left and right transverse processes are present in the normal dog (open arrowheads).

## Spina Bifida

Spina bifida is a defect in the normal embryologic development of the neural tube, characterized by failure of the vertebral arches/lamina to close over the spinal cord [8]. This is recognized by a duplication of the spinous process to the left/right sides of the midline on the ventrodorsal radiograph or absence of normally formed spinous processes (Figure 12.17). Typically, this malformation is not associated with neurologic defects and the underlying meninges and spinal cord are presumed normal. If instead, the meninges protrude through the open vertebral arch, the defect is referred to as meningocele, and if the meninges and neural tissue extend into the opening, it is referred to as meningomyelocele [8]. Radiographs cannot determine the degree of meningeal/neural involvement, which usually relies on MRI, though CT with a myelogram would accurately assess the degree of neural involvement (Figure 12.18).

# Uncommon, Diffuse Bone Diseases

## Osteosclerosis

Osteosclerosis is defined by a diffuse increase in opacity of long bone and vertebral medullary cavities (Figure 12.19). This radiographic appearance is occasionally seen in young or older patients, and may be attributed to multiple disease processes, though the cause is not always identified. *Osteopetrosis* is a rarely reported inherited bone disease caused by abnormal osteoclast function, resulting in osteosclerosis in young patients. Osteosclerosis has been described in cats infected by feline leukemia virus and also described as a paraneoplastic change [9].

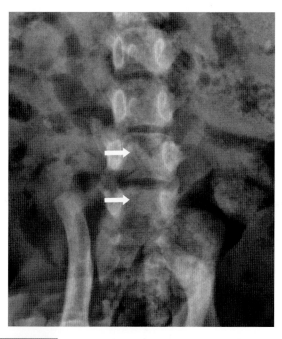

**FIGURE 12.17** VD radiograph of a dog with spina bifida. There is incomplete formation of the L6/7 lamina with lack of distinct spinous process (arrows).

## Congenital Hypothyroidism

This rare congenital disorder in dogs and cats is caused by an abnormality somewhere along the hypothalamic-pituitary-thyroid axis, resulting in decreased production of thyroid hormones. Most commonly, it is due to dysgenesis of the thyroid gland [10, 11]. As thyroid hormone is necessary for normal bone development, all bones are equally affected, with animals displaying disproportionate dwarfism with delayed epiphyseal maturation and epiphyseal dysgenesis [11]. In the spine, the vertebrae will have a shortened appearance and are often decreased in opacity (Figure 12.20). There may be secondary degenerative changes to the spinal articular joints.

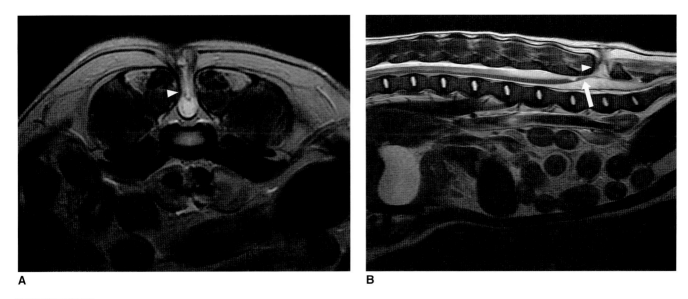

**FIGURE 12.18**   Transverse (**A**) and sagittal (**B**) T2W MRI images of a dog with spina bifida and a meningomyelocele. This is the same dog as Figure 12.17. The subarachnoid space protrudes through this defect (arrowheads). Note that the nerve roots of the cauda equina extend into this defect (arrow).

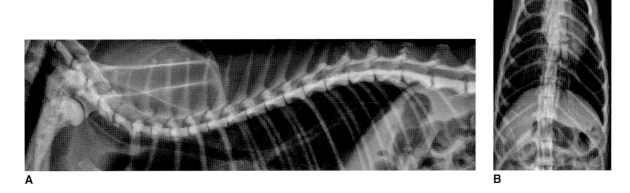

**FIGURE 12.19**   Lateral (**A**) and VD (**B**) radiographs of a cat with generalized osteosclerosis. There is diffuse increased opacity of the medullary bone, including the ribs and humeri.

## Osteogenesis Imperfecta

Osteogenesis imperfecta is a well-documented but rare heritable bone disease that results in diffuse skeletal maldevelopment, sometimes referred to as "brittle bone disease" [12, 13]. The cause is a defect in the genes that encode the precursor molecules to collagen type 1, which makes up 90% of the organic substance of bone. Defects in this matrix reduce

overall bone mineralization. These weakened bones are predisposed to folding fractures and are frequently malformed. Patients will commonly appear stunted. Radiographically, there is diffuse decrease in opacity of the vertebrae, and endplates and cortical bone will appear thin (Figure 12.21). Fractures and malformation of the spine are typical. Because this is a diffuse disease, similar changes are expected in the long bones.

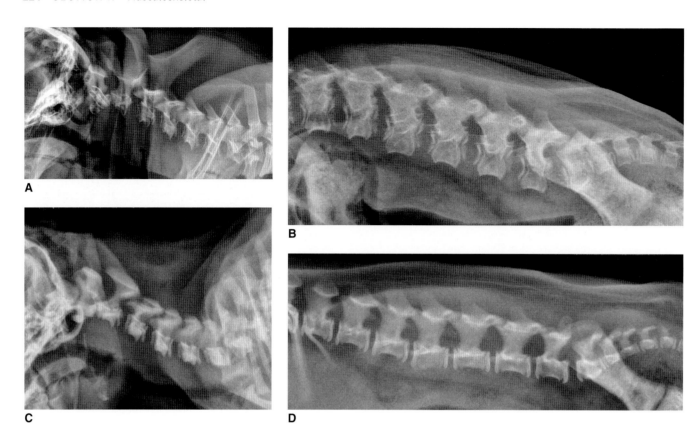

**FIGURE 12.20** Lateral cervical (**A**) and lumbar (**B**) radiographs of a dog affected by congenital hypothyroidism with cervical (**C**) and lumbar (**D**) radiographs from a normal age-matched dog. There is generalized decreased bone opacity and small epiphyses of the affected dog when compared to the normal dog.

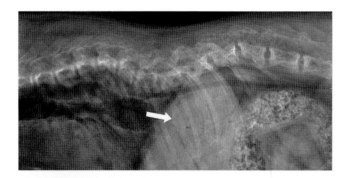

**FIGURE 12.21** Lateral radiograph of a dog with osteogenesis imperfecta. There is decreased bony opacity diffusely. Multiple rib fractures (arrow) are present and spinal deformations (short vertebrae, lordosis) from previous folding fractures.

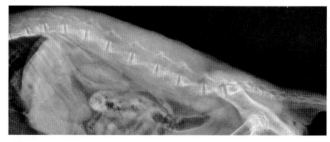

**FIGURE 12.22** Lateral radiograph of a cat with nutritional hyperparathyroidism. Notice that all bones are decreased in opacity relative to adjacent soft tissues, resulting in poor osseous contrast.

## Nutritional Secondary Hyperparathyroidism

Patients fed a diet with inappropriate levels of calcium and vitamin D are at risk of nutritional hyperparathyroidism. The resultant mobilization of calcium from osseous structures results in vertebrae which are more lucent than expected (Figure 12.22). The overall appearance is similar to osteogenesis imperfecta, but the conditions are readily differentiated when a complete diet history is collected.

# Intervertebral Disc Diseases

## Discospondylitis

Discospondylitis is infection (usually bacterial) of the intervertebral disc. The infection typically spreads to the disc through a hematogenous route, though rarely infections may be fungal in etiology and caused by local infections (such as those caused by epidural infections or migrating grass awns; Figure 12.23) [14]. The infection starts in the cartilaginous endplate of the vertebral body, and is recognized radiographically when lysis of the osseous endplate develops [14]. The bacterial source is most commonly in the urinary tract or prostrate, as

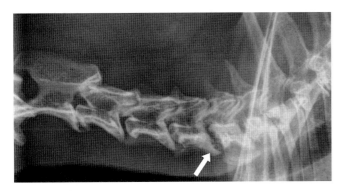

**FIGURE 12.23**   Lateral cervical radiograph showing C5–6 discospondylitis (arrow). There is ventral bony proliferation and widening of the disc space due to irregular endplate lysis.

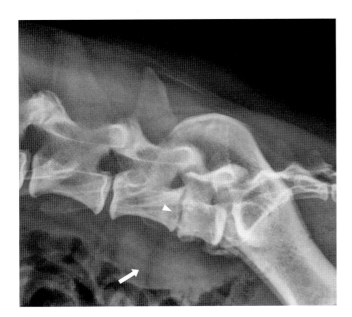

**FIGURE 12.24**   Lateral radiograph of a dog with L6–7 discospondylitis. Disc collapse has occurred with narrowing of the disc space. The endplates of L6–7 are sclerotic but lysis is subtle (arrowhead). There is ventral soft tissue swelling (arrow).

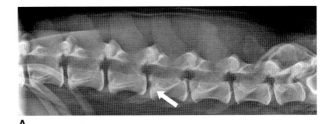

**A**

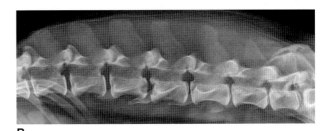

**B**

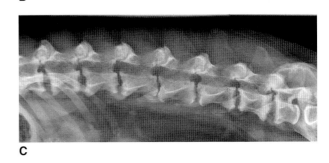

**C**

**FIGURE 12.25**   Lateral radiographs showing progressive discospondylitis. On original radiographs (**A**), there is mild endplate lysis at L3–4 (arrow). This is more pronounced on radiographs acquired 5 months later (**B**). This patient was immunocompromised and developed multiple areas of discospondylitis on radiographs 2 years later (**C**).

bacterial infections in this area may enter the bloodstream and lodge in the vertebrae via venous drainage of the caudal abdomen that flows through the venous sinuses.

Radiography is the most common screening method for discospondylitis. The osseous endplates demonstrate permeative or moth-eaten lysis causing an irregular margin (Figure 12.24). The adjacent vertebral body responds by bony deposition and a region of increased opacity. With time, the intervertebral disc space will collapse (Figure 12.25). Bony proliferation occurs at the margin of the vertebral bodies, with an appearance similar to spondylosis deformans. In juvenile dogs less than 6 months of age, intervertebral disc narrowing may occur before endplate lysis [15].

The sensitivity of radiographs for discospondylitis is relatively low, as significant (50% or more) bone loss must occur before the characteristic endplate lysis is seen. For that reason, CT is a more sensitive test for early or mild discospondylitis as it is more sensitive to mild bone loss and bony fragmentation (Figure 12.26).

MRI is also a sensitive test for discospondylitis, and will display osseous abnormalities before they are apparent on radiographs and soft tissue abnormalities before seen on CT (Figure 12.27) [14]. Because of the regional inflammation, affected endplates are STIR hyperintense and contrast enhance [16, 17]. There is also regional soft tissue contrast enhancement, extending further from the disc space than seen with degenerative intervertebral discs. Lysis of endplates is best recognized on T1-weighted sequences [17]. The disc itself is usually STIR/T2 hyperintense, and larger/more amorphous than typically seen with the well-defined, rounded appearance of the nucleus pulposus in a normal dog. If infection has spread into the adjacent vertebral canal (termed spinal empyema), diffuse or rim enhancement may be seen in the epidural space, as well as disruption and signal change in the typically homogenous epidural fat [18].

## Intervertebral Disc Degeneration and Herniation

Intervertebral disc degeneration is common in older dogs and is a complex, multifactorial process that affects all components of the intervertebral disc [19, 20]. It occurs as a form of

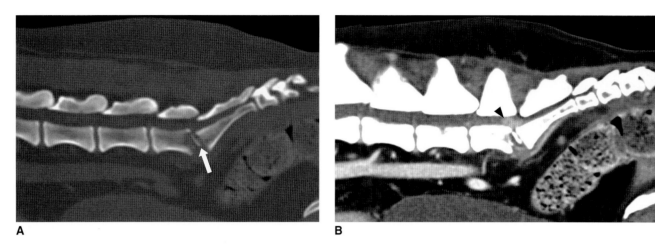

**FIGURE 12.26** Sagittal CT images in a bone window/level (**A**) and postcontrast sagittal image (**B**) of a dog with L7–S1 discospondylitis. There is endplate lysis and a fragment (arrow) at this site. The regional soft tissues contrast enhance (arrowhead).

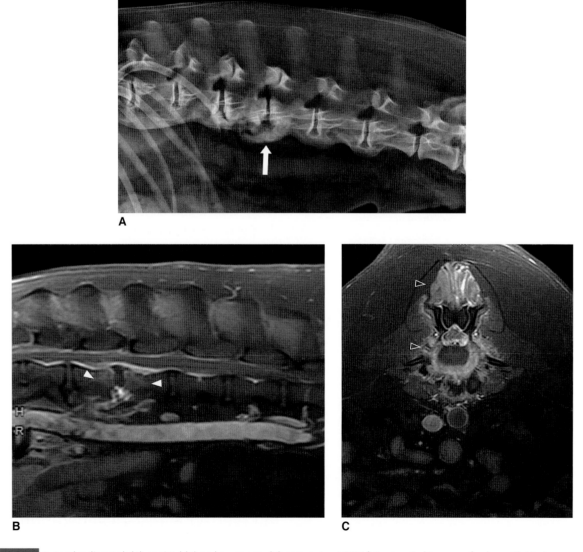

**FIGURE 12.27** Lateral radiograph (**A**), sagittal (**B**) and transverse (**C**) postcontrast T1W fat-saturated images of a dog with L3–4 discospondylitis. There is active spondylosis deformans (arrow; it is less well defined than adjacent spondylosis deformans) but no endplate lysis is seen. Contrast enhancement on MRI shows enhancement of the regional soft tissues (open arrowheads) and of the endplates (closed arrowheads) which is confirmatory for discospondylitis.

either chondroid metaplasia (more common in chondrodystrophic dogs) or fibrous metaplasia (more common in nonchondrodystrophic dogs), that ultimately results in decreased hydration of the nucleus pulposus and reduction in the hydroelastic properties of the disc [19]. Chondrodystrophic dogs may have these degenerative changes as early as 2 months of age, with nonchondrodystrophic dogs usually undergoing these changes later in life, from 7 years of age or older. Discs undergoing chondroid metaplasia will commonly mineralize over time which can be appreciated on radiographs, with up to 90% of dachshunds having at least one mineralized intervertebral disc [19].

Because of the loss of their normal resilient hydroelastic properties and damage to the annulus fibrosis, affected discs may eventually extend into the intervertebral canal. *Herniation* is the term for any disc material extending into the vertebral canal. If there is sudden herniation of degenerative/calcified nucleus pulposus completely through a ruptured annulus fibrosis, it is referred to as *extrusion*. This is also referred to as Hansen type I extrusion, and usually results in neurologic impairment and pain. The disc material may disperse and be difficult to identify (sometimes called Funkquist type III disc extrusion).

Alternatively, disc herniation may be a slower process, referred to as *protrusion* or Hansen type II disc herniation. This is more commonly associated with fibroid degeneration, and a gradual shift of the nucleus pulposus and thickened annulus fibrosis into the vertebral canal, and usually seen in older, large-breed dogs.

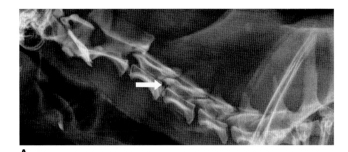

**A**

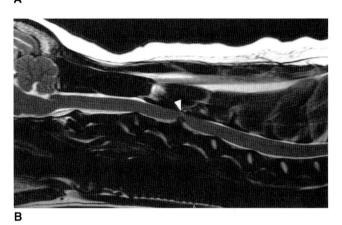

**B**

**FIGURE 12.28**   Lateral radiograph (**A**) and sagittal (**B**) T2W images of the cervical region in a dog with C3–4 disc extrusion. There is mineralization of the C3–4 disc which extends into the vertebral canal (arrow) on radiographs. MRI demonstrates the spinal cord compression by this extrusion (arrowhead).

## Survey Radiography of Disc Disease

Survey radiographs are insensitive to signs of disc degeneration as they cannot separately evaluate the components of the intervertebral disc. Disc narrowing is the major radiographic finding with disc degeneration. This does not necessarily imply disc herniation is present. Narrowing should not be confused radiographically with artifactual narrowing from obliquity, which may occur if the spine has some degree of lateral flexion (see Chapter 6). Artifactual disc narrowing may also occur if the disc of interest is at the edge of the radiographic field, as oblique beam geometry will falsely result in this impression.

If chondroid metaplasia is present, disc mineralization may be seen radiographically within the intervertebral disc space (Figure 12.28). With disc extrusion, mineralization may be seen in the intervertebral foramen on the lateral radiograph. Gas may be seen within the intervertebral space due to vacuum phenomenon (gas accumulation in an area of negative pressure created by disc extrusion). Gas within the disc space is relatively sensitive (but not specific) in identifying the site of acute disc extrusion [21]. Spondylosis deformans is associated with Hansen type II disc herniation. In dogs with neurologic dysfunction from disc herniation, survey radiography may be suggestive of likely sites for disc herniation, but is not specific enough to make a surgical decision (i.e., what location requires decompressive surgery). With some cases of disc degeneration, endplate resorption occurs due to herniation of disc material into the endplate (termed Schmorl's nodes). If extensive, the appearance may mimic discospondylitis.

## Myelography for Intervertebral Disc Disease

Before the advent of CT and MRI, myelography was the imaging gold standard to determine sites of intervertebral disc herniation causing neurologic symptoms. Noniodinated contrast material is injected into the subarachnoid space, allowing identification of spinal cord margins to be seen. Lumbar subarachnoid injections (at the level of L4–5 or L5–6 disc spaces) are most common as the contrast agent fills the subarachnoid space in ascending fashion. The injection is terminated before contrast agent reaches the brain, reducing the risk of postprocedure seizures. Injections into the cerebellomedullary cistern (at the atlantooccipital space) may be performed for suspected cervical intervertebral disc herniations. In that case, contrast agent may preferentially enter the calvarium rather than flow caudally past a site of resistance (such as a disc herniation compressing the subarachnoid space). For that reason, lumbar injections are often the preferred site regardless of cervical versus thoracolumbar lesion localization.

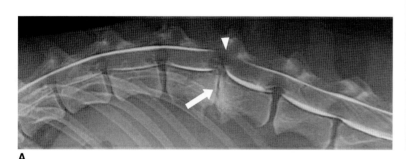

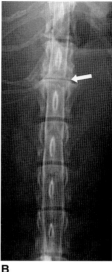

**FIGURE 12.29** Lateral (**A**) and VD (**B**) myelogram of a dog with L1–2 disc extrusion. Note the narrowed disc space and sclerosis (arrow) at L1–2. The ventral subarachnoid space is displaced dorsally, and both ventral and dorsal subarachnoid spaces are narrowed on the lateral projection (arrowhead). Herniation is present at L2–3, but note the dorsal subarachnoid space remains wide with no spinal cord compression.

Disc herniation narrows and deviates the adjacent subarachnoid space, with the pattern dependent on severity and location of the disc herniation within the spinal canal (Figure 12.29). On the lateral projection, the ventral subarachnoid space is typically deviated focally dorsally and thinned at the most affected site. On the ventrodorsal projection, right or left sidedness of the extrusion is determined by determining whether the left or right subarachnoid space is undergoing more severe axial displacement and thinning. If the herniation is entirely ventral, the spinal cord may actually appear widened on the ventrodorsal projection, as the disc herniation results in abaxial displacement of both the left and right subarachnoid spaces. This results in the false impression of an intramedullary lesion, so correlation of all projections is necessary for correct identification of lesion localization. Similarly, if the extrusion is lateralized, without a ventral component, the spinal cord may actually appear widened on the lateral projection due to abaxial displacement of the ventral and dorsal subarachnoid spaces (Figure 12.30). Oblique myelogram projections are often more helpful than the ventrodorsal projection when determining sidedness of disc herniation for surgical purposes and are always recommended.

## CT and CT Myelography of Intervertebral Disc Disease

Computed tomography is a sensitive test for disc degeneration, readily detecting the characteristic findings of disc narrowing, mineralization, and vaccum phenomenon. Acquiring thin slices (1 mm or less) provides better resolution when reformatting in sagittal, dorsal, and oblique planes. Sagittal planes are particularly helpful in evaluating intervertebral disc width and dorsal planes are useful when counting vertebrae prior to neurosurgical procedures.

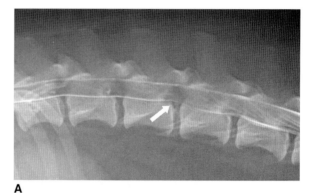

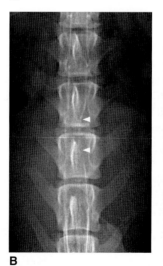

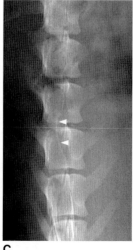

**FIGURE 12.30** Lateral (**A**), VD (**B**) and oblique (**C**) myelogram images of a dog with left lateralized disc extrusion at L2–3. There is severe rightward deviation and narrowing of the subarachnoid space at L2–3 on the VD and oblique images (arrowheads). Note the spinal cord appears only mildly impinged ventrally on the lateral projection (arrow), underestimating the degree of spinal cord compression. The L2–3 disc is also mineralized.

CT has largely replaced myelography in dogs with acute disc extrusion as the major modality used to determine the site and side of extrusion prior to surgery. CT findings of acute disc extrusion are increased attenuation within the vertebral canal, causing loss of normal epidural fat attenuation, and displacement and narrowing of the spinal cord silhouette (Figure 12.31). CT is as accurate as myelography in chondrodystrophic dogs with acute disc extrusion and has the added advantages of being noninvasive and a faster procedure (typically between 4 and 8 minutes compared to 30 minutes or more for myelography). Though MRI remains the gold standard for spinal imaging, CT results in similar surgical planning decisions when directly compared to MRI in these cases. For this reason, even in facilities that have both CT and MRI, CT is often the first test selected for chondrodystrophic patients that are suspected to have acute disc herniation.

Unfortunately, in some cases with acute disc extrusion (especially if nonmineralized), and in most cases of Hansen type II disc herniation, CT is not sufficiently sensitive to detect the site of herniation and develop a surgical plan. In these cases, CT may be performed after injection of intrathecal contrast medium, increasing the ability of this test to detect disc extrusion (Figure 12.32). Even small volumes of contrast are detectable on CT, so a diagnosis may be achieved even in cases where a radiographic myelogram may have been nondiagnostic.

## MRI for Intervertebral Disc Disease

Magnetic resonance imaging is the gold standard to identify disc degeneration and herniation due to its superior soft tissue contrast compared to radiography and CT. As nucleus pulposus

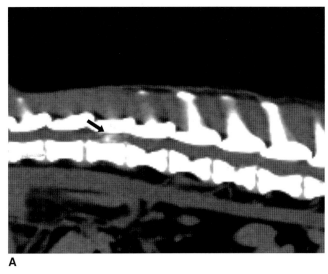

**A**

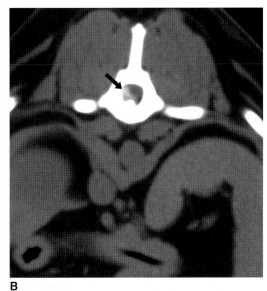

**B**

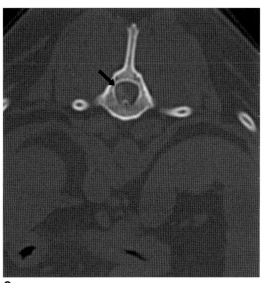

**C**

**FIGURE 12.31**    Sagittal (**A**) and transverse soft tissue window/level (**B**) and bone window/level (**C**) CT images of a dog with disc extrusion. There is amorphous increased attenuation material (arrow) in the vertebral canal representing extruded disc material and/or hemorrhage. This is more difficult to appreciate on the bone window/level images, illustrating the importance of using different window/level settings when evaluating for disc extrusion on CT images.

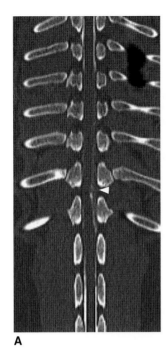
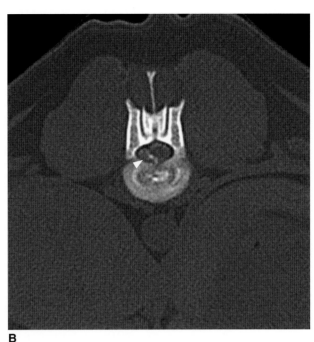

**A**    **B**

**FIGURE 12.32**  Dorsal (**A**) and transverse (**B**) CT postmyelogram images of a dog with a T12–13 left ventral disc extrusion. Note the rightward displacement and thinning of the subarachnoid space by the extradural material (arrowhead).

dehydration progresses as part of the degenerative process, it loses the normally intense T2 signal, becoming more T2 hypointense (Figure 12.33) [19]. There may also be degenerative changes in the adjacent vertebrae. As an early change, the fatty component of the vertebral bodies increases, resulting in increased T1 and T2 signal that should not be confused for inflammation. Later changes result in increased mineral content and sclerosis of the vertebrae, resulting in decreased T1 and T2 signal.

Evaluation for herniated material and spinal cord compression is best carried out through multiple different sequences and imaging planes. Broadly speaking, herniation of the intervertebral disc is recognized by broad-based decreased signal extending into the vertebral canal dorsal to the adjacent intervertebral disc space as seen on both T2- and T1-weighted images. Spinal cord displacement and narrowing are most readily identified on transverse images. The appearance of type I intervertebral disc extrusions generally differs from type II discs. Hemorrhage may accompany an acute type I disc extrusion, and can result in localized decrease in signal in T2-weighted images, complicating interpretation by masking the actual disc extrusion itself (Figure 12.34). Type I disc extrusions may have variable degree of spinal cord contusion as recognized by increased T2 signal in the spinal cord. Type II disc herniation, in contrast, has more localized dorsal extension of the disc into the canal, and spinal cord contusion is not expected.

Intravenous contrast agent is not usually required to diagnose intervertebral disc herniations (either type I or type II), but contrast enhancement may be seen in many cases, especially if acute, but should not be misinterpreted as a mass or neoplastic lesion (Figure 12.35). Increased T2 intensity in the spinal cord may be seen with acute disc extrusions, and represents cord edema or inflammation. Ascending/descending myelomalacia

is a serious but uncommon sequela to disc extrusion and may be recognized by more widespread increased T2 signal in the cord (Figure 12.36).

Acute extrusions of normal or only minimally degenerate nucleus pulposus may occur in dogs and cats, often associated with strenuous exercise or trauma [22]. Two such syndromes are recognized. The first is acute noncompressive nucleus pulposus extrusions (ANNPEs), sometimes called high-velocity, low-volume disc extrusion or Hansen type III disease. These lesions are not identified on radiography or CT, and myelography may be normal or show only minimal cord swelling. On MRI, these are recognized by focal cord contusion (T2 hyperintensity), reduction in volume of the adjacent intervertebral disc space, and possible small-volume extradural material (Figure 12.37). These may have some contrast enhancement but no spinal cord compression (Figure 12.38) [22].

Another type of minimally or nondegenerative extrusion has been reported in dogs. A hydrated nucleus pulposus extrusion occurs when the entire pulposus extrudes, resulting in a large mass effect and compression of the spinal cord requiring surgery (Figure 12.39). These result in a large focal area of T2 increased signal, that have occasionally been incorrectly referred to as "discal cysts" and are most common in the cervical area [23, 24].

## Spondylosis Deformans

Spondylosis deformans is defined radiographically by smooth bony proliferation extending from a vertebral endplate toward the adjacent vertebral endplate (Figure 12.40). Spondylosis deformans is most easily recognized on a lateral radiograph

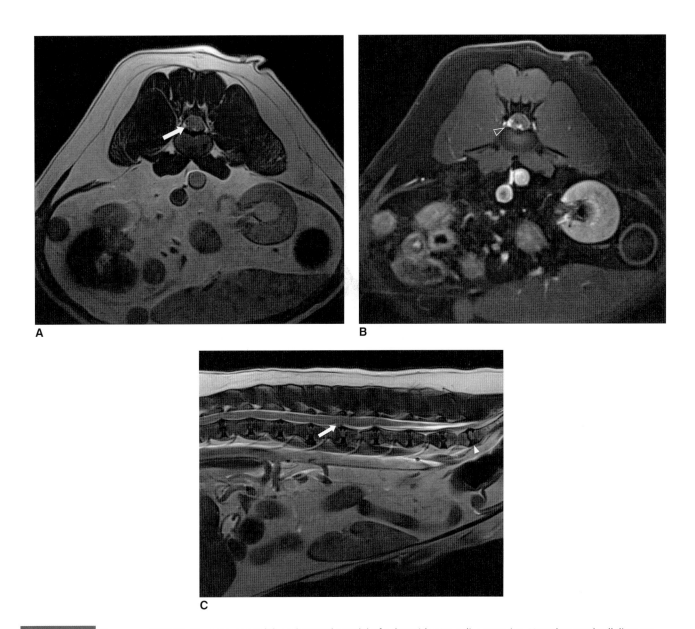

**FIGURE 12.33** Transverse T2W (**A**), T1 postcontrast (**B**), and sagittal T2W (**C**) of a dog with a L3–4 disc extrusion. Note that nearly all discs are variably T2W hypointense, indicating degeneration. The lumbosacral disc has a more normal hyperintense signal to the nucleus pulposus (closed arrowhead). There is T2W hypointese material (arrow) with regional contrast enhancement (open arrowhead) material in the ventral vertebral canal.

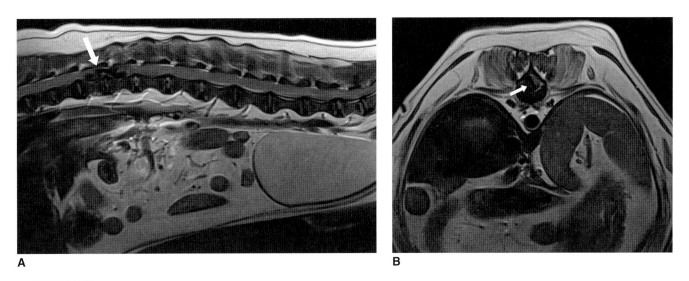

**FIGURE 12.34** Sagittal (**A**) and transverse (**B**) T2W images of a disc extrusion with hemorrhage at T12–13. The spinal cord is severely compressed by a large amount of T2 hypointense material (arrow) consistent with disc and hemorrhage.

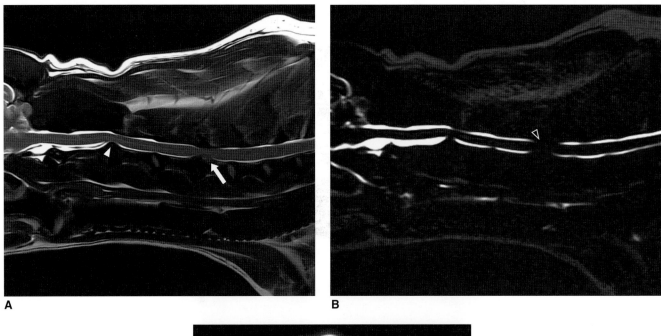

A

B

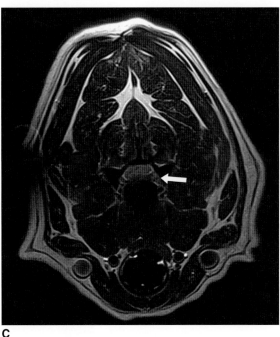

C

**FIGURE 12.35** Sagittal T2W (**A**), heavily T2W (**B**), and transverse T2W (**C**) of the cervical spine with an acute disc extrusion at C4–5 (arrow) and a chronic disc herniation at C2–3 (closed arrowhead). Note that there is loss of CSF signal (open arrowhead) at the acute site while the CSF signal is more retained at the more chronic site. There is significant spinal cord compression at C4–5.

where the ventral spondylosis is distinctly identified, but spondylosis can also be lateralized and requires a ventrodorsal projection to identify (Figure 12.41). It is a noninflammatory condition resulting from degeneration of the fibrous attachments of the intervertebral discs to the endplates, with secondary osseous proliferation [25].

The etiology of spondylosis deformans is unknown. It is unknown if spondylosis deformans is caused by intervertebral disc degeneration. It has been associated with Hansen type II disc herniation, but is also seen with healthy intervertebral discs [25, 26]. In general, spondylosis deformans is considered

an incidental finding, and not expected to cause any clinical signs, though if widespread it could result in some perceived stiffness or lack of spinal flexibility.

Spondylosis deformans is a common radiographic finding in many dogs, but is particularly common in the midthoracic region and thoracolumbar and lumbosacral junctions. It is typically limited to the region of the intervertebral disc but in very severe cases, excessive spondylosis deformans-like proliferation may be contiguous between a large number of sites (Figure 12.42). This excessive, flowing spondylosis deformans has been referred to as diffuse idiopathic skeletal

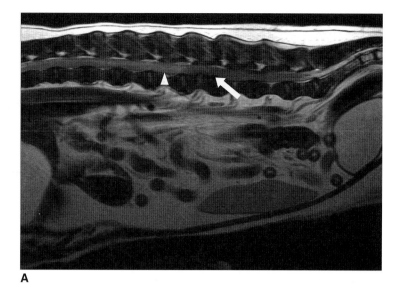

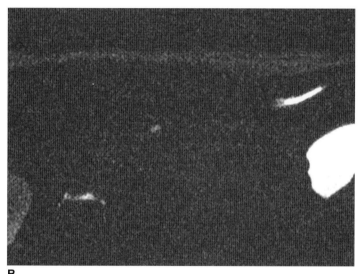

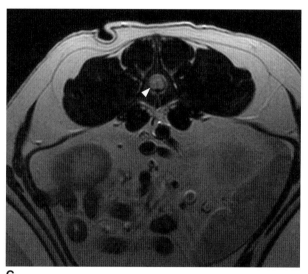

**FIGURE 12.36**   Sagittal T2W (**A**), heavily T2W (**B**), and transverse image (**C**) of a dog with myelomalacia from disc extrusion. There is disc extrusion in the vertebral canal (arrow) but severe loss of CSF signal diffusely on the heavily T2W image. The spinal cord also has increased T2 signal over a large area (arrowheads).

hyperostosis, named after a similar condition in humans, but this term has not been completely defined in veterinary literature. In some patients, there may be interruption of the spondylosis deformans with a fracture-like appearance (Figure 12.42).

On cross-sectional imaging, spondylosis may be seen dorsolaterally, and can narrow the intervertebral foramen. This does not typically result in clinical signs, but discomfort and nerve entrapment may occur, particularly at the lumbosacral junction. Contrast enhancement of spondylosis may be seen on MRI, and should not be mistaken as discospondylitis; the clinical significance of contrast-enhancing spondylosis deformans is unknown.

Spondylosis deformans has a range of severity, from very mild proliferation at the margins of one or both adjacent endplates, to severe flowing spondylosis deformans that extends completely ventral to a disc space. Spondylosis invariably has smooth margins, so the presence of irregular or active proliferation should alert the viewer that the proliferation could be associated with a process other than spondylosis deformans.

## Spinal Osteoarthritis

Geriatric canine patients frequently develop osteophyte formation of the spinal synovial articular process joints. Osteoarthritis is particularly common in the lumbar spine but also seen in the cervical or midthoracic regions. Patients with spinal osteoarthritis have increased proliferation along the articular processes, best appreciated on lateral projections,

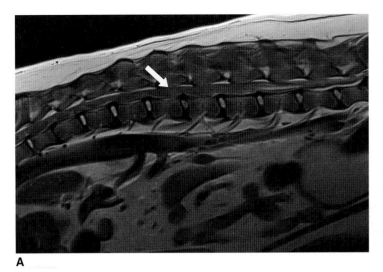

**A**

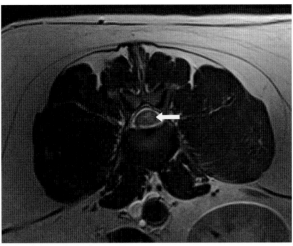

**B**

**FIGURE 12.37** Sagittal T2W (**A**) and transverse (**B**) images of a dog with acute noncompressive disc extrusion. There is focal increased signal in the spinal cord (arrow) but no external compression.

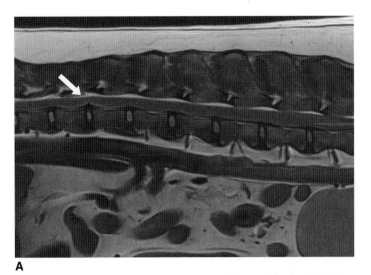

**A**

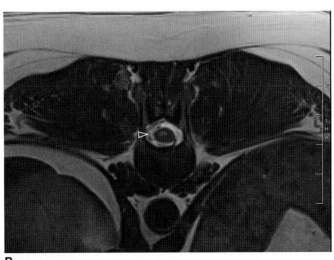

**B**

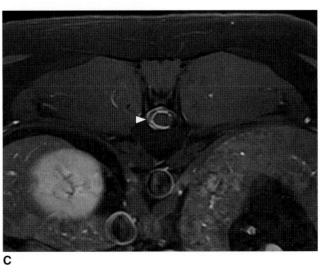

**C**

**FIGURE 12.38** Sagittal T2W (**A**), transverse T2W (**B**) and transverse postcontrast T1W fat-saturated image (**C**) of a dog with acute noncompressive disc extrusion. There is focal increased signal in the spinal cord (arrow) and a large amount of regional contrast enhancement (closed arrowhead). No spinal cord compression is present. There is mixed signal on T2 images within the epidural fat as a result of inflammation and extruded material (open arrowhead).

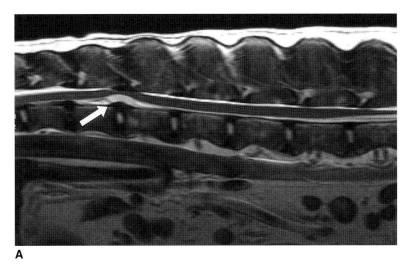

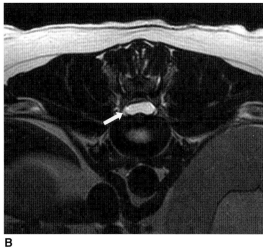

**FIGURE 12.39**    Sagittal (**A**) and transverse (**B**) T2W images of a dog with a hydrated nucleus pulposus extrusion ("discal cyst") at T13–L1. There is a large hyperintense structure (arrow) dorsally displacing and compressing the spinal cord.

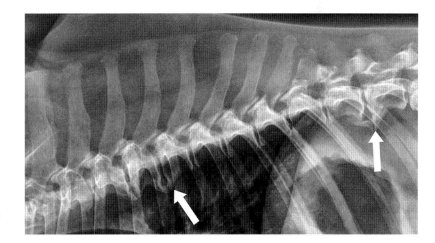

**FIGURE 12.40**    Lateral radiograph of a dog with moderate focal spondylosis of the thoracic spine. There is smooth bridging ventrally at multiple sites in the thoracic spine (arrows).

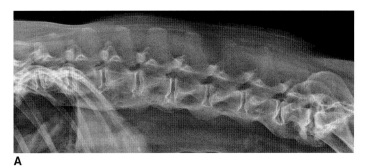

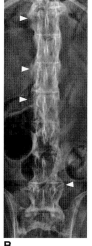

**FIGURE 12.41**    Lateral (**A**) and VD (**B**) radiographs of severe spondylosis deformans of the lumbar spine. Some of this proliferation is seen extending laterally on the VD projection (arrowheads).

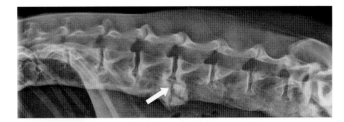

**FIGURE 12.42** Lateral radiograph of a dog with severe spondylosis deformans. There is an area of interruptions of this spondylosis deformans (arrow).

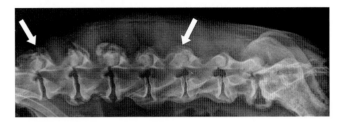

**FIGURE 12.43** Lateral radiograph of a dog with severe osteoarthritis of multiple articular facet joints (arrows, and all facets between the arrows) and moderate ventral spondylosis deformans.

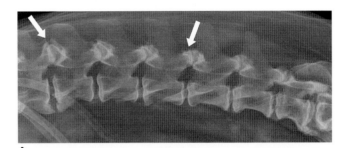

**A**

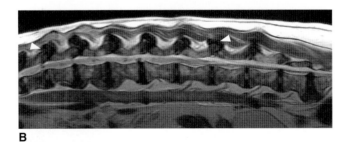

**B**

**FIGURE 12.44** Lateral radiograph (**A**) and sagittal T2W images (**B**) of a dog with spinal osteoarthritis. There are osteophytes seen on radiographs (between arrows) and MRI (between arrowheads).

though lateralized osteophytes may be seen on ventrodorsal images (Figure 12.43). T2- and T1-weighted images best demonstrate osteophytes with MRI (Figure 12.44). Spinal osteoarthritis is rarely clinically significant, but joint degeneration plays a role in dorsolateral spinal cord compression in dogs with cervical spondylomyelopathy, as the bony and soft tissue proliferation associated with osteoarthritis results in cord impingement.

# Cervical Spondylomyelopathy

Cervical spondylomyelopathy is a complex disease in large- and giant-breed dogs and results in cervical spinal cord compression. Its etiology is complex, reflected in the many different names for this disease process including wobbler syndrome, caudal cervical spondylomyelopathy, cervical stenotic myelopathy, and cervical malformation/malarticulation syndrome [27]. There are two different clinical entities grouped under the term "cervical spondylomyelopathy," each with unique morphologic abnormalities and anamnesis.

*Disc-associated cervical spondylomyelopathy* occurs in middle-aged or older large-breed dogs, especially Doberman pinschers. It does not have a strict definition, but is usually broadly considered as ventral compression of the spinal cord by a protruding intervertebral disc, though there can be concurrent osseous stenosis of the vertebral canal or ligamentum flavum hypertrophy [27, 28]. It usually occurs at C5–6 and C6–7.

*Osseous-associated cervical spondylomyelopathy* occurs in young adult giant-breed dogs, especially Great Danes. Osseous malformations, particularly enlargement of the vertebral arches or the articular facets, causes dorsal and/or lateral compression of the spinal cord. These malformations are most likely congenital in origin but in older dogs, facet osteoarthritis results in enlargement of the facets and plays a role in compression [27]. The malformations usually occur in the caudal cervical spine, but malformations occur as far cranial as C2–3 [29].

The disc- and osseous-associated versions of cervical spondylomyelopathy have complex pathogenesis. Signalment, history, and imaging findings can overlap, so that one dog may have elements of both. Large- and giant-breed dogs may display some of the morphologic abnormalities of cervical spondylomyelopathy when the neck is imaged for reasons other than neurologic disease, yet do not demonstrate clinical signs [30, 31].

Dogs with osseous spondylomyelopathy will have enlarged and increased opacity of the articular processes (Figure 12.45). On ventrodorsal projections, mediolateral narrowing of the vertebral canal may be apparent. Though some morphologic abnormalities of cervical spondylomyelopathy are seen on survey radiographs, radiographs alone are insufficient to confirm spinal cord compression and myelography is required. Dogs with disc-associated spondylomyelopathy often demonstrate narrowing of the caudal cervical disc spaces on radiographs, especially C5–6 and C6–7 (Figure 12.46). The vertebral bodies, especially C5, may have a triangular shape and there may be malalignment of vertebrae (vertebral "tipping") or vertebral canal stenosis. As part of the myelogram, traction projections are sometimes performed, as relief of spinal cord compression with traction may determine the type of surgical procedure performed (Figure 12.47).

CT more accurately defines the osseous abnormalities seen with disc-associated and osseous cervical spondylomyelopathy,

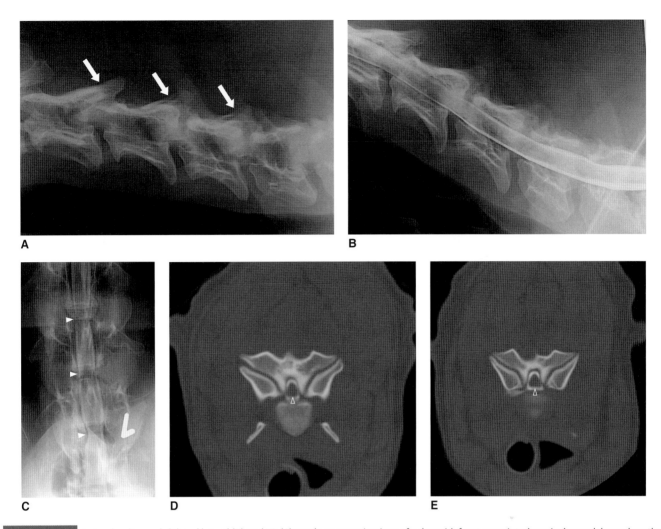

**FIGURE 12.45** Lateral radiograph (**A**) and lateral (**B**) and VD (**C**) myelogram projections of a dog with facet-associated cervical spondylomyelopathy. On the lateral radiograph, the C3–4 through C5–6 articular processes are large (arrows). No significant compression is seen on the lateral myelogram projection (**B**) but severe mediolateral compression is seen by the large facets at C3–4, C4–5, and C5–6 (**C**; closed arrowheads). Myelogram CTs at the level of C3–4 (**D**) and C5–6 (**E**) show the severe narrowing of the spinal cord by the large facets (open arrowhead).

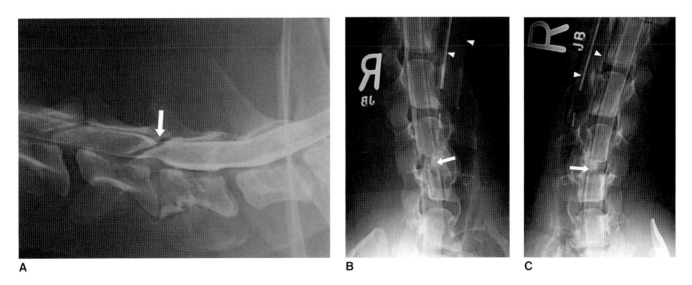

**FIGURE 12.46** Lateral (**A**) and oblique (**B,C**) myelogram images of a dog with spinal cord compression due to disc-associated spondylomyelopathy at C5–6. The spinal cord has an hour-glass shape (arrow) and there is deviation and narrowing of the ventral and dorsal subarachnoid space from disc herniation ventrally and soft tissue proliferation/thickening dorsally. The endotracheal tube is adjacent to the spine on the oblique projection (arrowhead) and should not be confused with margins of contrast agent.

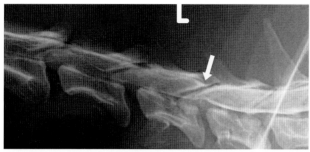

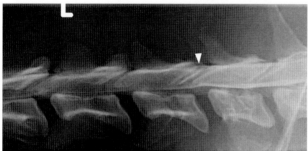

**FIGURE 12.47** Lateral (**A**) and lateral with traction (**B**) myelogram images of a dog with spinal cord compression due to disc-associated spondylomyelopathy at C5–6. The deviation and narrowing of the dorsal and ventral subarachnoid space (arrow) becomes less severe with traction (arrowhead).

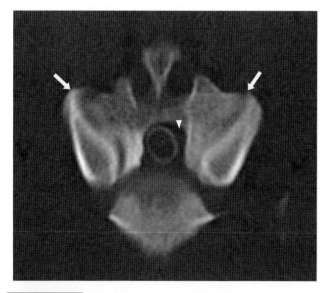

**FIGURE 12.48** Transverse CT myelogram image of osseous-associated spondylomyelopathy. The enlarged articular processes (arrows) are causing spinal cord compression. Notice that there is a gap (arrowhead) between the subarachnoid space and the articular processes, presumably from soft tissue proliferation adjacent to the articular processes, contributing to compression.

but still requires myelography (Figure 12.48) or MRI to determine the site of greatest spinal compression. Spinal cord atrophy is appreciated as a diffuse narrowing of the spinal cord and symmetric diffuse widening of the adjacent subarachnoid space, resulting in decreased cross-sectional area of the spinal cord.

MRI is the gold standard for imaging cervical spondylomyelopathy, as it allows noninvasive assessment of both osseous- and disc-associated malformations and the impact on the spinal cord and other soft tissues (Figure 12.49). Increased T2 signal in the spinal cord represents spinal cord edema or white and gray matter degenerative changes [27, 32]. Protrusive disc material and osseous malformations are readily identified. While traction MRI has been described, it is not commonly performed due to the challenges of maintaining traction for the lengthy duration of an MRI scan [32, 33]. MRI also evaluates for other concurrent soft tissue abnormalities which may contribute to compression, such as hypertrophy of the dorsal longitudinal ligament or intravertebral canal synovial cysts arising from the articular process joints (Figure 12.50).

# Spinal Fractures and Traumatic Subluxation/Luxation

The spine is well protected from minor trauma but significant trauma such as a vehicular impact or fall from great height can result in fracture or luxation. Fractures may be significantly displaced, resulting in an obvious radiographic abnormality. Fissures cause a thin linear lucency within the vertebrae, but are nondisplaced and therefore difficult to recognize radiographically. Similarly, vertebral luxation may cause obvious displacement of one vertebral segment compared to the next, but subluxation may cause subtle or intermittent displacement that is not recognized radiographically (Figure 12.51). Compression fractures cause shortening of one vertebrae compared to adjacent vertebrae (Figure 12.52).

Recognition of spinal trauma on radiographs requires careful patient positioning. Vertebrae have a complex shape with superimposition of other osseous structures (such as scapulae or rib heads) complicating radiographic interpretation. Even slight axial rotation of spinal radiographs complicates or prevents recognition of fractures or subtle subluxation. For these reasons, normal spinal radiographs do not completely rule out the presence of fracture or subluxation after a traumatic incident (Figure 12.53).

Despite this limitation, radiographs remain a useful first-line imaging test to screen for major spinal trauma, with further imaging (such as CT) pursued if fracture needs to be definitively ruled out. First performing a lateral projection (with the patient in lateral recumbency) screens for obvious fracture or subluxation. If clinical concern for spinal trauma persists after the lateral projection (such as significant pain or neurologic deficits), further patient positioning could aggravate a spinal injury, so positioning the patient in dorsal recumbency is avoided. A horizontal beam

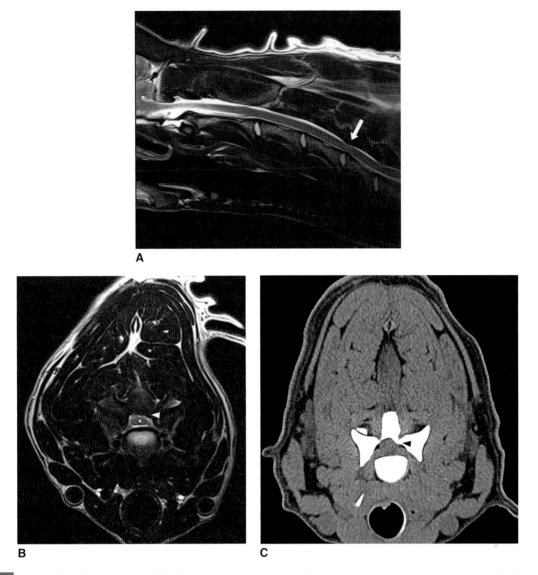

**FIGURE 12.49** Sagittal T2W (**A**), transverse T2W (**B**), and transverse CT image (**C**) of a dog with cervical spondylomyelopathy from vertebral malformation. There is thickening of the lamina and pedicles at C4–5 (arrowead) resulting in spinal cord compression (arrow) and increased cord signal consistent with gliosis. Notice that the CT image does not have intrathecal contrast; diagnosis of spinal cord compression requires either MRI or a myelogram to be performed.

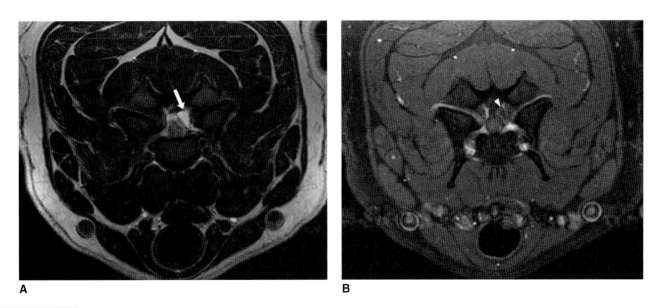

**FIGURE 12.50** Transverse T2W (**A**) and postcontrast T1W (**B**) images of the caudal cervical spine. There is a large cyst arising from the left articular facets (arrow) resulting in spinal cord compression. This structure has rim enhancement (arrowhead).

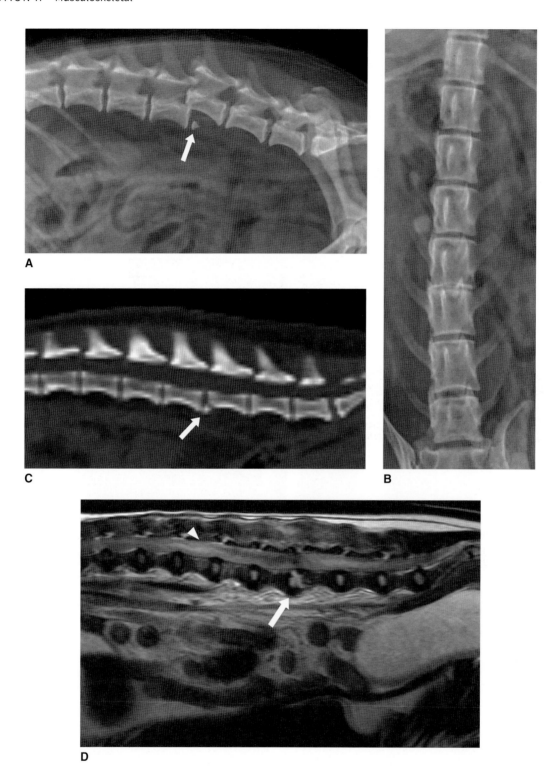

**FIGURE 12.51** Lateral (**A**) and ventrodorsal (**B**) radiographs, sagittal CT (**C**) and sagittal T2W MRI (**D**) of a dog with a traumatic spinal fracture and luxation. The luxation is more severe on the radiographs compared to CT and MRI where it is reduced. The luxation is not readily apparent on the VD compared to the lateral radiographs, an example of the importance of two radiographic projections. The fracture fragment (arrow) is seen on all modalities but is less apparent on the MRI. The spinal cord is severely T2 hyperintense, consistent with severe cord inflammation and damage (arrowhead).

ventrodorsal projection (with the patient remaining in lateral recumbency) allows evaluation of the orthogonal projection without the need to reposition the patient, and is the recommended method to achieve a ventrodorsal projection in the spinal trauma patient.

Pathologic fractures occur when underlying disease weakens bone, resulting in fracture. This typically occurs due to aggressive bone disease, such as primary or metastatic neoplasia, causing bone lysis and weakening the bone (Figure 12.54). Pathologic fractures in the spine are often

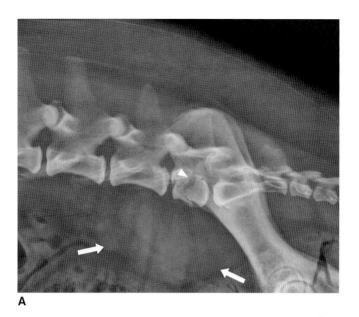

**A**

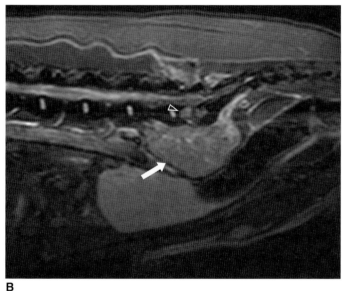

**B**

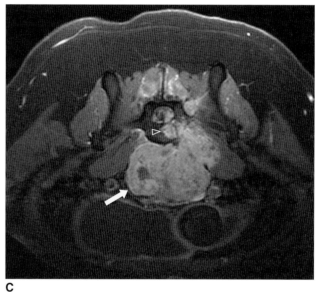

**C**

**FIGURE 12.52** Lateral radiograph (**A**), sagittal STIR (**B**), and transverse T1W postcontrast MRI (**C**) images of a pathologic L7 compression fracture due to primary bone neoplasia. On radiographs, L7 is decreased in length and fracture margins are seen (closed arrowhead) and there is a large mass effect ventral to the vertebrae (arrow). The contrast-enhancing mass is more apparent on the MRI; note the STIR intensity in the vertebral body (open arrowhead), but fracture margins are not well seen.

compression-type fractures, as the surrounding soft tissues and other adjacent unaffected osseous structures maintain overall alignment of the adjacent vertebral segments. Bone loss may not be apparent radiographically, particularly in the thoracic spine where ribs overlap the vertebral body (Figure 12.55).

Though subluxation at the lumbosacral junction occurs secondary to trauma, lumbosacral instability can also result from regional congenital malformations. Lumbosacral subluxation is particularly common in dogs with transitional vertebrae, either sacralized L7 or lumbarized S1, as these anatomic malformations predispose to instability. Lumbosacral subluxation is recognized as malalignment of the opposed L7/S1 endplates on lateral radiographs. Gentle flexion and extension of the pelvic

limbs may result in an abnormal angle of the sacrum relative to the lumbar spine. Though a definitive diagnosis of cauda equina compression requires myelogram, CT, or MRI, malalignment between the sacrum and the most caudal lumbar vertebra suggests the possibility in the patient with compatible clinical signs.

CT is a sensitive test for detecting small fissures or non-displaced fragments that may not be seen on radiographs (Figure 12.56). CT is often performed in a patient with normal survey radiographs, but a spinal fracture is suspected based on continued spinal pain or due to the severity of the initial traumatic insult. CT better characterizes fractures previously identified on radiographs and is required prior to attempted surgical spinal stabilization. CT is a more rapid diagnostic test

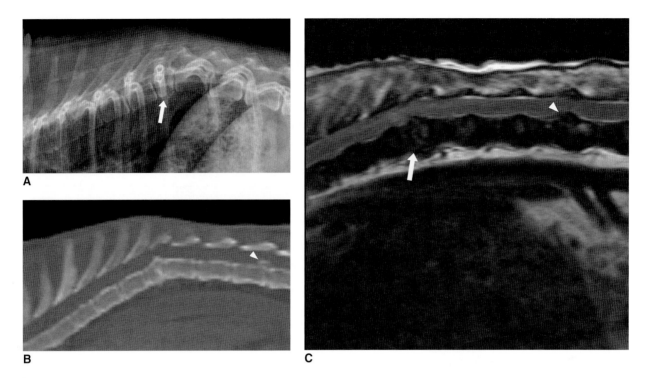

**FIGURE 12.53** Radiograph (**A**), CT (**B**), and MRI (**C**) of a dog with a traumatic compression fracture (arrow). No fracture is actually seen, but there has been a shortening of the vertebral body; this should not be confused with a congenital malformation. On CT and MRI images, shortening and malformation of the vertebral segment are more apparent. There is a chronic disc herniation seen more caudally (arrowhead).

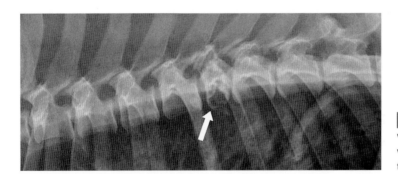

**FIGURE 12.54** Pathologic fracture of a midthoracic vertebral body (arrow). Notice there is more lysis of this vertebral body, indicating underlying pathology, compared to the dog with a traumatic fracture in Figure 12.53.

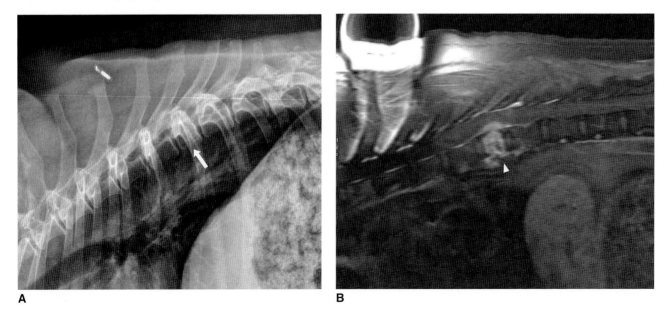

**FIGURE 12.55** Lateral radiograph (**A**) and sagittal postcontrast T1W (**B**) image of a dog with a pathologic compression fracture of a midthoracic vertebral segment, consistent with a shortening of the vertebral body (arrow). Lysis is not appreciated on the lateral projection, in part due to superimposition of the ribs. The MRI shows extensive contrast enhancement due to the underlying osseous neoplasm (arrowhead).

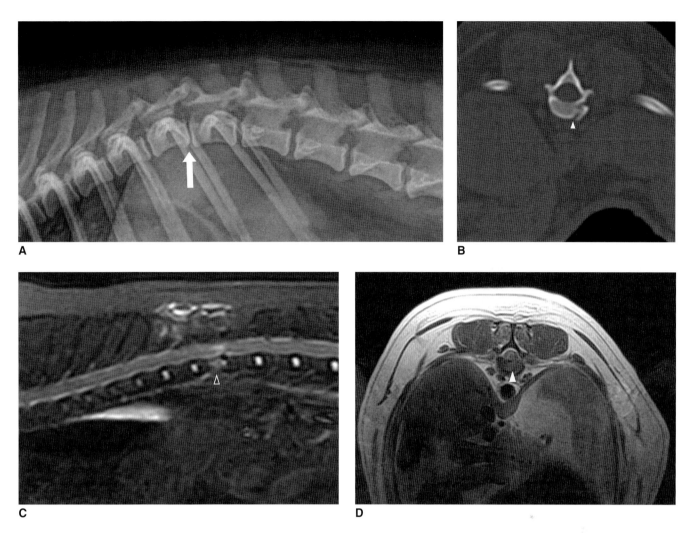

**FIGURE 12.56** Lateral radiograph (**A**), transverse CT (**B**), sagittal STIR MRI (**C**), and transverse T2W MRI (**D**) of a dog with a T12 vertebral body fracture. The fracture is not seen on radiographs, though the T12–13 disc space is narrow (arrow). The fracture fragments are distinct on CT (closed arrowhead) and somewhat distinct on transverse MRI images (closed arrowhead). On the STIR, there is diffuse increased signal in the vertebral body (open arrowhead) but the fracture margins are not seen.

than MRI, and often performed under light sedation or even no sedation in the comatose patient.

Though CT is sensitive to osseous pathology, it has limited ability to detect pathology within the spinal cord or spinal nerve roots. If spinal cord deficits are present in a patient with a history of trauma, MRI is the better test for evaluation of the spinal cord. In a patient with spinal fracture, MRI and CT serve a complementary purpose. CT better defines osseous pathology and assists with surgical planning, and MRI provides information regarding spinal cord trauma which can affect prognosis and eventual recovery.

# Vertebral Neoplasia

Osteosarcoma is the most common primary vertebral tumor in dogs. Its radiographic features are similar to those in the appendicular skeleton, displaying aggressive forms of bone lysis and periosteal response affecting a single vertebral segment (Figure 12.57). Metastatic neoplasia to the spine is common, particularly with urogenital carcinomas (Figure 12.58), and may have a multifocal appearance with multiple vertebrae affected. While vertebral neoplasia typically has a mix of lysis and bony proliferation, some tumors may predominantly cause lysis (Figure 12.59). Primary and metastatic spinal neoplasia demonstrate significant regional soft tissue thickening extending beyond the margins of the vertebrae and contrast enhancement when imaged with CT or MRI.

Osseous round cell tumors have a different radiographic appearance from primary bone tumors such as osteosarcoma. Plasma cell tumors affect only one vertebral segment but, unlike other primary bone tumors, are nearly entirely lytic with very little or absent proliferative response. Multiple myeloma similarly causes severe bone loss without osseous proliferation, but affects the spine diffusely, resulting in a "punched-out" appearance in numerous vertebral segments (Figure 12.60). MRI and CT are more sensitive than radiography for the detection of early

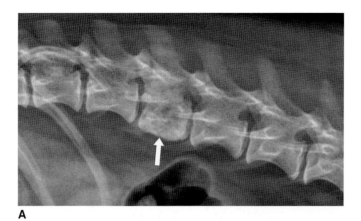

**A**

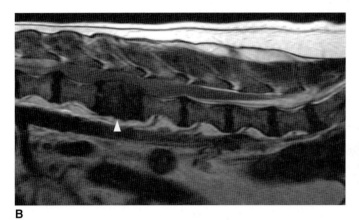

**B**

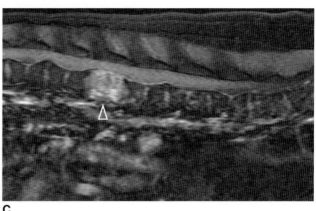

**C**

**FIGURE 12.57** Radiograph (**A**) and sagittal T2W (**B**) and postcontrast T1W (**C**) images of a L3 osteosarcoma. On the radiograph, the affected bone has mixed proliferation (arrow) and lysis. The MRI shows diffuse enhancement (open arrowhead) on postcontrast images and decreased signal on T2 images (closed arrowhead) due to mineral deposition.

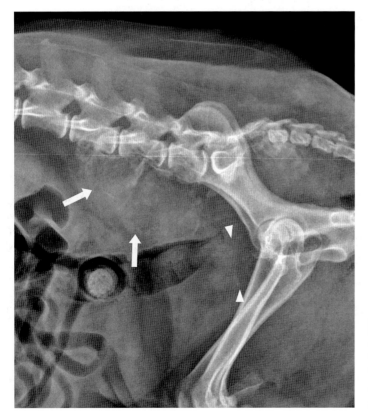

**FIGURE 12.58** Lateral radiograph of a metastatic prostatic carcinoma to the lumbar spine. There is mixed lysis of L5, with a ventral mass effect (arrow) that is partially mineralized. The prostate is also mildly large and mineralized (between arrowheads). The ventral soft tissue mass involves L5, L7 and the sacrum with areas of lysis and proliferation being noted.

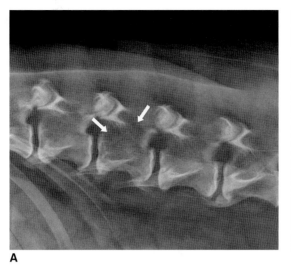
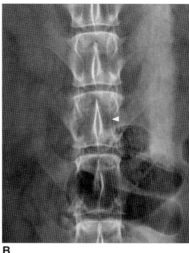

**FIGURE 12.59**   Lateral (**A**) and ventrodorsal (**B**) radiographs of a metastatic pheochromocytoma to L3. The metastasis is moth eaten and permeative lytic in nature (arrow). The arrowhead indicates the medial margin of the left vertebral pedicle; this is absent on the right side due to lysis by the tumor.

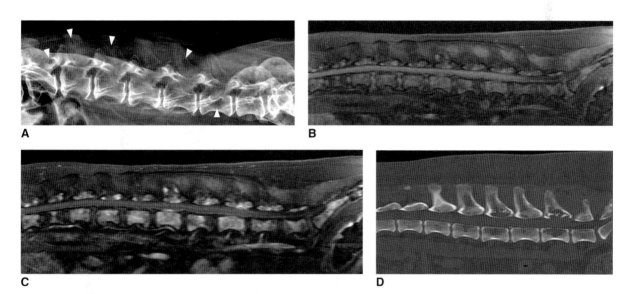

**FIGURE 12.60**   Radiograph (**A**), sagittal T1W precontrast (**B**) and postcontrast (**C**) MRI and sagittal CT (**D**) image of a dog with multiple myeloma. On radiographs, there are multifocal areas of decreased bone density (arrowheads; contrast on radiograph artifactually enhanced to better show areas of subtle lysis). On MRI, the vertebrae diffusely heterogeneously enhance. The CT better displays the areas of lysis through the laminae, spinous processes, and bodies.

or subtle primary bone tumors, and better able to define the soft tissue component of the tumor and resultant compression of the spinal cord.

# Intradural Spinal Cord Diseases

Magnetic resonance imaging provides the most detailed information regarding disease within the dura mater that affects the spinal cord. Though myelography or CT may identify the location of intradural lesions, MRI provides the most information about spinal cord pathology and better prioritizes differential diagnoses [34].

## Spinal Cord Tumors

Spinal cord tumors may be intramedullary or intradural extramedullary in location. In cats, lymphoma is the most common intramedullary spinal cord neoplasm. In dogs, primary intramedullary spinal cord tumors are rare. Glioma is

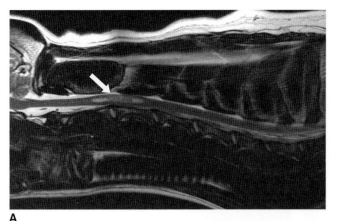

A

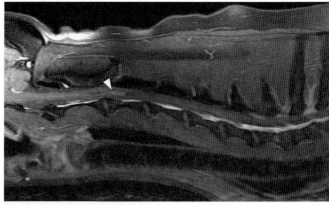

B

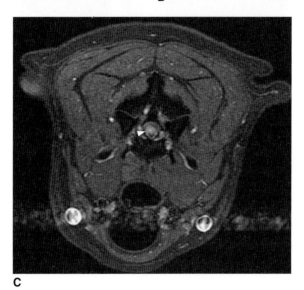

C

**FIGURE 12.61** Sagittal T2W (**A**), postcontrast T1W (**B**), and transverse postcontrast T1W (**C**) MRI images of a dog with a spinal cord glial cell tumor. The mass is mildly contrast enhancing (arrow) and T2 hyperintense (arrowhead).

the most common primary spinal cord tumor type, though a variety of other tumor types has been reported (Figure 12.61). Metastatic cord neoplasia is infrequently reported, with hemangiosarcoma and urogenital carcinoma the most common. On MRI, intramedullary spinal cord tumors center on the spinal cord, do not contact the pial surface, and usually contrast enhance with variable amounts of regional edema (Figure 12.62).

Intradural extramedullary tumors are more common than intramedullary tumors. These tumors are located within the dura mater but outside the parenchyma of the spinal cord and typically cause a characteristic widening of the adjacent subarachnoid space on myelography or MRI (Figure 12.63). Meningioma, nerve sheath tumors, and lymphoma are the tumors most likely to cause an intradural-extramedullary appearance on imaging. While there is overlap in the appearance of these

tumors, meningiomas tend to stay localized to the intradural location, and nerve sheath tumors may extend more peripherally through the intervertebral foramen along the course of spinal nerve roots. Lymphoma may affect numerous adjacent spinal cord/nerve root segments. In young, large-breed dogs, nephroblastoma (also called intradural extramedullary tumor of young dogs) has a characteristic location at the thoracolumbar junction.

## Spinal Inflammatory Diseases

Inflammatory disease of the spinal cord may be focal or diffuse. Primary inflammatory disease of the spinal cord is uncommon, with a variety of causes, including fungal granulomas, bacterial emboli, and immune-mediated disease such as granulomatous meningoencephalitis. Focal inflammatory lesions may appear

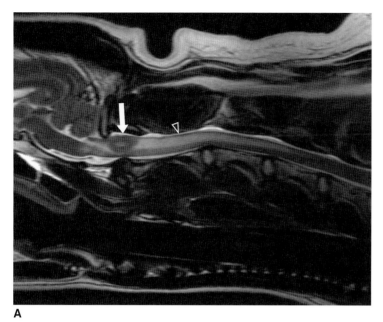
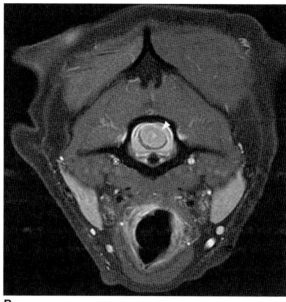

**A**                                                                                               **B**

**FIGURE 12.62**   Sagittal T2W (**A**) and transverse postcontrast T1W (**B**) MRI images of a dog with a spinal cord histiocytic sarcoma. The mass is T2 hypointense (arrow) but contrast enhancing (closed arrowhead), taking up a large percentage of the spinal cord diameter on the transverse image. There is a large amount of regional edema as seen on T2-weighted images (open arrowhead).

similar to primary or metastatic intramedullary neoplasms, resulting in a focal contrast-enhancing mass (Figure 12.64). Diffuse inflammatory diseases may cause significant extensive meningeal enhancement with variable spinal cord parenchymal enhancement (Figure 12.65).

## Spinal Cord Vascular Incidents

Ischemic events within the spinal cord are common in dogs. The most common cause is fibrocartilagenous emboli which arise from the nucleus pulposus of an adjacent intervertebral disc, but bacterial emboli, parasitic emboli, fat emboli, neoplastic emboli, and thrombi affecting the spinal cord have been reported. Dogs with ischemic myelopathy have an acute, focal nonprogressive hindlimb or tetraparesis from spinal cord dysfunction. This presentation may be similar to those with acute disc disease, though dogs with ischemic myelopathy typically do not display spinal pain.

Myelography reveals the presence of an intramedullary lesion, reflecting the concurrent cord edema which accompanies an ischemic event. With MRI, there is focal T2 hyperintensity within a spinal cord segment with no or minimal contrast enhancement (Figure 12.66). The imaging appearance of ischemic myelopathy may be difficult to differentiate from

ANNPE even with MRI, but there are distinguishing features of each [35]. Dogs with ischemic myelopathy typically have more extensive T2 hyperintensity in the spinal cord (spanning several vertebral segments) than dogs with ANNPE, where the area of T2 hyperintensity is more focally located at one vertebral segment. Ischemic myelopathy lacks the regional meningeal and epidural enhancement usually seen with disc extrusions.

## Arachnoid Diverticulum

Spinal arachnoid diverticula (previously called arachnoid cysts) are a focal dilation of the subarachnoid space, which can result in compression when large [36]. They most commonly occur in the cervical region of large-breed dogs and the thoracolumbar region in small-breed dogs, but may occur anywhere along the length of the spine. They most commonly involve the dorsal subarachnoid space, and are sometimes seen in association with other adjacent spinal cord disease (such as stenosis, vertebral malformations, or disc protrusions). On myelography, these cause focal expansion of the subarachnoid space, often with rounded margins (Figure 12.67). With MRI, they are recognized as a focal dilation of the subarachnoid space without regional enhancement (Figure 12.68).

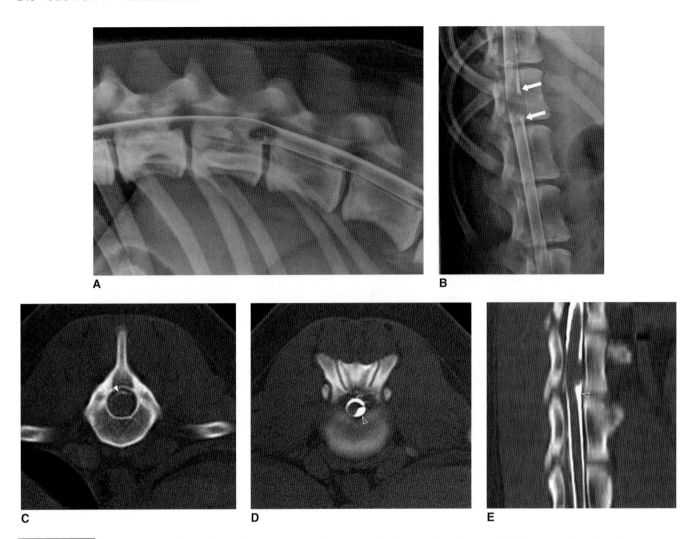

**FIGURE 12.63** Lateral (**A**) and oblique (**B**) myelogram radiograph, transverse CT (**C,D**), and oblique sagittal reformat (**E**) of a dog with nephroblastoma. The intradural-extramedullary nature of the mass is most apparent on the oblique image by the adjacent golf tee sign (arrows). This is less apparent on the lateral radiograph. At the level of the mass, only a small amount of subarachnoid contrast is present (closed arrowhead), but caudal to the mass the subarachoid space is expanded (open arrowhead), resulting in the golf tee appearance.

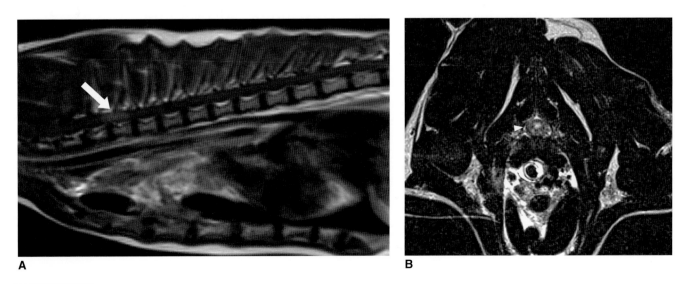

**FIGURE 12.64** Sagittal postcontrast T1W (**A**) and transverse T2W (**B**) MRI images of a *Cryptococcus* granuloma in the spinal cord of a cat. The mass is contrast enhancing (arrow) and T2 hyperintense (arrowhead).

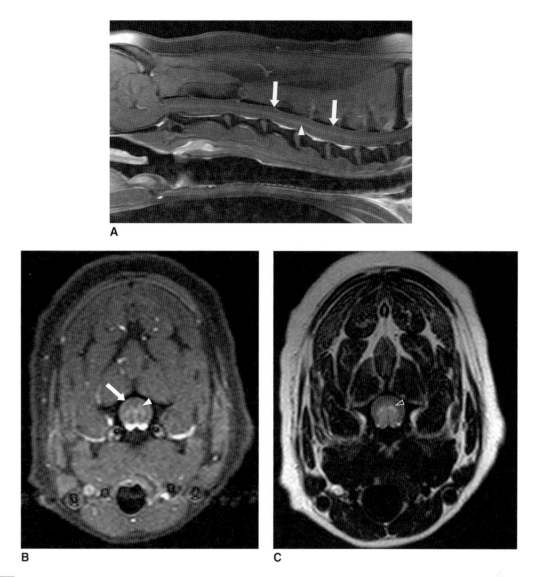

**FIGURE 12.65** Sagittal (**A**) and transverse (**B**) postcontrast T1W and transverse T2W (**C**) images of a meningoencephalitis of unknown origin. There is regional contrast enhancement of the meninges (arrow). The spinal cord has ill-defined contrast enhancement (closed arrowhead) and T2 hyperintensity (open arrowhead).

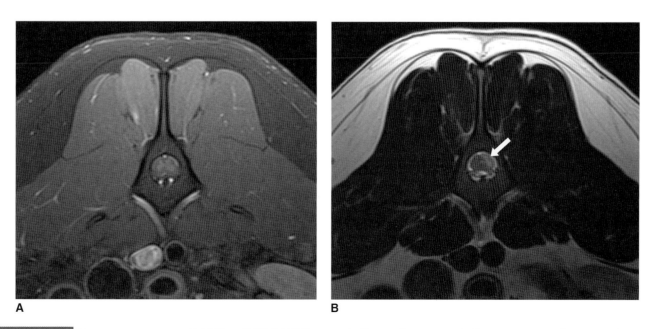

**FIGURE 12.66** Transverse postcontrast T1W (**A**) and T2W (**B**) MRI images of a fibrocartilagenous embolism. No contrast enhancement is seen (**A**), but there is a focal lateralized T2 hyperintensity (arrow).

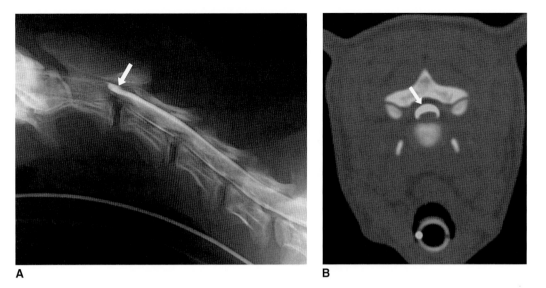

**FIGURE 12.67** Lateral myelogram (**A**) and postmyelogram CT (**B**) images of a dog with an arachnoid diverticulum. There is focal widening of the dorsal subarachnoid space (arrow) causing spinal cord compression.

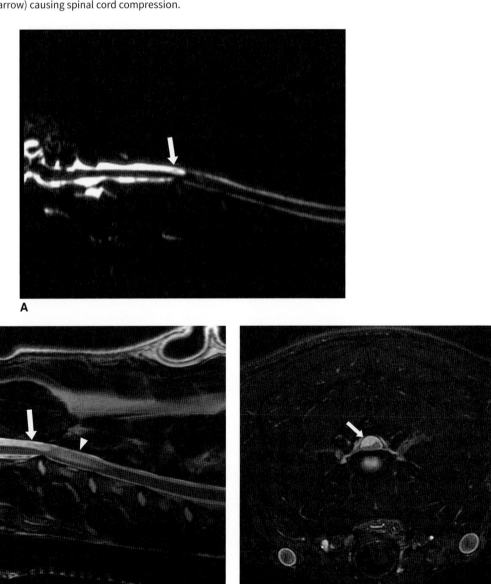

**FIGURE 12.68** Sagittal heavily T2W (**A**), sagittal T2W (**B**), and transverse fat-saturated T2W (**C**) MRI images of a dog with an arachnoid diverticulum. There is focal dilation of the dorsal subarachnoid space with a rounded caudal margin (arrow). There is T2 hyperintensity in the spinal cord (arrowhead) "downstream" consistent with edema.

# References

1. Fluckiger, M.A., Damur-Djuric, N., Hassig, M. et al. (2006). A lumbosacral transitional vertebra in the dog predisposes to cauda equina syndrome. *Vet. Radiol. Ultrasound* 47 (1): 39–44.

2. Fluckiger, M.A., Steffen, F., Hassig, M., and Morgan, J.P. (2017). Asymmetrical lumbosacral transitional vertebrae in dogs may promote asymmetrical hip joint development. *Vet. Comp. Orthop. Traumatol.* 30 (2): 137–142.

3. Ryan, R., Gutierrez-Quintana, R., Haar, G.T., and De Decker, S. (2019). Relationship between breed, hemivertebra subtype, and kyphosis in apparently neurologically normal French Bulldogs, English Bulldogs, and Pugs. *Am. J. Vet. Res.* 80 (2): 189–194.

4. Ryan, R., Gutierrez-Quintana, R., Ter Haar, G., and De Decker, S. (2017). Prevalence of thoracic vertebral malformations in French bulldogs, Pugs and English bulldogs with and without associated neurological deficits. *Vet. J.* 221: 25–29.

5. Gutierrez-Quintana, R., Guevar, J., Stalin, C. et al. (2014). A proposed radiographic classification scheme for congenital thoracic vertebral malformations in brachycephalic "screw-tailed" dog breeds. *Vet. Radiol. Ultrasound* 55 (6): 585–591.

6. Lin, J.L. and Coolman, B.R. (2009). Atlantoaxial subluxation in two dogs with cervical block vertebrae. *J. Am. Anim. Hosp. Assoc.* 45 (6): 305–310.

7. Bertram, S., Ter Haar, G., and De Decker, S. (2018). Caudal articular process dysplasia of thoracic vertebrae in neurologically normal French bulldogs, English bulldogs, and Pugs: prevalence and characteristics. *Vet. Radiol. Ultrasound* 59 (4): 396–404.

8. Song, R.B., Glass, E.N., and Kent, M. (2016). Spina bifida, meningomyelocele, and meningocele. *Vet. Clin. North Am. Small Anim. Pract.* 46 (2): 327–345.

9. Hanel, R.M., Graham, J.P., Levy, J.K. et al. (2004). Generalized osteosclerosis in a cat. *Vet. Radiol. Ultrasound* 45 (4): 318–324.

10. Bojanic, K., Acke, E., and Jones, B.R. (2011). Congenital hypothyroidism of dogs and cats: a review. *N. Z. Vet. J.* 59 (3): 115–122.

11. Greco, D.S. (2006). Diagnosis of congenital and adult-onset hypothyroidism in cats. *Clin. Tech. Small Anim. Pract.* 21 (1): 40–44.

12. Seeliger, F., Leeb, T., Peters, M. et al. (2003). Osteogenesis imperfecta in two litters of dachshunds. *Vet. Pathol.* 40 (5): 530–539.

13. Enderli, T.A., Burtch, S.R., Templet, J.N., and Carriero, A. (2016). Animal models of osteogenesis imperfecta: applications in clinical research. *Orthop. Res. Rev.* 8: 41–55.

14. Ruoff, C.M., Kerwin, S.C., and Taylor, A.R. (2018). Diagnostic imaging of discospondylitis. *Vet. Clin. North Am. Small Anim. Pract.* 48 (1): 85–94.

15. Kirberger, R.M. (2016). Early diagnostic imaging findings in juvenile dogs with presumed diskospondylitis: 10 cases (2008–2014). *J. Am. Vet. Med. Assoc.* 249 (5): 539–546.

16. Harris, J.M., Chen, A.V., Tucker, R.L., and Mattoon, J.S. (2013). Clinical features and magnetic resonance imaging characteristics of diskospondylitis in dogs: 23 cases (1997–2010). *J. Am. Vet. Med. Assoc.* 242 (3): 359–365.

17. Carrera, I., Sullivan, M., McConnell, F., and Goncalves, R. (2011). Magnetic resonance imaging features of discospondylitis in dogs. *Vet. Radiol. Ultrasound* 52 (2): 125–131.

18. De Stefani, A., Garosi, L.S., McConnell, F.J. et al. (2008). Magnetic resonance imaging features of spinal epidural empyema in five dogs. *Vet. Radiol. Ultrasound* 49 (2): 135–140.

19. Brisson, B.A. (2010). Intervertebral disc disease in dogs. *Vet. Clin. North Am. Small Anim. Pract.* 40 (5): 829–858.

20. Bergknut, N., Smolders, L.A., Grinwis, G.C. et al. (2013). Intervertebral disc degeneration in the dog. Part 1: anatomy and physiology of the intervertebral disc and characteristics of intervertebral disc degeneration. *Vet. J.* 195 (3): 282–291.

21. Lamb, C.R., Nicholls, A., Targett, M., and Mannion, P. (2002). Accuracy of survey radiographic diagnosis of intervertebral disc protrusion in dogs. *Vet. Radiol. Ultrasound* 43 (3): 222–228.

22. De Decker, S. and Fenn, J. (2018). Acute herniation of nondegenerate nucleus pulposus: acute noncompressive nucleus pulposus extrusion and compressive hydrated nucleus pulposus extrusion. *Vet. Clin. North Am. Small Anim. Pract.* 48 (1): 95–109.

23. Manunta, M.L., Evangelisti, M.A., Bergknut, N. et al. (2015). Hydrated nucleus pulposus herniation in seven dogs. *Vet. J.* 203 (3): 342–344.

24. Beltran, E., Dennis, R., Doyle, V. et al. (2012). Clinical and magnetic resonance imaging features of canine compressive cervical myelopathy with suspected hydrated nucleus pulposus extrusion. *J. Small Anim. Pract.* 53 (2): 101–107.

25. Kranenburg, H.C., Voorhout, G., Grinwis, G.C. et al. (2011). Diffuse idiopathic skeletal hyperostosis (DISH) and spondylosis deformans in purebred dogs: a retrospective radiographic study. *Vet. J.* 190 (2): e84–e90.

26. Levine, G.J., Levine, J.M., Walker, M.A. et al. (2006). Evaluation of the association between spondylosis deformans and clinical signs of intervertebral disk disease in dogs: 172 cases (1999–2000). *J. Am. Vet. Med. Assoc.* 228 (1): 96–100.

27. da Costa, R.C. (2010). Cervical spondylomyelopathy (wobbler syndrome) in dogs. *Vet. Clin. North Am. Small Anim. Pract.* 40 (5): 881–913.

28. De Decker, S., da Costa, R.C., Volk, H.A., and Van Ham, L.M. (2012). Current insights and controversies in the pathogenesis and diagnosis of disc-associated cervical spondylomyelopathy in dogs. *Vet. Rec.* 171 (21): 531–537.

29. Cooper, C., Gutierrez-Quintana, R., Penderis, J., and Goncalves, R. (2015). Osseous associated cervical spondylomyelopathy at the C2-C3 articular facet joint in 11 dogs. *Vet. Rec.* 177 (20): 522.

30. Martin-Vaquero, P. and da Costa, R.C. (2014). Magnetic resonance imaging features of Great Danes with and without clinical signs of cervical spondylomyelopathy. *J. Am. Vet. Med. Assoc.* 245 (4): 393–400.

31. da Costa, R.C., Parent, J.M., Partlow, G. et al. (2006). Morphologic and morphometric magnetic resonance imaging features of Doberman Pinschers with and without clinical signs of cervical spondylomyelopathy. *Am. J. Vet. Res.* 67 (9): 1601–1612.

32. da Costa, R.C., Parent, J., Dobson, H. et al. (2006). Comparison of magnetic resonance imaging and myelography in 18 Doberman Pinscher dogs with cervical spondylomyelopathy. *Vet. Radiol. Ultrasound* 47 (6): 523–531.

33. Penderis, J. and Dennis, R. (2004). Use of traction during magnetic resonance imaging of caudal cervical spondylomyelopathy ("wobbler syndrome") in the dog. *Vet. Radiol. Ultrasound* 45 (3): 216–219.

34. Masciarelli, A.E., Griffin, J.F., Fosgate, G.T. et al. (2017). Evaluation of magnetic resonance imaging for the differentiation of

inflammatory, neoplastic, and vascular intradural spinal cord diseases in the dog. *Vet. Radiol. Ultrasound* 58 (4): 444–453.

35. Specchi, S., Johnson, P., Beauchamp, G. et al. (2016). Assessment of interobserver agreement and use of selected magnetic resonance imaging variables for differentiation of acute noncompressive nucleus pulposus extrusion and ischemic myelopathy in dogs. *J. Am. Vet. Med. Assoc.* 248 (9): 1013–1021.

36. Mauler, D.A., De Decker, S., de Risio, L. et al. (2014). Signalment, clinical presentation, and diagnostic findings in 122 dogs with spinal arachnoid diverticula. *J. Vet. Intern. Med.* 28 (1): 175–181.

# Thorax

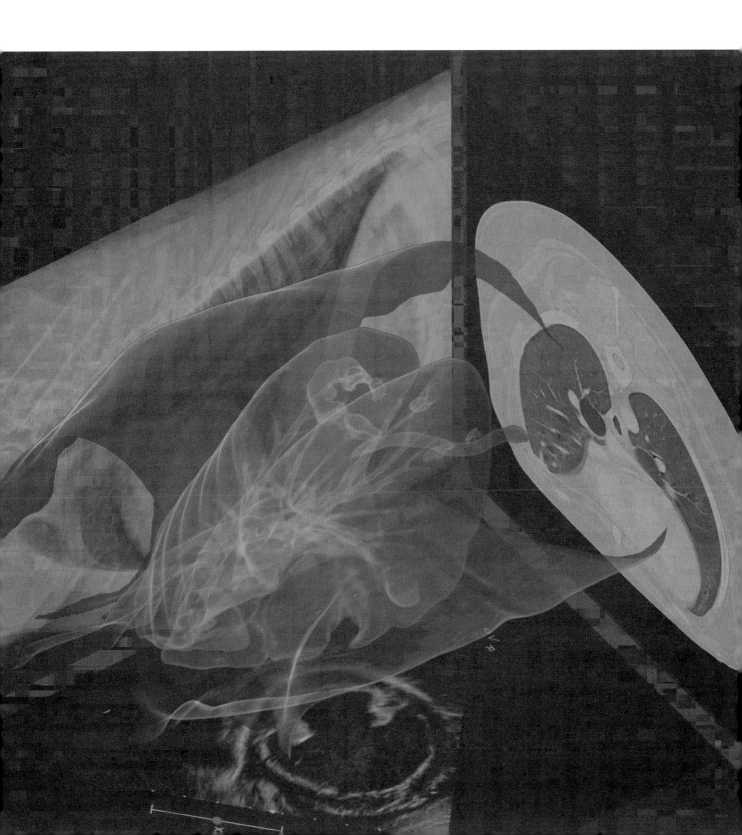

# CHAPTER 13

# Anatomy, Variants, and Interpretation Paradigm

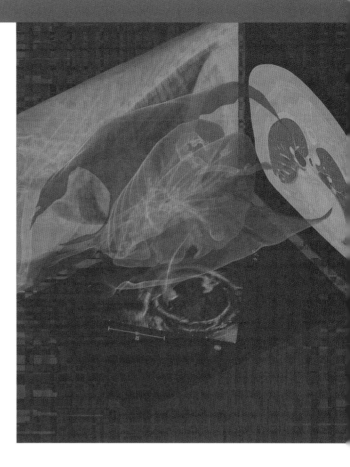

**Clifford R. Berry[1] and Elizabeth Huyhn[2]**

[1] Department of Molecular Biomedical Sciences, College of Veterinary Medicine, North Carolina State University, Raleigh, NC, USA
[2] VCA West Coast Specialty and Emergency Animal Hospital, Fountain Valley, CA, USA

## Overview

The thorax is ideally suited for radiographic imaging as it provides excellent subject contrast (gas compared with soft tissue), thereby providing excellent radiographic contrast. Thoracic radiographs are inexpensive, rapid to do, and still considered a first line test to survey the intra- and extrathoracic structures.

Currently, three-view thoracic radiographs are considered the standard of care in veterinary medicine for the evaluation of the thorax [1–4]. These include the right lateral, left lateral, and either the dorsoventral or ventrodorsal radiographs of the thorax. When describing the right and left lateral radiographs, these images refer to the recumbent side of the dog or cat when placed down against the x-ray table. The correct point of entrance to point of exit of the x-ray beam naming of the radiograph would be left to right lateral image (right lateral) and right to left lateral image (left lateral). The ventrodorsal and dorsoventral images appropriately describe the point of entrance to the point of exit of the x-ray beam as with standard x-ray labeling nomenclature. For example, with the dog in dorsal recumbency, a ventrodorsal image is made such that the ventral aspect of the patient is the entrance point of the x-ray beam and the dorsal aspect of the patient is the exit point of the x-ray beam.

The chapters involving the thorax will introduce radiographic concepts for interpretation. It is important to understand that all of the nuances associated with the interpretation of thoracic radiographs in small animals will not be covered, as one cannot see the infinite examples of thoracic diseases, much less normal variations. The purpose of this chapter is to review normal radiographic anatomy of the thorax, thoracic variants, and "fake-outs," and present an interpretation paradigm for the routine evaluation of the thorax.

*Atlas of Small Animal Diagnostic Imaging*, First Edition. Edited by Clifford R. Berry, Nathan C. Nelson, and Matthew D. Winter.
© 2023 John Wiley & Sons, Inc. Published 2023 by John Wiley & Sons, Inc.
Companion website: www.wiley.com/go/berry/atlas

# Thoracic Radiographs – Basic Principles

High-quality thoracic radiographs are the end goal for all thoracic imaging studies. High-quality radiographs require appropriate technique, positioning, and anatomy. For the technique, a high kVp and low mAs are used [5], which will provide the best latitude or overall image gray scale. However, for most digital radiography (computed radiography [CR] or digital radiography [DR]) scenarios, the dynamic range is wide enough, and the processing algorithms mature enough to result in high-quality images without significant technique manipulation between patients.

The most common mistake is photon starvation (underexposure) of the DR or CR plate, resulting in quantum mottle associated with the image. At the other extreme, one can oversaturate (expose) the digital plate which results in absence of information (no vessels, airways, etc.) in areas of the lung, specifically the right cranial lung lobe cranial to the cardiac silhouette and the accessory lung lobe caudal to the cardiac silhouette on the lateral images. Once a mAs (typically 1–3 mAs for the thorax) has been decided, the clinician should use the highest mA station so that the fastest time can be used to obtain the desired low mAs. This will decrease the likelihood of respiratory motion and artifact.

The thoracic radiograph should be taken on peak inspiration [6]. This is important for the overall cardiothoracic ratio and detection of pulmonary changes not associated with expiration (Figure 13.1). On expiratory radiographs, there is enlargement of the cardiothoracic ratio (cardiac silhouette appears larger relative to the thoracic volume) and an unstructured interstitial pulmonary pattern is often present [7]. These changes could result in the false-positive diagnosis of cardiomegaly and pulmonary edema (Figure 13.1A–D). On inspiration, the diaphragmatic crura will cross the thoracic spine at T11–T12 (or further caudal) and there will be an increase in size to the accessory lung lobe, resulting in a larger radiolucent triangle formed between the caudal border of the cardiac silhouette, the ventral border of the caudal vena cava and the cranial border of the central diaphragm when compared with expiratory radiographs, (Figure 13.1A–D).

In some medium- and large-breed dogs, there will be a radiolucent triangle noted with separation between the cardiac silhouette and the cupula of the ventral diaphragm. In some of the smaller dog breeds, the cardiac silhouette will be in contact with the cranial diaphragm on the lateral and ventrodorsal radiographs on inspiration as well as expiration. These images will still be inspiratory as a dog will breathe (tidal volume changes) by moving its diaphragmatic crura and not the entire diaphragm. If the lateral image was made on expiration, the diaphragmatic crura will be seen at the T8 vertebral body. Similarly, on the ventrodorsal radiograph, the cupula of the diaphragm will be located at the T6–T7 vertebral bodies

and there will be cranial displacement of the costophrenic pulmonary angle to the sixth to eighth intercostal spaces (Figure 13.2). Differences in inspiration and expiration in dogs are found in Table 13.1.

In cats, all films are typically made on inspiration with the diaphragmatic crura extending caudal to the level of T12–T13 and the cupula (dome) of the diaphragm being caudally displaced to the level of T10. There is usually a separation between the caudal cardiac silhouette and the cranial diaphragm seen on both the lateral and ventrodorsal images (Figure 13.3). This is because cats move all aspects of the diaphragm (crura and cupula) in a caudal direction during inspiration.

Technique and positioning of the thoracic radiographs are accomplished through experience and trial and error. Unfortunately, some veterinarians do not take the time to quality control this aspect of thoracic radiography and thereby do not obtain high-quality images on a consistent basis. The right and left lateral recumbent radiographs are made such that the sternum and vertebral column align with each other in the same plane parallel to the x-ray table top (Figure 13.4). The right and left rib heads at the vertebrae should overlap. The thoracic limbs should be taped cranially so that they do not superimpose over the cranial thorax. This is most easily accomplished if the pelvic limbs are taped and pulled caudally as well. A triangular radiolucent sponge can also be placed under the sternum to elevate the sternum away from the x-ray table top so that it is in the same sagittal plane as the vertebral column and parallel to the x-ray table top. This is needed for medium- and large-breed dogs. In dogs with a barrel-shaped thorax, one may need to rotate the sternum toward the table in order to get the sternum horizontal with the thoracic spine and parallel to the table top of the x-ray unit.

The collimation of the x-ray machine will dictate the anatomy that is projected onto the imaging device. The image should be centered along the caudal border of the scapula (middle of the cardiac silhouette) and include the thoracic inlet cranially, the 13th rib caudally, the spinous processes of the thoracic vertebrae dorsally, and the sternum ventrally. In smaller dogs and cats, collimation helps reduce x-ray scatter and thereby eliminates degradation of the x-ray image due to film fog from the scatter radiation as well as decreasing overall scatter radiation to any personnel who are in the x-ray room at the time of the exposure. However, the goal would be to position the dog or cat such that everyone is out of the x-ray room at the time of the exposure [8]. In giant-breed dogs, one might have to split the thorax into cranial and caudal halves with overlap in the middle of the image to ensure complete assessment of the thorax (Figure 13.5).

Other radiographic projections of the thorax include oblique, horizontal beam, and "humanoid" projections. Oblique projections are typically obtained with the patient in ventral or dorsal recumbency and obliqued to the right or left so that rib or pleural space abnormalities can be highlighted (Figure 13.6). Use of horizontal beam projections can only be accomplished if the tube head can be rotated from a vertical

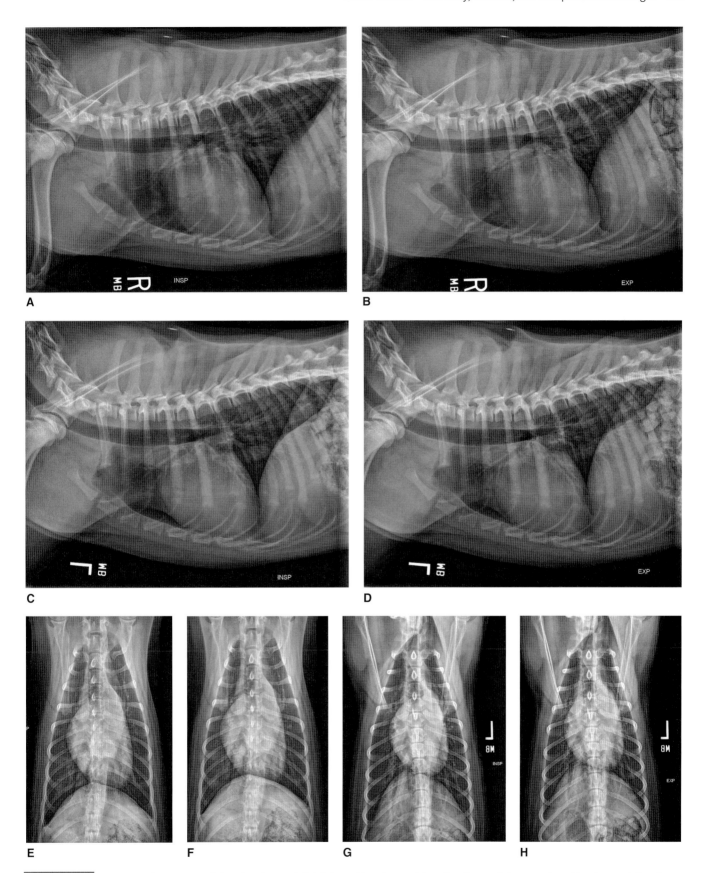

**FIGURE 13.1** Right lateral inspiratory (**A**) and expiratory (**B**), left lateral inspiratory (**C**) and expiratory (**D**), ventrodorsal inspiratory (**E**) and expiratory (**F**), and dorsoventral inspiratory (**G**) and expiratory (**H**) thoracic radiographs of a normal 5-year-old medium-sized mixed-breed dog.

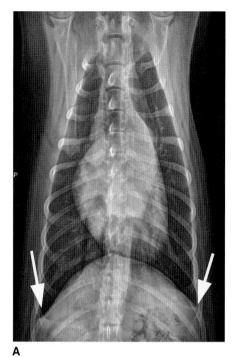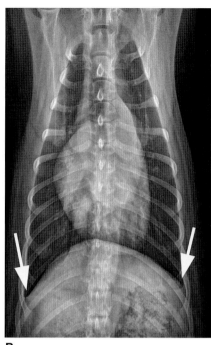

A          B

**FIGURE 13.2** Ventrodorsal inspiratory (**A**) and expiratory (**B**) thoracic radiographs of a 5-year-old medium-sized mixed-breed dog. Notice the differences between the position of the cupula and the diaphragmatic crura and relative size of the thoracic volume compared to the size of the cardiac silhouette. In expiration, the crura and costophrenic angle (white arrows) are displaced cranially.

**TABLE 13.1** Differences in peak inspiration and expiration based on lateral and ventrodorsal radiographs.

| Image | Inspiration | Expiration |
|---|---|---|
| Right and left laterals | Separation of ventral cardiac silhouette from sternum; postcardiac triangle larger with flattened diaphragm; relative and absolute cardiac size are decreased (smaller cardiothoracic ratio); minimal or no contact between cardiac silhouette and diaphragm; diaphragmatic crura caudal to the level of T10; relatively flat angle (horizontal) of the caudal vena cava; soft tissue opaque lesion conspicuity is best in the nondependent lung lobes | Lack of separation of the cardiac silhouette and sternum; overlap between the cardiac silhouette and cranial diaphragm; diaphragmatic crura to level of T8 (cranial to T10); relative and absolute cardiac size are increased (larger cardiothoracic ratio); postcardiac triangle smaller with curved diaphragm; dorsal angle of the caudal vena cava; recumbent atelectasis will decrease overall lesion conspicuity |
| Ventrodorsal/dorsoventral image | Elongation of the cardiac silhouette; separation of the cardiac silhouette from the cupula of the diaphragm; caudal positioning of the costophrenic angles of the lungs along the lateral margins of the thorax at the level of the 9th and 10th intercostal spaces; increased detail associated with the caudal lobar pulmonary vasculature | Smaller length of the cardiac silhouette; overlap between the cardiac silhouette and diaphragm; cranial positioning of the costophrenic angles of the lung at the level of the 6th intercostal space; decreased detail of the caudal lobar pulmonary vasculature |

to a horizontal position with the patient placed in lateral or ventral/dorsal recumbency (Figure 13.7). This view is obtained to confirm pneumothorax or to shift pleural fluid away from a given area to determine if an intrathoracic mass is present [9]. The "humanoid" view is a special radiographic projection, taken from the dorsal recumbent position, where rather than extending the thoracic limbs cranially, they are pulled caudally alongside the thorax. This will shift the right and left scapulae in a caudal and lateral position relative to the cranial thorax and thereby produce better visualization of the left and right cranial lung lobes (Figure 13.8).

# Thoracic Radiographic Anatomy

## Computed Tomographic Anatomy of the Thorax

Knowledge of thoracic anatomy is power when it comes to interpretation of thoracic radiographs. Conventional orthogonal radiographs provide a two-dimensional representation of

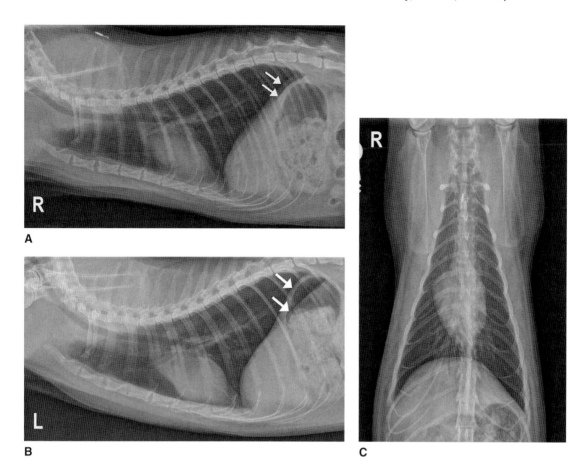

**FIGURE 13.3**   Right lateral (**A**), left lateral (**B**), and ventrodorsal (**C**) thoracic radiographs of a normal 5-year-old domestic shorthair cat. Notice the difference in position between the diaphragmatic crura on the lateral radiographs (white arrows).

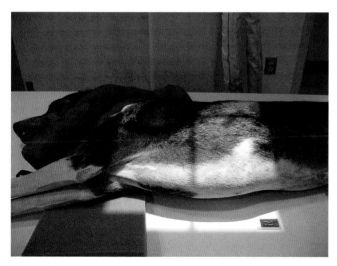

**FIGURE 13.4**   Right lateral recumbent positioning of a dog for a right lateral radiograph. Notice that the collimator light extends from the thoracic inlet caudally to the cranial abdomen (caudal border of the 13th rib) and extends dorsal from the spinous processes of the thoracic spine to the sternum ventrally.

a three-dimensional object with images taken at 90° relative to each other so that one can triangulate the anatomy. However, due to border effacement and summation, interpretation is hampered by geometric changes of the thorax and superimposition of

three-dimensional structures, making the radiographic images a "summary" image of the original anatomy (Figure 13.9).

*Border effacement* is where two objects of the same radiographic opacity are in contact with each other, resulting in a loss of border distinction for each of the objects (Figure 13.10). *Summation* is the added radiographic opacity of two superimposed structures that are not in contact with each other (Figure 13.11).

Computed tomography provides a three-dimensional approach to radiographic anatomy of the thorax. The initial volumetric data set acquired of the thorax represents raw data that can be reformatted into one of the standard anatomic planes (transverse, sagittal, dorsal). Transverse images can be used to review normal thoracic anatomy as thin section slices of the thorax presented in a lung (WW/WL: 2000/−700), soft tissue (400/100), and bone window (2000/1000) with contrast medium to highlight the intravascular space (Figure 13.12) [10]. One should review these images in the sagittal and dorsal plane images to better understand the relationships of the structures of the thorax as well as the complexities of individual lung lobes and bronchial anatomy (Figure 13.13).

## Right Lateral Radiograph
Patient positioning dictates the appearance of the radiographic anatomy of the thorax. The radiographic anatomy changes between the laterals and between ventrodorsal and dorsoventral images,

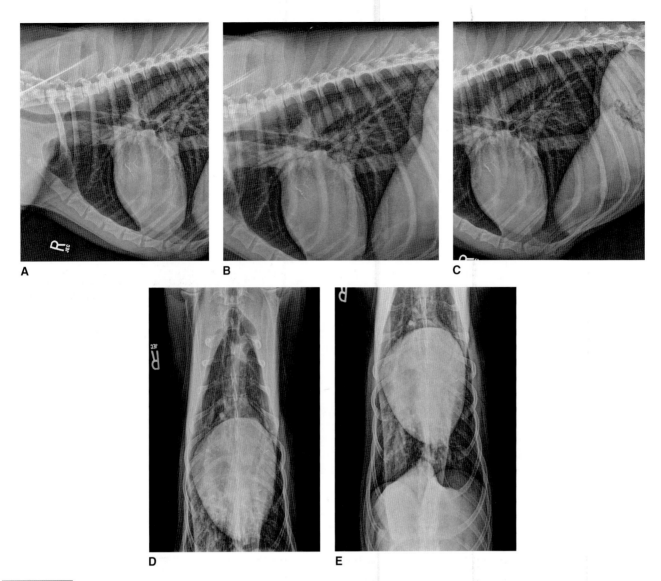

**FIGURE 13.5** Right lateral (**A,B,C**) and ventrodorsal (**D,E**) thoracic radiographs of a 7-year-old greyhound. The added soft tissue opacity noted in the right caudal thorax is due to superimposed skinfolds and not pulmonary pathology. This was confirmed on the left lateral images. Additionally, on the right lateral images there is mineralization noted to the aortic root and potentially the coronary arteries.

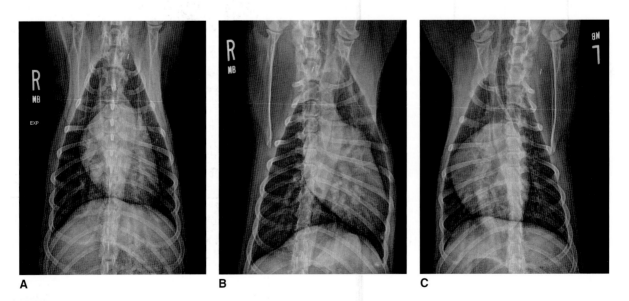

**FIGURE 13.6** Ventrodorsal (**A**), ventrodorsal left oblique (**B**), and ventrodorsal right oblique (**C**) thoracic radiographs of an 8-year-old medium-sized mixed-breed dog. When the sternum is obliqued to the left side of the dog, the main pulmonary artery appears prominent; when the sternum is obliqued to the right side of the dog, the right atrium and right side of the cardiac silhouette appear enlarged. This emphasizes the need for straight VD positioning as shown in (**A**) (sternum and vertebral column superimposed).

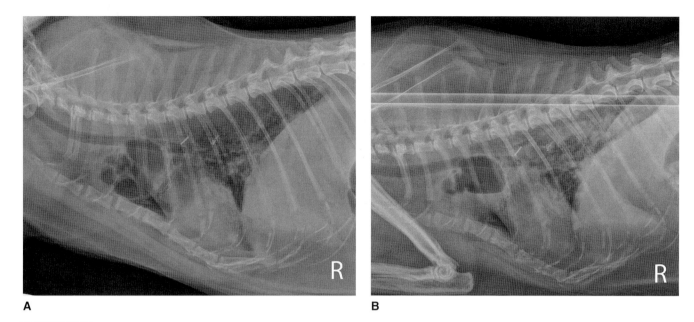

**A**     **B**

**FIGURE 13.7**   Right lateral (**A**) and horizontal beam (**B**) thoracic radiographs of a 15-year-old domestic shorthair cat with a large cavitated mass of the cranial subsegment of the left cranial lung lobe. On the right lateral radiograph, the intralesional fluid portion cannot be appreciated. On the horizontal beam radiograph, the intralesional fluid portion is further characterized by a fluid line oriented parallel to the sternum and x-ray table. The metallic hemoclips are from a prior lobectomy and lung lobe resection for a pulmonary carcinoma.

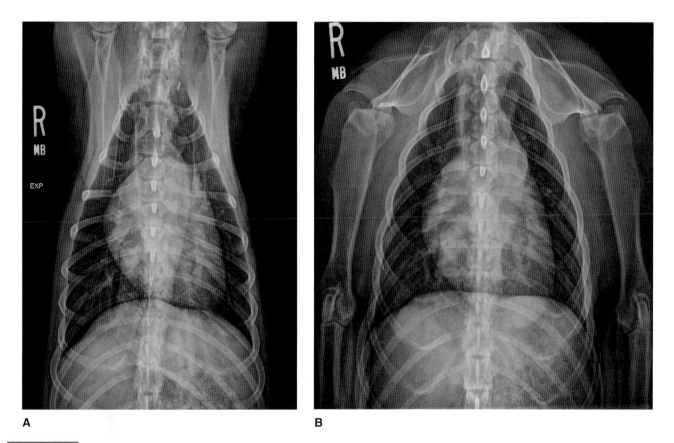

**A**     **B**

**FIGURE 13.8**   Ventrodorsal (**A**) and "humanoid" ventrodorsal (**B**) thoracic radiographs of an 8-year-old medium-sized mixed-breed dog. In the "humanoid" image, the scapulae are no longer superimposed over the right and left cranial lung lobes.

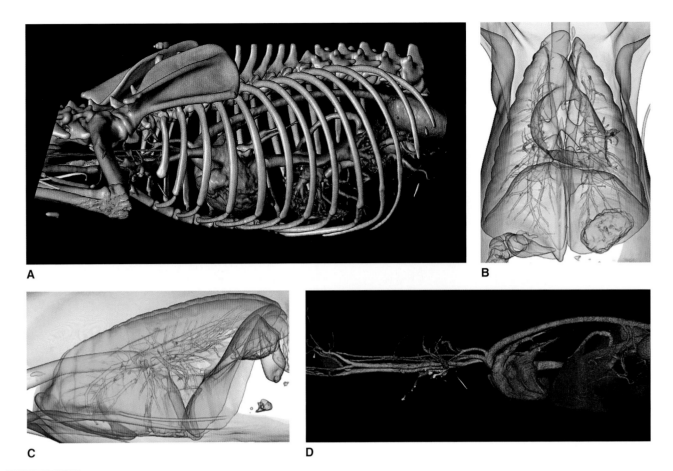

**A**

**B**

**C**

**D**

**FIGURE 13.9** Three-dimensional reconstruction of the thorax in sagittal plane including the osseous structures of the thorax and cardiovascular structures (**A**), in dorsal (**B**) and sagittal (**C**) planes delineating the air-filled structures of the thorax, in sagittal plane including the cardiovascular structures of the cervical region and thorax (**D**).

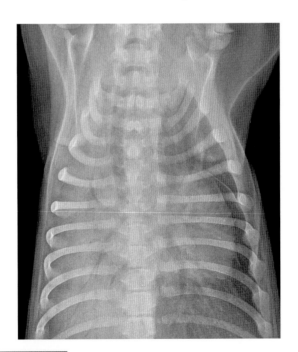

**FIGURE 13.10** Ventrodorsal thoracic radiograph of a 3-month-old Rottweiler. There is a diffuse alveolar pulmonary pattern of the right lung, border effacing and limiting the complete evaluation of the cardiac silhouette and pulmonary vasculature. Several pleural fissure lines are noted along the left side of the inner thoracic wall. The widening of the costochondral junctions is more prominent on the left than the right due to the leftward rotation of the sternum relative to the thoracic vertebral column.

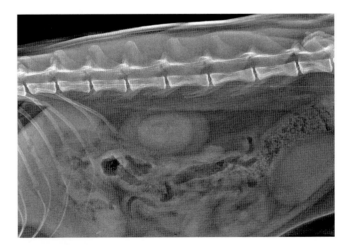

**FIGURE 13.11** Right lateral abdominal radiograph of a cat. There is summation of the left and right kidneys. Note the soft tissue opaque oval made by the caudal pole of the right kidney (cranially located) and the cranial pole of the left kidney (caudally located). The relative radiolucency noted in the center of the kidneys is secondary to fat deposition in the renal sinus at the renal hilum.

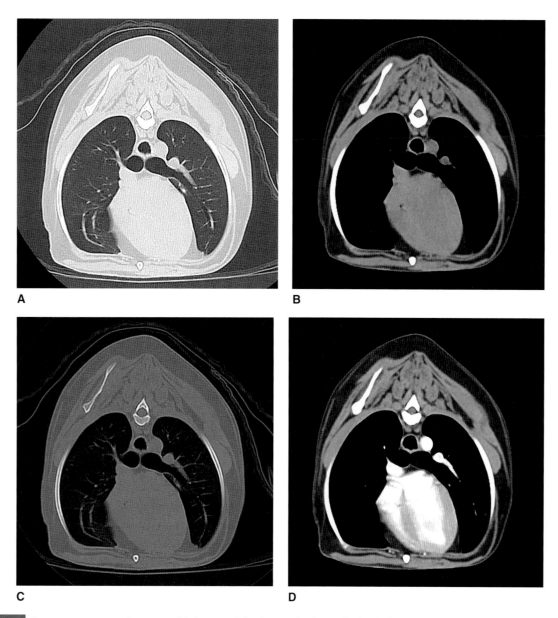

**FIGURE 13.12** Transverse computed tomographic images of the thorax of a dog at the level of the heart in the lung window (**A**), soft tissue window (**B**), bone window (**C**), and soft tissue window (**D**) after intravenous contrast administration.

particularly for medium- and large-sized dogs. In right lateral radiographs, the right thoracic limb will appear smaller than the left and will be in a more caudal position. The cardiac silhouette is in the ventral two-thirds of the middle thorax and has an oval or egg-shaped appearance. The cardiac silhouette is located dorsal to the sternum without separation from the sternum (except for deep-chested breeds and sight hounds). The right and left diaphragmatic crura parallel each other with the right crus being cranial to the left (Table 13.2). This is because the dependent (right) lung is less aerated, and the gravity-dependent abdominal contents displace the right side of the diaphragm cranially. The dorsal border of the caudal vena cava will become confluent with the right diaphragmatic crus (cranial crus) at the level of the caval foramen. In addition, the caudal vena cava will terminate cranially at the level of the caudal border of the cardiac silhouette where the caudal vena

cava becomes confluent with the right atrium (Figure 13.14). The fundic and body portions of the stomach will contain gas and are located caudal to the left crus (caudal crus).

With respect to the cranial lobar vasculature and bronchi, the right cranial lung lobe bronchus is the first radiolucent circle located superimposed over the carina (terminal portion of the trachea) on the right lateral image (Figure 13.15). One can then trace the right cranial lobe bronchus in a cranioventral direction with the pulmonary artery being dorsal and the pulmonary vein being ventral to the bronchus. The pulmonary artery and vein are equal in diameter to each other and should not be larger than the thinnest point of the proximal portion of the right fourth rib (Figure 13.16). In right lateral recumbency, the right cranial lung lobe bronchus is initially dorsal to the left cranial lobe bronchus, but then the two airways cross and the left cranial lobe bronchus becomes dorsal and cranial to the

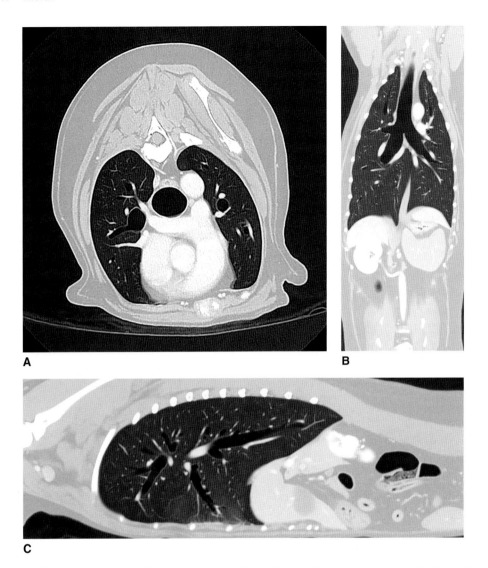

**A**  **B**  **C**

**FIGURE 13.13** Computed tomographic study of the thorax of a dog in lung window in the transverse plane (**A**), dorsal plane (**B**), and sagittal plane (**C**) images.

| TABLE 13.2 | Differences between right and left lateral thoracic radiographs in medium- and large-breed dogs. These changes are not seen routinely in the small breeds or cats. | |
|---|---|---|
| **Anatomic differences** | **Right lateral** | **Left lateral** |
| Cardiac silhouette | Oval or egg shaped | Circular/round |
| Crura | Right crus cranial; crura parallel to each other | Left crus cranial; crura diverge away from each other starting at the level of the caudal vena cava |
| Caudal vena cava | Dorsal border blends with cranial crus; the cranial end of the caudal vena cava ends at the cardiac silhouette | Dorsal border blends with caudal crus (passes over cranial crus); the cranial end of the caudal vena cava is superimposed over the caudal aspect of the cardiac silhouette |
| Gas in fundus/body of the stomach | Caudal to left crus | Caudal to the left crus but more conspicuous over the caudodorsal thorax |
| Cardio-sternal distance | Decreased and normally seen in juxtaposition with each other | Increased and away from each other |
| Cranial lobar bronchi and vessels | Criss-cross over each other cranial to the cardiac silhouette; right cranial bronchus, artery, and vein are dorsal to the left cranial subsegmental bronchus | Parallel to each other cranial to the cardiac silhouette; the left cranial subsegmental bronchus, artery, and vein are cranial and dorsal relative to the right cranial bronchus and vessel pair |

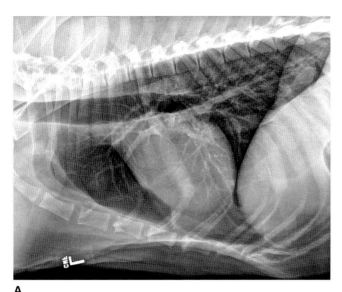 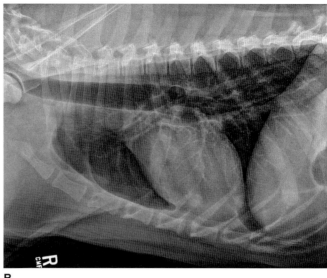

**A**                                                                                    **B**

**FIGURE 13.14**   Left lateral (**A**) and right lateral (**B**) thoracic radiographs from a large mixed-breed dog. The cardiac silhouette is oval on the right lateral radiograph and round on the left lateral radiograph. On the left lateral, the cardiac silhouette apex is noted to rotate away from the sternum. This gap between the ventral border of the cardiac silhouette and the sternum should not be mistaken for a pneumothorax. The right diaphragmatic crus is located cranial to the left diaphragmatic crus on the right lateral radiograph. The left diaphragmatic crus is located cranial to the right diaphragmatic crus on the left lateral radiograph. The intrathoracic caudal vena cava is confluent with the right diaphragmatic crus on both lateral radiographs.

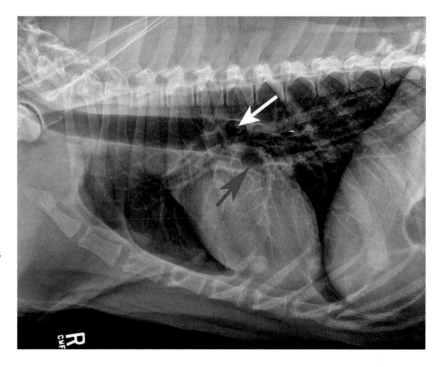

**FIGURE 13.15**   Right lateral thoracic radiographs from the same dog as in Figure 13.14. The right cranial lung lobe bronchus (white arrow) is the first radiolucent circle superimposed over the carina. The left cranial lobe bronchus exits the ventral aspect of the carina (red arrow) and immediately bifurcates into cranial and caudal subsegments.

right cranial lobe bronchus cranial to the cardiac silhouette (Figure 13.17).

In addition, if one traces the ventral margin of the trachea caudal to the opening of the right cranial lobe bronchus, a radiolucent gap will intersect the line so that there is a bronchus exiting the carina in a ventral direction (Figure 13.18). This is the common opening into the left cranial lobe bronchus. Within several millimeters of exiting the carina, the left

cranial bronchus will divide into the cranial and caudal subsegments. The cranial subsegmental bronchus can be traced in a cranial direction and overlaps the right cranial lung lobe bronchus, prior to crossing into a dorsal position relative to the right cranial lobe bronchus. The caudal subsegment of the left cranial bronchus extends ventrally over the middle of the cardiac silhouette and can be visualized on the right lateral projection. Occasionally, the right middle bronchus might be

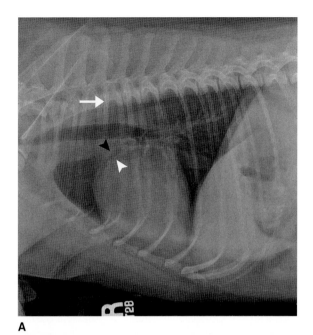

A

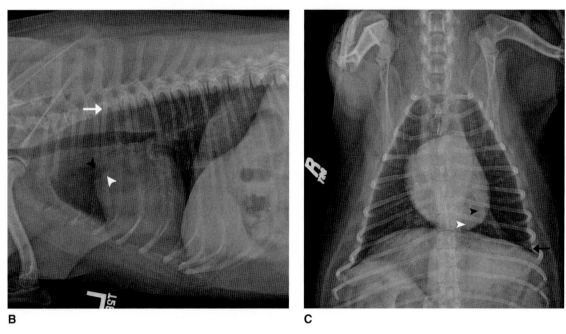

B                                      C

**FIGURE 13.16**    Right lateral (**A**), left lateral (**B**), and ventrodorsal (**C**) thoracic radiographs of a dog. The pulmonary artery (black arrowhead) and pulmonary vein (white arrowhead) are normal and symmetric. The pulmonary arteries and veins do not measure greater than the width of the fourth rib (white arrow) on the lateral radiographs and do not measure greater than the length of the ninth rib (black arrow) on the ventrodorsal radiograph.

visualized along the caudal border of the cardiac silhouette on the right lateral image but is more commonly seen on the left lateral image.

When the dog or cat is in right lateral recumbency, a lesion in the left lung will be better visualized due to better aeration of the nondependent lung lobes. In addition, there will be atelectasis of the right lung lobe and thereby border effacement with soft tissue opaque lesions (Figure 13.19) [11]. However, radiolucent lesions in the right lung lobe might be better visualized on the right lateral for the same reasoning. Lesion conspicuity

in the right cranial lung lobe where it wraps around the cranial aspect of the cardiac silhouette (just caudal to the cranioventral mediastinal reflection) and the right accessory lung lobes caudal to the cardiac silhouette are less influenced by recumbency due to the central position of these lobes.

**Left Lateral Radiograph**    In the left lateral image, the left diaphragmatic crus is displaced cranial to the right crus due to the fact that the dog's abdominal contents are

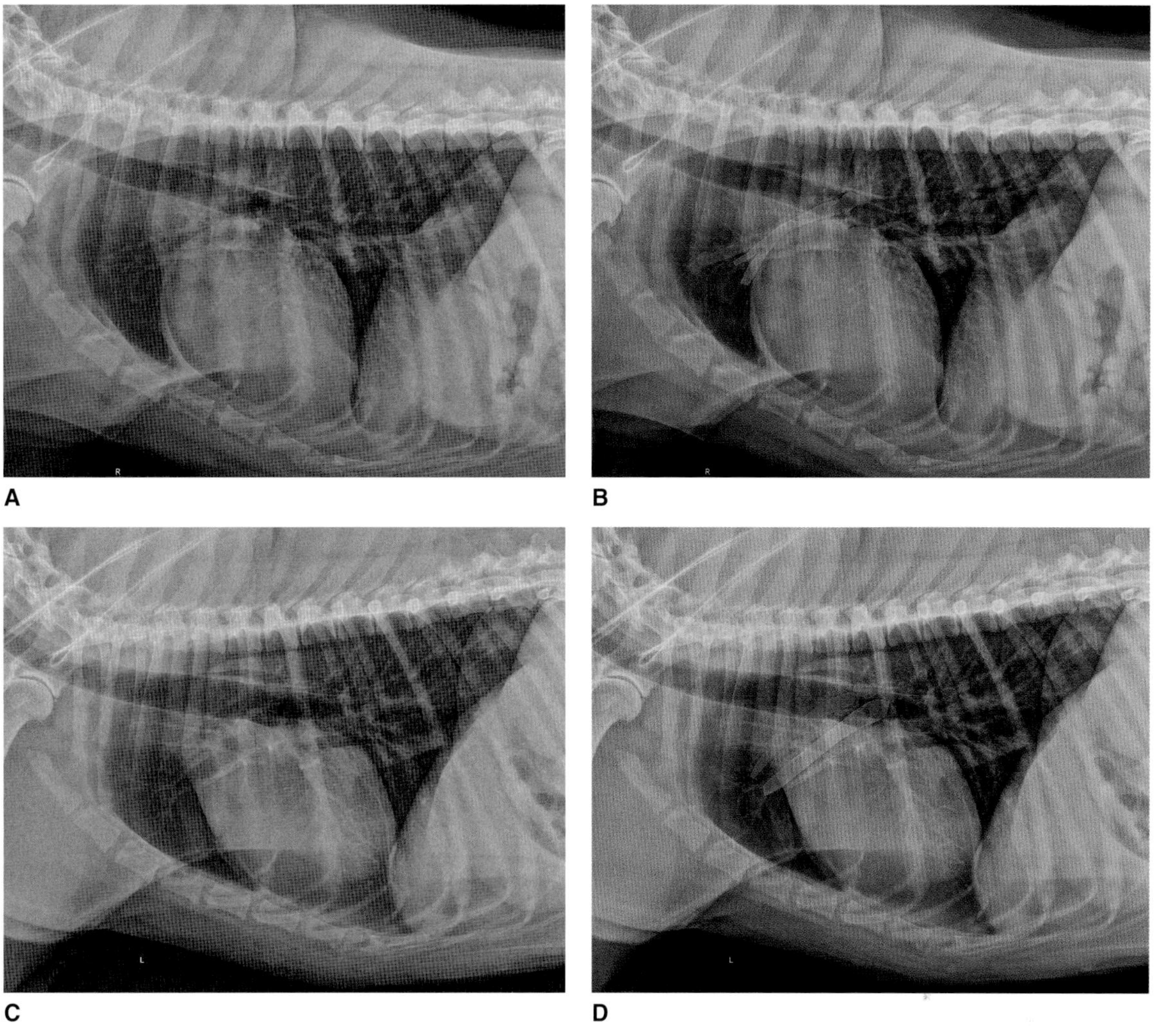

**A**

**B**

**C**

**D**

**FIGURE 13.17**  Right and left lateral thoracic radiographs from a 7-year-old golden retriever. (**A**) Right lateral radiograph. (**B**) Right lateral radiograph with the right cranial bronchus highlighted in yellow and the left cranial bronchus highlighted in green. The two airways cross each other at the cranial aspect of the heart base. (**C**) Left lateral radiograph. (**D**) Left lateral radiograph with the right cranial bronchus highlighted in yellow and the left cranial bronchus highlighted in green. The two airways parallel each other over the region of the heart base.

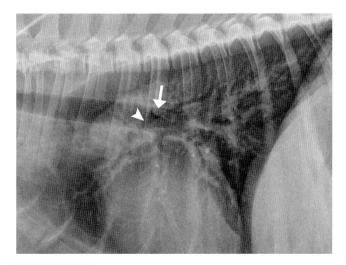

**FIGURE 13.18**  Collimated right lateral thoracic radiograph of a dog. At the opening of the right cranial lobe bronchus (white arrow), a radiolucent gap will intersect the line so that there is a bronchus (white arrowhead) exiting the carina in a ventral direction.

cranially displaced along the dependent left side (down side of the patient) secondary to gravity and atelectasis of the left lung lobes. Any gas within the fundus or body of the stomach will be seen caudal to the left crus. From the level of the diaphragmatic cupula, the right crus and left crus diverge away from each other dorsally (Figure 13.20). The cardiac silhouette elevates away from the sternum secondary to aeration of the right middle lung lobe and should not be mistaken for a pneumothorax. The silhouette will also have more of a rounded or circular shape. The caudal vena cava is seen superimposed over the caudal aspect of the cardiac silhouette and extends caudally over the left crus, becoming confluent with the right crus at the caval foramen. The left and right cranial lung lobe bronchi will parallel each other, with the left cranial lobe bronchus (cranial subsegment) being in a dorsal and cranial position relative to the right cranial lung lobe bronchus (that appears larger due to magnification). The right middle lung lobe bronchus is seen over the mid to caudal aspect of the cardiac silhouette.

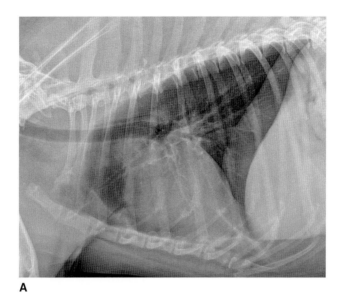

**A**

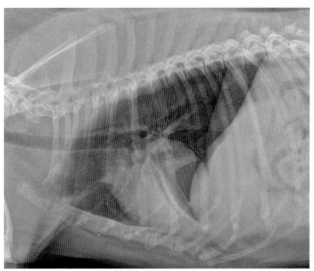

**B**

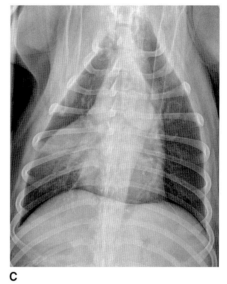

**C**

**FIGURE 13.19** Right lateral (**A**), left lateral (**B**), and ventrodorsal (**C**) thoracic radiographs of a dog with a right middle lung lobe aspiration pneumonia. This is best visualized on the left lateral image with a lobar sign and a central air bronchogram. This lesion is not seen on the right lateral, but is clearly visualized on the ventrodorsal image with border effacement of the right side of the cardiac silhouette.

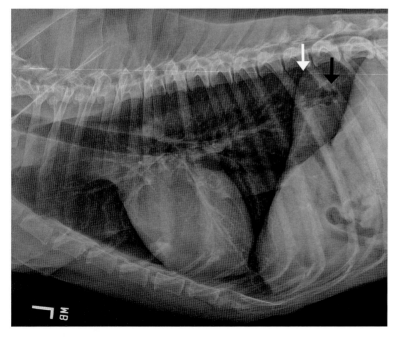

**FIGURE 13.20** Left lateral thoracic radiograph of a dog. The left diaphragmatic crus (white arrow) is located cranial to the right diaphragmatic crus. The mild accumulation of gas in the gastric fundus (black arrow) is seen superimposed over the left diaphragmatic crus.

Because the animal is in left lateral recumbency, a lesion in the right lung will be better visualized due to atelectasis of the left lung lobe and thereby border effacement with soft tissue opaque lesions. However, radiolucent lesions in the left lung lobe might be better visualized on the left lateral for the same reasoning.

There are several variants and "fake-outs" (normal radiographic changes seen that are not equated with pathology) that can be seen on left lateral radiographs when compared with the right lateral image. On the left lateral radiograph, it is common to see a focal area of pleural thickening between the right middle and right caudal lung lobes superimposed over the caudal aspect of the cardiac silhouette (Figure 13.21). Although the incidence of this finding has not been reported, in

the authors' experience this is routinely seen in approximately 40% of normal thoracic radiographic studies, particularly in older dogs, and should not be mistaken for a pleural effusion. This finding is not commonly seen in cats. In addition, gas can be seen in the thoracic esophagus at the level of the heart base or fluid seen in the caudal thoracic esophagus just cranial to the esophageal hiatus on the left lateral image (Figure 13.22).

**Ventrodorsal Radiograph** Differences between the dorsoventral (DV) and ventrodorsal (VD) images primarily involve the positioning and shape of the diaphragm, visualization of the caudal lung lobes, cardiac shape, and superimposition of the scapula over the cranial thorax.

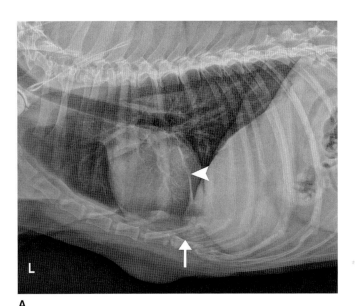

A

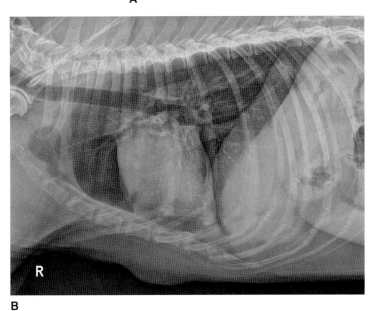

B

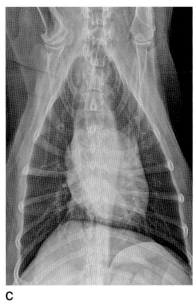

C

**FIGURE 13.21** Left lateral (**A**), right lateral (**B**), and ventrodorsal (**C**) thoracic radiographs of a dog. On the left lateral radiograph, there is pleural thickening (white arrowhead) between the right middle and right caudal lung lobes and increased conspicuity of the pericardial and/or middle mediastinal fat (white arrow), which are commonly mistaken for pleural effusion. On the right lateral and ventrodorsal radiographs, there is no evidence of pleural fissures.

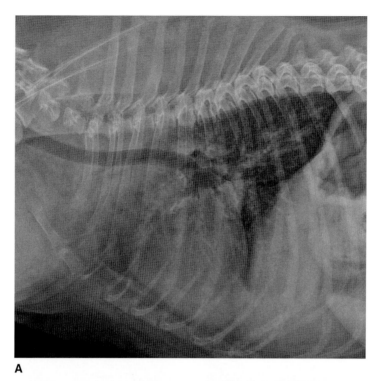

A

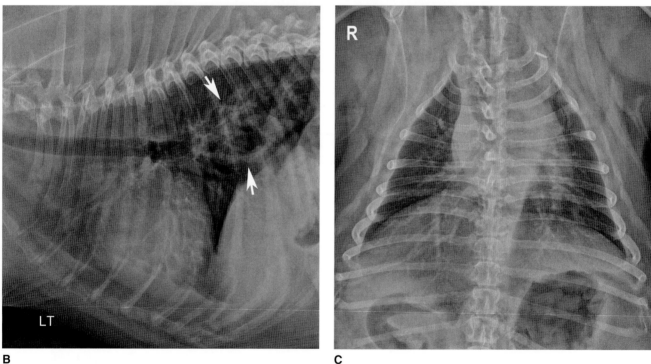

B

C

**FIGURE 13.22** Right lateral (**A**), left lateral (**B**), and ventrodorsal (**C**) thoracic radiographs of a brachycephalic dog. There is focal gas and soft tissue opacity in the region of the caudal thoracic esophagus consistent with a sliding hiatal hernia as seen on the left lateral radiograph (white arrows). This is not seen on the right lateral or ventrodorsal radiographs.

In the VD image, there are three surfaces seen on the thoracic side of the diaphragm forming three convex borders. The cupula (dome) of the diaphragm is central and cranial. Each diaphragmatic crus forms a convex surface on its respective side of the thoracic diaphragm. These are located cranial to the respective right or left side and caudal to the cupula (Figure 13.23). In some dogs and cats, there will be better separation between the cardiac silhouette and the cupula of the diaphragm as the accessory lung lobe is more elongated and apparent. This results in better visualization of the caudal

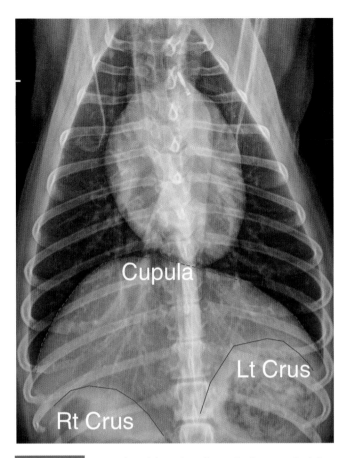

**FIGURE 13.23**   Ventrodorsal thoracic radiograph of a normal adult dog. There are three convex surfaces noted along the diaphragm that include the right and left diaphragmatic crura (labeled and red lines) and the cupula of the diaphragm (red dashed line and labeled; central and cranial).

vena cava. Changes in the descending thoracic aorta and great vessels may be more apparent on the DV image compared with the VD image (Figure 13.24).

In the VD image, the airways should be traced from their origin in the carina and caudal trachea (superimposed over or to the right of the spinous processes of the thoracic spine; Figure 13.25). The trachea terminates at the carina, with the bifurcation into the right and left principal bronchi. The right cranial lung lobe bronchus is the first branch from the right principal bronchus and extends in a cranioventral direction. The right middle bronchus originates from the ventrolateral aspect of the continuation of the right caudal lobar bronchus. Next, the accessory lung lobe bronchus originates in a ventromedial position along the right caudal lung lobe bronchus. The right caudal lobe bronchus then continues into the right caudal lung lobe in a caudodorsal direction (Figure 13.26).

The left cranial lung lobe bronchus branches from the left principal bronchus in a ventrolateral direction and then, within several millimeters, bifurcates into the cranial and caudal subsegments of the left cranial lung lobe. The left caudal lung lobe bronchus then continues caudal and dorsal into the left caudal lung lobe (Figure 13.27).

With respect to the cranial and caudal bronchi, the pulmonary arteries are lateral, and the pulmonary veins are medial or "central" along the midline (Figure 13.28), as "veins are located ventral and central to the bronchus." Remember pulmonary "*veins are ventral* (lateral radiograph) *and central* (VD/DV radiograph)." The caudal lobar pulmonary arteries and veins should be equal in size and taper peripherally as well as the airways. The normal pulmonary artery and vein should

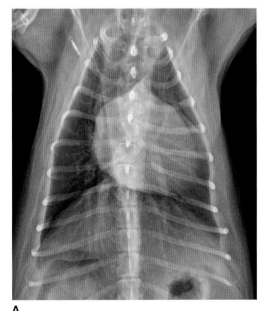

A

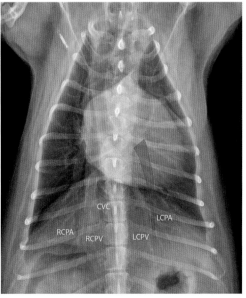

B

**FIGURE 13.24**   Dorsoventral radiograph without labels (**A**) and with labels (**B**) from a normal dog. The caudal lung lobe vasculature is labeled: RCPA – right caudal pulmonary artery; RCPV – right caudal pulmonary vein; LCPA – left caudal pulmonary artery; LCPV – left caudal pulmonary vein; and CVC – caudal vena cava. There is fat noted between the cranial and caudal subsegmental fissure of the left cranial lung lobe at the left fourth intercostal space.

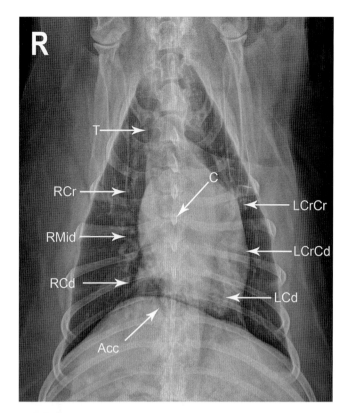

**FIGURE 13.25** Ventrodorsal thoracic radiograph of a normal dog. Note the right accessory lung lobe bronchus branches from the craniomedial aspect of the right caudal lung lobe bronchus. T, trachea; RCr, right cranial lung lobe bronchus; RMid, right middle lung lobe bronchus; RCd, right caudal lung lobe bronchus; Acc, accessory lung lobe bronchus; C, carina; LCrCr, cranial subsegment of the left cranial lung lobe bronchus; LCrCd, caudal subsegment of the left cranial lung lobe bronchus; LCd, left caudal lung lobe bronchus.

form a square as their margins are summated with the right and left ninth ribs (Figure 13.29).

**Dorsoventral Radiograph**  In the DV image, the cardiac shape is foreshortened due to the geometry of a more upright cardiac silhouette (Figure 13.30). In some deep-chested dogs, such as the Doberman pinscher, the cardiac silhouette can appear circular as one is looking dorsoventrally at the upright heart (Figure 13.31). There is decreased space between the cardiac silhouette and the cranial border of the cupula of the diaphragm. Additionally, the caudal lung lobe pulmonary vasculature can be better visualized due to being better aerated or inflated when compared to a VD image. Lesion conspicuity in the caudal lung lobes will be better on the DV radiograph due to lack of atelectasis of the caudal lung lobes as would be seen in a dog or cat in dorsal recumbency (Figure 13.32).

In a correctly positioned VD or DV image, the thoracic vertebrae and sternum should be superimposed and the right and left thoracic walls should be spaced evenly from the thoracic vertebrae at the same level (cranial, middle, or caudal thorax).

Collimation of the VD and DV images includes the thoracic inlet cranially, the cranial abdomen caudally (entire lung field and diaphragm should be included on the image), and the thoracic walls laterally. For the VD radiograph, when the animal is placed in dorsal recumbency a positioning trough is typically used (Figure 13.33).

## Feline Thorax

The feline thorax is more triangular and elongated in shape compared to the canine thorax (Figure 13.34). The lung lobe anatomy is the same as the canine, with six total lung lobes. The bronchial anatomy can be more difficult to identify, as the bronchial markings in a cat are less prominent than in a dog. The cardiac silhouette is an elongated ellipse on lateral radiographs, and one does not see the anatomic variations between right and left lateral images as one does in the dog. On both right and left lateral radiographs, the diaphragmatic crura are usually superimposed over each other and the cupula and crura move caudal on inspiration with separation of the cardiac silhouette from the cupula. Thoracic radiographs are typically taken on peak inspiration without the expiratory issues that can be seen in small-breed dogs.

Radiographic variations seen in the cat thorax include fat deposition ventral to the cardiac silhouette, cranial angulation of the cardiac silhouette, more prominence to the airways (presumed to be secondary to fibrosis), and a redundant aorta or aortic "knob" (Figure 13.35) [12].

# Variations of Thoracic Anatomy

Normal variations of thoracic structures present the potential for misdiagnosis (false positive). There is large variation in the size and shape of the thorax based on the different dog breeds (Figure 13.36). In addition, there are a potential number of variations that can occur within each breed. These variations are typically normal anatomy, but they can represent age-related changes or incidental findings that are not pathologic or related to the current clinical presentation of the animal.

The variants will be divided into the four compartments that form the basis for the interpretation paradigm of the thorax: extrathoracic structures, pleural space, pulmonary parenchyma, and the mediastinum (cranial, middle, and caudal).

## Extrathoracic Structures

The most common extrathoracic variants include musculoskeletal changes that are specific to the age of the patient. Young animals will have open physes (radiolucent lines) of the long bones and the endplates of vertebral bodies that should not be

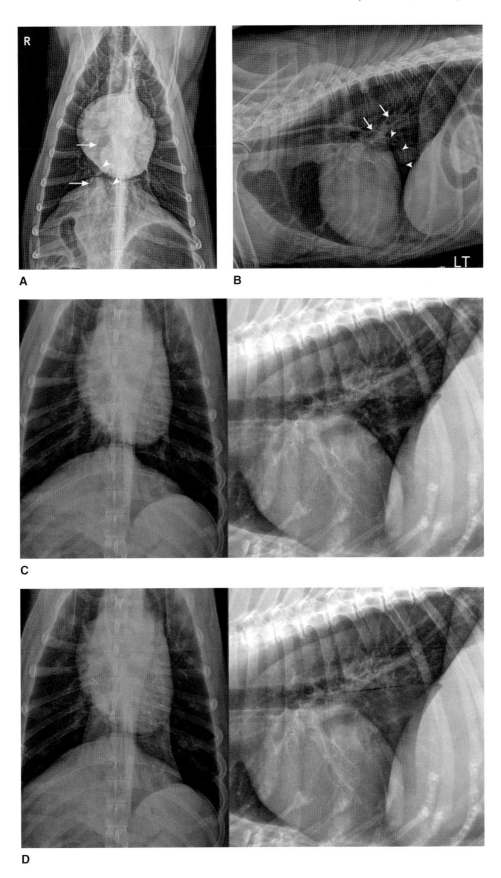

**FIGURE 13.26** Ventrodorsal (**A**) and left lateral (**B**) thoracic radiographs from a dog. The right accessory lung lobe bronchus (white arrowheads) originates in a ventromedial position along the right caudal lung lobe bronchus (white arrows). The right caudal lobe bronchus then continues into the right caudal lung lobe in a caudodorsal direction. There is ventral spondylosis deformans noted at T6–7. Gas-distended stomach and small intestinal segments are noted. Ventrodorsal and left lateral radiographs from a dog (different from **A** and **B**) where the accessory lung lobe is clearly visualized (**C** – no drawings; **D** – schematic with accessory lobe shown).

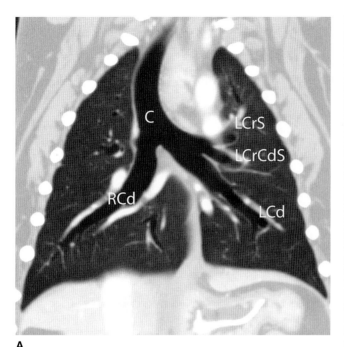

**A**

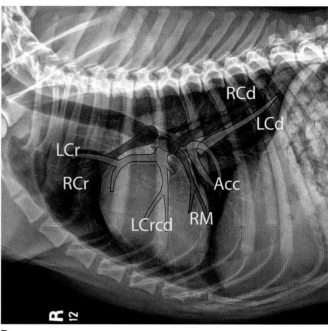

**B**

**FIGURE 13.27** (**A**) Dorsal plane reconstructed CT of the thorax from a dog. C, carina; LCrS, left cranial subsegment of the left cranial bronchus; RCd, right caudal; LCrCdS, left caudal subsegment of the left cranial lung lobe; LCd, left caudal bronchus. (**B**) Right lateral radiograph from a normal dog with the outline of the airways from the trachea. RCr, right cranial; LCr, left cranial subsegment of the left cranial lung lobe; LCrcd, left caudal subsegment of the left cranial lung lobe; RM, right middle; RCd, right caudal; Acc, accessory lung lobe; LCd, left caudal.

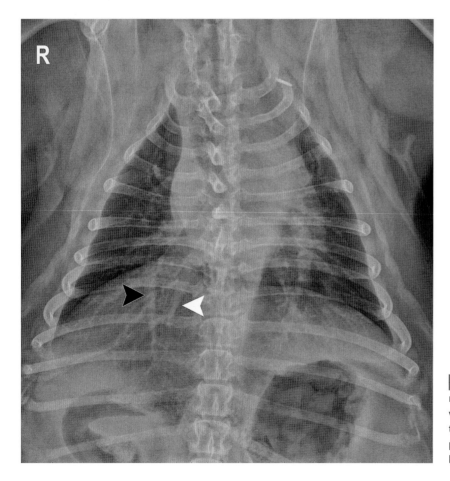

**FIGURE 13.28** Ventrodorsal thoracic radiograph of a dog. The right caudal pulmonary vein (white arrowhead) is located medial or central to the air-filled bronchus and the right caudal pulmonary artery (black arrowhead) is located lateral to the air-filled bronchus.

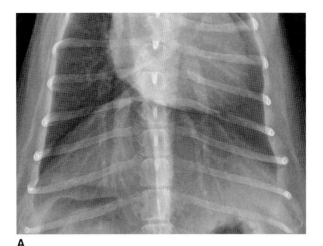

**A**

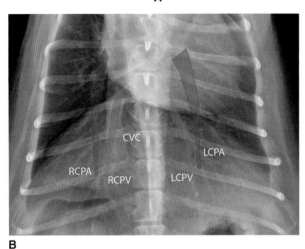

**B**

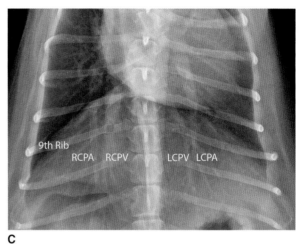

**C**

**FIGURE 13.29** Close-up dorsoventral thoracic radiographic images from a normal dog. (**A**) No labels. (**B**) With labels for the following vessels: RCPA, right caudal pulmonary artery; RCPV, right caudal pulmonary vein; LCPA, left caudal pulmonary artery; LCPV, left caudal pulmonary vein; CVC, caudal vena cava. (**C**) The summation squares (red and blue) are shown between the vessel and the ninth rib. This is considered normal.

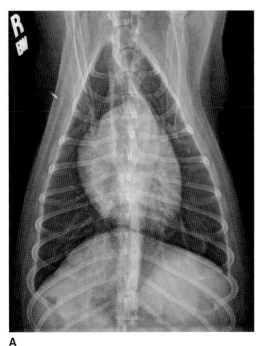

**A**

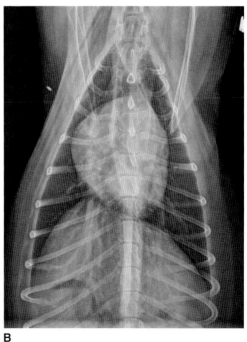

**B**

**FIGURE 13.30** Ventrodorsal (**A**) and dorsoventral (**B**) radiographs of a dog. On the dorsoventral radiograph, the cardiac silhouette is foreshortened compared to the cardiac silhouette on the ventrodorsal radiograph. On the dorsoventral image, the caudal lobar pulmonary vessels can be traced further into the peripheral aspect of the caudal lung lobes.

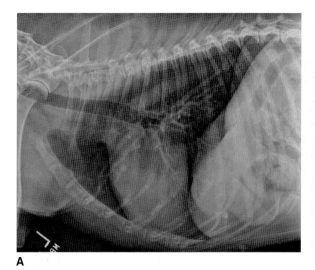
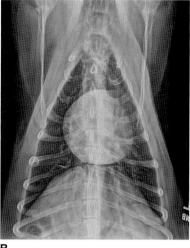

**A**

**B**

**FIGURE 13.31** Left lateral (**A**) and dorsoventral (**B**) thoracic radiographs of a Doberman pinscher. Note the upright appearance of the cardiac silhouette on the left lateral radiograph and the rounded appearance of the cardiac silhouette on the dorsoventral radiograph. There is a healed rib fracture noted at the peripheral aspect of the right sixth rib on the dorsoventral view.

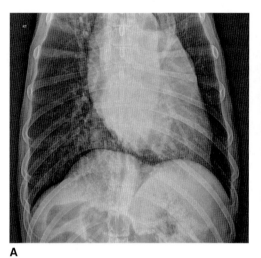
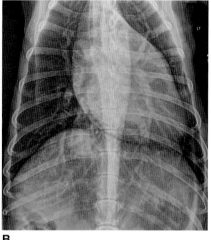

**A**

**B**

**FIGURE 13.32** Caudally collimated dorsoventral (**A**) and ventrodorsal (**B**) thoracic radiographs of a dog. The round, soft tissue opaque pulmonary nodule is best seen on the dorsoventral projection when compared to the ventrodorsal projection. This is because of better aeration of the caudal lobes on the dorsoventral view and magnification of the soft tissue nodule.

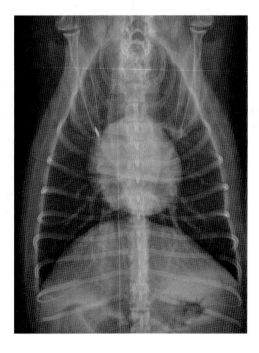

**FIGURE 13.33** Ventrodorsal thoracic radiograph of a dog in a trough. Note the well-defined, linear, mineral opaque trough artifact over the right parasagittal thorax and through the cranial abdomen.

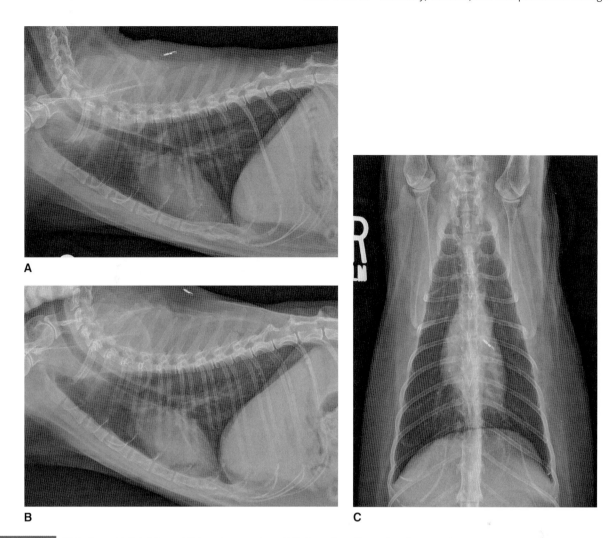

**FIGURE 13.34**   Right lateral (**A**), left lateral (**B**), and ventrodorsal (**C**) thoracic radiographs of a normal cat.

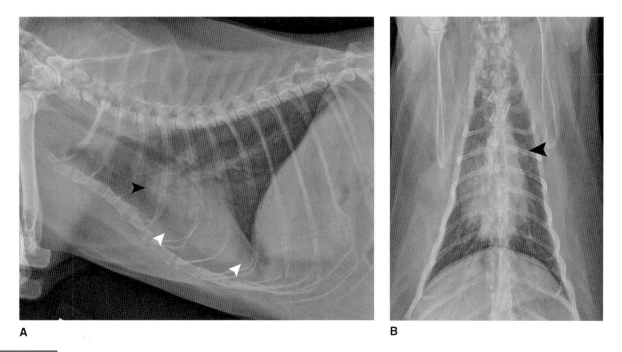

**FIGURE 13.35**   Right lateral (**A**) and ventrodorsal (**B**) thoracic radiographs of a geriatric cat with a prominent aortic arch (black arrowhead) and middle mediastinal fat deposition (white arrowheads).

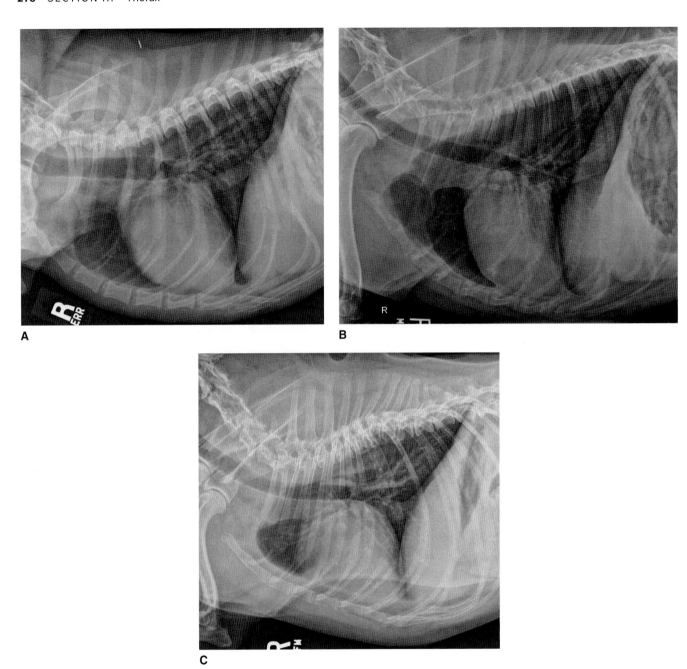

**FIGURE 13.36** Right lateral thoracic radiographs of a dachshund (**A**), Doberman pinscher (**B**), and bulldog (**C**).

mistaken for fracture lines (Figure 13.37). One common mistake occurs at the apophysis of the supraglenoid tubercle in dogs by misinterpreting that area of incomplete ossification for an avulsion fracture fragment (Figure 13.38).

There can be vertebral anomalies associated with the brachiocephalic breeds (Figure 13.39). These include several potential anomalies associated with the normal development of the vertebral bodies: block vertebrae, butterfly vertebrae (ventral and median aplasia), dorsal hemivertebrae (ventral aplasia), ventral wedge-shaped (ventral hypoplasia), lateral hemivertebrae (lateral aplasia), lateral wedge-shaped (lateral hypoplasia), dorsolateral hemivertebrae (ventrolateral aplasia) (Figure 13.40) [13], and spina bifida occulta lesions of the spinous processes and dorsal lamina (Figure 13.41) [14]. Anomalous developments seen

in any dog or cat breed also include transitional vertebral segments at the cervicothoracic or thoracolumbar junctions [15]. The vertebral segment at the junction will contain components of the cranial and caudal vertebral segments.

The sternum is also subject to developmental anomalies. Most commonly, there is a decrease in the overall sternebral number from the normal of eight (manubrium, six sternebrae, and xiphoid process; Figure 13.42). A *pectus excavatum* anomaly is dorsal deviation of the caudal sternum into the thorax. A *pectus carinatum* anomaly is ventral deviation of the caudal sternum away from the thorax (Figure 13.43).

In older dogs, degenerative changes associated with the musculoskeletal structures are common. These include osteoarthrosis of the costochondral cartilages, sternum, cubital

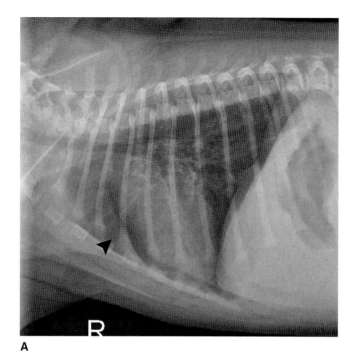

A

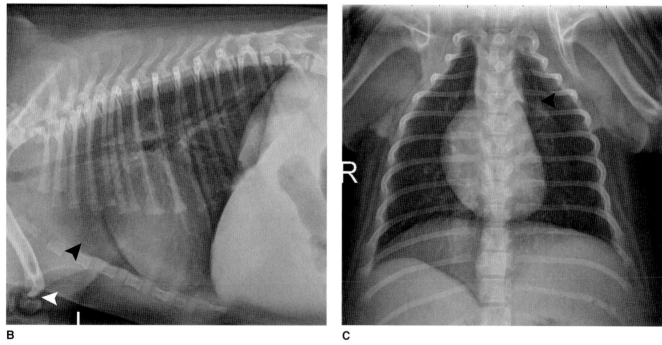

B

C

**FIGURE 13.37**   Right lateral (**A**), left lateral (**B**), and ventrodorsal (**C**) thoracic radiographs of a young dog. There is a persistent thymus (black arrowhead), causing increased cranial mediastinal soft tissue opacity on the lateral projections and a triangular-shaped, soft tissue opaque "sail sign" on the ventrodorsal projection. Multiple open physes (white arrowhead) are present.

joints, and humeral joints as evidenced by periarticular osteophyte formation, enthesophytes, and subchondral sclerosis (Figure 13.44). Degenerative changes of the costochondral junctions (CCJs) include expansile enlargement of the CCJs with irregular degrees of mineralization (Figure 13.45). The costal cartilages will normally mineralize early in the patient's life. The intersternebral and intervertebral disc spaces are made up of the same fibrocartilaginous material (inner nucleus pulposus and outer annulus fibrosis). Sternebral degenerative

changes will look similar with disc space narrowing, endplate sclerosis, and spondylosis deformans (Figure 13.46).

Chondrodystrophic breeds (dachshund and bassett hound) can have an extrapleural sign at the level of the parietal–visceral pleural interface due to the CCJs. These are most evident on ventrodorsal radiographs (Figure 13.47), but can also be seen on lateral projections. Dogs with excessive degenerative changes of the CCJ can also have similar findings on a ventrodorsal image.

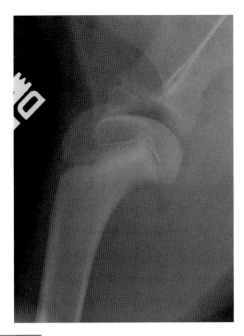

**FIGURE 13.38** Lateral shoulder radiograph of a normal 5-month-old mixed-breed dog. Note the incomplete ossification of the supraglenoid tubercle of the craniodistal scapula.

The cranial abdomen can have several "fake-outs." First, since we are taking thoracic radiographs on peak inspiration (in theory), we can expect the caudoventral margin of the liver to extend beyond the costal arch. This is described as a Roentgen sign of hepatomegaly in many textbooks. However, particularly in small-breed dogs, this can be seen routinely and should not be interpreted in isolation as hepatic enlargement. In addition, in deep-chested dogs such as the Doberman, the liver volume appears small and should not be misinterpreted as microhepatia. When evaluating the cranial abdomen, specifically the stomach, remember that on a right lateral radiograph, fluid will be in the pylorus and it will appear as a round structure along the ventral margin of the gastric silhouette (Figure 13.48). This should not be mistaken for a foreign body (ball) in the stomach.

## Pleural Space

The most common variants include the presence of thin pleural fissure lines, particularly noted over the cardiac silhouette between the right middle and caudal lung lobes on the left

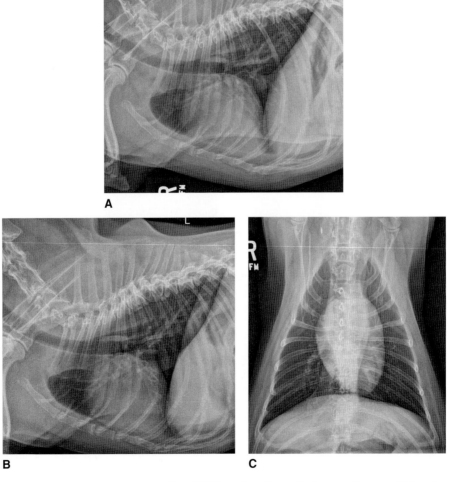

A

B

C

**FIGURE 13.39** Right lateral (**A**), left lateral (**B**), and ventrodorsal (**C**) thoracic radiograph of a normal 9-year-old female spayed bulldog. Note the breed-related congenital thoracic vertebral anomalies, further characterized by butterfly vertebrae and ventral wedge-shaped defects.

| **NORMAL VERTEBRA** | **SEGMENTATION DEFECTS** |
|---|---|
| 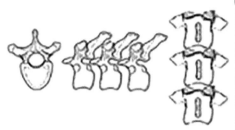 | 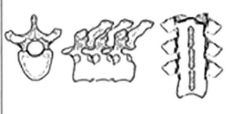 |
| | BLOCK VERTEBRA |

## VERTEBRAL BODY FORMATION DEFECTS

| Ventral aplasia | Ventral hypoplasia |
|---|---|
| 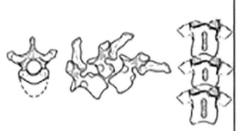 | 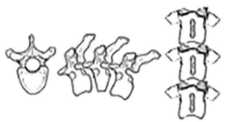 |
| DORSAL HEMIVERTEBRA | VENTRAL WEDGE-SHAPE |
| Lateral aplasia | Lateral hypoplasia |
| 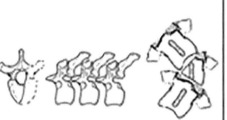 | 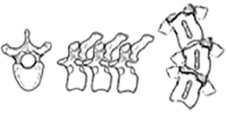 |
| LATERAL HEMIVERTEBRA | LATERAL WEDGE-SHAPE |
| Ventro-lateral aplasia | Ventral and median aplasia |
| 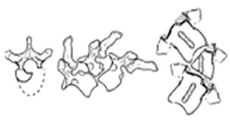 | 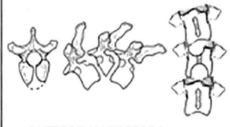 |
| DORSO-LATERAL HEMIVERTEBRA | BUTTERFLY VERTEBRA |

**FIGURE 13.40**   Schematic drawing of the radiographic appearance of the different vertebral malformations seen in brachycephalic dogs [13].

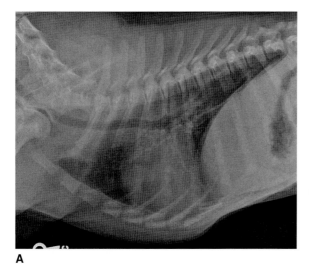
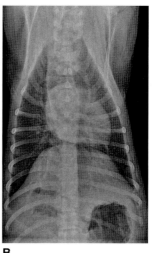

**A**                                                                      **B**

**FIGURE 13.41** Right lateral (**A**) and ventrodorsal (**B**) thoracic radiograph of a young dog. There is spina bifida occulta of the spinous process of T1, only seen on the ventrodorsal radiograph.

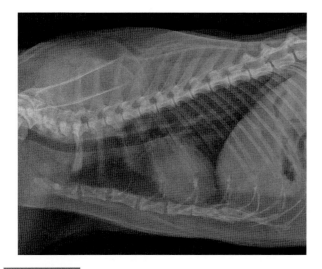

**FIGURE 13.42** Left lateral thoracic radiograph of a geriatric cat with incidentally seven sternebral segments.

lateral projection (Figure 13.49). Additionally, some dogs will have normal pleural fissure lines on the ventrodorsal view (Figure 13.50). These should not be mistaken for focal pleural effusion as there is no widening of the fissure or retraction of the lung lobe away from the thoracic wall. An extrapleural sign is a focal area of increased opacity along the peripheral aspect of the lung lobe that can be a normal variant or a potential indicator of disease. Cats will deposit fat in the pleural space and mediastinum ventral to the cardiac silhouette (Figure 13.51). This should not be mistaken as generalized cardiomegaly on a VD radiograph. Occasionally a dog will deposit fat between the right cranial and right middle lung lobe that appears as a curvilinear structure on a VD image (Figure 13.52). Rarely, a cholesterol inclusion cyst can be seen on thoracic radiographs with the mineralized structure being inside the pleural cavity (Figure 13.53).

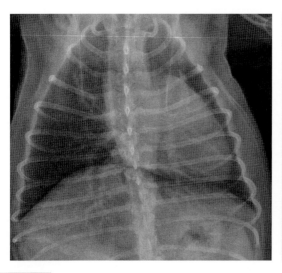
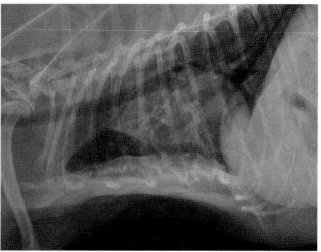

**FIGURE 13.43** Ventrodorsal and right lateral thoracic radiographs of a dog with pectus excavatum.

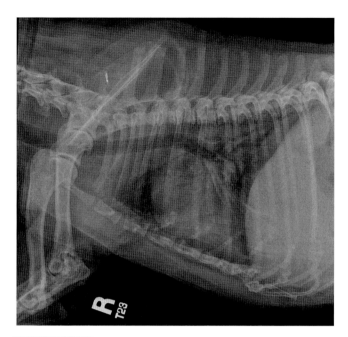

**FIGURE 13.44**   Right lateral thoracic radiograph of a dog with humeral and elbow osteoarthrosis as well as degenerative changes of the sternum and costochondral junction.

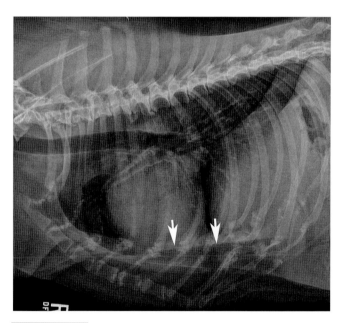

**FIGURE 13.45**   Right lateral thoracic radiograph of a dog with smoothly marginated osteoproliferation of the costochondral junction, consistent with degenerative changes. This curvature creates an extrapleural sign at the level of the costochondral junction (white arrows).

## Pulmonary Parenchyma

An expiratory radiograph will negatively impact your interpretation skills in two ways. First, the cardiac silhouette will look big relative to the overall thoracic volume and second, the lungs will appear "whiter" or more opaque than normal. If you only take right lateral radiographs of small dogs (for instance, with a clinical presentation of a cough) and the radiograph

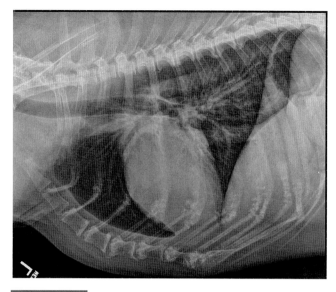

**FIGURE 13.46**   Right lateral thoracic radiograph of a dog with degenerative changes of the sternum similar in appearance to degenerative disc changes such as disc space narrowing, endplate sclerosis, and spondylosis deformans.

is made on expiration, the dog will have an enlarged cardiac silhouette and pulmonary edema every time (both are "fake-outs"!). If you were to take the DV or VD, you would see that the thorax is really normal. Peak inspiratory radiographs and a three-view thorax will alleviate these potential problems (Figure 13.54) [16].

Atelectasis is the loss of lung volume within a lung lobe beyond the tidal volume end-expiration. It does not imply an etiology. A variety of pulmonary and pleural diseases can cause atelectasis of affected lung lobes. Plate-like atelectasis is a curvilinear to linear soft tissue opacity that is seen superimposed over the trachea on either a right or left lateral image and can be seen in the dog and cat (Figure 13.55) [17]. These areas represent atelectasis of anatomic sublobar fissures [18].

If the dog or cat is in lateral recumbency for an extended period of time (greater than several minutes), an ipsilateral mediastinal shift of the cardiac silhouette toward that side can be seen on the ventrodorsal image. Again, this is not secondary to specific lung pathology but secondary to recumbent atelectasis (Figure 13.56). If one waits 5–10 minutes with the dog in sternal recumbency and then flips back into dorsal recumbency for reevaluation of the thoracic radiograph, the mediastinal shift should have resolved. Any time there is atelectasis, you will see everything from a mild unstructured interstitial pulmonary pattern to an alveolar pulmonary pattern (particularly involving general anesthesia with 100% $O_2$). These pulmonary changes can, in fact, border efface with Roentgen abnormalities associated with the lung lobes in question, resulting in a false negative [11].

When the patient is under general anesthesia, the two most common radiographic changes seen include pulmonary atelectasis (typically ipsilateral) and a gas-filled esophagus (Figure 13.57).

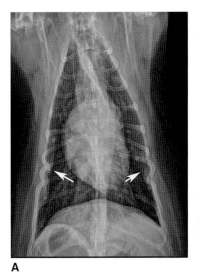 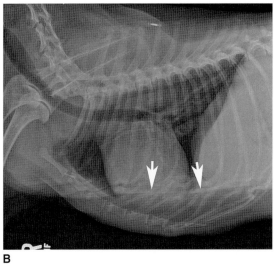

A                                                    B

**FIGURE 13.47** Ventrodorsal radiograph (**A**) of a basset hound with an incidental extrapleural sign and a right lateral radiograph (**B**) of a Shetland sheepdog with an incidental extrapleural sign secondary to degenerative changes of the costochondral junction (white arrows).

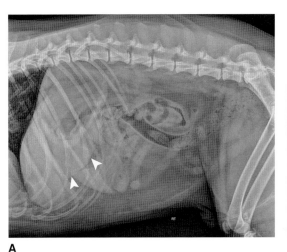 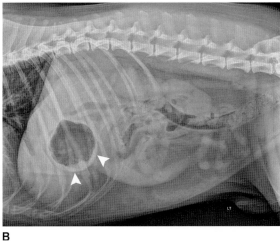

A                                                    B

**FIGURE 13.48** Right lateral (**A**) and left lateral (**B**) abdominal radiographs of a 5-year-old mixed-breed dog. On the right lateral radiograph, the pylorus (white arrowheads) is fluid filled. On the left lateral radiograph, the pylorus is gas filled. There are irregularly marginated vascular structures noted along the ventral abdominal wall that represent extrahepatic varices and acquired portosystemic shunts. The liver is small.

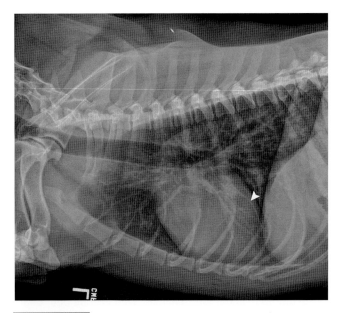 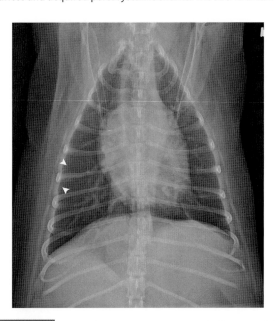

**FIGURE 13.49** Left lateral thoracic radiograph of a normal dog with a thin pleural fissure line (white arrowhead) between the right middle and caudal lung lobes.

**FIGURE 13.50** Ventrodorsal thoracic radiograph of a normal dog with thin pleural fissures between the right cranial and middle lung lobes and right middle and caudal lung lobes (white arrowheads).

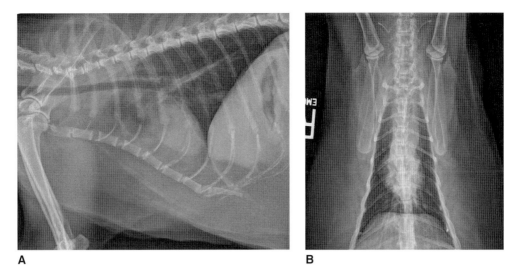

**FIGURE 13.51** Right lateral (**A**) and ventrodorsal (**B**) thoracic radiographs of an obese cat with increased mediastinal and pleural fat deposition.

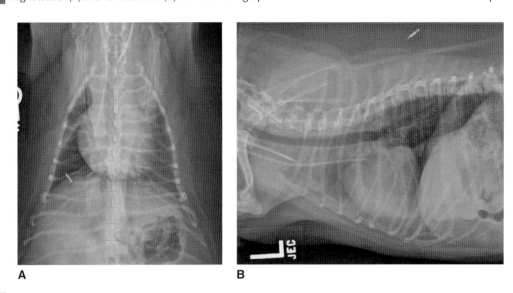

**FIGURE 13.52** Ventrodorsal (**A**) and left lateral (**B**) thoracic radiographs of an obese dog with fat deposition between the right cranial and right middle lung lobe that appears as a curvilinear structure on the ventrodorsal radiograph. This is not clearly delineated on the left lateral radiograph.

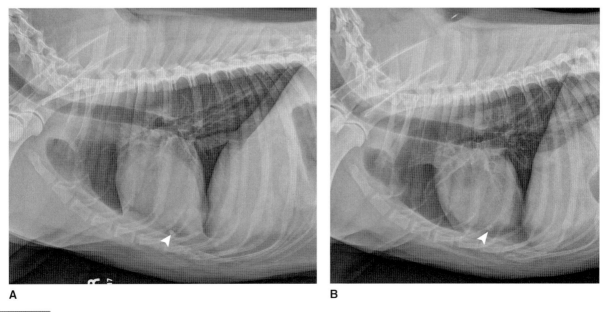

**FIGURE 13.53** Right lateral (**A**) and left lateral (**B**) thoracic radiographs of a dog with a left-sided pleural cholesterol inclusion cyst (white arrowhead), further characterized as a well-defined oval mineral opaque structure.

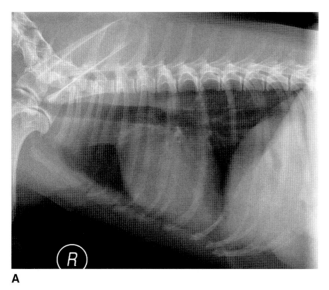
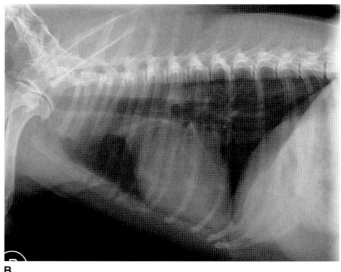

**FIGURE 13.54**    Right lateral expiratory (**A**) and inspiratory (**B**) thoracic radiographs of a normal adult Maltese dog. Note the difference in the opacity of the caudodorsal lungs on the expiratory and inspiratory radiographs.

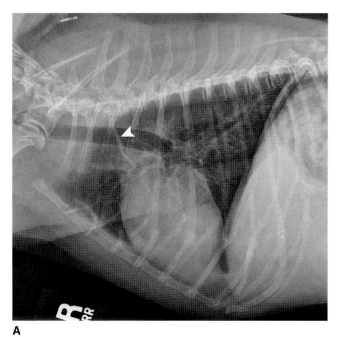
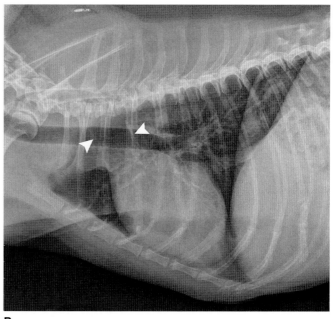

**FIGURE 13.55**    Right lateral (**A**) and left lateral (**B**) thoracic radiographs of a normal dog with plate-like atelectasis (white arrowheads).

As dogs age, there is a progression in the degree of unstructured interstitial pulmonary changes. These changes are presumed to be fibrosis and an age-related change. They would result in an overall increase in pulmonary opacity, more so than seen in the younger dog (Figure 13.58).

Cats will also experience collapse of the right middle lung lobe. This typically is associated with feline asthma and mucous plugging (Figure 13.59), but does not have to be [19]. In fact, you can have a normal thorax and still have right middle lung lobe collapse (Figure 13.60). The caudal subsegment of the left cranial lung lobe can also undergo atelectasis and collapse in cats with feline asthma. In the case of the right

middle lung lobe, a triangular soft tissue opacity will be noted that border effaces with the cardiac silhouette at 9 o'clock on the VD projection. There are primary pulmonary tumors that originate near the pulmonary hilum in cats and result in atelectasis of the lung lobe due to bronchial compression and resorption of the air within the affected lobe [20]. This is particularly true of bronchogenic carcinoma involving the right or left cranial lung lobes.

Pulmonary osteomas (i.e., osseous metaplasia, microlithiasis, pneumoliths, or heterotopic bone) are a "fake-out" for pulmonary nodules. Pulmonary osteomas are formed when type I pneumocytes produce osteoid, which accumulates and

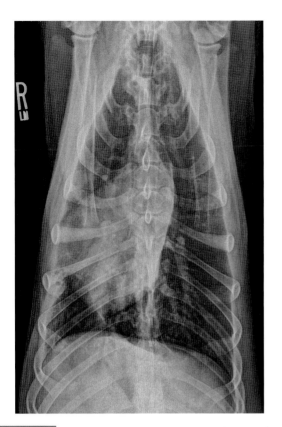

**FIGURE 13.56**   Ventrodorsal thoracic radiograph of a normal dog under general anesthesia with prolonged right lateral recumbency and ipsilateral shift of the middle mediastinum/cardiac silhouette.

calcifies with age (Figure 13.61). They are found ventrally in the thorax, are mineralized, and typically measure between 1 and 3 mm in diameter. They are also found more frequently in collies, boxers, and Shetland sheepdogs. Because of their size and opacity, they should not be mistaken for pulmonary nodules (which will be larger than 4–5 mm and soft tissue in opacity).

As dogs age, a common radiographic change includes mineralization of the central airways and trachea/carina. These changes can also be seen in dogs with Cushing syndrome [21]. The mineral pattern is very thin and linear in the airway walls whereas a geriatric mineralization pattern that might be seen in older dogs would be mineralization within the cartilaginous rings of the trachea. This can be quite eye-catching and should not be mistaken for a bronchial pulmonary pattern which implies airway wall thickening, not seen in central airway mineralization (Figure 13.62).

Another pulmonary hilar "fake-out" for the pulmonary parenchyma is the presence of blood vessels that are seen end-on in dogs and cats. These also should not be mistaken for pulmonary nodules. Pulmonary metastatic nodules must usually be at least >4–5 mm to visualize radiographically and are more commonly seen within the peripheral aspects of the lung lobes away from the hilum. The end-on pulmonary vessel is usually less than 5 mm in size and very radiopaque by nature of summation of the end-on vessel itself. Also, the end-on vessel will be adjacent to a circular bronchus and usually contiguous

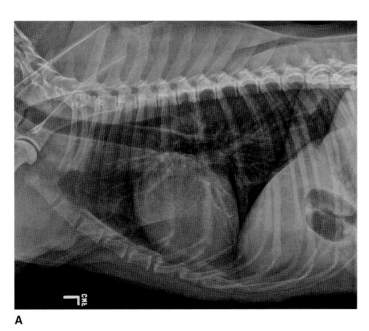

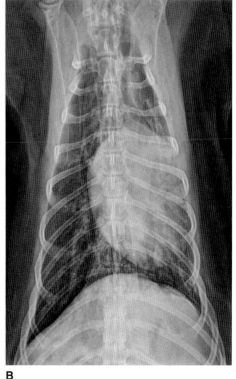

**A**                    **B**

**FIGURE 13.57**   Left lateral (**A**) and ventrodorsal (**B**) thoracic radiographs of a dog under general anesthesia. There is mild gas in the esophagus on the left lateral radiograph and left-sided pulmonary atelectasis and associated left-sided mediastinal shift secondary to prolonged recumbency and general anesthesia.

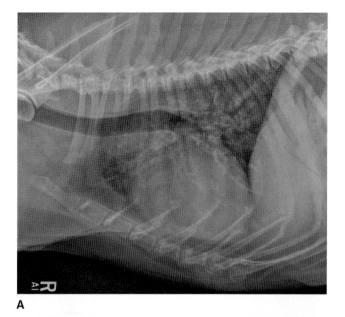

**A**

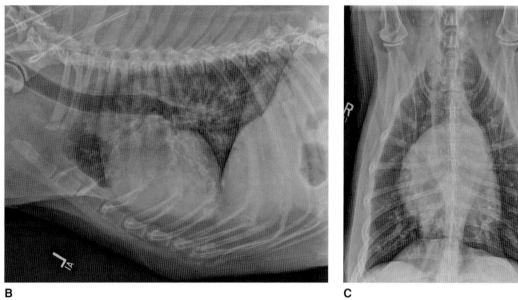

**B**

**C**

**FIGURE 13.58**   Right lateral (**A**), left lateral (**B**), and ventrodorsal (**C**) thoracic radiographs of a 10-year-old golden retriever with no clinical signs related to the respiratory system. There is a moderate diffuse bronchial pulmonary pattern. Differentials include age-related changes primarily, but pulmonary fibrosis or subclinical chronic lower airway disease are not excluded.

with the parent vessel (Figure 13.63). In some instances, superimposed ribs over pulmonary vasculature may cause an optical illusion that exaggerates the contrast between edges of differing shades of gray, contacting each other and causing edge detection called *Mach lines*.

Superimposed skinfolds can create the impression of a pneumothorax lateral to the skinfold itself (Figure 13.64). In addition, the left lateral projection can result in the cardiac silhouette becoming rounder and rotating away from the sternum due to atelectasis of the caudal subsegment of the left cranial lung lobe and inflation of the right middle lung lobe (Figure 13.65).

External structures superimposed over the thorax can give the impression of a pulmonary nodule (Figure 13.66). This is

particularly true for external skin tags, nipples, ectoparasites or extraneous debris on the skin. One should confirm the presence of these external structures by physical examination or one can apply positive contrast medium (liquid barium) to the external nodule and repeat the radiograph to confirm that the nodule is external and not pulmonary.

## The Mediastinum – Cranial

The trachea is the most obvious structure of the cranial mediastinum. The trachea is a radiolucent tube that extends from the larynx to the carina. It should be uniform in diameter throughout its course. Normally, the intrathoracic trachea ventrally

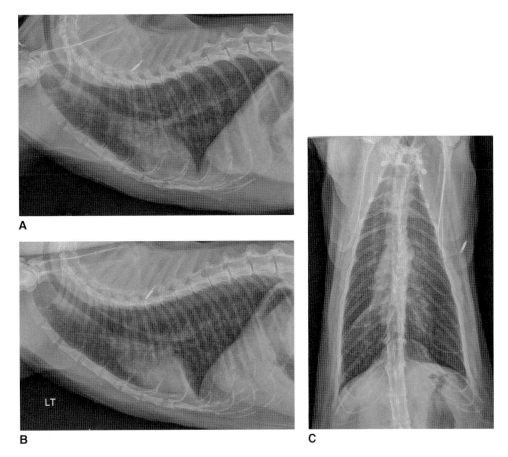

**FIGURE 13.59** Right lateral (**A**), left lateral (**B**), and ventrodorsal (**C**) thoracic radiographs of a cat with feline asthma and right middle lung lobe collapse, further characterized by a moderate diffuse bronchial pulmonary pattern and right middle alveolar pulmonary pattern.

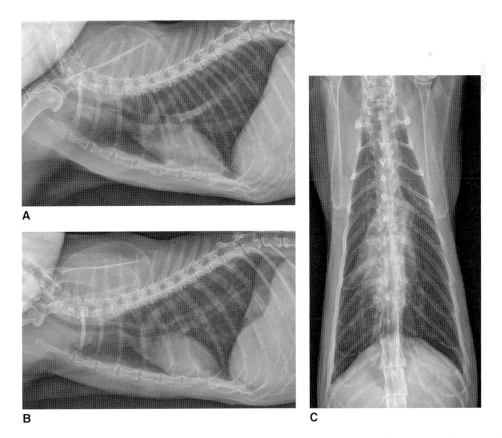

**FIGURE 13.60** Right lateral (**A**), left lateral (**B**), and ventrodorsal (**C**) thoracic radiographs of a cat with a structured interstitial pulmonary pattern. In addition, there is right middle lung lobe collapse, further characterized by a right middle alveolar pulmonary pattern with a rightward ipsilateral mediastinal shift.

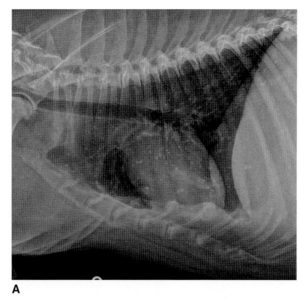

A

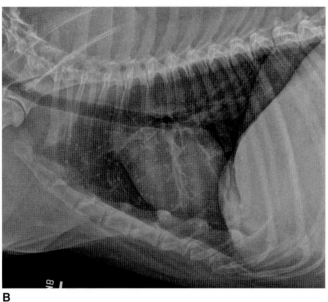

B

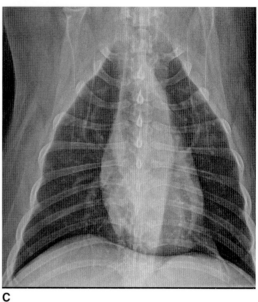

C

**FIGURE 13.61** Right lateral (**A**), left lateral (**B**), and ventrodorsal (**C**) thoracic radiographs of an 8-year-old Rottweiler. There are multifocal, ventrally distributed, well-defined, round, mineral opaque pulmonary foci, representing pulmonary osteomas. Multiple bronchial walls are incidentally mineralized. There is also an incidental extrapleural sign on the lateral radiographs, secondary to CCJ degenerative changes.

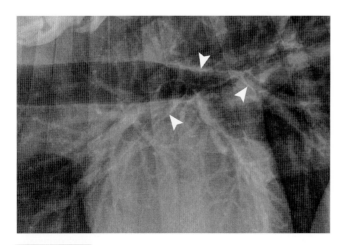

**FIGURE 13.62** A collimated right lateral radiograph of an adult dog with bronchial wall mineralization (white arrowheads).

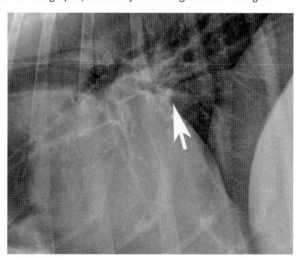

**FIGURE 13.63** Right lateral thoracic radiograph of an 11-year-old golden retriever. In the perihilar region, superimposed over the caudal pulmonary vessels and rib, there is a well-defined, round, soft tissue opaque nodule, consistent with an end-on vessel (white arrowhead).

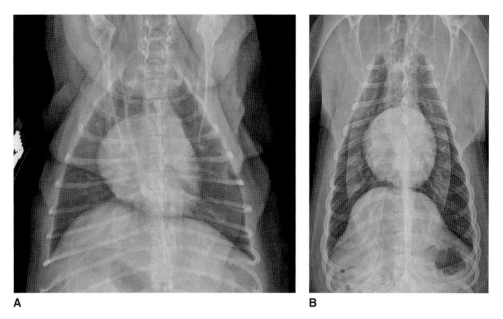

**FIGURE 13.64** (**A**) Ventrodorsal thoracic radiograph of a 13-year-old Labrador retriever. Multiple skinfolds are superimposed over the lateral thorax, particularly the left caudal thorax, giving the false impression of a pneumothorax. (**B**) Dorsoventral radiograph from a 7-year-old German shepherd with skinfolds oriented in a cranial to caudal direction along both sides of the cardiac silhouette. However, the pulmonary vasculature can be seen extending beyond the skinfolds consistent with summation and "fake-out."

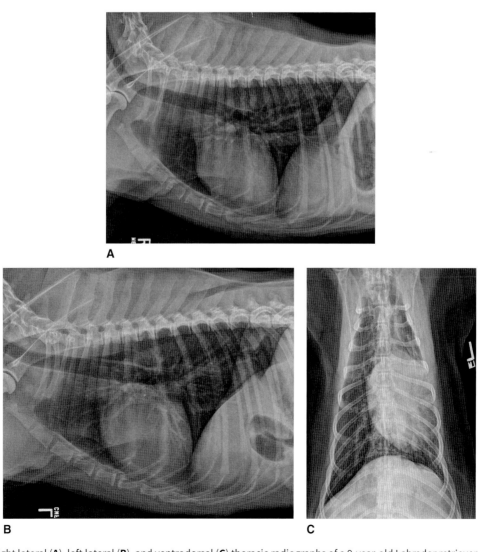

**FIGURE 13.65** Right lateral (**A**), left lateral (**B**), and ventrodorsal (**C**) thoracic radiographs of a 9-year-old Labrador retriever. The cardiac silhouette is more round on the left lateral radiograph when compared to the right lateral radiograph. There is left-sided pulmonary atelectasis seen on the ventrodorsal radiograph.

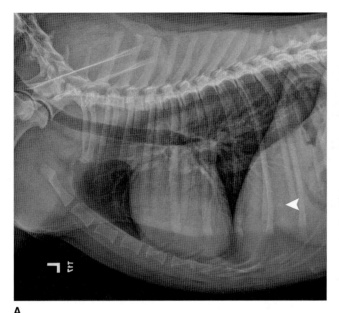
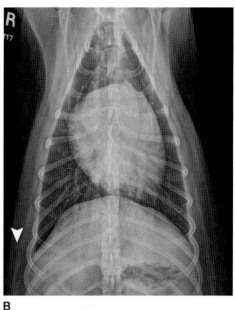

**A**          **B**

**FIGURE 13.66**   Left lateral (**A**) and ventrodorsal (**B**) thoracic radiographs of a 4-year-old Walker hound. There is a subcutaneous nodule (white arrowhead) within the right caudolateral thoracic body wall seen on the ventrodorsal radiograph, superimposed over the lung on the left lateral radiograph, causing the appearance of the pulmonary nodule.

diverges away from the thoracic spine in the cranial thorax on lateral radiographs. The trachea is found to the right of midline on a VD or DV radiograph (Figure 13.67). The tracheal diameter has been normalized to the thoracic inlet as a ratio, which is measured by a line drawn from the ventral aspect of the cranial endplate of the T1 vertebra to the dorsal aspect of the midbody of the manubrium, and a line drawn intersecting the height of the trachea at the same level (Figure 13.68). Normal ratios are ≥15% in nonbrachycephalic breed dogs, >16% in nonbulldog brachycephalic breed dogs, >12% in English bulldogs [22], 18% in domestic shorthair cats, and 20% in brachycephalic cats [23]. Some brachycephalic breeds are already hypoplastic by this standard and the tracheal diameter:thoracic inlet ratio of ≥12% is used [24].

The trachea can become dorsiflexed on lateral projections if the radiograph is made with the patient's head in a flexed position (Figure 13.69). However, on the VD radiograph there is no cranial mediastinal mass to account for the tracheal position. This is purely secondary to the neck positioning of the dog's head (flexion) at the time the radiograph was made and not a cranial mediastinal mass.

Additionally, there can be a redundant dorsal tracheal membrane superimposed over the trachea (Figure 13.70). This is considered by some a type I tracheal collapse but this is such a common finding that without additional testing (fluoroscopy or bronchoscopy), it is difficult to attribute any clinical significance to the redundant dorsal tracheal membrane [25]. Typically, the redundant membrane is seen superimposed over the dorsal trachea (50% of the luminal diameter). Redundant membranes greater than 50% of the tracheal diameter should be worked up for extrathoracic tracheal collapse if clinically warranted.

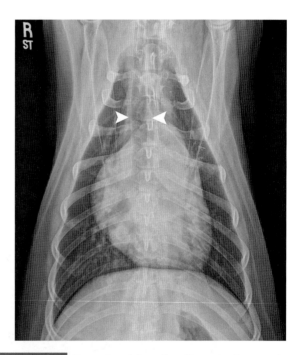

**FIGURE 13.67**   Ventrodorsal thoracic radiograph of a normal 8-year-old mixed-breed dog. The trachea is located slightly toward the right of the midline (between the white arrowheads).

On lateral and ventrodorsal radiographs, within the cranioventral mediastinal reflection in young dogs and cats, the thymus ("sail sign") can be visualized on the VD radiograph (Figure 13.71). The thymus is a triangular soft tissue opacity noted cranial to the cardiac silhouette that extends along the left side of the cranioventral mediastinal reflection. On the right lateral radiograph, the thymus appears as a thin radiopaque curvilinear structure just cranial to the cardiac silhouette.

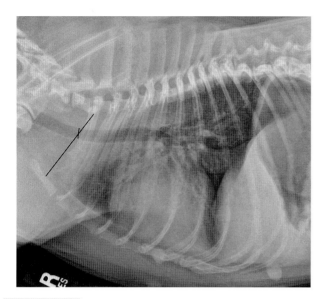

**FIGURE 13.68**  Right lateral thoracic radiograph of a normal 4-year-old bulldog. The tracheal diameter to thoracic inlet ratio is measured by a line drawn from the ventral aspect of the cranial endplate of the T1 vertebra to the dorsal aspect of the midbody of the manubrium, and a line drawn intersecting the height of the trachea at the same level. The distance of the tracheal diameter divided by the measurement of the thoracic inlet should be greater than or equal to 15% for normal dogs. In this case, the percentage is 12.5%, consistent with a hypoplastic trachea.

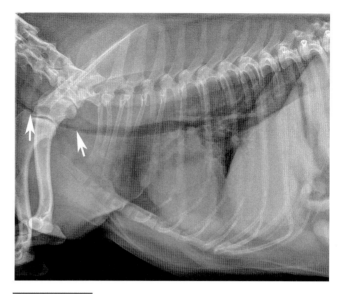

**FIGURE 13.70**  Left lateral thoracic radiograph of a normal 12-year-old Jack Russell terrier with an incidental redundant dorsal tracheal membrane (white arrows). This degree of a redundant membrane would be considered a type I tracheal collapse and should be evaluated for clinical significance using bronchoscopy.

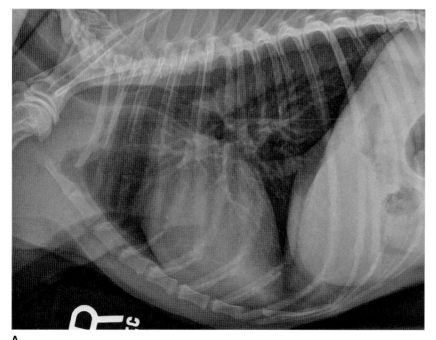

A

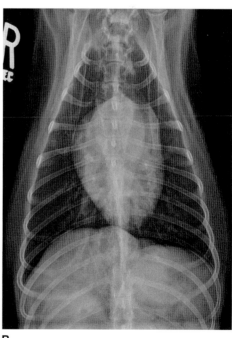

B

**FIGURE 13.69**  Right lateral (**A**) and ventrodorsal (**B**) thoracic radiograph of an 11-year-old miniature pinscher. There is dorsal deviation of the cranial intrathoracic trachea on the lateral radiograph, secondary to ventral neck and head positioning. There is no evidence of a cranial mediastinal mass, that would result in cranial mediastinal widening, noted on the ventrodorsal radiograph. Extending the head and neck will decrease this artifact.

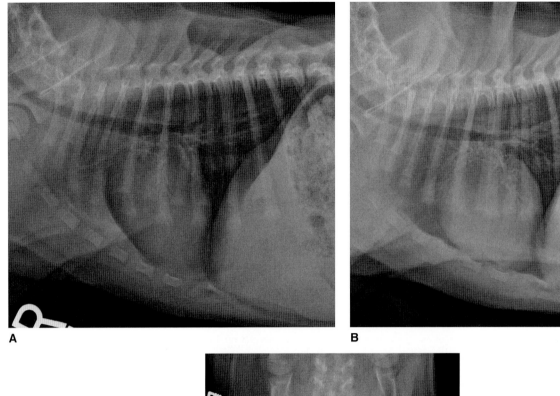

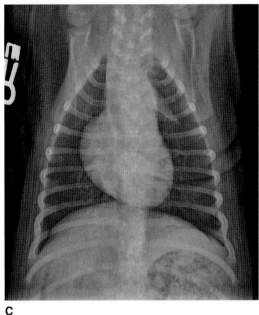

**FIGURE 13.71** Right lateral (**A**), left lateral (**B**), and ventrodorsal (**C**) thoracic radiographs of a normal 2-month-old mixed-breed dog with a thymus, further characterized by increased soft tissue opacity of the cranial mediastinum on the lateral radiographs and a "sail sign" of the left cranial mediastinum on the ventrodorsal radiograph.

In normal dogs, the mediastinal reflections are found cranial and caudal to the cardiac silhouette (Figure 13.72). In obese dogs, fat is deposited in the dorsal aspect of the cranial mediastinum, resulting in widening of the cranial mediastinum on the VD projection (Figure 13.73). Fat can also localize to the area of the cranioventral mediastinal reflection ventrally. These changes are atypical for obese cats, where fat accumulates in the midventral pleural and pericardial spaces (Figure 13.74) [26].

The normal esophagus is not typically seen on thoracic radiographs but can occasionally be seen on lateral thoracic radiographs (Figure 13.75), particularly the left lateral radiograph. Anatomically, it is located along the dorsal and left side of the trachea to the level of the carina, then continues on the left side of the thorax to the esophageal hiatus associated with the left central portion of the diaphragm. The esophagus is located equidistant between the descending thoracic aorta and the caudal vena cava on the lateral images in the caudal mediastinum.

Esophageal variants include a redundant esophagus at the level of the first intercostal space with ventral deviation of the caudal cervical/cranial thoracic esophagus below the level

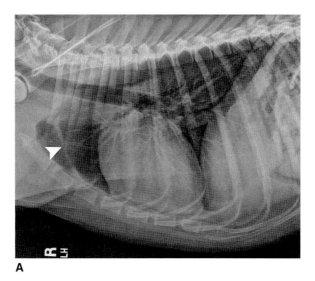

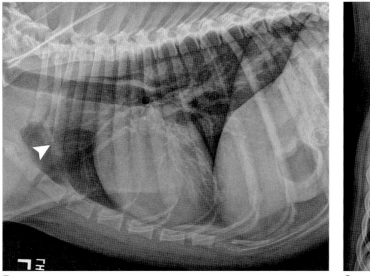

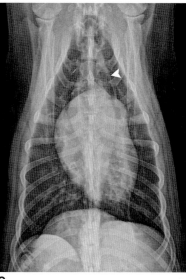

**FIGURE 13.72** Right lateral (**A**), left lateral (**B**), and ventrodorsal (**C**) thoracic radiographs of a normal 6-year-old Labrador retriever. The cranial mediastinal reflection (white arrowheads) is seen in the cranioventral thorax on the lateral radiographs and left craniolateral thorax on the ventrodorsal radiograph.

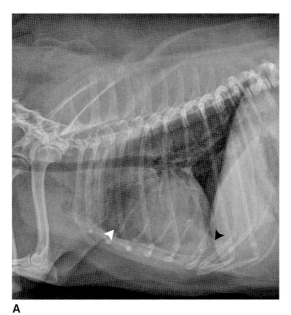

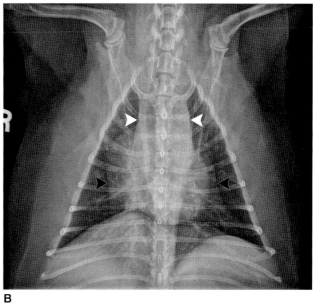

**FIGURE 13.73** Right lateral (**A**) and ventrodorsal (**B**) thoracic radiographs of an obese but otherwise normal 13-year-old mixed-breed dog. There is increased fat deposition in the cranial (white arrowheads) and middle (black arrowheads) mediastinum.

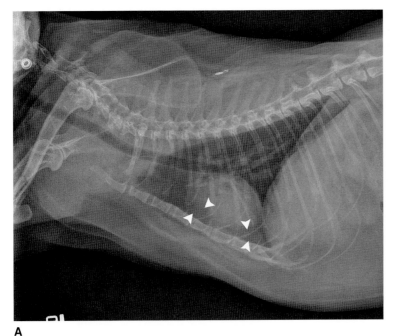
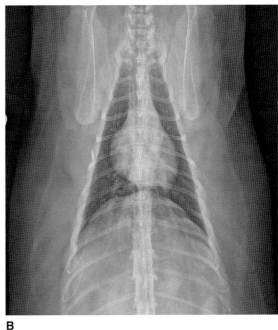

**A**

**B**

**FIGURE 13.74** Left lateral (**A**) and ventrodorsal (**B**) thoracic radiograph of an obese but otherwise normal 13-year-old Siamese cat. There is increased fat deposition in the middle mediastinum, surrounding the cardiac silhouette (white arrowheads).

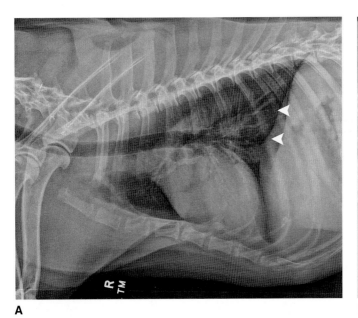
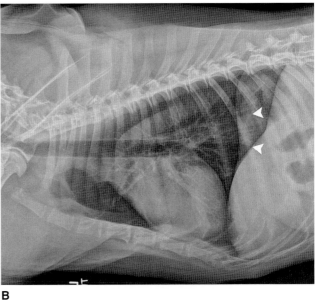

**A**

**B**

**FIGURE 13.75** Right lateral (**A**) and left lateral (**B**) thoracic radiographs of a normal 13-year-old mixed-breed dog with increased conspicuity of the caudal intrathoracic esophagus. The dorsal and ventral margin of the caudal intrathoracic esophagus can be seen (white arrowheads) located between the aorta dorsally and caudal vena cava ventrally.

of the trachea (Figure 13.76) [27, 28]. This variant is most commonly seen in bulldogs, other brachycephalic breeds, and shar peis. Additionally, there can be a focal accumulation of gas within the esophagus cranial to the heart base area seen on the left lateral projection (Figure 13.77). This should not be misinterpreted as an esophageal obstruction with gas accumulating in the oral side of the esophagus. This can result in combination of the ventral border of the esophagus and dorsal border of the trachea with border effacement between the two walls, called

the "tracheoesophageal stripe sign" (Figure 13.78). This can also be seen in cases of abnormal esophageal dilation.

## The Mediastinum – Middle

The cardiac silhouette is the most obvious soft tissue structure of the ventral aspect of the middle mediastinum. The normal cardiac silhouette is the summation shadow of all the coronary

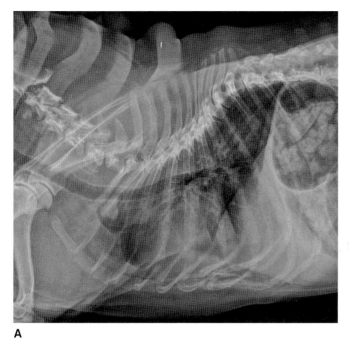

A

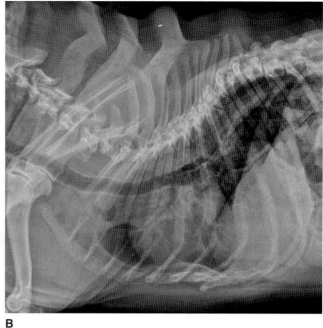

B

**FIGURE 13.76**   Right lateral (**A**) and left lateral (**B**) thoracic radiograph of a normal 3-year-old English bulldog. A gas-filled redundant esophagus is seen ventral to the trachea at the thoracic inlet on the lateral radiographs.

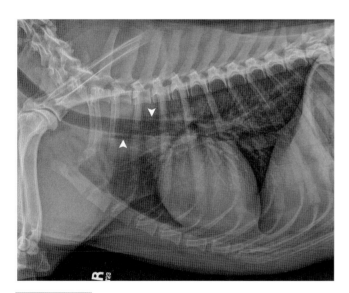

**FIGURE 13.77**   Right lateral thoracic radiograph of a normal 2-year-old Labrador retriever with mild cranial esophageal gas (white arrowheads).

vasculature, blood within the cardiac chambers, cardiac chambers and valves, myocardium, endocardium, epicardium, great vessels as they exit the respective outflow tracts, and pericardium. All the structures cannot be visualized unless positive contrast medium is administered as all structures are soft tissue opaque and therefore are border effaced with each other.

The size and shape are influenced by internal and external factors. Important internal factors include cardiac cycle and blood volume (Figure 13.79). In normal dogs, the primary external factor influencing the cardiac size and shape is the breed of dog being imaged. The normal cardiac silhouette on

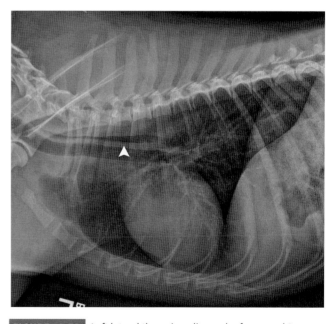

**FIGURE 13.78**   Left lateral thoracic radiograph of a normal 2-year-old mixed-breed dog. There is mild esophageal gas, creating the "tracheoesophageal stripe sign" (white arrowhead).

the lateral radiograph takes up 2.5–3.5 intercostal spaces wide and is two-thirds the height of the thoracic cavity height at the level of T8. The opacity of the cardiac silhouette is soft tissue, and the shape is oval on right lateral and VD radiographs and circular to round on left lateral and DV radiographs. Typically, the cardiac silhouette comes to a rounded point caudoventrally on lateral radiographs and along the caudal left side on VD or DV images; this point is the apex of the left ventricle (Figure 13.1A,C,E,G). The craniodorsal aspect of the heart on

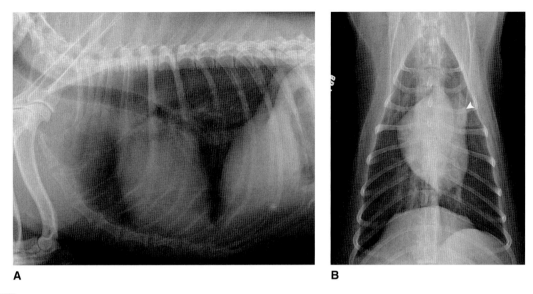

**A**  **B**

**FIGURE 13.79** Right lateral (**A**) and ventrodorsal (**B**) thoracic radiographs of a normal 8-year-old Cavalier King Charles spaniel. On the ventrodorsal radiograph, there is a soft tissue bulge in the region of the main pulmonary artery (white arrowhead), consistent with a normal variation of the cardiac cycle (radiograph obtained on systole).

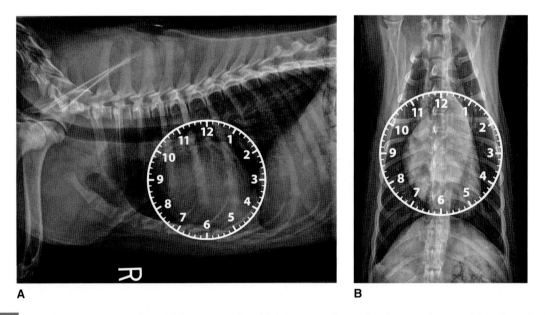

**A**  **B**

**FIGURE 13.80** Clock face analogy. Right lateral (**A**) and ventrodorsal (**B**) thoracic radiographs of a normal 5-year-old medium-sized mixed-breed dog. See Table 13.3 for a description of the positioning of the various cardiac structures related to the clock face. This works best for the dog and does not hold true for the cat.

lateral images and the cranial aspect of the heart on VD or DV images is the heart base and contains the great vessels superimposed over the right atrium.

It is difficult to characterize the shape of the heart as it relates to individual chambers or vessels. However, in general, one can use a clock face analogy on both lateral and VD/DV images and correlate shape and size changes in these areas to specific chambers or great vessels (Figure 13.80, Table 13.3). An example as to why this approach does not work very well is the right atrium. The right atrium extends from the craniodorsal to caudodorsal aspect of the cardiac silhouette on lateral radiographs. Yet, on the lateral radiograph, we generally

look at the area between 8 and 11 o'clock as being the right atrial position along the cranial surface of the cardiac silhouette. This area is really the area of the right auricle and there must be right auricular enlargement prior to being able to see a change in this region (Figure 13.81). The three-dimensional anatomy of the cardiac chambers and structures is complex and this simplistic approach to evaluating the cardiac silhouette using the clock face analogy does not always work. Again, it should be used as an approximation. The clock face analogy does not work very well for cats when compared with dogs. The normal vertebral heart score for the dog is 9.7±0.5 vertebral bodies [29, 30] based on an average dog size and across

**TABLE 13.3**   Clock face analogy.

| Lateral radiograph | 12–3 o'clock | Left atrium |
| --- | --- | --- |
| | 3–5 o'clock | Left ventricle |
| | 5–9 o'clock | Right ventricle |
| | 9–10 o'clock | Right auricle |
| | 10–11 o'clock | Great vessels |
| Ventrodorsal radiograph | 11–1 o'clock | Aortic arch |
| | 1–2 o'clock | Main pulmonary artery |
| | 3 o'clock | Left auricle |
| | 3–5 o'clock | Left ventricle |
| | 5–9 o'clock | Right ventricle |
| | 9–11 o'clock | Right atrium |

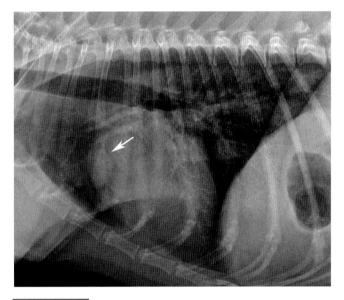

**FIGURE 13.81**   Right lateral thoracic radiograph of a 9-year-old mixed-breed dog. There is right auricular enlargement (white arrow) consistent with a mass or right auricular hernia (as was proven in this case on CT evaluation).

many different breeds [31–33]. This calculation may best be used in longitudinal studies of the cardiac silhouette in the same patient on the right lateral radiograph [34]. The normal vertebral heart score for the cat is 7.5 ± 0.3 [35].

Several variants related to the cardiac silhouette need to be considered. A large variation in the shape and size of the cardiac silhouette is noted in all the different dog breeds (Figure 13.82). This has resulted in breed-specific vertebral heart scores [31–33]. In small-breed dogs, the cardiac silhouette takes up more space relative to the overall thoracic volume when compared with large-breed dogs (except for the greyhound). Additionally, on a VD radiograph, thoracic obliquity can accentuate certain cardiac chambers, causing an impression of enlargement (Figure 13.83). If the sternum is obliqued to the left side, the area of the right atrium will appear artifactually enlarged. If the sternum is obliqued to the right side, the area of the main pulmonary artery will appear artifactually enlarged. Also, the cardiac cycle can result in different sizes of the cardiac silhouette and/or specific cardiac chambers (Figure 13.79). If the radiograph is made on diastole, which is most commonly the case, the cardiac silhouette will appear larger than if it is made on systole. If the VD radiograph is made on systole, the main pulmonary artery will appear artifactually enlarged. In cats, a normal vertebral heart scale does not preclude underlying heart disease [36]. On radiography, specific cardiac chamber enlargement is not always detected. In some instances, biatrial enlargement can be seen on the ventrodorsal or dorsoventral radiograph, representing a "Valentine heart" shape [37, 38].

A variant that has been seen in different dog breeds (not cats) is aortic root mineralization [39, 40]. This incidental idiopathic area of mineralization has not been associated with any conditions that might result in dystrophic or metastatic mineralization of the aortic sinus and ascending aorta (Figure 13.84).

As cats age, 30–40% will develop a "lazy heart" and a redundant aorta. The angle between the cardiac silhouette and the sternum on the lateral radiograph will decrease (Figure 13.85). The aorta will develop some more acute angles rather than having a natural curve in the aortic arch into the descending thoracic aorta. On the VD radiograph, the aortic arch will be seen end-on which is called an "aortic knob." This should not be mistaken for a pulmonary nodule in the left cranial lung lobe of the cat (Figure 13.85c).

## The Mediastinum – Caudal

The most common variant of the caudal mediastinum is associated with the esophagus. If there is fluid in the esophagus, it will appear soft tissue opaque and will be visualized on lateral projections between the descending thoracic aorta and the caudal vena cava (Figure 13.75). This change can also be seen, however, in dogs and cats with caudal esophagitis, reflux from the stomach, or soft tissue foreign bodies lodged in the caudal thoracic esophagus. The other esophageal variant is the presence of a hiatal hernia (Figure 13.86). These are typically seen on left lateral and/or VD images as soft tissue opacity just dorsal to the area of the expected lower esophageal sphincter on the lateral or rounded soft tissue opacity between the diaphragmatic crura on the VD radiograph. This finding is typically incidental but can be associated with regurgitation, reflux disease, and/or esophagitis [41].

The two conspicuous vessels seen in the caudal thorax on thoracic images are the descending thoracic aorta and the caudal vena cava. The thoracic aorta should be of a similar diameter throughout its course in the thorax [42]. The aortic arch can be seen at the heart base on the VD or DV image and then tapers toward the midline as the vessels continue caudally

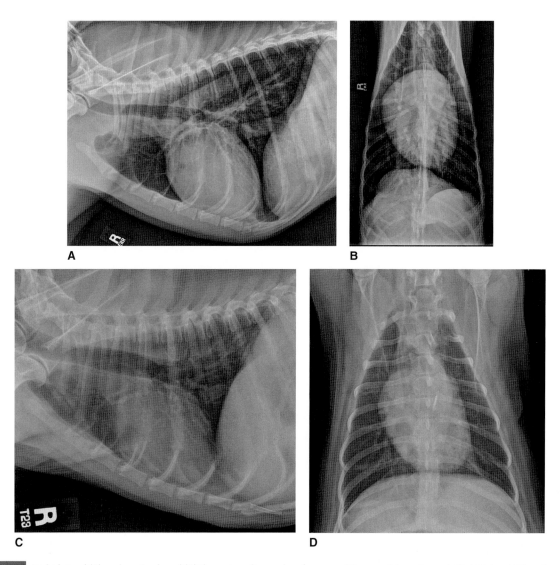

**FIGURE 13.82** Right lateral (**A**) and ventrodorsal (**B**) thoracic radiographs of a normal 3-year-old greyhound. Right lateral (**C**) and ventrodorsal (**D**) thoracic radiographs of a normal 5-year-old poodle.

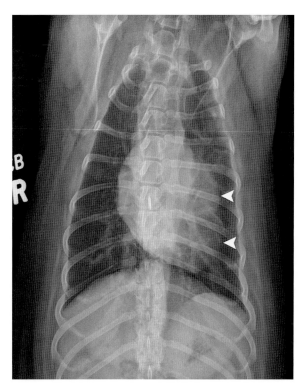

**FIGURE 13.83** Ventrodorsal thoracic radiograph of a normal 11-year-old pug. The radiograph is slightly oblique, causing an artifactual cardiac chamber enlargement (white arrowheads).

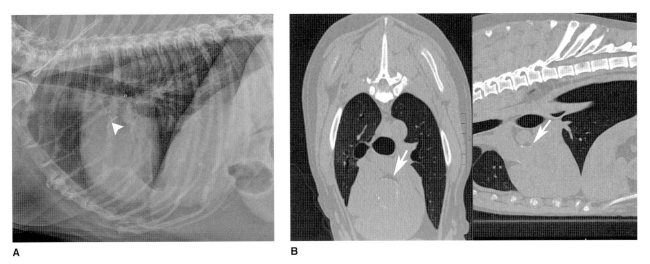

**FIGURE 13.84** (**A**) Left lateral thoracic radiograph of a normal 8-year-old mixed-breed dog with an incidental finding of aortic root mineralization (white arrowhead). (**B**) Transverse (left image) and sagittal reconstruction (right image) of a 4-year-old greyhound with an incidental finding of aortic root mineralization.

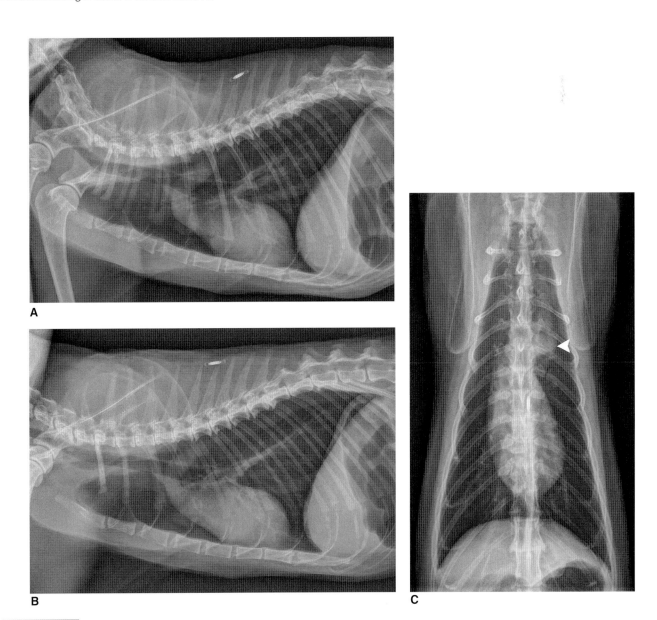

**FIGURE 13.85** Right lateral (**A**), left lateral (**B**), and ventrodorsal (**C**) thoracic radiographs of a normal 13-year-old domestic shorthair cat. The cardiac silhouette has a "lazy heart" appearance on the lateral radiographs. The aorta is redundant with an "aortic knob" on the ventrodorsal radiograph (white arrowhead).

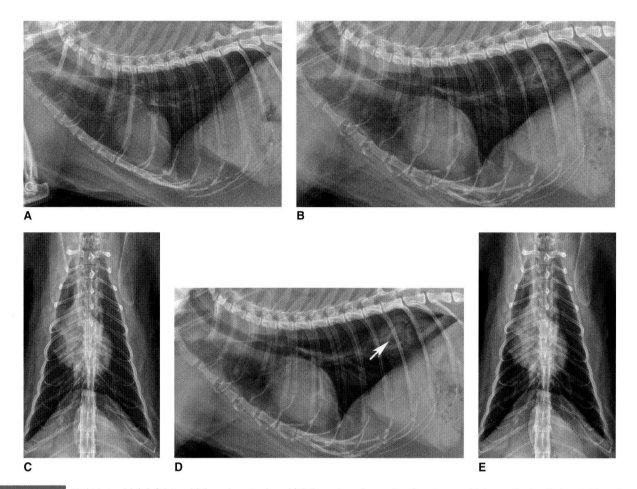

**FIGURE 13.86**   Right lateral (**A**), left lateral (**B**), and ventrodorsal (**C**) thoracic radiographs of an 8-year-old domestic shorthair cat. There is a sliding hiatal hernia noted on the left lateral and ventrodorsal images in the caudal dorsal thorax. (**D**) Left lateral with schematics. The dotted red line outlines the hiatal hernia. The white arrow denotes the gastric contents (fundus) superimposed over the caudal thorax. (**E**) Ventrodorsal image with dashed red line outlining the sliding hiatal hernia.

(Figure 13.87). The caudal portion of the thoracic aorta is less conspicuous due to a decrease in the overall lung volume that surrounds the vessel, thereby decreasing the contrast between a soft tissue opacity and gas. The caudal mediastinal space is contiguous with the retroperitoneal space at the aortic hiatus as seen just to the left of the midline associated with the dorsal aspect of the central diaphragm. In certain instances, pneumoretroperitoneum can be seen in conjunction with pneumomediastinum.

The caudal vena cava can have a variety of diameters depending on the degree of filling of the caudal vena cava with returning blood from the abdomen and pelvis/pelvic limbs or phases of respiration [43, 44]. The vessel may appear different in size and shape even on the same study (Figure 13.88). The caudal vena cava should not be two times greater in diameter than the thoracic aortic diameter at the same level of the cava. The cava can normally be thin. However, in concert with small pulmonary vessels and microcardia, hypovolemia or central vascular (extracellular fluid space) volume depletion should be considered (Figure 13.89) [44].

# Interpretation Paradigm

The thorax can be divided into four compartments that will each need to be evaluated. The interpretation paradigm for the thorax is found in Appendix II. The four compartments are the extrathoracic structures, the pleural space, the pulmonary parenchyma, and the mediastinum. The mediastinum can be divided into thirds (cranial, middle, and caudal) with the cardiac silhouette being located in the ventral middle mediastinum. Each of these compartments will serve as the basis for the next four chapters. Recognize that there are many diseases that involve multiple compartments. For example, a dog with mitral valve degenerative disease that is in left heart failure has the primary disease in the middle mediastinum (heart) with secondary involvement of the pulmonary parenchyma (enlarged pulmonary veins and cardiogenic pulmonary edema).

The divisions of the thorax are artificial and should be used to help evaluate thoracic radiographs, but in the end the entirety of the thorax needs to be considered when arriving at differential diagnoses for abnormal radiographic findings.

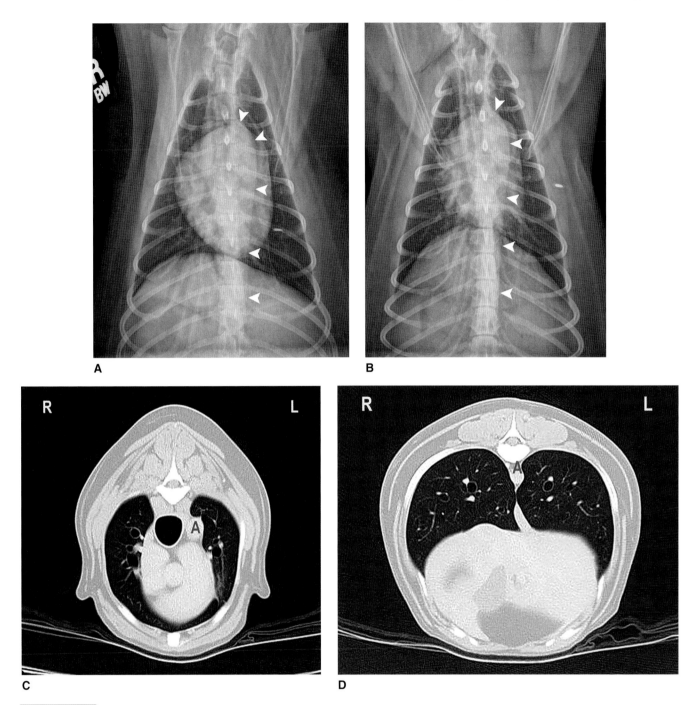

**FIGURE 13.87**   Ventrodorsal (**A**) and dorsoventral (**B**) thoracic radiographs of a normal 2-year-old Cavalier King Charles spaniel. The aortic arch and descending intrathoracic aorta can be seen parasagittal to the vertebral column (white arrowheads). On lateral projections, the cranial aspect of the aorta is better visualized due to the indentation into the dorsal and medial aspect of the left cranial lobe. As the descending aorta extends caudally, it shifts to a midline position and is not as well visualized on lateral images toward the dorsal diaphragmatic crura. Transverse CT images (**C**) and (**D**) showing the relationship of the descending thoracic aorta in the cranial thorax (A, aorta) compared with the caudal thorax where the aorta is in the caudal mediastinum and there are no pulmonary indentations. R, right; L, left.

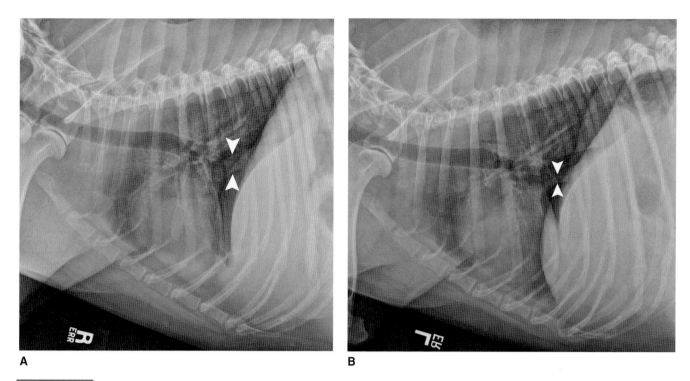

A          B

**FIGURE 13.88**   Right lateral (**A**) and left lateral (**B**) thoracic radiographs of a normal 9-year-old pit bull terrier with variably sized caudal vena cava (between the white arrowheads).

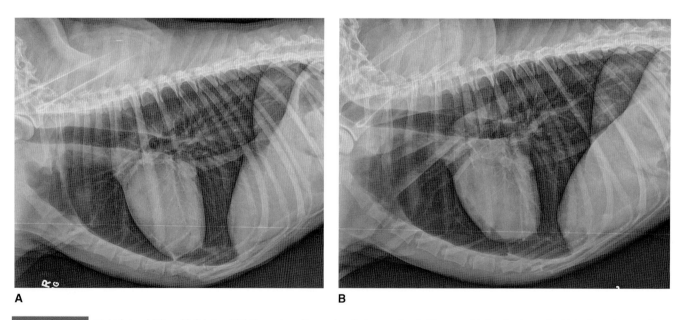

A          B

**FIGURE 13.89**   Right lateral (**A**) and left lateral (**B**) thoracic radiographs of a hypovolemic 11-year-old standard poodle. Note the microcardia causing elevation of the cardiac silhouette from the sternum, thin caudal vena cava, and decrease in size of the pulmonary arteries and veins.

# References

1. Pechman, J. (1987). Effect of dependency vs. nondependency on lung lesion visualization. *Vet. Radiol.* 28: 185–190.
2. Barthez, P., Hornof, W., Theon, A. et al. (1994). Receiver operating characteristic curve analysis of the performance of various radiographic protocols when screening dogs for pulmonary metastases. *J. Am. Vet. Med. Assoc.* 204: 237–240.
3. Ober, C.P. and Barber, D. (2006). Comparison of two- vs. three-view thoracic radiographic studies on conspicuity of structured interstitial patterns in dogs. *Vet. Radiol. Ultrasound* 47: 542–545.
4. Lang, J., Wortman, J., Glickman, L. et al. (1986). Sensitivity of radiographic detection of lung metastasis in the dog. *Vet. Radiol.* 27: 74–78.
5. Wolvekamp, W.T. (1995). Basic principles of thoracic radiography. *Vet. Q.* 17 (Suppl 1): S31–S32.
6. Silverman, S. and Suter, P.F. (1975). Influence of inspiration and expiration on canine thoracic radiographs. *J. Am. Vet. Med. Assoc.* 166: 502–510.
7. Chhoey, S., Lee, S.K., Je, H. et al. (2020). Effect of expiratory phase for radiographic detection of left heart enlargement in dogs with mitral regurgitation. *Vet. Radiol. Ultrasound* 61: 291–301.
8. Mauragis, D. and Berry, C.R. (2011). Small Animal Thoracic Radiography. https://todaysveterinarypractice.com/small-animal-thoracic-radiography.
9. Lynch, K.C., Oliveira, C.R., Matheson, J.S. et al. (2012). Detection of pneumothorax and pleural effusion with horizontal beam radiography. *Vet. Radiol. Ultrasound* 53: 38–43.
10. De Rycke, L.M., Gielen, I.M., Simoens, P.J., and van Bree, H. (2005). Computed tomography and cross-sectional anatomy of the thorax in clinically normal dogs. *Am. J. Vet. Res.* 66: 512–524.
11. Barletta, M., Almondia, D., Williams, J. et al. (2014). Radiographic evaluation of positional atelectasis in sedated dogs breathing room air versus 100% oxygen. *Can. Vet. J.* 55: 985–991.
12. Moon, M., Keene, B., Lessard, P., and Lee, J. (1993). Age related changes in the feline cardiac silhouette. *Vet. Radiol. Ultrasound* 34: 315–320.
13. Gutierrez-Quintana, R., Guevar, J., Stalin, C. et al. (2014). A proposed radiographic classification scheme for congenital thoracic vertebral malformations in brachycephalic "screw-tailed" dog breeds. *Vet. Radiol. Ultrasound* 55: 585–591.
14. Wilson, J.W., Kurtz, H.J., Leipold, H.W., and Lees, G.E. (1979). Spina bifida in the dog. *Vet. Pathol.* 16: 165–179.
15. Damur-Djuric, N., Steffen, F., Hässig, M. et al. (2006). Lumbosacral transitional vertebrae in dogs: classification, prevalence, and association with sacroiliac morphology. *Vet. Radiol. Ultrasound* 47: 32–38.
16. Nemanic, S., London, C.A., and Wisner, E.R. (2006). Comparison of thoracic radiographs and single breath-hold helical CT for detection of pulmonary nodules in dogs with metastatic neoplasia. *J. Vet. Intern. Med.* 20: 508–515.
17. Giglio, R.F., Winter, M.D., Reese, D.J. et al. (2013). Radiographic characterization of presumed plate-like atelectasis in 75 nonanesthetized dogs and 15 cats. *Vet. Radiol. Ultrasound* 54: 326–331.
18. Mendoza, P., Giglio, R.F., Olmo, C. et al. (2019). Anatomic characterization of pulmonary accessory fissures in canine cadavers. *Anat. Histol. Embryol.* 48: 157–163.
19. Corcoran, B.M., Foster, D.J., and Fuentes, V.L. (1995). Feline asthma syndrome: a retrospective study of the clinical presentation in 29 cats. *J. Small Anim. Pract.* 36: 481–488.
20. Woodring, J.H. (1988). Determining the cause of pulmonary atelectasis: a comparison of plain radiography and CT. *Am. J. Roentgenol.* 150: 757–763.
21. Berry, C.R., Hawkins, E.C., Hurley, K.J., and Monce, K. (2000). Frequency of pulmonary mineralization and hypoxemia in 21 dogs with pituitary-dependent hyperadrenocorticism. *J. Vet. Intern. Med.* 14: 151–156.
22. Harvey, C. and Fink, E. (1982). Tracheal diameter: analysis of radiographic measurements in brachycephalic and nonbrachycephalic dogs. *J. Am. Anim. Hosp. Assoc.* 18: 570–576.
23. Hammond, G., Geary, M., Coleman, E., and Gunn-Moore, D. (2011). Radiographic measurements of the trachea in domestic shorthair and Persian cats. *J. Feline Med. Surg.* 13: 881–884.
24. Regier, P.J., Grosso, F.V., Stone, H.K., and van Santen, E. (2020). Radiographic tracheal dimensions in brachycephalic breeds before and after surgical treatment for brachycephalic airway syndrome. *Can. Vet. J.* 61: 971–976.
25. Lindl Bylicki, B.J., Johnson, L.R., and Pollard, R.E. (2015). Comparison of the radiographic and tracheoscopic appearance of the dorsal tracheal membrane in large and small breed dogs. *Vet. Radiol. Ultrasound* 56: 602–608.
26. Litster, A.L. and Buchanan, J.W. (2000). Radiographic and echocardiographic measurement of the heart in obese cats. *Vet. Radiol. Ultrasound* 41: 320–325.
27. Reeve, E.J., Sutton, D., Friend, E.J., and Warren-Smith, C.M.R. (2017). Documenting the prevalence of hiatal hernia and oesophageal abnormalities in brachycephalic dogs using fluoroscopy. *J. Small Anim. Pract.* 58: 703–708.
28. Eivers, C., Chicon Rueda, R., Liuti, T., and Salavati Schmitz, S. (2019). Retrospective analysis of esophageal imaging features in brachycephalic versus non-brachycephalic dogs based on videofluoroscopic swallowing studies. *J. Vet. Intern. Med.* 33: 1740–1746.
29. Buchanan, J.W. and Bücheler, J. (1995). Vertebral scale system to measure canine heart size in radiographs. *J. Am. Vet. Med. Assoc.* 206: 194–199.
30. Buchanan, J.W. (2000). Vertebral scale system to measure heart size in radiographs. *Vet. Clin. North Am. Small Anim. Pract.* 30: 379–393. vii.
31. Birks, R., Fine, D.M., Leach, S.B. et al. (2017). Breed-specific vertebral heart scale for the dachshund. *J. Am. Anim. Hosp. Assoc.* 53: 73–79.
32. Jepsen-Grant, K., Pollard, R.E., and Johnson, L.R. (2013). Vertebral heart scores in eight dog breeds. *Vet. Radiol. Ultrasound* 54: 3–8.
33. Kraetschmer, S., Ludwig, K., Meneses, F. et al. (2008). Vertebral heart scale in the beagle dog. *J. Small Anim. Pract.* 49: 240–243.
34. Greco, A., Meomartino, L., Raiano, V. et al. (2008). Effect of left vs. right recumbency on the vertebral heart score in normal dogs. *Vet. Radiol. Ultrasound* 49: 454–455.
35. Litster, A.L. and Buchanan, J.W. (2000). Vertebral scale system to measure heart size in radiographs of cats. *J. Am. Vet. Med. Assoc.* 216: 210–214.

36. Guglielmini, C. and Diana, A. (2015). Thoracic radiography in the cat: identification of cardiomegaly and congestive heart failure. *J. Vet. Cardiol.* 17 (Suppl 1): S87–S101.

37. Winter, M.D., Giglio, R.F., Berry, C.R. et al. (2015). Associations between 'valentine' heart shape, atrial enlargement and cardiomyopathy in cats. *J. Feline Med. Surg.* 17: 447–452.

38. Oura, T.J., Young, A.N., Keene, B.W. et al. (2015). A valentine-shaped cardiac silhouette in feline thoracic radiographs is primarily due to left atrial enlargement. *Vet. Radiol. Ultrasound* 56: 245–250.

39. Schwarz, T., Sullivan, M., Störk, C.K. et al. (2002). Aortic and cardiac mineralization in the dog. *Vet. Radiol. Ultrasound* 43: 419–427.

40. Douglass, J.P., Berry, C.R., Thrall, D.E. et al. (2003). Radiographic features of aortic bulb/valve mineralization in 20 dogs. *Vet. Radiol. Ultrasound* 44: 20–27.

41. Phillips, H., Corrie, J., Engel, D.M. et al. (2019). Clinical findings, diagnostic test results, and treatment outcome in cats with hiatal hernia: 31 cases (1995–2018). *J. Vet. Intern. Med.* 33: 1970–1976.

42. Lehmkuhl, L.B., Bonagura, J.D., Biller, D.S., and Hartman, W.M. (1997). Radiographic evaluation of caudal vena cava size in dogs. *Vet. Radiol. Ultrasound* 38: 94–100.

43. Tuplin, M.C., Romero, A.E., and Boysen, S.R. (2017). Influence of the respiratory cycle on caudal vena cava diameter measured by sonography in healthy foals: a pilot study. *J. Vet. Intern. Med.* 31: 1556–1562.

44. Kwak, J., Yoon, H., Kim, J. et al. (2018). Ultrasonographic measurement of caudal vena cava to aorta ratios for determination of volume depletion in normal beagle dogs. *Vet. Radiol. Ultrasound* 59: 203–211.

# CHAPTER 14

# Extrathoracic Structures

**Clifford R. Berry[1] and Federico R. Vilaplana Grosso[2]**

[1] Department of Molecular Biomedical Sciences, College of Veterinary Medicine, North Carolina State University, Raleigh, NC, USA
[2] Department of Small Animal Clinical Sciences, College of Veterinary Medicine, University of Florida, Gainesville, FL, USA

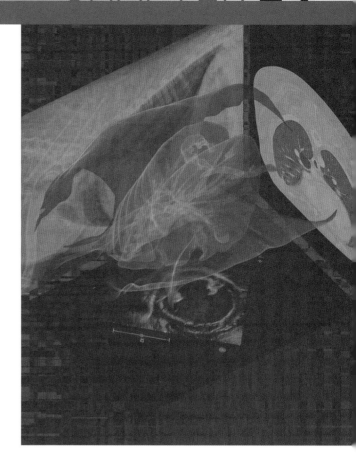

## Overview

The first area to be evaluated using the thoracic interpretation paradigm is the extrathoracic structures. These include the soft tissue and osseous structures of the thoracic limbs, cervical and thoracic spine, sternum and ribs, diaphragm, the organs of the cranial abdomen and the peritoneal space. This chapter reviews the normal radiographic appearance and abnormalities associated with each extrathoracic structure.

## Thoracic Limbs

Depending on the size of the dog, there will be a variable amount of the thoracic limb present on the radiographic images. In smaller dogs and cats, the proximal antebrachium through the scapula will be seen and are superimposed over each other on lateral projections. In larger dogs, the scapula and glenohumeral joint may be the only portion of the thoracic limb visualized. Common abnormalities associated with the thoracic limbs include traumatic injury and degenerative joint disease of the glenohumeral or elbow joints. The degenerative change is seen as osteophyte formation of the periarticular structures. For the glenohumeral joint, this would include the caudal aspect of the glenoid cavity and the caudal aspect of the humeral head (Figure 14.1). Other common abnormalities would be fractures related to trauma (Figure 14.2).

Aggressive changes of the osseous structures of the thoracic limb should not be missed. Primary bone tumors are commonly seen in the proximal humeral metaphysis and can have aggressive areas of osteolysis and osteoproliferation (Figure 14.3). Primary tumors of the scapula are less common but should not be missed when evaluating the scapula on lateral images even though they are superimposed. Confirmation of laterality can be done using the ventrodorsal (VD) or dorsoventral (DV) radiograph (Figure 14.4). Palisading periosteal reaction along the diaphyseal cortices of the humeri can be seen in dogs with hypertrophic osteopathy (see Chapter 10).

*Atlas of Small Animal Diagnostic Imaging*, First Edition. Edited by Clifford R. Berry, Nathan C. Nelson, and Matthew D. Winter.
© 2023 John Wiley & Sons, Inc. Published 2023 by John Wiley & Sons, Inc.
Companion website: www.wiley.com/go/berry/atlas

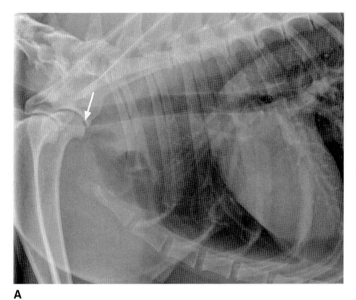
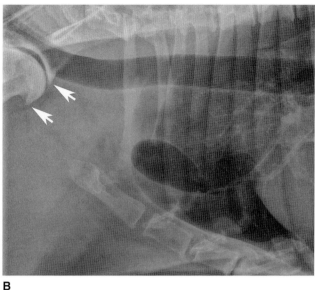

A

B

**FIGURE 14.1** (**A**) Five-year-old Labrador with an incidental finding of a focal subchondral defect in the caudal humeral head (white arrow). (**B**) Ten-year-old German shepherd with degenerative periarticular osteophytes of the caudal glenoid cavity and humeral head (white arrows).

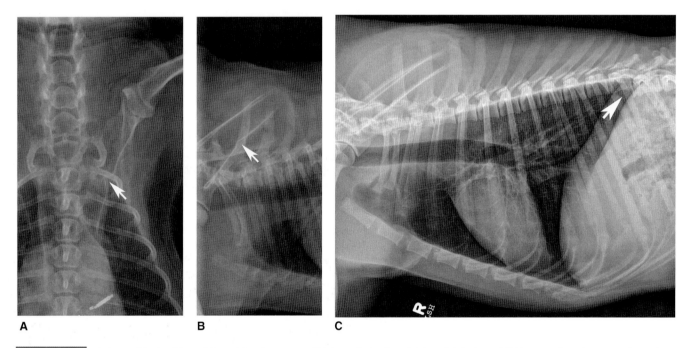

A

B

C

**FIGURE 14.2** Six-year-old mixed-breed dog with acute trauma (hit by car). On the VD (**A**) and right lateral (**B**) images there is a comminuted scapular fracture with the spine of the scapula being displaced and angled. (**C**) A 15-month-old Labrador with acute trauma. The right lateral thoracic image is shown and there is ventral displacement (luxation) of the caudal thoracic spine at T11–12 with a caudal ventral endplate fracture of T11 (white arrow). Also notice the pulmonary vessels and the cardiac silhouette are small, consistent with hypovolemia.

# Thoracic Wall, Vertebral Column, Ribs, and Sternum

A radiolucent space is noted between all thoracic vertebrae and all sternebrae except between S7 and the xiphoid process. This radiolucency represents the intervertebral disc and

intersternebral cartilage, respectively. In the thoracic vertebral location, the intervertebral disc is made up of an outer annulus fibrosis and an inner nucleus pulposus, being a fibrocartilaginous joint. A cartilaginous center is noted to the synchondrosis joint of the sternebral discs. Degenerative changes of the intervertebral disc and intersternebral spaces are the most common changes seen involving the vertebrae and the sternum. These changes include intervertebral disc/intersternebral

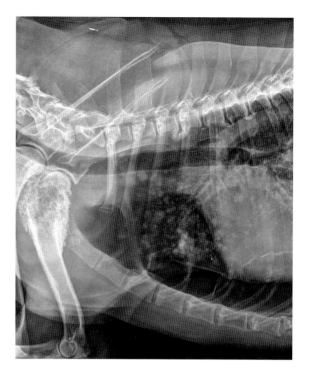

**FIGURE 14.3** Nine-year-old German shepherd with a proximal right humeral aggressive lesion. There is marked osteolysis and irregular periosteal reaction involving the proximal humeral diaphysis, metaphysis, and epiphysis consistent with a primary bone tumor. In addition, there are multiple pulmonary soft tissue nodules (variably sized) along with a pneumothorax as evidenced by dorsal elevation of the ventral lung lobes and the cardiac silhouette on this right lateral image. There are thickened pleural margins noted ventrally as evidenced by the irregular soft tissue opaque lines. Ventral spondylosis deformans is also noted in the cranial to midthoracic spine.

space narrowing, adjacent endplate sclerosis and ventral spondylosis deformans (intervertebral disc space) or ventral/dorsal osseous proliferation (sternal cartilaginous degenerative change). These areas of osteoproliferation are smoothly marginated, are located at the edge of the vertebral body and sternal segment, and do not appear aggressive (Figure 14.5).

The vertebral bodies of the thoracic spine articulate with the ribs on both the right and left sides. The ribs are uniform in mineral opacity and articulate ventrally with the costal cartilage at the costochondral junction (Figure 14.6). The costal cartilage will mineralize early on in the animal's life so that a uniform mineral opaque structure is present that articulates with the sternum or with other costal cartilages caudally. The costochondral junctions can undergo enlargement and degenerative changes, creating an extrapleural sign (Box 14.1, Figure 14.7). Bassett hounds routinely have an extrapleural sign on lateral, ventrodorsal or dorsoventral radiographs (Figure 14.8).

Aggressive lesions of the vertebral bodies, disc spaces, ribs, and sternum are characterized by osteolysis and cortical disruption. Vertebral body tumors can be lytic and result in vertebral body collapse and a compression fracture (Figure 14.9). Discospondylitis is an infection of the intervertebral disc space. The radiographic features of discospondylitis include intervertebral disc space narrowing/collapse, endplate lysis of the caudal and cranial aspects of the vertebral bodies at the intervertebral disc space, and osseous proliferation associated with the vertebral bodies in an attempt to wall off the infectious agent (Figure 14.10) [1]. Infections of the intersternebral disc spaces have similar radiographic abnormalities. *Nocardia* and

*Actinomyces* sp. infections have been described involving the sternum, vertebrae, pleural space, and the different lung lobes, particularly the accessory lung lobe (Figure 14.11). Primary tumors or secondary soft tissue tumors with sternebral involvement also occur (Figure 14.12).

Common rib abnormalities include fractures and tumors. Acute rib fractures can be seen as breaks in the cortices of the rib with displacement of one margin of the fracture relative to the other (Figure 14.13). Chronic rib fractures are characterized by varying degrees of callus formation and healing (Figure 14.13). Chronic rib fractures can also be seen in dogs and cats with *thoracic bellows* secondary to chronic pulmonary or pleural space abnormalities (Figure 14.14).

Rib tumors can occur anywhere along the osseous portion of the rib and the most common rib tumor is an osteosarcoma. Radiographic features of rib tumors are summarized in Box 14.2. The lesion is aggressive with an expansile appearance that results in cortical lysis (Figures 14.15 and 14.16). Varying degrees of osseous proliferation may be present with an aggressive amorphous appearance. A pleural effusion may or may not be present (Figure 14.17). Metastasis of the primary rib tumor to the lungs can occur. Secondary or metastatic neoplasia of the vertebrae and ribs is common in adenocarcinomas that have osseous metastatic changes (Figure 14.18). A differential for this pattern of metastasis is multiple myeloma (Figure 14.19).

Thoracic wall masses may also be present. Most commonly these are lipomas. Differentials for a thoracic wall mass would include all differentials for a space-occupying mass such as neoplasia, abscess/infection, hemorrhage, or hematoma.

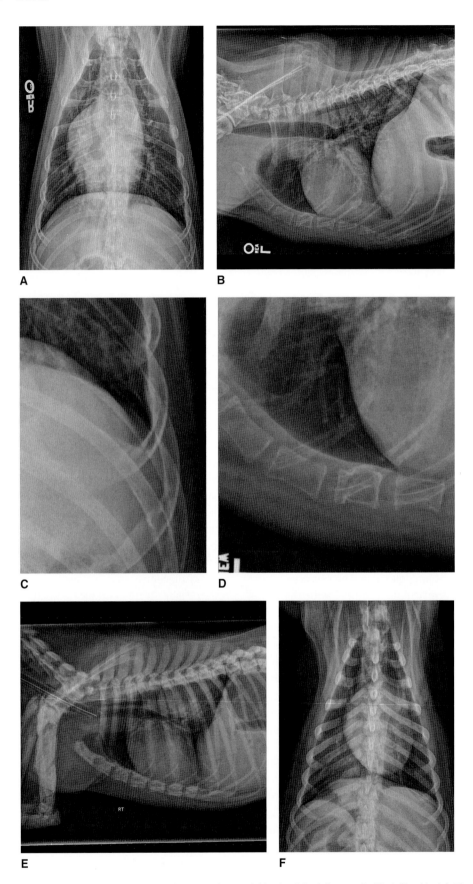

**FIGURE 14.4** Ten-year-old Labrador with an aggressive lesion in the caudal body of the left scapula (ill-defined lysis). There are multiple areas of osseous expansion and extrapleural signs involving the ribs (**A,B**, with close-ups in **C,D**). In addition, there is a compression, pathologic fracture of the fourth sternebrae. These changes were all secondary to a primary osteosarcoma of the left scapula with metastatic disease to other osseous structures including the ribs and sternum. In (**E**) and (**F**), there is a right-sided pulmonary mass in this 12-year-old MN Havenese. This was a primary lung tumor. In addition, there is extreme periosteal reaction that is smooth along all the bones included in the images. These reactions are consistent with hypertrophic osteopathy.

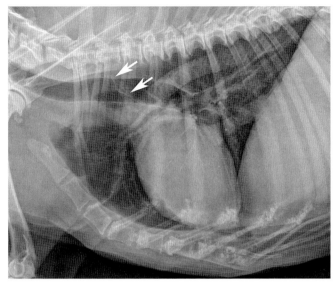
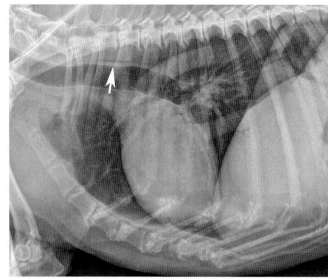

**A**      **B**

**FIGURE 14.5**   Ten-year-old MN boxer with multifocal areas of degenerative change. These include glenohumeral, elbow, costochondral, intersternebral, sternocostal, and intervertebral disc degenerative changes. These changes are seen on both the right (**A**) and left lateral (**B**) images and primarily consist of osteoproliferative changes without aggressive areas of lysis or osseous destruction. Notice there is a small amount of gas present within the cranial thoracic esophagus on the left lateral image (**B**; white arrow). This results in a "tracheoesophageal stripe sign" (combination of the dorsal wall of the trachea and the ventral wall of the esophagus that border efface with each other). On the right lateral image, there is a focal linear area of plate-like atelectasis (white arrow) superimposed over the trachea, that represents atelectasis along subpleural margins of the right and/or left cranial lung lobes.

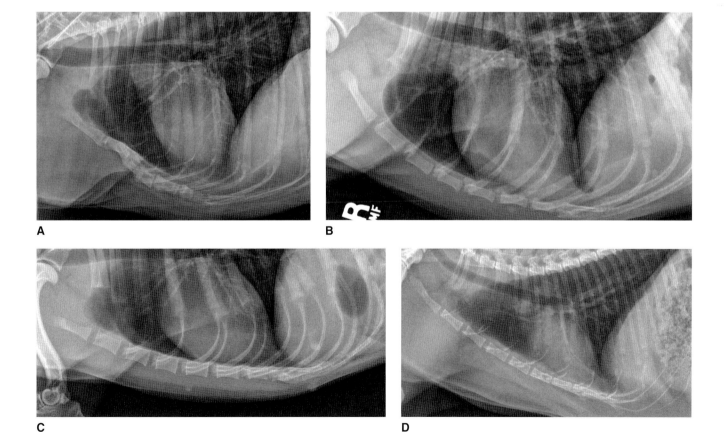

**A**      **B**

**C**      **D**

**FIGURE 14.6**   Right lateral images from various dogs (**A–C**) and a cat (**D**). (**A**) Seven-year-old dog with congenital malformation of the sternum including elongation of the manubrium, fusion of the second, third, fourth, and fifth sternebral segments. These are considered incidental findings. (**B**) Two-year-old dog with mineralization of the costal cartilages and normal sternebral development. Note the lack of complete mineralization of the first set of costal cartilages that can be a common finding in younger dogs and cats. (**C**) Similar changes seen in a different dog that was 3 years old. (**D**) Normal sternal and costal cartilage appearance in an 11-year-old cat.

## Box 14.1 The Extrapleural Sign.

Defined as the indentation of the pleural space by an extrathoracic structure resulting in added opacity over the lung fields at the indentation. The most common cause of an extrapleural sign is secondary to costochondral changes seen in chondrodystrophic dog breeds such as the bassett hound.

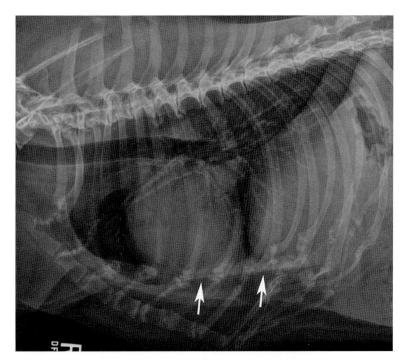

**FIGURE 14.7**   Right lateral radiograph from a 9-year-old bassett hound. Note the costochondral degenerative changes with irregular mineralization and indentation of the pleural space such that an extrapleural sign is noted along the ventral caudal thorax (white arrows). Degenerative ventral spondylosis deformans is noted in the cranial thoracic vertebrae.

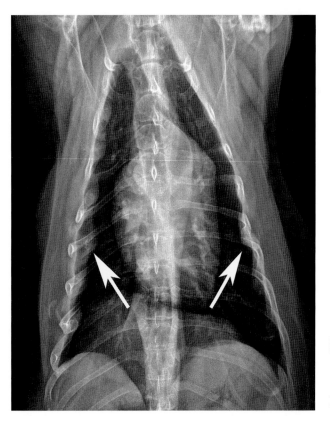

**FIGURE 14.8**   Ventrodorsal radiograph from an 8-year-old bassett hound. There is increased soft tissue opacity noted along the lateral margins of the thorax because of the indentation from the costochondral junctions (white arrows). Benign soft tissue mineralization is noted lateral to the right seventh intercostal space.

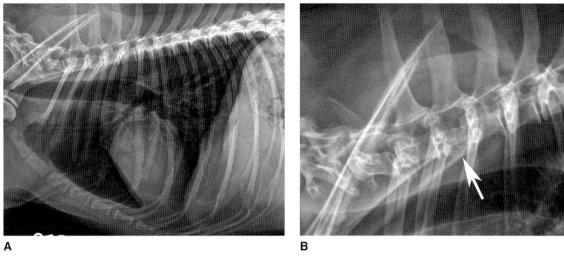

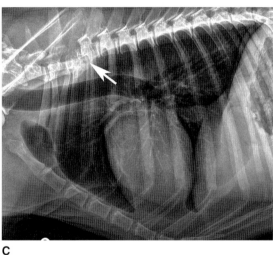

**FIGURE 14.9** Right lateral thoracic (**A**) and close-up (**B**) radiographs from a 7-year-old German shepherd with a compression fracture of T2 (white arrow). This was secondary to a primary bone tumor. In (**A**) there is a decrease in size of the pulmonary vasculature and cardiac silhouette consistent with hypovolemia. (**C**) Compression fracture luxation of T2 with dorsal displacement of the caudal thoracic vertebral column relative to T2 (white arrow). There is osteolysis of T2 with lysis of the lamina and spinous process. This was secondary to a primary bone tumor (osteosarcoma). There is a decrease in pulmonary vascular and cardiac silhouette size consistent with hypovolemia.

# Diaphragm

The diaphragm consists of three parts: the central dome or cupula, and the right and left diaphragmatic crura. The right and left crura insert along the ventral aspect of the L3 and L4 vertebral bodies, resulting in a thinner cortex when compared with the surrounding lumbar vertebral bodies (Figure 14.20). The cranial surface of the diaphragm is easily visualized due to the lung–soft tissue interface. The caudal surface of the diaphragm is not visualized due to border effacement with the liver, gall bladder, and stomach (see Chapter 13 for differences in appearances of the diaphragmatic crura on orthogonal radiographic projections). Ventrally, the caudal border of the diaphragm (cupula, centrally) can be visualized due to fat within the falciform ligament (Figure 14.21). A large amount of fat is often seen in obese

cats in the falciform ligament, the lateral and dorsal thoracic wall and in the pleural space surrounding the cardiac silhouette.

Diaphragmatic integrity is usually assessed based on smooth pleural surfaces and lack of cranial displacement of abdominal organs/viscera into the pleural space in the area of a ruptured diaphragm. Diaphragmatic rupture is the most common abnormality of the diaphragm seen (Figure 14.22). Ruptures of the diaphragm tend to involve the lateral margins (crura) of the diaphragm. The radiographic features of a diaphragmatic rupture are summarized in Box 14.3. True congenital hernias of the lateral aspect of the diaphragm are rare. Although uncommon, a central defect in the normal formation of the cupula portion of the diaphragm (*septum transversum*) will lead to a peritoneopericardial diaphragmatic hernia (Figures 14.23 and 14.24). The radiographic features of a peritoneopericardial diaphragmatic hernia are summarized in Box 14.4.

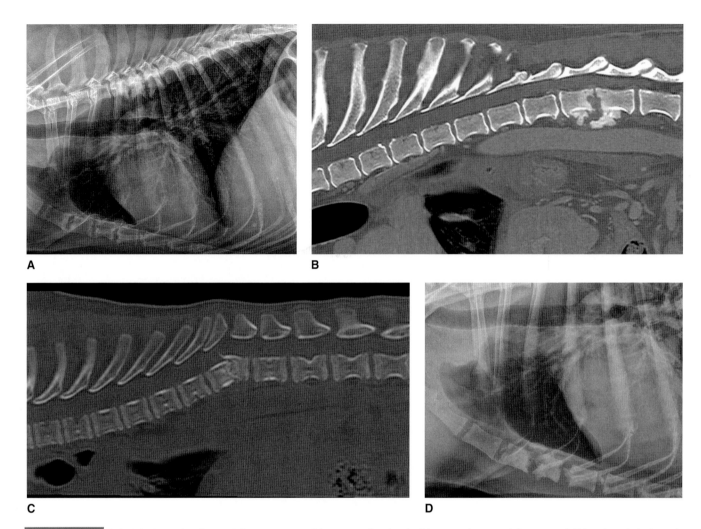

A    B

C    D

**FIGURE 14.10** (**A**) Right lateral radiograph from a 7-year-old German shepherd with several areas of discospondylitis. There is lysis and osteoproliferation associated with the endplates of T4–5 and T5–6. Collapse of the intervertebral disc spaces is present. (**B,C**) Sagittal reconstructions from CT studies from two different dogs with discospondylitis. In (**B**) there is collapse of the T12–13 intervertebral disc space with endplate lysis and ventral periosteal proliferation that is irregular extending from the endplate to the midbody of each vertebra. In (**C**) there is collapse of the T9–10 intervertebral disc space, endplate lysis and subluxation of T10 relative to T9 with angulation being noted at the site. There is some sclerosis noted within the T9 and T10 vertebral bodies. (**D**) There is lysis of the endplates noted between the third and fourth sternal segments with surrounding osteosclerosis and ill-defined periosteal reaction. This was secondary to *Aspergillus* sp. infection.

Diaphragmatic thickening has been described in dogs and cats with muscular dystrophy (Figure 14.25). Other features of muscular dystrophy in dogs and cats include hyperinflation, gastroesophageal intussusceptions, hiatal hernias, and aspiration pneumonia.

Diaphragmatic asymmetry can be an indicator of a phrenic nerve abnormality on a given side with cranial displacement of that crus on all radiographic projections. This can be confirmed by lack of motion of the affected crus using fluoroscopy. Diaphragmatic tenting can be seen in dogs and cats that are hyperinflated as the soft tissue curvilinear attachments of the ventral aspect of the diaphragm with the costal arches (Figure 14.26).

In addition, abdominal masses that are right or left sided or central in position can displace the area of the diaphragm involved cranially. In extremely obese dogs with Pickwickian syndrome, the diaphragm is cranially displaced due to a lack of ventilation (as seen on comparative inspiratory and expiratory radiographs). Diaphragmatic eventration is a focal abnormality of the diaphragm where the diaphragmatic muscle has thinned or torn but the pleural and peritoneal margins remain intact (Figure 14.27).

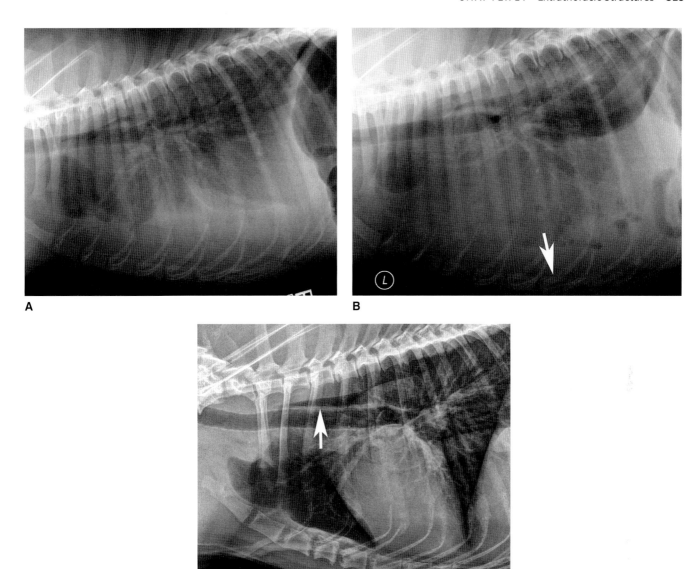

**FIGURE 14.11** *Actinomyces* infection with accessory lung lobe mass, pleural effusion with gas (abscess on the left lateral) and smooth periosteal reaction noted along the dorsal aspect of the seventh sternebrae ((**A**) – right lateral, (**B**) – left lateral with white arrow over S7). (**C**) Left lateral radiograph from a dog with intersternebral infections at S3–4 and S4–5. Endplate lysis, irregularity, and sclerosis are present. There is mild soft tissue thickening noted dorsal to these areas along the ventral pleural margins. A focal accumulation of gas is present, resulting in a tracheal esophageal stripe sign (white arrow; soft tissue linear shadow of the dorsal wall of the trachea and ventral wall of the esophagus that are border effaced due to both being soft tissue opacity).

# Cranial Abdomen

The cranial abdomen that is evaluated on thoracic radiographs includes the liver, tail of the spleen, the stomach, and possibly the kidneys and transverse colon. In addition, the overall serosal detail of the cranial abdomen can be assessed. Severe abdominal effusion or cranial abdominal masses (such as hepatic) can result in cranial displacement of diaphragm and an overall decrease in thoracic volume even though an attempt was made to obtain the radiographs on peak inspiration

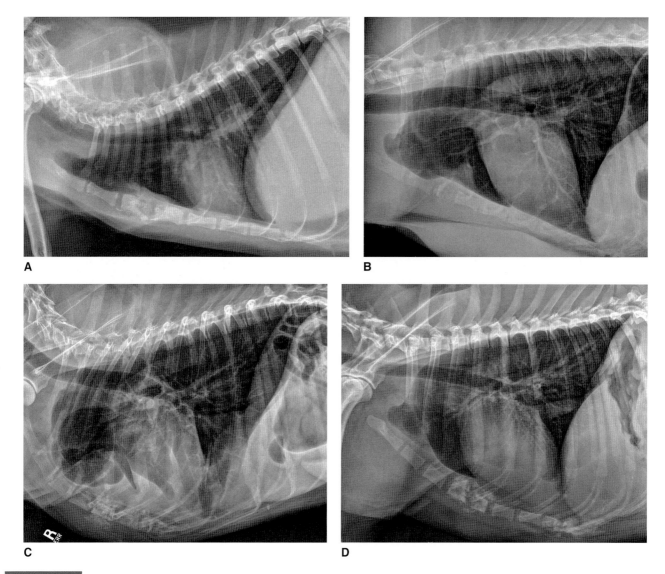

**FIGURE 14.12** Multiple lateral thoracic radiographic examples of neoplastic and infectious processes involving the sternum. (**A**) Focal soft tissue mass with osteolysis and proliferation of the third sternebrae. Changes involving the fourth sternebrae are also noted. There is focal soft tissue opacity along the floor of the thoracic cavity/pleural space at the sternal abnormalities. These were secondary to a fibrosarcoma with invasion of the sternebrae and thorax. (**B**) There is lysis and collapse of the third sternebral segment. A focal soft tissue mass is noted extending into the ventral thorax. These changes were secondary to an osteosarcoma of the third sternebral segment. (**C**) A focal osteoproliferative lesion of the fifth sternebral segment with an associated ventral pleural mass and pleural effusion. (**D**) There is a focal soft tissue mass effect with involvement of the fourth and fifth sternebral segments. There is osteolysis and osteoproliferation of these sternebrae and ill-defined periosteal reaction surrounding the sternal segments that are involved. This tumor was a histiocytic sarcoma.

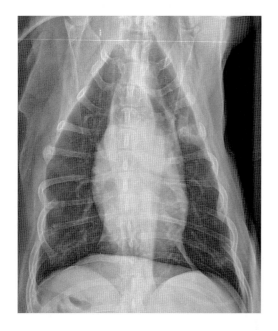

**FIGURE 14.13** Ventrodorsal image from a dog with generalized osteopenia secondary to chronic Cushing disease. There are multiple rib fractures that are acute (sharply marginated without periosteal reaction) and chronic fractures (ill-defined margins, callus formation) and extrapleural signs noted on both the left and right sides.

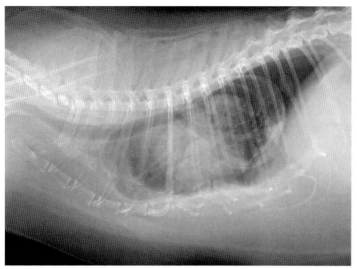
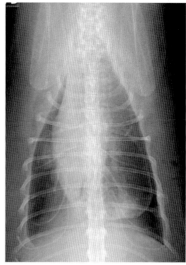

**A**        **B**

**FIGURE 14.14** Thoracic bellows with chronic rib fractures resulting from a chronic pleural effusion (chylothorax) with a restrictive pleuritis and thickening of the visceral pleura, particularly surrounding the left caudal lung lobe. The lung lobe is restricted by the pleural thickening so that it will not reinflate when the air is withdrawn from the pleural space (pneumothorax). Several gas opacities are noted adjacent to the left side of the thorax consistent with prior thoracocentesis.

---

**Box 14.2** Radiographic Features of Primary Rib Tumors.

1. Extrapleural sign at the site of the lesion
2. Aggressive expansile osseous changes with cortical lysis
3. Varying degrees of osteoproliferation, often with an aggressive amorphous appearance

4. ± Pleural effusion
5. Intra- and extrathoracic extension with soft tissue mass effect

---

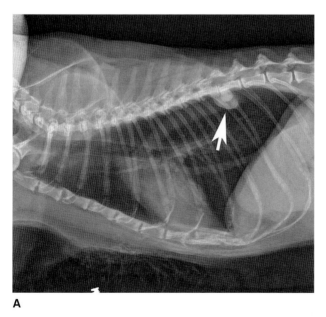
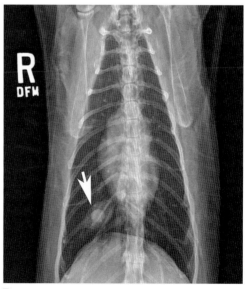

**A**        **B**

**FIGURE 14.15** Right lateral (**A**) and ventrodorsal (**B**) thoracic radiographs. Focal osteosclerotic lesion associated with the dorsal body of the right 10th rib from an 11-year-old DSH (white arrows). There is smooth periosteal proliferation surrounding the central mineral opaque structures associated with the rib. This was resected and determined to be an osteosarcoma in this cat. There is no radiographic evidence of pulmonary metastatic disease.

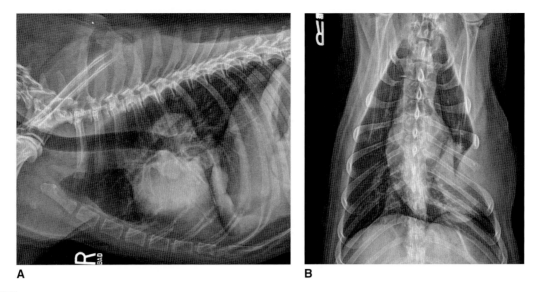

**FIGURE 14.16** Right lateral (**A**) and ventrodorsal (**B**) thoracic radiographs from an 8-year-old dog with a left thoracic wall mass. There is complete lysis associated with the left fifth rib centrally with a mass effect extending into the left pleural space. A lobulated soft tissue mass was also present within the caudal segment of the left cranial lung lobe and the ventral segment of the left caudal lobe. The rib mass was determined to be an osteosarcoma with multiple pulmonary metastatic lesions.

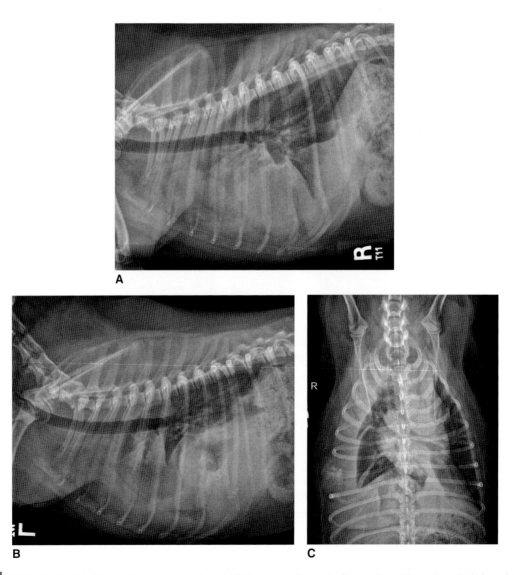

**FIGURE 14.17** Right lateral (**A**), left lateral (**B**), and ventrodorsal (**C**) thoracic radiographs from a dog with a right-sided pleural effusion (retractions of the lung lobes, multiple pleural fissure lines, soft tissue opacity border effacing the cardiac silhouette and the diaphragm). There is an irregular ill-defined area of osteoproliferation associated with the right eighth rib with areas of lysis at the level of the described changes. The rib mass was resected and was an osteosarcoma on histology.

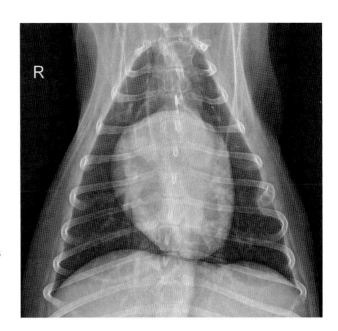

**FIGURE 14.18** Ventrodorsal thoracic radiograph from a 10-year-old terrier that presented for a transitional cell (urothelial) carcinoma. There is a focal expansile, osteolytic lesion of the left sixth rib with an extrapleural sign. An ultrasound-guided aspirate of this lesion was determined to be carcinoma on cytology, presumed to be metastatic from the known urogenital neoplasm.

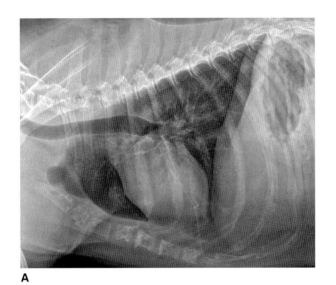

**A**

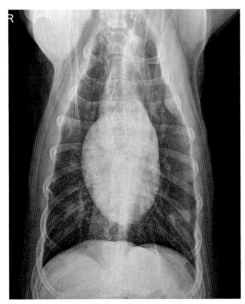

**B**

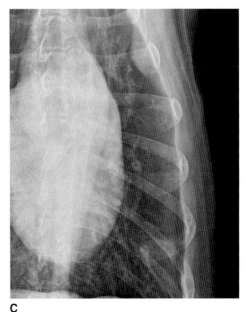

**C**

**FIGURE 14.19** Right lateral (**A**), ventrodorsal (**B**), and close-up ventrodorsal (**C**) thoracic radiographs from a 5-year-old Shetland sheepdog. There are multiple osteolytic lesions of the thoracic spine, sternum, and ribs. On the close-up, ventrodorsal image there are numerous expansile, osteolytic lesions associated with the left ribs. An extrapleural sign is present involving the left third rib secondary to an expansile lesion. These changes were confirmed to be multiple myeloma.

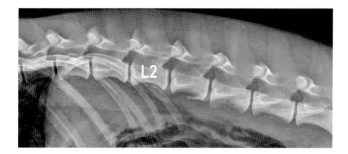

**FIGURE 14.20**    Lateral lumbar spine radiograph from a dog that shows the ill-defined appearance of the L3 and L4 vertebral bodies (L2 is marked), compared with the ventral bodies of the adjacent lumbar vertebra. These are normal changes, seen primarily in dogs, associated with the attachment of the diaphragmatic crura to the ventral aspect of L3 and L4.

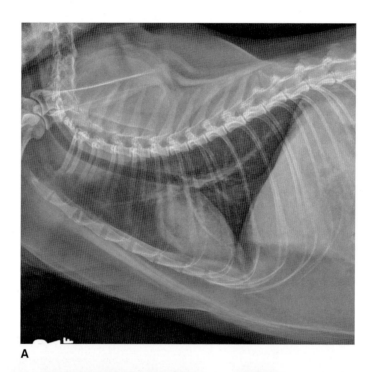

A

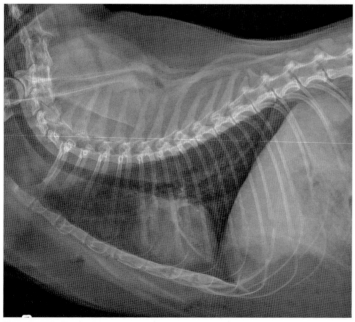

B

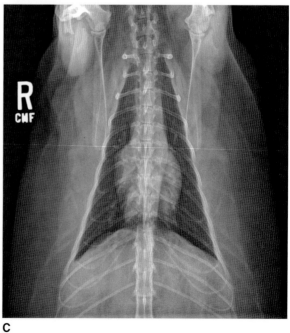

C

**FIGURE 14.21**    Right lateral (**A**), left lateral (**B**), and ventrodorsal thoracic (**C**) radiographs from an obese cat. There is fat deposition within the falciform ligament (such that the caudal surface of the diaphragm can be seen), the ventral pleural space surrounding the cardiac silhouette and the lateral and dorsal soft tissues of the thoracic wall.

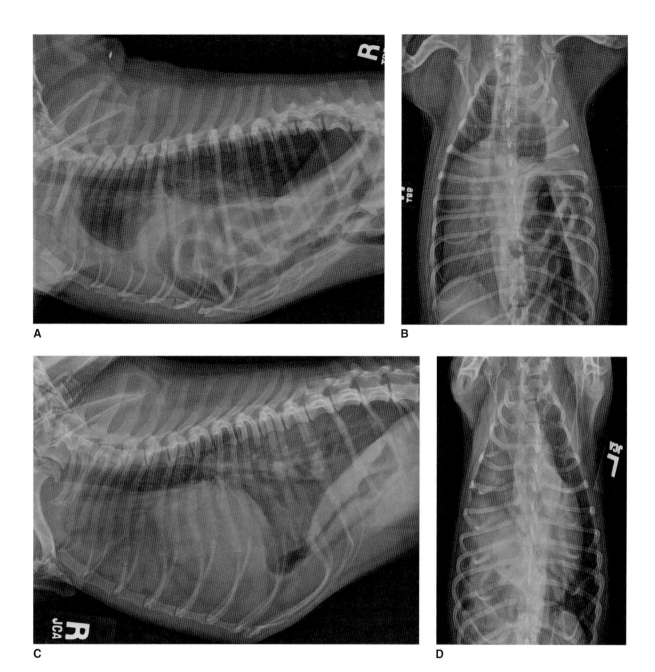

**FIGURE 14.22** Two cases of posttrauma diaphragmatic ruptures. Case 1: Right lateral (**A**) and ventrodorsal (**B**) images from a dog post trauma. There is disruption of the left diaphragm with cranial displacement of small bowel that is abnormally gas distended. There is a contralateral mediastinal shift of the cardiac silhouette on the ventrodorsal image. There is a mild volume of left-sided pleural effusion with some atelectasis of the left lung lobes. Case 2: Right lateral (**C**) and ventrodorsal (**D**) images from a dog post trauma. There is a right-sided diaphragmatic rupture with cranial displacement of liver, fat, small intestines (fluid filled and best seen on the right lateral), and stomach. There is a leftward contralateral mediastinal shift of the cardiac silhouette. Chronic rib fractures are noted involving the left 7th–11th ribs with callus formation.

---

## Box 14.3 Radiographic Features of A Diaphragmatic Rupture.

1. Space-occupying mass effect in the right or left pleural space, resulting in separation of the lungs away from the thoracic wall

2. Contralateral mediastinal shift of the cardiac silhouette away from the displaced abdominal viscera in the pleural space

3. Cranial displacement of the gastric axis

4. Loss of visualization or absence of normal abdominal structures in the cranial abdomen

5. Border effacement of the diaphragmatic margins with abdominal viscera

6. ± Pleural effusion

7. Appearance of abdominal structures in the thorax

8. Loss of normal margins of the diaphragm with abnormal bulges in the area of defect

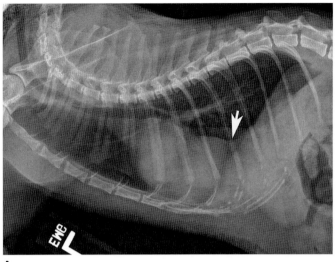
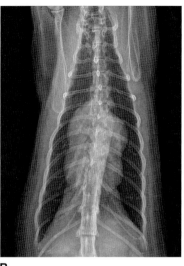

**A**                                                **B**

**FIGURE 14.23**   Right lateral (**A**) and ventrodorsal (**B**) thoracic images from a 4-year-old DSH. There is a soft tissue mass effect that border effaces the caudal cardiac silhouette and cranial border of the diaphragm. There is a dorsal peritoneal pericardial mesothelial remnant (white arrow on the lateral image) noted ventral to the caudal vena cava margin. These changes are consistent with a peritoneal pericardial diaphragmatic hernia. On thoracic ultrasound, a liver lobe and gall bladder were noted in the caudal aspect of the pericardium adjacent to the heart. Abnormalities of the caudal sternum are not seen (incidental finding of a fused manubrium and second sternebral segment).

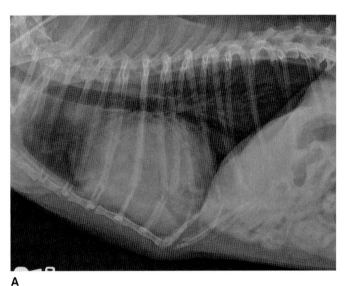
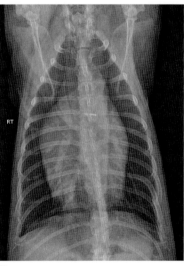

**A**                                                **B**

**FIGURE 14.24**   Peritoneal pericardial diaphragmatic hernia in a dog. There is differential soft tissue and fat opacity within the enlarged cardiac silhouette (generalized enlargement). There is dorsal elevation of the trachea. There is microhepatia noted in the cranial abdomen. Ventral spondylosis deformans is noted at the thoracolumbar junction.

---

## Box 14.4 Radiographic Features of A Peritoneopericardial Diaphragmatic Hernia.

1. Confluence between the caudal cardiac silhouette and the cranial aspect of the diaphragm

2. Cranial displacement of the gastric axis

3. Differential opacities within the cardiac silhouette that may include fat, soft tissue structures (spleen), and/or gastrointestinal tract with fluid/gas

4. Enlargement of the cardiac silhouette with abnormal shapes that do not correspond with specific chamber enlargement patterns

5. Presence of the dorsal peritoneopericardial mesothelial remnant (DPMR) ventral to or superimposed over the caudal vena cava in the cat

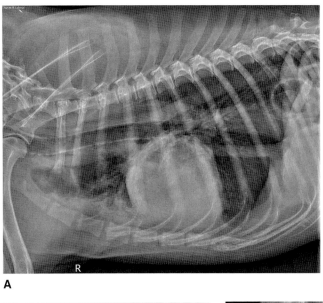

**A**

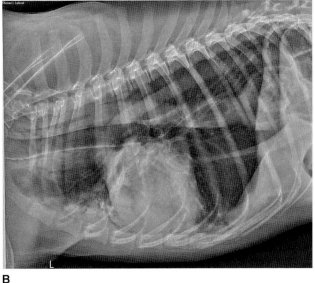

**B**

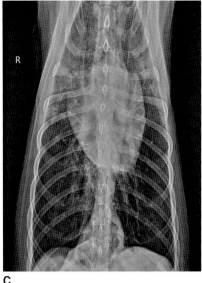

**C**

**FIGURE 14.25**   Right lateral (**A**), left lateral (**B**), and ventrodorsal (**C**) radiographs from a German shepherd with muscular dystrophy. There is a gastroesophageal intussusception, pneumomediastinum, fluid-filled esophagus, focal alveolar pulmonary pattern within the ventral aspect of the right and left cranial lung lobes, and hyperinflation of the lung lobes. Source: Courtesy of Dr Christine Gremillion.

(Figure 14.28). Hepatic masses are generally focal and result in caudal displacement of the gastric axis. Differentials for hepatic masses include primary tumors such as adenoma (hepatoma), hepatocellular carcinoma, or hemangiosarcoma. Secondary tumors of the liver include any of the round cell neoplasms such as lymphoma or histiocytic sarcoma or metastatic neoplasia.

A pneumoperitoneum should be evaluated for on both lateral and ventrodorsal/dorsoventral images. Recognition of a pneumoperitoneum would include gas between the liver and the abdominal surface of the diaphragm, gas outlining any cranial abdominal structure, and small gas bubbles present in the cranioventral abdomen that are not contained within the gastrointestinal tract (Figure 14.29).

Changes in opacity within the liver include gas within the gall bladder and bile ducts (emphysematous cholecystitis),

rounded mineral opacities in the gall bladder, and curvilinear mineral opacities present throughout the hepatic parenchyma that represent dystrophic mineralization of the biliary tree (Figure 14.30). Liver changes primarily deal with microhepatia, hepatomegaly or focal hepatic mass(es) (Figure 14.31). Hepatomegaly can be difficult to identify on thoracic radiographs as the radiographs were made on peak inspiration, meaning that the caudoventral margin of the liver extends beyond the costal arch and may even extend beyond the margin of collimation. If hepatomegaly is suspected, abdominal radiographs should be obtained. The most common reason for microhepatia in the dog is congenital macroscopic extra- or intrahepatic portosystemic shunts. In these dogs, the gastric axis is shifted cranially.

Evaluation of the stomach primarily involves changes in size, position, and opacity. A gastric dilation volvulus can be

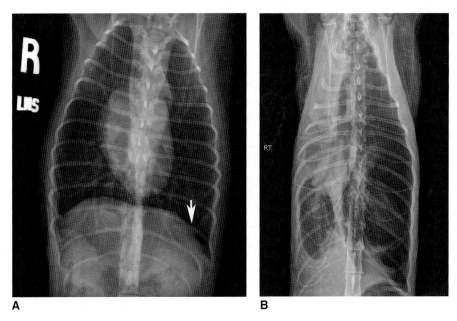

**FIGURE 14.26** Two ventrodorsal radiographs from different cases with some degree of tenting of the ventral margins of the diaphragm. (**A**) Hyperinflation in a dog from an upper airway obstruction. Curvilinear soft tissue opacities are noted along the left border of the diaphragm at their attachments with the costal cartilages (white arrow). A thymic remnant (sail sign) is seen along the left lateral side of the cranial mediastinum just cranial to the cardiac silhouette. (**B**) A tension pneumothorax in a cat post trauma with a severe left-sided pneumothorax. There is flattening and tenting of the left margins of the diaphragm. There is a rightward contralateral mediastinal shift of the remaining thoracic structures with varying degrees of atelectasis of the lung lobes. A mild to moderate right-sided pleural effusion is also present.

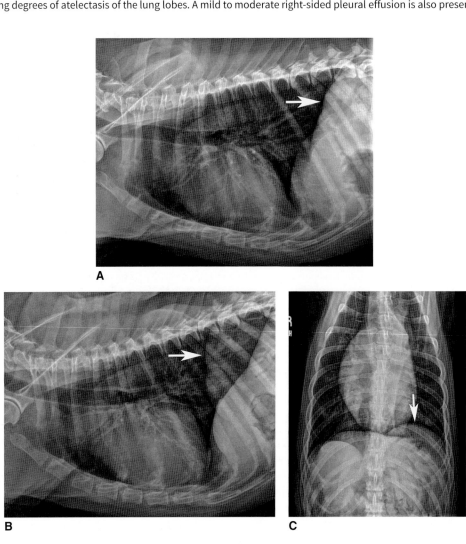

**FIGURE 14.27** Right lateral (**A**), left lateral (**B**), and ventrodorsal (**C**) radiographs from a golden retriever with diaphragmatic eventration (see text for details; white arrows). There is a cranial bulge in the left diaphragmatic crus on all three images. This was secondary to tearing or thinning of the diaphragmatic musculature but an intact pleural and peritoneal mesothelial lining so that actual herniation of abdominal contents into the pleural space was not present.

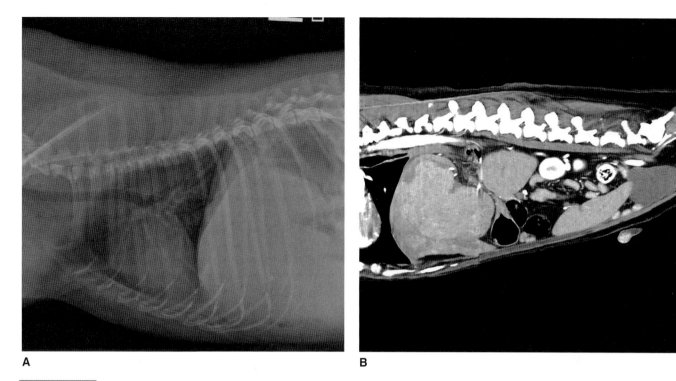

**FIGURE 14.28**   (**A**) Right lateral thoracic image where the radiograph is expiratory in nature due to a large hepatic mass with cranial displacement diaphragm and caudal displacement of the gastric silhouette. (**B**) Sagittal CT reconstruction of a central hepatic mass (with contrast enhancement) displacing the diaphragm cranially.

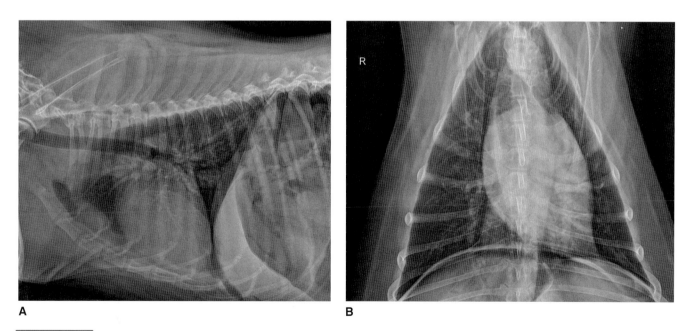

**FIGURE 14.29**   Right lateral (**A**) and ventrodorsal (**B**) radiographs from a dog with a pneumoperitoneum secondary rupture of an intestinal tumor. There is a large amount of gas within the peritoneal space caudal to the diaphragm and outlining various abdominal structures. There is moderate enlargement of the sternal lymph node consistent with abdominal disease (soft tissue opacity within the cranial thorax dorsal to the second and third sternebrae).

seen on thoracic radiographs (Figure 14.32; see Chapter 25). Foreign bodies can be seen within the stomach, and one should always compare the right and left laterals for visualization of the pylorus and gas surrounding any abnormalities within the pylorus on the left lateral view (Figure 14.33; see Chapter 25).

# Summary

The extrathoracic structures represent a large component of the thoracic radiograph and need to be assessed individually and thoroughly. The ability to detect radiographic abnormalities is

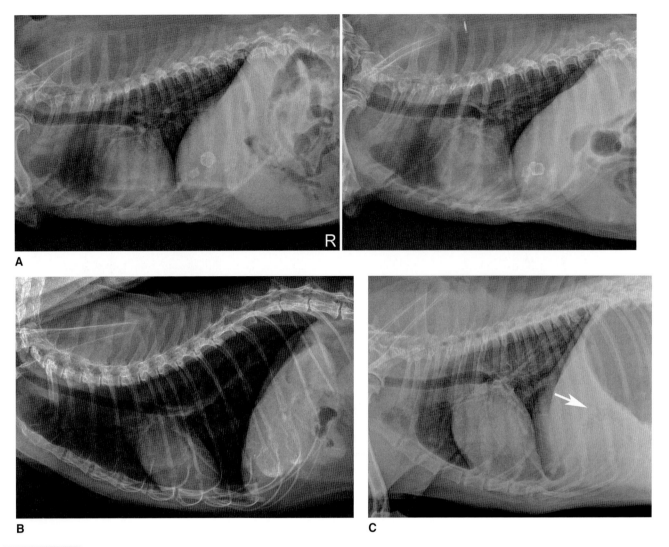

**FIGURE 14.30** Three examples of varying opacities (abnormal) within the hepatic parenchyma from different cases. (**A**) Several large mineral opaque calculi are present within the gall bladder. (**B**) Multiple curvilinear mineral opacities present within the liver in this cat consistent with mineralization of the biliary tree. There is also mineral opaque material noted in the ventral aspect of the gall bladder. (**C**) Multifocal gas opacities (white arrow) seen superimposed over the hepatic silhouette consistent with a hepatic abscess from a dog.

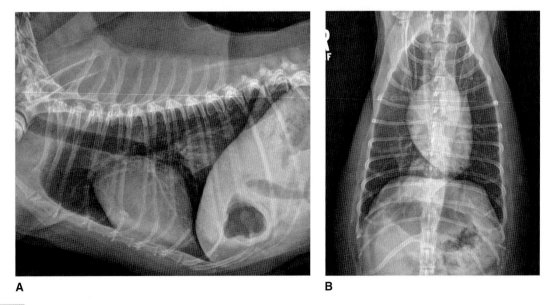

**FIGURE 14.31** Left lateral (**A**) and ventrodorsal (**B**) thoracic radiographs from a poodle with microhepatia. The liver is small with cranial displacement of the gastric axis. On the ventrodorsal image, the hepatic parenchyma takes up 1.5 intercostal spaces between the diaphragm and the gastric silhouette. There is a medial right caudal lung lobe mass also present that was diagnosed as a pulmonary adenocarcinoma.

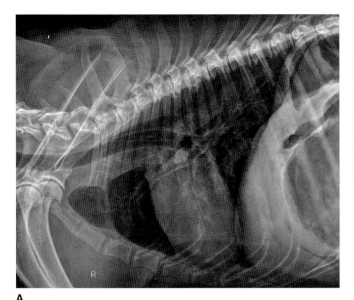

A

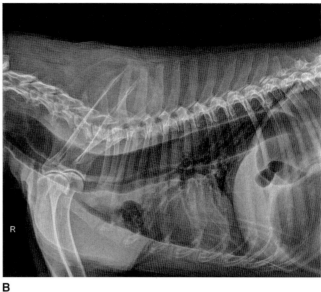

B

**FIGURE 14.32**   Right lateral thoracic radiographs from two different dogs with gastric dilatation volvulus. (**A**) The stomach is gas distended and the pylorus is dorsal and the fundic portion of the stomach is ventral. There is gastric wall thickening and a pneumoperitoneum present. The cardiac silhouette, pulmonary vasculature, and caudal vena cava are small, consistent with hypovolemia. There is some gas noted in the thoracic esophagus dorsal to the trachea at the heart base. Ventral spondylosis deformans of the thoracic spine and degenerative changes of the glenohumeral joints are present. (**B**) Similar changes are noted involving the stomach. There is generalized gas distension of the cervical and thoracic esophagus with ventral displacement of the trachea and cardiac silhouette. Focal unstructured interstitial pulmonary changes are present in the cranioventral thorax. Multiple skinfold artifacts are present superimposed over the mid to caudal thorax.

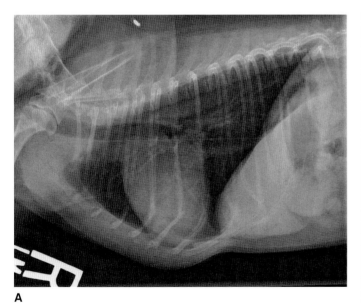

A

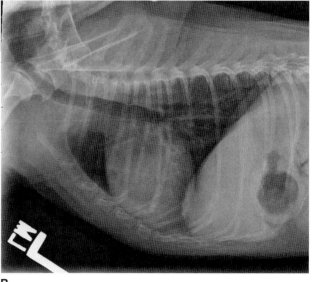

B

**FIGURE 14.33**   Right lateral (**A**) and left lateral (**B**) thoracic radiographs from a dog. On the right lateral, there is fluid within the pylorus creating a rounded soft tissue opacity that might be mistaken for a foreign body or cranial abdominal mass. On the left lateral, there is gas in the pylorus consistent with normal air distribution in the right side of the stomach. A pyloric "ball" is not seen.

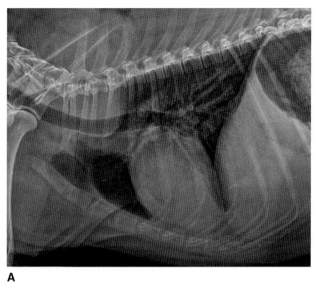
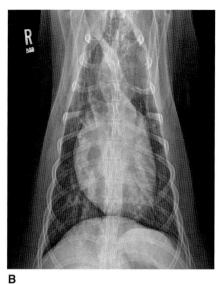

**A**  **B**

**FIGURE 14.34**   Right lateral (**A**) and ventrodorsal (**B**) radiographs from a dog with rib tumor. There is a focal soft tissue opacity noted that displaces the trachea on the right lateral view. On the ventrodorsal image, there is a missing rib (complete lysis) noted dorsally near the vertebral body (second left rib) with a mass effect and rightward deviation of the trachea and cranial mediastinum.

based on careful inspection of these structures. Of all the structures, lesions within the ribs are usually the most difficult to identify as these lesions can be purely lytic and missing information on the radiograph is easy to overlook (Figure 14.34).

# Reference

1.   Kirberger, R.M. (2016). Early diagnostic imaging findings in juvenile dogs with presumed diskospondylitis: 10 cases (2008–2014). *J. Am. Vet. Med. Assoc.* 249 (5): 539–546.

# CHAPTER 15

# Pleural Space

**Clifford R. Berry[1] and Elodie E. Huguet[2]**

[1] Department of Molecular Biomedical Sciences, College of Veterinary Medicine, North Carolina State University, Raleigh, NC, USA
[2] Department of Small Animal Clinical Sciences, College of Veterinary Medicine, University of Florida, Gainesville, FL, USA

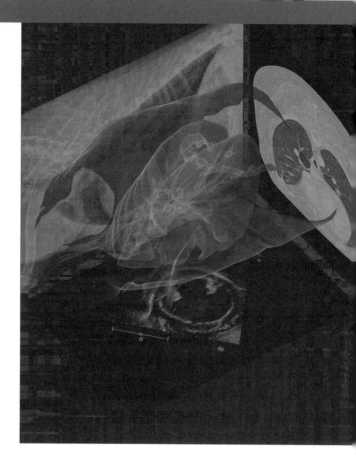

## Overview

The pleural space is a potential space in the right and left hemithorax created by the serosal mesothelial lining of the thoracic cavity. The pleural space is located on both the right and left sides of the thorax and is bounded by the parietal pleura, along the inside of the thoracic body wall, diaphragm and mediastinum and the visceral pleura covering the surface of the lungs [1–7]. The right and left visceral pleurae reflect at the pulmonary hilum and join with the parietal pleurae, which forms the mediastinum (the space between the right and left pleural cavities) [1–7]. This chapter describes the normal pleural space and abnormalities of the pleural space.

## Pleural Anatomy and Physiology

The normal pleural cavities represent a potential space, and in the healthy animal, a small amount of pleural fluid is spread over the pleural surface to facilitate the sliding motion between the visceral and parietal pleura as the lungs expand and contract during normal respiration.

The visceral pleura lines the lung lobes, including the surface of the lung lobes that form the interlobar fissures (the space between different lung lobes on each side of the thorax), so that the visceral pleurae of adjacent lung lobes are in contact with each other. These interlobar fissures have a specific anatomic

*Atlas of Small Animal Diagnostic Imaging*, First Edition. Edited by Clifford R. Berry, Nathan C. Nelson, and Matthew D. Winter.
© 2023 John Wiley & Sons, Inc. Published 2023 by John Wiley & Sons, Inc.
Companion website: www.wiley.com/go/berry/atlas

location for the divisions between the right cranial and right middle, right middle and right caudal, cranial and caudal subsegments of the left cranial and between the left cranial and left caudal lung lobes (Box 15.1; Figure 15.1). In addition, there is a special fold of pleura in the accessory lung lobe called the *plica vena cava* that incorporates the caudal vena cava from the level of the diaphragm to its insertion in the caudal aspect of the right atrium along the caudodorsal margin of the cardiac silhouette. *The normal pleural space is not visualized on thoracic radiographs in the dog and cat.*

# Abnormalities of the Pleural Space

Some basic questions that could be asked about the pleural space would include the following.

- Is there a pleural effusion?
- Is there a pneumothorax?
- Is there a diaphragmatic rupture (covered in the section on the thorax, Chapter 14)?
- Is there a pleural mass or extrapleural sign?

Each of these changes has specific Roentgen signs and will be reviewed.

## Pleural Effusion

Abnormal fluid accumulation within the pleural space is called a *pleural effusion*. In order to be detected on thoracic radiographs, a certain threshold of fluid needs to be present.

The Roentgen signs of pleural effusion are summarized in Box 15.2. In acute pleural effusions, the most common Roentgen signs will include retraction of the lung lobes away from the thoracic wall, a decrease in the overall volume present within each lung lobe, leaf-like appearance of the lung lobe, presence of soft tissue between the thoracic wall (parietal pleural surface) and the visceral pleural surface along the lung lobes, widened interlobar fissures, dorsal elevation of the trachea, and border effacement of the cardiac silhouette and the cranial surface of the diaphragm, particularly ventrally (Figures 15.2–15.4). On a ventrodorsal image, one is more likely to see the interlobar fissures; however, the cardiac silhouette is not border effaced due to the dorsal recumbent positioning and the fluid will collect in the dorsal aspect of the pleural space. However, on a dorsoventral radiograph where the animal is in sternal recumbency, the fluid will collect in the ventral pleural space and thereby result in border effacement of the cardiac silhouette and cranial diaphragmatic cupula (Figure 15.5).

Radiographically, one cannot differentiate between the different causes of pleural effusion (transudate, modified transudate, and exudate). If the effusion is unilateral, then the type of effusion is most likely an exudate, resulting in blockage of normal mediastinal fenestrations between the right and left pleural spaces as noted normally in dogs and cats (Figure 15.6). The most common exudates would include pus, chyle, hemorrhage or a neoplastic effusion. In chronic exudative effusions, particularly pyothorax and chylothorax, the visceral pleural surface can become thickened, resulting in a rounded lung lobe (called a *restrictive pleuritis*; Box 15.3, Figures 15.7 and 15.8). This thickening of the visceral pleura can also block the normal mediastinal fenestrations and restrict the lung lobe from reexpanding when the effusion is removed, also known as a *pleural peel sign*. Additionally, there can be chronic rib fractures

---

**Box 15.1** Location of Interlobar Fissures Based on Intercostal Spaces (ICS). See Figure 15.1G for Anatomic Localization.

**Ventral**

*Right*
Fissure between right cranial and right middle lung lobes – 5th ICS
Fissure between right middle and right caudal lung lobes – 7th ICS

*Left*
Fissure between the cranial and caudal subsegments of the left cranial lung lobes – 4th ICS
Fissure between the left cranial and left caudal lung lobes – 6th ICS

**Dorsal**

*Right*
Fissure between right cranial and right caudal lung lobes – 6th ICS

*Left*
Fissure between the left cranial and left caudal lung lobes – 6th ICS

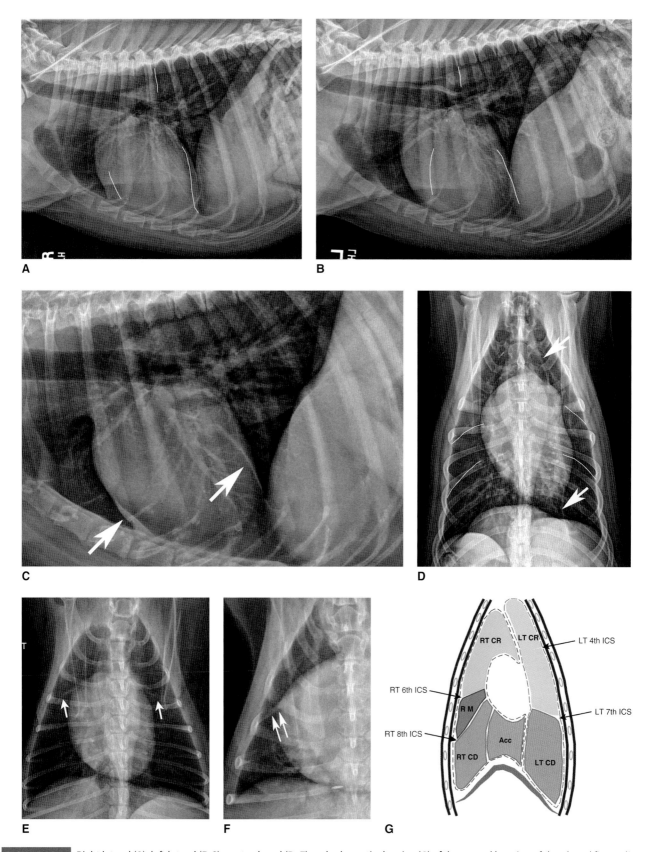

**FIGURE 15.1** Right lateral (**A**), left lateral (**B,C**), ventrodorsal (**D–F**) and schematic drawing (**G**) of the normal location of the pleural fissure lines (white lines on the images) that would be visualized when a pleural effusion or pneumothorax is present in the dog or cat. The pleural fissure lines are in a similar location in the dog and cat (see Box 15.1). In (**C**) there are two fissure lines present (white arrows). The first fissure line is between the right cranial and right middle lung lobes and is not routinely seen. The caudal fissure line is between the right middle and right caudal lung lobe and represents mild effusion, pleural thickening or the pleural fissure being oriented tangential to the x-ray beam and thereby creating a soft tissue opacity. In (**E**) and (**F**), ventrodorsal radiographs from normal dogs document pleural fat localization with the interlobar fissures between the right cranial and right middle and the interlobar fissure between the cranial subsegment and caudal subsegment of the left cranial lung lobe (white arrows). (**G**) Schematic drawing of the location of each of the ventral interlobar fissures relative to the different lung lobes in a dog or a cat.

## Box 15.2 Roentgen Signs of Pleural Effusion.

1. Retraction of lung lobes away from the parietal pleura (thoracic wall)
2. Presence of pleural fissure lines with widening of the peripheral aspect of the interlobar fissures at specific anatomic locations
3. Border effacement of the cardiac silhouette

4. Border effacement of the diaphragm
5. Blunting of the costophrenic angle on the ventrodorsal image
6. Scalloping of the ventral lung margins on the lateral radiographs
7. Border effacement of the ventral cranial mediastinal line

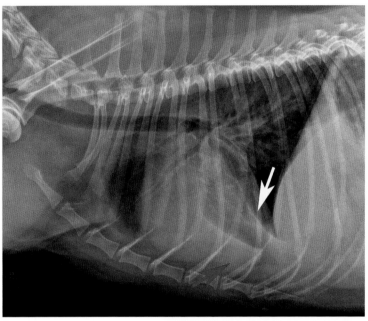

A

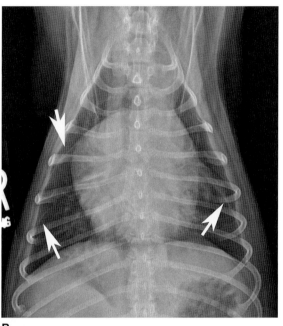

B

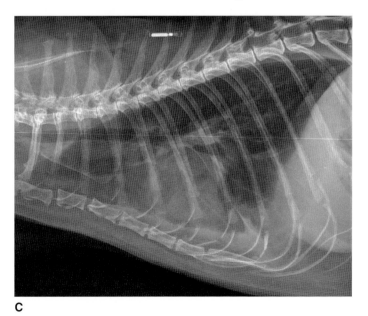

C

**FIGURE 15.2**   Mild pleural effusion: (**A**) right lateral and (**B**) ventrodorsal images from a dog with hypoproteinemia. The effusion results in border effacement of the ventral cardiac silhouette and cranioventral margin of the diaphragm and separation of the interlobar fissures with soft tissue opacity (red and white arrows). (**C**) Right lateral radiograph from a cat with a mild to moderate pleural effusion. Similar features are noted as described for the dog. In this cat, the effusion was determined to be a modified transudate.

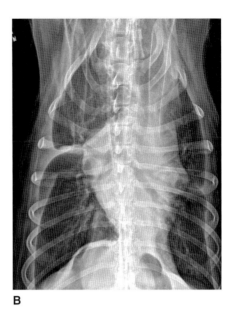

**FIGURE 15.3**  Moderate pleural effusion: right lateral (**A**) and ventrodorsal images (**B**) with multiple pleural fissure lines and retraction of the lung lobes away from the thoracic wall. The cardiac silhouette can be visualized on the VD image and is not enlarged. There is a pneumoperitoneum present consistent with prior surgical intervention. Multiple catheters are in place.

associated with a chylothorax that is secondary to a *thoracic bellows effect* (Figure 15.9).

In evaluating the thorax for a pleural effusion, one should look for certain secondary changes in thoracic structures that might explain the effusion. First, be sure to evaluate all of the ribs for any areas of expansile lesions that are aggressive in nature (lots of lysis) as pleural masses can cause a pleural effusion (Figure 15.10). The aggressive lesion could also originate from the thoracic spine or sternum. Evaluate the cardiac silhouette for the presence of a mediastinal shift that might indicate a mass lesion in one side of the hemithorax. Additionally, a diaphragmatic rupture can result in pleural effusions and if significant cranial abdominal organ displacement is present, this can result in a mediastinal (contralateral) shift away from the abdominal viscera. A thoracic ultrasound might be indicated in order to evaluate the pleural space for a mass or abdominal contents.

Evaluate the major airways, particularly the right middle, left cranial, and right cranial bronchi. If the airway appears twisted or pinched off at the pulmonary hilum, then a lung lobe torsion should be considered as the cause of the pleural effusion. Cardiomegaly secondary to right heart disease or a pericardial effusion can result in right heart failure and ascites and a pleural effusion in the dog or just a pleural effusion in the cat. Evaluate the position of the carina on the lateral radiographs in a cat. If the carina is located at the seventh intercostal space (abnormal caudal position), then the possibility of a cranial mediastinal mass should be considered (Figure 15.11).

There are many different causes of pleural effusion, some of which include hypoproteinemia, pancreatitis, fluid overload, trauma, right heart failure in a dog, congestive heart failure in a cat, mediastinal or pleural masses, lung lobe torsion, chylothorax, pyothorax (tends to be unilateral and young cats), coagulopathy, vasculitis, diaphragmatic translocation of abdominal effusions, and diaphragmatic ruptures. If a pleural effusion is identified, one should tap and drain the fluid then repeat the thoracic radiographs to determine if there are any Roentgen signs that would support a specific etiology as the cause of the effusion. If chest tubes are placed, follow-up thoracic radiographs are indicated to document chest tube placement.

## Pneumothorax

The Roentgen signs associated with a pneumothorax (gas within the pleural space) are like those described for pleural effusion, except rather than a soft tissue opacity separating the visceral and parietal pleural surfaces, a gas opacity will be present and contrast with radiopaque lungs (Box 15.4). The most common Roentgen findings of a pneumothorax include retraction of the lung lobes away from the parietal pleural surfaces with visualization of the visceral pleural surface of the lung lobe, separation of the cardiac silhouette from the sternum, and gas will be present in the pleural space, as characterized by the absence of pulmonary vessels and airways normally seen in fully inflated lung lobes contacting the parietal pleural space (Figure 15.12). The visceral pleural surface of the lungs will be seen at the level of the pneumothorax, depending on the degree of pneumothorax that is present. As the pneumothorax progresses, more extensive and increased degrees of atelectasis are seen within the lung lobes.

The most common cause of a pneumothorax is trauma. In a tension pneumothorax, the opening into the pleural space acts as a one-way valve and air continues to accumulate, typically

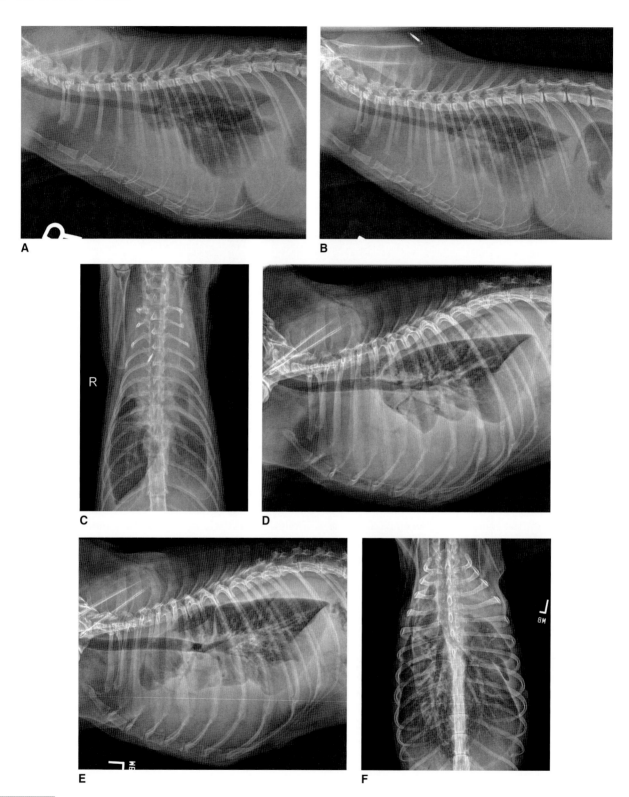

**FIGURE 15.4** Right lateral (**A**), left lateral (**B**), and ventrodorsal radiographs (**C**) from a cat with a severe pleural effusion secondary to a chylothorax. There is retraction of all lung lobes away from the thoracic walls with multiple pleural fissures lines filled with soft tissue opacity. On the ventrodorsal image, there is collapse of the right cranial and left cranial segments of the left cranial lung lobes with air bronchograms noted centrally. The cardiac silhouette and diaphragm are border effaced by the pleural fluid. On the ventrodorsal image, there is enlargement of the caudal lobar pulmonary vessels due to preferential shunting of blood to the lung lobes that are aerated for oxygenation of the blood. Right lateral (**D**), left lateral (**E**), and dorsoventral (**F**) views from a dog with a cranial mediastinal mass and severe pleural effusion. There are similar changes noted as for the cat related to the pleural space. An unstructured interstitial pulmonary pattern is present throughout the lung lobes consistent with partial atelectasis from the pleural effusion. Additionally, there is an air bronchogram within the right cranial lung lobe on the left lateral projection consistent with complete collapse of the right cranial lobe. On the ventrodorsal image, there is caudal and medial displacement of the left cranial lung lobe. The cranial mediastinal mass was a thymoma with a left-sided distribution.

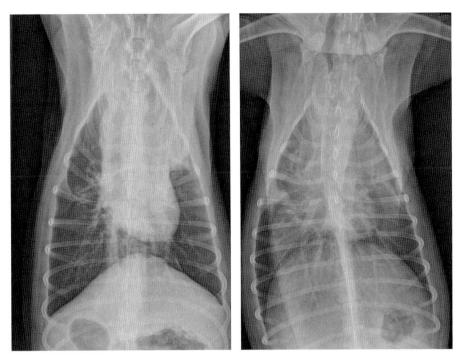

**FIGURE 15.5** Ventrodorsal (left) and dorsoventral (right) from a dog with a mild to moderate pleural effusion. The effusion was secondary to a cranial mediastinal mass within the left cranioventral mediastinal reflection. The fine needle aspirate was consistent with a thymoma. On the VD image, the pleural fluid is in the dorsal thorax (dorsal recumbency) and the cardiac silhouette and cranial mediastinal mass can be visualized. On the DV image, the pleural fluid is in the ventral thorax and border effaces the cardiac silhouette and the cranial mediastinal mass such that they are not visualized.

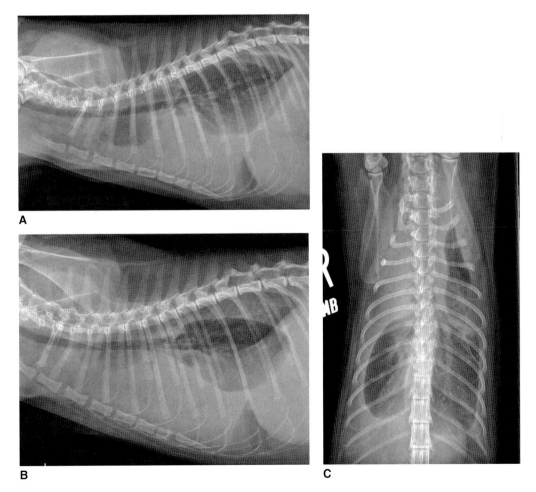

**FIGURE 15.6** Moderate to severe right-sided pleural effusion and a mild left-sided pleural effusion with rounding of the caudal lung lobes consistent with a predominantly unilateral effusion. This cat (right lateral, left lateral, and ventrodorsal images (**A–C**)) had an exudate consistent with a pyothorax on cytology of the pleural fluid. The right cranial and right middle lung lobes are collapsed as noted on the left lateral and ventrodorsal images.

**Box 15.3** Roentgen Signs of A Chronic Pleural Effusion (Restrictive Pleuritis).

1. Rounding and retraction of the lung lobes away from the thoracic wall
2. Thickened soft tissue lines outlining the lung lobes (called pleural peel)
3. Border effacement of the cardiac silhouette
4. Border effacement of the diaphragm
5. Can be unilateral, particularly if a pyothorax
6. Chronic rib fractures (thoracic bellows effect)

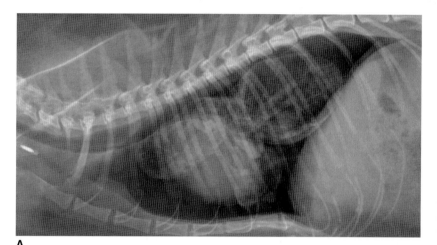

A

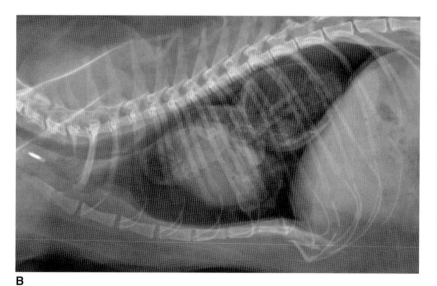

B

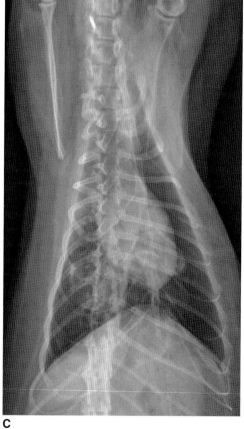

C

**FIGURE 15.7** A cat that has a history of a chronic chylothorax. In this cat (right lateral, left lateral, and ventrodorsal images (**A–C**)), there is a bilateral severe pneumothorax with rounding of the visceral pleural margins of the lung lobes consistent with *restrictive pleuritis* and *pleural peel*. All lung lobe margins are rounded and thickened with dorsal elevation of the cardiac silhouette away from the sternum. There is enlargement of the sternal lymph node. Dorsal elevation of the trachea is also noted. The pneumothorax is presumed to be iatrogenic after the pleural effusion was removed secondary to leakage from one of the lung lobes after trauma related to the thoracocentesis. Progression to a tension pneumothorax is possible but did not occur in this cat.

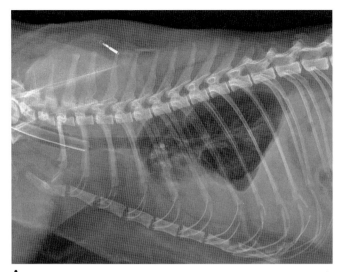

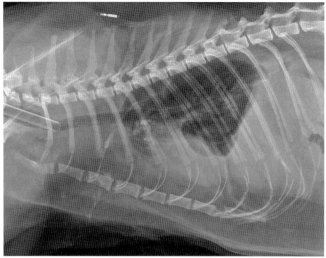

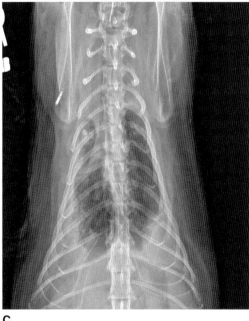

**FIGURE 15.8** Right lateral (**A**), left lateral (**B**), and ventrodorsal (**C**) images from a 7-year-old DSH with a chronic chylothorax and bilateral pleural effusion. There is severe thickening of the visceral pleural margins of the lung lobes particularly noted caudodorsally on the ventrodorsal image (consistent with a *pleural peel*). There are multiple cranial lobar broncholiths also seen.

on one side. This results in extreme atelectasis of the affected lung lobes, a contralateral mediastinal shift away from the side of the tension pneumothorax, and flattening of the diaphragm on the side of the tension pneumothorax (Figure 15.13).

## Extrapleural Sign and Pleural Mass(es)

As explained in the extrathoracic chapter (Chapter 14), an extrapleural sign is added soft tissue opacity in the lung field that is secondary to indentation of the lung by an extrapleural structure that extends into the thorax (Figure 15.14). The most common normal extrapleural sign is associated with chondrodystrophic breeds and the indentation at the costochondral junction (Figure 15.14). Pleural masses are a result of primary (mesothelioma, lipoma, sarcoma) or metastatic disease (carcinomatosis) within the pleural space (Figure 15.15). The most common metastatic diseases would be lymphoma in the cat and bronchogenic carcinoma in the dog. Rarely, there can be periosteal proliferation (hypertrophic osteopathy type of reaction) associated with the ribs in conditions of primary or secondary pleural tumors.

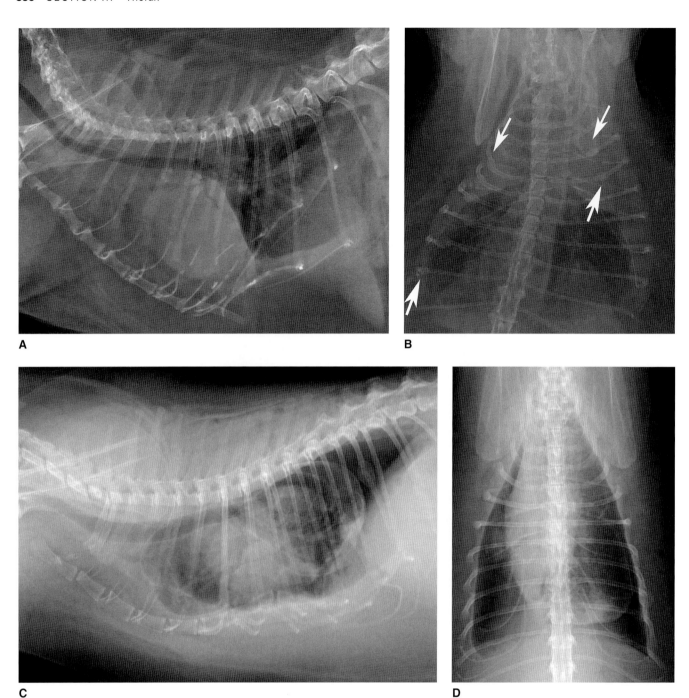

**FIGURE 15.9** *Thoracic bellows* effect seen in two different cats ((**A,B**) and (**C,D**) – right lateral and ventrodorsal images for each). In cat 1, there is a bilateral pleural effusion and multiple healing rib fractures (white arrows). Multiple air bronchograms are noted in the right and left cranial lung lobes on both projections. The pleural effusion was a chylothorax. In cat 2 (**C,D**), there is a bilateral pneumothorax with severe rounding of the lung lobes and a *pleural peel* consistent with a *restrictive pleuritis*. In addition, on peak inspiration there is dynamic narrowing of the thorax in the ventrodorsal view with an apparent dynamic pectus excavatum noted on the lateral view. Left-sided subcutaneous emphysema is present consistent with prior thoracocentesis.

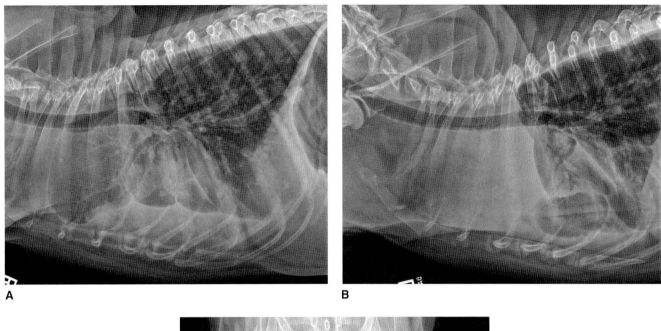

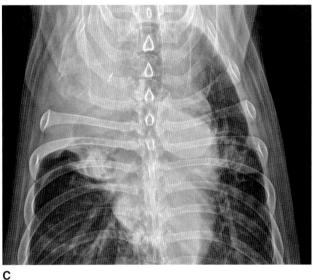

**FIGURE 15.10**   A three-view thorax (right lateral, left lateral, and dorsoventral views (**A–C**)) from a 10-year-old mixed-breed dog that presented for respiratory distress. There is an expansile, osteolytic lesion associated with the fourth right rib that results in a mass within the right cranial thorax. A bilateral pleural effusion is present. There are multiple pulmonary nodules noted consistent with pulmonary metastatic disease. The primary diagnosis on histology was osteosarcoma of the rib with pleural and pulmonary metastasis.

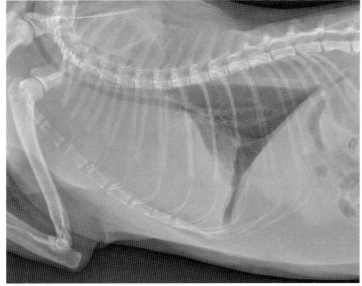

A

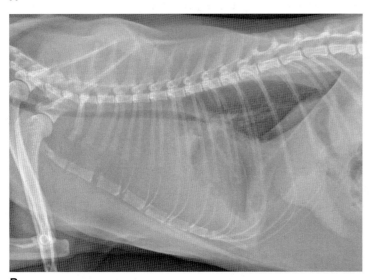
B

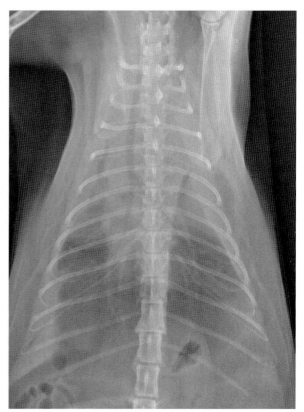
C

**FIGURE 15.11**   Right lateral (**A**), left lateral (**B**), and dorsoventral (**C**) radiographs from a 9-year-old DSH that presented for respiratory distress. There is a mild to moderate bilateral pleural effusion. There is a cranial mediastinal mass with dorsal elevation of the trachea, caudal displacement of the carina (to the seventh intercostal space) and the cardiac silhouette. Fine needle aspirates of the cranial mediastinal mass and pleural fluid were consistent with lymphoma.

---

## Box 15.4 Roentgen Signs of A Pneumothorax.

1. Separation of the cardiac silhouette from the sternum by gas

2. Presence of radiopaque thin lines in the ventral thorax

3. Retraction of the lung lobes away from the parietal pleural margins

4. Gas present between the lung lobes and between the parietal and visceral pleural surfaces

5. Absence of pulmonary vasculature and airways in the area of retraction

6. Identification of the visceral pleural surface

7. General increase in overall lung opacity secondary to atelectasis

8. In a tension pneumothorax, there will be flattening of one of the hemidiaphragms and a contralateral mediastinal shift away from the side of the tension pneumothorax (see text for details)

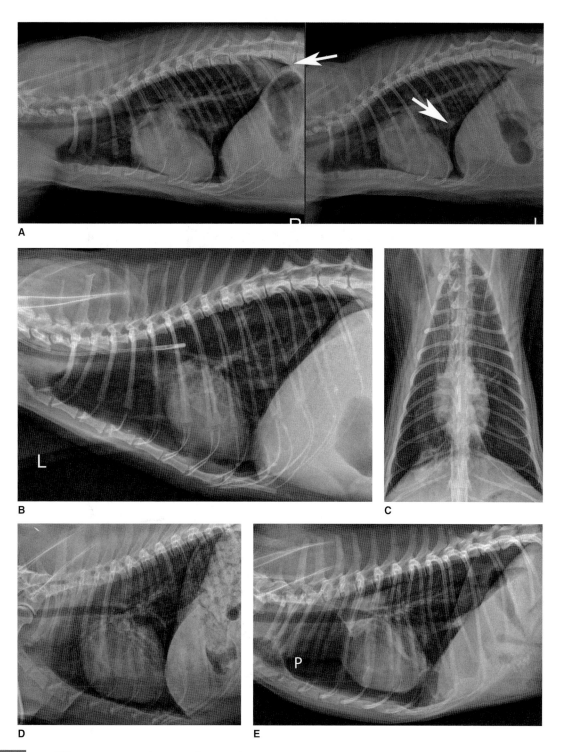

**FIGURE 15.12** Five different patients with varying degrees of pneumothorax. All cases were secondary to trauma. In cat 1 (right and left lateral images (**A**)), there is mild retraction of the caudal lung lobes from the diaphragm (white arrows). Additionally, there is a focal alveolar pulmonary pattern associated with the caudodorsal lung lobe consistent with a pulmonary contusion. The cardiac silhouette is enlarged with atrial and ventricular enlargement and an indentation along the caudal border of the cardiac silhouette. This cat was determined to have hypertrophic cardiomyopathy on echocardiography. In cat 2 (left lateral and ventrodorsal images (**B,C**)), there is retraction of the lung lobes away from the thoracic wall. There is visualization of the lateral margins of the visceral pleural surface of the lung lobes. This space is filled with air consistent with a pneumothorax. There is mild dorsal elevation of the cardiac silhouette on the left lateral. In dog 1 (left lateral only (**D**)), there is a mild pneumothorax with dorsal elevation of the cardiac silhouette away from the sternum and pleural air is present within this space consistent with a pneumothorax. In dog 2 (left lateral and ventrodorsal images (**E,F**)), there is retraction of the lungs away from the thoracic walls and elevation of the cardiac silhouette away from the sternum consistent with a moderate pneumothorax (P). There is an unstructured interstitial pulmonary pattern within the atelectatic lung lobes; however, this change in the peripheral lung lobes is consistent with the degree of the bilateral pneumothorax. In dog 3 (right lateral and dorsoventral images (**G,H**)), there is a mild to moderate bilateral pneumothorax. However, there is a generalized severe unstructured interstitial to early alveolar pulmonary pattern noted throughout the lung lobes. These changes are consistent with pulmonary contusions in this trauma case and would be considered severe. There is a focal bulla seen in the lateral aspect of the right cranial lung lobe at the fifth right rib on the dorsoventral view. A metal opaque structure (foreign body) is noted in the cranial abdomen.

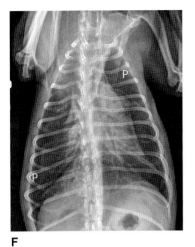

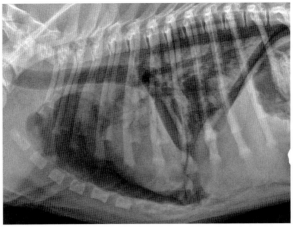

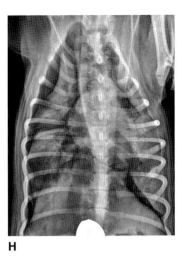

**F**   **G**   **H**

**FIGURE 15.12**   (Continued)

# Summary

The pleural space is a normal anatomic space that is not visualized on thoracic radiographs in normal dogs and cats. Obese animals can lay down fat in the pleural space. The most common abnormalities of the pleural space in small animals include pleural effusion, pneumothorax or diaphragmatic ruptures. A working knowledge of the Roentgen signs related to these common abnormalities is critical when reviewing thoracic radiographs of the dog and cat.

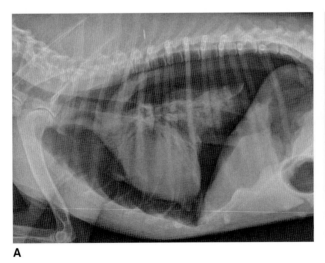

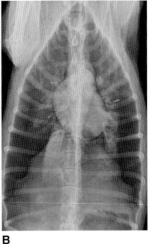

**A**   **B**

**FIGURE 15.13**   Three examples of a tension pneumothorax. In dog 1 (right lateral and dorsoventral images (**A,B**)), there is a severe bilateral pneumothorax with collapse of the lung lobes (atelectasis) centrally. The cardiac silhouette is elevated dorsally. There are soft tissue curved structures seen along the sternum on the lateral view consistent with muscle attachments to the costal cartilages. On the dorsoventral image, there is "tenting" of the diaphragm with central positioning of the cardiac silhouette (due to the bilateral pneumothorax) consistent with a tension pneumothorax. In cat 1 (dorsoventral and right lateral views (**C,D**)), there is a unilateral severe pneumothorax with leftward shift of the cardiac silhouette and collapse of the right lung lobes. These changes are consistent with a unilateral tension pneumothorax. In cat 2 (right lateral and ventrodorsal images (**E,F**)), there is a severe unilateral left-sided pneumothorax with a rightward contralateral mediastinal shift away from the central mediastinum. In addition, there is a right-sided pleural effusion with rounding of the right caudal lung lobe. On the ventrodorsal view, there is "tenting" of the left side of the diaphragm. The effusion was determined to be a pyothorax post thoracocentesis.

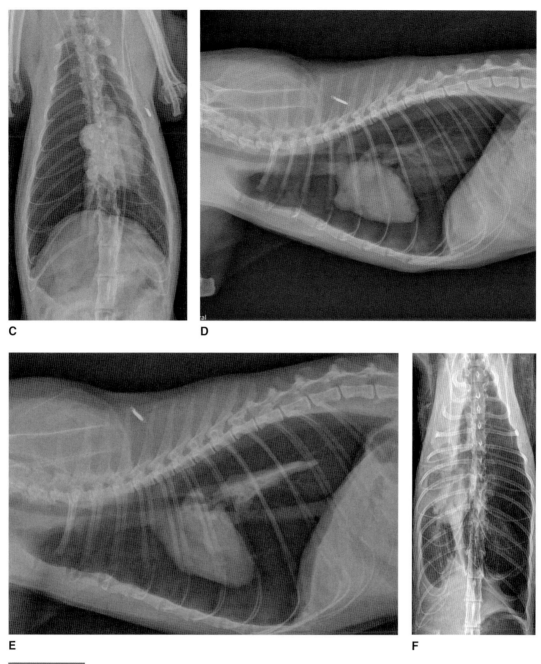

C

D

E

F

**FIGURE 15.13**   (Continued)

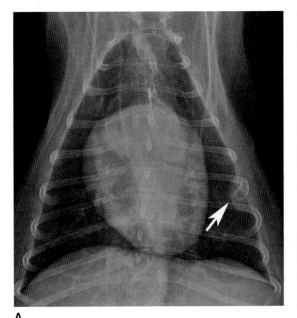
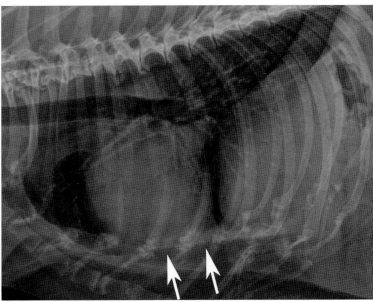

A

B

**FIGURE 15.14**   Examples of extrapleural signs. In (**A**), there is a metastatic lesion of the left sixth rib with a soft tissue indentation into the lung field. On fine needle aspirate, the osteolytic, expansile rib lesion was consistent with a carcinoma (presumed to be metastatic from renal cell carcinoma documented in this dog). In (**B**), there is a linear soft tissue opaque line noted at the costal chondral junction (white arrows) on this right lateral projection from a bassett hound.

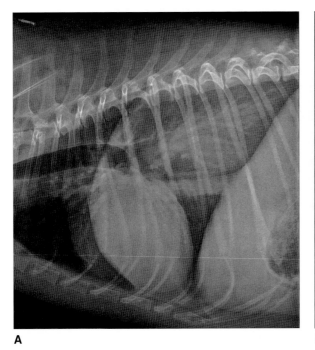
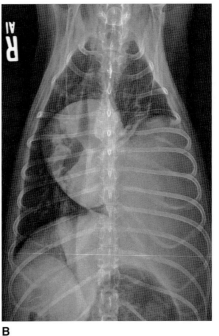

A

B

**FIGURE 15.15**   An example of an intrathoracic (pleural-based) lipoma in a 11-year-old Jack Russell terrier (right lateral and ventrodorsal images (**A,B**)). There is a large fat opaque mass noted within the caudal left pleural space with rightward displacement of the lung lobes and the cardiac silhouette. Compression atelectasis secondary to the mass effect is noted on both projections. The diaphragmatic margin is border effaced on the ventrodorsal image due to the thickness of the mass attenuating the x-rays of the primary beam. The mass also exhibits a mass effect with straightening of the left ribs over the mass compared to the caudal direction of the right ribs on the ventrodorsal radiograph.

# References

1. Thrall, D.E. (2018). Canine and feline pleural space. In: *Textbook of Veterinary Diagnostic Imaging*, 7e (ed. D.E. (e.) Thrall). St Louis, MO: Elsevier.

2. Hecht, S. (2020). Thorax (excluding the heart). In: *Diagnostic Radiology in Small Animal Practice*, 2e (ed. S. Hecht). Great Easton, Essex: 5m Books.

3. Garcia Real, M.I. (2014). *Atlas of Radiographic Interpretation in Small Animals*. Zaragoza, Spain: Grupo Asis.

4. Bradley, K. (2019). Radiology of the thorax. In: *BSAVA Manual of Canine and Feline Radiography and Radiology* (ed. A. Holloway and F. McConnell). Gloucester, UK: BSAVA.

5. Frame, M. and King, A. (2008). The pleural space. In: *BSAVA Manual of Canine and Feline Thoracic Imaging* (ed. T. Schwarz and V. Johnson). Gloucester, UK: BSAVA.

6. Kealy, J.K., McAllister, H., and Graham, J.P. (2010). *Diagnostic Radiology and Ultrasonography of the Dog and Cat*, 5e. St Louis, MO: Elsevier.

7. Mai, W. (2008). Pleura. In: *BSAVA Manual of Canine and Feline Thoracic Imaging* (ed. T. Schwarz and V. Johnson). Gloucester, UK: BSAVA.

# CHAPTER 16

# Pulmonary Parenchyma

**Clifford R. Berry[1] and Elodie E. Huguet[2]**

[1] Department of Molecular Biomedical Sciences, College of Veterinary Medicine, North Carolina State University, Raleigh, NC, USA

[2] Department of Small Animal Clinical Sciences, College of Veterinary Medicine, University of Florida, Gainesville, FL, USA

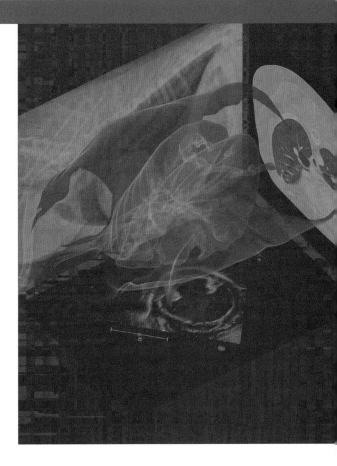

## Overview

The normal pulmonary parenchyma can be a challenge for interpretation. This is because of the substantial breed variations in dogs and also, the technical aspect of taking the thoracic radiograph impacts overall lung opacity and thereby may preclude accurate interpretation. It is imperative that the practitioner obtains well-positioned, thoracic radiographs of high diagnostic quality that are made on peak inspiration. An interpretation paradigm will be used in this chapter that tries to simplify the approach to interpretation of the lungs. This paradigm should serve as a starting point for evaluating thoracic radiographs. Continued evaluation of thoracic radiographs will refine the interpretation paradigm as the practitioner grows in experience and the art of pulmonary interpretation.

## Warnings and Obstacles

The infinite number of nuances of pulmonary interpretation makes it impossible to show all examples for the different radiographic presentations for each disease process.

It is important to recognize several caveats about the pulmonary parenchyma and a description of pulmonary changes. The first is that pulmonary pattern recognition is not necessarily the endgame in interpretation of the lungs. Second, pulmonary patterns do not equate with histology, although pulmonary patterns were originally ascribed to histology. This is no longer the case, as different diseases can have mixed pulmonary patterns. The pulmonary patterns represent nonspecific changes that could be caused by multiple different etiologies. However, certain etiologies do occur with certain lung patterns, thereby providing a differential diagnosis list. Third,

*Atlas of Small Animal Diagnostic Imaging*, First Edition. Edited by Clifford R. Berry, Nathan C. Nelson, and Matthew D. Winter.
© 2023 John Wiley & Sons, Inc. Published 2023 by John Wiley & Sons, Inc.
Companion website: www.wiley.com/go/berry/atlas

often lung patterns are mixed, and one needs to decide the dominant lung pattern to look up a specific set of differentials.

Finally, there are descriptive terms used in veterinary medicine that have not been defined and thereby should be avoided. Additionally, when looking up differentials, these terms are not used in current veterinary textbooks for creating differential lists. The first term is *infiltrate*, which refers to a nonspecific increase in pulmonary opacity from many possible etiologies. The term has, in fact, been discarded from the human pulmonary radiology literature because a definition has never been agreed upon. Infiltrate is a histologic description and since radiology is not histology, it should not be used. The second term is *consolidation*. This has been used to describe an increased opacity that involves a portion of or an entire lung lobe without volume loss within the affected lung lobe. This term is really an act of two businesses merging to form a larger corporation and has nothing to do with the lung. The Fleishner Society has defined consolidation as just an increase in opacity within the lung, so it is also non-specific [1]. The third term is the use of combinations such as *broncho-interstitial* pulmonary pattern. Again, this term does not have a differential list associated with it in the textbooks. There are plenty of diseases that can result in both an unstructured interstitial and bronchial pulmonary pattern; however, one must choose what the dominant pattern is, as this will dictate the differential diagnosis and next steps for reaching a final diagnosis.

# Anatomy and Physiology

There are six lung lobes present in the dog and cat (Figures 16.1 and 16.2) [2–15]. The pulmonary parenchyma is characterized by a background gray appearance that gets its overall opacity from the airspace within the alveoli, major and minor airways, the circulating blood, blood vessels and capillary beds of the pulmonary circulation. The blood supply to the lung is twofold, including the pulmonary circulation carrying deoxygenated blood from the right ventricle in the pulmonary arteries to the lungs, pulmonary capillaries and then returning oxygenated blood to the left atrium via the pulmonary veins. The bronchoesophageal artery (branch of the thoracic aorta at the level of the right fourth intercostal artery) carries oxygenated blood to the airways. The venous drainage of the bronchial blood supply enters the azygos vein before entering the cranial vena cava or right atrium.

The trachea extends from the larynx (Figure 16.3) through the thoracic inlet to its bifurcation into the right and left principal bronchi at the terminal trachea that is called the *carina*. Immediately off the right principal bronchus is the right cranial lung lobe (RB1) that extends in a cranioventral direction over the base of the cardiac silhouette [12]. The right cranial lung lobe has a dorsal and ventral aspect. The dorsal aspect is in contact with the craniodorsal mediastinal structures along its medial side. Caudally, the right cranial lung lobe is in contact

with the right caudal lung lobe dorsally and the right middle lung lobe and cardiac silhouette ventrally. The ventral aspect of the right cranial lung lobe is separated from the left cranial lung lobe by the *cranioventral mediastinal reflection*. The right cranial lung lobe extends from the right to the left side of the thorax cranial to the cardiac silhouette (Figure 16.4). The right middle lung lobe bronchus extends from the right caudal bronchus in a ventral location and has a triangular shape. This lung lobe does not go above the carina as noted on the lateral views. The caudal border of the right middle lung lobe approximates the caudal border of the cardiac silhouette (Figure 16.5). The right caudal lobe bronchus continues caudally as seen on the lateral projections in the caudodorsal lung field. The right caudal lung lobe also has a dorsal and ventral component and meets the mediastinal structures on the medial side of the lung and the diaphragmatic surface caudally.

The accessory lobe bronchus originates from the right caudal lung lobe bronchus in a ventromedial position and extends from the right to left side of the thorax caudal to the cardiac silhouette (Figure 16.4). The accessory lung lobe wraps around the caudal vena cava at the *plica vena cava*. This lobe extends to the left side of the thorax. The left lateralmost extent of the accessory lung lobe is the *caudoventral mediastinal reflection* as seen on ventrodorsal or dorsoventral radiographs (Figure 16.6). The dorsal border of the accessory lung lobe can be seen between the esophagus and the caudal vena cava (Figure 16.6).

The left lung is smaller than the right and is made up of the left cranial and left caudal lung lobes. The left cranial lung lobe is divided into cranial and caudal subsegments. The cranial subsegment extends cranioventrally to the thoracic inlet and in some dogs can extend over to the right side of the thorax (called the *lingula*; Figure 16.7). The left cranial lung lobe bronchus extends ventrally from the left lobe principal bronchus at the bifurcation of the trachea. This bronchus immediately divides into cranial and caudal subsegments (Figure 16.8). Dorsally, the left lung lobes contain an impression along the medial aspect as an indentation of the descending thoracic aorta. This impression is deeper in the cranial thorax and the descending thoracic aorta continues caudal and medial to a midline position by the time the aorta enters the abdomen at the aortic hiatus of the diaphragm. In some dogs, the descending thoracic aorta is more clearly visible cranially compared to the caudal thoracic aorta (Figure 16.9).

# Atelectasis

The term *atelectasis* implies volume loss within a given lung lobe. The degree of air volume loss correlates with the degree of atelectasis. There are physiologic and pathologic factors that result in the loss of normal air volume from an affected lung lobe. Atelectasis should be viewed as a nonspecific change that can be caused by multiple etiologies (different diseases) that affect the lungs, mediastinum, and pleural space. Acute

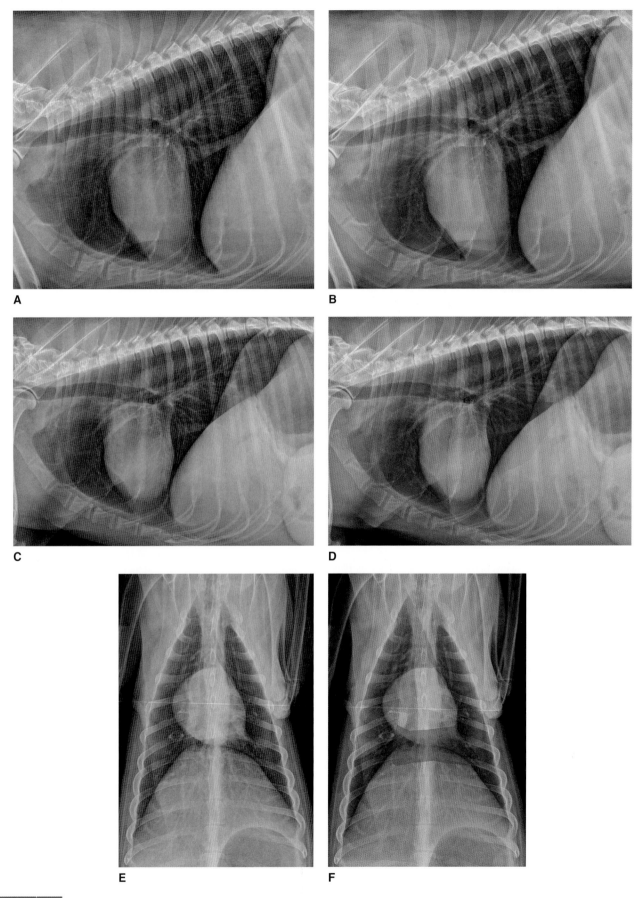

**FIGURE 16.1** Right lateral, left lateral, and dorsoventral radiographs from a normal adult dog (**A,C,E**). In (**B**), the left cranial (yellow) and left caudal (green) lung lobes are highlighted. In (**D**), the right cranial (light blue), right middle (yellow), right caudal (green), and accessory (dark blue) lung lobes are highlighted. In (**F**), all lung lobes are highlighted in the different colors (RCr, orange; LCr, light blue; RMid, yellow; RCd, pink; Acc, dark blue; LCd, green).

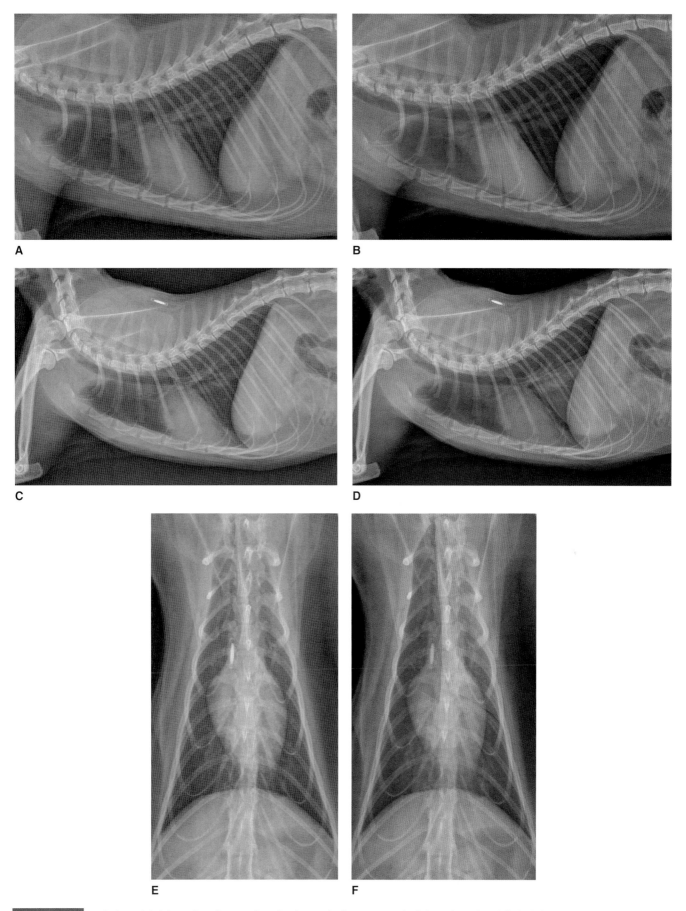

**FIGURE 16.2** Right lateral, left lateral, and ventrodorsal radiographs from a normal adult cat (**A,C,E**). In (**B**), the left cranial (yellow) and left caudal (dark blue) lung lobes are highlighted. In (**D**), the right cranial (red), right middle (blue), right caudal (green), and accessory (yellow) lung lobes are highlighted. In (**F**), all lung lobes are highlighted in the different colors (RCr, dark blue; LCr, yellow; RMid, orange; RCd, green; Acc, pink; LCd, light blue).

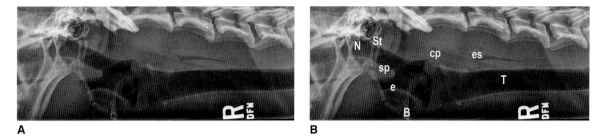

**FIGURE 16.3** Normal canine larynx without (**A**) and with (**B**) labels. N, nasopharynx; St, stylohyoid; sp., soft palate; e, epiglottis; B, basihyoid; cp, cricopharynx; es, esophagus; T, trachea.

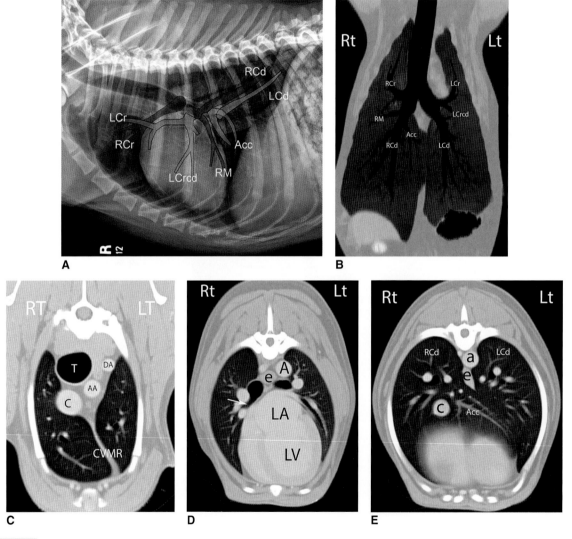

**FIGURE 16.4** Bronchial anatomy in the dog. CT images were obtained post intravenous contrast medium administration. (**A**) Right lateral radiograph with the different airways highlighted in different colors (RCr, right cranial; LCr, cranial subsegment of the left cranial; LCrcd, caudal subsegment of the left cranial lobe; RM, right middle; Acc, accessory; RCd, right caudal; LCd, left caudal). (**B**) MinIP dorsal plane reconstructed image of the thorax highlighting the airways. Abbreviations as before. (**C**) Transverse CT image of the cranial thorax with the right cranial lung lobe and left cranial lung lobe noted. The mediastinal reflection between the two lobes is the cranioventral mediastinal reflection (CVMR). C, cranial vena cava; AA, ascending aorta; DA, descending aorta ; T, trachea. (**D**) Transverse CT image of the midthorax at the left atrium (LA) and left ventricle (LV) just caudal to the carina and tracheal bifurcation. The right middle bronchus originates from the ventrolateral aspect of the right caudal lobe bronchus (white arrow). The caudal subsegment of the left cranial lobe bronchus is noted extending in a dorsal to ventral direction within the left lung. e, esophagus; A, aorta. (**E**) Transverse CT image of the caudal thorax between the cardiac silhouette and the abdomen with a portion of the diaphragm and liver noted in the ventral aspect of the image. C, caudal vena cava; e, esophagus; a, descending thoracic aorta; RCd, right caudal lobe; Acc, accessory lobe; LCd, left caudal lung lobe.

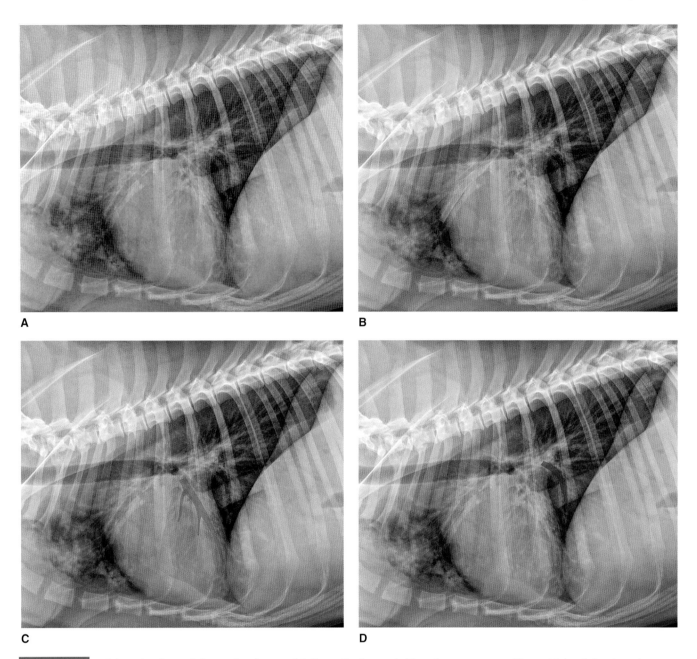

**FIGURE 16.5**   Left lateral radiograph from a dog that was febrile and had a cough. There is an unstructured interstitial and alveolar pulmonary pattern noted within the right cranial and left cranial lung lobes (**A**). (**B**) The right cranial (yellow) and left cranial (green) bronchi are highlighted. (**C**) The right middle bronchus and right middle lobe are highlighted (red). (**D**) The accessory lobe bronchus and the accessory lung lobe are highlighted (blue).

atelectasis will result in an ipsilateral mediastinal shift of the cardiac silhouette toward the area of atelectasis (Figure 16.10). As the atelectasis becomes chronic, hyperinflation of the surrounding lung lobes may shift the cardiac silhouette back into a *levocardia* position, with the apex of the cardiac silhouette pointing in a leftward and caudal direction (Figure 16.10).

Common causes of atelectasis include prolonged lateral recumbency and/or anesthesia, particularly with a $FiO_2$ of 100% [16–18]. *Plate-like atelectasis* has been reported in dogs and cats as a focal linear collapse of a portion of the lung lobe specifically localized to a sublobar fissure (Figure 16.10) [19].

# Interpretation Paradigm

A systematic approach to the evaluation of the lung is necessary so that all aspects of the lung fields are evaluated. There is a normal background opacity that is a result of the blood, blood vessels, capillary beds, airways, and interstitium (supporting connective tissue; Figure 16.11). Once an abnormality is identified, one must ask whether the abnormality is an increase in opacity, a decrease in opacity or both. Increased and decreased opacity will determine which part of the decision tree one goes

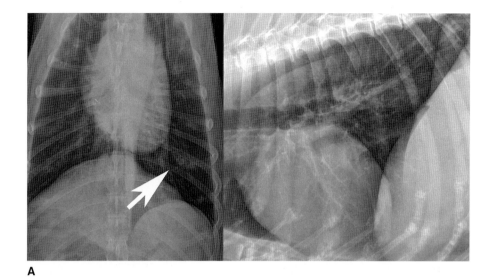

**A**

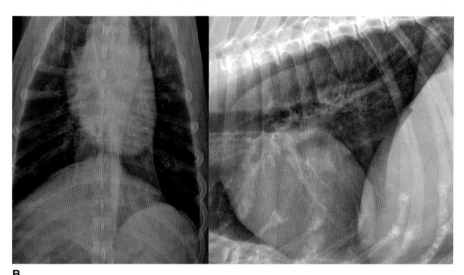

**B**

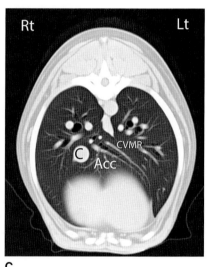

**C**

**FIGURE 16.6** Ventrodorsal (**A**) and left lateral (**B**) radiographs where the caudoventral mediastinal reflection is seen on the ventrodorsal (white arrow) and the accessory lung lobe is visualized as the more radiolucent area below the esophagus on the left lateral. These areas are highlighted in green in (**B**). (**C**) CT transverse image documenting the accessory lung lobe bronchus (center bronchus) with the accessory pulmonary artery being dorsal to the bronchus and the pulmonary vein being ventral to the bronchus. Acc, accessory lung lobe; CVMR, caudoventral mediastinal reflection; C, caudal vena cava.

down in describing a specific pattern and formulating a differential diagnosis.

If decreased opacity, the first question is whether the change is focal, multifocal, or generalized (Box 16.1). If focal, is the opacity structured into a circular lesion or lobar? If circular, then differentials would include pulmonary bulla, pneumatocele, or hematocele (Figure 16.12). If lobar (triangular), then is the decreased opacity due to regional oligemia (from decreased blood flow) or trapping of gas within the pulmonary parenchyma? The most common causes of lobar decreased opacity include bullous lobar emphysema (Figure 16.13) or pulmonary thromboembolism (Figure 16.14). If multifocal, then the distribution will be random throughout the lung lobes and the appearance circular as in multiple cavitated nodules, bullae (Figure 16.15) or lobar as in pulmonary thromboembolic disease. The above reasons for decreased opacity

have an uncommon prevalence. The most common reason for decreased opacity is hypovolemia regardless of the cause, which is generalized with all lung lobes being equally affected (Figure 16.16). In addition, in hypovolemic patients, the cardiac silhouette and caudal vena cava can be small (Figure 16.17).

The increased opacity decision tree also starts with distribution and specifically where the lesion is located (position in lung lobes and which lung lobes are involved). The first question is focal, multifocal, or generalized? Focal would involve one lung lobe, multifocal would involve more than one lung lobe and generalized would involve all lung lobes.

Anatomically, it is important to think of the thorax in terms of cranial and ventral opposed to caudal and dorsal distributions. A bronchopneumonia will be gravity dependent and cranioventral in distribution. Pulmonary edema (cardiogenic or noncardiogenic) will be caudodorsal in distribution.

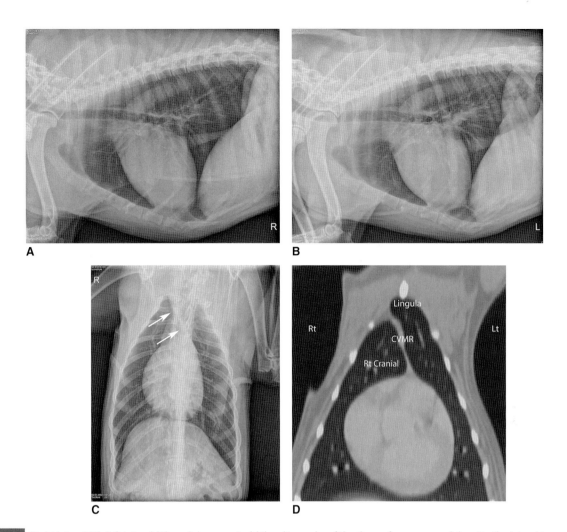

**FIGURE 16.7** Right lateral (**A**), left lateral (**B**), and dorsoventral (**C**) radiographs of the thorax from a normal dog. On the lateral images, the cranialmost radiolucency is the rightward extent of the cranial aspect of the left cranial lung lobe and is called the *lingula*. The right cranial lung lobe ventrally extends from right to left in contact with the cardiac silhouette. The cranioventral mediastinal reflection is the soft tissue opaque oblique line between the right cranial and left cranial lung lobe on the dorsoventral radiograph (white arrows). (**D**) Dorsal plane reconstructed image from a normal dog where the left cranial lung lobe is seen extending to the right and cranial to the right cranial lung lobe (lingula). The right cranial lobe extends from right to left cranial to the cardiac silhouette. The fat and soft tissue attenuating oblique line seen between the left and right cranial lung lobes is the cranioventral mediastinal reflection (CVMR).

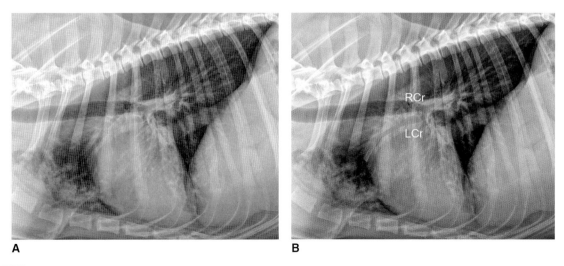

**FIGURE 16.8** Right lateral projection from the same dog as in Figure 16.5. Without (**A**) and with (**B**) highlighted areas for the right cranial (yellow) and left cranial (green – cranial and caudal subsegmental airways drawn in) lung lobes. The opening into the right cranial bronchus on a right lateral image is represented by a radiolucent circle over the area of the carina. The bronchus then angles cranioventrally into the right cranial lobe. If one traces the ventral wall of the trachea past this opening, there is an opening into the left cranial bronchus that is seen as parallel lines directed ventrally, then almost immediately splits into a cranial and caudal subsegmental bronchus.

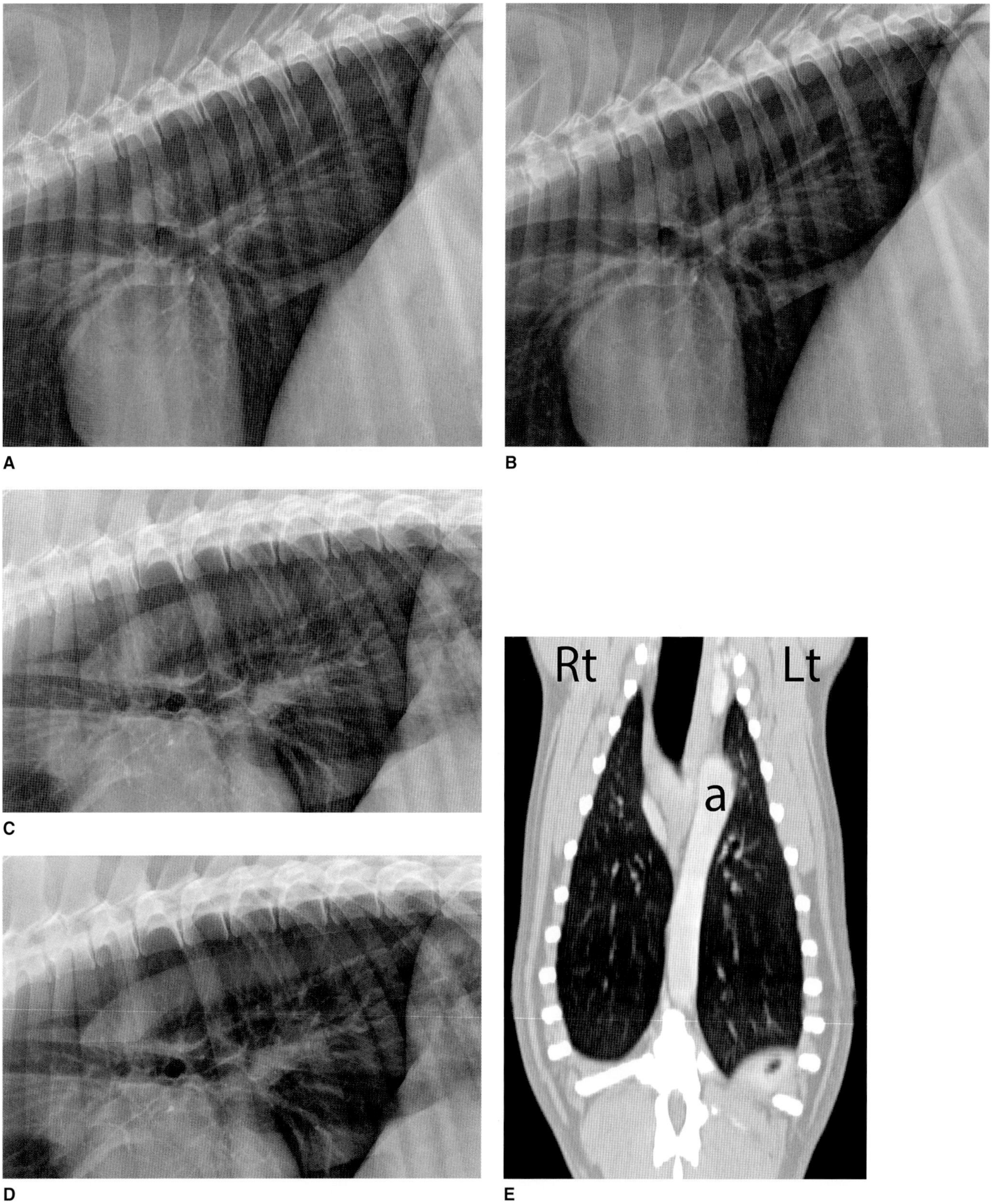

**FIGURE 16.9** Right lateral (**A**) and left lateral (**C**) radiographs from two different dogs where the cranial descending thoracic aorta is better visualized than the caudal descending thoracic aorta due to the contact with impression of the aortic arch and cranial descending thoracic aorta within the left cranial lung lobe. In (**B**) and (**D**), the aortic shadow is highlighted. (**E**) Dorsal plane reformatted CT image post intravenous contrast medium administration documenting the descending thoracic aorta (a) extending into the medially located aortic impression in the left cranial lung lobe. As the aorta continues caudally, it angles to a more midline position whereby the aorta is not highlighted in an aortic impression in the left caudal lung lobe but located in the caudal dorsal mediastinum between the right and left caudal lung lobes.

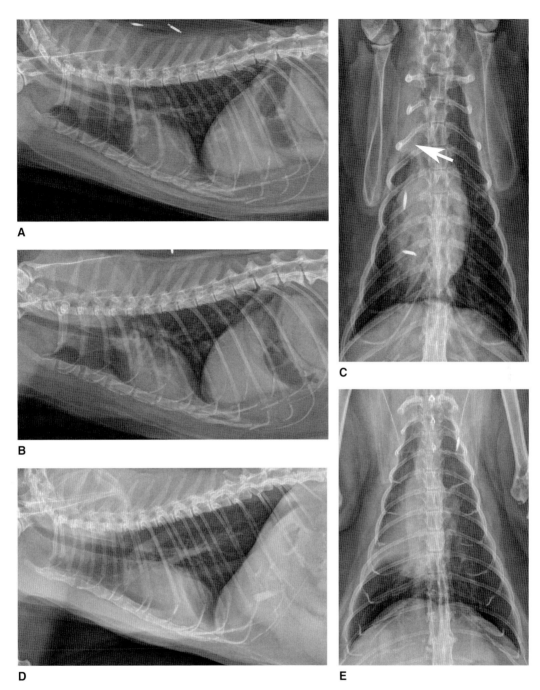

**FIGURE 16.10** Atelectasis of different lung lobes from three different cats. Right lateral, left lateral, and ventrodorsal images (**A–C**) of an older cat with a cough. There is collapse of the right cranial lung lobe (white arrow (**C**)). In addition, there are many cavitated pulmonary nodules noted throughout the pulmonary parenchyma. This cat had a bronchogenic carcinoma of the right cranial lung lobe with metastatic disease. In the second cat, there are two sets of radiographs taken 1 year apart. Left lateral (**D**) and ventrodorsal (**E**) images documenting collapse of the right middle lung lobe and a focal lobar sign associated with the right middle lobe on the left lateral view. There is a rightward mediastinal shift toward the affected lobe (ipsilateral mediastinal shift) implying volume loss within the lesion. One year later, the collapse is still present within the right middle lung lobe. However, the right cranial and right caudal lung lobes have hyperinflated and the mediastinal shift is no longer present (**F,G**). On both sets of images, mineralization is noted within the liver and gall bladder. Right lateral, left lateral, and ventrodorsal images (**H–J**) from a cat with a history of a cough and weight loss. In this cat, there is a mass within the left caudal lung lobe with associated volume loss. There is a leftward, ipsilateral mediastinal shift. On the lateral images, there is only one airway and set of vessels noted extending into the right caudal lung lobe. These changes are consistent with a pulmonary mass resulting in atelectasis of the affected lung lobe. Carcinoma was identified cytologically from ultrasound-guided fine needle aspirates. Metastatic lesions were not seen on this thoracic study. In (**K**), there is a focal curvilinear soft tissue opacity noted at the level of the trachea and second intercostal space (white arrow). This is an example of *plate-like atelectasis* in this dog that is most likely an incidental finding.

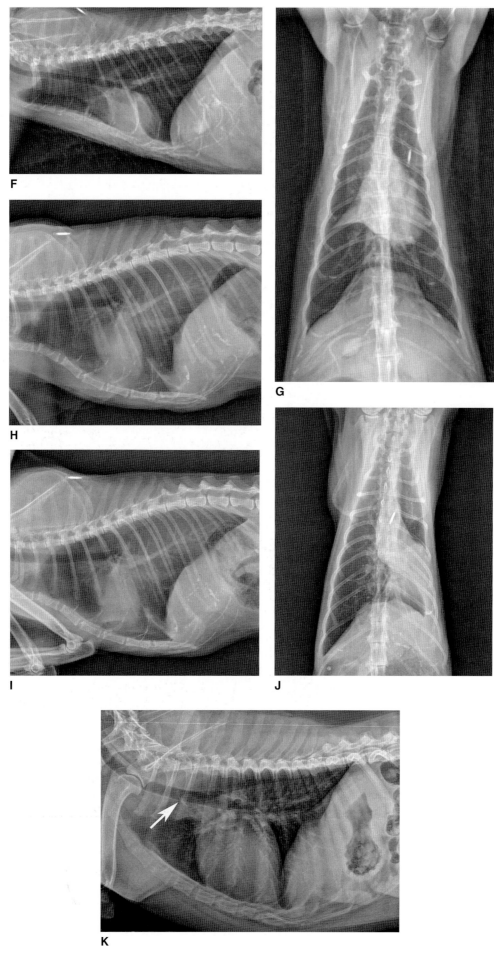

F

H

I

G

J

K

**FIGURE 16.10** (Continued)

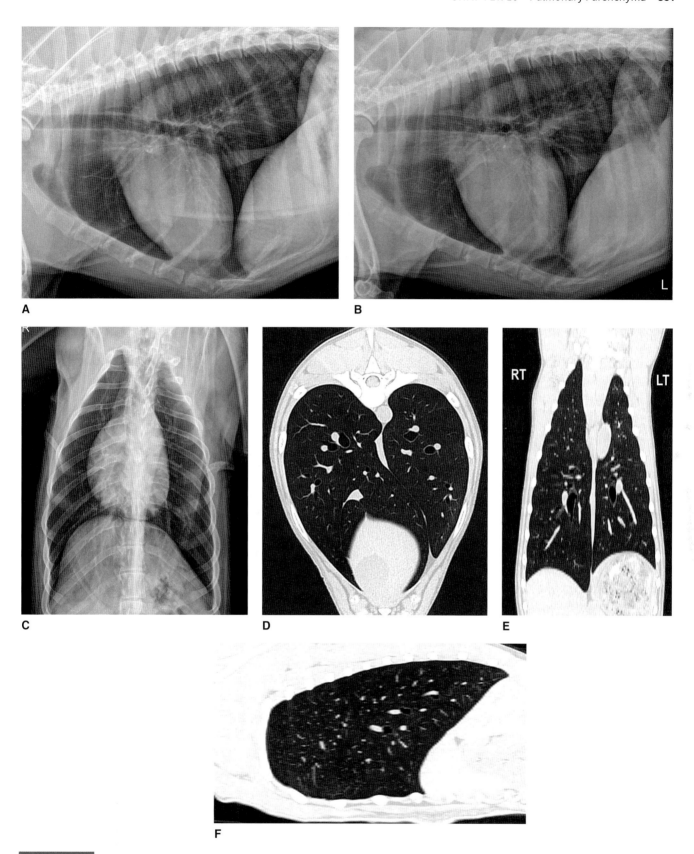

**FIGURE 16.11**   Normal lung opacity from an adult dog with right lateral (**A**), left lateral (**B**), and dorsoventral (**C**) radiographs. The overall opacity is a background dark gray with visualization of the pulmonary vessels into the periphery of the lung lobes. In addition, the airways can be visualized dividing into secondary and in some cases tertiary bronchi. Multiplanar reconstructed CT images from a different dog with a normal thorax. The images include transverse (**D**), dorsal (**E**), and sagittal (**F**) plane images post intravenous contrast medium administration. The background attenuation is increased relative to air with a normal HU value around −700 HU. Airways and vessels can be seen in the peripheral aspect of all lung lobes.

**Box 16.1** Decision Tree with Differentials for Decreased Opacity Associated with The Pulmonary Parenchyma.

1. **Focal**
   *Circular* – DDX: bulla, pneumatocele, hematocele, cavitated mass (primary pulmonary tumor)
   *Lobar (triangular shape): lobar oligemia (small vessels)* – DDX: pulmonary thromboembolic disease, lobar emphysema (congenital)

2. **Multifocal**
   *Circular* – DDX: bullae, pneumatocele, hematocele, paragonimiasis (parasitic), chemotherapy
   *Lobar* – DDX: pulmonary thromboembolic disease

3. **Generalized (with microcardia and small caudal vena cava)** – DDX: emphysema, hypovolemia, cardiogenic or hemorrhagic shock, anemia, Addison disease

The position of the mediastinum should then be evaluated assuming the ventrodorsal/dorsoventral radiographs are straight in their positioning. An *ipsilateral* mediastinal shift will result in the cardiac silhouette moving toward the area of increased opacity, usually secondary to loss of air volume within the lung lobe (called *atelectasis*; Figure 16.18). A *contralateral* mediastinal shift will result in the cardiac silhouette being displaced away from the increased opacity, which typically is a mass or creates a mass effect (Figure 16.19).

Next is defining the pulmonary pattern. The easiest approach to learning pulmonary patterns is to run a list of possibilities from easiest to identify to the hardest to identify (Box 16.2). These include:

- pulmonary mass
- alveolar pulmonary pattern
- bronchial pulmonary pattern
- vascular pulmonary pattern
- structured interstitial pulmonary pattern
- unstructured interstitial pulmonary patterns.

One always must bear in mind that the pulmonary abnormality identified can be a combination of several pulmonary patterns and a differential list must be created for each pattern. Also, unstructured interstitial pulmonary pattern and alveolar pulmonary pattern in the same patient most likely represents different degrees of severity of the same disease process. One can progress to the other (unstructured interstitial to alveolar) as the disease process worsens and one can regress as the disease responds to treatment (alveolar to unstructured interstitial; Figure 16.20).

The easiest pattern to identify is a *pulmonary mass*. A mass is greater than 3 cm in diameter and has a smooth rounded border (Figure 16.21). Pulmonary masses can be cavitated and/or mineralized (Figure 16.22). The process of cavitation involves the central portion of the mass outgrowing its blood supply and becoming necrotic fluid. The mass then invades a bronchus, and the fluid drains out of the mass and is replaced by air. Pulmonary abscesses in small animals can also have a gas-cavitated mass appearance but this is less

common. Depending on the location of the mass, the mass can border efface with the cardiac silhouette or diaphragm and is usually a uniform soft tissue opacity. The most common mass in the dog is found in the left caudal lung lobe and is secondary to a primary lung tumor (bronchogenic, bronchoalveolar or squamous cell carcinomas; Figure 16.23). Masses in the right middle lung lobe in dogs have been shown to most commonly be histiocytic sarcoma (Figure 16.24). In cats, pulmonary (bronchogenic carcinoma most common) masses can occur in the hilum and obstruct a central bronchus, resulting in an atelectatic lung lobe (see Chapter 19). Additionally, *lung–digit syndrome* occurs where the pulmonary bronchogenic carcinoma metastasizes to the digits (see Chapter 19). Often these cats present clinically for a thoracic or pelvic limb lameness and not clinical signs related to thoracic disease. In some pulmonary interpretation paradigms, pulmonary masses are characterized as a structured interstitial pulmonary pattern. This implies that these masses originate from the interstitium, which is the least common origin for a pulmonary mass. The mass could be alveolar, bronchial, or interstitial in cell origin. Also, the term pulmonary mass is very descriptive and implies a large (greater than 3 cm), rounded and soft tissue opaque lesion.

The next pulmonary pattern that is easy to identify is the *alveolar pattern* (Box 16.3). There are five aspects of an alveolar pulmonary pattern: a uniform soft tissue opacity with the presence of air bronchograms (Figure 16.25), a lobar sign, border effacement of the affected lung lobe with the cardiac silhouette or diaphragm, depending on the lung lobe involved and position within the lung lobe, and border effacement of the small structures within the affected portion of the lung lobe, including the pulmonary vessels and serosal border of the bronchi. Three of the five must be present to be an alveolar pattern. Border effacement of the small structures and outer serosal wall of the bronchi must be present to represent an alveolar pulmonary pattern. *Air bronchograms*, although considered the hallmark of alveolar disease, do not always have to be present and in a minority of cases will not be present. Total atelectasis of a lung lobe would be considered an alveolar pattern but does not necessarily contain a central air bronchogram (Figure 16.26).

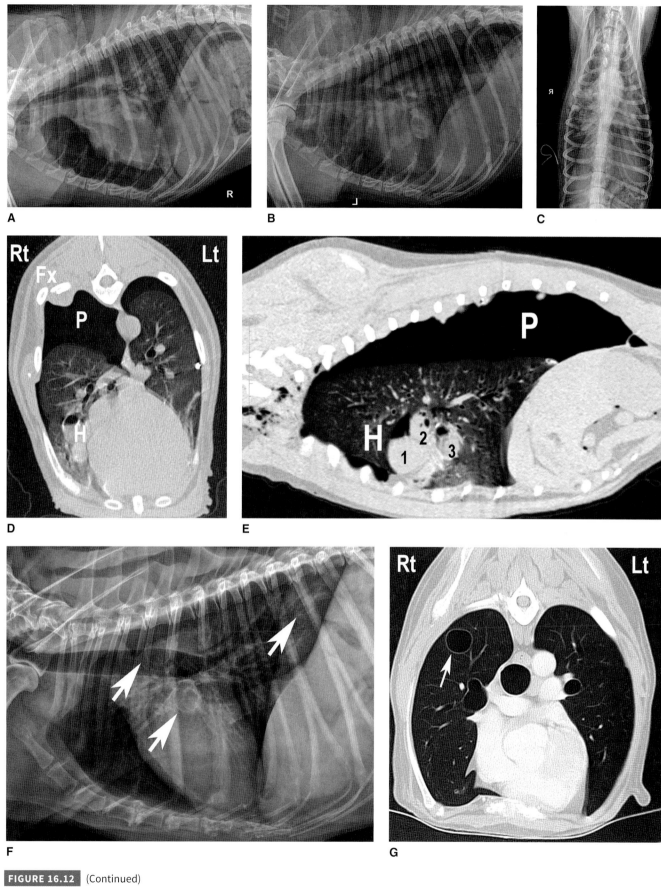

**FIGURE 16.12**   (Continued)

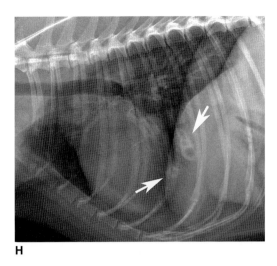

**H**

**FIGURE 16.12** Representative dogs that had traumatic injuries with varying degrees of radiolucency associated with the pulmonary parenchyma. Images from dog 1 (**A–E**) document a pneumomediastinum, pneumothorax, and multiple hematoceles (H1,2,3) noted within the right middle and cranial lung lobes. Multiple right-sided rib fractures are present with localized pleural hemorrhage. On the radiographs, the hematoceles are best seen on the left lateral image. On the CT images, subcutaneous emphysema, a pneumothorax (P) and multiple hematoceles (H1,2,3) and a pneumoperitoneum (**E**) are identified. In the second dog (**F,G**) there are a number of pulmonary bulla present on both the left lateral (white arrows) and the transverse CT image (white arrow). In the third dog (**H**), there are several hematoceles present.

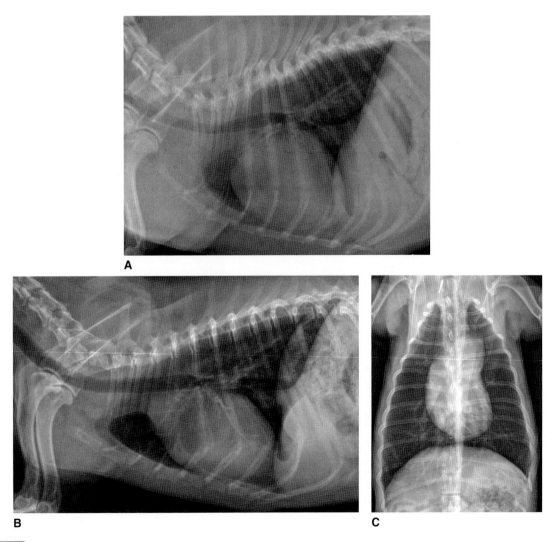

**A**

**B**                                        **C**

**FIGURE 16.13** Increased radiolucency is noted in two dogs within the pulmonary parenchyma. In a dog with right ventricular enlargement and a pulmonic stenosis on echocardiography (**A**), there is decreased vessel size noted caudodorsally. In the second dog (left lateral (**B**) and dorsoventral (**C**) images), there is hyperlucency noted within several different lung lobes. There is right ventricular enlargement and enlargement of the main pulmonary artery. These changes are consistent with a severe pulmonic stenosis with poststenotic dilation (confirmed on echocardiography with a pressure gradient greater than 120 mmHg) and pulmonary underperfusion.

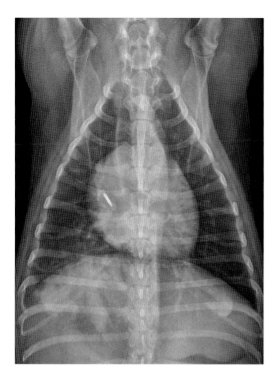

**FIGURE 16.14** Ventrodorsal image from a dog that was hypoxemic. There is increased lucency associated with the left hemithorax. An unstructured interstitial to alveolar pulmonary pattern is present within the right caudal lung lobe. At necropsy, pulmonary thromboemboli were noted within the pulmonary arteries to the left cranial and caudal lung lobes resulting in regional oligemia.

The most common lung lobe to undergo complete atelectasis is the right middle lung lobe which usually occurs in cats with feline allergic lung disease secondary to mucous plugging (Figure 16.27).

The next pulmonary pattern that could result in increased opacity is a *bronchial pulmonary pattern*. The hallmark feature of this disease is the presence of thickened small airways (rings and, less commonly, parallel lines; Figure 16.28). Typically, bronchial disease is a generalized disease, and the rings and parallel lines are found in the peripheral aspects (thinnest sections) of the lung parenchyma. The caveat includes the fact that the central airways are always prominent and should not be misinterpreted as a bronchial pattern. In addition, there are geriatric changes as well as disease conditions (Cushing syndrome) that might result in central bronchial mineralization (and can be quite eye catching; Figure 16.29). This should not be misinterpreted as a bronchial pulmonary pattern. The term "peribronchial" cuffing has been used in veterinary medicine, but it is extremely rare in that the increased pulmonary opacity forms a concentric separate circle surrounding a thickened bronchus centrally. When switching from analog radiographic film to a digital system, one can also see the airway walls more clearly, but this is not a bronchial pulmonary pattern.

A bronchial pulmonary pattern is determined by thickening of the airway walls and the finding of midzone and peripheral interlobar airway walls (rings and parallel lines). Inappropriate radiographic technique (such as when radiographing the

abdomen) can also artefactually increase the conspicuity of the bronchi and can be misinterpreted as a bronchial pattern, falsely raising concerns for lower airway disease.

The next pulmonary pattern is the *vascular pulmonary pattern*. Increased opacity implies that the pulmonary arteries and/or veins are enlarged, thereby adding opacity to the lung lobes. The pulmonary artery and vein parallel each other and are equal in size. Pulmonary artery enlargement is seen in canine and feline heartworm disease (Figure 16.30). This disease process results in an endarteritis of the pulmonary arteries where the arteries will become enlarged, tortuous, and/or blunted (abruptly tapers). Enlargement of the pulmonary veins usually implies elevations of left ventricular and left atrial end-diastolic pressures and thereby increased pulmonary venous pressures (Figure 16.31). This is typically seen in dogs and cats with congestive left-sided heart failure. Enlargement of the pulmonary arteries and veins is usually secondary to volume overload of the pulmonary circulation. This could be secondary to overcirculation from left to right intra- or extracardiac congenital shunts, volume overload from excessive intravenous fluids, arteriovenous fistulas, or cats with congestive left-sided heart failure, (Figure 16.32).

A *structured interstitial pulmonary pattern* can be classified as *nodular* or *miliary*. Pulmonary nodules range in size from 0.5 to 3.0 cm, and are rounded and soft tissue in opacity (Figure 16.33). Fake-outs for pulmonary nodules include centrally located end-on pulmonary vessels (near the pulmonary hilum), ectoparasites, osteomas, degenerative costochondral junction changes, nipples, and cutaneous masses/nodules (Figure 16.34). Metastatic neoplasia is the primary differential diagnostic consideration for pulmonary nodules although other causes of nodules are not excluded (such as granulomas or abscesses). A miliary pulmonary pattern implies that there is a generalized increase in soft tissue opacity with a nodular background opacity shaped like "millet seeds" (Figure 16.35). Differentials would include fungal disease, lymphoma, or metastatic carcinoma.

The final cause of an increased opacity (essentially the left-over back door diagnosis) is the *unstructured interstitial pulmonary pattern* (Figure 16.36). The features of an unstructured interstitial pattern include an increase in soft tissue opacity with partial loss of normal vascular and bronchial markings but not complete border effacement. The pulmonary changes could also obscure but not border efface the cardiac silhouette and/or the diaphragm, depending on the location of the pulmonary abnormalities. The unstructured interstitial pattern could be further classified as moderate or severe. A mild unstructured interstitial pulmonary pattern can commonly be recognized but is not worth taking into consideration given that no therapy will be administered solely based on the presence of a mild unstructured interstitial pulmonary pattern (particularly generalized) as this could just be age-related change (pulmonary fibrosis), expiration, and underexposure. The severe unstructured interstitial pulmonary pattern is on its way to being alveolar, but air bronchograms are not yet present and one can still make out vessels in the affected pulmonary parenchyma.

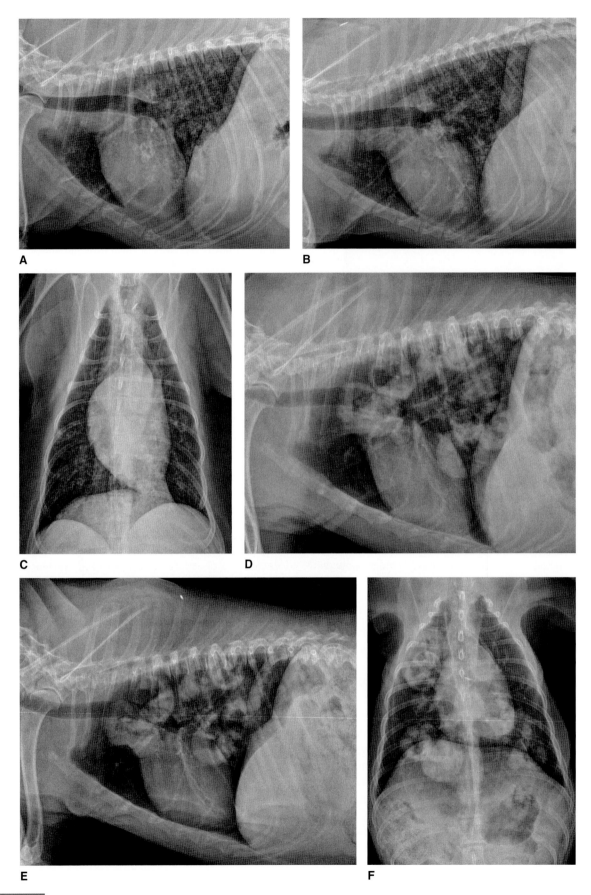

**FIGURE 16.15** Two different dogs with cavitated nodules and masses. In dog 1 (**A–C**), there is a generalized bronchial pulmonary pattern with multiple cavitated nodules noted throughout all lung lobes. This was secondary to pulmonary flukes (*Paragonimus kellicotti*). In the second dog (**D–F**), there are multiple pulmonary masses that are cavitated (mixed gas and soft tissue opacity). Metastatic carcinoma was documented in this case from a renal cell carcinoma. This dog had been undergoing chemotherapy, so it is presumed that the cavitation was present secondary to necrosis within the metastatic neoplasia.

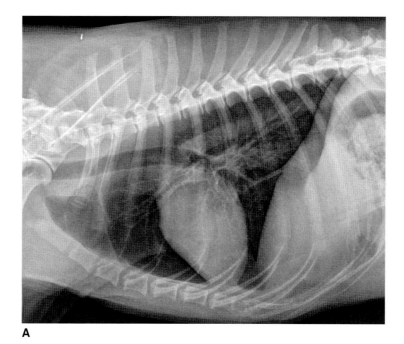

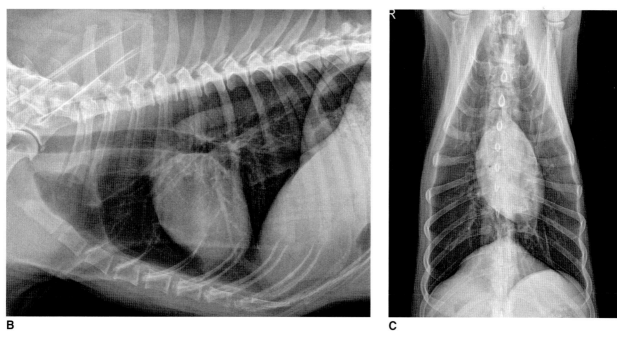

**FIGURE 16.16**   Right lateral, left lateral, and ventrodorsal radiographs (**A–C**) from a dog with hypovolemia. The pulmonary vessels, cardiac silhouette, and caudal vena cava are small from central volume depletion. Other differentials would be hypovolemia secondary to trauma, haemoabdomen from a bleeding tumor or Addison disease.

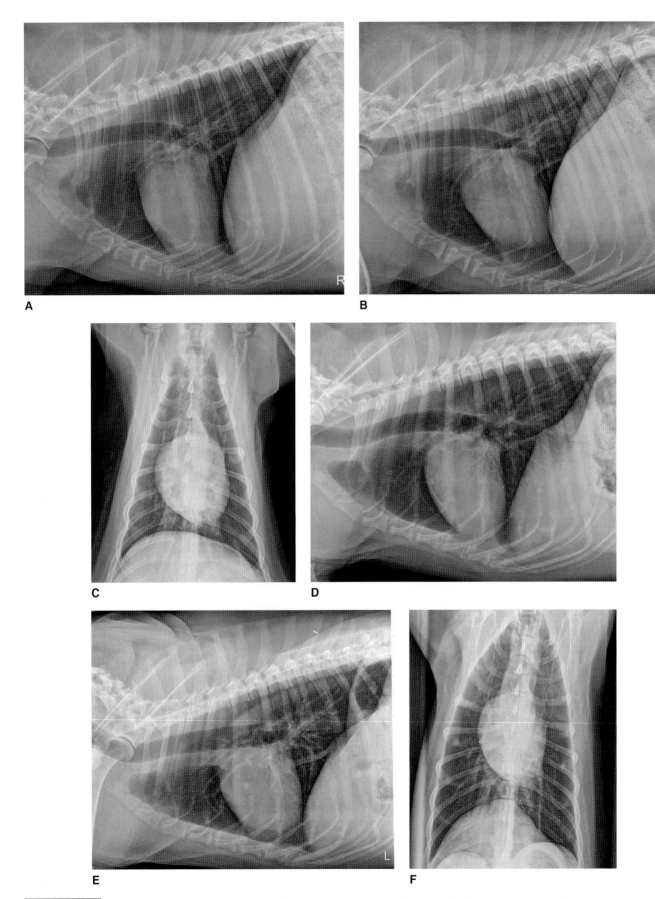

**FIGURE 16.17** Thoracic radiographs from two dogs with a hemoabdomen secondary to a bleeding splenic or hepatic tumor. In both dogs, the final histologic diagnosis was hemangiosarcoma. In the first dog (**A–C**), there is generalized decrease in size of the pulmonary vessels, cardiac silhouette, and caudal vena cava. There is decreased cranial abdominal detail due to the peritoneal effusion. Similar changes are noted in the second dog (**D–F**) except there are also small, variably sized, soft tissue, pulmonary nodules (structured interstitial pattern) noted consistent with metastatic disease.

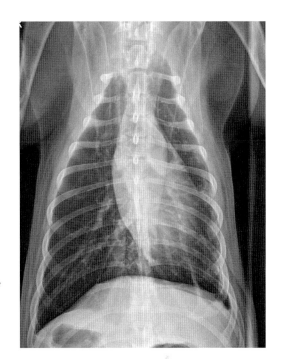

**FIGURE 16.18**   Ventrodorsal radiograph from a dog under general anesthesia. There is a leftward ipsilateral mediastinal shift and an unstructured interstitial pulmonary pattern noted in the peripheral aspect of the left and right cranial lung lobes. These changes are consistent with anesthesia-related atelectasis. Additionally, generalized esophageal distension can be seen in dogs and cats under general anesthesia.

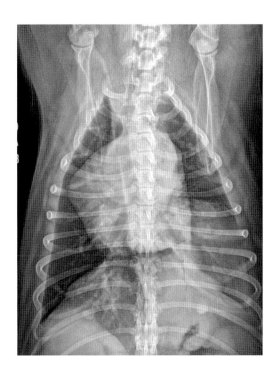

**FIGURE 16.19**   Ventrodorsal radiograph from a dog with a large mass in the left caudal lung lobe with contralateral displacement of the cardiac silhouette. The radiograph is slightly obliqued and there is an unusual bulge in the right atrium (9 o'clock position) that was determined to be fat within the pericardium on echocardiography.

## Box 16.2 Pulmonary Patterns.

1. Pulmonary mass (can be cavitated or mineralized)
2. Alveolar pulmonary pattern
3. Bronchial pulmonary pattern
4. Vascular pulmonary pattern
5. Structured interstitial
   a. Nodules
   b. Miliary
6. Unstructured interstitial

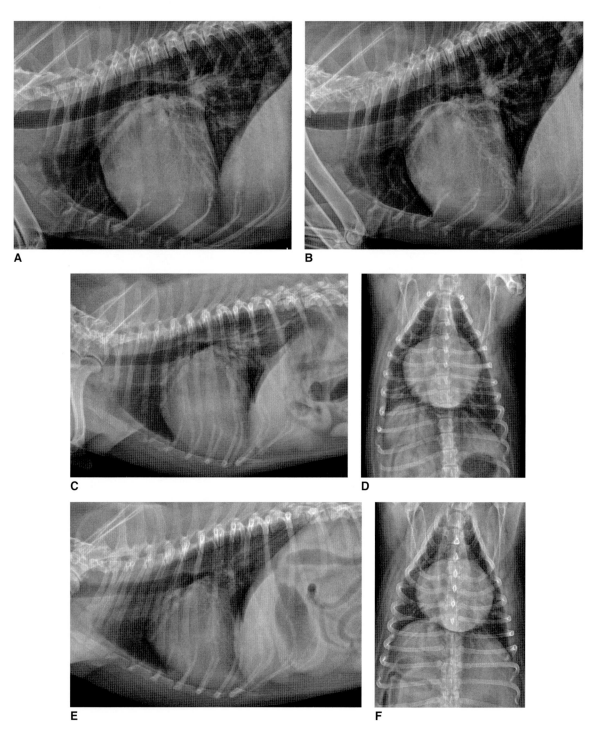

**FIGURE 16.20** Two different dogs before and after Lasix® administration for left heart failure (pulmonary edema). In the first dog, dilated cardiomyopathy was diagnosed based on echocardiographic assessment. On the initial left lateral (**A**), there is a generalized unstructured interstitial pulmonary pattern and pulmonary venous enlargement. The cardiac silhouette is enlarged with left-sided (ventricular and atrial) enlargement and dorsal elevation of the trachea. In the 24-h post Lasix administration left lateral (**B**), the pulmonary parenchyma is not as radiopaque, and the unstructured interstitial pulmonary pattern is less prominent. The cranial lobar pulmonary venous enlargement remains but is not as enlarged as on the prior radiograph. In the second dog, mitral valve degenerative disease with severe mitral regurgitation was noted on echocardiography. On the initial radiographs (left lateral (**C**) and dorsoventral (**D**)), there is moderate to severe left-sided cardiomegaly (ventricular and atrial) with dorsal displacement of the trachea, carina, and caudal bronchi. The left caudal lobe bronchus is compressed between the descending thoracic aorta and the enlarged left atrium. There is an alveolar pulmonary pattern noted in the right caudal lung lobe with an unstructured interstitial pattern in the right middle lung lobe on the dorsoventral view. The pulmonary veins are mildly enlarged compared with the corresponding pulmonary arteries. On the follow-up radiographs (left lateral (**E**) and dorsoventral (**F**)), there is dramatic reduction of the pulmonary edema with a mild unstructured pulmonary pattern present in the right caudal lung lobe. NOTES: the right caudal lung lobe is the most common lobe involved in developing pulmonary edema in dogs with mitral valve degenerative disease. This is because of the anatomic orientation of the right caudal lobar pulmonary vein (RC) relative to the centrally directed regurgitant jet (white arrow) between the left ventricle (LV) and atrium (LA) as noted in (**G**), a CT transverse image of the heart and caudal lobar pulmonary veins relative to left atrial entrance. C, caudal vena cava. In (**H**), a transverse CT image post intravenous contrast medium administration, there is moderate to severe left atrial enlargement with compression of the left caudal lobe bronchus between the enlarged left atrium (LA) and the descending thoracic aorta (Ao) as seen at the yellow arrow. The right caudal bronchus is normal (orange arrow). LV, left ventricle.

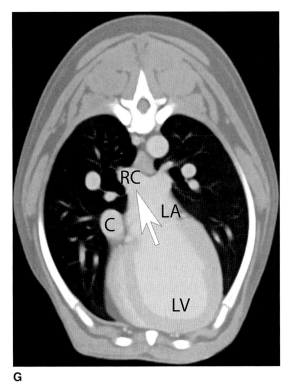

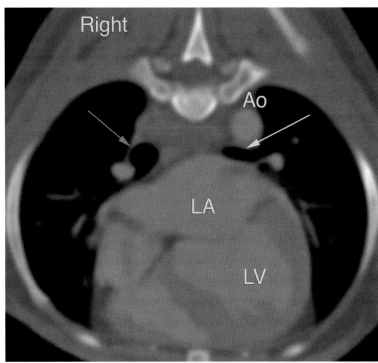

**G**   **H**

**FIGURE 16.20**   (Continued)

Mixed pulmonary patterns include a combination of decreased and increased opacity. This include hematoceles, pneumatoceles, cavitated lung nodules or masses (neoplasia or abscess formation), and a *vesicular* pulmonary pattern. A vesicular pulmonary pattern is a specific term to describe the type of pattern seen in a lung lobe torsion. The right middle lobe is the most common lobe to undergo a torsion in deep-chested dogs (Figure 16.37). Radiographic features of a lung lobe torsion are described in Box 16.4.

# Airspace and Bronchocentric Disease: an Alternative Approach

A different interpretation paradigm has been proposed [20]. In this paradigm, the opacity of the lung, the degree of lung expansion, and the anatomic distribution of the alterations are utilized to prioritize differentials. Increased opacity is further characterized as being solid (consolidation) or atelectasis and as either airspace or bronchocentric in pulmonary distribution.

In this scheme, consolidation refers to a lung lobe that is soft tissue opaque with loss of intralobar structures, has not lost volume and may or may not have air bronchograms within the affected lobe. In this scenario, *atelectasis* implies loss of air volume of the affected lung lobe with an ipsilateral mediastinal shift toward the affected lobe. Four different types of atelectasis have been described in human medicine: *relaxing, obstructive, adhesive,* and *cicatrizing.* These terms will not be defined here as often the etiology of the atelectasis may not be determined on the thoracic radiographs.

The term *airspace* has been applied to the lower airways and alveoli that contain air normally. This term can be applied to lesions that have been characterized as being consolidation, ground-glass opacity, nodules, and masses. This would correlate with alveolar, structured interstitial, unstructured interstitial, and mass pulmonary patterns in the previously described pulmonary interpretation paradigm.

Bronchocentric distribution implies thickening and abnormalities of the bronchovascular bundle (airways and corresponding blood vessels) in each of the lung lobes. This would correlate with bronchial and vascular pulmonary patterns in the previously described paradigm. At a certain level, these terms introduce an entire new level of complexity with overlap in their use and meaning, making the interpretation paradigm confusing. This interpretation paradigm, however, should not be totally discounted and has its merits. These include the same starting points with increased or decreased opacity, anatomic localization of the abnormal lung opacity, and presence or absence of a mediastinal shift being answered in both paradigms.

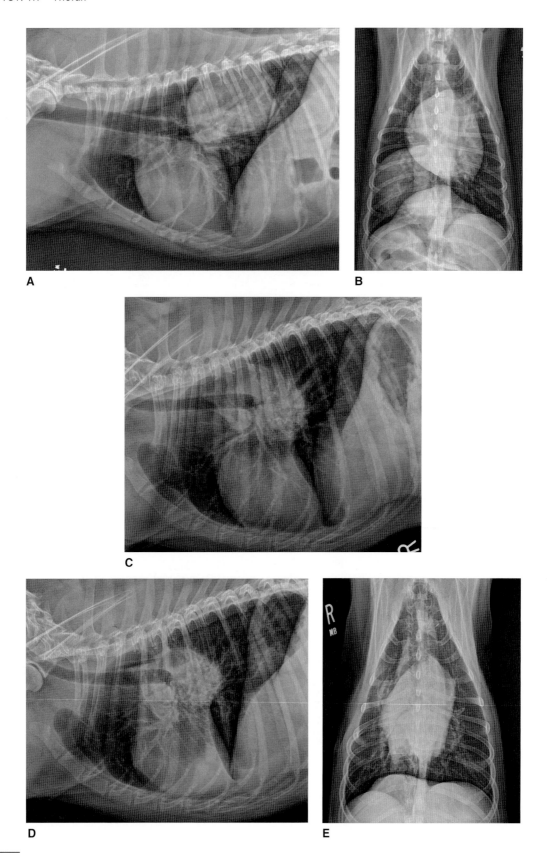

**FIGURE 16.21** Two dogs with pulmonary masses. In dog 1 (left lateral (**A**) and ventrodorsal (**B**) images), there is a right caudal pulmonary mass located caudal and dorsal within the lung lobe which measures 7.5 cm in diameter. In dog 2 (right lateral (**C**), left lateral (**D**), and ventrodorsal (**E**) images), there is a hilar mass that was documented to be pulmonary in origin at surgery even though the mass has characteristics of central tracheobronchial lymph node enlargement. There is peripheral atelectasis of the right middle lung lobe as seen on the left lateral view. Areas of central mineralization are noted within the pulmonary mass. Both tumors were bronchogenic carcinomas on histology.

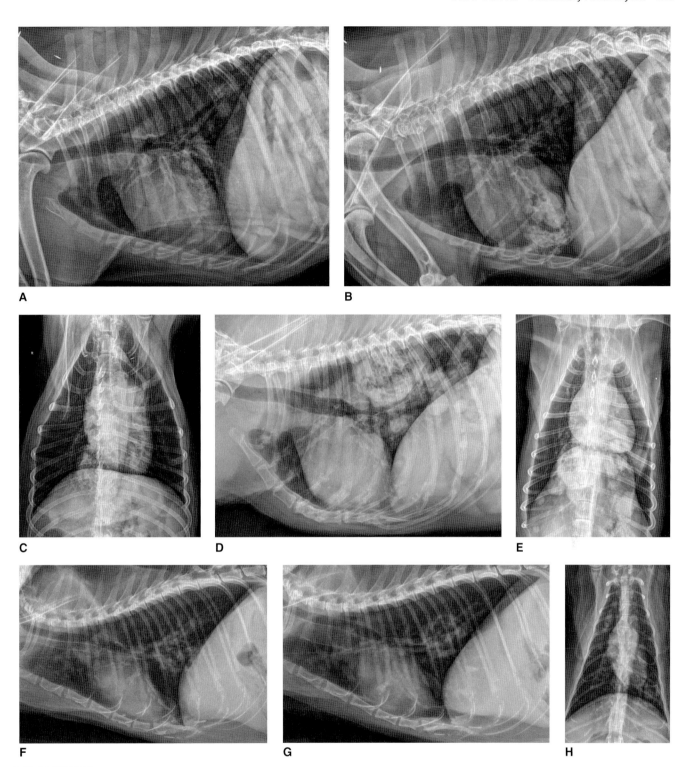

**FIGURE 16.22** Multiple pulmonary masses within the thorax of three dogs and one cat. In the first dog, (right lateral, left lateral, and ventrodorsal images (**A–C**)), there is a cavitated mass in the right middle lung lobe with multiple pulmonary nodules throughout the remainder of the lung lobes. A cavitated bronchoalveolar carcinoma was diagnosed at necropsy. In dog 2 (left lateral and dorsoventral images (**D,E**)), there is a large cavitated mass within the right caudal lung lobe and multiple variably sized pulmonary nodules noted predominantly in the caudal lung lobes. This was consistent with a primary lung tumor and metastatic pulmonary disease. On histology, the diagnosis was a bronchogenic carcinoma. In the cat (right lateral, left lateral, and dorsoventral images (**F–H**), there is a medium-sized cavitated pulmonary mass in the left caudal lung lobe. Other metastatic nodules are also noted within other lung lobes. The histologic diagnosis was bronchogenic carcinoma. In the last 2-year-old dog (right lateral, left lateral, and ventrodorsal radiographs (**I–K**)), there is a large central right caudal lung lobe mass with other pulmonary nodules and a right-sided unstructured interstitial to alveolar pulmonary pattern. At necropsy, mild to moderate tracheobronchial lymph enlargement was also identified. Histologic diagnosis was lymphomatoid granulomatosis.

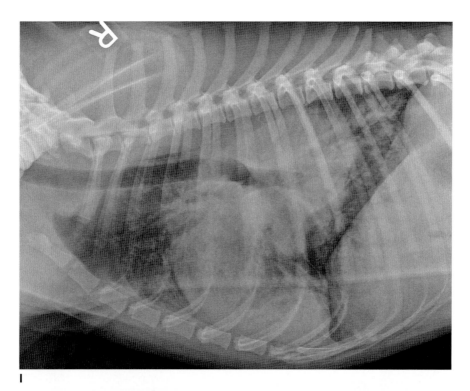

I

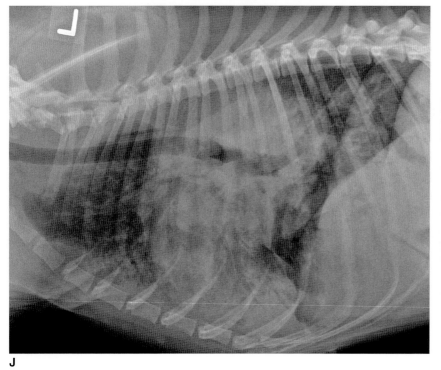

J

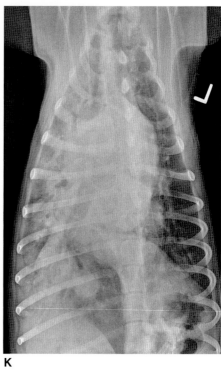

K

**FIGURE 16.22** (Continued)

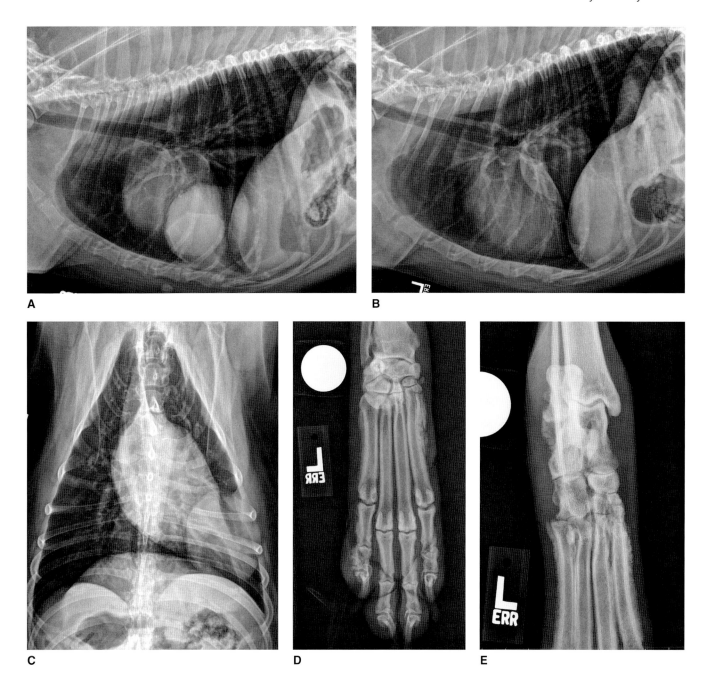

A

B

C

D

E

**FIGURE 16.23**  (**A-C**) In this dog, there is a large, left caudal and peripheral pulmonary mass with a peripheral pleural component (as noted on the ventrodorsal image). On other views (dorsopalmar manus/carpus (**D**) and dorsoplantar pes/tarsus (**E**)), an irregular palisading periosteal reaction is noted along the metacarpal, phalanges, metatarsal, and tarsal bones. These changes are consistent with hypertrophic osteopathy secondary to the pulmonary mass (cytologic diagnosis: carcinoma). The changes are axial and abaxial in location as is typical for hypertrophic osteopathy initially.

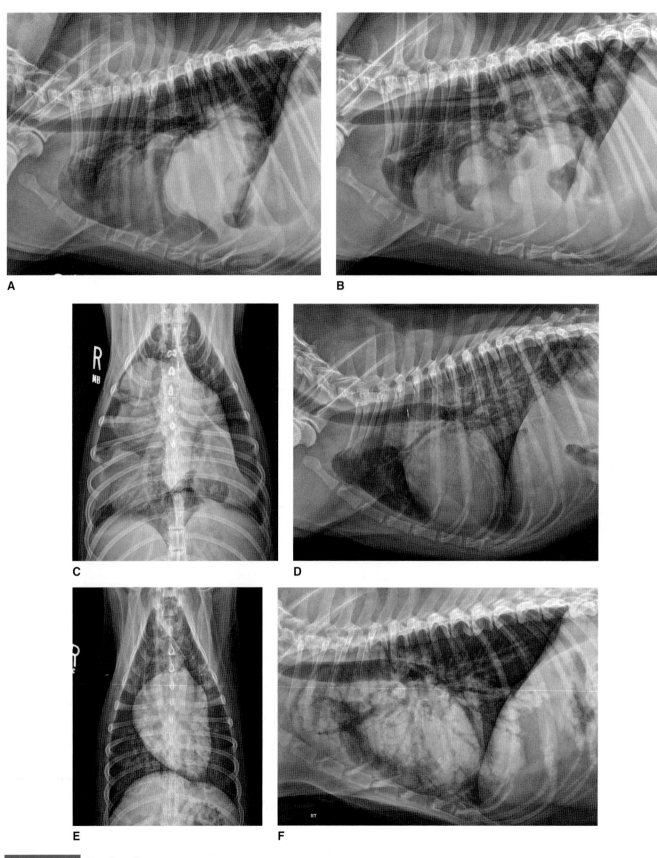

A

B

C

D

E

F

**FIGURE 16.24** (Continued)

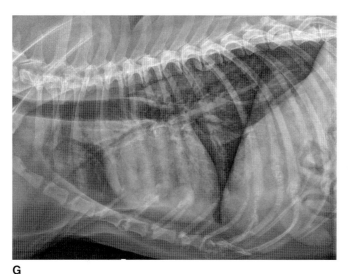
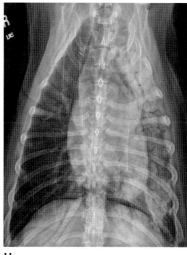

G

H

**FIGURE 16.24**  Variable presentations of histiocytic sarcoma. Although not shown, this lesion has been shown to involve the right middle lung lobe most commonly. In dog 1 (right lateral, left lateral, and ventrodorsal images (**A–C**)), there are multiple pulmonary nodules and masses, tracheobronchial lymph node enlargement, and pleural involvement (mass effect along right thoracic wall on ventrodorsal and pleural effusion). In dog 2 (left lateral and ventrodorsal images (**D,E**)), there is primarily an unstructured interstitial pulmonary pattern with a caudodorsal distribution. In dog 3 (right lateral, left lateral, and ventrodorsal images (**F–H**)), there is an alveolar pulmonary pattern within the left cranial and caudal lung lobes with pulmonary nodules noted in the right middle lobe on the left lateral view. The typical radiographic features of histiocytic sarcoma include pulmonary masses (with right middle involvement) and thoracic lymph node enlargement. In the second and third dogs in this Figure, atypical presentations are shown.

---

**Box 16.3** Roentgen Signs of An Alveolar Pulmonary Pattern.

1. Uniform soft tissue opacity
2. Air bronchograms (present 95% of the time)
3. Lobar sign
4. Border effacement of the cardiac silhouette and/or diaphragm

5. Border effacement of the small structures within the lung lobe such as the pulmonary vessels and the outer serosal wall of the airways (must be present)

---

# Tying It All Together

Anatomic localization and pulmonary patterns become important in formulating a differential diagnosis. Cranioventral distribution means that pneumonia from any cause is a primary differential. Caudodorsal distribution means that pulmonary edema (cardiogenic or noncardiogenic) from any cause is a primary differential. A prioritized differential list can only be made after the clinical signs, history, physical exam, and laboratory findings and signalment are taken into account. Repeat radiographs of the thorax can then be used to evaluate response to therapy. In dogs with an alveolar pulmonary or bronchial pulmonary pattern, the next step would be a transtracheal wash or bronchoalveolar lavage for obtaining cytology and fluid for

culture and antibiotic sensitivity if any bacteria are grown. A structured and unstructured interstitial does not lend itself to retrieving cells for cytologic evaluation.

Thoracic ultrasound and ultrasound-guided fine needle aspirations are useful for pulmonary masses and nodules that are peripheral in location. In addition, some interstitial pulmonary changes will exfoliate, and fine needle aspirates can be beneficial for providing a definitive diagnosis.

Differentials for pulmonary diseases are listed in Box 16.5 based on a pattern approach. Remember, thoracic radiographs do not equate with histology and next steps should be pursued to obtain a definitive diagnosis when appropriate. In certain cases, response to therapy (as documented on follow-up thoracic radiographs) and presumptive diagnoses are appropriate.

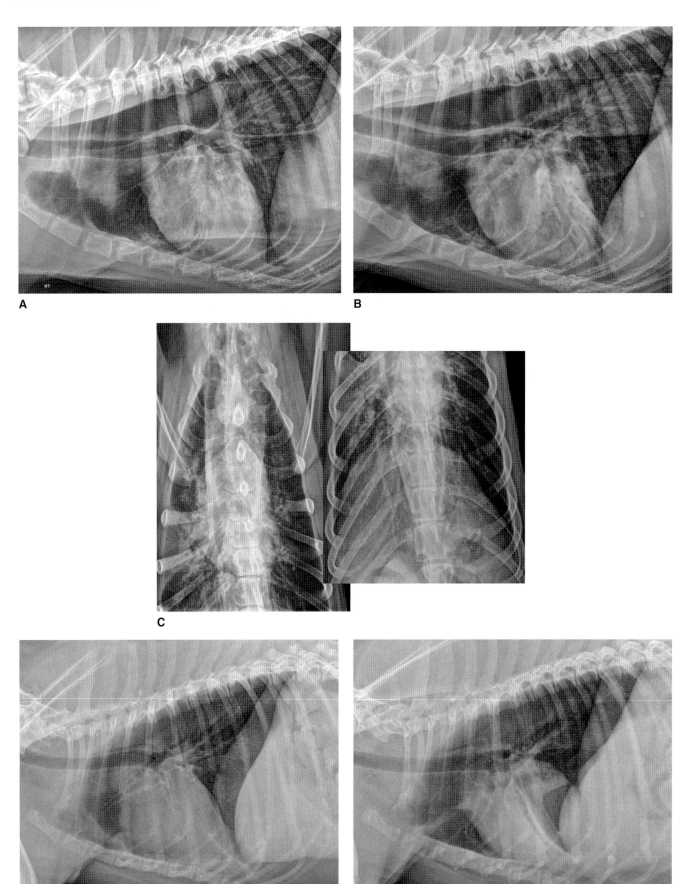

A

B

C

D

E

**FIGURE 16.25** (Continued)

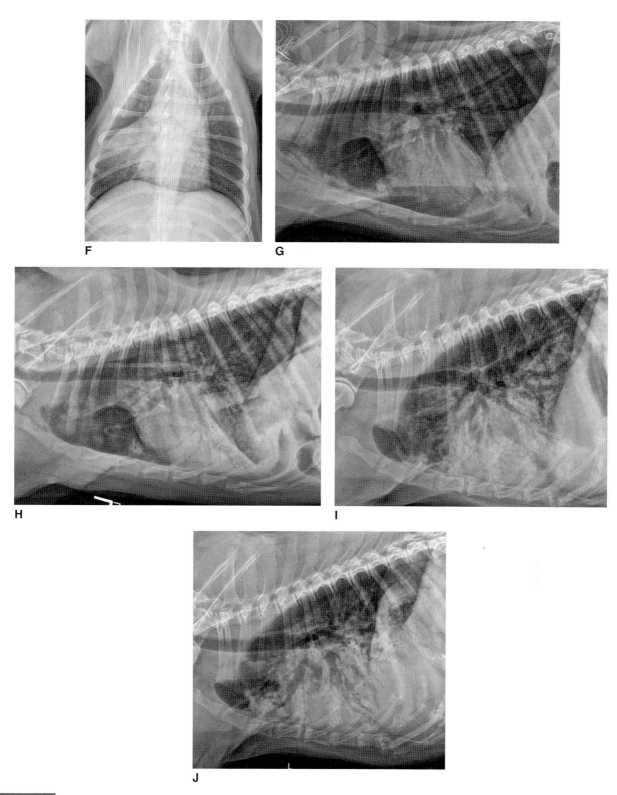

**FIGURE 16.25** Varying degrees of alveolar pulmonary patterns are shown in four different dogs, all with aspiration or bronchopneumonia. In dog 1 (right lateral, left lateral, and ventrodorsal views (**A–C**)), there is a generalized gas distension of the esophagus, an alveolar pulmonary pattern within the caudal subsegment of the left cranial lung lobe, best seen on the right lateral, an alveolar pattern within the right middle lung lobe, best seen on the left lateral image, and an ill-defined cranial mediastinal mass. These changes are consistent with a cranial mediastinal thymoma, a paraneoplastic syndrome of myasthenia gravis with a megaesophagus and an aspiration pneumonia. In dog 2 (right lateral, left lateral, and ventrodorsal views (**D–F**)), there is a focal right middle lung lobe aspiration pneumonia from vomiting. Notice that the affected lobe and pathology are not seen on the right lateral except as a thin pleural fissure line over the caudal ventral cardiac silhouette. On the left lateral, all the features of an alveolar pulmonary pattern can be identified. In dog 3 (right lateral and left lateral views (**G,H**)), there is a ventral alveolar pulmonary pattern within the right and left cranial and right middle lung lobes. Additionally, an unstructured interstitial pulmonary pattern is noted in the right caudal lung lobe on the left lateral and in a more central position than the peripheral alveolar patterns noted. In dog 4 (right lateral and left lateral views (**I,J**)), there is a ventral alveolar pulmonary pattern within the right and left cranial and right middle and caudal lung lobes. Additionally, there is some peripheral dilation of the airways consistent with a saccular bronchiectasis. In this last dog, the changes had a more chronic history and ciliary dyskinesia was diagnosed based on electron microscopy of the airway cilia.

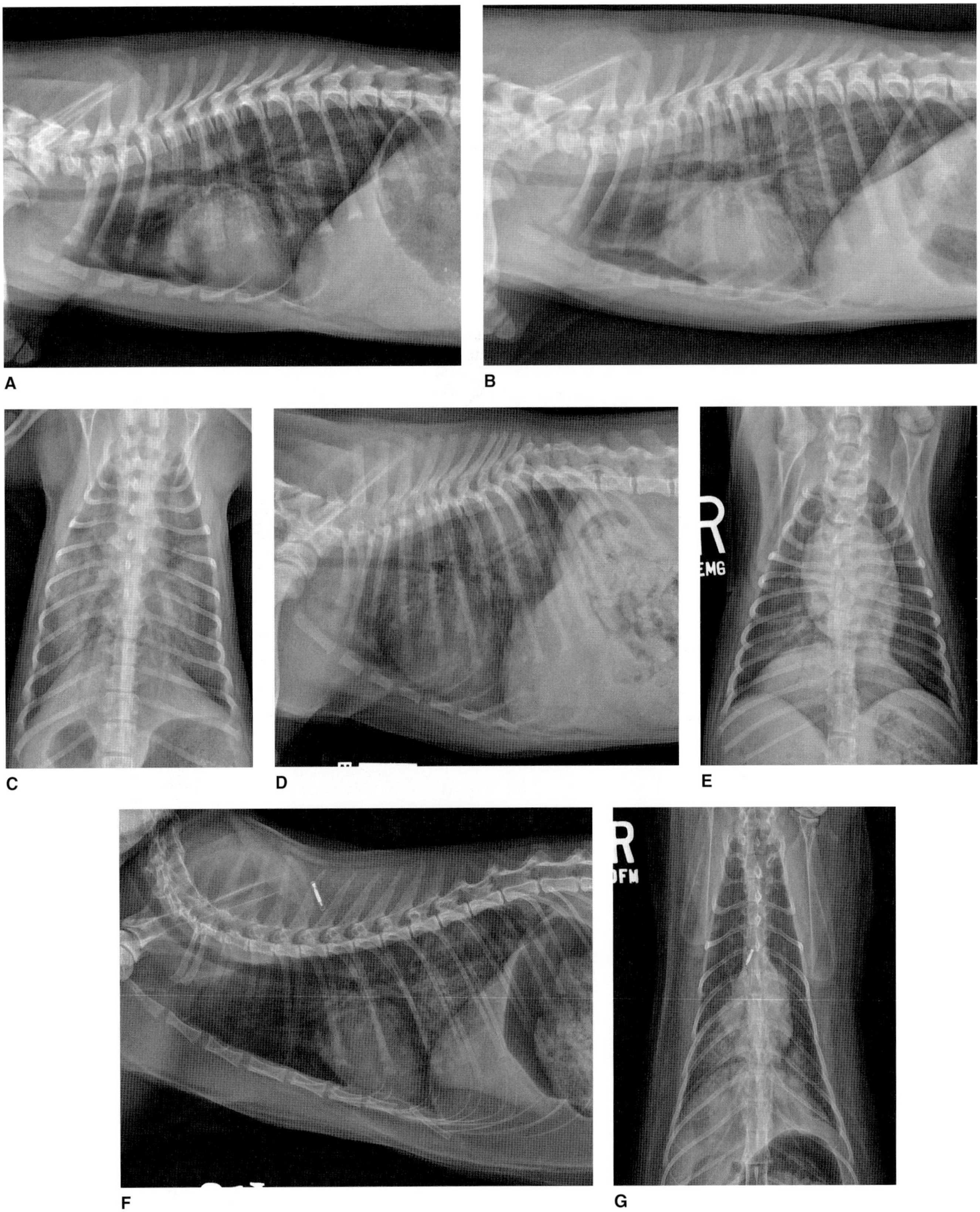

**FIGURE 16.26** Varying degrees of noncardiogenic pulmonary edema secondary to electric cord bites from two dogs and a cat. In dog 1 (right lateral, left lateral, and dorsoventral views (**A–C**)), there is a generalized moderate to severe unstructured interstitial pulmonary pattern. Similar changes are noted in dog 2 (right lateral and ventrodorsal views (**D,E**)), except the anatomic distribution is more caudodorsal. Additional thoracic vertebral anomalies are noted consistent with the bulldog breed. In the cat (third case, right lateral and ventrodorsal images (**F,G**)), there are unstructured interstitial to early alveolar pulmonary patterns noted in the caudodorsal lung fields. As neurogenic edema is a proteinaceous edema, it will take 3–5 days to resolve, whereas cardiogenic pulmonary edema is responsive to Lasix and typically clears in 24 hours post treatment.

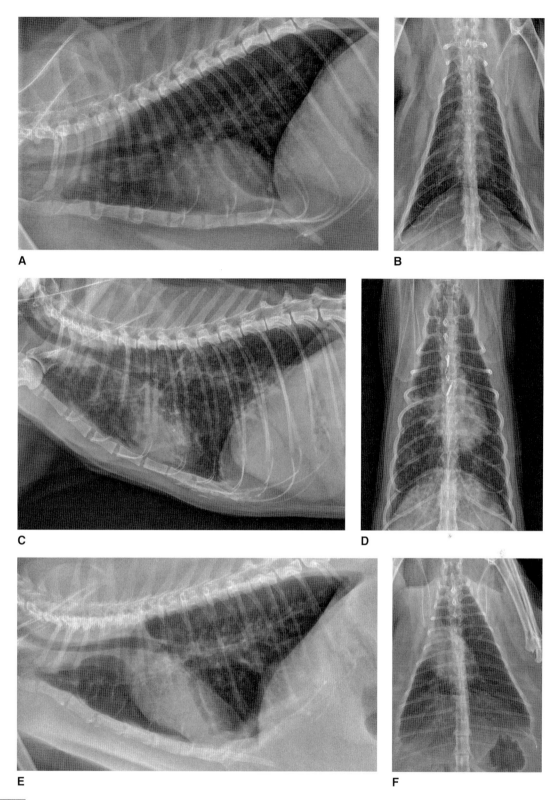

**FIGURE 16.27** Three examples of bronchial changes in different cats. All cats were diagnosed with *feline allergic lung disease* and responded to appropriate therapy with recurrence when off treatment. In cat 1 (left lateral and dorsoventral images (**A,B**)), there is a moderate bronchial pulmonary pattern that is generalized. There is collapse of the right middle lung lobe with a lobar sign on the left lateral view over the caudoventral aspect of the cardiac silhouette. The airway walls are thickened throughout. Several soft tissue nodules are noted consistent with mucous plugging of distal airways. In cat 2 (right lateral and ventrodorsal views (**C,D**)), there is a diffuse bronchial pulmonary pattern with some degree of unstructured interstitial pulmonary pattern between the thickened airway walls. There are several areas of plate-like atelectasis, emphysematous changes, and bronchiectasis. These changes are all consistent with chronic obstructive pulmonary disease. In cat 3 (left lateral and dorsoventral images (**E,F**)), there is a generalized severe bronchial pulmonary pattern. There is lobar collapse of the right cranial lung lobe with craniolateral deviation of the cardiac silhouette. A lobar sign is noted over the pulmonary hilum on the left lateral view consistent with the collapsed right cranial lung lobe and alveolar pulmonary pattern. The atelectasis in this case was secondary to mucous plugging. There is moderate enlargement of the right caudal pulmonary artery with some degree of better inflation of the left lung field on the dorsoventral view.

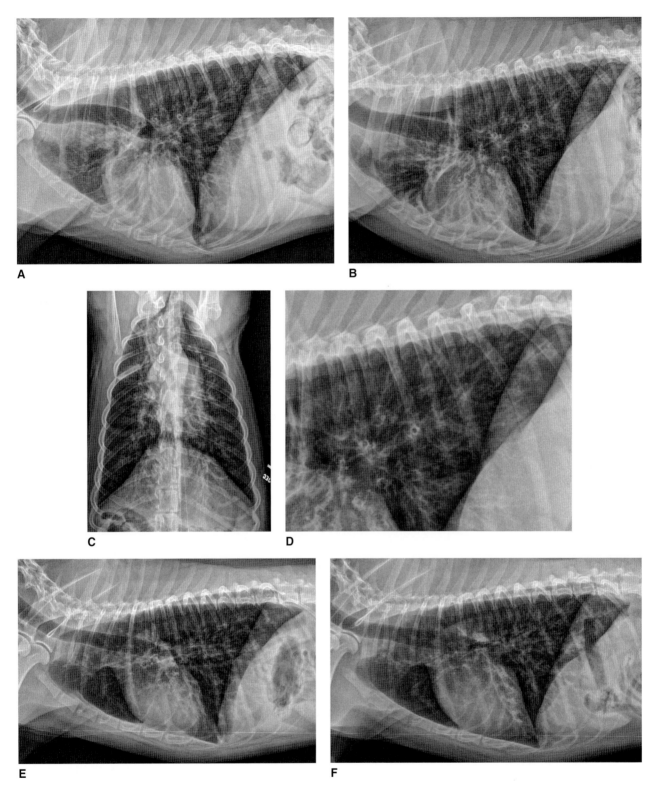

**FIGURE 16.28** Four different dogs with varying degrees of bronchial changes (including bronchiectasis in several cases). In dog 1 (right lateral, left lateral, dorsoventral, and close-up left lateral images (**A–D**)), there is a severe generalized bronchial pulmonary pattern with peripheral alveolar changes noted on the lateral images. The "rings and lines" can be traced out into the thin sections of the peripheral aspect of the different lung lobes. The final diagnosis was eosinophilic bronchopneumopathy. In dog 2 (right lateral, left lateral, and ventrodorsal images (**E–G**)), there is a moderate diffuse bronchial pulmonary pattern. The same diagnosis as the first dog was made. In dog 3 (right lateral, left lateral, and ventrodorsal images (**H–J**)), there is a diffuse bronchial pulmonary pattern with severe tubular bronchiectasis. Peripheral alveolar changes are noted on the laterals and there is an alveolar pulmonary pattern with some volume loss noted to the right middle lung lobe. On the ventrodorsal image, there is border effacement of the right side of the cardiac silhouette with the right middle lung lobe. This dog had ciliary dyskinesia with chronic bronchiectasis and recurrent pneumonias. In dog 4 (right lateral, left lateral, ventrodorsal, and CT images (**K–P**)), there is a bronchial pulmonary pattern with some degree of peripheral bronchiectasis noted on the radiographs. Multifocal soft tissue nodules are noted in the peripheral aspect of the lung lobes on the lateral images. The right middle lung lobe is atelectatic with loss of volume and an alveolar pulmonary pattern. The CT images document the severity of the bronchiectasis that cannot be visualized on the survey thoracic radiographs. The last image (**P**) is a 3-D oblique rendering of the right lung lobes, documenting the saccular nature of the bronchiectatic changes within these lung lobes. The soft tissue nodules were focal collections of pus within the saccular bronchiectatic airways.

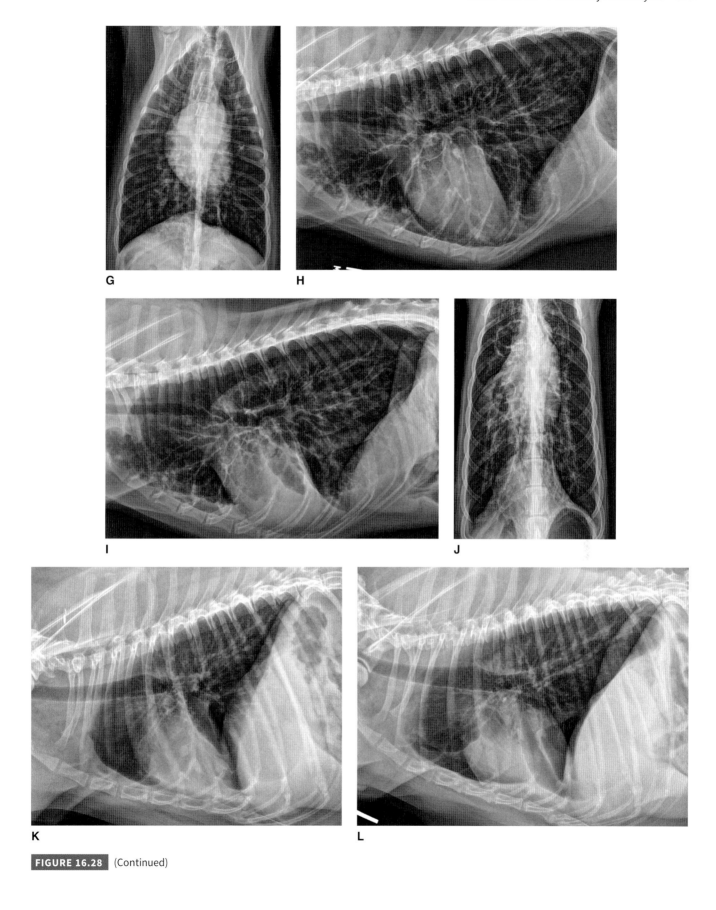

**FIGURE 16.28**    (Continued)

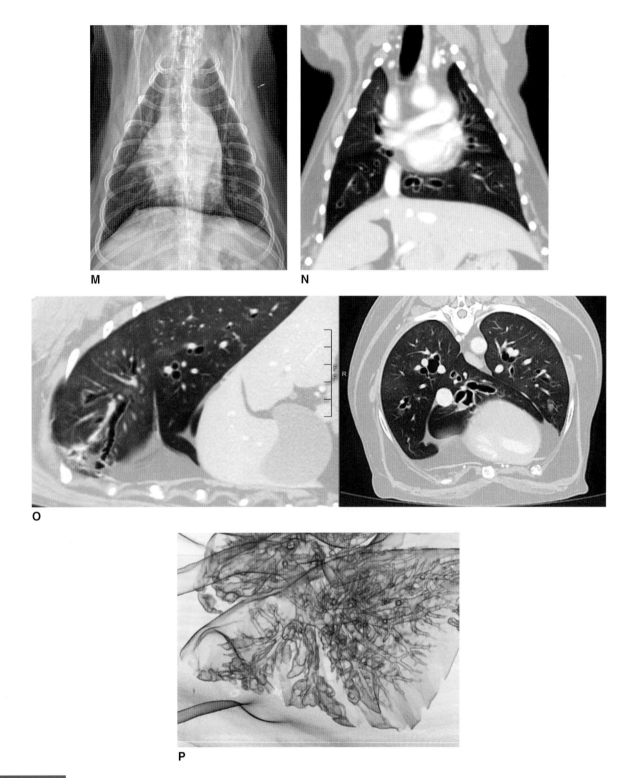

**FIGURE 16.28** (Continued)

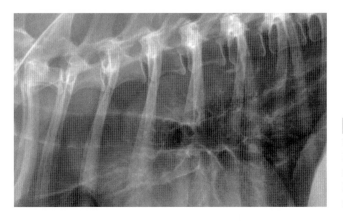

**FIGURE 16.29** Central airway mineralization without bronchial wall thickening. Central bronchiectasis is also seen in this geriatric dog. Differentials would include age related changes in a geriatric patient, Cushing disease or dystrophic mineralization secondary to chronic bronchitis (which is probably the case in this dog with the associated airway dilation).

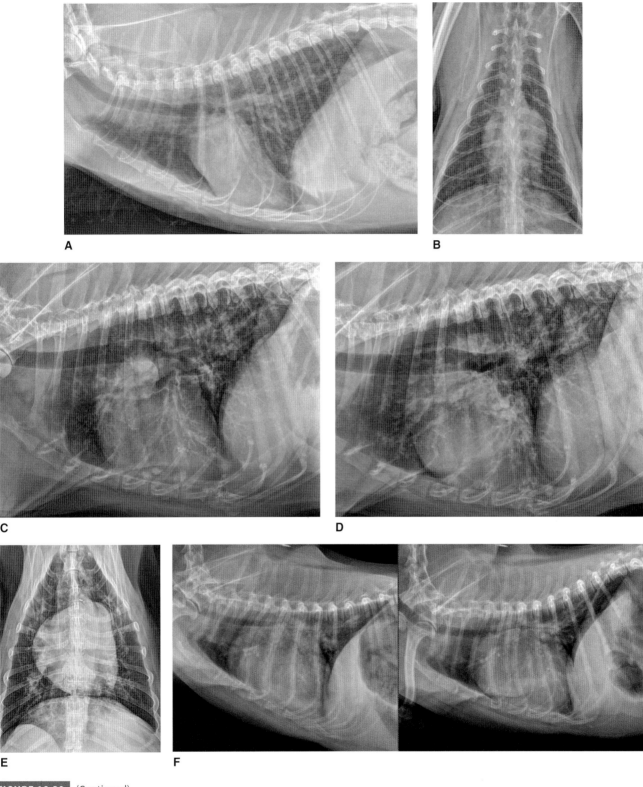

A

B

C

D

E

F

**FIGURE 16.30** (Continued)

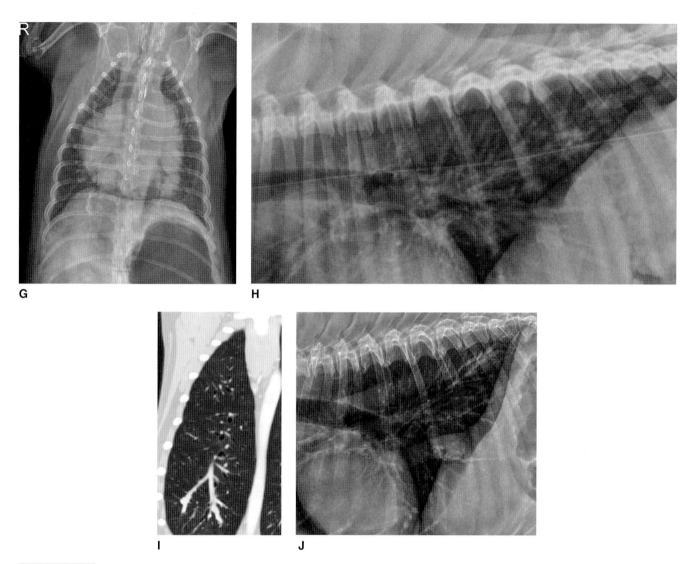

**FIGURE 16.30** Various radiographic abnormalities seen with heartworm disease in the dog and cat. In the initial set of images (right lateral and dorsoventral images (**A,B**)) from a cat that presented for a cough and vomiting, there is a generalized bronchial pulmonary pattern and enlargement and irregular margination (tortuosity) noted to the caudal lobar pulmonary arteries. There is blunting of the right caudal lobar artery. In dog 1 (right lateral, left lateral, and ventrodorsal images (**C–E**)), there is a generalized bronchial pulmonary pattern with enlargement of the pulmonary arteries noted throughout the lung fields. There is enlargement of the main pulmonary artery and the right and left caudal lobar pulmonary arteries seen on both the lateral and ventrodorsal images. There is right-sided cardiomegaly most pronounced on the ventrodorsal. Blunting and irregular margination of the left caudal pulmonary artery is present consistent with chronic thromboembolic disease. An underlying unstructured interstitial pulmonary pattern is also present. In dog 2 (right lateral, left lateral, and ventrodorsal images (**F,G**)) there is severe main pulmonary artery enlargement, right-sided cardiomegaly and severe caudal lobar pulmonary artery enlargement with tortuosity and blunting in the periphery. Several areas of pulmonary artery mineralization are noted consistent with chronic thromboembolic disease. In dog 3 (right lateral close-up and dorsal plane CT images (**H,I**)), there is enlargement of multiple pulmonary vessels in the periphery on the radiograph. On the dorsal plane reconstructed CT, there is enlargement, tortuosity, and saccular dilation noted to the pulmonary arteries in the right caudal lung lobe. In the final dog (right lateral image (**J**)), there are areas of multifocal dystrophic mineralization associated with prior heartworm disease post adulticide therapy. These changes do not rule out active disease.

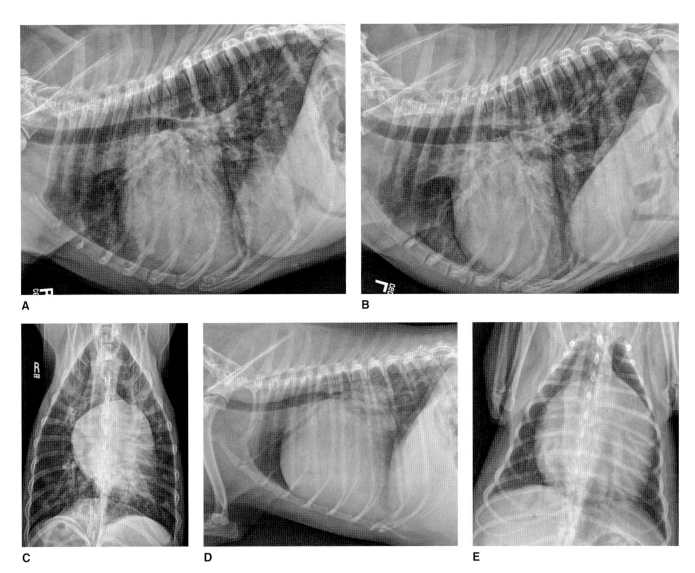

A

B

C

D

E

**FIGURE 16.31** Two dogs presenting with clinical signs related to acute onset of pulmonary edema. In dog 1 (right lateral, left lateral, and ventrodorsal images (**A–C**)), there is enlargement of the left side of the cardiac silhouette, pulmonary vein enlargement and a generalized unstructured interstitial pulmonary pattern. This dog had dilated cardiomyopathy and left heart failure. In dog 2 (left lateral and ventrodorsal images (**D,E**)), there is severe left-sided cardiomegaly, dorsal elevation of the trachea and carina, compression of the left caudal bronchus and an unstructured interstitial pulmonary pattern noted in the caudodorsal lung lobes. Severe mitral valve degenerative disease was diagnosed on echocardiography.

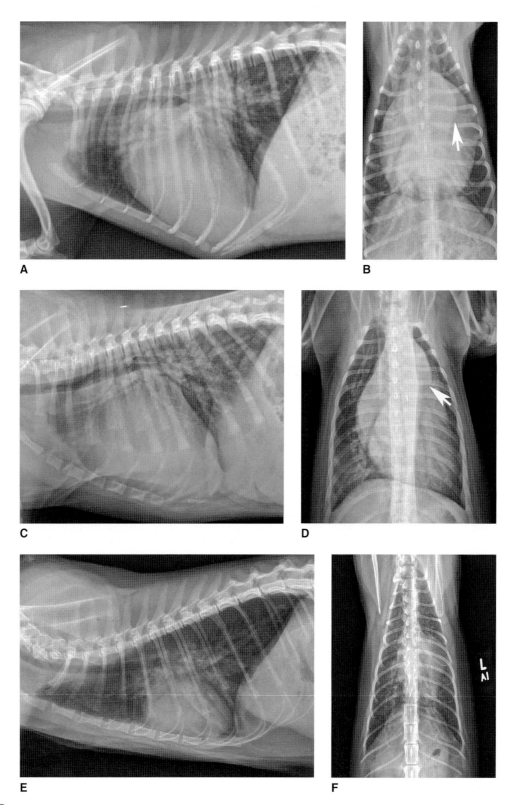

**FIGURE 16.32** Enlargement of the pulmonary arteries and veins in two dogs and a cat. In dog 1 (right lateral and dorsoventral images (**A**,**B**)) and dog 2 (right lateral and dorsoventral images (**C**,**D**)), there is severe left-sided cardiomegaly, pulmonary artery and venous distension, dorsal elevation of the trachea, an unstructured interstitial pulmonary pattern and a ductus diverticulum (white arrows) noted on the dorsoventral images consistent with left to right shunting patent ductus arteriosus. In the cat (right lateral and ventrodorsal images (**E**,**F**)), there is atrial enlargement with enlargement of the pulmonary artery and vein on the ventrodorsal image. An unstructured interstitial pulmonary pattern is present. These changes were consistent with primary or secondary myocardial disease with left heart failure and pulmonary edema. The cat was diagnosed with hypertrophic cardiomyopathy on the echocardiogram.

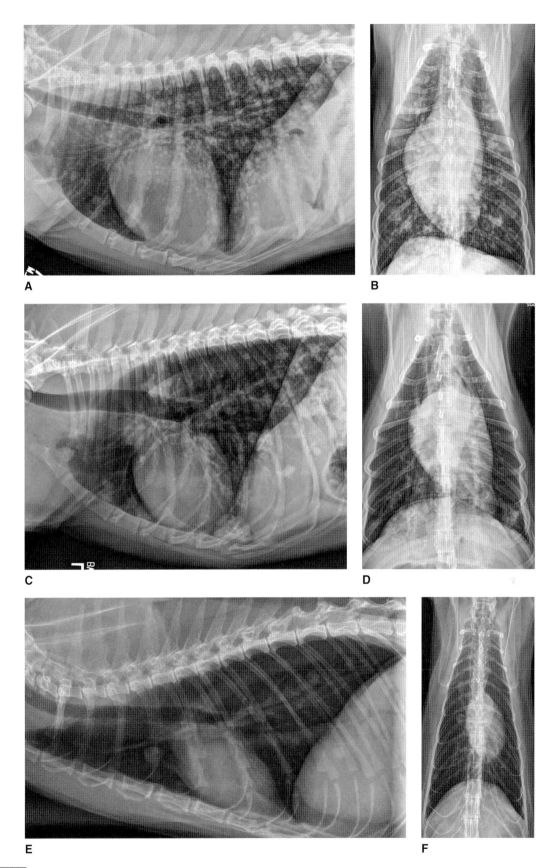

**FIGURE 16.33** Four examples of pulmonary metastatic disease. In dog 1, there are multiple small to varying sized pulmonary nodules (right lateral and ventrodorsal images (**A,B**)). Metastatic hemangiosarcoma was diagnosed at necropsy. In dog 2, variably sized pulmonary nodules are interspersed throughout all lung lobes (left lateral and ventrodorsal images (**C,D**)). Metastatic carcinoma from urothelial carcinoma was diagnosed. In cat 1 (right lateral and ventrodorsal images (**E,F**)), there are variably sized nodules noted consistent with metastatic disease. A primary mammary gland carcinoma was diagnosed. In dog 3, there are multiple pulmonary nodules and a diffuse right middle and right caudal unstructured interstitial pulmonary pattern (left lateral and ventrodorsal images (**G,H**)). All of the pulmonary changes were confirmed at necropsy to be metastatic disease from a renal cell carcinoma.

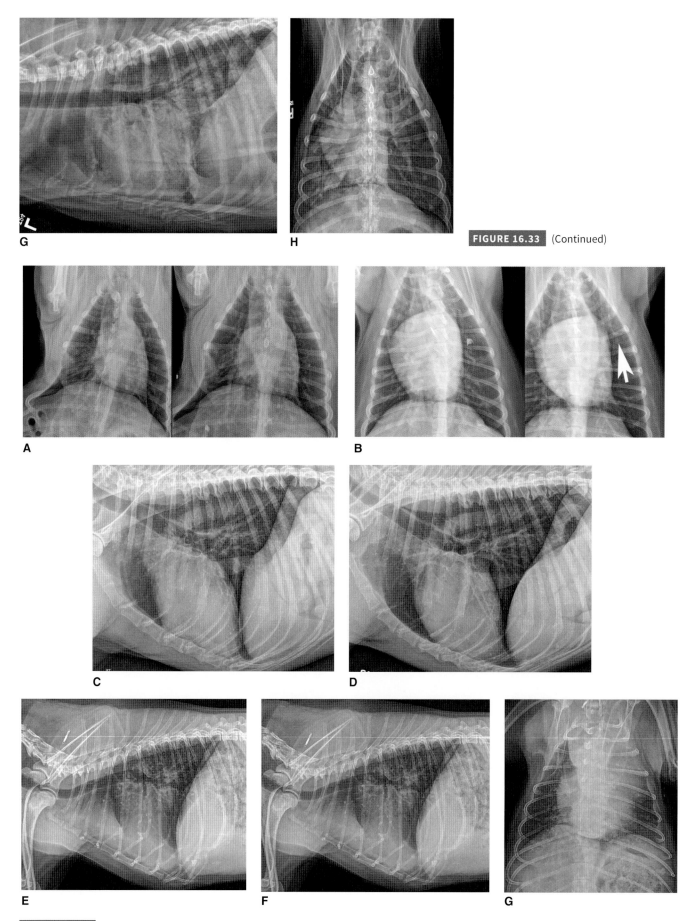

**FIGURE 16.33** (Continued)

**FIGURE 16.34** Several examples of other causes of "apparent" pulmonary nodules. In the first two dogs (all dorsoventral images (**A**,**B**)), there is pre- and postcontrast medium application (barium) on external nipples or skin tags. One can see that in dog 1, there are other pulmonary nodules present consistent with metastatic disease (primary was osteosarcoma from rib tumor with prior resection). In dog 2, the barium highlights a nipple that was apparent on the initial ventrodorsal as a possible pulmonary nodule. In dog 3 (right and left lateral images (**C**,**D**)) and dog 4 (right lateral, left lateral, and ventrodorsal images (**E–G**)), there are multiple small, mineralized, pulmonary osteomas. In addition, in the last dog there is a large left cranial lung lobe mass that was diagnosed on cytology as a carcinoma.

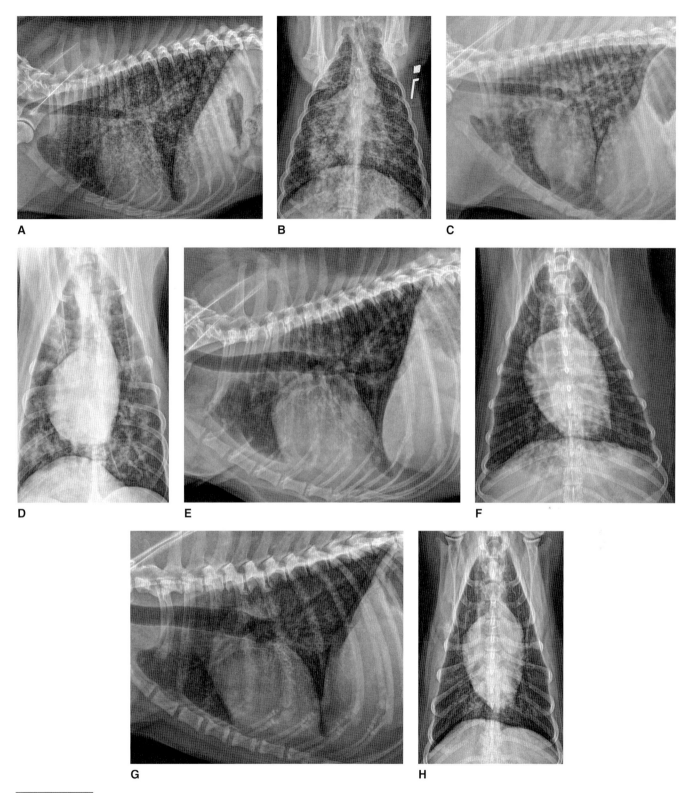

**FIGURE 16.35**   Multiple examples of miliary pulmonary patterns. The diagnoses in these cases were: dog 1 (**A,B**) – blastomycosis; dog 2 (**C,D**) – lymphoma; dogs 3 and 4 (**E–H**) – metastatic carcinoma.

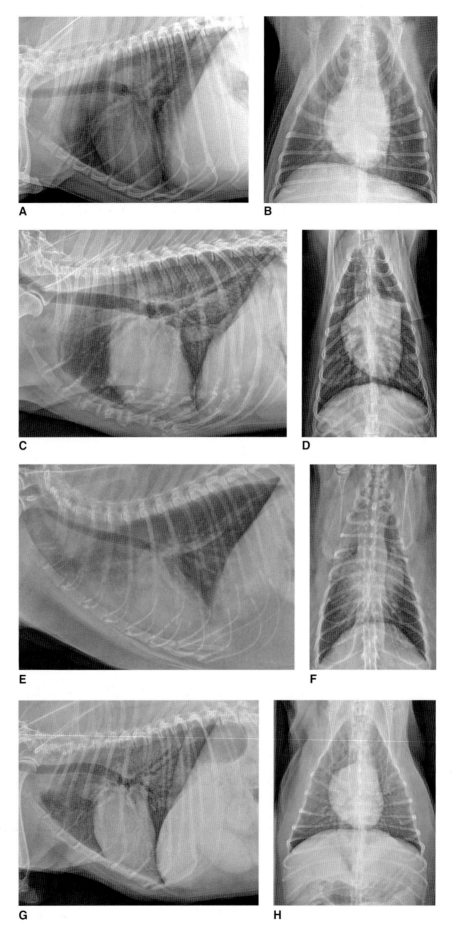

**FIGURE 16.36** Four examples (right lateral and ventrodorsal images for each) from three dogs and a cat with an unstructured interstitial pulmonary pattern. In the first two dogs (**A** and **B**, **C** and **D**) the diagnosis was pulmonary lymphoma (first dog also has thoracic lymph node enlargement). In the cat (**E**, **F**), the diagnosis was thoracic lymphoma (mild pleural effusion also evident; echocardiography of this cat was normal, and this was not left heart failure). In the final dog (**G**, **H**), the pattern is also noted to be mineralized. This last case was a dog with pulmonary mineralization secondary to chronic glucocorticoid administration.

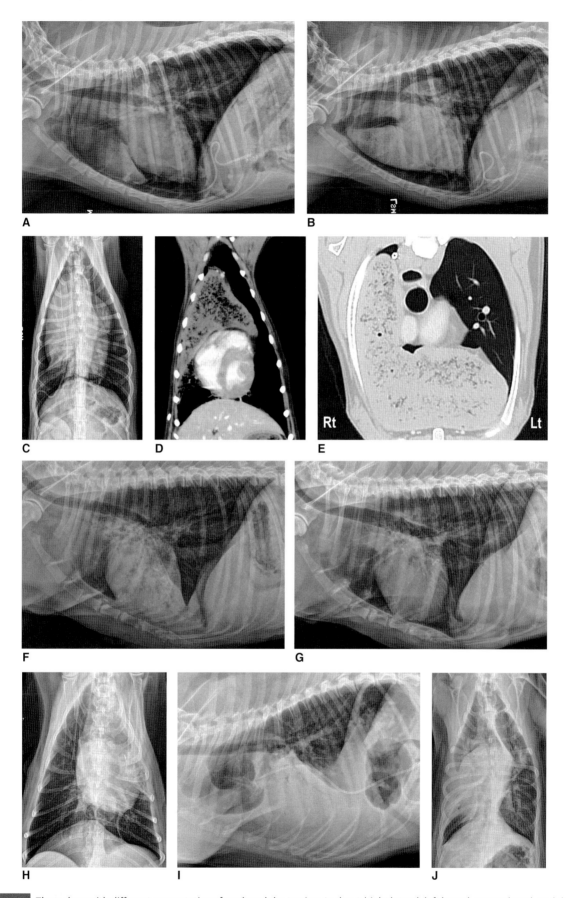

**FIGURE 16.37** Three dogs with different presentations for a lung lobe torsion. In dog 1 (right lateral, left lateral, ventrodorsal, and dorsal plane reconstructed and transverse CT images (**A–E**)), there is a large mass effect within the right cranial lobe, with a vesicular pulmonary pattern. There is a pneumothorax, and a chest tube has been placed. There is collapse of the right cranial bronchus at the pulmonary hilum. In dog 2 (right lateral, left lateral, and ventrodorsal images (**F–H**)), there is a vesicular pattern within the left cranial lung lobe with a mass effect. The bronchus of the left cranial tapers abruptly at the carina. In dog 3 (left lateral and ventrodorsal images (**I,J**)) there is a pleural effusion (predominantly right sided) with a mass effect in the right middle lung lobe and a central air bronchogram. The proximal bronchus is not seen.

---

**Box 16.4 Roentgen Signs Associated with Lung Lobe Torsion.**

1. Lobar involvement (uniform soft tissue opacity with central air bronchogram or vesicular pattern)
2. ± Pleural effusion
3. ± Mass effect within the affected lung lobe
4. Mediastinal shift away from the affected lobe
5. Blunting or twisting of the central portion of the affected lung lobe bronchus

---

**Box 16.5 Common Causes of Pulmonary Patterns in Dogs and Cats.**

Pulmonary Masses

Primary lung tumor

Granulomatous pneumonia (fungal, *Mycobacterium*, eosinophilic granulomatosis, lymphomatoid granulomatosis)

Histiocytic sarcoma

Metastatic neoplasia

Pulmonary Alveolar Pattern

Hemorrhage

Pneumonia (ventral distribution, right middle, canine more so than feline)

Neoplasia

Edema (caudodorsal [right-sided or bilateral] distribution, feline cardiogenic edema is variable, can be ventral, and multifocal)

Atelectasis (secondary to some other disease process; right middle lung lobe collapse, secondary mucous plugging common in cats with feline allergic lung disease)

Inflammatory syndromes (acute respiratory distresss syndrome)

Alveolar proteinosis

Lipid pneumonia

Noncardiogenic edema

Bronchial Pulmonary Pattern

Allergic lung disease (generalized, feline asthma)

Infectious (bacterial or parasitic)

Cardiogenic pulmonary edema (feline)

Disseminated neoplasia

Pulmonary Vascular Patterns – Increased Size
(A – artery; V – vein; B – both)

Fluid overload (B)

Left-to-right shunts (B)

Cardiogenic pulmonary edema – dogs (V)

Cardiogenic pulmonary edema – cats (B)

Heartworm disease and endarteritis (includes dirofiliarisis, angiostrongyliasis)
(A)

Aelurostrongyliasis – cats (A)

Thromboembolic disease (A)

Pulmonary hypertension and severe chronic obstructive lung disease (COPD) (A)

Structured Interstitial

Nodules

Metastatic disease (± cavitation), osteomas (small, mineralized), granulomas (bacterial, fungal, parasitic ±cavitation)

Miliary

Lymphoma, fungal, metastatic carcinoma

Unstructured Interstitial (Back Door Diagnosis by Ruling all Other Patterns Out)

Underexposure

Expiration

Obesity

Lymphoma

Cardiogenic and noncardiogenic edema

Hemorrhage

Neoplasia – metastatic disease

Toxicity

Venoocclusive disease

Upper airway obstruction

Fibrosis

Infectious (viral or fungal)

Bacterial pneumonia

Pulmonary mineralization

Lipid pneumonia

# References

1. Hansell, D.M., Bankier, A.A., MacMahon, H. et al. (2008). Fleischner Society: glossary of terms for thoracic imaging. *Radiology* 246 (3): 697–722.

2. Tidwell, A.S. (1992). Diagnostic pulmonary imaging. *Probl. Vet. Med.* 4 (2): 239–264.

3. Schwarz, L.A. and Tidwell, A.S. (1999). Alternative imaging of the lung. *Clin. Tech. Small Anim. Pract.* 14 (4): 187–206.

4. Habing, A., Coelho, J.C., Nelson, N. et al. (2011). Pulmonary angiography using 16 slice multidetector computed tomography in normal dogs. *Vet. Radiol. Ultrasound* 52 (2): 173–178.

5. Shimbo, G. and Takiguchi, M. (2021). CT morphology of anomalous systemic arterial supply to normal lung in dogs. *Vet. Radiol. Ultrasound* 62 (6): 657–665.

6. Thrall, D.E. (2018). Canine and feline lung. In: *Textbook of Veterinary Diagnostic Imaging*, 7e (ed. D.E. Thrall). St Louis, MO: Elsevier.

7. Szabo, D., Sutherland-Smith, J., Barton, B. et al. (2015). Accuracy of a computed tomography bronchial wall thickness to pulmonary artery diameter ratio for assessing bronchial wall thickening in dogs. *Vet. Radiol. Ultrasound* 56 (3): 264–271.

8. Silverman, S. and Suter, P.F. (1975). Influence of inspiration and expiration on canine thoracic radiographs. *J. Am. Vet. Med. Assoc.* 166 (5): 502–510.

9. Cannon, M.S., Wisner, E.R., Johnson, L.R., and Kass, P.H. (2009). Computed tomography bronchial lumen to pulmonary artery diameter ratio in dogs without clinical pulmonary disease. *Vet. Radiol. Ultrasound* 50 (6): 622–624.

10. Panopoulos, I., Auriemma, E., Specchi, S. et al. (2019). 64-multidetector CT anatomical assessment of the feline bronchial and pulmonary vascular structures. *J. Feline Med. Surg.* 21 (10): 893–901.

11. Samii, V.F., Biller, D.S., and Koblik, P.D. (1998). Normal cross-sectional anatomy of the feline thorax and abdomen: comparison of computed tomography and cadaver anatomy. *Vet. Radiol. Ultrasound* 39 (6): 504–511.

12. Amis, T.C. and McKierman, B.C. (1986). Systematic identification of the endobronchial anatomy during bronchoscopy in the dog. *Am. J. Vet. Res.* 47: 2549–2657.

13. Hornby, N.L. and Lamb, C.R. (2017). Does the computed tomographic appearance of the lung differ between young and old dogs? *Vet. Radiol. Ultrasound* 58 (6): 647–652.

14. Brinkman, E.L., Biller, D., and Armbrust, L. (2006). The clinical usefulness of the ventrodorsal versus dorsoventral thoracic radiograph in dogs. *J. Am. Anim. Hosp. Assoc.* 42 (6): 440–449.

15. Kirberger, R.M. and Avner, A. (2006). The effect of positioning on the appearance of selected cranial thoracic structures in the dog. *Vet. Radiol. Ultrasound* 47 (1): 61–68.

16. Barletta, M., Almondia, D., Williams, J. et al. (2014). Radiographic evaluation of positional atelectasis in sedated dogs breathing room air versus 100% oxygen. *Can. Vet. J.* 55 (10): 985–991.

17. Hunt, T.D. and Wallack, S.T. (2021). Minimal atelectasis and poorly aerated lung on thoracic CT images of normal dogs acquired under sedation. *Vet. Radiol. Ultrasound* 62 (6): 647–656.

18. Winegardner, K., Scrivani, P.V., and Gleed, R.D. (2008). Lung expansion in the diagnosis of lung disease. *Compend. Contin. Educ. Vet.* 30 (9): 479–489.

19. Giglio, R.F., Winter, M.D., Reese, D.J. et al. (2013). Radiographic characterization of presumed plate-like atelectasis in 75 nonanesthetized dogs and 15 cats. *Vet. Radiol. Ultrasound* 54 (4): 326–331.

20. Scrivani, P.V. (2009). Nontraditional interpretation of lung patterns. *Vet. Clin. North Am. Small Anim. Pract.* 39 (4): 719–732.

# CHAPTER 17

# Mediastinum

Silke Hecht

Department of Small Animal Clinical Sciences, College of Veterinary Medicine, University of Tennessee, Knoxville, TN, USA

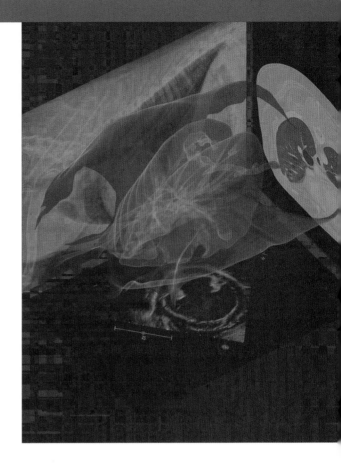

## Normal Anatomy

The mediastinal space is located between the right and left mediastinal pleura which is a continuation of the costal parietal pleura and marks the medial border of the left and right pleural sacs, respectively [1–3]. It is bordered dorsally by the spine and ventrally by the sternum (Figure 17.1). Cranially, the mediastinal space connects to the deep fascial planes of the neck musculature. Caudally, the ventral aspect of the mediastinal space is bordered by the diaphragm, while its dorsal aspect connects to the retroperitoneal space via the aortic hiatus. Organs contained within the mediastinal space include the heart, vessels (aorta, azygous vein, cranial and caudal vena cava [CVC], brachiocephalic trunk and left subclavian artery, main pulmonary arteries and veins, and smaller vessels), trachea and proximal mainstem bronchi, esophagus, lymphatic structures (thoracic duct, lymph nodes, thymus) as well as the vagus nerve and other smaller nerves. Additional structures within the mediastinal space include musculature (most notably the M. longus colli in the cranial thorax) and a variable amount of fat. Although the majority of the mediastinum is located roughly in the midsagittal plane of the thorax, there are exceptions.

- The cranioventral portion extends obliquely from right cranial (termed the *cranial mediastinal reflection*) to left caudal across the midline, resulting in shift of the thymus or thymic remnant into the left cranial hemithorax (Figure 17.2A).
- The caudoventral mediastinal recess extends from the plica of the CVC on the right across the midline and forms a pocket to accommodate leftward extension of the accessory lung lobe (ALL) (Figure 17.2B). The left border of this extension is termed the *caudal mediastinal reflection*.

The mediastinum can be categorized into a dorsal part and a ventral part using the tracheal bifurcation or heart base as an anatomic marker (Figure 17.3A). The mediastinum can also

*Atlas of Small Animal Diagnostic Imaging*, First Edition. Edited by Clifford R. Berry, Nathan C. Nelson, and Matthew D. Winter.
© 2023 John Wiley & Sons, Inc. Published 2023 by John Wiley & Sons, Inc.
Companion website: www.wiley.com/go/berry/atlas

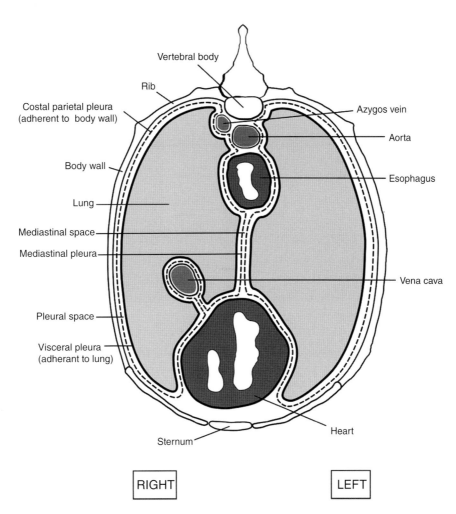

**FIGURE 17.1** Schematic transverse image of the thorax at the level of the heart. The parietal pleura, which covers the inner margin of the thoracic wall, continues into the mediastinal pleura which separates the left and right pleural cavities. The mediastinal pleural layers contain the mediastinal space. *Source:* Drawing courtesy of Dr Elodie Huguet.

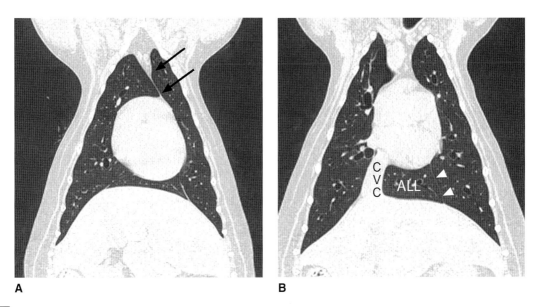

**FIGURE 17.2** Dorsal multiplanar reconstructed computed tomographic images of the normal thorax in a 16-year-old cocker spaniel. (**A**) The cranial aspect of the mediastinum crosses midline in a right-cranial to left-caudal direction (arrows). (**B**) The caudal mediastinum is bordered on the right by the caudal vena cava (CVC) and forms a pocket bordered to the left by the caudal mediastinal reflection (arrowheads) to accommodate leftward extension of the accessory lung lobe (ALL). Note also widening of the middle mediastinum to accommodate the heart.

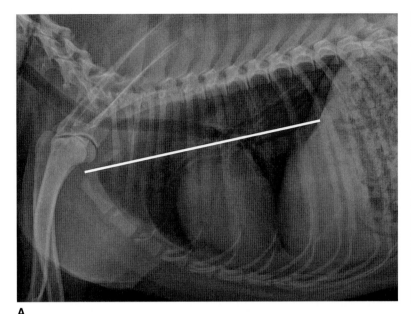
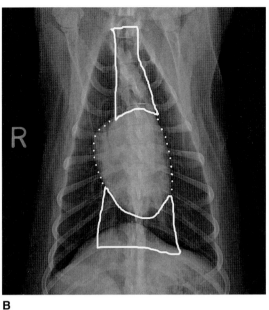

**A**   **B**

**FIGURE 17.3**   Right lateral (**A**) and ventrodorsal (**B**) radiographs demonstrating subdivision of the mediastinum into dorsal and ventral (**A**) as well as cranial, middle, and caudal (**B**).

be subdivided into cranial, middle, and caudal (Figure 17.3B). The cranial mediastinum extends from the thoracic inlet to the cranial margin of the heart. The middle mediastinum is occupied by the cardiac silhouette and is significantly widened. The caudal mediastinum extends from the heart to the diaphragm.

# Normal Radiographic Anatomy

As for any radiographic study of the thorax, the mediastinum should be evaluated on orthogonal views [2–4]. While the ventrodorsal (VD) view is generally considered superior for evaluation of the mediastinal structures, especially in the ventral aspect of the thorax, a dorsoventral (DV) view may aid in the evaluation of more dorsally located structures such as tracheobronchial lymph nodes and esophagus [5, 6]. On lateral thoracic radiographs, several mediastinal organs are visible (see later in this chapter), but most of the mediastinum itself is not seen as a distinct structure or compartment. The cranial mediastinal reflection may be apparent cranial to the heart and dorsal to the sternum as a curvilinear soft tissue opacity band which may contain a variable amount of fat (Figure 17.4A). On VD and DV radiographs, the mediastinal space is mostly located on the midline and superimposed with the spine and sternum. Similar to the lateral view, the cranial mediastinal reflection may be seen and appears as an obliquely oriented soft tissue opacity band in the right cranial thorax (Figure 17.4B), and the caudal mediastinal reflection which borders the left margin of the caudal mediastinum may be visible as a soft tissue opacity band of variable width (Figure 17.4C).

Overall, the width of the cranial mediastinum should not exceed twice the width of the spine in dogs (Figure 17.5A) although a large amount of fat deposits may result in significant mediastinal widening. In cats, the cranial mediastinum rarely exceeds the width of the spine (Figure 17.5B).

Of the organs and structures located in the mediastinum, only a few are visible on radiographs in normal animals as the others are either too small to be discernible (e.g., normal lymph nodes) or have the same (soft tissue) opacity as adjacent mediastinal structures, resulting in silhouetting (e.g., cranial mediastinal vessels). The following mediastinal structures are seen (Figures 17.6–17.9).

1. Cardiac silhouette
2. Trachea
3. CVC
4. Aorta
5. (± Variable amount of gas in esophagus, particularly on left lateral)
6. (± Variable amount of mediastinal fat)
7. (± Thymus in young animals)

# Mediastinal Abnormalities and Disorders

This chapter will discuss mediastinal shift, mediastinal fluid accumulation, masses, lymphadenopathy, pneumomediastinum, and esophageal and tracheal disorders. The heart is covered in a separate chapter.

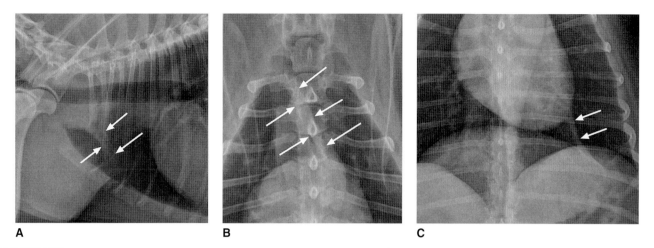

**FIGURE 17.4** The cranial mediastinal reflection appears as a curvilinear soft tissue opacity band on lateral (**A**) and ventrodorsal (**B**) radiographs (arrows). The caudal mediastinal reflection borders the left margin of the caudal mediastinum and is visible as a soft tissue opacity band of variable width on ventrodorsal views (arrows; **C**).

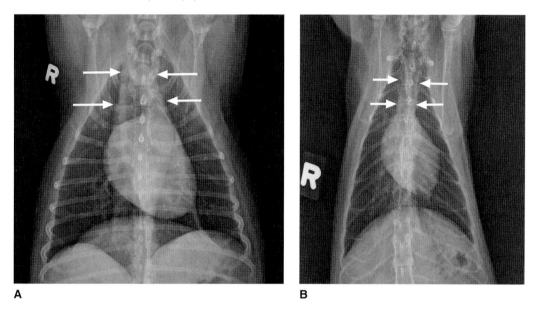

**FIGURE 17.5** Ventrodorsal radiographs of the cranial thorax in a normal dog (**A**) and cat (**B**). While the cranial mediastinum (arrows) in normal dogs may reach twice the width of the vertebral column it usually does not extend significantly beyond the spinal margins in cats.

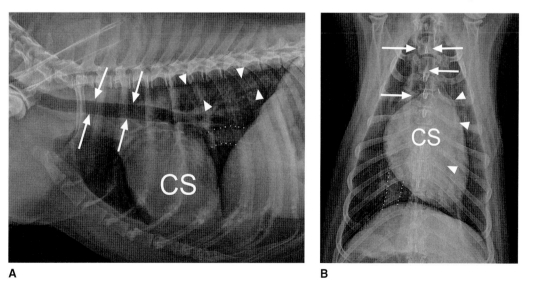

**FIGURE 17.6** Lateral (**A**) and ventrodorsal (**B**) radiographs indicating mediastinal structures visible in normal animals: cardiac silhouette (CS), trachea (arrows), aorta (arrowheads), caudal vena cava (dotted outline). Note also mediastinal fat deposits delineating the ventral margin of the heart on the lateral view.

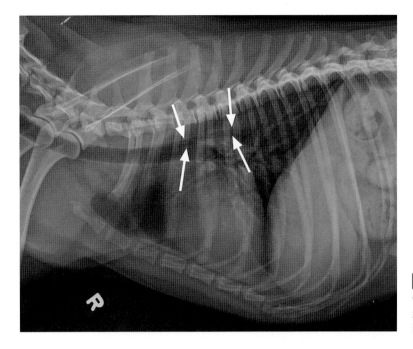

**FIGURE 17.7** Lateral view of the thorax in a 9-year-old mixed-breed dog demonstrating a small amount of gas within the thoracic esophagus (arrows) which is an incidental finding.

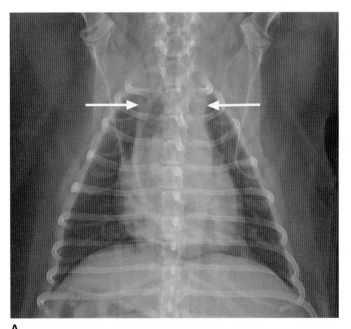

A

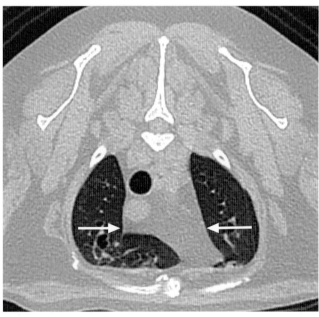

B

**FIGURE 17.8** Ventrodorsal thoracic radiograph (**A**) and transverse CT image cranial to the heart (**B**) demonstrating accumulation of a large amount of fat in the cranial mediastinum in a 13-year-old Pekingese resulting in cranial mediastinal widening (arrows).

## Mediastinal Shift

While mediastinal shift is not a disorder of the mediastinum per se, it is a very common finding in animals. A mediastinal shift is recognized on VD/DV views based on displacement of mediastinal structures (most notably the heart) into the left or right hemithorax [4, 7]. It can occur secondary to pull or push forces. The most common example of pull forces is pulmonary volume loss (atelectasis) due to lateral recumbency. This is a very common incidental finding and is frequently noted when obtaining radiographs under sedation or anesthesia (Figure 17.10). Other examples of pull forces include volume loss of a lung lobe secondary to bronchial obstruction (Figure 17.11) and decreased lung volume due to prior lung lobectomy (Figure 17.12). Any kind of space-occupying lesion within the thorax can result in a push force and cause mediastinal shift. Examples include severe lateralized pneumothorax or pleural effusion, abnormal contents in the thoracic cavity due to diaphragmatic hernia (Figure 17.13), thoracic masses (Figure 17.14), and deformities of the thoracic wall and/or sternum (Figure 17.15).

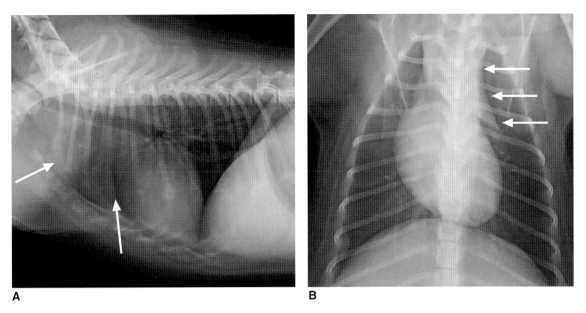

**FIGURE 17.9** Lateral (**A**) and ventrodorsal (**B**) radiographs of the thorax in a puppy. The thymus is seen as a triangular soft tissue opacity structure in the cranioventral mediastinum (arrows), resulting in a classic "sail sign" on the VD view (**B**). *Source:* Courtesy of Dr Janina Bartels, University of Tennessee.

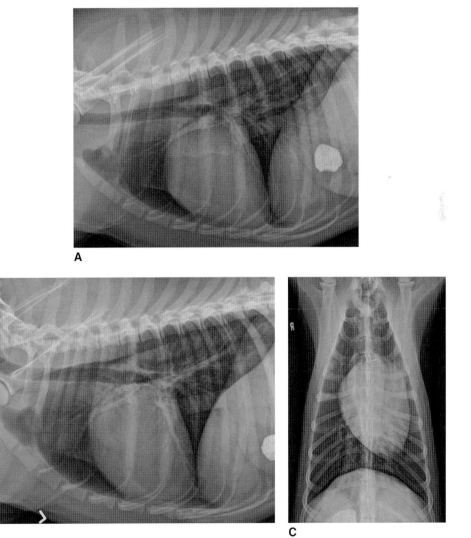

**FIGURE 17.10** Right lateral (**A**), left lateral (**B**), and VD (**C**) views of the thorax in a normal 2-year-old Bouvier de Flanders. The dog had been sedated and positioned on its left side for several minutes prior to obtaining the VD view radiograph. (**A,B**) The lateral views are unremarkable. (**C**) On the VD view the cardiac silhouette is shifted into the left hemithorax. Note also diffusely increased opacity of the atelectatic caudal subsegment of the left cranial lung lobe. The large mineral opaque structure within the stomach is consistent with ingestion of a rock which was incidental.

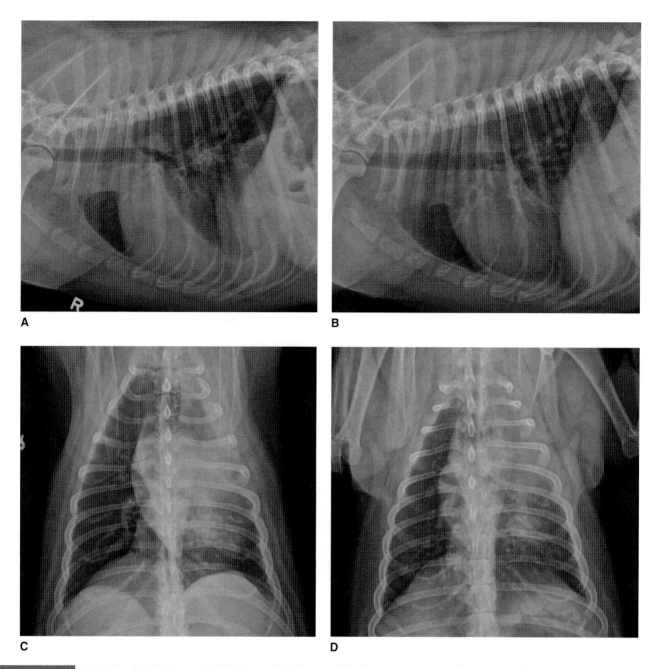

**FIGURE 17.11** Right lateral (**A**), left lateral (**B**), VD (**C**), and DV (**D**) views of the thorax in an 8-year-old mixed-breed dog presented with lower airway disease. (**A**) There is faint increased opacity in the plane of the cranial thorax following the expected margins of the left cranial lung lobe. This lobe appears decreased in volume. (**B**) The radiographic changes are similar but less pronounced than on the right lateral view. (**C**, **D**) The left cranial lobar bronchus is not visible due to obstruction with a mucous plug. The secondary volume loss of this lung lobe results in leftward mediastinal shift and diffuse soft tissue opacity of the left cranial lung lobe.

## Mediastinal Fluid Accumulation

Fluid accumulation within the mediastinum is mostly seen in conjunction with pleural effusion [8] and may in those cases not always be recognized due to overlying fluid opacity within the pleural space. Similarly, if mediastinal effusion is present along with a mediastinal mass (see below), it may not be recognized as a separate entity. Hemorrhagic effusion within the mediastinum may develop, e.g., secondary to trauma, invasive neoplasia, coagulopathy and vascular pathology, or may be idiopathic [9–14]. Other possible causes of mediastinal fluid accumulation include but are not limited to inflammation (mediastinitis, perforating esophageal foreign body, pyothorax, others), chylous effusion, and transudate [8, 15].

Radiographically, depending on the underlying cause and nature of effusion, the mediastinum appears generally, multifocally or focally of soft tissue opacity and widened on the VD view (Figure 17.16; see also Figures 17.26 and 17.72). Tracheal narrowing may be observed secondary to compression by surrounding fluid (Figure 17.17).

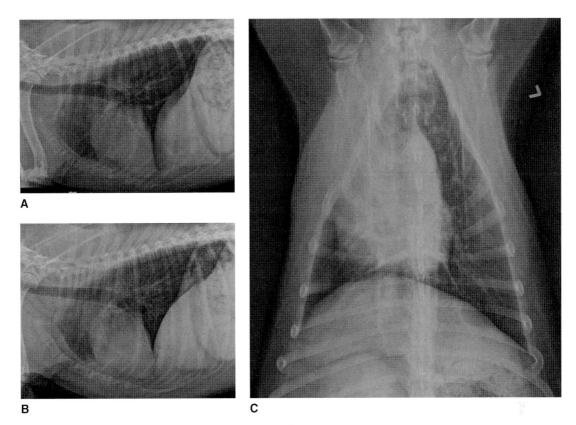

**FIGURE 17.12** Right lateral (**A**), left lateral (**B**), and VD (**C**) views of the thorax in a 7-year-old Weimaraner following prior right cranial lung lobectomy for treatment of pulmonary carcinoma. (**A,B**) The lateral views are unremarkable although on close inspection only one pair of pulmonary vessels is seen supplying the right cranial and middle lung field on the left lateral view. (**C**) On the VD view there is rightward mediastinal shift and increased soft tissue opacity to the right cranial thorax.

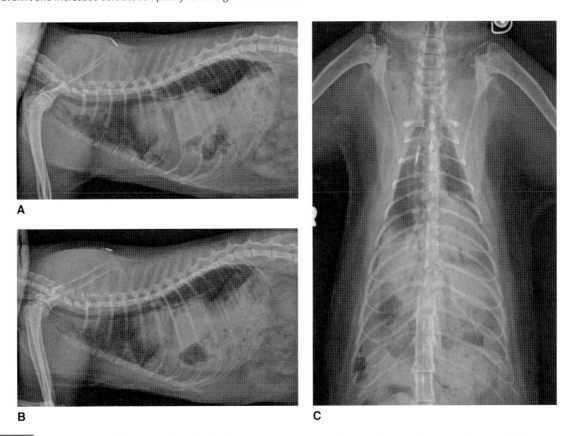

**FIGURE 17.13** Right lateral (**A**), left lateral (**B**), and VD (**C**) views of the thorax in a 4-year-old DSH cat who was found outside and suspected to have been hit by car. (**A,B**) On the lateral views abdominal viscera are present in the thoracic cavity and the diaphragm is discontinuous. In addition to the diaphragmatic hernia, mild pneumothorax and pulmonary contusions are also evident. (**C**) On the VD view the cardiac silhouette is pushed into the left hemithorax.

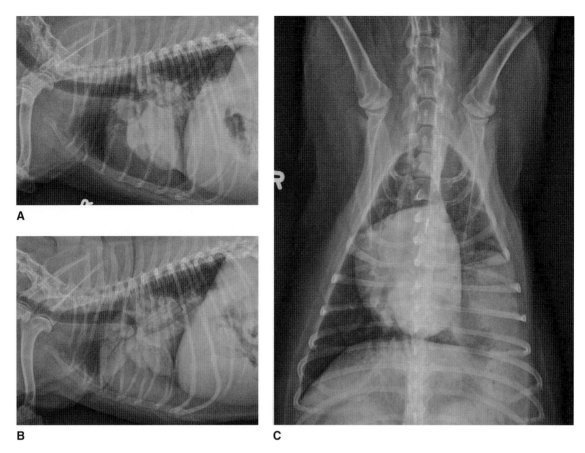

**FIGURE 17.14** Right lateral (**A**), left lateral (**B**). and VD (**C**) views of the thorax in an 11-year-old cocker spaniel with a large pulmonary mass (adenocarcinoma) of the left caudal lung lobe which pushes the cardiac silhouette toward the right on the VD view (**C**). Note also obliteration of the left caudal lobar bronchus on this view. Additional smaller pulmonary nodules are consistent with metastatic disease in this patient.

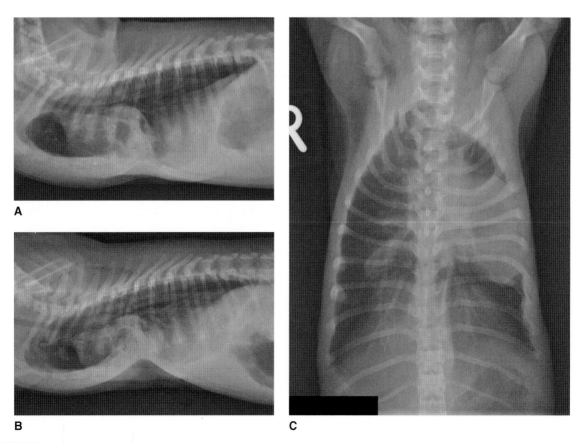

**FIGURE 17.15** Right lateral (**A**), left lateral (**B**), and VD (**C**) views of the thorax in a 3-month-old Pekingese. (**A,B**) On the lateral views there is displacement of caudal sternebral segments dorsally beyond the costochondral junctions, consistent with pectus excavatum. (**C**) On the VD view the cardiac silhouette is completely displaced into the left hemithorax.

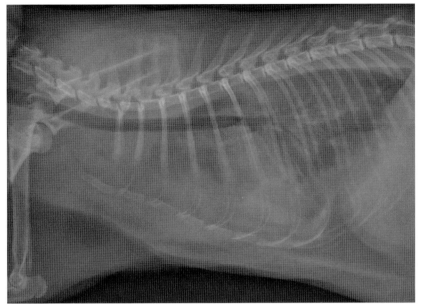

A

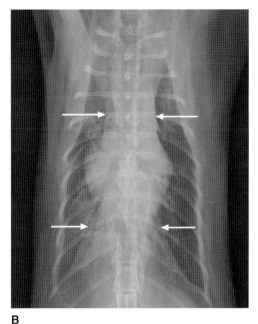

B

**FIGURE 17.16** Right lateral (**A**) and ventrodorsal (**B**) views of the thorax in a 7-month-old DSH cat with mediastinal effusion due to a systemic inflammatory disease process, the underlying etiology of which was not elucidated. (**A**) On the lateral view there is diffuse increased opacity throughout the entire thorax with poor delineation of the cardiac silhouette. Additionally, mild pleural effusion recognized by scalloping and retraction of lung margins from the sternum and spine and diffuse patchy increased opacity to the lung fields is evident. (**B**) The VD view reveals diffuse generalized widening of the mediastinum which is of soft tissue opacity and silhouettes with cranial and caudal margins of the cardiac silhouette as well as the diaphragm (arrows). There is also more focal widening of the cranial mediastinum from the thoracic inlet to the third intercostal space, consistent with cranial mediastinal mass or lymphadenopathy. Pleural effusion (indicated by retraction of the right lung from the thoracic wall and right-sided pleural fissure lines) as well as multifocal unstructured interstitial to alveolar pulmonary patterns are again noted.

# Mediastinal Masses and Lymphadenopathy

Mediastinal masses and enlarged lymph nodes within the mediastinum manifest as variably sized and shaped mass lesions which may partially obscure and displace normal mediastinal structures on the lateral view and will result in focal or multifocal mediastinal widening on the VD/DV view. Concurrent thoracic abnormalities such as pleural effusion may be encountered and may make identification of a mediastinal mass difficult. Even though enlarged mediastinal lymph nodes may resemble mediastinal masses of different origin, differentiation between an enlarged mediastinal lymph node and other types of mediastinal mass is crucial to establish an appropriate list of differential diagnoses and appropriately plan the additional diagnostic workup of a patient. A decision tree is shown in Figure 17.18 to help with the interpretation of focal or multifocal mass lesions.

Although normal mediastinal lymph nodes are not visible radiographically, one has to be familiar with their location to recognize thoracic lymphadenopathy. Additionally, it is important to know their tributary areas as lymph node enlargement may be related to primary disease processes in their draining region. Three groups of lymph nodes are located within the mediastinum [1] (Figure 17.19).

- The sternal lymph nodes are in broad-based contact with the cranial sternum (typically, second to third sternebrae) and drain part of the thoracic wall, the thymus, cranial mammary complexes, pleura, and peritoneum.

- The cranial mediastinal lymph nodes are located ventral to the thoracic trachea and drain certain musculoskeletal components of the neck and thoracic wall, mediastinal structures, and pleura.

- The tracheobronchial lymph nodes are located around the tracheal bifurcation and are primarily responsible for drainage of the lung and bronchi and to a lesser degree the caudal mediastinal structures and the diaphragm.

Enlargement of a single lymph node or group of lymph nodes is commonly related to neoplasia and less likely an inflammatory process in the tributary area. Occasionally, and especially for the tracheobronchial lymph nodes, enlargement of a single lymph node or group of lymph nodes can be associated with a systemic disease process such as round cell neoplasia (e.g., lymphoma) or fungal disease [16–18]. Radiographically, there will be a well- or ill-defined increased soft tissue opacity in the expected location of the respective lymph node group (Figures 17.20–17.23). In case of enlargement of two or all three groups of thoracic lymph nodes (Figure 17.24), disseminated neoplasia (lymphoma or other

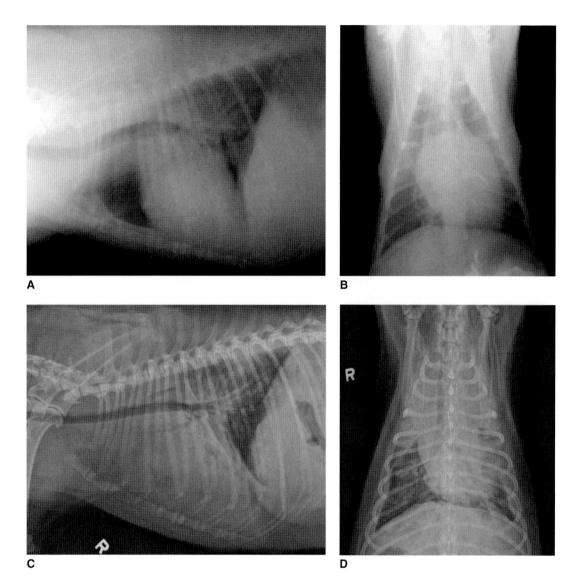

**FIGURE 17.17** Right lateral (**A,C**) and ventrodorsal (**B,D**) radiographs of the thorax in a 12-year-old miniature poodle with dyspnea, thrombocytopenia, and disseminated intravascular coagulopathy (DIC). Initial radiographs (**A,B**) were obtained by the referring veterinarian at the initial onset of clinical signs 2 days prior to recheck radiographs obtained at the referral institution (**C,D**). (**A,B**) Initial radiographs show increased opacity in the perihilar region with a J-shaped course of the caudal trachea, consistent with tracheobronchial lymphadenopathy. No significant pleural, pulmonary or cranial mediastinal abnormalities are observed at this point. On recheck radiographs (**C,D**) there are additional findings of pleural effusion, multifocal unstructured interstitial to alveolar pulmonary infiltrates, and increased opacity to the cranial mediastinum with loss of visualization of the cranial cardiac margin and diffuse circumferential tracheal narrowing indicative of mediastinal effusion. Postmortem examination revealed necrotizing lymphadenitis and interstitial pneumonia with multiorgan hemorrhage including mediastinal bleeding.

round cell neoplasia) and fungal disease are the most likely differential diagnoses [16, 17].

In many cases, mediastinal masses can be categorized based on their location. However, it is important to realize that exceptions to these general rules exist and that mediastinal malignancies as well as benign mass lesions (e.g., abscesses, granulomas, or hematomas) may be encountered in various locations.

## Cranioventral
These masses are the most common type within the mediastinum. They are located dorsal to the sternum and cranial to the cardiac silhouette. Dependent on their size and location, they may be silhouetting with and/or displacing

the heart and cranial mediastinal vessels, and/or they may be displacing and compressing the trachea [2, 4, 7]. On the VD view, these masses are associated with a variable degree of mediastinal widening. On lateral views, they may lead to confusion with sternal lymphadenopathy; however, they typically can be distinguished due to their more acute angle with the sternum rather than broad-based contact, their larger size, and a differing location compared to the sternal lymph nodes. Concurrent pleural effusion may be present due to impairment of venous or chylous return to the heart or vascular invasion by the mass [8, 14, 19].

The most common etiologies of a cranial mediastinal mass are thymoma (Figure 17.25) and (thymic) lymphoma

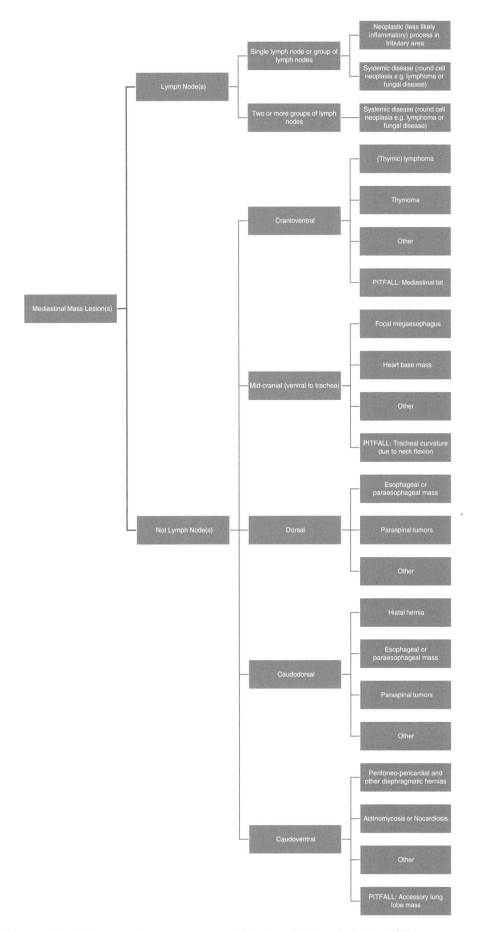

**FIGURE 17.18** Decision tree for soft tissue opacity mass or masses within the mediastinum including pitfalls.

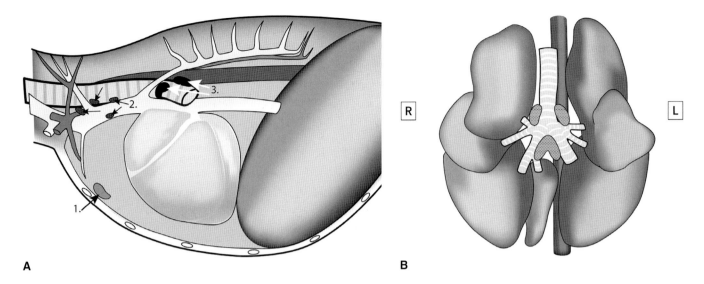

**A**

**B**

**FIGURE 17.19** (**A**) Schematic lateral view of the thorax showing location of sternal (1), cranial mediastinal (2) and tracheobronchial (3) lymph nodes. (**B**) Dorsal schematic image of the lungs showing arrangement of tracheobronchial lymph nodes around the tracheal bifurcation. *Source:* Drawings courtesy of Dr Elodie Huguet.

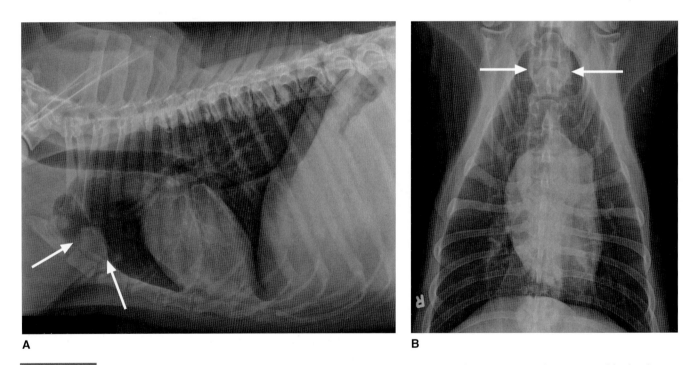

**A**

**B**

**FIGURE 17.20** Sternal lymphadenopathy secondary to neoplastic disease in the tributary area (peritoneal cavity) in a 6-year-old Labrador retriever. On the lateral view (**A**), a focal well-demarcated broad-based soft tissue opacity mass is identified dorsal to the second sternebra (arrows). On the VD view (**B**), the cranial mediastinum is mildly focally widened (arrows). Note loss of serosal margin detail in the abdomen consistent with peritoneal effusion. Based on laboratory findings (severe leukocytosis with predominant lymphocyte population and many lymphoblasts both in the peripheral circulation and the abdominal effusion), a diagnosis of acute lymphoid leukemia was made.

(Figure 17.26) [16, 20–22]. Other tumor types (e.g., ectopic thyroid carcinoma, hemangiosarcoma or histiocytic sarcoma; Figure 17.27) as well as benign masses (abscess, granuloma) are also possible [14, 23, 24].

Even though a definitive diagnosis based on radiographic findings is not possible, concurrent imaging or laboratory findings may allow prioritization of the list of differential diagnoses. For example, FeLV-positive status in a young cat with a cranial

mediastinal mass is most consistent with lymphoma [25]. Several paraneoplastic syndromes (myasthenia gravis, polymyositis, hypercalcemia, dermatitis) have been described in association with thymomas, and the concurrent observation of a cranial mediastinal mass with megaesophagus is highly suggestive of this condition [20, 21].

While not apparent on radiographs, ultrasonographic findings of a heterogeneous mass or internal cysts are also

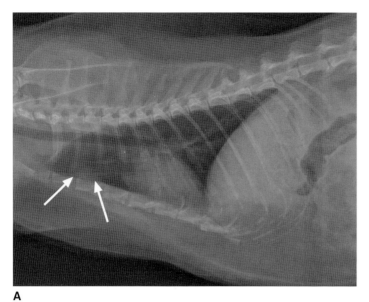
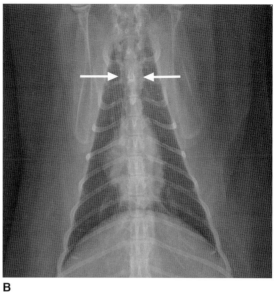

**FIGURE 17.21** Sternal lymphadenopathy secondary to peritoneal neoplasia (carcinomatosis) in a 10-year-old domestic shorthair cat. On the right lateral view (**A**), an ovoid soft tissue opacity mass is present dorsal to the third sternebra (arrows) which results in mild focal cranial mediastinal widening on the VD view (**B**; arrows). Note granular lack of serosal margin detail in the visible abdomen consistent with effusion and carcinomatosis.

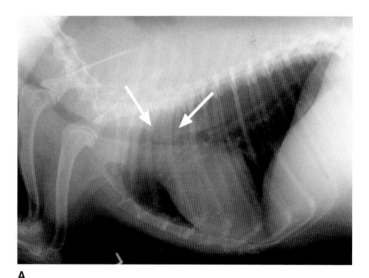
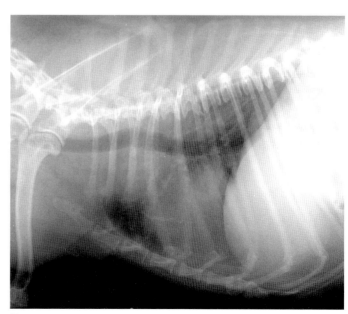

**FIGURE 17.22** Cranial mediastinal lymphadenopathy due to metastatic disease from a tracheal mast cell tumor. (**A**) The initial left lateral view at presentation shows a lobulated tracheal mass with near complete obliteration of the lumen (arrows). (**B**) Recheck radiograph 5 months following surgical resection of the mass and adjuvant chemotherapy reveals a focal soft tissue mass resulting in dorsal displacement of the trachea cranial to the heart base, consistent with an enlarged cranial mediastinal lymph node.

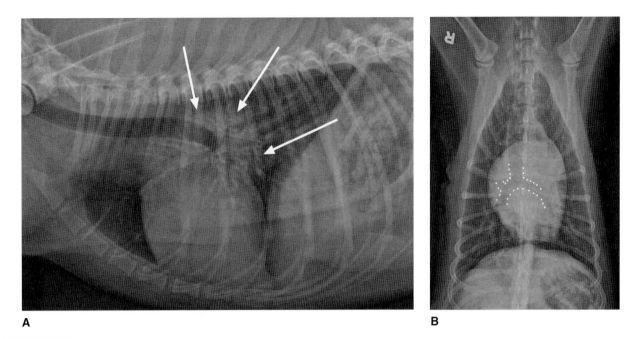

**FIGURE 17.23** Tracheobronchial lymphadenopathy in an 11-year-old mixed-breed dog with fungal disease (blastomycosis). Note increased opacity in the perihilar region with J-shaped course of the caudal trachea on the right lateral view ((**A**) arrows) and lateral deviation of the main stem bronchi (indicated by dotted lines) with increased soft tissue opacity between these bronchi on the VD view resembling a "double opacity" or "bow-legged cowboy" sign (**B**).

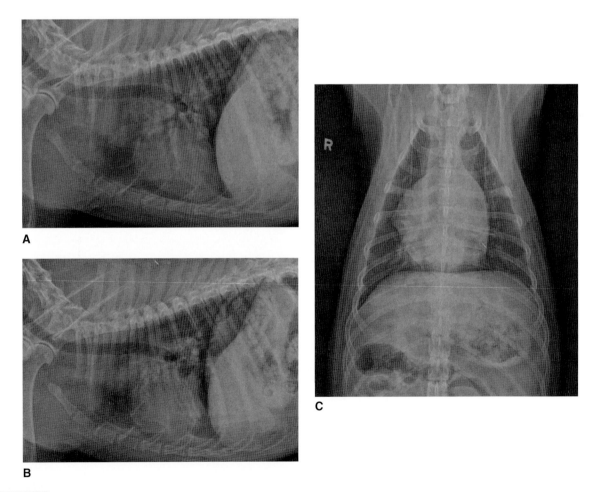

**FIGURE 17.24** Generalized thoracic lymphadenopathy in an 11-year-old mixed-breed dog diagnosed with lymphoma. Right lateral (**A**), left lateral (**B**), and ventrodorsal (**C**) radiographs of the thorax show focal areas of increased soft tissue opacity attributed to the sternal, cranial mediastinal, and tracheobronchial lymph nodes.

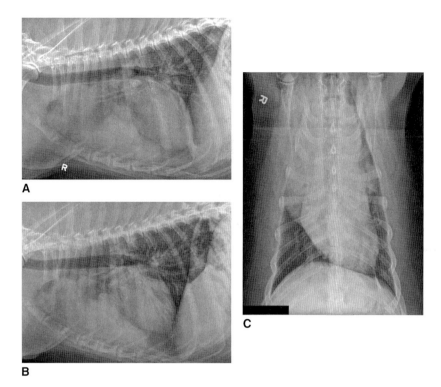

**FIGURE 17.25**  Large cranial mediastinal mass in an 8-year-old German shepherd dog. Right lateral (**A**) and left lateral (**B**) views show a lobulated soft tissue opacity mass occupying the cranial ventral thorax and displacing the cardiac silhouette caudally. On the ventrodorsal view (**C**), the mass is located on the midline, is more extensive and abutting the thoracic wall on the right side, and silhouettes with the cranial margin of the cardiac silhouette. Ultrasound-guided fine needle aspiration and surgical biopsy yielded a diagnosis of thymoma.

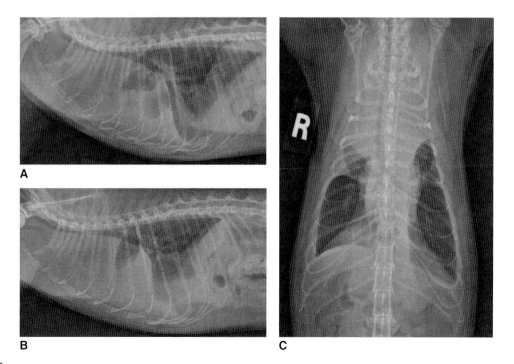

**FIGURE 17.26**  Cranial mediastinal mass and pleural effusion in a 2-year-old FeLV-positive domestic longhair cat. On the lateral views (**A**,**B**) there is a large, homogeneous, soft tissue opacity mass within the cranioventral thorax, the cranial margin of the cardiac silhouette is obscured, and the trachea is displaced dorsally and compressed. Additional findings include scalloped fluid opacity to the ventral thorax, retraction of the lung lobes and pleural fissure lines consistent with pleural effusion. On the VD view (**C**), there is marked widening of the cranial mediastinum and silhouetting of the cranial thoracic mass with the cranial margin of the cardiac silhouette. Retraction of the lung from the thoracic wall (especially right-sided) and pleural fissure lines are again identified. Widening of the caudal mediastinum is noted which suggests concurrent mediastinal effusion. Cytology of pleural effusion yielded a diagnosis of lymphoma.

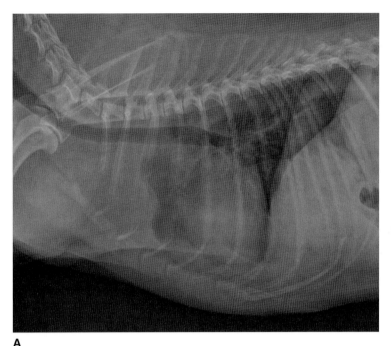
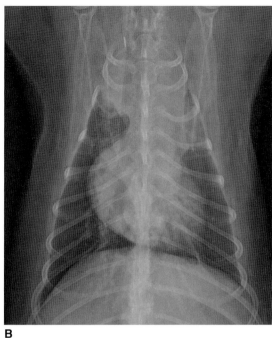

**A**   **B**

**FIGURE 17.27**  Left lateral (**A**) and ventrodorsal (**B**) radiographs of the thorax in an 8-year-old Shetland sheepdog showing a cranial mediastinal mass. The cytologic diagnosis was histiocytic sarcoma.

most consistent with thymoma [26–28]. Based on the author's experience, mild thymic enlargement in an adult dog with maintenance of the overall normal thymic shape is occasionally seen in patients with lymphoma (Figure 17.28). Cranial mediastinal cysts are an occasional finding in cats and are typically found incidentally without clinical signs which would be expected with malignant lesions (Figure 17.29) [29, 30]. Deposition of a large amount of fat within the mediastinum will result in mediastinal widening on the VD view (see Figure 17.8) which may lead to an erroneous diagnosis of a cranial mediastinal mass. However, a distinction is usually possible as the cranial margin of the heart will contrast with fat and remain clearly visible on lateral views while it will be obscured in cases of cranial mediastinal masses (Figure 17.30).

**Midcranial**  There is overlap in the differential diagnoses for midcranial and cranial dorsal thoracic masses. Severe focal esophageal enlargement (e.g., focal megaesophagus such as seen secondary to vascular ring anomaly or an esophageal mass) may be visible dorsally as well as ventrally to the trachea on lateral views and will appear as a cranial mediastinal mass lesion of variable size and echogenicity on VD/DV views (Figure 17.31; see also "Esophagus" section below) [31, 32]. A heart base mass (e.g., chemodectoma) is typically located immediately cranioventral to the tracheal bifurcation and results in dorsal displacement and J-shaped course of the intrathoracic trachea on lateral views and rightward displacement of the trachea on VD/DV views (Figures 17.32 and 17.33) [4]. It is important to note that survey radiographs are fairly specific but not very sensitive in the detection of heart base masses in dogs [33].

**Dorsal**  Mass lesions in the dorsal mediastinum most commonly originate from the esophagus (e.g., neoplasia or foreign body; see below), the paraesophageal tissues (e.g., abscess), or the spinal and paraspinal tissues [32, 34] (Figure 17.34). Aortic lesions are typically not expected to result in radiographic changes. However, aneurysms and dissecting hematomas have been described in small animals [35–37] and may result in dorsal mediastinal abnormalities (see Figure 17.60).

**Caudodorsal**  In addition to the options listed above, hiatal hernia is another differential diagnosis for a caudodorsal mediastinal mass lesion [38, 39]. A hiatal hernia is defined by a protrusion of any abdominal structure other than the esophagus into the thoracic cavity through the esophageal hiatus [40]. These may be encountered in dogs and cats and are of variable clinical significance [38, 41–45]. Sliding hiatal hernias (type I hiatal hernias) where the gastroesophageal junction migrates cranially are most common, and manifest as soft tissue and/or gas opacity structures in the caudal dorsal mediastinum immediately cranial to the diaphragm. Unlike true caudodorsal mediastinal masses, they may only intermittently be visible on serial radiographs (Figure 17.35). In paraesophageal hernias, abdominal contents herniate through the esophageal hiatus next to the gastroesophageal junction which remains in normal position (Figure 17.36). These hernias can be subdivided into type II (herniation of portion of the fundus), type III (combination of types I and II), and type IV (presence of a structure other than the stomach within the hernia sac) [40].

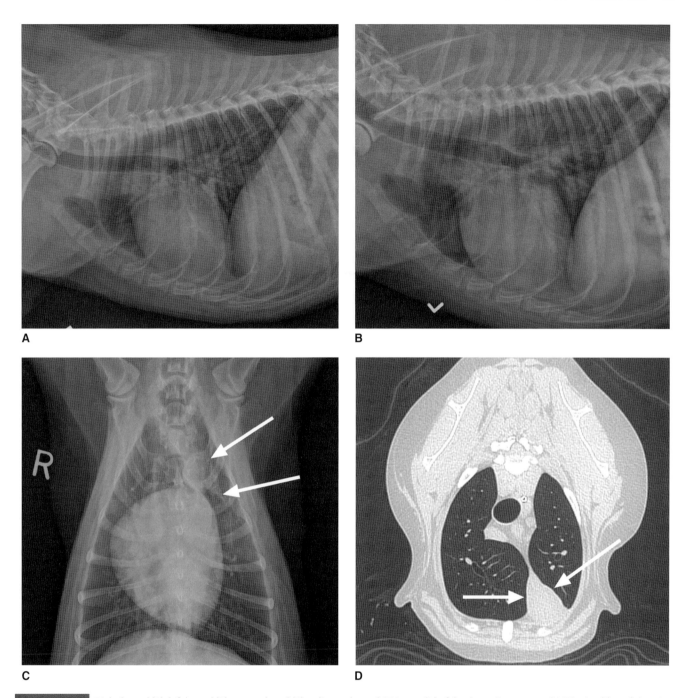

**FIGURE 17.28**    Right lateral (**A**), left lateral (**B**), ventrodorsal (**C**) radiographs and CT image (**D**) of the thorax in a 6-year-old MC mixed-breed dog. On the lateral views (**A,B**), there is faint increased opacity to the cranial mediastinum. On the VD view (**C**) and the CT image (**D**), there is enlargement and rounding of the thymic remnant (arrows), concerning for neoplastic infiltration. Ultrasound-guided tissue sampling yielded a diagnosis of lymphoma.

**Caudoventral**    Some congenitally predisposed diaphragmatic hernias, including peritoneal-pericardial diaphragmatic hernias and "true" (peritoneal-pleural) diaphragmatic hernias, may result in a caudal ventral mediastinal mass due to protrusion of abdominal viscera into the caudal ventral thorax. Although these types of hernias may have associated clinical signs if herniated organs become incarcerated or otherwise compromised, most commonly they seem to be diagnosed as incidental findings. In peritoneal-pericardial diaphragmatic hernias, there is

congenital connection between the peritoneal and pericardial cavities [46, 47]. Radiographic abnormalities include enlargement and abnormal shape of the cardiac silhouette, abdominal organs within the pericardial sac, an indistinguishable border of the ventral diaphragm, and abnormal mostly soft tissue opacity structures between the caudal ventral margin of the cardiac silhouette and the diaphragm (Figure 17.37) [39].

In "true" (peritoneal-pleural) diaphragmatic hernias, there is incomplete formation of the diaphragm, allowing

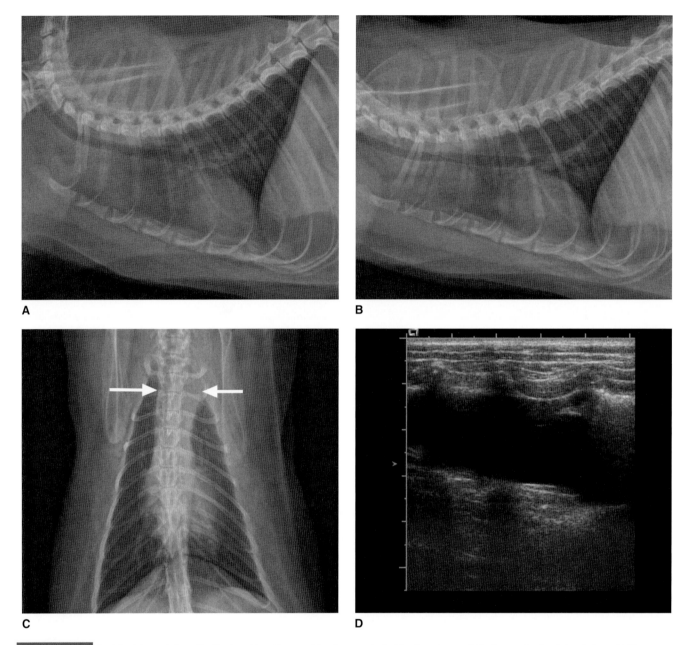

**FIGURE 17.29** Incidental cranial mediastinal cyst in a 9-year-old cat presented with chronic nasal discharge. On the lateral views (**A,B**), there is faint increased opacity to the cranial mediastinum. On the VD view (**C**), there is mild cranial mediastinal widening (arrows). Ultrasound examination (**D**) confirms the cystic nature of the cranial mediastinal lesion which appears anechoic and well circumscribed.

protrusion of abdominal viscera through the resultant defect (Figure 17.38) [26, 39, 48]. The exact nature of a congenital diaphragmatic hernia may on occasion remain elusive (Figure 17.39). True caudal ventral mediastinal masses of either neoplastic or inflammatory etiology are rare. However, pyogranulomas due to actinomycosis or nocardiosis appear to have a predilection for this location (Figure 17.40) [49]. The ALL is located between the right and left caudal lung lobes and is bordered cranially by the heart and caudally by the diaphragm. Due to its location, abnormalities of this lobe (e.g., mass) may mimic an actual caudoventral mediastinal mass or even a diaphragmatic hernia (Figure 17.41) [50].

## Pneumomediastinum

Gas accumulation within the mediastinum most commonly occurs secondary to some sort of traumatic event. Blunt thoracic trauma may lead to leakage of air from the alveoli into the pulmonary interstitium and subsequent diffusion into the mediastinum [51]. Tracheal injury is another fairly common cause of pneumomediastinum and may be secondary to perforating injury or iatrogenic (e.g., due to overinflated endotracheal cuff, following endoscopy, or following removal of a tracheal foreign body) [52, 53]. Gas within the soft tissues of the neck (e.g., secondary to bite wounds) can dissect along fascial

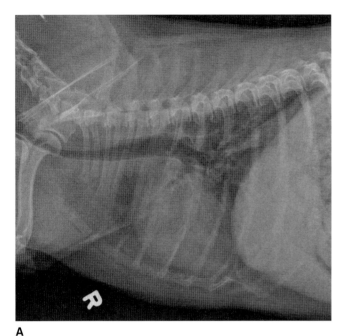
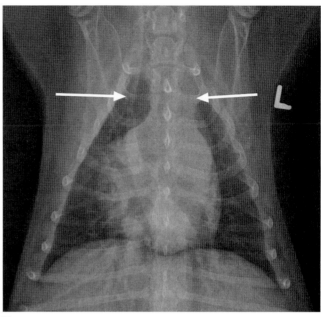

**A**          **B**

**FIGURE 17.30**  Thoracic radiographs in a 13-year-old West Highland white terrier presented for coughing. On the VD view (**B**), there is widening of the cranial mediastinum (arrows) which could be mistaken for a soft tissue mass. On the lateral view (**A**), the cranial margin of the cardiac silhouette is clearly visible and there is no evidence of a cranial mediastinal mass. A fusiform soft tissue opacity in the plane of the dorsal trachea is consistent with a redundant tracheal membrane. A diffuse unstructured interstitial and bronchial pattern and mild hepatomegaly are also identified.

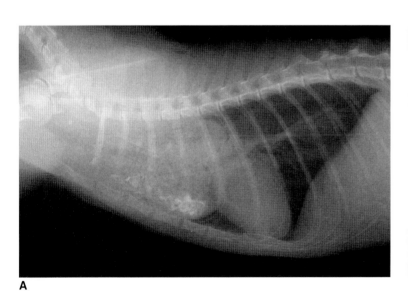
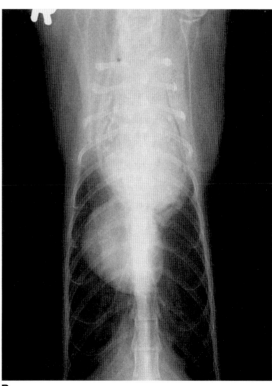

**A**          **B**

**FIGURE 17.31**  "Mass" within the cranial mediastinum in a 2-year-old domestic shorthair cat with focal megaesophagus secondary to a vascular ring anomaly (persistent right aortic arch). The severely dilated cranial thoracic esophagus contains a mixture of granular ingesta and mineral material and on the right lateral view (**A**) occupies the mediastinum both ventrally and dorsally to the trachea. The cervical esophagus is gas distended, and the esophagus is not visible caudal to the fifth intercostal space. On the VD view (**B**), the focal esophageal dilation appears as a heterogeneous soft tissue opacity mass in the cranial mediastinum, slightly more severe left-sided.

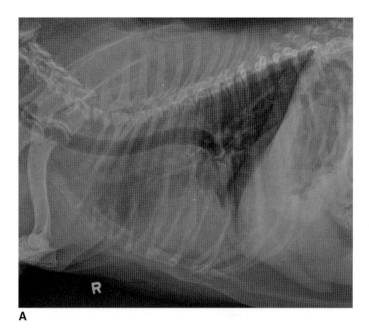

A

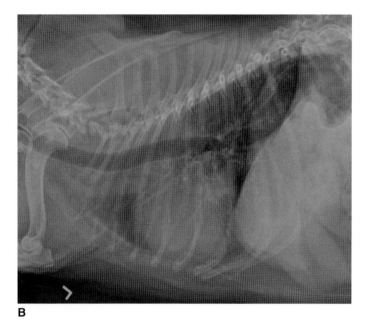

B

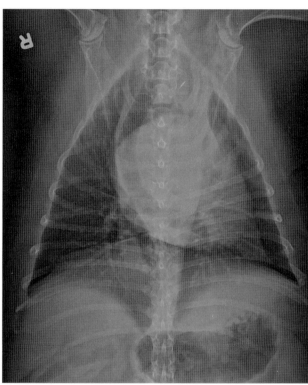

C

**FIGURE 17.32**   Heart base mass (chemodectoma, suspected) in an 11-year-old English bulldog. On the right lateral view (**A**) a mass is associated with the midcranial mediastinum (ventral to the trachea), resulting in dorsal displacement and focal J-shaped course of the midcervical trachea. On the left lateral view (**B**), the mass is less evident. On the VD view (**C**). there is marked focal rightward deviation of the intrathoracic trachea due to the mass.

planes and cause pneumomediastinum [54]. Pneumomediastinum secondary to other pulmonary diseases, esophageal rupture or mediastinal infection with gas-producing bacteria, and spontaneous pneumomediastinum are also reported [55–61].

Radiographically, pneumomediastinum is best visualized on lateral views and, if moderate or severe, is characterized by increased visibility of mediastinal structures that are ordinarily not seen (azygous vein, cranial mediastinal vessels, outer margin of esophagus and trachea) [4] (Figures 17.42–17.44). Accumulation of gas in an unexpected multifocal or "bubbly"

pattern or in an unusual location should raise concern for esophageal tear, infection with gas-producing bacteria (mediastinitis), or other uncommon conditions (Figure 17.45; see also Figure 17.79).

The mediastinal space communicates with the neck and the retroperitoneal space, and pneumomediastinum may result in subcutaneous emphysema or pneumoretroperitoneum and vice versa (Figure 17.46). Pneumomediastinum may also progress to pneumothorax, but pneumothorax will not cause pneumomediastinum.

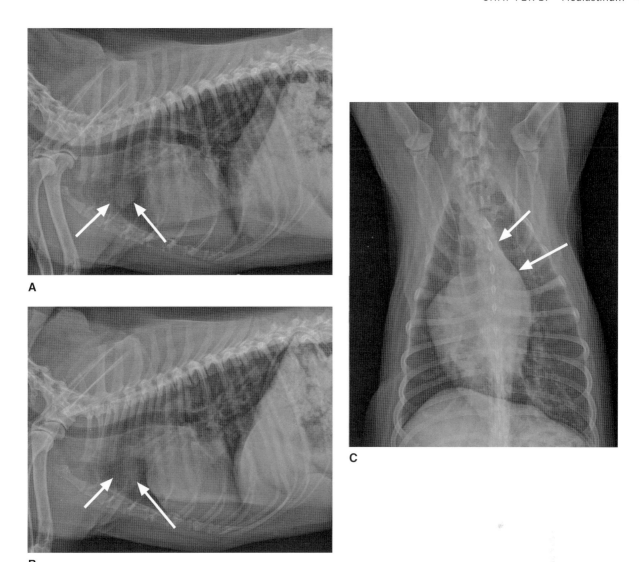

**A**

**B**

**C**

**FIGURE 17.33**   Heart base mass with metastasis in an 11-year-old mixed-breed dog. On both lateral views (**A,B**) there is a soft tissue opacity mass ventral to the trachea immediately cranial to the tracheal bifurcation, resulting in focal dorsal deviation and J-shaped course of the trachea. Additionally, there is a round soft tissue opacity slightly ventral to the expected location of a cranial mediastinal lymph node (arrows). Multifocal mixed pulmonary patterns are also noted. On the VD view (**C**), there is a focal soft tissue opacity mass (arrows) silhouetting with the left cranial cardiac margin and resulting in rightward displacement of the caudal trachea. Necropsy yielded a diagnosis of invasive chemodectoma with metastasis to regional lymph nodes. Histopathology of the lung was consistent with infarction and neutrophilic and histiocytic bronchopneumonia.

# Esophagus

The normal esophagus is not visible on survey radiographs of the thorax in dogs and cats. However, a small amount of intraluminal gas is commonly present (see Figure 17.7), and occasionally an indistinct linear soft tissue opacity is seen in normal animals dorsal to the CVC, representing a mild fluid accumulation within the esophagus [62, 63].

The imaging modalities commonly used to evaluate a patient for suspected esophageal disorders are survey radiographs and positive contrast esophagography. This technique involves oral administration of positive contrast medium (typically, barium sulfate suspension) and, dependent on indication, subsequent administration of barium sulfate paste, barium mixed with canned food, and barium mixed with kibble. Iodinated contrast media are not commonly used but nonionic iodinated contrast media may be the best choice if esophageal perforation is suspected. Static radiographs following contrast medium administration may aid in identification of a (focal) megaesophagus, esophageal foreign body or mass but are inadequate to evaluate dynamic abnormalities and swallowing disorders [32].

## Megaesophagus

Generalized esophageal dilation (generalized megaesophagus) can occur secondary to multiple conditions including endocrine, congenital, toxic, autoimmune and other causes or

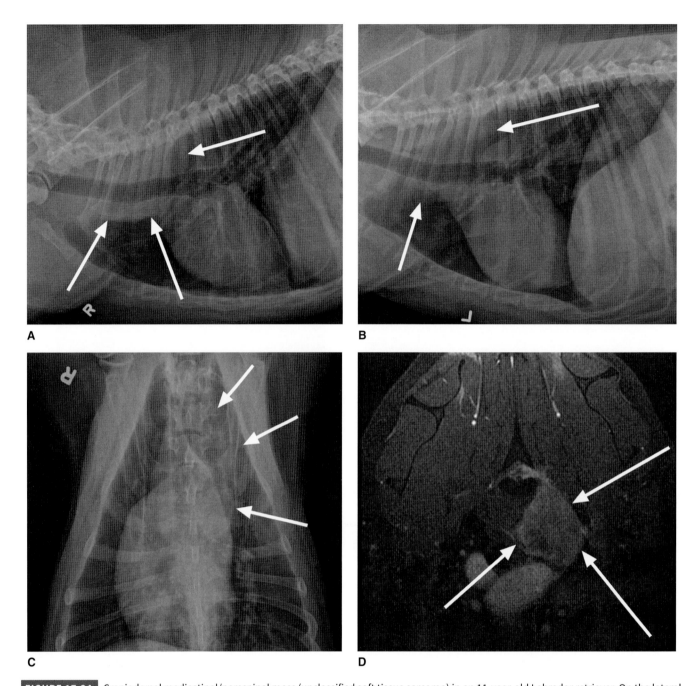

**FIGURE 17.34** Craniodorsal mediastinal/paraspinal mass (unclassified soft tissue sarcoma) in an 11-year-old Labrador retriever. On the lateral views (**A,B**) there is increased soft tissue opacity to the cranial dorsal thorax from the thoracic inlet to the cranial aspect of the fourth thoracic vertebra (arrows) with mild ventral displacement of the cranial thoracic trachea best seen on the right lateral view (**A**). On the VD view (**C**), there is asymmetric left-sided widening of the cranial mediastinum (arrows). Transverse T1-weighted MR image (with fat saturation) (**D**) following contrast medium administration shows a contrast-enhancing mass (arrows) left ventral to the cranial thoracic spine with extension into the vertebral canal.

may be idiopathic [64]. A diagnosis is usually made on survey radiographs where the dilated esophagus appears as a tubular structure in the dorsal mediastinum which may contain gas, fluid, food or a combination of those. On the lateral view, the trachea and heart may be displaced ventrally, and summation of the dorsal tracheal wall with the ventral wall of the esophagus commonly results in a linear opacity margin, termed the "tracheo-esophageal stripe sign." The VD view is often unrewarding, but generalized widening of the mediastinum may

be observed. Concurrent aspiration pneumonia is frequently observed [32, 62] (Figures 17.47 and 17.48). Gas dilation of the esophagus is occasionally noted in patients with dyspnea or if radiographs were obtained under heavy sedation or anesthesia, and care must be taken to always correlate radiographic findings with clinical presentation when making a diagnosis of true megaesophagus (Figure 17.49).

A focal esophageal dilation may result from either increased intraluminal pressure (e.g., secondary to chronic

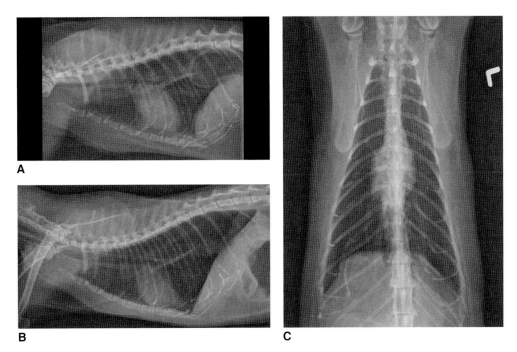

**FIGURE 17.35** Sliding hiatal hernia in a 10-year-old cat incidentally discovered during workup of nasal disease. On the right lateral image (**A**), part of the gas-filled stomach protrudes from the abdomen into the caudal dorsal mediastinum. On the left lateral view (**B**), only a focal soft tissue opacity is noted in the location of the previously seen hiatal hernia, which may represent a remaining small part of the stomach or fluid in the esophagus. No abnormalities are identified on the VD view (**C**).

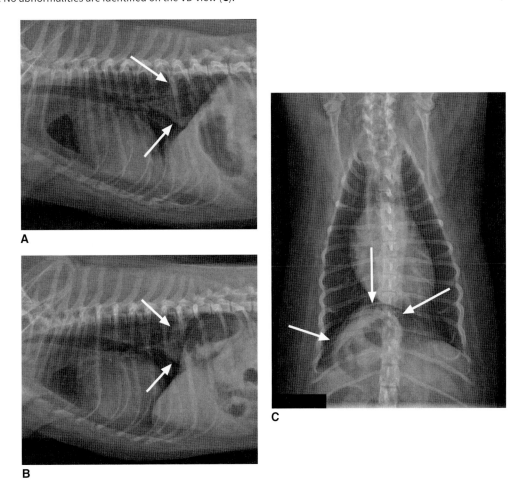

**FIGURE 17.36** Paraesophageal hiatal hernia in a 5-year-old shi tzu. (**A,B**) Both lateral views show a heterogeneous mixed soft tissue and gas opacity in the caudal dorsal mediastinum immediately cranial to the diaphragm (arrows). (**C**) On the VD view there is herniation of gas-filled abdominal content (part of stomach ± small intestine) into the caudal mediastinum (arrows) to the right of the midline and thus to the right of the expected location of the gastroesophageal junction. Surgical exploration confirmed a congenital connection between aortic and esophageal hiatus and paraesophageal hiatal hernia.

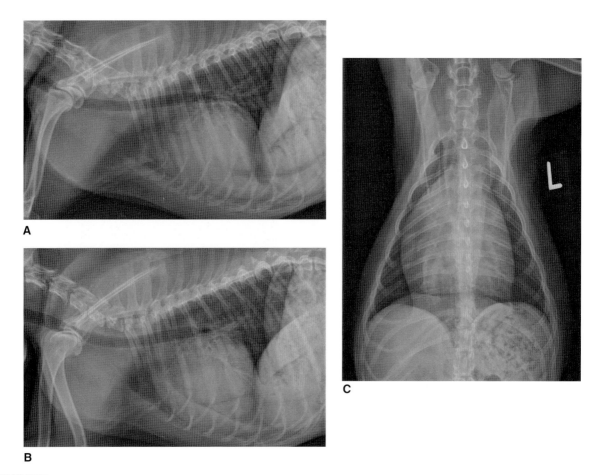

**FIGURE 17.37** Incidental finding of a peritoneal-pericardial diaphragmatic hernia in an 11-year-old miniature schnauzer presented for workup of neurologic signs. (**A,B**) The lateral views demonstrate enlargement with abnormal shape and opacity of the cardiac silhouette, lack of clear demarcation of the ventral diaphragm, and herniation of the majority of liver parenchyma into the ventral pericardial sac. (**C**) On the VD view, enlargement of the cardiac silhouette is the predominant radiographic finding, and no left liver is identified within the abdomen.

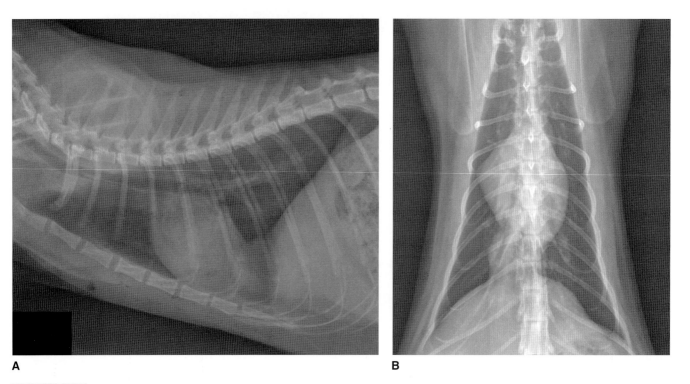

**FIGURE 17.38** "True" (peritoneal-pleural) diaphragmatic hernia with herniation of falciform fat in a 4-year-old cat presented with anemia. On the left lateral view (**A**), there is a smoothly marginated caudal ventral thoracic mass lesion which is in broad-based contact with the underlying diaphragm and mostly of fat opacity. The lesion is located slightly to the right of midline on the VD view (**B**).

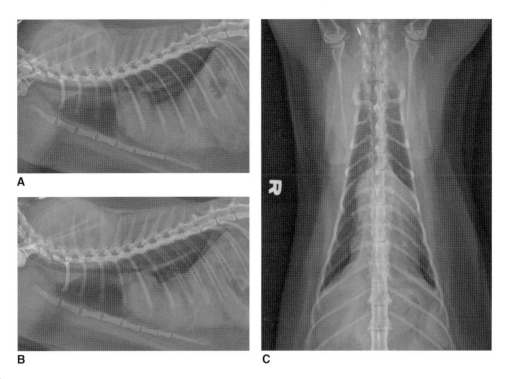

**FIGURE 17.39** Incidental finding of a congenital diaphragmatic hernia in a 4-year-old cat presented with neurologic signs. On the lateral (**A,B**) and VD (**C**) views, soft tissue opaque material occupies the space between the caudal ventral cardiac silhouette and the ventral half of the diaphragm with lack of distinction between those structures. Determination of the exact type of hernia (peritoneal-pericardial vs peritoneal-pleural) is difficult in this case. *Source:* Courtesy of Dr William H. Adams.

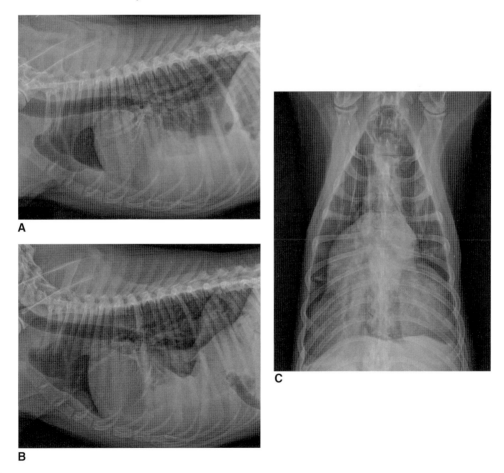

**FIGURE 17.40** *Actinomyces* pyogranuloma in the caudal ventral mediastinum in a 4-year-old Labrador retriever. (**A,B**) On the lateral views there is a homogeneous soft tissue opacity mass between the caudal ventral cardiac margin and the diaphragm obscuring the margins of these structures. Focal increased soft tissue opacity is also noted within the cranial ventral mediastinum dorsal to the third and fourth sternebrae. (**C**) On the VD view, the mass silhouettes with the caudal margin of the cardiac silhouette, is centered on the midline and extends into both the left and right hemithorax. *Source:* Courtesy of Dr William H. Adams.

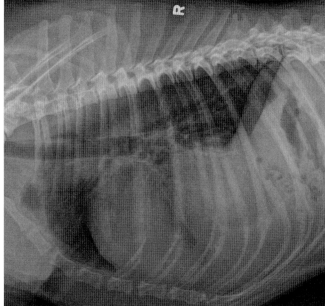

**A**

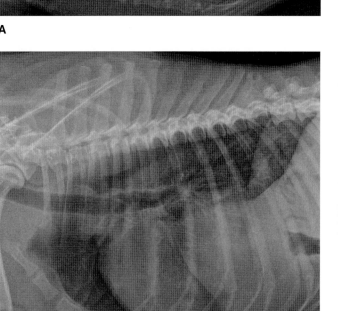

**B**

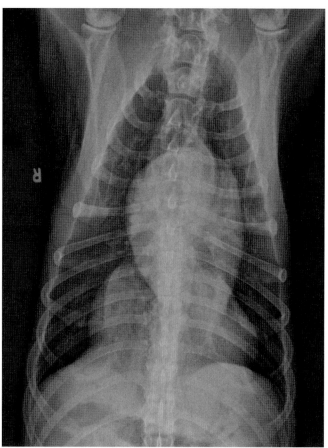

**C**

**FIGURE 17.41** Right lateral (**A**), left lateral (**B**), and ventrodorsal (**C**) thoracic radiographs showing an accessory lung lobe mass (pulmonary carcinoma) in a 10-year-old boxer. The mass is located on the midline between the caudal cardiac margin and the diaphragm and silhouettes with the latter.

partial obstruction) or external traction. A common cause of significant focal megaesophagus in the cranial thorax is a vascular ring anomaly in which the esophagus and trachea become encircled by vasculature secondary to developmental anomalies of the aortic arches [65]. Persistent right aortic arch (PRAA) is the most common form in small animals, but other anomalies including aberrant subclavian arteries and double aortic arch are reported [31, 66–70]. The esophageal constriction is located at the level of or immediately cranial to the heart base.

Radiographically, there is severe esophageal distension cranial to the site of the vascular ring anomaly (Figure 17.50; see also Figure 17.31). This may be more severe in cases of PRAA than other vascular ring anomalies. Caudally, the esophagus is commonly normal although generalized dilation may be found in some cases. The abnormal position of the aorta in PRAA may be recognized on the VD view based on leftward deviation of the trachea (Figure 17.50). As described for generalized mega-esophagus, aspiration pneumonia is a common concurrent finding in focal megaesophagus as well. In most cases, a focal

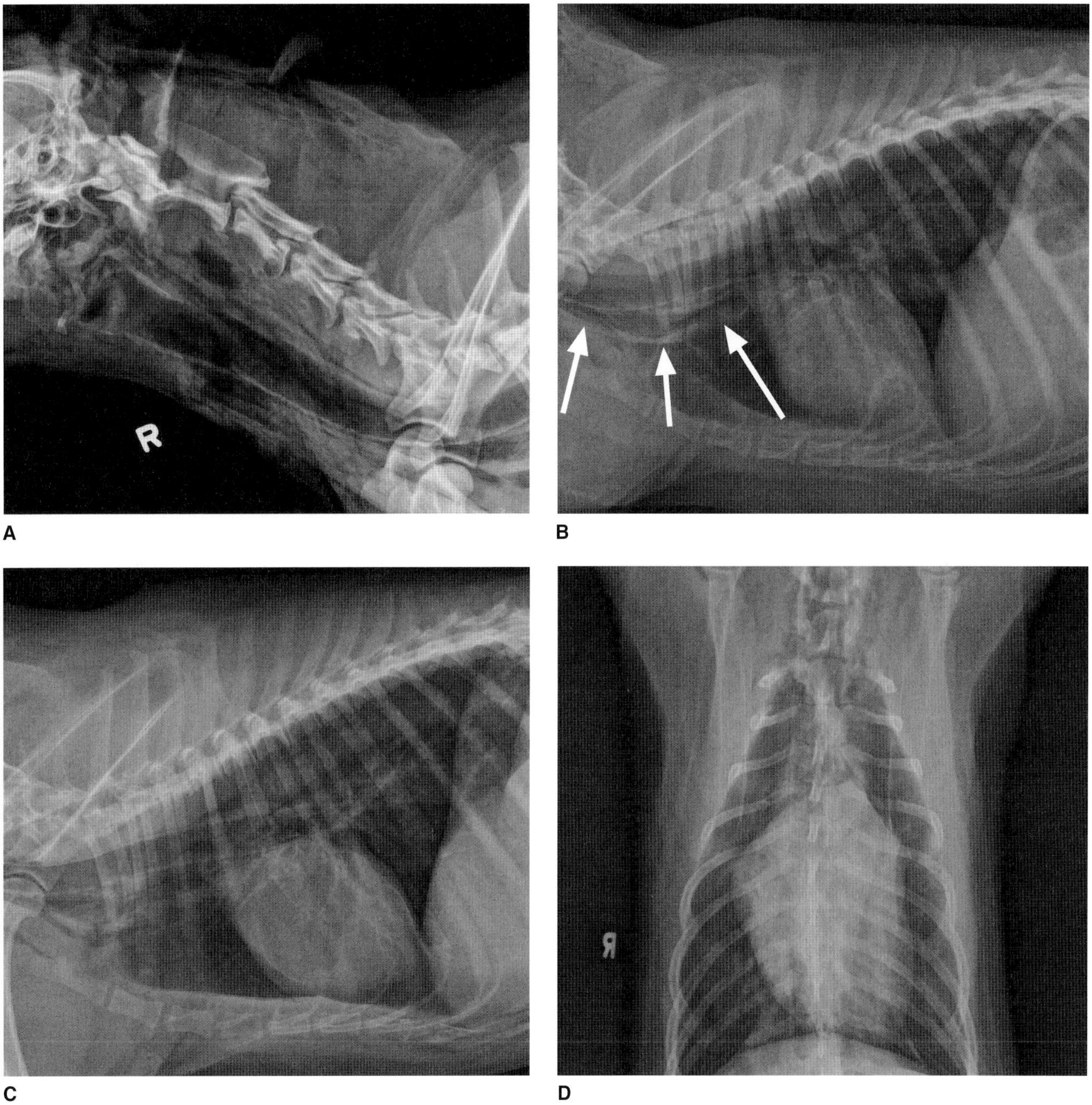

**FIGURE 17.42** Lateral view of the neck (**A**), right lateral (**B**), left lateral (**C**), and ventrodorsal (**D**) radiographs of the thorax in a 5-year-old old coonhound who sustained bite wounds to the neck. (**A**) There are gas inclusions within the soft tissues of the neck and extending along fascial planes. (**B–D**) Gas tracks along fascial planes into the mediastinum and highlights margins of cranial mediastinal organs which are normally not visible (outer ventral wall of trachea and cranial mediastinal vessels; arrows in (**B**).

megaesophagus is easily diagnosed on survey radiographs, especially in cases of vascular ring anomaly. Administration of positive contrast medium (esophagography) may be helpful in select cases (Figure 17.51) but carries an added risk of aspiration pneumonia.

A potential pitfall in the diagnosis of a focal megaesophagus is esophageal redundancy which is often an incidental finding in brachycephalic dogs such as shar peis and bulldogs

and which appears as a tortuous diverticulum at the thoracic inlet [32] (Figure 17.52).

## Esophageal Stricture

Esophageal stricture is usually the result of injury/insult to the mucosal lining of the esophagus followed by scarring, fibrosis,

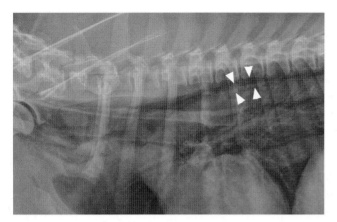

A

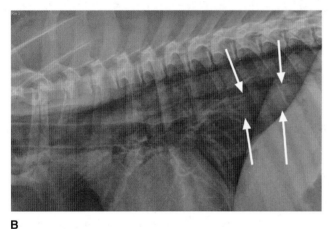

B

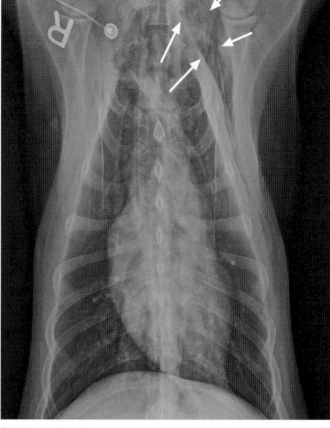

C

**FIGURE 17.43** Cropped right lateral (**A**), left lateral (**B**), and ventrodorsal (**C**) thoracic radiographs in a 2-year-old Rhodesian ridgeback presented with recent-onset seizures. Pneumomediastinum in this patient was unexpected and of undetermined cause. Linear gas opacities are present within the mediastinum resulting in visualization of the outer wall of the trachea, the cranial mediastinal vessels, the esophagus (arrows; **B**) and the azygous vein (arrowheads; **A**). On the VD view (**C**) mild emphysema is noted cranial to the thoracic inlet and best seen medial to the left scapula (arrows).

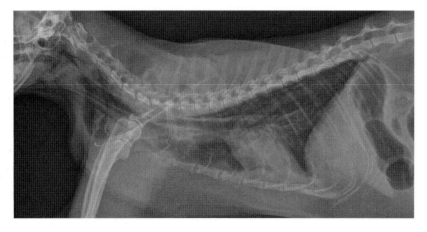

**FIGURE 17.44** Single right lateral view of the neck and thorax in a 12-year-old cat with iatrogenic pneumomediastinum following endoscopic biopsies of a laryngeal mass. There are gas inclusions associated with the soft tissues of the neck which track along the fascial planes and extend into the mediastinal space. There is increased visualization of the outer margin of the trachea and linear soft tissue bands dorsal to the aorta likely representing the azygous vein and thoracic duct.

and resultant luminal narrowing [71, 72]. Possible etiologies include gastroesophageal reflux/esophagitis, prior esophageal foreign body, and other injuries. Stricture secondary to an esophageal neoplasm is also possible. Survey radiographs are often normal or may show dilation of the esophagus proximal to the stricture. Esophagography allows identification of luminal narrowing as well as mucosal irregularities, if present (Figures 17.53 and 17.54).

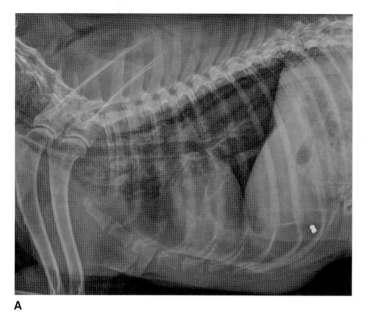
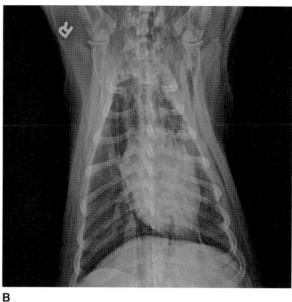

**A**  **B**

**FIGURE 17.45** Right lateral (**A**) and ventrodorsal (**B**) thoracic radiographs in a 5-year-old Australian cattle dog, 2 days following inadvertent feeding tube placement outside the esophagus and within the cranial mediastinum. There are extensive irregularly marginated punctate gas inclusions associated with the soft tissues of the neck and the mediastinum with associated mediastinal effusion, consistent with mediastinitis. The bullet seen in the plane of the cranioventral abdomen on the lateral view was an incidental finding.

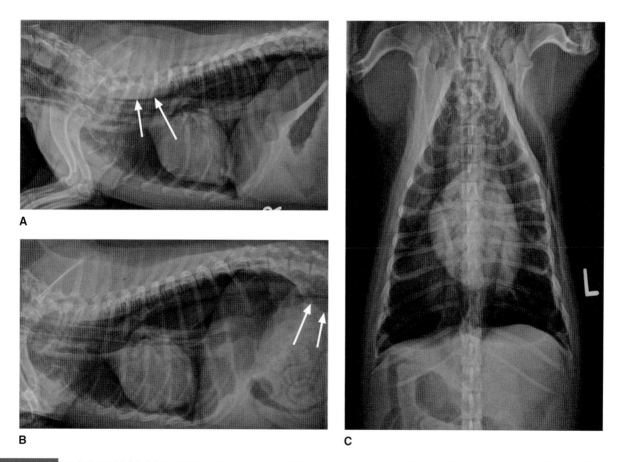

**A**

**B**  **C**

**FIGURE 17.46** Right lateral (**A**), left lateral (**B**), and ventrodorsal (**C**) thoracic radiographs in a 3-year-old mixed-breed dog with deep bite wounds to the neck and tracheal lacerations. There are extensive gas inclusions associated with the soft tissues of the neck, tracking along the fascial planes, and resulting in pneumomediastinum characterized by visibility of outer wall of trachea, ventral margin of the M. longus colli (**A**; arrows), cranial mediastinal vessels, esophagus, and azygous vein. Additionally, there is subcutaneous emphysema along the left thoracic wall and moderate pneumothorax. On the left lateral view, gas opacity is present in the plane of the retroperitoneal space consistent with extension of free mediastinal gas through the aortic hiatus (**B**; arrows). Note that the surgically confirmed tracheal tears are not visible radiographically.

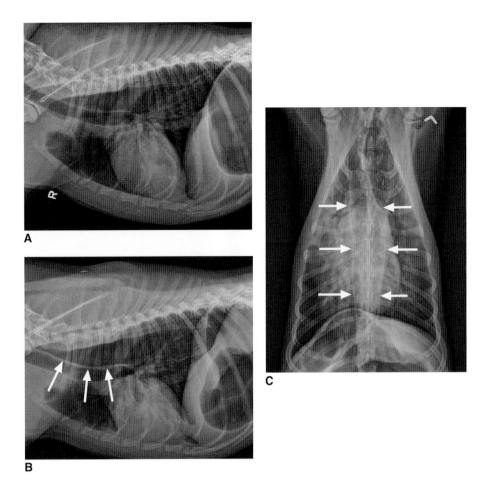

**FIGURE 17.47** Right lateral (**A**), left lateral (**B**), and ventrodorsal (**C**) thoracic radiographs in a 3-year-old Vizsla with megaesophagus and secondary aspiration pneumonia. On the lateral views (**A,B**) the gas-distended esophagus extends from the neck throughout the entire length of the thorax. The ventral wall of the cranial thoracic esophagus silhouettes with the dorsal wall of the trachea, resulting in a "tracheal stripe sign" (arrows; **B**). Patchy alveolar patterns with air bronchograms are associated with the ventral aspect of the right cranial, right middle and left cranial lung lobes. On the VD view (**C**), the entire mediastinum is widened by the gas-filled tubular esophagus (arrows).

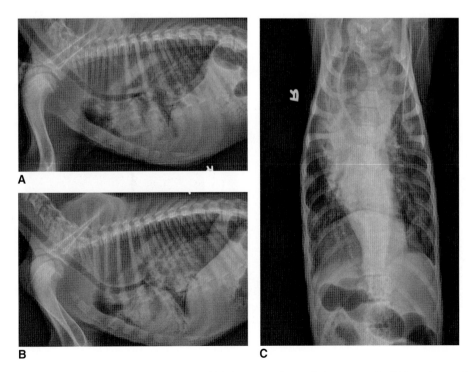

**FIGURE 17.48** Right lateral (**A**), left lateral (**B**), and ventrodorsal (**C**) thoracic radiographs in a 4-month-old Great Dane with congenital megaesophagus and secondary aspiration pneumonia. (**A,B**) On the lateral views the thoracic esophagus is severely generally distended with gas and fluid and displaces the trachea ventrally. (**C**) On the VD view there is diffuse mediastinal widening. Alveolar patterns are associated with the ventral aspect of right cranial, right middle, left cranial, and both caudal lung lobes.

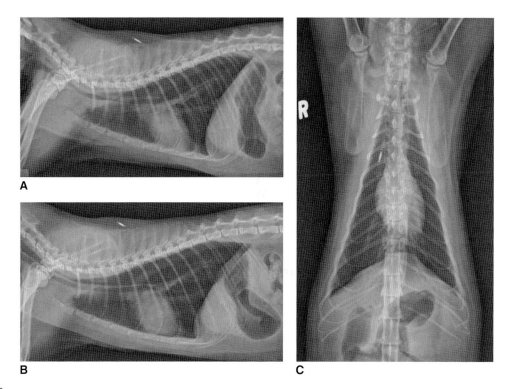

**FIGURE 17.49** Right lateral (**A**), left lateral (**B**), and ventrodorsal (**C**) thoracic radiographs in a 6-year-old DSH cat with upper airway obstruction due to a mass lesion of the nasal planum. The generalized esophageal dilation in this patient was attributed to dyspnea rather than an esophageal motility disorder as there was no history of regurgitation or vomiting.

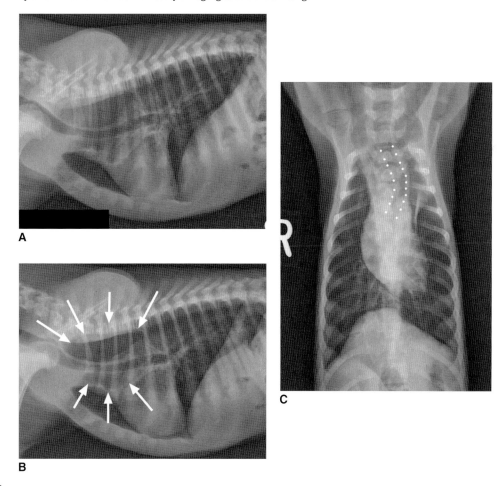

**FIGURE 17.50** Focal megaesophagus in a 9-week-old mixed-breed dog due to a vascular ring anomaly (persistent right aortic arch). On the lateral views (**A,B**) there is focal gas distension of the esophagus seen mostly dorsally to and resulting in ventral displacement of the cranial thoracic trachea (arrows; **B**). Part of the dilated esophagus is also seen ventral to the trachea and overlying with cranial mediastinal vessels (arrows; **B**). On the VD view (**C**), there is widening of the cranial mediastinum and focal leftward displacement of the cranial thoracic trachea (indicated by dotted lines) consistent with persistent right aortic arch.

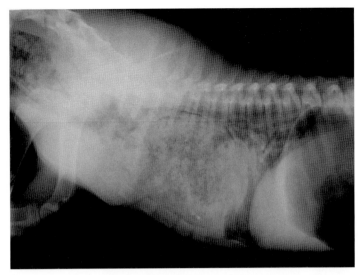

A

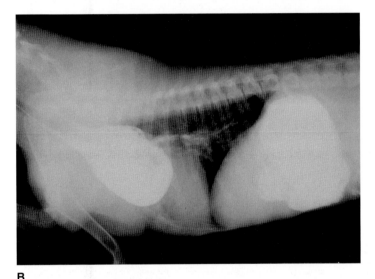

B

**FIGURE 17.51** Focal megaesophagus in a 4-month-old Australian cattle dog due to a vascular ring anomaly (persistent right aortic arch). On the initial lateral view (**A**) the cervical and cranial thoracic esophagus is severely distended with granular ingesta, and the intrathoracic portion overlies and obscures the cardiac silhouette. Gaseous distension of the stomach is consistent with aerophagia. An esophagram performed later (**B**) shows severe distension of the cranial intrathoracic esophagus with positive contrast medium. The esophagus is of normal diameter caudal to the focal esophageal narrowing at the level of the fourth pair of ribs.

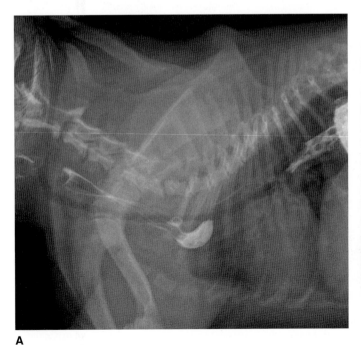

A

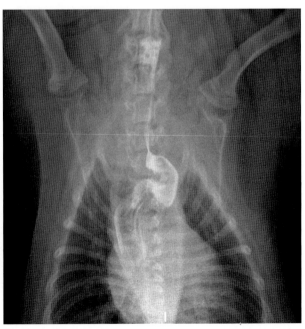

B

**FIGURE 17.52** Incidental finding of esophageal redundancy in a young English bulldog presented after choking on a chicken bone. Lateral (**A**) and VD (**B**) views show a focal tortuous course and dilation of the esophagus at the thoracic inlet. *Source:* Courtesy of Dr Anthony Fischetti.

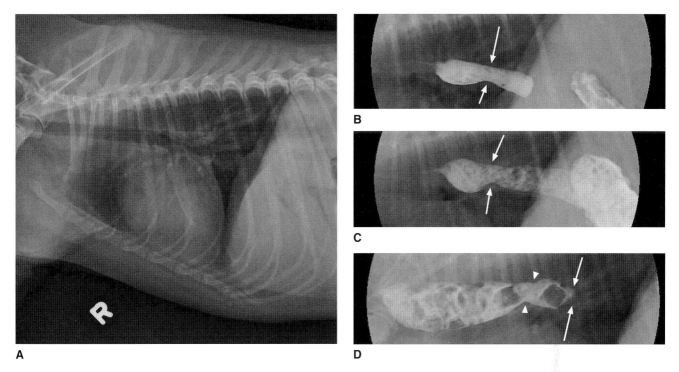

**FIGURE 17.53** Right lateral thoracic radiograph (**A**) and fluoroscopic esophagography images (**B–D**) in a 3-year-old mixed-breed dog with prior diagnosis of severe esophagitis and subsequent development of an esophageal stricture. (**A**) No abnormalities are detected on the survey radiograph. (**B–D**) Following oral administration of barium sulfate suspension (**B**) and canned food mixed with barium sulfate suspension (**C**), there is mild focal narrowing of the esophageal lumen caudal to the tracheal bifurcation (arrows), but contrast material passes to reach the stomach. Kibble mixed with barium sulfate suspension (**D**) is unable to pass the stricture (arrows), and there is a new finding of esophageal dilation orad to the stricture site. A second lesser degree severity stricture is observed at the level of the tracheal bifurcation (arrowheads).

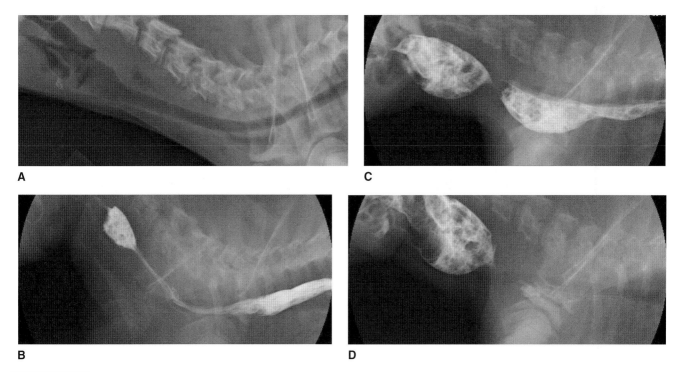

**FIGURE 17.54** Right lateral radiograph of the neck (**A**) and fluoroscopic esophagography images (**B–D**) in a 3-month-old mixed-breed dog with regurgitation since birth. (**A**) On the survey radiograph the esophagus is multifocally irregularly dilated with gas. (**B–D**) Following oral administration of barium sulfate suspension (**B**) and canned food mixed with barium sulfate suspension (**C**), there is marked focal narrowing of the midesophageal lumen, but material passes. Kibble mixed with barium sulfate suspension (**D**) is unable to pass the stricture and results in proximal esophageal dilation. A reason for the esophageal stricture in this puppy was not identified.

## Esophageal Foreign Body

Esophageal foreign bodies are a common presenting complaint in canine and, to a lesser degree, feline emergency patients [73–77]. A diagnosis on survey radiographs is straightforward if the foreign body is of mineral, bone, or metal opacity (Figure 17.55). However, cloth, cartilage, plastic/rubber, and other materials of soft tissue opacity are more difficult to detect. Heterogeneous gas inclusions within the foreign material, ventral displacement of the trachea on the lateral views, esophageal dilation proximal to the obstructive lesion, and mediastinal widening on the VD view may aid in establishing a diagnosis (Figure 17.56). In questionable cases, esophagography is helpful (Figure 17.57), and the diagnosis is typically possible on static radiographic images following barium sulfate suspension administration.

Complications due to presence of the foreign body or following surgical removal include hemorrhage, esophageal perforation, development of an esophageal fistula and stricture [78–80]. Information on pneumomediastinum, mediastinal effusion, and esophageal strictures can be found above.

## Esophageal Mass

Esophageal tumors are rare. Several different tumors have been reported to affect the esophagus, including squamous cell carcinoma, smooth muscle tumors (leiomyoma, leiomyosarcoma), fibrosarcoma, and others [81, 82]. Survey radiographs may show a variably sized and usually soft tissue opaque mass in the expected location of the esophagus in the dorsal mediastinum; however, esophagography is often needed to identify a lesion and

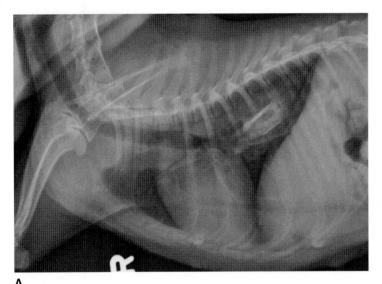

**A**

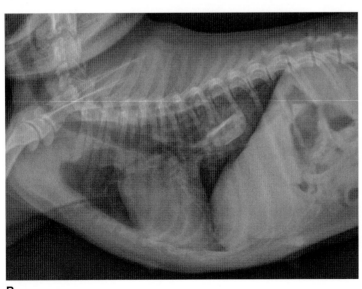

**B**

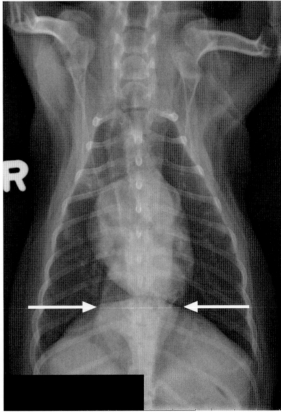

**C**

**FIGURE 17.55** Right lateral (**A**), left lateral (**B**), and ventrodorsal (**C**) radiographs of the thorax in a 5-year-old Chihuahua with an esophageal foreign body (chicken bone). (**A,B**) On the lateral views, the bone opacity foreign body is clearly visible within the caudal dorsal esophagus. (**C**) On the VD view, the foreign body is superimposed over the spine. Caudal mediastinal widening is the predominant radiographic finding (arrows).

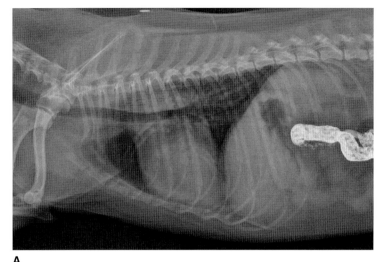

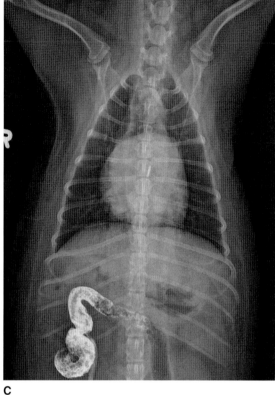

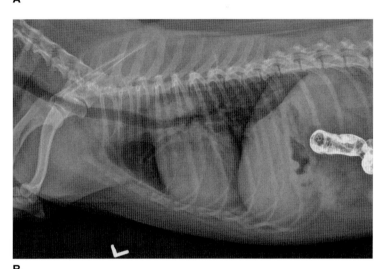

**FIGURE 17.56** Right lateral (**A**), left lateral (**B**), and ventrodorsal (**C**) radiographs of the thorax in a 5-year-old Shih Tzu. There is a granular to linear mostly soft tissue opacity structure with interspersed gas opacities associated with the thoracic esophagus from approximately the level of the third through seventh thoracic vertebrae. This lesion results in ventral displacement and compression of the caudal trachea and mainstem bronchi on the lateral views. A piece of chicken jerky was removed endoscopically.

confirm esophageal origin (Figures 17.58 and 17.59). In addition to the identification and classification of the mass, esophagography may also aid in diagnosis of complications associated with the tumor (ulceration, stricture, perforation). Esophageal sarcomas secondary to *Spirocerca lupi* infestation have been reported in indigenous areas [83, 84]. Radiographic abnormalities include an esophageal mass usually in the caudal esophagus, spondylitis, and undulation of the aortic border [36, 83, 85] (Figure 17.60).

## Hiatal Abnormalities

Hiatal hernias in which abdominal contents protrude through the esophageal hiatus were covered under "Caudal dorsal mediastinal masses" above (see also Figures 17.35 and 17.36). Gastroesophageal intussusception (GEI) is a rare condition that usually affects young dogs (generally less than 1 year, with

most less than 3 months), with a higher incidence reported in males and German shepherd dogs [86–92]. GEI is characterized by invagination of the stomach, and possibly other abdominal organs (spleen, pancreas, omentum, proximal duodenum), into the distal esophagus. Survey radiographs may show a soft tissue or heterogeneous mass in the caudal dorsal mediastinum (Figure 17.61A–C), and the stomach may be partially or completely absent from the cranial abdomen (Figure 17.61D).

# Trachea

The trachea extends from the cricoid cartilage of the larynx to its bifurcation into the mainstem bronchi dorsal to the heart base [3, 93]. The cervical trachea is oriented approximately parallel with the spine. While the thoracic trachea in barrel-chested

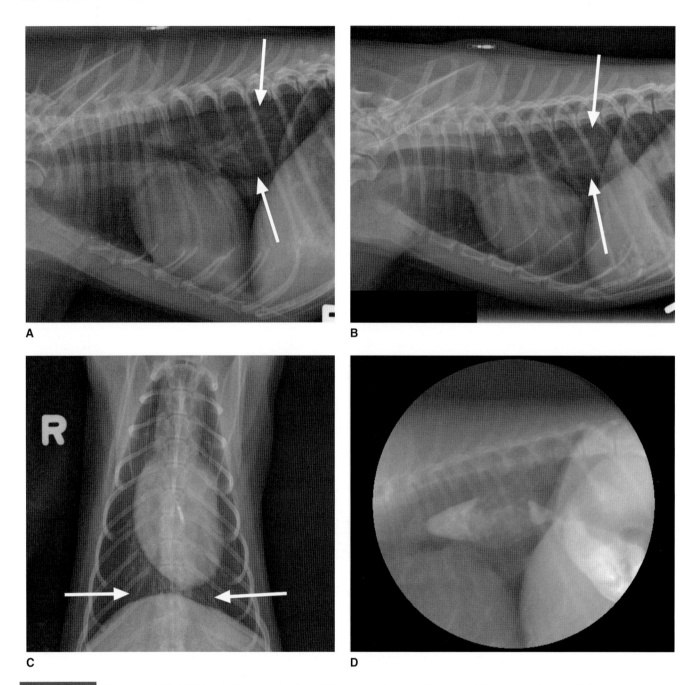

**FIGURE 17.57** Right lateral (**A**), left lateral (**B**), and ventrodorsal (**C**) radiographs of the thorax, and fluoroscopic image (**D**) during esophagography in a 9-year-old Maltese dog. (**A–C**) On the survey radiographs there is a very faint rounded soft tissue opacity in the plane of the caudal dorsal mediastinum (arrows). (**D**) During the esophagogram a large round intraluminal foreign body is clearly delineated. A large piece of carrot was removed endoscopically.

breeds is also almost parallel with the spine, there is mild cau-doventral deviation of the trachea from the thoracic inlet to the tracheal bifurcation in most dogs and cats (Figure 17.62A). If the neck is flexed when a thoracic radiograph is obtained, the stiff trachea assumes an undulating course within the cranial thorax, which should not be mistaken for a cranial mediastinal mass [94] (Figure 17.62B). On the VD view, the trachea typically is located close to and slightly to the right of midline (Figure 17.62C). Due to superimposition with the spine and mediastinal structures, most tracheal disorders are best evaluated on lateral views. The trachea is of similar diameter throughout and slightly smaller than the larynx. Published reference values for a normal ratio of tracheal diameter to thoracic inlet are $0.20 \pm 0.03$ for non-brachycephalic dogs, $0.16 \pm 0.03$ for nonbulldog brachycephalic dogs, and $0.13 \pm 0.04$ for bulldogs [95]. The tracheal wall is of soft tissue opacity, but mineralization of tracheal rings is a com-mon incidental finding, especially in older and large-breed dogs (Figure 17.63). Due to its location and mobility, tracheal displacement or compression due to masses originating from surrounding tissues (e.g., cranial mediastinum, heart base or esophagus) is common (see above).

This section will cover primary tracheal disorders.

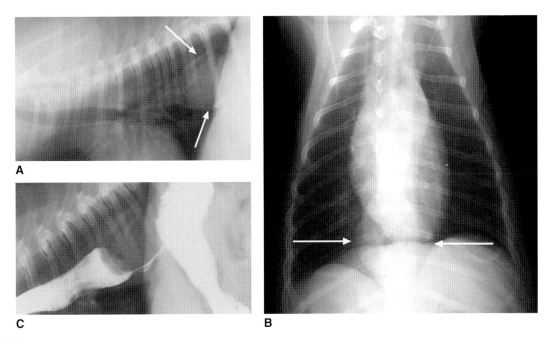

**FIGURE 17.58** Cropped right lateral (**A**), ventrodorsal (**B**), and esophagography (**C**) radiographs in an older mixed-breed dog with an esophageal mass (leiomyoma). On survey radiographs (**A,B**), a caudal dorsal homogeneous soft tissue opacity mass is located cranial to the diaphragm (arrows). (**C**) Esophagography demonstrates a smoothly marginated exophytic mural mass. *Source:* Courtesy of Dr William H. Adams.

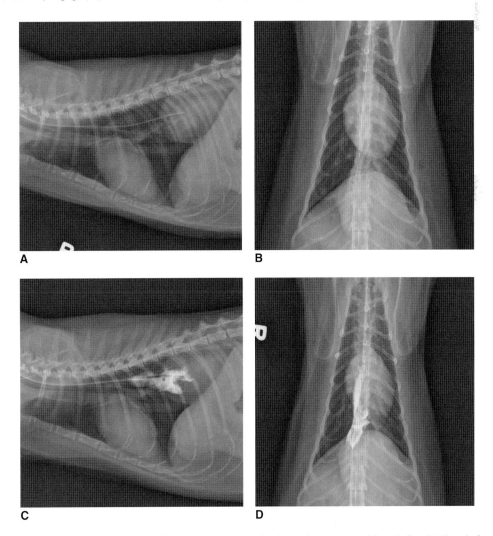

**FIGURE 17.59** Right lateral (**A,C**) and ventrodorsal (**B,D**) radiographs of the thorax in an 8-year-old cat before (**A,B**) and after (**C,D**) administration of positive contrast medium into an esophageal tube. (**A,B**) Survey radiographs show a large caudal dorsal mediastinal mass. (**C,D**) Contrast medium administration and subsequent ultrasonographic examination via a transdiaphragmatic approach confirmed an esophageal mass. The patient was diagnosed with multicentric lymphoma; samples of the esophageal mass were not obtained.

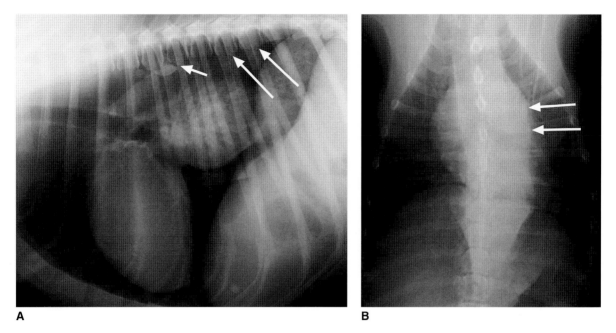

**FIGURE 17.60** Left lateral (**A**) and dorsoventral (**B**) radiographs of the thorax in an adult dog with spirocercosis. (**A**) The lateral view shows a large caudal dorsal esophageal mass and faint irregular periosteal reaction associated with several ventral vertebral bodies (arrows), consistent with spondylitis. (**B**) An additional finding on the DV view is an undulating contour of the lateral margin of the aorta due to aneurysm formation (arrows). *Source:* Courtesy of Dr Chee Kin Lim.

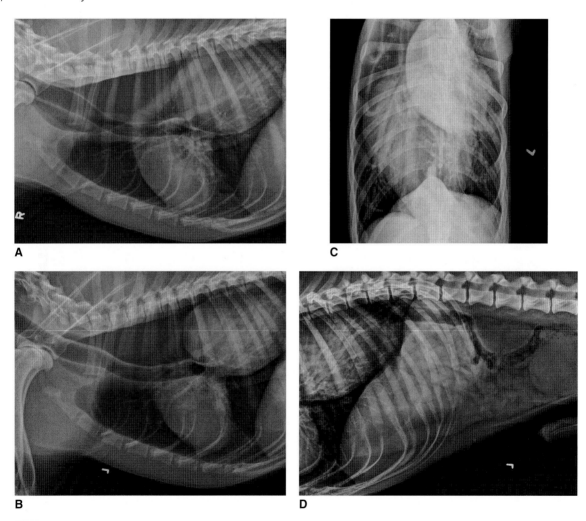

**FIGURE 17.61** Gastroesophageal intussusception in a 2-year-old German shepherd dog. Right lateral (**A**), left lateral (**B**), and ventrodorsal (**C**) radiographs of the thorax demonstrate marked generalized dilation of the esophagus with gas and a very large sharply marginated soft tissue opacity mass lesion within the caudal esophageal lumen. The trachea is displaced ventrally by the dilated esophagus. Ill-defined alveolar patterns are associated with the right middle and caudal subsegment of left cranial lung lobe on the lateral views, consistent with aspiration pneumonia. (**D**) The left lateral view of the cranial abdomen demonstrates absence of the stomach within the abdomen and extension of the colon into the esophageal hiatus.

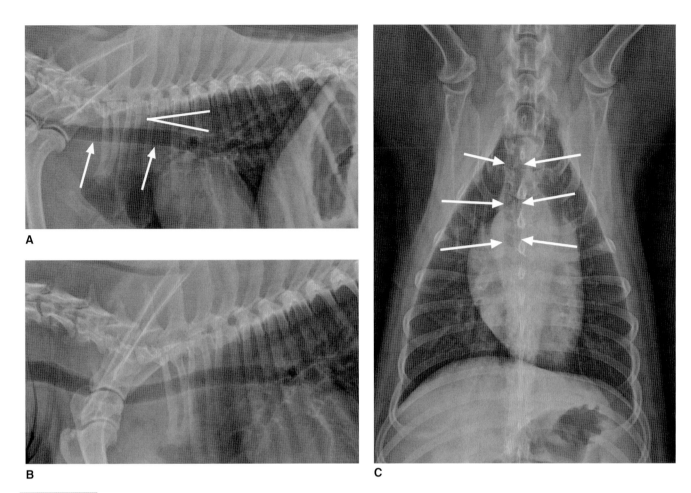

**FIGURE 17.62**   Normal thorax in a 7-year-old Staffordshire terrier. On the cropped right lateral view (**A**), the air-filled trachea (arrows) deviates from and forms an angle with the spine, consistent with breed conformation. On the cropped left lateral view (**B**), there is mild dorsal curvature of the thoracic trachea which is an incidental variant due to flexion of the neck during radiographic exposure. On the VD view (**C**), the trachea (arrows) is superimposed with and slightly to the right of the cranial thoracic spine.

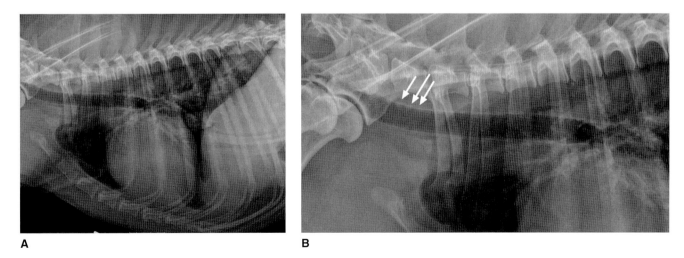

**FIGURE 17.63**   Lateral view of the thorax (**A**) and magnified image of the trachea (**B**) in a 10-year-old Labrador retriever. There is incidental mineralization of the tracheal rings (arrows).

# Tracheal Collapse

Tracheal collapse is a very common disorder in (small-breed) dogs [96–101] and is rare in cats [102]. It is the result of tracheal chondromalacia and is characterized by static or dynamic narrowing of the tracheal lumen and/or mainstem bronchi.

Collapse can occur anywhere along the length of the trachea and tracheal bifurcation. Static collapse is easily diagnosed on lateral radiographs of the neck and thorax as typically severe persistent narrowing of the tracheal lumen [93] (Figures 17.64 and 17.65). Dynamic collapse is best evaluated using fluoroscopy [103]. Although inspiratory and expiratory radiographs may also aid in the assessment of patients suspected to be affected by tracheal collapse, exact timing of radiographic exposure with maximum inspiration, expiration, and cough limits the

diagnostic yield of this technique. Dynamic cervical tracheal collapse typically occurs during inspiration. Dynamic intrathoracic and mainstem bronchial collapse typically occurs during expiration or coughing (Figures 17.66 and 17.67). The role of a "redundant" dorsal tracheal membrane in dogs with tracheal collapse is still poorly understood. This term has been used for a fusiform soft tissue opacity commonly seen along the dorsal trachea in the caudal neck and cranial thoracic region on thoracic radiographs which is attributed to focal flaccidity and indentation of the dorsal tracheal membrane by the esophagus (Figures 17.68 and 17.69). It is a frequent incidental finding especially when seen in large-breed dogs; however, in dogs with tracheal collapse, the dorsal tracheal membrane occupies a larger percentage of tracheal circumference and thus may be a factor in the disease process [98].

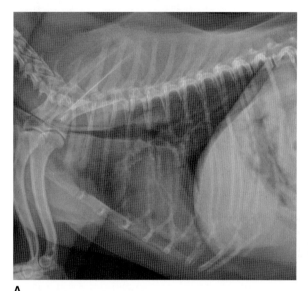

A

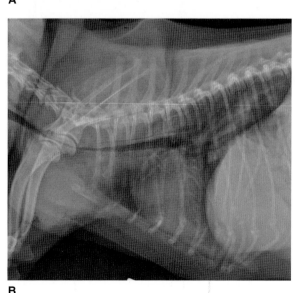

B

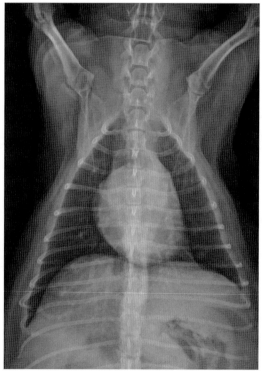

C

**FIGURE 17.64** Static tracheal collapse in a 10-year-old Chihuahua. Better seen on the right lateral (**A**) and left lateral (**B**) than on the VD view (**C**), there is consistent severe narrowing of the tracheal lumen in the caudal neck and cranial thorax. A small amount of gas is present in the esophagus dorsal to the trachea.

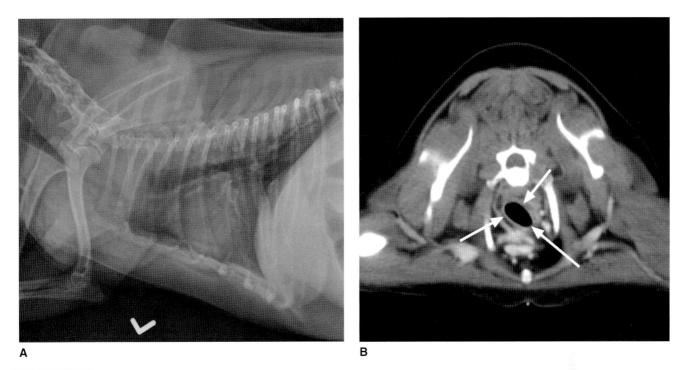

**FIGURE 17.65** Static tracheal collapse in a 13-year-old Yorkshire terrier. The left lateral (**A**) view documents complete collapse of the caudal cervical and cranial thoracic trachea with obliteration of the lumen. Transverse CT image (**B**) at the level of the thoracic inlet shows abnormal flattening of the trachea (arrows) despite positive pressure ventilation, consistent with chondromalacia.

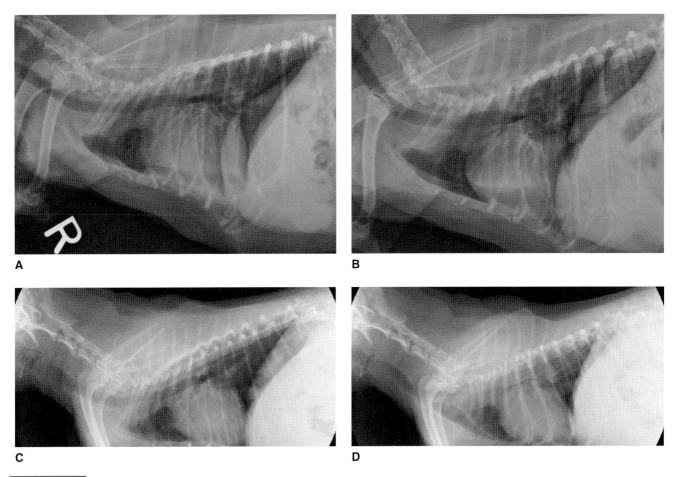

**FIGURE 17.66** Dynamic intrathoracic tracheal and mainstem bronchial collapse in a 13-year-old Maltese. On standard right (**A**) and left (**B**) lateral views, there is no evidence of tracheal or mainstem bronchial collapse. Dynamic fluoroscopic images obtained during inspiration (**C**) and expiration (**D**) show complete collapse of the intrathoracic trachea and mainstem bronchi on expiration.

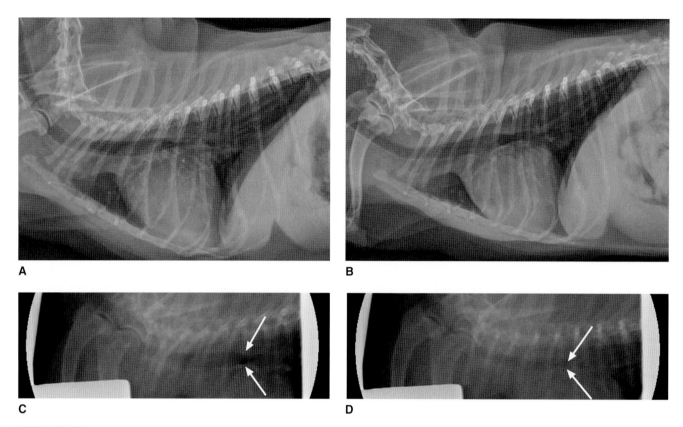

**A**   **B**

**C**   **D**

**FIGURE 17.67**   Dynamic mainstem bronchial collapse in a 14-year-old toy poodle. On standard right (**A**) and left (**B**) lateral views, there is no evidence of tracheal or mainstem bronchial collapse. Dynamic fluoroscopic images obtained during inspiration (**C**) and coughing (**D**) show complete collapse of the mainstem bronchi during cough (arrows).

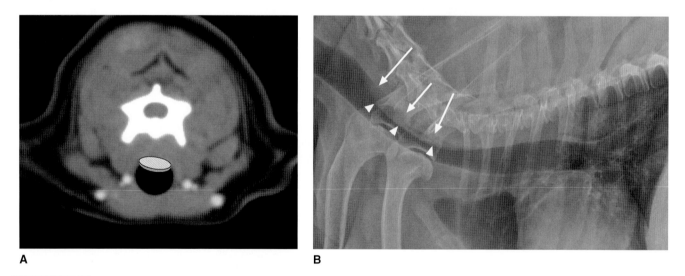

**A**   **B**

**FIGURE 17.68**   Redundant tracheal membrane. (**A**) Schematic image using a modified transverse CT image of the caudal neck in a dog to illustrate the "redundant tracheal membrane" concept. The dorsal tracheal membrane and esophagus (indicated as striated oval structure dorsal to the esophagus) fold into the dorsal tracheal lumen which will result in a fusiform soft tissue opacity band superimposed with the dorsal aspect of the trachea on a lateral thoracic radiograph (arrowheads; **B**). Note that the actual dorsal tracheal wall (arrows) remains visible.

## Tracheal Stenosis

Focal narrowing of the tracheal lumen most commonly occurs as a sequela to tracheal trauma (e.g., overinflation of endotracheal cuff, bite wound or endotracheal foreign body) [54, 104–108]. Cervicothoracic radiographs will show circumferential narrowing of the tracheal lumen which should not be mistaken for a tracheal mass (Figure 17.70).

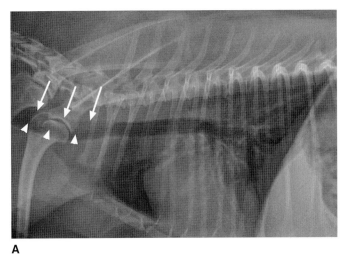

**A**          **B**

**FIGURE 17.69**   Right lateral (**A**) radiograph of the thorax and craniocaudal view of the ventral neck/thoracic inlet ("skyline view") (**B**) in a 10-year-old Chihuahua. (**A**) A fusiform soft tissue opacity is associated with the dorsal trachea (arrowheads), partially obscuring its lumen, while the dorsal tracheal wall is clearly visible (arrows). (**B**) The skyline view confirms that this opacity corresponds to a "redundant" tracheal membrane (arrows).

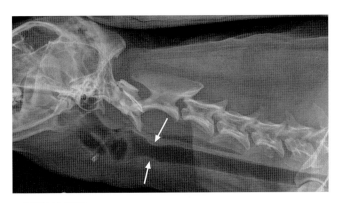

**FIGURE 17.70**   Tracheal stenosis in a 12-year-old Siberian husky presented with inspiratory stridor. The lateral view of the neck demonstrates approximately 50% reduction in diameter of the most cranial trachea caudal to the cricoid cartilage (arrows). This was of undetermined etiology in this patient.

## Tracheal Hypoplasia

In tracheal hypoplasia, there is a generalized reduction in tracheal diameter. This is a congenital condition and is a common feature in patients afflicted with brachycephalic airway obstruction, especially bulldogs [109–111]. Animals typically present at a very young age. Radiographs reveal generalized narrowing of the tracheal lumen, either subjectively or compared to published reference values (see above) (Figure 17.71). Concurrent aspiration pneumonia at time of diagnosis is common.

## Diffuse Tracheal Narrowing

In addition to tracheal hypoplasia, other conditions which may result in diffuse tracheal narrowing include mediastinal effusion (see Figure 17.17) and thickening of the tracheal wall secondary

to edema, inflammation, hemorrhage, or, less commonly, diffuse neoplasia [9, 10, 26, 93] (Figures 17.72 and 17.73). As these are acquired conditions, affected animals typically present at a higher age and with a different history from animals affected by tracheal hypoplasia

## Tracheal Foreign Body

Aspiration of foreign material is an occasional presenting complaint in dogs (especially young and hunting breeds) and cats [112–116]. Affected animals typically present with acute onset of severe dyspnea and/or cough. A diagnosis is usually straightforward as the gas column within the trachea contrasts with the intraluminal foreign body (Figure 17.74). As foreign bodies tend to lodge in the area of the carina due to the abrupt narrowing in airway diameter at this level, particular attention should be paid to this region when evaluating thoracic radiographs [93].

## Tracheal Mass

Masses arising from the tracheal wall are most commonly neoplastic in etiology and include lymphoma, chondrosarcoma, adenocarcinoma, squamous cell carcinoma, leiomyoma, polyps, and benign osteochondral tumors [81, 82]. Inflammatory tracheal masses (granulomas) are infrequently reported as a primary problem [117, 118] but are a common sequela following endotracheal stent placement [119]. Similar to tracheal foreign bodies, masses originating from the tracheal wall and extending into the lumen are usually easily visualized due to contrast with adjacent intraluminal air (Figure 17.75; see also Figure 17.22). However, a diagnosis may be more challenging if the mass is obscured by overlying soft tissue structures such as aorta or esophagus (Figure 17.76).

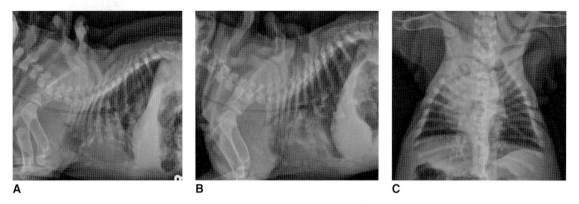

**FIGURE 17.71** Right lateral (**A**), left lateral (**B**), and ventrodorsal (**C**) thoracic radiographs in a 10-week-old English bulldog puppy with hypoplastic trachea and secondary aspiration pneumonia. (**A,B**) On both lateral views severe generalized tracheal narrowing is evident. (**C**) There is also a generalized unstructured interstitial and bronchial pattern with multifocal ventrally distributed alveolar infiltrates.

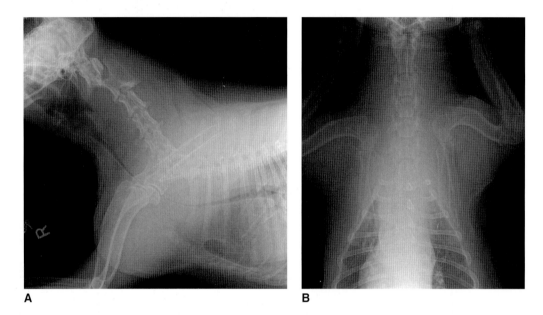

**FIGURE 17.72** Right lateral (**A**) and ventrodorsal (**B**) thoracic radiographs in a middle-aged Labrador retriever with intramural tracheal hemorrhage due to rodenticide toxicity. There is severe diffuse narrowing of the trachea seen on both views. Increased opacity and widening of the cranial mediastinum suggest concurrent mediastinal effusion. *Source:* Courtesy of Dr Matthew Baron.

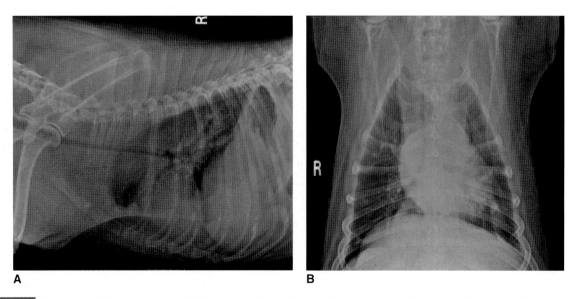

**FIGURE 17.73** Right lateral (**A**) and ventrodorsal (**B**) thoracic radiographs showing severe generalized tracheal narrowing in an 11-year-old boxer due to tracheitis. Tracheal bronchoscopy found generalized reduction in airway diameter by 60–75%, with mucosal irregularity and hyperemia. Bronchoalveolar lavage yielded a diagnosis of septic suppurative inflammation. Additional radiographic findings in this patient include mediastinal widening, mild pleural effusion, and ventrally distributed alveolar patterns likely representing foci of pneumonia.

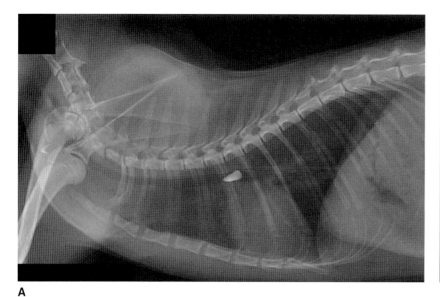

**A**

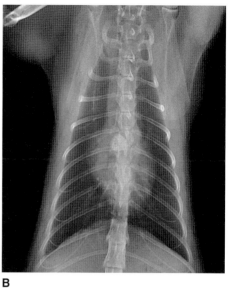

**B**

**FIGURE 17.74** Left lateral (**A**) and ventrodorsal (**B**) thoracic radiographs in a 9-month-old cat showing a mineral opaque foreign body in the caudal trachea immediately cranial to the cranial bifurcation. A rock was retrieved endoscopically. *Source:* Courtesy of Big Springs Veterinary Hospital, Maryville, Tennessee.

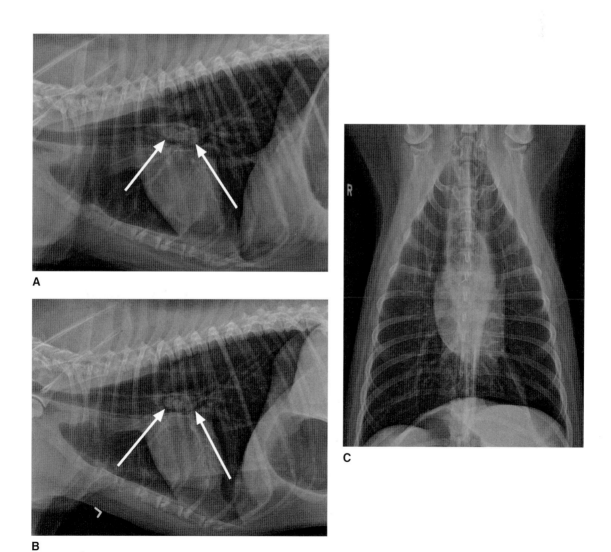

**FIGURE 17.75** Right lateral (**A**), left lateral (**B**), and ventrodorsal (**C**) thoracic radiographs in a 9-year-old Labrador retriever. Both lateral views (**A,B**) allow identification of a lobulated tracheal mass (arrows), while the ventrodorsal view (**C**) is unhelpful. Bronchoscopic biopsy yielded a diagnosis of anaplastic sarcoma.

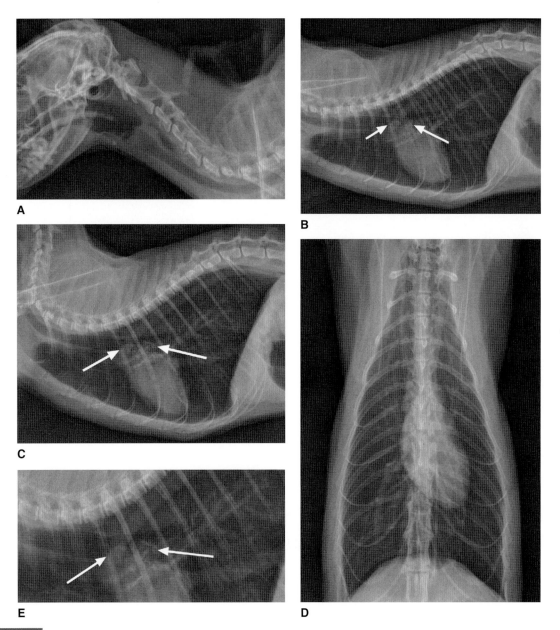

**FIGURE 17.76** Lateral view of the neck (**A**), right lateral (**B**), left lateral (**C**), and ventrodorsal views of the thorax (**D**), and magnified lateral view of the tracheal bifurcation (**E**) in a 10-year-old cat with severe respiratory difficulties. (**A**) Overdistension of the pharynx is consistent with severe dyspnea and airway obstruction. (**B, C, E**) A focal soft tissue opacity mass is located within the trachea immediately cranial to the heart base and extending toward the tracheal bifurcation (arrows). Superimposition of the aortic arch makes mass identification difficult. (**B–D**) Hyperinflation of the lungs seen on all three thoracic views is consistent with dyspnea. Endoscopic and subsequent postmortem biopsy was consistent with tracheal and primary bronchial adenocarcinoma.

## Tracheal Trauma (Rupture/Tear/ Avulsion/Perforation)

A tracheal rupture or tear is usually traumatic in etiology (e.g., bite wound), although other causes, including iatrogenic injury, are possible. Radiographically, affected animals present with pneumomediastinum (see above; see Figures 17.42–17.46), gas inclusions within fascial planes, subcutaneous emphysema, and commonly associated pneumothorax (Figure 17.77). Intrathoracic tracheal avulsion is an uncommon condition reported in

cats [120–123]. It results from blunt traumatic hyperextension of the neck and/or thorax which leads to stretching and ultimately rupture of the trachea. The airway lumen is often maintained by either an intact tracheal adventitia or by thickened mediastinal tissue, and diverticula may form. Reported cases involved the intrathoracic trachea; the author has seen one case in the cervical region (Figure 17.78). Focal small perforation of the trachea secondary to a foreign body or parasite migration is rare but may result in soft tissue swelling and/or gas inclusions within the adjacent tissues (Figure 17.79).

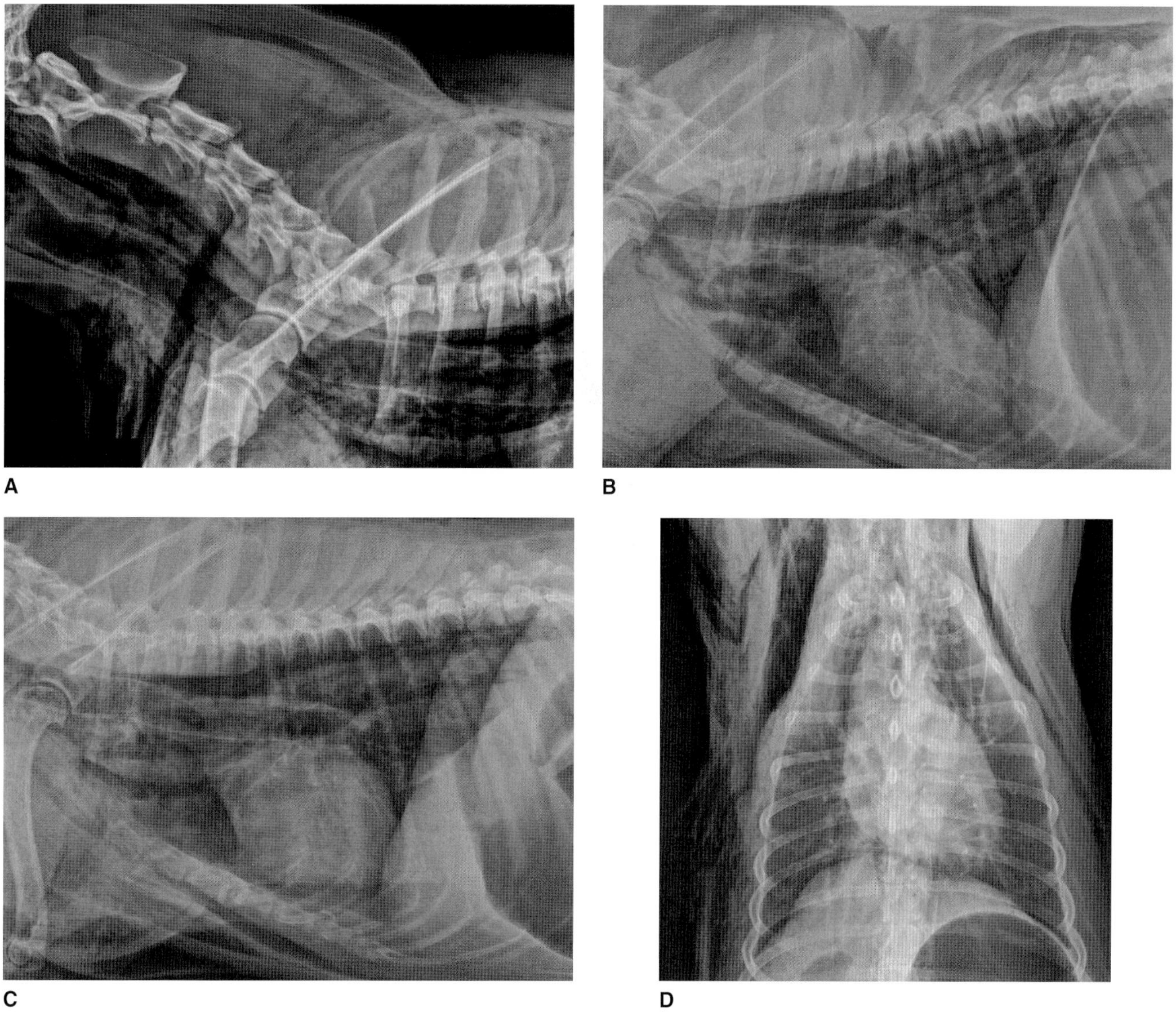

A

B

C

D

**FIGURE 17.77** Presumptive tracheal injury/tear in a 9-year-old golden retriever that had undergone anesthesia and endotracheal intubation 3 days before. Lateral view of the neck (**A**) and right lateral (**B**), left lateral (**C**), and ventrodorsal (**D**) thoracic radiographs show extensive gas inclusions within the soft tissues of the neck and dissecting along fascial planes, subcutaneous emphysema, pneumomediastinum, and mild pneumothorax. The source of air leakage is not identified but was suspected to be a tracheal injury, possibly from overinflation of the endotracheal cuff.

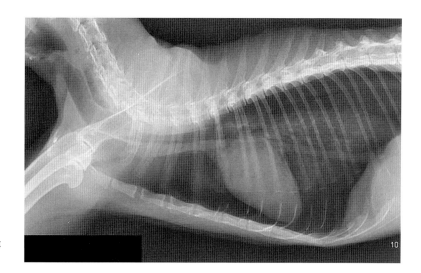

**FIGURE 17.78** Right lateral thoracic radiograph in a 12-year-old cat with tracheal avulsion. There is severe widening and unusual contour of the cervical trachea. The thoracic caudal trachea is of normal diameter and contour. Surgical exploration found complete rupture between two tracheal rings with intact adventitial coverage resulting in a "balloon-like" appearance of the airway rather than pneumomediastinum. Pneumothorax is, however, present.

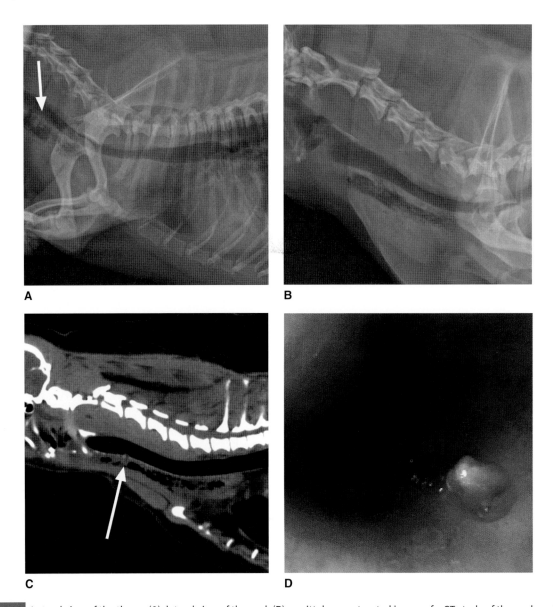

A

B

C

D

**FIGURE 17.79** Lateral view of the thorax (**A**), lateral view of the neck (**B**), sagittal reconstructed image of a CT study of the neck and thorax (**C**), and endoscopic image (**D**) in a patient with punctate tracheal perforation due to aberrant Cuterebra larva migration. (**A**) Multiple punctate gas opacity foci are present ventral to the trachea in the caudal neck and cranial thoracic area. There is a faint focal irregular thickening of the ventral cervical tracheal wall (arrow). (**B**) There is improved visualization of the unusual focal emphysematous region within the soft tissues of the neck and extending into the mediastinum, but the suspected tracheal lesion is not clearly seen. (**C**) In addition to abnormalities noted on radiographs, there is a hypoattenuating tract extending from the tracheal lumen to the emphysematous region within the neck (arrow). At this point, a perforating foreign body was suspected. (**D**) Endoscopy yielded a diagnosis of tracheal perforation by an aberrant Cuterebra larva which was subsequently successfully retrieved via cutaneous stab incision. *Source:* Courtesy of Dr Lee Emery.

# References

1. Evans, H.E. and de Lahunta, A. (2013). *Miller's Anatomy of the Dog*. St Louis, MO: Elsevier Saunders.

2. Suter, P.F. and Lord, P.F. (1984). *Thoracic Radiography. Thoracic Diseases of the Dog and Cat*. Wettswil: Peter F. Suter.

3. Thrall, D.E. and Robertson, I.D. (2011). *Atlas of Normal Radiographic Anatomy & Anatomic Variants in the Dog and Cat*. St Louis, MO: Elsevier Saunders.

4. Thrall, D.E. (2013). The mediastinum. In: *Textbook of Veterinary Diagnostic Radiology*, 6e (ed. D.E. Thrall), 550–570. St Louis, MO: Elsevier Saunders.

5. Brinkman, E.L., Biller, D., and Armbrust, L. (2006). The clinical usefulness of the ventrodorsal versus dorsoventral thoracic radiograph in dogs. *J. Am. Anim. Hosp. Assoc.* 42: 440–449.

6. Kirberger, R.M. and Avner, A. (2006). The effect of positioning on the appearance of selected cranial thoracic structures in the dog. *Vet. Radiol. Ultrasound* 47: 61–68.

7. Mitten, R.W. (1982). Radiology of mediastinal diseases. *Vet. Clin. North Am. Small Anim. Pract.* 12: 193–211.

8. Mellanby, R.J., Villiers, E., and Herrtage, M.E. (2002). Canine pleural and mediastinal effusions: a retrospective study of 81 cases. *J. Small Anim. Pract.* 43: 447–451.

9. Berry, C.R., Gallaway, A., Thrall, D.E., and Carlisle, C. (1993). Thoracic radiographic features of anticoagulant rodenticide toxicity in 14 dogs. *Vet. Radiol. Ultrasound* 34: 391–396.

10. Blocker, T.L. and Roberts, B.K. (1999). Acute tracheal obstruction associated with anticoagulant rodenticide intoxication in a dog. *J. Small Anim. Pract.* 40: 577–580.

11. Espino, L., Vazquez, S., Failde, D. et al. (2010). Localized pleural mesothelioma causing cranial vena cava syndrome in a dog. *J. Vet. Diagn. Invest.* 22: 309–312.

12. Mason, G.D., Lamb, C.R., and Jakowski, R.M. (1990). Fatal mediastinal hemorrhage in a dog. *Vet. Radiol.* 31: 214–216.

13. Rickman, B.H. and Gurfield, N. (2009). Thymic cystic degeneration, pseudoepitheliomatous hyperplasia, and hemorrhage in a dog with brodifacoum toxicosis. *Vet. Pathol.* 46: 449–452.

14. Slensky, K.A., Volk, S.W., Schwarz, T. et al. (2003). Acute severe hemorrhage secondary to arterial invasion in a dog with thyroid carcinoma. *J. Am. Vet. Med. Assoc.* 223: 649–653, 636.

15. Gendron, K., Christe, A., Walter, S. et al. (2014). Serial CT features of pulmonary leptospirosis in 10 dogs. *Vet. Rec.* 174: 169–176.

16. Blackwood, L., Sullivan, M., and Lawson, H. (1997). Radiographic abnormalities in canine multicentric lymphoma: a review of 84 cases. *J. Small Anim. Pract.* 38: 62–69.

17. Geyer, N.E., Reichle, J.K., Valdes-Martinez, A. et al. (2010). Radiographic appearance of confirmed pulmonary lymphoma in cats and dogs. *Vet. Radiol. Ultrasound* 51: 386–390.

18. Legendre, A.M. (2006). Blastomycosis. In: *Infectious Diseases of the Dog and Cat*, 3e (ed. C.E. Greene), 569–576. St Louis, MO: Saunders.

19. Myers, N.C. 3rd, Engler, S.J., and Jakowski, R.M. (1996). Chylothorax and chylous ascites in a dog with mediastinal lymphangiosarcoma. *J. Am. Anim. Hosp. Assoc.* 32: 263–269.

20. Aronsohn, M.G., Schunk, K.L., Carpenter, J.L., and King, N.W. (1984). Clinical and pathologic features of thymoma in 15 dogs. *J. Am. Vet. Med. Assoc.* 184 (11): 1355–1362.

21. Atwater, S.W., Powers, B.E., Park, R.D. et al. (1994). Thymoma in dogs: 23 cases (1980–1991). *J. Am. Vet. Med. Assoc.* 205: 1007–1013.

22. Gabor, L.J., Malik, R., and Canfield, P.J. (1998). Clinical and anatomical features of lymphosarcoma in 118 cats. *Aust. Vet. J.* 76: 725–732.

23. Patnaik, A.K., MacEwen, E.G., Erlandson, R.A. et al. (1978). Mediastinal parathyroid adenocarcinoma in a dog. *Vet. Pathol.* 15: 55–63.

24. Yoon, H.Y., Kang, H.M., and Lee, M.Y. (2014). Primary cranial mediastinal hemangiosarcoma in a young dog. *Ir. Vet. J.* 67: 15.

25. Vail, D.M. (2007). Feline lymphoma and leukemia. In: *Small Animal Clinical Oncology*, 4e (ed. S.J. Withrow and D.M. Vail), 733–756. St Louis, MO: Saunders.

26. Hecht, S. and Penninck, D. (2015). Thorax. In: *Atlas of Small Animal Ultrasonography* (ed. D. Penninck and M.A. d'Anjou), 81–110. Ames, IA: Wiley Blackwell.

27. Patterson, M.M. and Marolf, A.J. (2014). Sonographic characteristics of thymoma compared with mediastinal lymphoma. *J. Am. Anim. Hosp. Assoc.* 50: 409–413.

28. Tidwell, A.S. (1998). Ultrasonography of the thorax (excluding the heart). *Vet. Clin. North Am. Small Anim. Pract.* 28: 993–1015.

29. Reichle, J.K. and Wisner, E.R. (2000). Non-cardiac thoracic ultrasound in 75 feline and canine patients. *Vet. Radiol. Ultrasound* 41: 154–162.

30. Zekas, L.J. and Adams, W.M. (2002). Cranial mediastinal cysts in nine cats. *Vet. Radiol. Ultrasound* 43: 413–418.

31. Buchanan, J.W. (2004). Tracheal signs and associated vascular anomalies in dogs with persistent right aortic arch. *J. Vet. Intern. Med.* 18: 510–514.

32. Gaschen, L. (2013). The canine and feline esophagus. In: *Textbook of Veterinary Diagnostic Radiology*, 6e (ed. D.E. Thrall), 500–521. St Louis, MO: Elsevier Saunders.

33. Guglielmini, C., Baron Toaldo, M., Quinci, M. et al. (2016). Sensitivity, specificity, and interobserver variability of survey thoracic radiography for the detection of heart base masses in dogs. *J. Am. Vet. Med. Assoc.* 248: 1391–1398.

34. Rizzo, S.A., Newman, S.J., Hecht, S., and Thomas, W.B. (2008). Malignant mediastinal extra-adrenal paraganglioma with spinal cord invasion in a dog. *J. Vet. Diagn. Invest.* 20: 372–375.

35. Boulineau, T.M., Andrews-Jones, L., and Van Alstine, W. (2005). Spontaneous aortic dissecting hematoma in two dogs. *J. Vet. Diagn. Invest.* 17: 492–497.

36. Kirberger, R.M., Stander, N., Cassel, N. et al. (2013). Computed tomographic and radiographic characteristics of aortic lesions in 42 dogs with spirocercosis. *Vet. Radiol. Ultrasound* 54: 212–222.

37. Lenz, J.A., Bach, J.F., Bell, C.M., and Stepien, R.L. (2015). Aortic tear and dissection related to connective tissues abnormalities resembling Marfan syndrome in a Great Dane. *J. Vet. Cardiol.* 17: 134–141.

38. Lorinson, D. and Bright, R.M. (1998). Long-term outcome of medical and surgical treatment of hiatal hernias in dogs and cats: 27 cases (1978–1996). *J. Am. Vet. Med. Assoc.* 213: 381–384.

39. Randall, E.K. and Park, R.D. (2013). The diaphragm. In: *Textbook of Veterinary Diagnostic Radiology*, 6e (ed. D.E. Thrall), 535–549. St Louis, MO: Elsevier Saunders.

40. Kohn, G.P., Price, R.R., Demeester, S.R., et al. (2013). Guidelines for the Management of Hiatal Hernia. www.sages.org/publications/guidelines/guidelines-for-the-management-of-hiatal-hernia.

41. Guiot, L.P., Lansdowne, J.L., Rouppert, P., and Stanley, B.J. (2008). Hiatal hernia in the dog: a clinical report of four Chinese shar peis. *J. Am. Anim. Hosp. Assoc.* 44: 335–341.

42. Kirkby, K.A., Bright, R.M., and Owen, H.D. (2005). Paraoesophageal hiatal hernia and megaoesophagus in a three-week-old Alaskan malamute. *J. Small Anim. Pract.* 46: 402–405.

43. Levine, J.S., Pollard, R.E., and Marks, S.L. (2014). Contrast videofluoroscopic assessment of dysphagic cats. *Vet. Radiol. Ultrasound* 55: 465–471.

44. Miles, K.G., Pope, E.R., and Jergens, A.E. (1988). Paraesophageal hiatal hernia and pyloric obstruction in a dog. *J. Am. Vet. Med. Assoc.* 193: 1437–1439.

45. Rahal, S.C., Mamprim, M.J., Muniz, L.M., and Teixeira, C.R. (2003). Type-4 esophageal hiatal hernia in a Chinese Shar-pei dog. *Vet. Radiol. Ultrasound* 44: 646–647.

46. Banz, A.C. and Gottfried, S.D. (2010). Peritoneopericardial diaphragmatic hernia: a retrospective study of 31 cats and eight dogs. *J. Am. Anim. Hosp. Assoc.* 46: 398–404.

47. Burns, C.G., Bergh, M.D., and McLoughlin, M.A. (2013). Surgical and nonsurgical treatment of peritoneopericardial diaphragmatic hernia in dogs and cats: 58 cases (1999–2008). *J. Am. Vet. Med. Assoc.* 242: 643–650.

48. Voges, A.K., Bertrand, S., Hill, R.C. et al. (1997). True diaphragmatic hernia in a cat. *Vet. Radiol. Ultrasound* 38: 116–119.

49. Sivacolundhu, R.K., O'Hara, A.J., and Read, R.A. (2001). Thoracic actinomycosis (arcanobacteriosis) or nocardiosis causing thoracic pyogranuloma formation in three dogs. *Aust. Vet. J.* 79: 398–402.

50. Lora-Michiels, M., Biller, D.S., Olsen, D. et al. (2003). The accessory lung lobe in thoracic disease: a case series and anatomical review. *J. Am. Anim. Hosp. Assoc.* 39: 452–458.

51. Simmonds, S.L., Whelan, M.F., and Basseches, J. (2011). Nonsurgical pneumoperitoneum in a dog secondary to blunt force trauma to the chest. *J. Vet. Emerg. Crit. Care* 21: 552–557.

52. Mitchell, S.L., McCarthy, R., Rudloff, E., and Pernell, R.T. (2000). Tracheal rupture associated with intubation in cats: 20 cases (1996–1998). *J. Am. Vet. Med. Assoc.* 216: 1592–1595.

53. Zambelli, A.B. (2006). Pneumomediastinum, pneumothorax and pneumoretroperitoneum following endoscopic retrieval of a tracheal foreign body from a cat. *J. S. Afr. Vet. Assoc.* 77: 45–50.

54. Basdani, E., Papazoglou, L.G., Patsikas, M.N. et al. (2016). Upper airway injury in dogs secondary to trauma: 10 dogs (2000–2011). *J. Am. Anim. Hosp. Assoc.* 52: 291–296.

55. Agut, A., Talavera, J., Buendia, A. et al. (2015). Imaging diagnosis – spontaneous pneumomediastinum secondary to primary pulmonary pathology in a Dalmatian dog. *Vet. Radiol. Ultrasound* 56: E54–E57.

56. Cariou, M.P. and Lipscomb, V.J. (2011). Successful surgical management of a perforating oesophageal foreign body in a cat. *J. Feline Med. Surg.* 13: 50–55.

57. Jones, B.R., Bath, M.L., and Wood, A.K. (1975). Spontaneous pneumomediastinum in the racing Greyhound. *J. Small Anim. Pract.* 16: 27–32.

58. Maes, S., Van Goethem, B., Saunders, J. et al. (2011). Pneumomediastinum and subcutaneous emphysema in a cat associated with necrotizing bronchopneumonia caused by feline herpesvirus-1. *Can. Vet. J.* 52: 1119–1122.

59. Stephens, J.A., Parnell, N.K., Clarke, K. et al. (2002). Subcutaneous emphysema, pneumomediastinum, and pulmonary emphysema in a young schipperke. *J. Am. Anim. Hosp. Assoc.* 38: 121–124.

60. Thomas, E.K. and Syring, R.S. (2013). Pneumomediastinum in cats: 45 cases (2000–2010). *J. Vet. Emerg. Crit. Care* 23: 429–435.

61. Yun, S., Lee, H., Lim, J. et al. (2016). Congenital lobar emphysema concurrent with pneumothorax and pneumomediastinum in a dog. *J. Vet. Med. Sci.* 78: 909–912.

62. Kleine, L.J. (1971). Radiographic examination of the esophagus in dogs and cats. *Vet. Clin. North Am.* 4: 663–687.

63. Stickle, R.L. and Love, N.E. (1989). Radiographic diagnosis of esophageal diseases in dogs and cats. *Semin. Vet. Med. Surg. (Small Anim.)* 4: 179–187.

64. Mace, S., Shelton, G.D., and Eddlestone, S. (2013). Megaesophagus in the dog and cat. *Tierarztl Prax Ausg K Kleintiere Heimtiere* 41: 123–131; quiz 132.

65. VanGundy, T. (1989). Vascular ring anomalies. *Compendium* 11: 35–48.

66. Bottorff, B. and Sisson, D.D. (2012). Hypoplastic aberrant left subclavian artery in a dog with a persistent right aortic arch. *J. Vet. Cardiol.* 14: 381–385.

67. House, A.K., Summerfield, N.J., German, A.J. et al. (2005). Unusual vascular ring anomaly associated with a persistent right aortic arch in two dogs. *J. Small Anim. Pract.* 46: 585–590.

68. Joly, H., d'Anjou, M.A., and Huneault, L. (2008). Imaging diagnosis – CT angiography of a rare vascular ring anomaly in a dog. *Vet. Radiol. Ultrasound* 49: 42–46.

69. Muldoon, M.M., Birchard, S.J., and Ellison, G.W. (1997). Long-term results of surgical correction of persistent right aortic arch in dogs: 25 cases (1980–1995). *J. Am. Vet. Med. Assoc.* 210: 1761–1763.

70. Pownder, S. and Scrivani, P.V. (2008). Non-selective computed tomography angiography of a vascular ring anomaly in a dog. *J. Vet. Cardiol.* 10: 125–128.

71. Adamama-Moraitou, K.K., Rallis, T.S., Prassinos, N.N., and Galatos, A.D. (2002). Benign esophageal stricture in the dog and cat: a retrospective study of 20 cases. *Can. J. Vet. Res.* 66: 55–59.

72. Sellon, R.K. and Willard, M.D. (2003). Esophagitis and esophageal strictures. *Vet. Clin. North Am. Small Anim. Pract.* 33: 945–967.

73. Deroy, C., Corcuff, J.B., Billen, F., and Hamaide, A. (2015). Removal of oesophageal foreign bodies: comparison between oesophagoscopy and oesophagotomy in 39 dogs. *J. Small Anim. Pract.* 56: 613–617.

74. Gianella, P., Pfammatter, N.S., and Burgener, I.A. (2009). Oesophageal and gastric endoscopic foreign body removal: complications and follow-up of 102 dogs. *J. Small Anim. Pract.* 50: 649–654.

75. Jankowski, M., Spuzak, J., Kubiak, K. et al. (2013). Oesophageal foreign bodies in dogs. *Pol. J. Vet. Sci.* 16: 571–572.

76. Leib, M.S. and Sartor, L.L. (2008). Esophageal foreign body obstruction caused by a dental chew treat in 31 dogs (2000–2006). *J. Am. Vet. Med. Assoc.* 232: 1021–1025.

77. Pratt, C.L., Reineke, E.L., and Drobatz, K.J. (2014). Sewing needle foreign body ingestion in dogs and cats: 65 cases (2000–2012). *J. Am. Vet. Med. Assoc.* 245: 302–308.

78. Cohn, L.A., Stoll, M.R., Branson, K.R. et al. (2003). Fatal hemothorax following management of an esophageal foreign body. *J. Am. Anim. Hosp. Assoc.* 39: 251–256.

79. Fox, S.M., Allan, F.J., Guilford, W.G. et al. (1995). Broncho-oesophageal fistula in two dogs. *N. Z. Vet. J.* 43: 235–239.

80. Keir, I., Woolford, L., Hirst, C., and Adamantos, S. (2010). Fatal aortic oesophageal fistula following oesophageal foreign body removal in a dog. *J. Small Anim. Pract.* 51: 657–660.

81. Withrow, S.J. (2007a). Cancer of the larynx and trachea. In: *Small Animal Clinical Oncology*, 4e (ed. S.J. Withrow and D.M. Vail), 515–517. St Louis, MO: Saunders.

82. Withrow, S.J. (2007b). Esophageal cancer. In: *Small Animal Clinical Oncology*, 4e (ed. S.J. Withrow and D.M. Vail), 477–478. St Louis, MO: Saunders.

83. van der Merwe, L.L., Kirberger, R.M., Clift, S. et al. (2008). *Spirocerca lupi* infection in the dog: a review. *Vet. J.* 176: 294–309.

84. Ranen, E., Lavy, E., Aizenberg, I. et al. (2004). Spirocercosis-associated esophageal sarcomas in dogs. A retrospective study of 17 cases (1997–2003). *Vet. Parasitol.* 119: 209–221.

85. Kirberger, R.M., van der Merwe, L.L., and Dvir, E. (2012). Pneumoesophagography and the appearance of masses in the caudal portion of the esophagus in dogs with spirocercosis. *J. Am. Vet. Med. Assoc.* 240: 420–426.

86. Lockwood, A., Radlinksy, M., and Crochik, S. (2010). Gastroesophageal intussusception in a German shepherd. *Compend. Contin. Educ. Vet.* 32: E1–E4.

87. Mathis, K.R., Nykamp, S.G., Ringwood, B.P., and Martin, D.M. (2013). What is your diagnosis? Gastroesophageal intussusception. *J. Am. Vet. Med. Assoc.* 242: 465–467.

88. Nagel, C.M., Montgomery, J.E., and O'Connor, B.P. (2014). What is your diagnosis? Gastroesophageal intussusception. *J. Am. Vet. Med. Assoc.* 244: 279–280.

89. Pietra, M., Gentilini, F., Pinna, S. et al. (2003). Intermittent gastroesophageal intussusception in a dog: clinical features, radiographic and endoscopic findings, and surgical management. *Vet. Res. Commun.* 27 (Suppl 1): 783–786.

90. Roach, W. and Hecht, S. (2007). What is your diagnosis? Gastroesophageal intussusception. *J. Am. Vet. Med. Assoc.* 231: 381–382.

91. Shibly, S., Karl, S., Hittmair, K.M., and Hirt, R.A. (2014). Acute gastroesophageal intussusception in a juvenile Australian Shepherd dog: endoscopic treatment and long-term follow-up. *BMC Vet. Res.* 10: 109–114.

92. Torad, F.A. and Hassan, E.A. (2015). Gastroesophageal intussusception in a 50-day-old German shepherd dog. *Top. Companion Anim. Med.* 30: 22–24.

93. Alexander, K. (2013). The pharynx, larynx, and trachea. In: *Textbook of Veterinary Diagnostic Radiology*, 6e (ed. D.E. Thrall), 489–499. St Louis, MO: Elsevier Saunders.

94. Kneller, S.K. (2002). The larynx, pharynx, and trachea. In: *Textbook of Veterinary Diagnostic Radiology*, 4e (ed. D.E. Thrall), 323–329. Philadelphia: W.B. Saunders.

95. Harvey, C.E. and Fink, E.A. (1982). Tracheal diameter – analysis of radiographic measurements in brachycephalic and non-brachycephalic dogs. *J. Am. Anim. Hosp. Assoc.* 18: 570–576.

96. Johnson, L. (2000). Tracheal collapse. Diagnosis and medical and surgical treatment. *Vet. Clin. North Am. Small Anim. Pract.* 30: 1253–1266, vi.

97. Johnson, L.R. and Pollard, R.E. (2010). Tracheal collapse and bronchomalacia in dogs: 58 cases (7/2001–1/2008). *J. Vet. Intern. Med.* 24: 298–305.

98. Lindl Bylicki, B.J., Johnson, L.R., and Pollard, R.E. (2015). Comparison of the radiographic and tracheoscopic appearance of the dorsal tracheal membrane in large and small breed dogs. *Vet. Radiol. Ultrasound* 56: 602–608.

99. Marolf, A., Blaik, M., and Specht, A. (2007). A retrospective study of the relationship between tracheal collapse and bronchiectasis in dogs. *Vet. Radiol. Ultrasound* 48: 199–203.

100. Salisbury, S.K., Forbes, S., and Blevins, W.E. (1990). Peritracheal abscess associated with tracheal collapse and bilateral laryngeal paralysis in a dog. *J. Am. Vet. Med. Assoc.* 196: 1273–1275.

101. Tappin, S.W. (2016). Canine tracheal collapse. *J. Small Anim. Pract.* 57: 9–17.

102. Hendricks, J.C. and O'Brien, J.A. (1985). Tracheal collapse in two cats. *J. Am. Vet. Med. Assoc.* 187: 418–419.

103. Macready, D.M., Johnson, L.R., and Pollard, R.E. (2007). Fluoroscopic and radiographic evaluation of tracheal collapse in dogs: 62 cases (2001–2006). *J. Am. Vet. Med. Assoc.* 230: 1870–1876.

104. Corcoran, B.M. (1989). Post traumatic tracheal stenosis in a cat. *Vet. Rec.* 124: 342–343.

105. Gordon, W. (1973). Surgical correction of tracheal stenosis in a dog. *J. Am. Vet. Med. Assoc.* 162: 479–480.

106. Kahane, N. and Segev, G. (2014). Long-term outcome of conventional endotracheal tube balloon dilation of tracheal stenosis in a dog. *Can. Vet. J.* 55: 1241–1244.

107. Smith, M.M., Gourley, I.M., Amis, T.C., and Kurpershoek, C. (1990). Management of tracheal stenosis in a dog. *J. Am. Vet. Med. Assoc.* 196: 931–934.

108. Tattersall, J. and Pratschke, K.M. (2002). What is your diagnosis? Endoscopy demonstrated marked tracheal stenosis at the avulsed proximal tracheal segment. *J. Small Anim. Pract.* 43 (333): 370–331.

109. Bedford, P.G. (1982). Tracheal hypoplasia in the English bulldog. *Vet. Rec.* 111: 58–59.

110. Lodato, D.L. and Hedlund, C.S. (2012). Brachycephalic airway syndrome: pathophysiology and diagnosis. *Compend. Contin. Educ. Vet.* 34: E3.

111. Riecks, T.W., Birchard, S.J., and Stephens, J.A. (2007). Surgical correction of brachycephalic syndrome in dogs: 62 cases (1991–2004). *J. Am. Vet. Med. Assoc.* 230: 1324–1328.

112. Davies, C.M. (1989). Tracheal foreign body in a German shepherd dog. *Vet. Rec.* 125: 648–649.

113. Johns, S., Sellon, R., Spencer, E., and Tucker, M. (2014). Tracheal foreign body and pneumonia in a cat: a near missed diagnosis. *J. Am. Anim. Hosp. Assoc.* 50: 273–277.

114. Le Roux, A.B. and Cahn, D. (2016). What is your diagnosis? Tracheal foreign body (possibly a wood stick) with secondary pneumonia in the accessory lung lobe. *J. Am. Vet. Med. Assoc.* 248: 879–881.

115. Lotti, U. and Niebauer, G.W. (1992). Tracheobronchial foreign bodies of plant origin in 153 hunting dogs. *Compend. Contin. Educ. Vet.* 14: 900–905.

116. Tivers, M.S. and Moore, A.H. (2006). Tracheal foreign bodies in the cat and the use of fluoroscopy for removal: 12 cases. *J. Small Anim. Pract.* 47: 155–159.

117. Adamama-Moraitou, K.K., Soubasis, N., Pardali, D. et al. (2015). Recurrent intraluminal eosinophilic tracheal granuloma in a Siberian husky. *Vet. Q.* 35: 116–122.

118. Kotani, T., Horie, M., Yamaguchi, S. et al. (1995). Lungworm, Filaroides osleri, infection in a dog in Japan. *J. Vet. Med. Sci.* 57: 573–576.

119. Rosenheck, S., Davis, G., Sammarco, C.D., and Bastian, R. (2017). Effect of variations in stent placement on outcome of endoluminal stenting for canine tracheal collapse. *J. Am. Anim. Hosp. Assoc.* 53: 150–158.

120. Griffiths, L.G., Sullivan, M., and Lerche, P. (1998). Intrathoracic tracheal avulsion and pseudodiverticulum following pneumomediastinum in a cat. *Vet. Rec.* 142: 693–696.

121. Schmierer, P.A., Schwarz, A., Bass, D.A., and Knell, S.C. (2014). Novel avulsion pattern of the left principal bronchus with involvement of the carina and caudal thoracic trachea in a cat. *J. Feline Med. Surg.* 16: 695–698.

122. White, R.N. and Burton, C.A. (2000). Surgical management of intrathoracic tracheal avulsion in cats: long-term results in 9 consecutive cases. *Vet. Surg.* 29: 430–435.

123. White, R.N. and Milner, H.R. (1995). Intrathoracic tracheal avulsion in three cats. *J. Small Anim. Pract.* 36: 343–347.

# CHAPTER 18

# Cardiovascular System

**Elodie E. Huguet[1], Sandra Tou[2], and Clifford R. Berry[3]**

[1] Department of Small Animal Clinical Sciences, College of Veterinary Medicine, University of Florida, Gainesville, FL, USA
[2] Department of Clinical Sciences, College of Veterinary Medicine, North Caroline State University, Raleigh, NC, USA
[3] Department of Molecular Biomedical Sciences, College of Veterinary Medicine, North Carolina State University, Raleigh, NC, USA

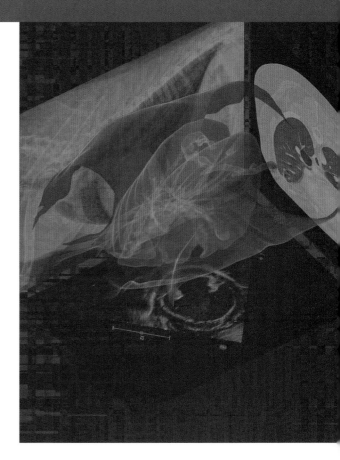

## Introduction

The heart is a dynamic three-dimensional structure requiring various imaging modalities with excellent temporal and spatial resolution for the diagnosis, staging, and monitoring of cardiovascular diseases. Current imaging modalities, such as radiography, echocardiography, nuclear scintigraphy, computed tomography (CT), and magnetic resonance imaging (MRI), provide a noninvasive way to assess the cardiovascular system in both a static and dynamic manner.

Radiography is most widely available and provides a practical way to screen for morphologic alterations of the cardiovascular structures and the presence of left- and/or right-sided congestive heart failure. However, the absence of radiographic abnormalities does not rule out underlying cardiac disease. Echocardiography is considered the test of choice to comprehensively evaluate the structure and function of the heart.

While echocardiography has many inherent safety and diagnostic advantages, it is limited in its capability of assessing the surrounding tissues within the thoracic cavity. Therefore, a more complete evaluation of the cardiovascular system is routinely achieved by combining radiographic and echocardiographic findings.

Many new technologic advances and developments have provided novel ways to assess the anatomy and function of the cardiovascular system, including new software applications and validated studies for echocardiography, nuclear scintigraphy (positron emission tomography [PET]), CT, and MRI. The use of contrast agents with routine or cross-sectional imaging modalities aids in the detection of pathology. Original positive contrast selective angiographic techniques with fluoroscopy and digital subtraction angiography (DSA) have been, for the most part, replaced by noninvasive, higher resolution three-dimensional imaging techniques. However, the use of positive contrast selective angiography with fluoroscopy and/or DSA maintains an important role in the guidance of interventional procedures and will be briefly discussed in this chapter.

Alterations in the movement of blood in the cardiovascular structures (heart, arteries, capillaries, veins) may lead to multiple Roentgen abnormalities that collectively can be used to synthesize an imaging diagnosis. For instance, variations in blood velocity, normal laminar flow, and direction can result in detectable dilation of cardiac chambers and vessels with third spacing of fluid (pleural effusion or pulmonary edema). Subsequently, the systemic delivery of oxygen and nutrients to various tissues may be impaired, resulting in clinical signs. An understanding of the normal three-dimensional anatomy of the cardiovascular system and dynamics of blood circulation is important in the interpretation of all imaging modalities.

The following sections in this chapter will discuss the imaging characteristics of the normal canine and feline cardiovascular system, as well as abnormal variations for the identification of cardiovascular diseases.

# Normal Anatomy

The heart is the driving force (pump) of the circulatory system. Through coordinated extrinsic and intrinsic neurogenic stimuli and muscular contractions, the heart pushes blood through a closed network of blood vessels to provide the body with a continuous supply of oxygen and nutrients. Blood circulates in the four chambers of the heart: the right atrium (*atrium dextrum*), right ventricle (*ventriculus dexter*), left atrium (*atrium sinistrum*), and left ventricle (*ventriculus sinister*). Deoxygenated blood from the systemic circulation returns to the right atrium via the cranial and caudal vena cava, coronary, and azygous veins. The right atrium pushes blood through the tricuspid valve during atrial systole (ventricular enddiastole) into the right ventricle. During ventricular systole, the right ventricle pushes the deoxygenated blood into the main pulmonary artery through the pulmonary valve. Blood continues through the pulmonary arteries into a fine network of capillary pulmonary beds surrounding the alveoli. Here, blood becomes oxygenated and enters the left atrium via the pulmonary veins. It then moves into the left ventricle through the mitral valve during ventricular diastole. During ventricular systole, the blood is pumped into the systemic and coronary circulation through the aorta. Each atrium has a small blind pouch, called the auricle.

One-way passage of blood through the different chambers of the heart is controlled by four valves, all synchronized to open and close at distinct intervals during each cardiac cycle. The cardiac cycle and all the details are summarized in Appendix 18.1. The atrioventricular valves allow passage of blood from the atria to the ventricles during diastole and prevent backflow of blood during systole. Small fibrous bands, called the *chordae*

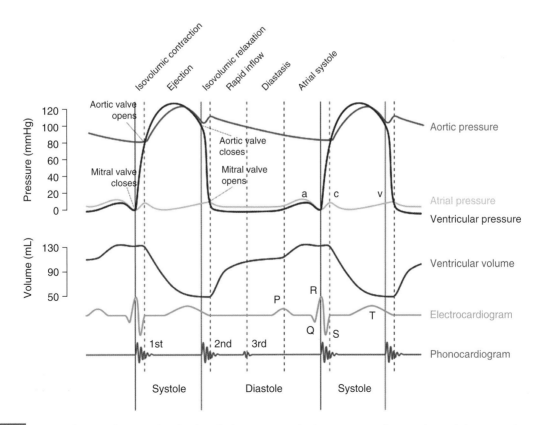

**APPENDIX 18.1**   Wiggers diagram documenting the electrical, pressure, and volume curves, valve opening and closures and associated heart sounds during the normal cardiac cycle.

Source: Daniel Chang MD / Wikimedia Commons / CC BY-SA 4.0.

*tendineae*, arise from papillary muscles along the ventricular wall and extend to the atrioventricular valves to prevent valvular prolapse during systole when the left and right ventricular pressures are increased. The left atrioventricular or mitral valve separates the left ventricle and left atrium. The mitral valve is larger than the right atrioventricular or tricuspid valve (separating the right ventricle and right atrium). As its name indicates, the tricuspid valve is composed of three leaflets, called the septal, parietal, and angular leaflets. In comparison, the mitral valve is bicuspid and includes two leaflets (septal and parietal). Blood exiting the right and left ventricles is controlled by the pulmonary and aortic semilunar valves, respectively. The pulmonary and aortic valves have a similar morphology and consist of three semilunar leaflets. The pulmonary valve has right, left, and septal semilunar leaflets, whereas the aortic valve has right, left, and intermediate (noncoronary) semilunar leaflets. The aortic and pulmonic sinuses represent a focal dilation of the proximal ascending aorta and main pulmonary artery, respectively, at the base of the heart. The aortic sinus contains opening into the right and left coronary arteries (right and left semilunar leaflets, respectively).

The pulmonary valve controls passage of blood from the right ventricle into the main pulmonary artery, which then divides into the left and right pulmonary arteries. The main pulmonary artery contacts the left lateral wall of the more centrally located aortic sinus and ascending aorta (Figure 18.1). A small ligamentous remnant of the *ductus arteriosus* (fetal embryology), called the *ligamentum arteriosum*, connects the aorta to the main pulmonary artery at the level of the bifurcation into the left and right pulmonary arteries. The left pulmonary artery is ventral to the left principal bronchus and divides into the left cranial and caudal lobar branches. The left cranial lobar branch further divides into smaller cranial and caudal segmental branches. The right pulmonary artery courses in a left to right direction ventral to the trachea and is ventral to the right principal bronchus and divides into right cranial, middle, and caudal branches. The branches of the caudal lobar pulmonary arteries are dorsolateral to the caudal lobar bronchi, which are then ventromedially bordered by the branches of the caudal lobar pulmonary veins, best seen on a ventrodorsal or dorsoventral projection (Figure 18.2). The cranial lobar arteries have a similar arrangement, respectively consisting of the arterial branch, cranial lobar bronchus, and branch of the pulmonary veins in a craniodorsal to caudoventral direction, best viewed on a lateral radiograph (Figure 18.3). Most of the pulmonary veins have separate openings for oxygenated blood to enter the left atrium. The right and left caudal lobar veins enter the left atrium in a caudodorsal position, with the right cranial vein being more upright. The right and left cranial lobar pulmonary veins enter the left atrium along its craniolateral border on the right and left sides respectively.

Oxygenated blood is distributed into the systemic circulation by the aorta. The aorta is the thickest blood vessel to withstand the higher pressure of blood (120 mmHg during systole; Table 18.1) entering the systemic circulation. The aorta consists of a short ascending portion, the aortic arch, and descending thoracic aorta that continues through the diaphragm as the abdominal aorta. Deoxygenated blood from the pelvic limbs, pelvis, and abdomen is returned to the heart by the caudal vena cava and azygos vein. Deoxygenated blood from the head and thoracic limbs is transported to the heart by

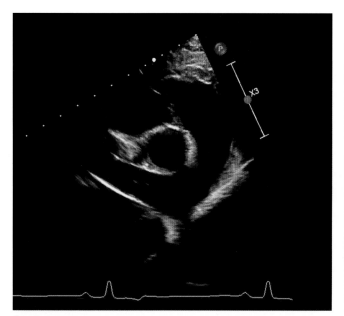

**A**

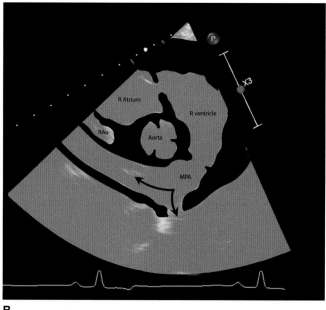

**B**

**FIGURE 18.1**  Right parasternal short axis view of the heart base documenting the aortic sinus (central position) surrounded by the main pulmonary artery, which then divides dorsally into the right and left main pulmonary arteries.

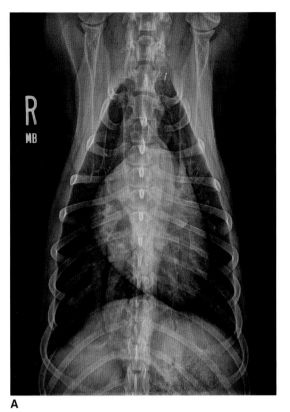
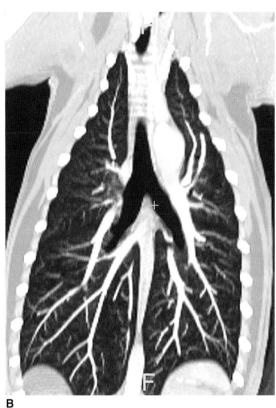

**A**                                    **B**

**FIGURE 18.2**   (**A**) Dorsoventral radiograph of a canine thorax with highlighted caudal lobar pulmonary arteries (red) and caudal lobar pulmonary veins (blue). (**B**) Corresponding dorsal plane reconstructed computed tomographic image in a lung window (maximum intensity projection) at the level of the caudal lobar pulmonary arteries and veins.

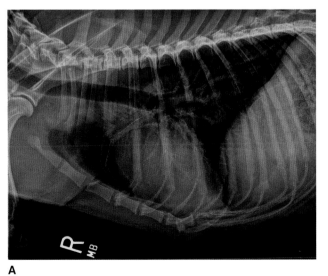
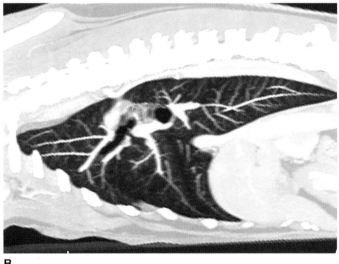

**A**                                    **B**

**FIGURE 18.3**   (**A**) Right lateral radiograph of a canine thorax with highlighted cranial lobar pulmonary arteries (red) and caudal lobar pulmonary veins (blue). (**B**) Corresponding right parasagittal plane reconstructed, computed tomographic image in a lung window (maximum intensity projection) at the level of the right cranial lobar pulmonary arteries and veins.

the cranial vena cava. The azygos vein also drains the bronchial venous circulation in the right atrium.

Blood to the myocardium is supplied by the coronary arteries. The left and right coronary arteries arise from the supravalvular (sinus) region of the ascending aorta (Figure 18.4). The left coronary artery originates from the left sinus of the aorta and divides into two or, in many cases, three major branches called the circumflex, paraconal interventricular,

| TABLE 18.1 | Normal systolic/diastolic pressures of the various chambers and great vessels of the heart for the dog and cat. | |
|---|---|---|
| **Cardiac chamber/vessel** | **Systole (mmHg)** | **Diastole (mmHg)** |
| Right atrium | 3–5 | 0 |
| Right ventricle | 25 | 0 |
| Main pulmonary artery | 25 | 10–15 |
| Left atrium | 3–5 | 0 |
| Left ventricle | 120 | 0 |
| Aorta | 120 | 80 |

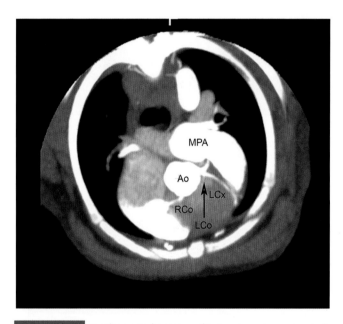

**FIGURE 18.4**  Cardiac-gated angiographic images using computed tomography at the level of the aortic sinus (Ao) and main pulmonary artery (MPA), showing the right coronary artery (RCo), left coronary artery (LCo), and the circumflex artery (LCx).

and septal branches. The circumflex artery is in the coronary groove and can be traced along the caudodorsal aspect of the heart as it extends toward the apex of the heart. The circumflex artery principally supplies the left atrium, auricle, and ventricle. Small branches from the circumflex artery also supply blood to the right atrium. Part of the blood supply to the right and left ventricles is provided by the paraconal interventricular artery which extends ventrally and to the right of the heart in the paraconal interventricular groove. In many dogs and cats, the septal branch originates from the paraconal interventricular artery and runs deep into the interventricular musculature to supply the papillary muscles, as well as most of the interventricular septum. The right coronary artery is shorter than the left coronary artery and originates from the right sinus at the ascending aortic sinus. The right coronary extends along

the right side of heart in a cranioventral direction into the coronary groove to supply blood to the right atrium and ventricle. All blood flow into the myocardium extends from an epicardial to endocardial direction and occurs during atrial and ventricular diastole.

The heart is surrounded by a thin fibrous and serous layer called the pericardium. These layers form the pericardial cavity which contains a small amount of physiologic fluid. Surrounding the pericardium is the pericardial mediastinal pleura. Within the mediastinum, the cardiac silhouette is centrally located with its apex positioned near the caudal sternum and cranial diaphragm. The long axis of the heart is slightly obliqued in a craniodorsal to caudoventral direction with the apex being rotated to the left of midline on a ventrodorsal or dorsoventral radiograph (called the normal *levocardia* position).

Variations in the size and positioning of the cardiac silhouette exist between the different dog and cat breeds. In older cats, the axis of the cardiac silhouette may be positioned in a more horizontal relationship relative to the sternum, also referred to as a "lazy heart" position [1]. Associated with this change in orientation, the aortic arch may be become elongated, redundant or tortuous (Figure 18.5). This change in cardiac silhouette orientation is caused by thickening of the endothelium and the tunica intima and media of the ascending aorta, aortic arch and proximal aspect of the descending aorta as the cat ages.

# Radiographic Evaluation

Routine evaluation of the cardiac silhouette consists of three standard radiographic projections: left lateral, right lateral, ventrodorsal or dorsoventral (Figure 18.6). A dorsoventral projection should also be considered as part of the standard radiographic series to increase the conspicuity of the caudal lobar vessels and lesions in the caudodorsal lung lobes, due to magnification of these structures in the dorsal thoracic cavity, as well as better inflation of the caudal lung lobes with the patient in ventral recumbency.

Overall, straight patient positioning is essential for recognition of the normal cardiac anatomy. When possible, radiographs should be acquired before echocardiography to avoid atelectasis from prolonged lateral recumbency and wet-hair artifact due to the application of acoustic gel or alcohol. Additionally, for appropriate evaluation of the ventrodorsal and dorsoventral projections, the positioning must be such that the sternum overlaps and is summated with the thoracic vertebrae and spinous processes. To reduce the superimposition of the appendicular musculature with the cranial thoracic region, the thoracic limbs should be pulled cranially, best with both thoracic limbs taped together (Figure 18.7).

Due to inherent high contrast within the thoracic cavity associated with the presence of air within the lungs, thoracic

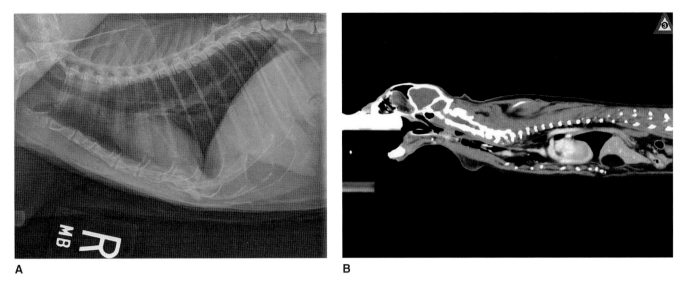

**FIGURE 18.5** Radiographic (**A**) and computed tomographic (**B**) images of an older feline patient with a "lazy heart" and redundant aorta, representing normal age-associated variants.

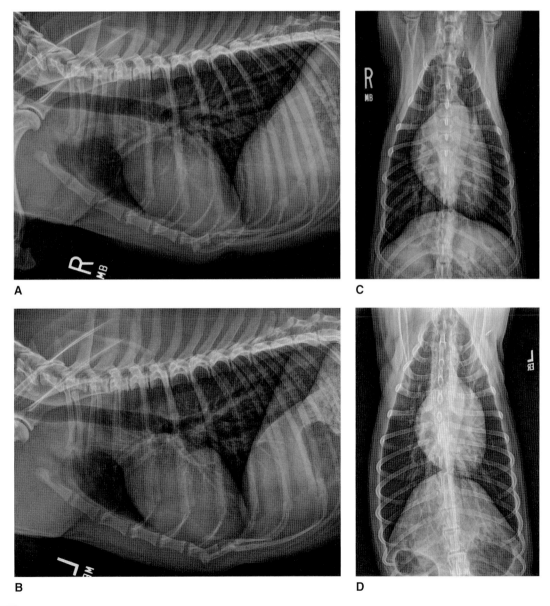

**FIGURE 18.6** Normal right lateral (**A**), left lateral (**B**), ventrodorsal (**C**) and dorsoventral (**D**) projections of a normal canine thorax.

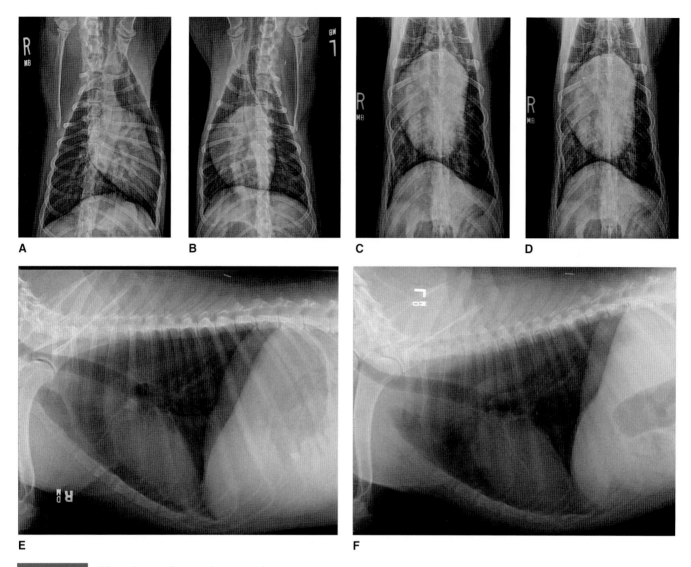

**FIGURE 18.7** Obliqued ventrodorsal radiographs of a dog with the spine displaced to the left (**A**) and to the right (**B**). Ventrodorsal radiographs of a normal canine heart and lateral radiographs of a normal feline heart respectively acquired during diastole (**C,D**) and systole (**E,F**).

radiographs should be obtained using a high peak kilovoltage (kVp) and low milliampere-second (mAs) technique. To maximize contrast and decrease atelectasis, the radiographic exposure should be made at peak inspiration. Due to border effacement of the myocardium with blood within the cardiac chambers and fluid within the pericardial space, interpretation of the heart relies on the recognition of morphologic changes to the size and shape of the cardiac silhouette. On the dorsoventral projection, there is increased contact of the cupula of the diaphragm with the apex of the cardiac silhouette, and the cardiac silhouette has a more upright position with a rounded appearance (Figure 18.8). The normal cardiac silhouette has a smooth contour or margin, and any alterations to the cardiac silhouette can be localized to specific cardiac chambers or the great vessels in the dog based on their relative positioning. On the ventrodorsal/dorsoventral projections, the clock face analogy is commonly used to illustrate the location of the different cardiac chambers in relation to the peripheral margins of the heart (Figure 18.9; Table 18.2).

A similar approach can be applied to the cardiac silhouette on the lateral projections (Figure 18.10). This approach is not as readily applicable to the anatomic description of the feline cardiac silhouette.

The size of the cardiac silhouette in the absence of pathology varies greatly between different dog breeds [1–7]. Dogs with a barrel-shaped chest may have a cardiac silhouette with a larger appearance than dogs with a narrow deep-shaped chest. In large-breed dogs, the cardiac silhouette may have an elongated contour on lateral radiographs and a rounded appearance on ventrodorsal or dorsoventral radiographs. As a subjective assessment of the cardiac silhouette size, the cranial to caudal length of the cardiac silhouette should not exceed 3.5 intercostal spaces on lateral projections. In addition, the height of the cardiac silhouette should not exceed two-thirds of the height of the thoracic cavity on lateral projection. The width of the cardiac silhouette should not exceed one-half the width of the thoracic cavity on the ventrodorsal or dorsoventral projection.

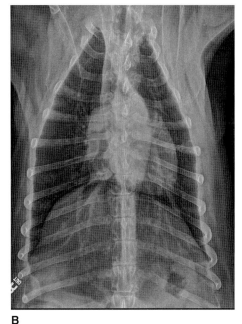

**FIGURE 18.8**   Ventrodorsal (**A**) and dorsoventral (**B**) radiographs of a normal canine thorax with normal rounding of the cardiac silhouette and increased diaphragmatic contact.

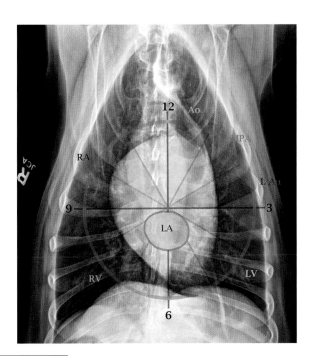

**FIGURE 18.9**   Illustrations of the clock face analogy for location of the cardiac chambers in dogs on ventrodorsal/dorsoventral projections.

| TABLE 18.2 | Clock face analogy for interpretation of the changes in shape, margin, and size of the cardiac silhouette in the dog. | |
| --- | --- | --- |
| **View** | **Clock position on the cardiac silhouette** | **Area/margin highlighted** |
| VD/DV | 11–1 | Aortic arch |
| | 1–2 | Main pulmonary artery (MPA) |
| | 3 | Left auricle |
| | 4–5 | Left ventricle |
| | 5–9 | Right ventricle |
| | 9–11 | Right atrium |
| Right lateral | 12–3 | Left atrium |
| | 3–5 | Left ventricle |
| | 5–8 | Right ventricle |
| | 8–10 | Right auricle/atrium |
| | 10–12 | Heart base structures (aorta and MPA) |

VD/DV, ventrodorsal or dorsoventral view.

A more objective assessment of the cardiac silhouette uses the vertebral heart size or score (VHS) measurement, with some breed conformation variations having been reported. Using the VHS method, the long axis of the cardiac silhouette is measured from the ventral border of the carina to the apex of the cardiac silhouette at its longest distance on right lateral radiograph. The short axis is next measured at the widest point of the cardiac silhouette, perpendicular to the long axis. Both measurements are then individually scaled to the thoracic vertebral column, starting at the cranial endplate of T4. The number of vertebral bodies corresponding to the length of the short and long axes of the cardiac silhouette are summed together to provide the VHS (Figure 18.11). Out of 100

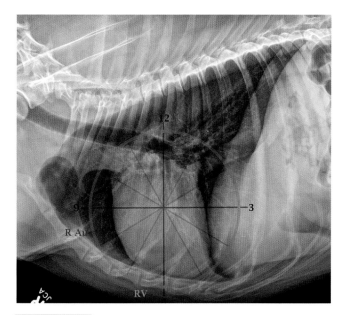

**FIGURE 18.10** Illustrations of the clock face analogy for location of the cardiac chambers in dogs on lateral projections.

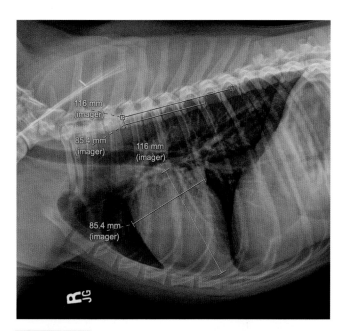

**FIGURE 18.11** Vertebral heart score measurement of a normal canine's cardiac silhouette. The width and apicobasal lengths in relation to the length of the vertebral bodies starting from T4 are added to obtain the vertebral heart score on right lateral projections.

dogs with normal hearts, 98% of population had VHS less than 10.5 (9.7±0.5).

The VHS of various dog breeds have been described and are listed in Table 18.3. This value may represent a clinically relevant maximum VHS to identify cardiomegaly in various dog breeds. However, a normal value does not exclude the possibility of cardiac abnormalities. A similar measurement method has been proposed in cats. In another study, a mean±SD vertebral heart score of 7.5±0.3 was measured in 100 healthy

cats. In the same study, the long axis of the cardiac silhouette was scaled to the sternum, starting at the cranial endplate of S2, and equaled the length of three sternebrae. On right lateral and ventrodorsal radiographs, the length of the manubrium has been correlated to the size of the cardiac silhouette in dogs by expressing the sum of the cardiac short axis length and long axis length as a ratio over the length of the manubrium in both small-breed (≤12 kg) and large-breed (≥16 kg) dogs. In large-breed dogs, ratios of 4.8±0.5 and 5.4±0.6 were measured on right lateral and ventrodorsal projections, respectively. In comparison, ratios of 5.3±0.8 and 5.3±0.9 were measured in small-breed dogs on right lateral and ventrodorsal projections, respectively.

Fewer variations in heart size exist between breed of cats. However, obese patients may deposit fat around their pericardium, resulting in a nonpathologic increase in size of the cardiac silhouette, particularly on the ventrodorsal/dorsoventral views. The normal feline heart is ovoid to almond shaped and subjectively measures between 2 and 2.5 intercostal spaces in width on lateral projections. On ventrodorsal and dorsoventral projections, the cardiac silhouette should be less than 50% of the overall thoracic width.

Evaluation of the cranial and caudal lobar branches of the pulmonary arteries and veins is made by assessing their relative size and shape. Normal lobar pulmonary veins and arteries follow a generally straight path as they gradually taper in the periphery of the lung field. The size of the lobar pulmonary vessels may be assessed by comparing cranial lobar vessel diameter to the width of the fourth rib on lateral projections and caudal lobar vessels dimensions to the width of the ninth rib on ventrodorsal or dorsoventral projection. Normal lobar pulmonary arteries and veins should be approximately the same size as the rib used as a reference. Additionally, pulmonary lobar arteries and veins associated with a particular lung lobe should be similar in size (Figure 18.12).

# Echocardiography

There are many excellent textbooks and articles related to veterinary echocardiography. In this text, a summary will be presented with the intention of providing a better understanding of the three-dimensional nature of the cardiac silhouette and anatomic relationships between the cardiac structures. Two-dimensional echocardiography is used for a dynamic structural and functional evaluation of the heart related to the electrocardiogram. A complete evaluation of the cardiovascular structures includes multiple standard echocardiographic views with the patient positioned in right or left lateral recumbency, while imaging the heart from the patient's recumbent side (right or left parasternal locations, respectively). Routine echocardiographic views are listed in Table 18.4.

Time-motion mode (M-mode) echocardiography allows the continuous display of an "icepick" view through the heart

**TABLE 18.3**  VHS and associated references for different dog breeds.

| Breed | Recumbency | VHS (mean±SD) | Reference |
|---|---|---|---|
| Pug | Right | 10.7±0.9 | Jepsen-Grant et al. [8] |
| Pomeranian | Right | 10.5 ± 0.9 | Jepsen-Grant et al. [8] |
| Yorkshire terrier | Right | 9.9 ± 0.6 | Jepsen-Grant et al. [8] |
| Dachshund | Right | 9.7 ± 0.5 | Jepsen-Grant et al. [8] |
| | Right | 10.3 (range 9.25–11.55) | Birks et al. [16] |
| | | 10.1 (range 8.7–11.31) | |
| | Left | | Birks et al. [16] |
| Bulldog | Right | 12.7 ± 1.7 | Jepsen-Grant et al. [8] |
| Shih tzu | Right | 9.5 ± 0.6 | Jepsen-Grant et al. [8] |
| Lhasa apso | Right | 9.6 ± 0.8 | Jepsen-Grant et al. [8] |
| Boston terrier | Right | 11.7 ± 1.4 | Jepsen-Grant et al. [8] |
| Chihuahua | Right | 10.0±0.6 | Puccinelli et al. [9] |
| Cavalier King Charles spaniel | Right | 10.6±0.5 | Lamb et al. [10] |
| German shepherd | Right | 9.7±0.8 | Lamb et al. [10] |
| Boxer | Right | 11.6±0.8 | Lamb et al. [10] |
| Doberman | Right | 10.0±0.6 | Lamb et al. [10] |
| Poodle | Right | 10.1±0.5 | Fonsecapinto and Iwasaki [11] |
| | Right | 9.72±0.7 | Azevedo et al. [17] |
| Turkish shepherd | Left | 9.7±0.7 | Gulanber et al. [12] |
| Whippet (show) | Left | 10.5±0.6 | Bavegems et al. [13] |
| | Right | 10.8±0.6 | |
| Whippet (racing) | Left | 11.1±0.4 | Bavegems et al. [13] |
| | Right | 11.4±0.4 | |
| Greyhound | Left/right | 10.5±0.1 | Marin et al. [14] |
| Rottweiler | Left/right | 9.8±0.1 | Marin et al. [14] |
| Beagle | Left | 10.2±0.4 | Kraetschmer et al. [15] |
| | Right | 10.5±0.4 | |
| Iranian native dog | Left | 9.4±0.6 | Ghadiri et al. [19] |
| | Right | 9.4±0.54 | |
| American pit bull terrier | Right | 10.9±0.4 | Cardoso et al. [20] |
| Indian mongrel dog | Right | 9.7±0.7 | Kumar et al. |
| Labrador retriever | Left | 10.3±0.1 | Gugjoo et al. [22] |
| | Right | 10.4±0.1 | |
| | Left | 10.2±0.2 | Bodh et al. [18] |
| | Right | 10.4±0.2 | |
| Spitz | Left | 10.0±0.1 | Bodh et al. [18] |
| | Right | 10.21±0.1 | |
| Belgian Malinois | Right | 9.6±0.5 | Almeida et al. [23] |

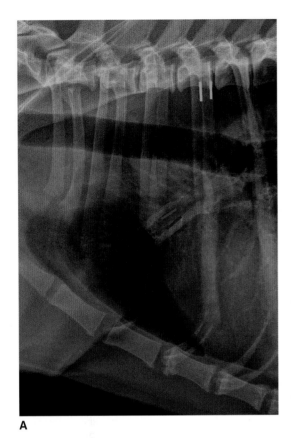

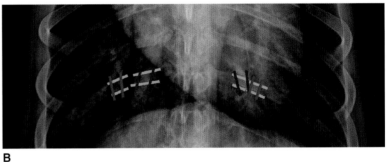

**A**

**B**

**FIGURE 18.12** Measurement of the lobar pulmonary vessels by comparing the cranial lobar vessel diameter to the width of the fourth rib on lateral projections (**A**) and caudal lobar vessels dimensions to the width of the ninth rib on ventrodorsal or dorsoventral projections (**B**). The margins of the lobar pulmonary veins are outlined in blue, the lobar pulmonary arteries in red, and the reference rib in green.

such that structures within that view are assessed over time. Using M-mode, the ventricular size can be measured during systole (LVIDs) and diastole (LVIDd) at the level of the chordae tendineae in dogs. From these measurements, the systolic function of the left ventricle can be extrapolated from a measurement known as fractional shortening (%), calculated as follows: ([LVIDd − LVIDs]/LVIDd) × 100. Normal fractional shortening values are 25–45% in dogs and 30–55% in cats. The disproportionate shape of the right ventricle limits reliable chamber measurements and is estimated to be one-third the dimension of the left ventricle. Additionally, the interventricular septum (IVS) thickness can be measured in systole (IVSs) and diastole (IVSd), as well as the left ventricular free wall thickness in systole (LVWs) and diastole (LVWd). To assess the size of the left atrium, the diameters of the aorta and the left atrium are measured from the right-sided short-axis view at the level of the aortic cusps during early diastole (Figure 18.13). Calculation of the left atrium to aorta (LA:Ao) ratio may suggest left atrium enlargement is greater than 1.5. The size of the right atrium should be similar to the size of the left atrium.

Color flow Doppler is used to determine the direction and velocity of blood flow using a color-coded map. The characteristic of the color signal can suggest normal laminar or turbulent blood flow based on the pulse-repetition frequency

(PRF) or the velocity scale. Quantitative measurements of blood velocities over time can be acquired using spectral Doppler. These velocity measurements are routinely measured at the mitral, tricuspid, pulmonic, and aortic valves (all velocities should be 1 m/s with the aortic valve outflow velocity being up to 1.6 m/s) and can be used to measure the pressure gradient between the chambers it separates using the modified Bernoulli equation (pressure gradient = 4 × [maximum or peak velocity][2]).

# Alternative Imaging Modalities

The use of nuclear medicine to diagnose cardiac disease is small animals remains limited. Nuclear scintigraphy uses an intravenously administered radiopharmaceutical to trace blood flow through the cardiovascular structures to localize anatomic abnormalities, identify ventilation and pulmonary perfusion abnormalities, quantitate function, or assess for collateral blood flow. The combination of positron emission tomography with computed tomography (PET-CT) provides excellent three-dimensional spatial and temporal resolution for the localization of radiopharmaceutical uptake of PET metabolic radiotracers within the myocardium.

**TABLE 18.4**   Routine echocardiographic views for dogs and cats.

| | View | Structures in view | Indication |
|---|---|---|---|
| **Right parasternal views**: With the patient in right lateral recumbency, the probe is positioned at the level of the costochondral junction in the third to sixth intercostal spaces | Right parasternal long axis 4-chamber view | Left and right atrioventricular valves, ventricles and atria | – Mitral valve abnormalities (prolapse) |
| | Right parasternal long axis left ventricular outflow tract view | Aorta, aortic cusps, interventricular septum, and the anterior mitral valve movement in systole | – Subaortic stenosis<br>– Abnormalities of the aortic valve<br>– Anterior motion of the mitral valve<br>– Heart base tumors |
| | Right parasternal short-axis views<br>*Five standard images are obtained in a transverse plane* | – Left ventricle and papillary muscles<br>– Left ventricle at the level of the chordae tendineae<br>–Mitral valve, the left atrium and aorta<br>– Right ventricular outflow tract and the pulmonic valve<br>– Pulmonary artery branches, the right auricle and caudal vena cava | |
| **Left caudal (apical) parasternal views**: With the patient in left lateral recumbency, the probe is placed between the left 5th and 7th intercostal spaces in proximity to the sternum | Left apical 4-chamber view | Mitral and tricuspid valves | – Atrioventricular valve insufficiency |
| | Left apical 5-chamber view | Left ventricular outflow tract, aorta, left and right ventricles and atria | – Abnormalities of the ventricular outflow tract and aorta |
| | Long axis 2-chamber view | Left ventricle, mitral valve and left atrium | |
| | Long axis left ventricular outflow tract view | Left ventricle, mitral valve, left ventricular outflow tract and aortic root | |
| **Left cranial parasternal views**: With the patient in left lateral recumbency, the probe is positioned between the left third and fourth intercostal spaces between the sternum and costochondral junction | Left long axis views<br>*Three standard images are obtained in a longitudinal plane* | – Left ventricular outflow tract, aortic valve and aortic root<br>– Left ventricle and the right atrium, tricuspid valve, and right ventricular inflow tract<br>– Right ventricular outflow tract, pulmonary valve and main pulmonary artery | – Heart base tumor and aortic valve abnormalities.<br>– Right atrial/auricular masses<br>– Patent ductus arteriosus and pulmonic stenosis |
| | Short axis view | Aortic root and right ventricular inflow and outflow tracts | |
| **Subcostal view:** With the patient in dorsal recumbency, the probe is placed under the costal arch, just dorsal to the xyphoid | Long axis 4-chamber view | Aorta, left and right ventricles and atria | |

The greatest imaging advances have been in the development of new techniques and software in cardiac and vascular imaging with CT and MRI. Contrast agents can be used with CT and MRI to increase the conspicuity of blood flow within the cardiovascular structures. Cardiac-gated MRI reduces motion artifacts with the continuous acquisition of a single slice over the duration of the cardiac cycle (Figure 18.14).

The function and dynamic morphology of the heart can be assessed. The function of the heart may be evaluated with fluoroscopy and can be used to guide interventional procedures. The conspicuity of the cardiac chambers and great vessels is increased with intravenous or arterial catheterization for targeted injection of positive contrast medium at specific sites, also referred as selective angiography (Figure 18.15).

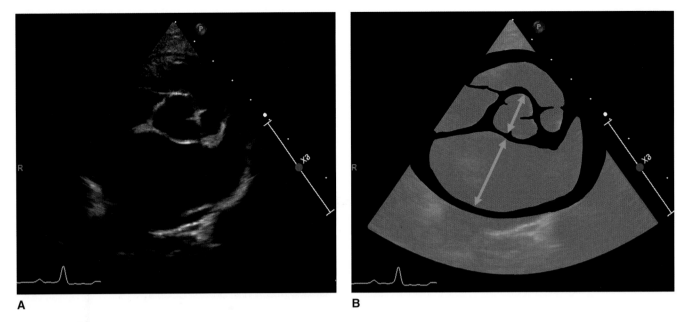

**FIGURE 18.13** Right-sided short axis view at the level of the aortic cusps during early diastole (**A**) with illustration (**B**) showing measurement of the left atrium to aorta (LA:Ao) ratio.

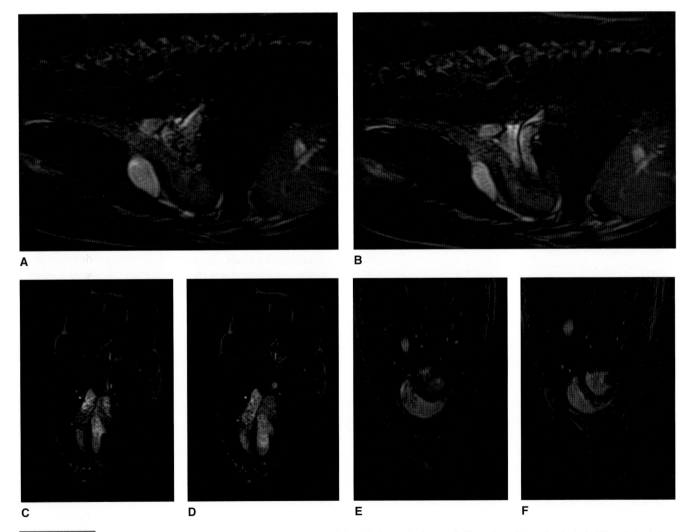

**FIGURE 18.14** Cardiac-gated MRI images in sagittal, transverse, and dorsal planes during peak diastole and systole. Systole (**A**) and diastole (**B**) in a sagittal plane. Systole (**C**) and diastole (**D**) in a transverse plane. Systole (**E**) and diastole (**F**) in a dorsal plane.

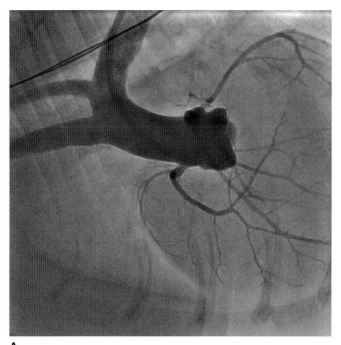
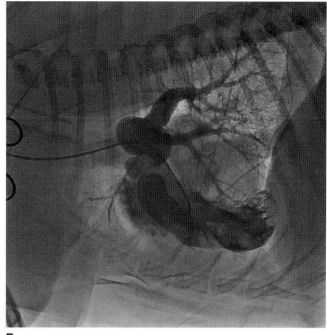

**A**          **B**

**FIGURE 18.15**   Selective angiography of the aortic root (**A**) and a severely dilated main pulmonary artery due to pulmonic stenosis (**B**), done under fluoroscopic guidance.

# Interpretation Paradigm of The Cardiac Structures in Diagnostic Imaging

## Is the Cardiac Silhouette Large, Small or Normal in Size?

The size of the cardiovascular structures is routinely evaluated on thoracic radiographs and is described earlier. In rare instances, *situs inversus* can be recognized by identifying right to left inversed orientation of the cardiac silhouette and associated great vessels in a transverse plane (Figure 18.16). The positioning of the cardiac apex to the right of midline (*dextrocardia* position) can be present without situs inversus. An online library of normal thoracic radiographs in different dog breeds is available at the following link: **http://media.news.health.ufl.edu/misc/vetmed/gvi/DogBreeds**.

In dogs, a cardiac silhouette greater than 3.5 intercostal spaces or two-thirds the height and 50% of the width of the thoracic cavity is consistent with cardiomegaly. Additionally, a VHS greater than 10.5 is consistent with cardiomegaly in most dog breeds. The increased size of the cardiac silhouette causes an eventual mass effect associated with dorsal displacement of the trachea at the level of the carina. In more advanced stages of left, right or generalized cardiomegaly, the trachea will be parallel to the spine, and enlargement of the

left atrium results in compression and narrowing of the left principal bronchus, and if severe left atrial enlargement is present, there will also be compression of the right caudal and accessory lung lobe bronchi. The relationship of the left atrium and principal bronchi is best visualized on cross-sectional imaging (Figure 18.17).

Microcardia may also be seen on thoracic radiographs with hypovolemia, such as due to dehydration, blood loss or Addison disease. While maintaining a normal contour, the cardiac silhouette is subjectively decreased in size with reduction in the 45° angle relative to the sternum. In addition, the pulmonary vessels will be small, resulting in diffuse hyperlucency of the pulmonary parenchyma (Figure 18.18). With severe hypovolemia, persistent narrowing of the caudal vena cava will be seen on all radiographic projections obtained.

## Is Cardiomegaly Due to Left- or Right-Sided Enlargement or Generalized as with Pericardial Disease?

On thoracic radiographs, alterations to the size and shape of the cardiac silhouette may suggest left- and/or right-sided cardiomegaly. Enlargement of the left atrium is associated with a soft tissue bulge along the caudodorsal aspect of the cardiac silhouette on lateral projections. This results in elongation of the cardiac silhouette with straightening of the

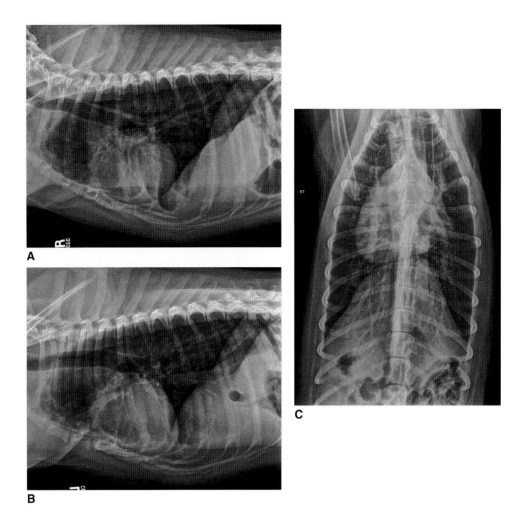

**FIGURE 18.16** Right lateral, left lateral, and dorsoventral radiographs (**A–C**) of a dog with situs inversus. On the dorsoventral radiograph, note the right to left inversed orientation of the cardiac silhouette and associated great vessels, as well as the intraabdominal organs. On the lateral images, note the complete reversal of the diaphragmatic orientation and the anatomy of the primary bronchi centrally. An alveolar pulmonary pattern is noted in the right middle lung lobe that is best seen in this dog on the right lateral view due to the situs inversus abnormality. In conjunction with the presence of bronchiectasis, bronchopneumonia, and chronic sinusitis, the dog was diagnosed with Kartagener syndrome.

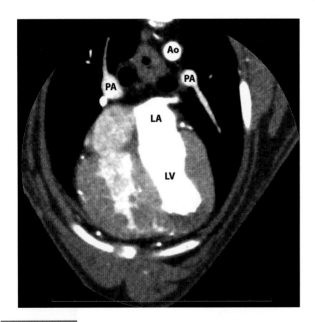

**FIGURE 18.17** Computed tomographic and angiographic image of a normal canine heart in a transverse plane showing the position of the left principal bronchus between the aorta (Ao) and left atrium (LA) and ventricle (LV). The left and right pulmonary arteries (PA) are seen coursing lateral to their respective principal bronchi.

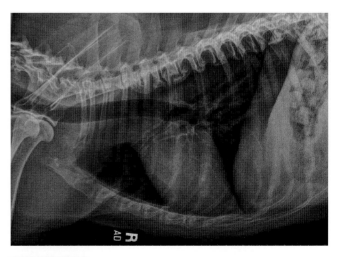

**FIGURE 18.18** Right lateral radiograph of a dog with a small cardiac silhouette, thinning of the pulmonary vasculature and narrowing of the caudal vena cava due to hypovolemia.

caudal border. On ventrodorsal and dorsoventral projections, enlargement of the left atrium is correlated to the presence of a focal increase in soft tissue opacity caudal to the tracheal bifurcation, causing widening of the principal bronchi, also called a "bow-legged cowboy" sign (Figure 18.19A,B). A well-defined region of increased soft tissue opacity with a double wall appearance may be seen caudal to the tracheal bifurcation on the ventrodorsal or dorsoventral projection with severe left atrial enlargement (Figure 18.19C). Subsequent enlargement of the left auricle is also recognized on ventrodorsal and dorsoventral projections by the presence of an elongated soft tissue bulge at the 3 o'clock position along

the cardiac silhouette with moderate and severe left atrial enlargement (Figure 18.19D). It is expected to see enlargement of the main body of the left atrium with left auricular enlargement.

Radiography is less sensitive for right-sided cardiomegaly, with detectable changes seen when at least moderate right-sided chamber enlargement is present. Right-sided cardiomegaly is characterized as rounding of the cranial and right lateral border of the cardiac silhouette with a leftward shift of the cardiac apex on ventrodorsal or dorsoventral images (Figure 18.20). Rounding of the right lateral margins has been suggested to give the cardiac silhouette a "reverse-D"

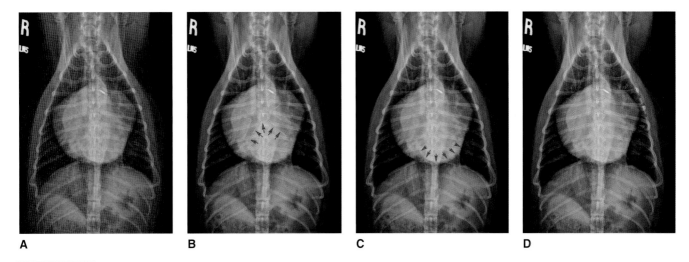

**FIGURE 18.19** Dorsoventral radiograph of a dog with severe left-sided cardiomegaly without annotations (**A**), showing splaying of the principal bronchi (e.g., "bow-legged cowboy" sign) (**B**), double wall appearance of the left atrium (**C**) and left auricular enlargement (**D**). In (**D**), the abnormality to be highlighted is outlined in blue arrows.

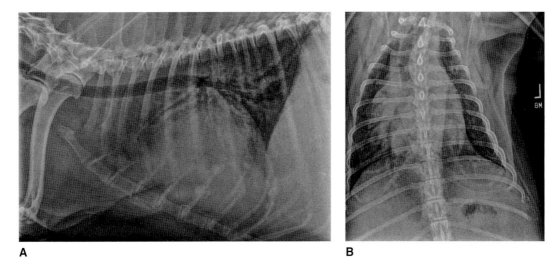

**FIGURE 18.20** Right lateral (**A**) and ventrodorsal (**B**) radiographs of a dog with moderate right-sided cardiomegaly, characterized by rounding of the cranial and right lateral border of the cardiac silhouette with a leftward shift of the cardiac apex on the ventrodorsal projection (e.g., "reverse D" appearance).

appearance on these images. On ventrodorsal and dorsoventral projections, a distinct bulge may be seen along the right cranial cardiac margin (9–10 o'clock position) in the region of the right atrium (Figure 18.21A). Enlargement of the right auricle may also be associated with a soft tissue bulge along the craniodorsal aspect of the cardiac silhouette on the lateral projections, particularly the left lateral view (Figure 18.21B). On thoracic radiographs, the presentation of a pericardial effusion depends on the amount of fluid within the pericardial space; however, a pericardial effusion should be considered when the cardiac silhouette is moderately to severely enlarged with a globoid appearance (Figure 18.22).

Evidence of cardiomegaly may not always be present in cats with echocardiographic evidence of cardiac chamber abnormalities. Some cats with left-sided cardiomegaly have widening of the base of the heart on ventrodorsal and dorsoventral projections, giving the heart a "valentine-shaped" appearance (Figure 18.23A). In some cats, left atrial enlargement results in a focal concavity along the dorsal aspect of the cardiac silhouette on lateral projections (Figure 18.23B). Concurrent right-sided cardiomegaly is often associated with generalized shape changes of the cardiac silhouette in cats. In some cases, a left ventricular bulge is seen along the caudal aspect of the cardiac silhouette with left ventricular wall thickening or chamber

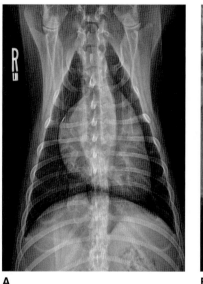
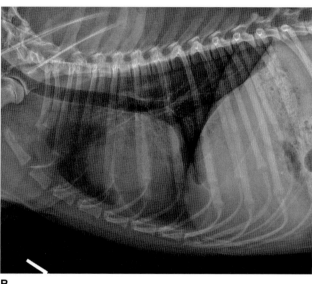

**FIGURE 18.21**   (**A**) Ventrodorsal projection of a dog with right atrial enlargement, characterized by the presence of a large soft tissue opaque bulge at the 9–10 o'clock position in the region of the right atrium along the cardiac silhouette. (**B**) Left lateral projection of a dog with a large soft tissue bulge along the craniodorsal aspect of the cardiac silhouette, representing enlargement of the right auricle.

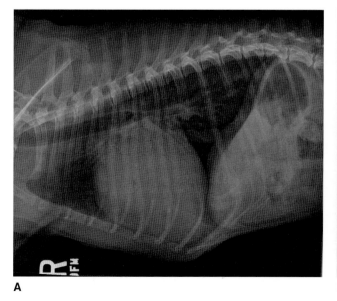
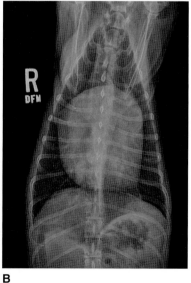

**FIGURE 18.22**   Right lateral (**A**) and ventrodorsal (**B**) projections of a severely enlarged cardiac silhouette with a globoid appearance in a dog due to presence of severe pericardial effusion from a left atrial tear.

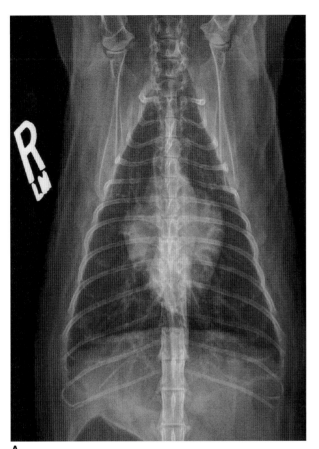

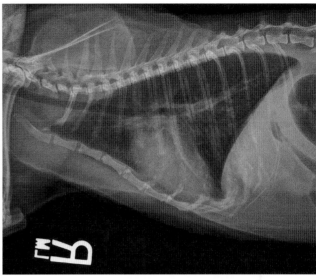

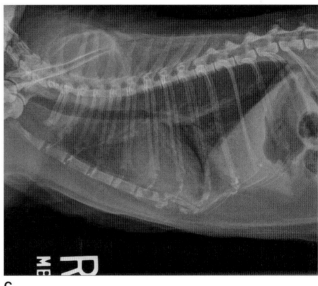

**FIGURE 18.23**   (**A**) Ventrodorsal radiographs of a cat with severe left-sided cardiomegaly and associated widening of the heart base, resulting in a "valentine-shaped" appearance. (**B**) Right lateral projection of the same cat with presence of a focal concavity along the dorsal aspect of the cardiac silhouette secondary to the presence of severe left-sided cardiomegaly. (**C**) Right lateral projection of a different cat with left ventricular enlargement, characterized by the presence of a left ventricular bulge along the caudal aspect of the cardiac silhouette.

enlargement (Figure 18.23C). In both cats and dogs, echocardiography remains the gold standard to assess all the cardiac chambers, including their structural and functional integrity.

## Are the Pulmonary Vessels Enlarged?

Enlargement of the pulmonary vessels may be seen with arterial enlargement and/or venous congestion. Enlargement of both the pulmonary lobar arteries and veins may be seen with increased intravascular volume from intravenous fluid overload. Some disease processes such as left to right shunts may also cause generalized pulmonary artery and venous distension (Figure 18.24). In cats, both pulmonary arteries and veins may be enlarged when in congestive heart failure (Figure 18.25).

Pulmonary venous distension alone is primarily seen in association with left-sided heart failure from mitral valve insufficiency secondary to mitral valvular degenerative disease. Pulmonary arterial enlargement with tortuosity and truncation with lack of pulmonary artery visualization is seen in dogs and cats with heartworm disease (Figure 18.26).

## Is There Evidence of Enlargement of the Great Vessels?

Direct size and indirect pressure measurements of the caudal vena cava, main pulmonary artery, pulmonary veins, and aorta can be obtained with echocardiography. Using radiography,

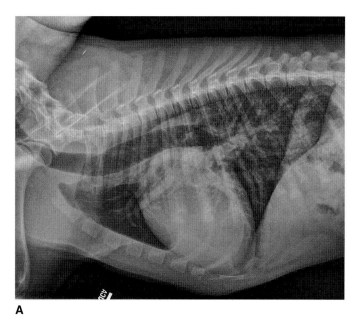

**A**

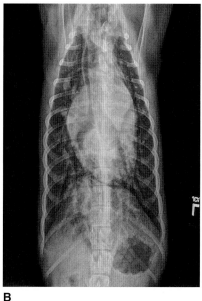

**B**

**FIGURE 18.24** Left lateral (**A**) and dorsoventral (**B**) projections of a dog with a left to right patent ductus arteriosus and associated generalized pulmonary artery and venous distension.

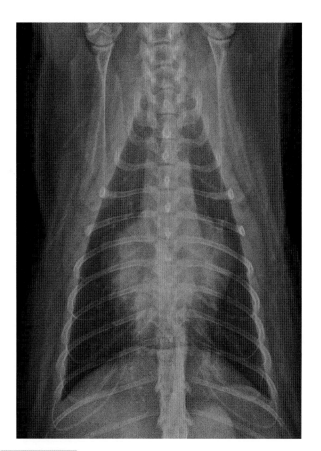

**FIGURE 18.25** Ventrodorsal projection of a cat in congestive heart failure with both pulmonary artery and venous distension.

increased size of the vessels may result in distinct soft tissue bulges along the cardiac silhouette, each of which is discussed in detail in the following sections and described in Tables 18.5

and 18.6. Mineralization of the aortic root and sinuses can be seen on rare occasions in dogs and has been described as an incidental finding (Figure 18.27).

## Is There Radiographic Evidence of Left- or Right-Sided Congestive Heart Failure?

When assessing the cardiovascular structures, identification of fluid within the pulmonary parenchyma, pleural space, pericardium, and peritoneal space may suggest congestive heart failure from pressure and/or volume overload. Left-sided pressure or volume overload can lead to elevated enddiastolic left ventricular pressures, left atrial pressures and then elevations in pulmonary venous pressures. This results in pulmonary edema. Evidence of pulmonary edema is most readily assessed with thoracic radiographs. In dogs, cardiogenic pulmonary edema is most often seen as an unstructured interstitial pulmonary pattern with a caudodorsal distribution, which may then progress into an alveolar pattern based on the severity and degree of edema present (Figure 18.28). In cats, cardiogenic pulmonary edema can also have a variable and even a ventral pulmonary distribution. Infrequently, severe, chronic left atrial enlargement secondary to severe mitral valve regurgitation may result in endocardial splitting, left atrial rupture, and development of a hemorrhagic pericardial effusion (see Figure 18.22).

Other features of right-sided congestive heart failure, which may be detected with radiographs or ultrasound, include the presence of pleural effusion, ascites, and hepatomegaly.

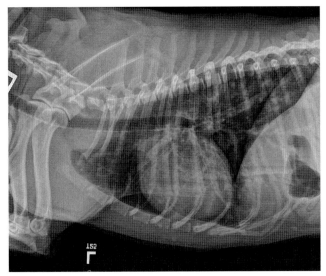 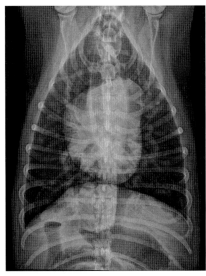

A                                                                              B

**FIGURE 18.26** Left lateral (**A**) and ventrodorsal (**B**) projections of a dog with heartworm disease, characterized by the presence of severe right-sided cardiomegaly and main pulmonary artery enlargement due to pulmonary hypertension. Additionally, the lobar pulmonary arteries are tortuous and truncated.

**TABLE 18.5** Summary of congenital heart diseases in dogs and cats.

| Disease | Pathophysiology | Cardiomegaly | Aorta/MPA enlargement | Congestive heart failure | Pulmonary arteries (PA) and pulmonary veins (PV) |
|---|---|---|---|---|---|
| Left to right patent ductus arteriosus (PDA) | Overcirculation of left heart and pulmonary circulation | Left atrial enlargement with eccentric hypertrophy of the left ventricle | Enlarged aorta (descending) and MPA | ± Left heart failure | Both PA and PV enlarged |
| Right to left PDA | Pulmonary hypertension | Concentric hypertrophy of the right ventricle | Enlarged aorta (descending) and MPA | ± Right heart failure | Enlarged centrally (PA), but taper peripherally; can be small (PA and PV) |
| Subaortic stenosis (SAS) | Left ventricular outflow tract obstruction with left ventricular pressure overload | Concentric hypertrophy of the left ventricle | Aortic bulge (ascending aorta and aortic arch) | ± Left heart failure | Normal |
| Pulmonary stenosis (PS) | Right ventricular outflow tract obstruction with right ventricular pressure overload | Concentric hypertrophy of the right ventricle | Enlarged MPA | ± Right heart failure | ± Small pulmonary arteries |
| Tricuspid valve dysplasia (TVD) | Right atrial and ventricular volume overload | Right atrial enlargement with eccentric hypertrophy of the right ventricle | Normal | ± Right heart failure | Normal |
| Mitral valve dysplasia (MVD) | Left atrial and ventricular volume overload | Left atrial enlargement with eccentric hypertrophy of the left ventricle | Normal | ± Left heart failure | PV enlarged |
| Left to right ventricular septal defect (VSD) | Overcirculation of the left heart and pulmonary circulation | Left atrial and ventricular enlargement | Normal | ± Left heart failure | Both PA and PV enlarged |

(Continued)

TABLE 18.5 (Continued)

| Disease | Pathophysiology | Cardiomegaly | Aorta/MPA enlargement | Congestive heart failure | Pulmonary arteries (PA) and pulmonary veins (PV) |
|---|---|---|---|---|---|
| Tetralogy of Fallot | Large ventricular septal defect, dextroposition of the aorta and pulmonic stenosis with right ventricular hypertrophy and pulmonary arterial and venous undercirculation | Concentric hypertrophy of the right ventricle | Normal | Rarely results in right heart failure | Small PA and PV |
| Left to right atrial septal defect (ASD) | Right-sided volume overload ± pulmonary hypertension | Right atrial and ventricular enlargement | ± MPA enlargement if pulmonary hypertension is present | ± Right heart failure | Normal |
| Mitral valve stenosis (MS) | Obstruction of transmitral blood flow with left atrial pressure overload | Left atrial | Normal | ± Left heart failure | PV enlarged |

MPA, main pulmonary artery; left heart failure, pulmonary venous enlargement, and/or pulmonary edema; right heart failure, pleural effusion, caudal vena cava enlargement, hepatomegaly, and ascites.

**TABLE 18.6** Summary of acquired heart diseases in dogs and cats.

| Disease | Pathophysiology | Cardiomegaly | Aorta/MPA enlargement | Congestive heart failure | Pulmonary arteries (PA) and pulmonary veins (PV) |
|---|---|---|---|---|---|
| Degenerative mitral valve disease (DMVD) | Mitral valve insufficiency with left-sided volume overload | Left atrial enlargement with eccentric hypertrophy of the left ventricle | Normal | ± Left heart failure | PV enlarged |
| Degenerative tricuspid valve disease (DTVD) | Tricuspid valve insufficiency with right-sided volume overload | Right atrial enlargement with eccentric hypertrophy of the right ventricle | Normal | ± Right heart failure | Normal |
| Endocarditis – aortic or mitral valve | Left-sided volume overload | Left atrial enlargement with eccentric hypertrophy of the left ventricle | Normal | ± Left heart failure | PV > PA or both enlarged |
| Hypertrophic cardiomyopathy | Inherited myocardial failure with left-sided pressure overload | Left atrial enlargement with concentric hypertrophy of the left ventricle | Normal | ± Left heart failure | PV (and PA) enlarged |
| Dilated cardiomyopathy | Myocardial failure with compensatory volume overload (primarily left-sided) | Most commonly see eccentric hypertrophy of the left ventricle, but may involve all chambers | Normal | ± Left heart failure | PV enlarged |
| Arrhythmogenic right ventricular cardiomyopathy (ARVC) | Myocardial failure with compensatory volume overload (primarily right-sided) | Most often normal. May see eccentric hypertrophy of the right ventricle or all chambers in advanced cases | Normal | ± Right heart failure | Normal |
| Feline restrictive cardiomyopathy (RCM) | Myocardial fibrosis, primarily of the left ventricle | Left atrial enlargement | Normal | ± Left heart failure | PV (and PA) enlarged |

TABLE 18.6 (Continued)

| Disease | Pathophysiology | Cardiomegaly | Aorta/MPA enlargement | Congestive heart failure | Pulmonary arteries (PA) and pulmonary veins (PV) |
|---|---|---|---|---|---|
| Pulmonary hypertension/ cor pulmonale | Increased pulmonary vascular pressure due to lower airway or pulmonary vascular diseases | Right atrial enlargement with concentric hypertrophy of the right ventricle | MPA enlargement | ± Right heart failure with cor pulmonale; high pressure pulmonary edema has been reported | Small or blunted PA with throm- boembolisms Enlarged and tortuous PA with heartworm disease |

MPA, main pulmonary artery; left heart failure, pulmonary venous enlargement and/or pulmonary edema; right heart failure, pleural effusion, caudal vena cava enlargement, hepatomegaly, and ascites.

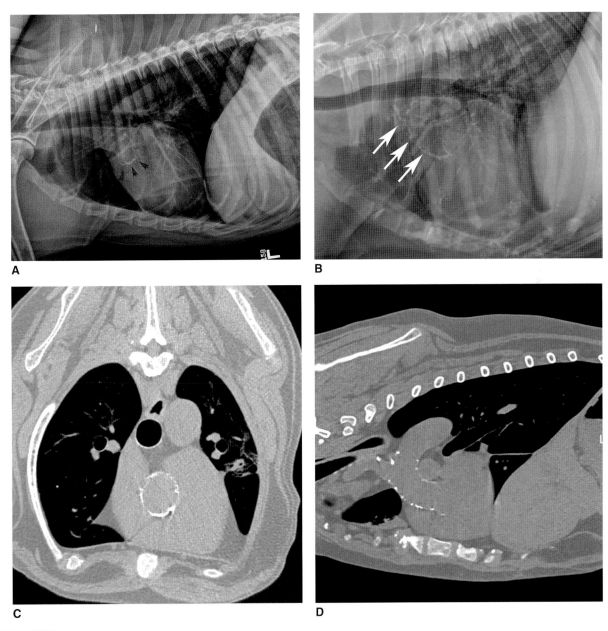

**FIGURE 18.27** Examples from two different dogs with aortic root and arch mineralization. In (**A**), a left lateral radiograph of a dog with mineralization of the aortic root and sinuses (arrows), representing an incidental finding. In (**B**), a second dog with extensive aortic root mineralization (white arrows) noted on the right lateral radiograph. CT images including transverse (**C**) and reconstructed sagittal plane (**D**) images from the second dog showing the extent of the dystrophic mineralization of the aorta.

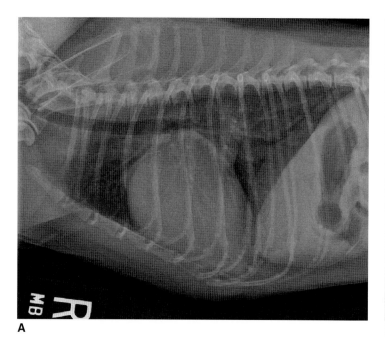
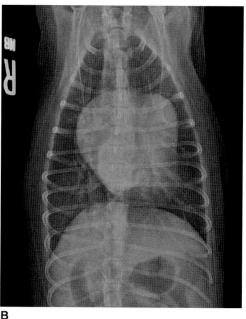

**A**

**B**

**FIGURE 18.28** Left lateral (**A**) and ventrodorsal (**B**) radiographs of a dog with severe degenerative mitral valve disease and a caudodorsally distributed unstructured interstitial to alveolar pulmonary pattern, representing cardiogenic pulmonary edema due to left-sided heart failure.

# Congenital Cardiovascular Diseases

## Left to Right Shunting Patent Ductus Arteriosus (PDA)

Left to right PDAs and subaortic stenosis are considered the most common congenital cardiac defects in dogs. In the left to right shunting PDA, the ductus arteriosus fails to close after birth which results in shunting of blood from the aorta (high pressure) into the pulmonary artery (low pressure). The pulmonary circulation and left-sided cardiac chambers become volume overloaded, resulting in eccentric hypertrophy of the left ventricle. Recirculation of blood through the heart also causes volume overload (overcirculation) of the pulmonary arteries and veins, with bulges at the level of the descending thoracic aorta (*ductus diverticulum*) and main pulmonary artery at the level of the PDA, and if severe left atrial enlargement is present, the left auricle will be enlarged (left fourth intercostal space on the VD or DV image). Left sided-congestive heart failure is seen in dogs with left to right shunting PDAs (Figure 18.29).

## Right to Left Shunting PDA

If the pulmonary arterial pressure exceeds aortic pressure, blood flow through the PDA will be reversed. Concentric hypertrophy of the right ventricle is seen in response to pressure overload. The left atrium and ventricle are

pulmonary vasculature and are thereby relatively small in size (Figure 18.30). In addition, a ductus diverticulum will be seen on the ventrodorsal/dorsoventral view at the fourth left intercostal space.

## Subaortic Stenosis (SAS)

Stenosis at the level of the left outflow tract occurs in the subvalvular region of the left ventricular outflow tract in the majority of dogs with SAS. SAS is the second most prevalent congenital disorder in the dog and is uncommon in cats. Pressure overload results from obstruction of the left ventricular outflow tract. Concentric hypertrophy of the left ventricular wall occurs in response to the increased left ventricular pressure. The left ventricle becomes less distensible and volume underloaded. Undercirculation of the coronary vasculature results in reduced myocardial perfusion and may cause arrhythmias. As the coronary supply extends from the epicardium to the endocardium, loss of normal endocardial blood supply results in fibrosis and dystrophic mineralization in severe cases (Figure 18.31).

## Pulmonic Stenosis (PS)

Pulmonic stenosis is the third most common congenital disorder in dogs and is uncommon in cats. Stenosis occurs at the level of the pulmonary valve and is usually associated with fusion of the valvular commissures and thickening of the free edges of the leaflets. Narrowing of the pulmonary valve obstructs passage of blood through the right ventricular outflow tract

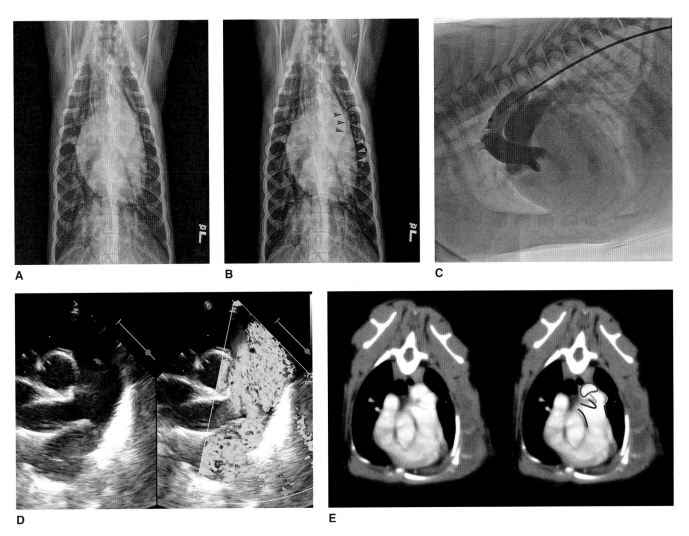

**FIGURE 18.29** Ventrodorsal (**A**) and dorsoventral (**B**) radiographs of a dog with a left to right PDA, characterized by enlargement of the aorta (red arrowheads), main pulmonary artery (blue arrowheads) and left auricle (green arrowheads), also described as the "three-knuckle" sign. Variable degrees of left-sided cardiomegaly and pulmonary venous and arterial enlargement are seen due to overcirculation. The ductus arteriosus of the same dog is directly visualized with selective angiography under fluoroscopic guidance (**B**). Additionally, digital subtraction angiography (**C**), echocardiography (**D**) and CTA (**E**) can be used to identify the shunting vessel.

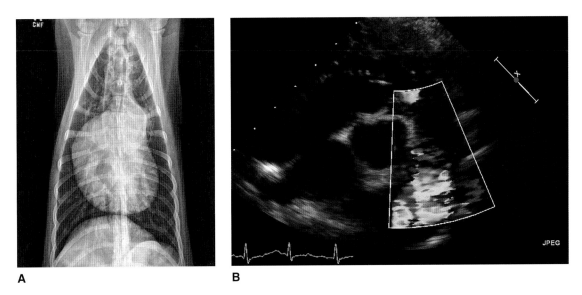

**FIGURE 18.30** (**A**) Ventrodorsal radiograph of a dog with a right to left patent ductus arteriosus and associated right-sided cardiomegaly and severe enlargement of the main pulmonary artery. The ductus diverticulum is superimposed over the main pulmonary artery enlargement. In addition to direct visualization of the PDA, echocardiography (**B**) is used to identify the reversal of blood flow (blue direction away from the transducer with some aliasing) through the ductus arteriosus (right to left direction).

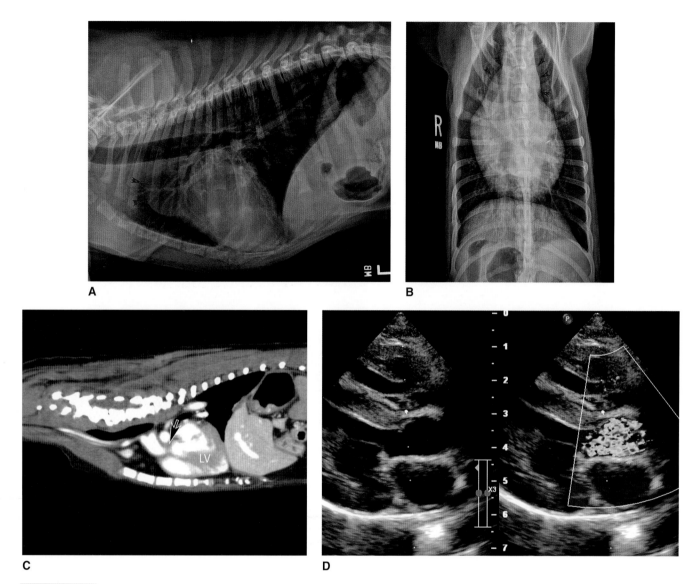

**FIGURE 18.31** (**A**) Radiographic findings seen with SAS include left-sided cardiomegaly with dilation of the aortic arch (blue arrowheads). In mild cases, no radiographic abnormalities may be apparent. (**B**) Similar left-sided cardiomegaly and dilation of the aortic arch is seen on computed tomography. (**C**) CTA reconstructed in a sagittal plane with narrowing of the left ventricular outflow tract (black arrow) and thickening of the left ventricle (LV). (**D**) Echocardiography reveals concentric hypertrophy of the left ventricular wall and subvalvular stenosis in the left ventricular outflow tract. The degree of stenosis present directly correlates to the peak flow velocity (pressure gradient) across with the aortic valve using spectral Doppler. In many cases, aortic regurgitation is also observed at the aortic valve using color flow Doppler evaluation or continuous wave spectral Doppler.

with a consequent increase in right ventricular pressure. The increased blood pressure within the right ventricle results in concentric hypertrophy of the right ventricle, reducing compliance and filling of the right ventricle (Figure 18.32). Dogs with PS may be concurrently diagnosed with a right to left shunting patent foramen ovale.

## Tricuspid Valve Dysplasia (TVD)

Tricuspid valve dysplasia is most commonly seen in large-breed dogs (Labrador retrievers) and is more prevalent than mitral valve dysplasia. Normal closure of the tricuspid valve is altered by malformation and thickening of the tricuspid valve leaflets. The chordae tendineae may be shortened and restrict closure of the tricuspid valve by hindering normal leaflet apposition. Subsequently, regurgitation of blood into the right atrium occurs, resulting in severe enlargement of the right atrium secondary to volume overload (Figure 18.33). The right ventricle also becomes enlarged due to eccentric hypertrophy. Rarely, stenosis of the tricuspid valve is seen in dogs with TVD.

Another form of TVD, known as *Ebstein anomaly*, is characterized as abnormal ventral displacement of the tricuspid valve due to basal attachment of the tricuspid valve annulus into the right ventricle.

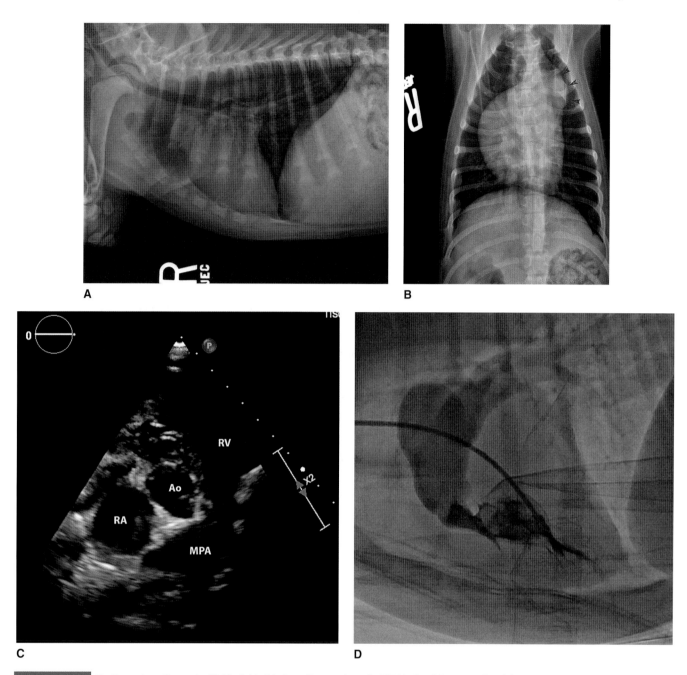

A

B

C

D

**FIGURE 18.32**   On thoracic radiographs (**A,B**), right-sided cardiomegaly and a MPA bulge (blue arrowheads) is consistent with the diagnosis of PS. Radiographic changes associated with right-sided congestive heart failure, such as ascites and hepatomegaly, may be seen in more advanced cases. Due to pulmonary undercirculation, the pulmonary arteries and veins are decreased in size. (**C**) A definitive diagnosis is made with echocardiography by direct identification of a stenotic pulmonic valve with subsequent right ventricular hypertrophy and enlargement. The severity of the stenosis is proportional to the peak velocity of blood flow measured across the pulmonary valve with spectral continuous wave Doppler. Using color Doppler, pulmonic and tricuspid regurgitation may be concurrently identified. (**D**) Selective angiography is commonly done for identification of the pulmonic stenotic lesion and the degree of poststenotic dilation prior to balloon valvuloplasty.

## Mitral Valve Dysplasia (MVD)

Like TVD, MVD is characterized by malformation and thickening of the mitral valve leaflets. The chordae tendineae may be shortened or thickened, restricting normal closure of the mitral valve. Mitral valve insufficiency and systolic regurgitation of blood into the left atrium result in volume overload and left atrial and ventricular enlargement (Figure 18.34). Stenosis of the mitral valve is less frequently identified in dogs and cats with MVD. In addition to hypertrophic cardiomyopathy (HCM), MVD is the most common cause of mitral regurgitation in cats. Severe mitral valve insufficiency and volume overload may lead to pulmonary venous congestion and left-sided congestive heart failure.

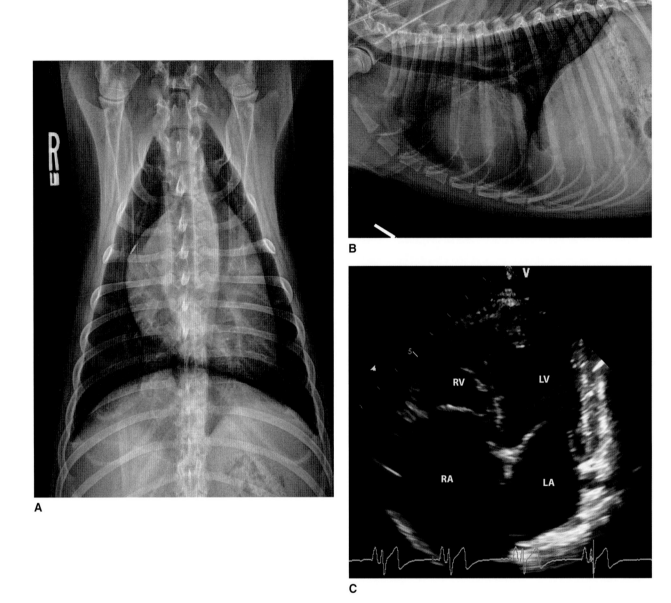

**FIGURE 18.33** On thoracic radiographs (**A,B**), moderate to severe right atrial enlargement is apparent when tricuspid valve regurgitation can be seen secondary to tricuspid valve dysplasia. The right atrium is usually larger than the right ventricle. Enlargement of the caudal vena cava with hepatic venous congestion may also precede right-sided congestive heart failure (presence of ascites and/or pleural effusion). Echocardiography (**C**) shows thickening of the tricuspid valve leaflets and shortening or fusion of the chordae tendineae with valvular insufficiency characterized by the presence of a regurgitant jet using color flow Doppler.

## Left to Right Ventricular Septal Defect (VSD)

Ventricular septal defect is a common congenital cardiac disorder in cats (Figure 18.35) and is a subset of the broader category of endocardial cushion defects, that might involve the atrial septum, ventricular septum, and the tricuspid and mitral valves. A single orifice, usually perimembranous in origin, spans the interventricular wall in the subvalvular region of the tricuspid valve and beneath the aortic valve. Due to the increased

pressure in the left ventricle, blood is shunted from the left ventricle to the right ventricle. Therefore, there is overcirculation of the pulmonary vasculature with volume overload of the right ventricle, left atrium, and ventricle. Eccentric hypertrophy of the left ventricle is seen in response to the increased blood volume. Due to the increased compliance of the right ventricular wall in comparison to the left ventricular and volume overload, the right ventricle can also undergo eccentric hypertrophy. Cardiogenic edema associated with left-sided congestive heart failure may result from pulmonary overcirculation.

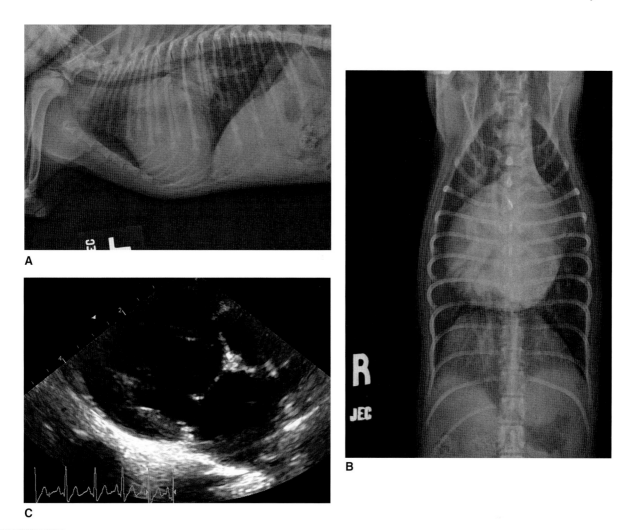

**FIGURE 18.34**   Left-sided cardiomegaly is commonly seen with MVD (**A**,**B**). In more advanced cases with severe volume overload, cardiac decompensation is seen, characterized by the presence of pulmonary venous distension and cardiogenic pulmonary edema. Evaluation of the mitral valve and quantification of left atrial and ventricular enlargement are best achieved with echocardiography (**C**). Evidence of mitral valve malformation includes reduced motion and thickening of the mitral valve leaflet, shortening of the chordae tendineae, and abnormal changes to the papillary muscles. M-mode echocardiography may show concordant mitral valve leaflet motion due to fusion.

*Eisenmenger syndrome* is when a left to right shunting VSD starts to shunt right to left due to pulmonary hypertension and elevations in right ventricular pressures.

## Tetralogy of Fallot

Tetralogy of Fallot is a complex of four congenital abnormalities (Figure 18.36), which include:

- a right to left shunting interventricular septal defect
- right ventricular concentric hypertrophy
- pulmonic stenosis
- dextroposition (overriding) of the aorta over the right and left ventricular outflow tracts.

The presence of a perimembranous interventricular defect impairs the stability of the septal wall, resulting in dextroposition of the aorta and narrowing of the right ventricular outflow tract due to higher blood pressures present within the left atrial and ventricular chambers. Increased blood pressure within the right ventricle secondary to the PS results in concentric hypertrophy of the right ventricular wall and dysrhythmias.

The size of the interventricular septal defect and the degree of PS affect the hemodynamic consequences of tetralogy of Fallot. With mild PS, left to right shunting of blood is seen through the VSD. Most commonly, the PS is severe, and higher systolic pressures within right ventricle in relation to the left ventricle result in reversed blood flow (right to left) through the VSD. Subsequently, there is decreased outflow of blood into the pulmonary vasculature with decreased amounts of blood

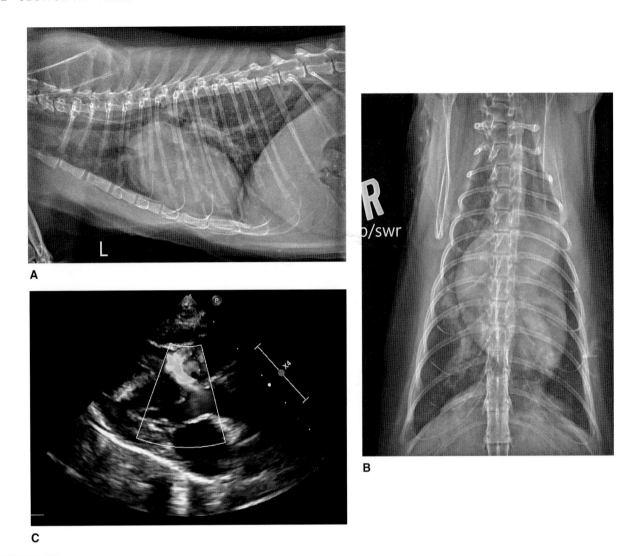

**FIGURE 18.35** In cats and dogs with ventricular septal defects, thoracic radiographs reveal left, right or generalized cardiomegaly with pulmonary arterial and venous dilation depending on the location of the VSD relative to the right ventricular outflow tract. In more advanced cases, pulmonary hypertension is also seen with left-sided congestive heart failure. Left lateral (**A**) and ventrodorsal (**B**) radiographs from a 2-year-old DSH with a right to left shunting VSD and pulmonary hypertension. There is cardiomegaly, enlargement of the pulmonary vasculature with tortuosity of the caudal lobar pulmonary arteries. There is enlargement of the main pulmonary artery noted on the ventrodorsal radiograph. Using echocardiography from a different cat (**C**), a left to right VSD is directly visualized, and Doppler interrogation of blood flow through the defect is used to characterize the defect as resistive (small) or non-resistive (large). Small resistive VSDs are more commonly seen in dogs. Additionally, the direction of blood flow helps to grade the severity of the VSD. With worsening pulmonary hypertension, shunt reversal can occur, resulting in conditions known as Eisenmenger complex. Echocardiography is also used to identify and quantify the degree of left, with or without concurrent right, atrial and ventricular enlargement.

returned to the left atrium from the pulmonary veins. Deoxygenated blood is circulated into the systemic circulation which results in cyanosis and secondary polycythemia.

Right-sided congestive heart failure is rarely seen with tetralogy of Fallot due to the compensatory shunting of blood through the VSD and into the systemic circulation.

## Left to Right Atrial Septal Defect (ASD)

Atrial septal defects originate from the failure of closure of three different embryologic sites. This results in *ostium secondum*, *ostium primum*, and *sinus venosus* ASDs (Figure 18.37).

Of these, ostium secondum defects are more common in dogs and occur centrally within the atrial septum, just above the atrioventricular valve in the region of the foramen ovale. In comparison, ostium primum defects are more common in cats and occur near the atrioventricular valves and may be combined with other *endocardial cushion defects*, such as mitral or TVD. The least common ASD is the sinus venosus defect near the junction with the pulmonary vein.

While small defects may have no hemodynamic effects, blood is shunted from the left atrium to the right atrium with larger shunts, causing volume overload of the right atrium and ventricle. Right-sided volume overload results in eccentric hypertrophy of the right atrium and ventricle. Pleural effusion,

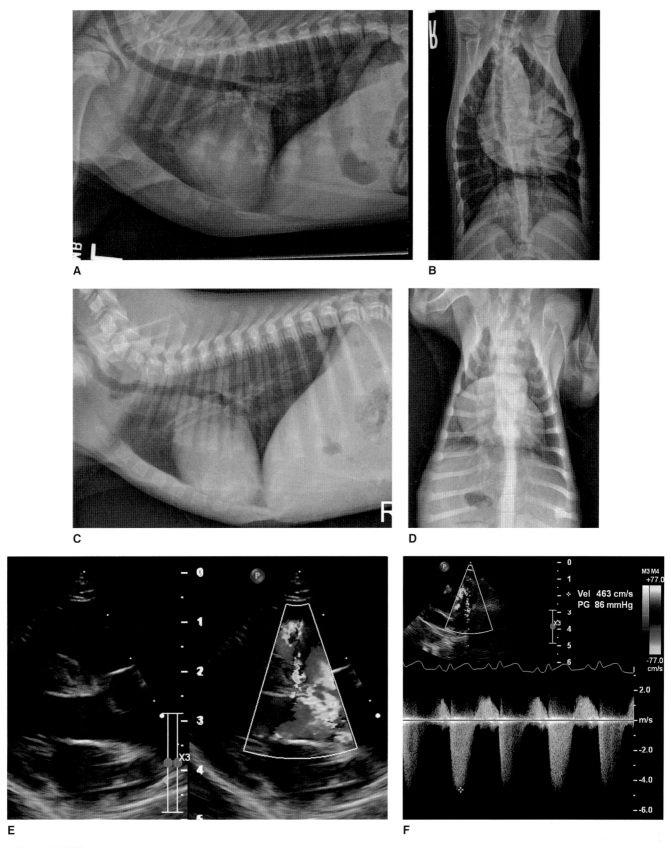

**FIGURE 18.36** (**A,B**) Radiographic findings for tetralogy of Fallot include right-sided cardiomegaly with decreased size of the pulmonary vessels due to arterial and venous undercirculation. (**C,D**) Right lateral and dorsoventral radiographs from a second dog with tetralogy of Fallot, with a more "boot"-shaped appearance to the cardiac silhouette on the dorsoventral image. (**E**) Echocardiography reveals a large septal defect, dextroposition of the aorta and pulmonic stenosis with right ventricular hypertrophy. Color Doppler is used to identify the direction of blood flow through the VSD. Spectral Doppler is used to measure the peak blood velocity across the pulmonary valve (**F**).

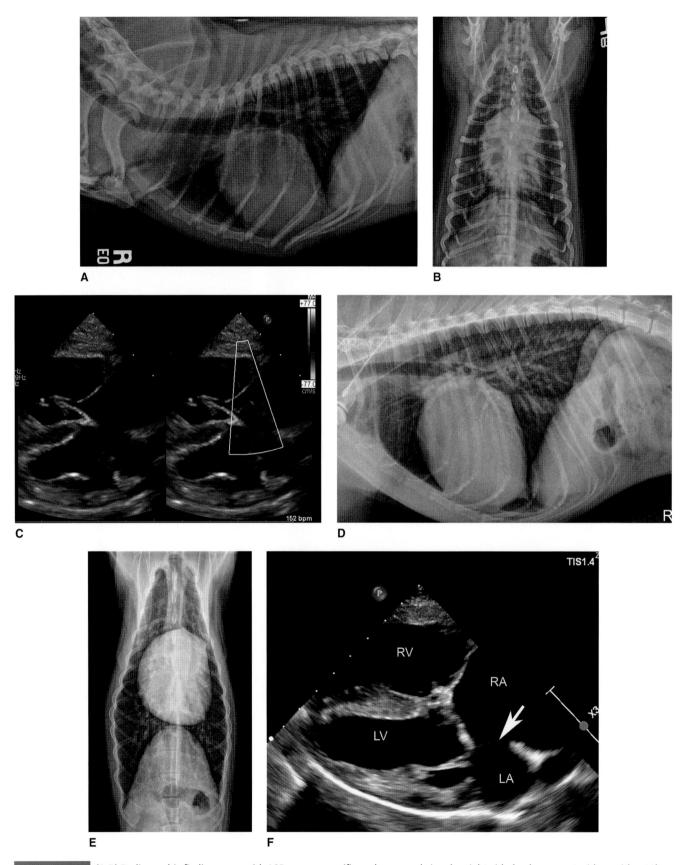

**FIGURE 18.37** (**A,B**) Radiographic findings seen with ASD are nonspecific and commonly involve right-sided enlargement with or without the present of right-sided congestive heart failure. When pulmonary hypertension is present, enlargement of the main pulmonary artery may also be identified. Echocardiography (**C**) helps to further assess the degree of right atrial and ventricular enlargement present. The ASD is best recognized with color Doppler to directly visualize communication between the right and left atriums. (**D,E**) Right lateral and ventrodorsal radiographs from a dog with a left to right shunting ASD. There is enlargement of the right atrium. (**F**) An ostium secondum defect is identified in a right parasternal long axis plane (white arrow; LA, left atrium; RA, right atrium; RV, right ventricle; LV, left ventricle). There is right ventricular and right atrial enlargement noted on the echo image.

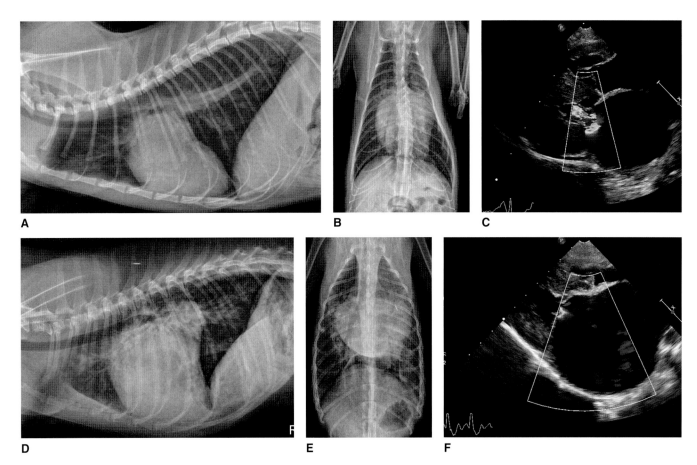

**FIGURE 18.38**   A cat (**A–C**) and a dog (**D–F**) with mitral stenosis. There is cardiomegaly with atrial enlargement noted on the cat radiographs (**A,B**) with pulmonary vessel enlargement (veins > arteries), and an unstructured interstitial pulmonary pattern noted in multifocal anatomic locations (cranial and caudal lung lobes). In (**C**), there is severe left atrial dilation and turbulent flow noted at the mitral valve during atrial systole. The left ventricle is also thickened. In the dog, there is severe left-sided cardiomegaly with dorsal elevation of the trachea and carina (**D,E**). There is severe left auricular enlargement. The pulmonary veins are mildly enlarged compared with their corresponding arteries and there is an unstructured interstitial pulmonary pattern that is generalized (but predominantly left sided). Similar change is noted on the right parasternal long axis image of the heart (**F**) with left atrial enlargement and a reversal of flow and aliasing seen at the central aspect of the mitral valve at atrial systole.

hepatic venous congestion, and ascites may succeed with progression into right-sided congestive heart failure. If concurrent pulmonic valve insufficiency and pulmonary hypertension are present, blood flow reversal can result in cases with excessive right atrial pressure.

## Mitral Valve Stenosis (MS)

Stenosis of the mitral valve occurs due to thickening and fusion of the mitral valve leaflets. Obstruction and increased resistance of transmitral blood flow result in increased left atrial pressure. Pulmonary venous congestion and left-sided

congestive heart failure are seen in more advanced cases (Figure 18.38).

## Cor Triatriatum Sinistrum/Cor Triatriatum Dextrum

Cor triatriatum is a rare congenital abnormality, characterized as abnormal division of the left atrium (*cor triatriatum sinistrum*) or right atrium (*cor triatriatum dextrum*), resulting in a total of three atrial chambers. The atrium is divided by a thick septum representing an embryologic remnant. The septum may be intact or fenestrated and may be associated with other congenital anomalies. While cor triatriatum is most often diagnosed early in life, it may go undetected in asymptomatic dogs and cats. Cor triatriatum sinistrum may result in left-sided volume overload and subsequent pulmonary venous congestion and pulmonary edema. Cor triatriatum dextrum is more common and may result in right-sided congestive heart failure, characterized by systemic venous congestion and ascites and/or pleural effusion (Figure 18.39).

## Persistent Right Aortic Arch (PRAA)

Persistent right aortic arch is the most common vascular ring anomaly in dogs and is also reported in cats (Figure 18.40). Under normal circumstances, the left aortic arch persists and gives rise to the brachiocephalic trunk and left subclavian artery. On rare occasions, the right aortic arch fails to regress and persists to become the functional aortic arch. The ascending aorta and aortic arch are then located to the right of the esophagus and trachea, while the main pulmonary artery maintains a normal position to the left and ventral to the esophagus and trachea. The ductus arteriosus, which connects the aorta to the main pulmonary artery, runs dorsal to the esophagus and trachea, resulting in entrapment of these structures.

## Aortic Coarctation

Coarctation of the aorta is an uncommon congenital heart defect in the dog and rare in the cat, with narrowing of a portion of the ascending aorta, aortic arch or descending thoracic aorta being noted (Figure 18.41). There is a focal dilation in the aorta that is usually distal to the stenotic or narrowed segment. Left ventricular concentric hypertrophy may be present due to increased aortic resistance, thereby increasing left ventricular pressures to maintain a normal systemic circulation.

## Congenital Pericardial Disease

The most common congenital pericardial disease is a peritoneal pericardial diaphragmatic hernia (PPDH) where the septum transversum of the central, ventral diaphragm fails to close and there is a communication between the peritoneal and pericardial spaces. Varying degrees of abdominal contents can then herniate into the pericardium. Radiographic diagnosis is based on cardiomegaly, unusual shape or contour changes to the cardiac silhouette, differential radiographic opacities within the pericardium and lack of visualization of the normal cranial abdominal viscera on the different radiographic projections (Figure 18.42).

A positive contrast peritoneogram or echocardiography can be used to confirm the diagnosis.

# Acquired Cardiovascular Diseases

## Degenerative Valvular Diseases

**Degenerative Mitral Valve Disease (DMVD)**  This condition is also referred to as *myxomatous valvular degeneration* or *endocardiosis*. DMVD is the most common acquired cardiac disorder in older dogs and is uncommon in cats. Chronic and progressive sterile structural changes to the mitral valve impair the function of the mitral valve and result in cardiac compensation followed by decompensation in more advanced cases.

Over time, the mitral valve becomes thickened and nodular in appearance. The chordae tendineae may also stretch and become elongated. Occasionally, chordae tendineae may rupture which results in flailing of a mitral valve leaflet and severe mitral valve insufficiency and overt pulmonary edema. Additionally, contracture of the mitral valve leaflet occurs with severe thickening of the mitral valve, hindering normal apposition of the mitral valves during diastole and resulting in regurgitation of blood into the left atrium. When added to the volume of blood returning from the lung, the regurgitated volume of blood into the left atrium results in left atrial volume overload. An increased volume of blood is subsequently ejected into the left ventricle, resulting in dilation or eccentric hypertrophy of the left ventricle. Left-sided volume overload may progress into congestion of the pulmonary veins and development of left-sided congestive heart failure, as evidenced by the presence of cardiogenic pulmonary edema (Figure 18.43).

Thoracic radiographs are important in the diagnosis of DMVD and are complementary to echocardiography. The absence of radiographic findings does not rule out early DMVD. In more advanced cases of DVMD, variable degrees of left atrial, ventricular, and auricular enlargement are observed. Compression of the left mainstem bronchus and, less frequently, the bronchus to the right caudal and accessory lobe is seen with severe left atrial enlargement. With pulmonary venous congestion, the pulmonary lobar veins are enlarged in comparison to the pulmonary lobar arteries and often precede the development of cardiogenic pulmonary edema. Evaluation of the structural and functional integrity of the mitral valve is best achieved with echocardiography. The mitral valve has a thickened appearance and may prolapse into the left atrium during systole. The mitral valve maintains a normal uniform echogenicity. Since variable amounts of blood are regurgitated back into the left atrium during systole, the fractional

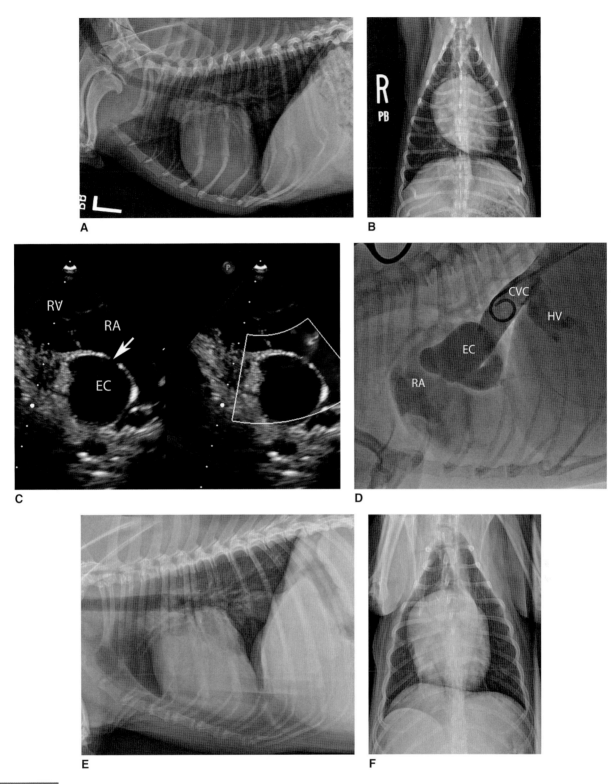

**FIGURE 18.39** On radiographs, variable degrees of left or right heart enlargement may be seen with cor triatriatum sinistrum or dextrum, respectively. Images (**A**) and (**B**) represent right lateral and ventrodorsal projections of a dog with cor triatriatum dextrum. Cardiac decompensation is also reported in more advanced cases. Echocardiography (**C**) and fluoroscopy (**D**) can be used to identify division of the right atrium by aberrant septum (RV, right ventricle; RA, right atrium; EC, extra right atrial chamber). On the echo image there is flow from the extra chamber into the right atrium during diastole. In (**D**) a pig tail catheter has been placed into the distended caudal vena cava (CVC) from a saphenous vein approach. There is enlargement of an extra chamber (EC) seen caudal to the right atrium that contains only a small amount of contrast medium (RA; superimposed over other cardiac structures that also contain some contrast medium). The hepatic veins (HV) are noted to be distended with reflux from the caudal vena cava due to the upstream obstruction at the cor triatriatum dextrum chamber. In a second dog with cor triatriatum dextrum, there is mild to moderate right atrial enlargement and marked enlargement of the caudal vena cava (**E**,**F**). On a right parasternal long axis echocardiographic still image (**G**), there is compression of the normal right atrium (RA) by the extra chamber (EC) from the cor triatriatum dextrum lesion. The EC also compresses the medial wall of the left atrium (RV, right ventricle; LV, left ventricle; LA, left atrium). A CTA was done in this dog due to the presence of a hepatic mass (HM). (**H**) There is marked enlargement of the caudal vena cava and the extra chamber is noted with cranial displacement of the normal right atrium during the initial phase after contrast medium intravenous administration.

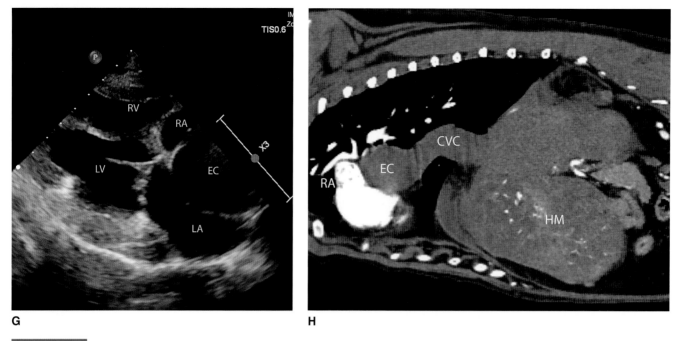

**G**

**H**

**FIGURE 18.39** (Continued)

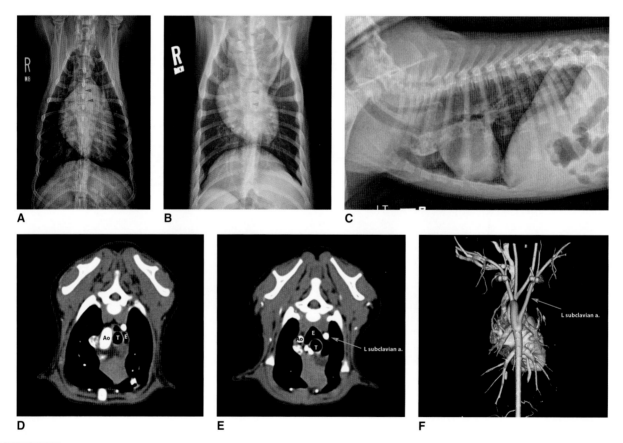

**A**

**B**

**C**

**D**

**E**

**F**

**FIGURE 18.40** Under normal circumstances, the trachea slightly curves to the right of the midline (blue arrowheads) on ventrodorsal or dorsoventral radiographs (**A**). When a PRAA is present (**B**), the trachea is more centrally located or deviated to the left of the midline (green arrowheads). Additionally, ventral deviation of the trachea will be present on lateral projections (**C**). An esophagram with positive contrast agent, such as a barium swallow, will enhance visualization of esophageal dilation cranial to the heart base due to extraluminal obstruction of the esophagus caused by the PRAA. Computed tomography angiography allows for further evaluation of the PRAA and identification of accompanying vascular anomaly for surgical planning. Images (**D**) and (**E**) (transverse CT images post intravenous contrast medium) show the aortic root (Ao) and arch on the right of the trachea (T) and esophagus (E), resulting in mild leftward displacement of the intrathoracic trachea. The left subclavian artery is seen coursing dorsally and left lateral, around the esophagus, before branching into the thoracic, vertebral, and axillary arteries. Cranial to the heart base, the caudal cervical and intrathoracic esophagus is moderately gas dilated. Image (**F**) is a 3D volume rendering of the vascular anatomy in the same dog.

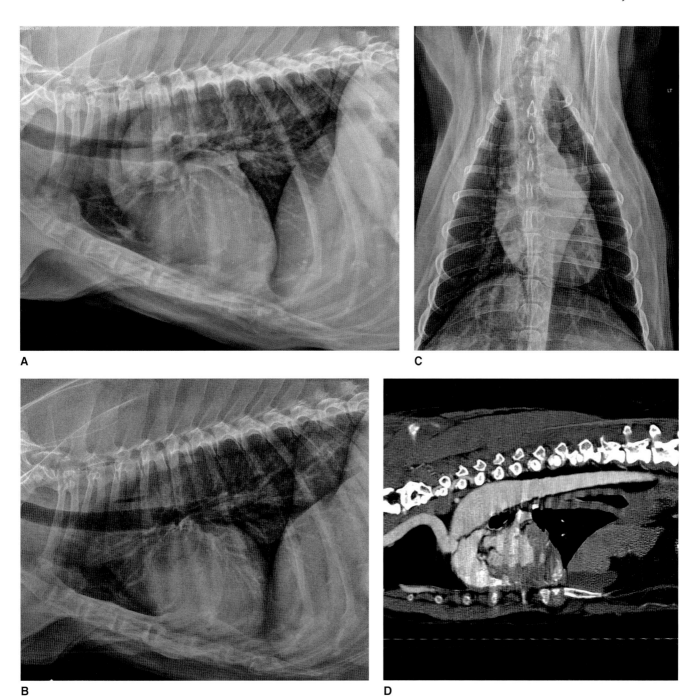

**A**

**B**

**C**

**D**

**FIGURE 18.41** Right lateral, left lateral, and ventrodorsal images (**A–C**) from a 10-year-old American pit bulldog with a descending aortic coarctation. There is a large bulge in the descending thoracic aorta noted on all projections. Sternal lymph node enlargement is also noted. Reconstructed sagittal plane CT (post intravenous contrast medium administration) (**D**) documents the focal aortic narrowing and poststenotic dilation of the aortic coarctation.

shortening is increased. Additionally, color Doppler is used to noninvasively confirm the present of mitral valve regurgitation. Congestive heart failure cannot be identified with echocardiography and requires thoracic radiographs to support a diagnosis.

Over time, in some dogs, DMVD can lead to pulmonary hypertension and enlargement of the main pulmonary artery.

## Degenerative Tricuspid Valve Disease (DTVD)

Degenerative tricuspid valve disease can be seen in conjunction with DMVD or as a single pathologic process. A pathophysiology like DMVD is considered in dogs with DTVD except involving the right side of the heart. While a small degree of tricuspid valve regurgitation is considered incidental, progressive and more advanced changes to the tricuspid valve may result in right-sided volume overload. Enlargement of the caudal vena cava and liver

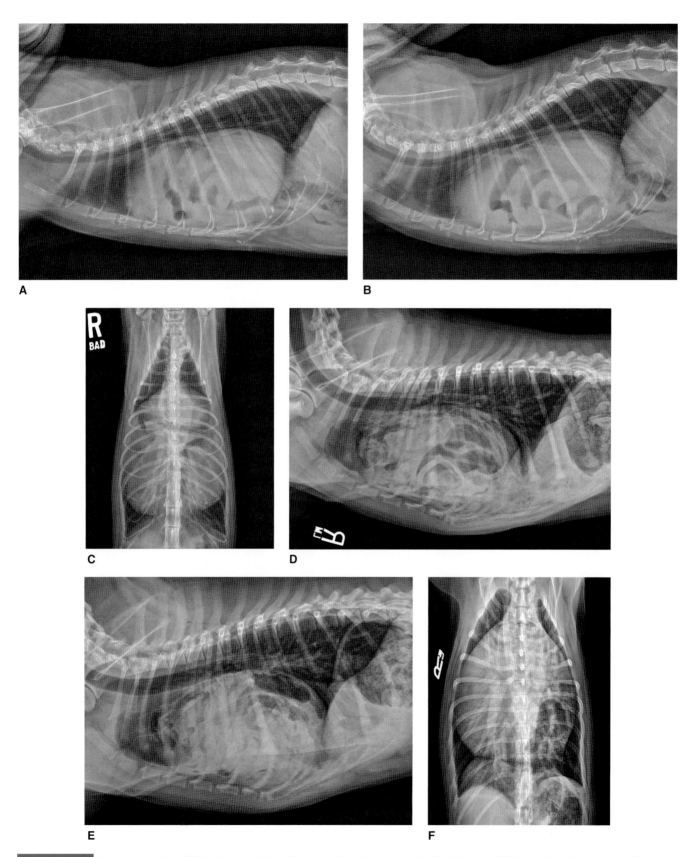

**FIGURE 18.42** Peritoneal-pericardial diaphragmatic hernias in a cat (**A–C**) and a dog (**D–F**). Right lateral, left lateral, and ventrodorsal images are presented for each case. In both the cat and dog, there is generalized enlargement of the cardiac silhouette with dorsal elevation of the trachea. There is differential opacity within the cardiac silhouette with fat, soft tissue, and gas opacities. There are multiple small intestinal segments noted. The cranial abdominal structures are cranially displaced with absence of normal hepatic silhouettes.

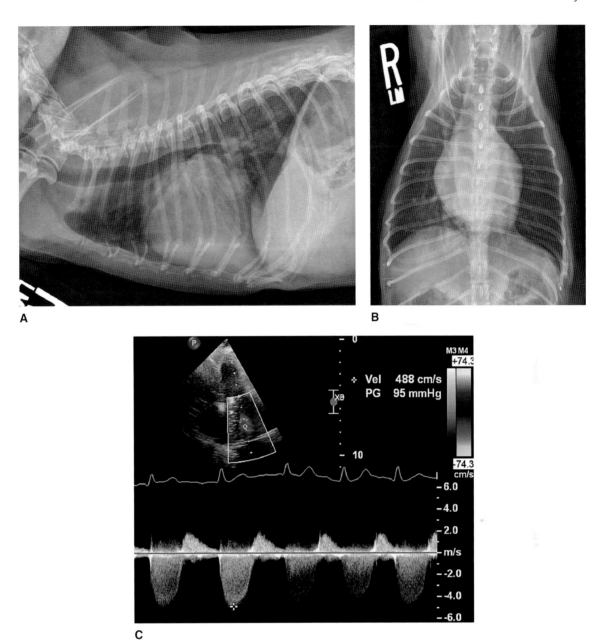

**FIGURE 18.43** Right lateral and ventrodorsal radiographs from a 12-year-old MN poodle (**A**, **B**). There is predominantly left-sided cardiomegaly with dorsal elevation of the trachea and carina. The cardiac silhouette is greater than 80% of the thoracic height and four intercostal spaces in width. There is an unstructured interstitial pulmonary pattern noted in the right caudal lung field on the ventrodorsal view. In (**C**), there is a left apical view of the heart with continuous wave Doppler spectral tracing of the mitral valve insufficiency with a peak velocity of 4.8 m/s.

precedes the development of ascites and pleural effusion seen with right-sided congestive heart failure (Figure 18.44).

On radiographs, right-sided cardiomegaly is identified in more advanced cases. The presence of ascites and/or pleural effusion is consistent with right-sided congestive heart failure. Echocardiography is the modality of choice to assess the structural integrity and function of the tricuspid valve. With DTVD, the tricuspid valve may be thickened and fails to close completely

during systole. Using color Doppler, a regurgitant jet into the right atrium is identified at the level of the tricuspid valve orifice.

**Endocarditis**  While seen more commonly in dogs, infective endocarditis may also be rarely identified in cats. Most commonly, infective endocarditis is characterized as bacterial infection of the aortic and mitral valve leaflets with

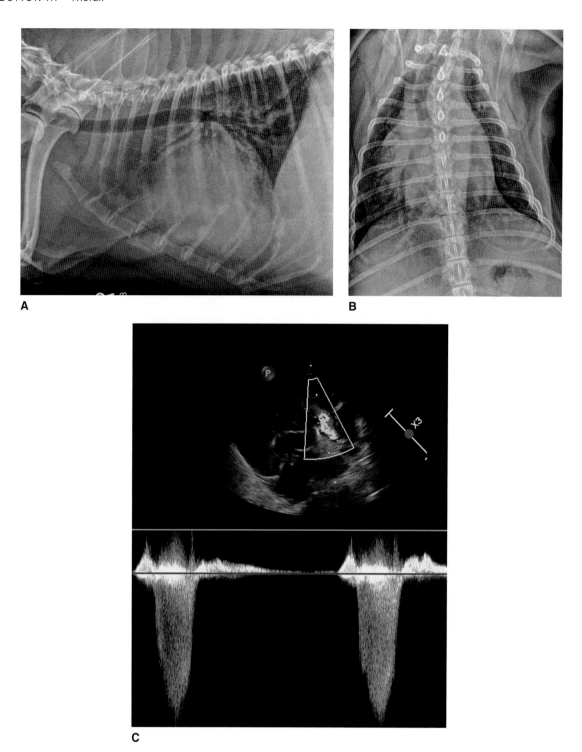

**FIGURE 18.44** Right lateral and ventrodorsal radiographs from a 10-year-old FN mixed-breed dog (**A,B**). There is predominantly right-sided cardiomegaly with atrial and ventricular enlargement. In (**C**), there is a right apical view of the heart with continuous wave Doppler spectral tracing of the tricuspid valve insufficiency with a peak velocity of 2.4 m/s.

gram-positive bacteria, such as streptococci and staphylococci. Gram-negative bacteria, such as *Escherichia coli*, are a less commonly identified cause of infective endocarditis. Occasionally, the myocardium or tricuspid valve may also be affected.

Infective endocarditis is most often a sequela to bacteremia, which often originates from a separate primary site of infection. Noninfective thrombi may serve as a nidus of

infection, seeding bacteria into the heart. Vegetative endocarditis of the heart valves results in significant nonreversible damage and dysfunction of the heart valves. Aortic and/or mitral valve insufficiency precedes left-sided congestive heart failure. With aortic insufficiency, the left ventricle experiences significant volume overload due to incoming blood from the left atrium and regurgitant blood flow from the aortic valve. The myocardium becomes dysfunctional as it is unable to meet the increased oxygen demand. Infected emboli may also shed from the affected heart valve into the systemic circulation, further spreading the infection. Infective endocarditis carries a poor prognosis and has been reported to be associated with subaortic stenosis.

On thoracic radiographs, left-sided cardiomegaly is most often seen with infective endocarditis of the aortic or mitral valve leaflets (Figure 18.45). Cardiac decompensation is commonly observed, by the presence of cardiogenic pulmonary edema. Small vegetative lesions of the heart valve may be difficult to identify with echocardiography. When present, the lesions may move independently from the normal valve motion. Vegetative nodules may be distinguished from DVMD lesions due to their increased echogenicity, abnormal thickening of the entire affected leaflet, and "cauliflower" appearance with mineralization when compared to unaffected valves. Echocardiographic evidence of left atrial and ventricular enlargement is often present. Color and spectral Doppler is used to identify and characterize the presence of valvular insufficiency. The absence of echocardiographic findings does not exclude the possibility of infective endocarditis in bacteremic patients.

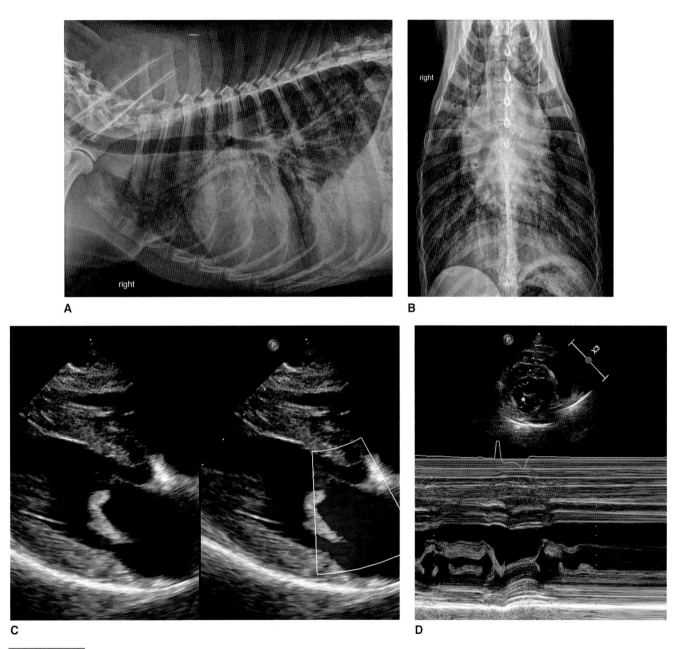

**FIGURE 18.45**   Right lateral and ventrodorsal radiographs from a 6-year-old MN golden retriever (**A,B**). There is predominantly left-sided cardiomegaly without significant enlargement. There is a generalized unstructured interstitial pulmonary pattern noted with pulmonary venous enlargement. In (**C**), there is a right long axis view of the heart with color Doppler documenting a markedly thickened and flail leaflet of the mitral valve extending back into the left atrium. In (**D**), an M-mode tracing documents marked thickening of the mitral valve leaflets without normal opening during diastole and closure during systole.

## Myocardial Diseases

**Hypertrophic Cardiomyopathy** Hypertrophic cardiomyopathy (HCM) is the most common primary myocardial disease in cats and predominantly affects the left ventricle. HCM is heritable in cats and prevalent in Maine coon and Norwegian forest cats. Progressively, the myocardium of the left ventricle becomes severely increased in thickness (concentric hypertrophy), reducing the size of the chamber lumen. During systole, the left ventricle is unable to eject an adequate volume of blood into the systemic circulation. Normal ventricular relaxation is impaired during diastole by the degree of mural wall thickening. To compensate for the decreased stroke volume, the heart rate increases, thereby further limiting refilling of the left ventricle during diastole. Since adequate volumes of blood are unable to circulate through the left ventricle, the left atrium becomes volume overloaded, leading to pulmonary venous dilation and left-sided heart failure. Thickening of the papillary muscles exacerbates the progression of left-sided congestive heart failure.

Systolic anterior motion (SAM) of the mitral valve results in mitral valve insufficiency and regurgitation. Additionally, the mitral valve is pulled into the left ventricular outflow tract, resulting in dynamic outflow obstruction of the left ventricle during systole. Concentric hypertrophy may also be secondary to other underlying factors, such as systemic arterial hypertension, hyperthyroidism, and aortic stenosis, that should be differentiated from HCM (Figure 18.46).

On thoracic radiographs, the cardiac silhouette may be variable in size. Radiographs are most useful in the identification of pulmonary venous distension and left-sided congestive heart failure, as characterized by the presence of pulmonary edema and/or pleural effusion. Echocardiography allows direct measurements of the ventricular wall and lumen.

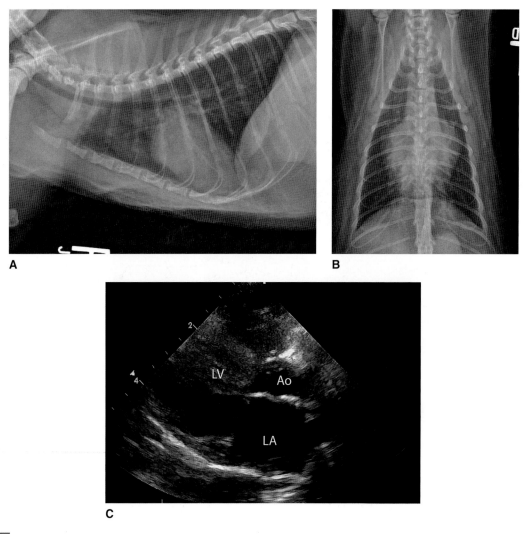

**A**

**B**

**C**

**FIGURE 18.46** Right lateral and ventrodorsal radiographs from a 5-year-old MN DSH can (**A,B**). There is predominantly cardiomegaly with enlargement of the cardiac base (atrial enlargement). The cardiac silhouette is greater than 75% of the thoracic height and 2.5 intercostal spaces in width. There is a mild generalized, unstructured interstitial pulmonary pattern noted. On the ventrodorsal view, there is a valentine-shaped appearance to the cardiac silhouette. In (**C**), there is a right parasternal long axis view of the heart documenting severe interventricular septal and left ventricular free wall thickening with lack of a lumen (LV) and enlargement of the left atrium (18–20 mm; LA). Ao, aortic sinus.

Severe ventricular wall and papillary muscle thickening is seen with severe HCM. The presence of left atrial and auricular enlargement is consistent with pressure and volume overload of the left atrium. Due to stasis of blood, echogenic blood flow (known as smoke) and thrombi may be identified within the left atrium or auricle.

## Dilated Cardiomyopathy (DCM)

Dilated cardiomyopathy is the most common cardiomyopathy in dogs and is overrepresented in certain breeds, particularly male dogs, such as Doberman pinscher, Irish wolfhound, and Great Dane. Most cases are diagnosed when around 6–8 years of age (range 3–12 years). As an exception, Portuguese water dogs are predisposed to a juvenile form of DCM and may present in congestive heart failure as early as 1 month of age. DCM is a progressive disease, which may go unrecognized until more advanced changes are present. Early stages may include left atrial and ventricular enlargement with the presence of cardiac arrhythmias.

The etiology of DCM is idiopathic and appears to have an inherited trait. Other known causes include taurine and carnitine deficiency. Taurine deficiency is a common cause of DCM in cats and American cocker spaniels. All the cardiac chambers can be affected, with the left side being the most severe. The affected chamber is increased in diameter and volume at the end of diastole along with systolic dysfunction. Severe enlargement and widening of the left atrium result in separation of the mitral valve leaflets and subsequent mitral valve insufficiency. When clinical, patients with DCM present in congestive heart failure or with a history of syncope or exercise intolerance.

On thoracic radiographs, generalized cardiomegaly is seen with progressive DCM (Figure 18.47). Cardiomegaly can be difficult to identify in Doberman pinschers due to their deep-chested conformation. The interpretation paradigm and provided link of the normal appearance of the cardiac silhouette in various dog breeds is a useful reference to aid with interpretation. In Dobermans, the only radiographic abnormality associated with the cardiac silhouette may be enlargement of the left atrium.

Echocardiography is a more sensitive modality to evaluate the size of the cardiac chambers. All four cardiac chambers may be enlarged on echocardiography; however, left atrial and ventricular enlargement often predominates.

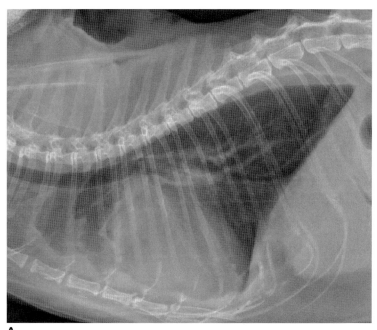
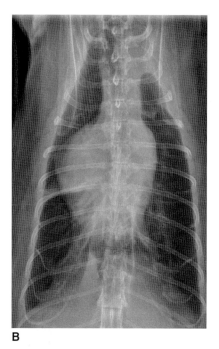

**A**   **B**

**FIGURE 18.47**   Dilated cardiomyopathy in a cat (**A**–**C**) and a dog (**D**–**F**). Right lateral and ventrodorsal images as well as M-Mode echocardiographic images (of the left ventricle right parasternal axis) are presented for each case. In the cat, there is marked enlargement of the cardiac silhouette with a pleural effusion and enlargement of the pulmonary vasculature and caudal vena cava. Dorsal elevation of the trachea and carina is noted. There is tenting of the diaphragm noted on the ventrodorsal radiograph. In (**C**), there is an M-mode representation of the left ventricle documenting a markedly dilated left ventricle with hypomotility and a low fractional shortening. There is thinning of the interventricular septum and the left ventricular free wall. In the dog (**D**, **E**), there is left-sided cardiomegaly with caudodorsal straightening of the caudal cardiac silhouette. There is an unstructured interstitial pulmonary pattern noted in the perihilar region. In (**F**), a representative M-mode slice through the ventricle is presented and the same features described for the cat in (**C**) are present for this Doberman (6-year-old MN). In (**G**), a right parasternal long axis view of the left ventricle and left atrium with color Doppler documents mitral valve regurgitation (aliasing jet) into the left atrium due to mitral valve annular dilation from the dilated cardiomyopathy.

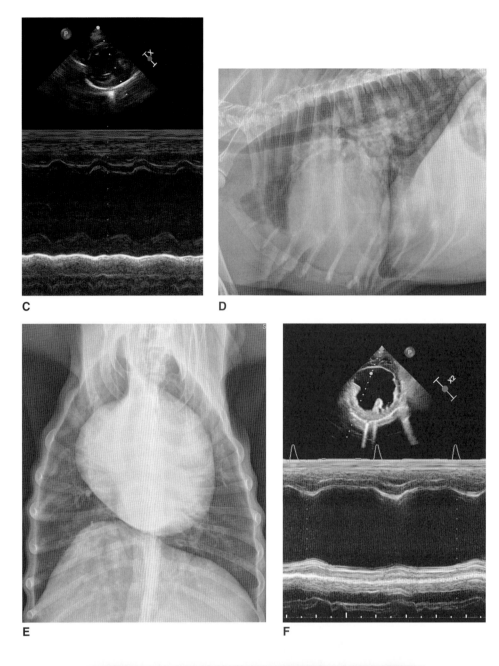

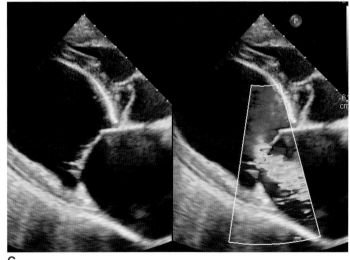

**FIGURE 18.47** (Continued)

### Arrhythmogenic Right Ventricular Cardiomyopathy (ARVC)

Also known as *boxer cardiomyopathy*, ARVC primarily affects the myocardium of the right ventricle but can also affect the left ventricle and atria. ARVC is a heritable disease in boxer dogs and is also identified in cats. Arrhythmias may precede echocardiographic evidence of chamber enlargement. Arrhythmias may range from intermittent premature ventricular depolarizations to sustained ventricular tachycardia. Occasionally, right-sided congestive heart failure will be noted on physical examination and radiographs.

No abnormalities may be present on thoracic radiographs and echocardiography (Figure 18.48). In more advanced cases, right-sided cardiomegaly and congestive heart failure may represent a nonspecific radiographic finding associated with the ARVC. Echocardiography may help to provide earlier evidence of chamber enlargement. ARVC is more reliably diagnosed using electrography to identify cardiac arrhythmias.

### Feline Restrictive Cardiomyopathy (RCM)

Restrictive cardiomyopathy is uncommon in cats and is difficult to

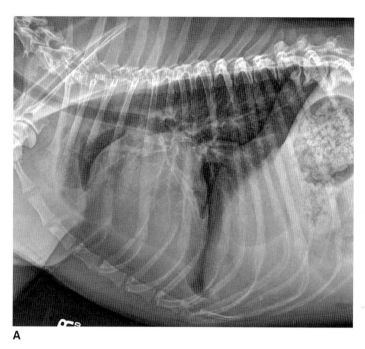

**A**

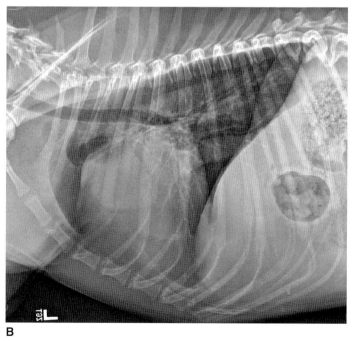

**B**

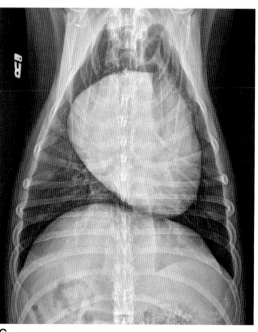

**C**

**FIGURE 18.48**    Right lateral, left lateral, and dorsoventral views (**A–C**) from a 7-year-old MN boxer with ARVC. There is right-sided cardiac enlargement with a mild pleural effusion. There is mild enlargement of the caudal vena cava and a decrease in cranial abdominal serosal detail as with ascites and right heart failure.

differentiate from UCM (described below). A definitive diagnosis is often best achieved with histopathology obtained at necropsy. RCM is characterized as diastolic dysfunction due to myocardial fibrosis and subsequent impaired filling of the left ventricle. Fibrosis of the papillary muscles and mitral valve may result in left-sided volume overload and congestive heart failure.

Severe left atrial enlargement is most often seen on thoracic radiographs (Figure 18.49). The pulmonary arteries and veins may also be enlarged and associated with cardiogenic pulmonary edema and/or pleural effusion in cases with left-sided congestive heart failure. Left atrial enlargement is often confirmed with echocardiography. The left ventricle may be distorted and increased in echogenicity, depending on the degree of fibrosis present. Structural and functional measurements of

the left ventricle are usually normal. The papillary muscles may be fused and associated with mitral valve insufficiency.

## Unclassified Cardiomyopathy (UCM)

Unclassified cardiomyopathy includes a diverse group of cardiomyopathies, which lack the characteristics of the other cardiomyopathies. Restriction of diastolic filling has been proposed as the underlying disease process but the true cause remains unknown. Most cases present in left-sided congestive heart failure and have severe left-sided or generalized cardiomegaly.

On thoracic radiographs, nonspecific left-sided or generalized cardiomegaly with evidence of pulmonary edema and/or pleural effusion is identified (Figure 18.50). Echocardiographic findings are also variable and may range from mild to severe

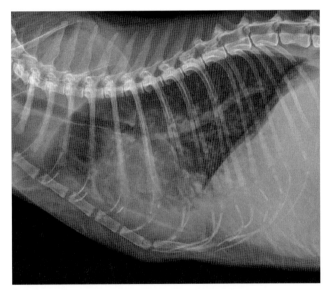

**A**

**B**

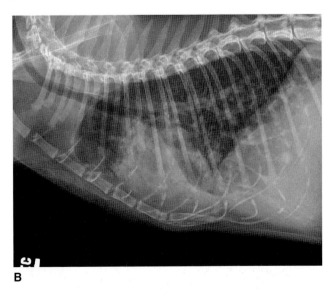

**C**

**FIGURE 18.49**　Right lateral, left lateral, and ventrodorsal views (**A–C**) from a 11-year-old MN DSH with RCM. There is generalized cardiac enlargement with a mild to moderate pleural effusion. There is mild enlargement of the pulmonary vasculature. In addition, there are multiple variably sized pulmonary nodules consistent with metastatic disease from a pancreatic carcinoma. The cardiac changes were independent of the pulmonary metastatic disease. There is a lack of serosal detail within the cranial abdomen consistent with an abdominal effusion.

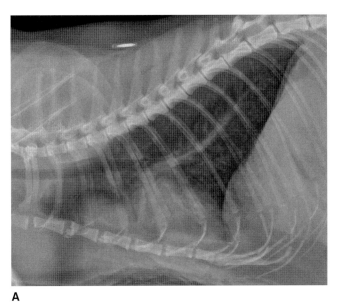

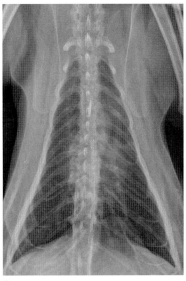

A                                                                    B

**FIGURE 18.50**   Right lateral and dorsoventral views (**A,B**) from a 5-year-old FN DSH with UCM. There is mild cardiac enlargement with a mild pleural effusion. A mild to moderate generalized bronchial pulmonary pattern is noted. There is a soft tissue opaque mass noted cranial to the cardiac silhouette. Changes within the heart on the echocardiogram were consistent with systolic and diastolic dysfunction. The cranial mediastinal mass was a branchial cyst. The bronchial pattern was unrelated to the underlying cardiac disease and consistent with feline allergic lung disease.

left-sided or generalized cardiomegaly with variable degrees of eccentric or concentric hypertrophy.

## Neoplastic Heart Diseases

Hemangiosarcoma and chemodectomas are the two most often identified cardiac neoplasms in dogs. Hemangiosarcoma is seen in dogs originating from the right auricle and atrium. Metastasis to other organs, such as the spleen or liver, is commonly reported. In comparison, chemodectomas and paragangliomas are localized to the heart base and rarely metastasize. When larger masses are identified at the heart base or right atrium or auricle, compression of blood flow into the right cardiac chambers results in distension of the vena cava, as well as right-sided congestive heart failure in more advanced cases. Additionally, pericardial effusion may be identified with masses originating from both the heart base and right atrium and auricle. In cats, lymphoma is the most frequently identified cardiac neoplasm and presents as direct infiltration of the myocardium.

Heart base and right atrial or auricular tumors can be indistinguishable on thoracic radiographs, particularly if a severe pericardial effusion is present. Soft tissue opaque masses at the base of the cardiac silhouette, causing dorsal and lateral displacement of the trachea, are most associated with chemodectomas or other heart base tumors (Figures 18.51 and 18.52). The cardiac silhouette may be enlarged with a globoid appearance due to presence of pericardial effusion. Obstruction of venous return to the right heart is evidenced by enlargement of the caudal vena cava. The presence of ascites and/or pleural

effusion is consistent with right-sided heart failure. Echocardiography is used to confirm the presence of pericardial effusion and mass lesions. Additionally, echocardiography allows subjective quantification of the amount of pericardial effusion, as well as assessment of the heart's contractility for evidence of cardiac tamponade. MRI may be of diagnostic benefit in the identification and localization of cardiac nodules that are not seen on echocardiography.

## Pericardial Diseases

**Pericardial Effusion**   Hemorrhage into the pericardial sac represents the most common cause of pericardial effusion in dogs and is most often associated with the presence of cardiac neoplasia. In comparison, cats may develop pericardial effusion due to left-sided congestive heart failure. Due with severe left-sided cardiomegaly, such as with advanced stages of DMVD, left atrial rupture can result in the acute development of pericardial effusion. Less commonly, pericardial effusion may be idiopathic in dogs.

On thoracic radiographs, the cardiac silhouette is enlarged with a globoid appearance (Figure 18.53). The cardiac silhouette is homogeneously soft tissue opaque with decreased conspicuity of the overlying pulmonary vessels. Echocardiography is the most convenient noninvasive method of identifying and subjectively quantifying pericardial effusion. Using echocardiography, cardiac masses may be identified as a cause for pericardial effusion.

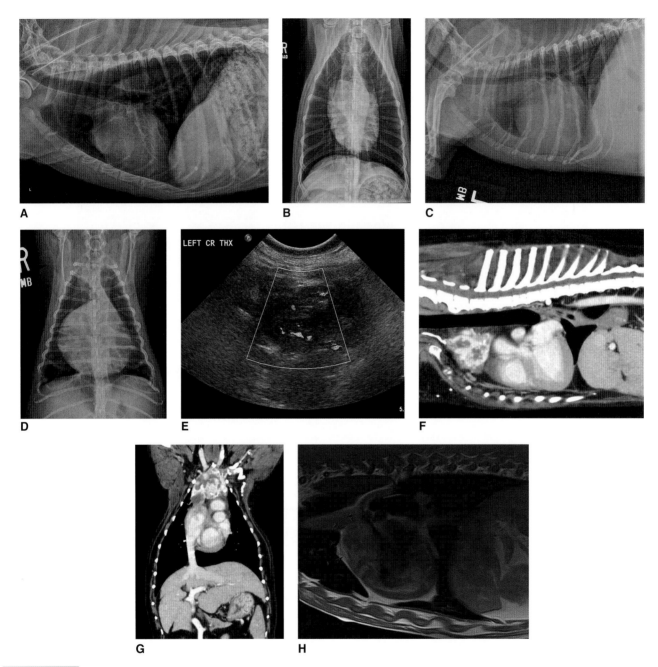

**FIGURE 18.51** (**A,B**) Right atrial or auricular masses can be difficult to recognize on thoracic radiographs, especially if small in size. The presence of a focal soft tissue mass in the region of the right atrium/auricle, occasionally resulting in focal dorsal displacement of the trachea, should raise concerns for a right atrial or auricular mass. (**C,D**) The cardiac silhouette may be enlarged with a globoid appearance due to presence of pericardial effusion. Obstruction of venous return to the right heart is evidenced by enlargement of the caudal vena cava. The present of ascites and/or pleural effusion is suggestive of right-sided heart failure. (**E**) Cardiac masses can be difficult to identify with echocardiography. The absence of a visible mass on echocardiography does not exclude the possibility of cardiac neoplasia. Echocardiography is used to confirm the presence of pericardial effusion. Additionally, it allows subjective quantification of the amount of pericardial effusion, as well as assessing the heart's contractility for evidence of cardiac tamponade. Computed tomography (**F,G**) and magnetic resonance (**H**) imaging are of diagnostic benefit in the identification and localization of cardiac masses.

## Restrictive Pericardial Disease

Usually seen as a complication of inflammatory diseases, restrictive pericardial disease is associated with thickening and fibrosis of the pericardium. The parietal and visceral pericardial layers may become adhered, obliterating the pericardial space. The pericardium loses elasticity and becomes less compliant or may even constrict in more advanced cases. Inflammatory processes, which may result in restrictive pericarditis, include chronic septic pericarditis, neoplasia, or recurrent idiopathic hemorrhagic pericardial effusion. The decreased compliance of the pericardium decreases normal diastolic filling of the ventricles, primarily the right ventricle. The increased diastolic pressures may result in right-sided congestive heart failure.

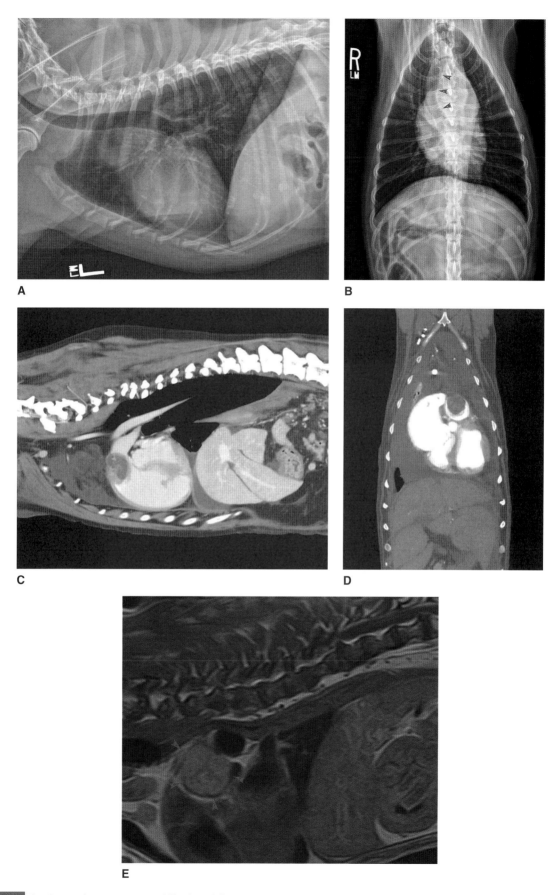

**FIGURE 18.52** (**A,B**) Heart base tumors are difficult to differentiate from right atrial and auricular masses on radiographs and may be recognized as soft tissue opaque masses at the base of the cardiac silhouette, causing focal rightward (blue arrowheads) and/or dorsal displacement of the trachea. Similar to right atrial and/or auricular masses, heart base masses may also be difficult to recognize on echocardiography. (**C,D**) Computed tomography provides a sensitive evaluation of heart base masses. (**E**) Magnetic resonance imaging can also be used to identify heart base masses (blue arrowheads).

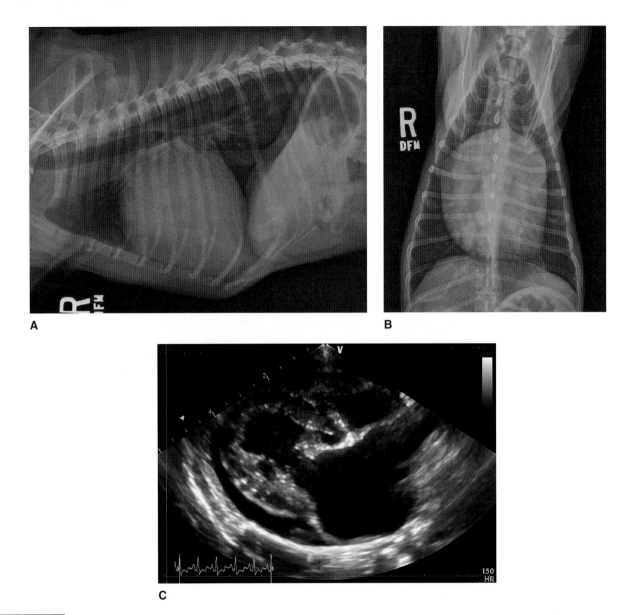

A

B

C

**FIGURE 18.53** (**A,B**) On thoracic radiographs, the cardiac silhouette is enlarged with a globoid appearance. The cardiac silhouette is homogeneously soft tissue opaque with decreased conspicuity of the overlying pulmonary vessels. (**C**) Echocardiography is the most convenient noninvasive method of identifying and subjectively quantifying pericardial effusion. In addition, it can support cardiac tamponade (pericardial pressures exceed right atrial and ventricular pressures) with right atrial and right ventricular diastolic free wall collapse.

Radiographic findings are nonspecific. Signs of right-sided congestive heart failure may be identified on thoracic radiographs without overt evidence of cardiomegaly.

Cardiac catheterization is required to confirm a diagnosis consistent with a restrictive pericarditis (step up in pressures within the right atrium and ventricle).

**Pneumopericardium** Pneumopericardium is the rare infiltration of air within the pericardial sac. Pneumopericardium may be a consequence of trauma, tracheal rupture, or surgery due to excessive positive pressure ventilation or abdominal surgery in animals with PPDH.

Air within the pericardial sac results in separation of the parietal and visceral layers of the epicardium with increased contrast of the cardiac structures (Figure 18.54).

## Pulmonary and Systemic Hypertension

**Pulmonary Hypertension** Pulmonary hypertension is due to increased pulmonary vascular resistance secondary to underlying lower airway disease or pulmonary artery disease or chronic mitral valve disease. Resultant increased pulmonary arterial pressures hinder normal emptying of the right ventricle and cause an increase in right ventricular pressure and concentric hypertrophy. Reduced cardiac output through pulmonary circulation results in hypoxemia and a compensatory increase in heart rate. Right-sided cardiac overload and distension of the vena cava precede the development of ascites and pleural effusion in more advanced cases with right-sided congestive heart

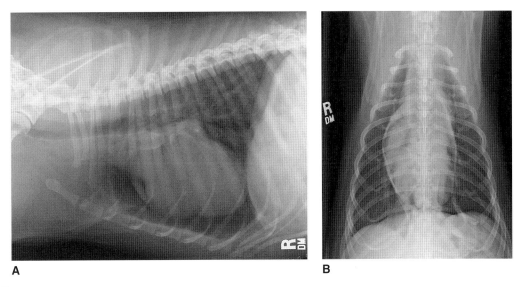

**FIGURE 18.54** (**A,B**) Pneumopericardium is characterized by the presence of gas within the pericardial sac, resulting in separation of the parietal and visceral layers of the epicardium with increased contrast of the cardiac structures.

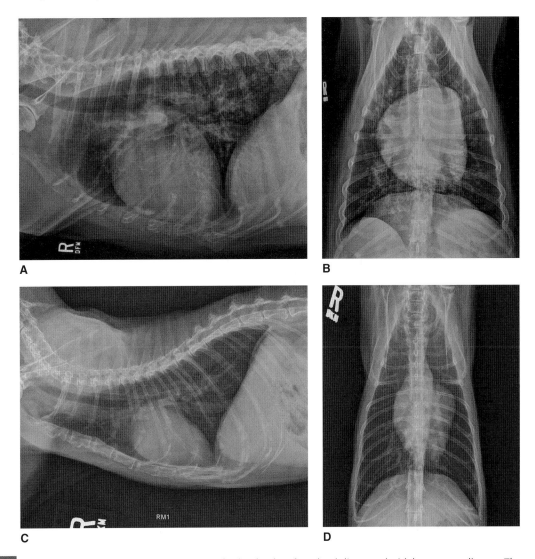

**FIGURE 18.55** Right lateral and ventrodorsal projections of a dog (**A,B**) and cat (**C,D**) diagnosed with heartworm disease. The cardiac silhouette is enlarged with rounding of the right cranial and lateral margin due to the presence of right cardiac chamber enlargement. A large bulge at the 2 o'clock position along the cardiac silhouette is suggestive of main pulmonary artery enlargement and is associated with enlargement, tortuosity, blunting, and mineralization of the lobar pulmonary arteries. A bronchial pattern combined with an unstructured interstitial pulmonary pattern and nodules is compatible with the presence of a eosinophilic bronchopneumopathy and granulomas. The nodules could also represent end-on enlarged pulmonary arteries. Right-sided pressure overload may result in right heart failure, characterized by the presence of caudal vena cava distension, hepatomegaly due to congestion, and ascites.

failure. Right heart failure due to pathologic processes resulting in pulmonary hypertension is known as *cor pulmonale*. Common causes include:

- heartworm (Figure 18.55)
- pulmonary thromboembolism (Figure 18.56)
- primary pulmonary/lower airway diseases (Figure 18.57)
- degenerative mitral valve disease (Figure 18.58).

**Systemic Hypertension** Systemic hypertension is most clinically significant with mitral regurgitation. Primary causes of hypertension are rare. Most commonly, systemic hypertension results from underlying renal diseases due to dysregulation of the renin-angiotensin-aldosterone system (RAAS) resulting in retention of sodium and water, thereby increasing systemic blood pressure. Increased intraglomerular pressures may result in irreversible renal damage. Other secondary

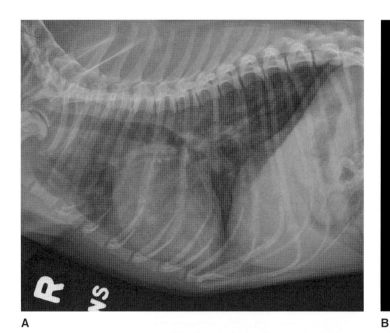

**A**

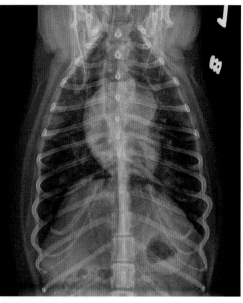

**B**

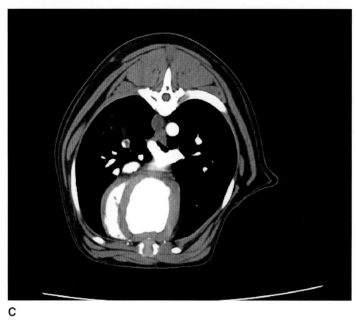

**C**

**FIGURE 18.56** Pulmonary thromboembolism may be a sequela of various disease entities, such as heartworm disease, hypercoagulability from underlying disseminated pulmonary thromboembolism, pituitary-dependent hyperadrenocorticism or other systemic diseases, and neoplasia. On radiographs (**A,B**), a predominantly peripherally distributed and multifocal unstructured interstitial to alveolar pattern is recognized in the acute stages due to congestion. If complete occlusion of the pulmonary arteries is present, regions of oligemia may be present. Computed tomography (**C**) allows direct visualization of the pulmonary thromboembolisms which are best identified during the arterial phase. With chronicity, pulmonary thromboemboli may increase in attenuation and mineralize; therefore, identification may be more difficult on postcontrast images.

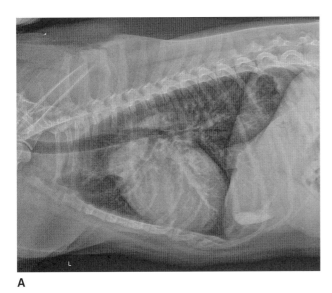
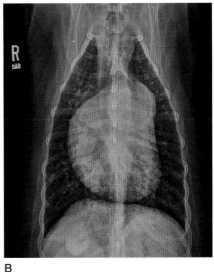

**A**

**B**

**FIGURE 18.57**   (**A,B**) The presence of a bronchial pattern in patients with respiratory signs raises concerns for bronchitis of allergic, inflammatory, or infectious etiologies. If chronic, evidence of pulmonary hypertension characterized by the presence of right-sided cardiomegaly, along with main (red arrowheads) and lobar pulmonary artery enlargement, may ensue. In this dog, there was a bronchial and an unstructured interstitial pulmonary pattern present. Even though the central pulmonary arteries are enlarged, the dog was negative for all heartworm tests. Severe pulmonary hypertension was noted on echocardiography. In dogs with chronic pulmonary fibrosis (West Highland white terriers), pulmonary hypertension can develop over time, resulting in right-sided cardiomegaly and main pulmonary artery enlargement.

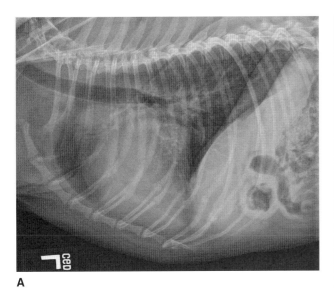
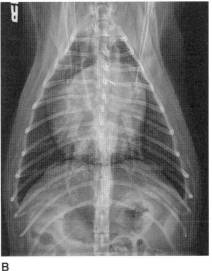

**A**

**B**

**FIGURE 18.58**   (**A,B**) The presence of right-sided cardiomegaly in this dog with concurrent presence of left-sided cardiomegaly and a history of prior cardiogenic pulmonary edema should raise concern for pulmonary hypertension secondary to DMVD, especially if associated with the presence of main and lobar pulmonary artery enlargement. These later radiographic changes do not have to be present in dogs with chronic DMVD and pulmonary hypertension.

causes of systemic hypertension include hyperadrenocorticism, hypothyroidism, hyperaldosteronism, diabetes mellitus or pheochromocytoma.

# Summary

The cardiac structures, pulmonary vessels, and great vessels are an integral component of interpretation of the normal thorax. The interpretation paradigm presented in this chapter should aid in the review of thoracic radiographs of the dog and cat. An understanding of the different phases of the cardiac cycle and respiratory cycle, as well as species and breed differences, will impact the interpretation of these structures. Different dog breeds and their normal conformations as well as the appearance of the cardiac structures can be found at **http://media.news.health.ufl.edu/misc/vetmed/gvi/ DogBreeds.**

# References

1. Moon, M., Keene, B.W., Lessard, P., and Lee, J. (1993). Age related changes in the feline cardiac silhouette. *Vet. Radiol. Ultrasound* 34 (5): 315–320.

2. Buchanan, J.W. and Bücheler, J. (1995). Vertebral scale system to measure canine heart size in radiographs. *J. Am. Vet. Med. Assoc.* 206: 194–194.

3. Schwarz, T., Sullivan, M., Störk, C. et al. (2002). Aortic and cardiac mineralization in the dog. *Vet. Radiol. Ultrasound* 43 (5): 419–427.

4. Douglass, J.P., Berry, C., Thrall, D. et al. (2003). Radiographic features of aortic bulb/valve mineralization in 20 dogs. *Vet. Radiol. Ultrasound* 44 (1): 20–27.

5. Litster, A.L. and Buchanan, J.W. (2000). Vertebral scale system to measure heart size in radiographs of cats. *J. Am. Vet. Med. Assoc.* 216 (2): 210–214.

6. Mostafa, A. and Berry, C.R. (2017). Radiographic assessment of the cardiac silhouette in clinically normal large-and small-breed dogs. *Am. J. Vet. Res.* 78 (2): 168–177.

7. Bahr, R. (2018). Canine and feline cardiovascular system. In: *Textbook of Veterinary Diagnostic Radiology*, 7e (ed. D.E. Thrall). St Louis, MO: Elsevier.

8. Jepsen-Grant, K., Pollard, R.E., and Johnson, L.R. (2013). Vertebral heart scores in eight dog breeds. *Vet. Radiol. Ultrasound* 54 (1): 3–8.

9. Puccinelli, C., Citi, S., Vezzosi, T. et al. (2021). A radiographic study of breed-specific vertebral heart score and vertebral left atrial size in Chihuahuas. *Vet. Radiol. Ultrasound* 62: 20–26.

10. Lamb, C.R., Wikeley, H., Boswood, A., and Pfeiffer, D. (2001). Use of breed-specific ranges for the vertebral heart scale as an aid to the radiographic diagnosis of cardiac disease in dogs. *Vet. Rec.* 148 (23): 707–711.

11. de Fonsecapinto, A.C.B. and Iwasaki, M. (2002). Radiographic methods in the cardiac evaluation dogs. *Vet. Noticias* 8 (1): 67–75.

12. Gulanber, E.G. (2005). Vertebral scale system to measure heart size in thoracic radiographs of Turkish shepherd (Kangal) dogs. *Turkish J. Vet. Anim. Sci.* 29 (3): 723–726.

13. Bavegems, V., van Caelenberg, A., Duchateau, L. et al. (2005). Vertebral heart size ranges specific for whippets. *Vet. Radiol. Ultrasound* 46 (5): 400–403.

14. Marin, L.M., Brown, J., McBrien, C. et al. (2007). Vertebral heart size in retired racing greyhounds. *Vet. Radiol. Ultrasound* 48 (4): 332–334.

15. Kraetschmer, S., Ludwig, K., Meneses, F. et al. (2008). Vertebral heart scale in the beagle dog. *J. Small Anim. Pract.* 49 (5): 240–243.

16. Birks, R., Fine, D., Leach, S. et al. (2017). Breed-specific vertebral heart scale for the dachshund. *J. Am. Anim. Hosp. Assoc.* 53 (2): 73–79.

17. Azevedo, G.M., Pessoa, G., Sousa, F., and Moura, L. (2016). Comparative study of the vertebral heart scale (VHS) and the cardiothoracic ratio (CTR) in healthy poodle breed dogs. *Acta Sci. Vet.* 44 (1): 7.

18. Bodh, D., Hoque, M., Saxena, A. et al. (2016). Vertebral scale system to measure heart size in thoracic radiographs of Indian Spitz, Labrador retriever and mongrel dogs. *Vet. World* 9 (4): 371.

19. Ghadiri, A.R., Avizeh, R., and Fazli, G.H. (2010). Vertebral heart scale of common large breeds of dogs in Iran. *Iran. J. Vet. Med* 4: 107–111.

20. Cardoso, M.J., Caludino, J.L., and Melussi, M. (2011). Measurement of heart size by VHS (vertebral heart size) method in healthy American pit bull terrier. *Ciência Rura* 41.1: 127–131.

21. Kumar, V. et al. (2011). Vertebral heart scale system to measure heart size in thoracic radiographs of Indian mongrel dog. *Indian J. Vet. Surg.*.

22. Gugjoo, M.B., Hoque, M., Saxena, A. et al. (2013). Vertebral scale system to measure heart size in dogs in thoracic radiographs. *Adv. Anim. Vet. Sci.* 1: 1–4.

23. Almeida, G., Almeida, M., Santos, A. et al. (2015). Vertebral heart size in healthy Belgian Malinois dogs. *J. Vet. Adv.* 5 (12): 1176–1180.

# CHAPTER 19

# Feline Thorax

**Martha M. Larson[1] and Clifford R. Berry[2]**

[1] Department of Small Animal Clinical Sciences, VA-MD College of Veterinary Medicine, Virginia Tech, Blacksburg, VA, USA
[2] Department of Molecular Biomedical Sciences, College of Veterinary Medicine, North Carolina State University, Raleigh, NC, USA

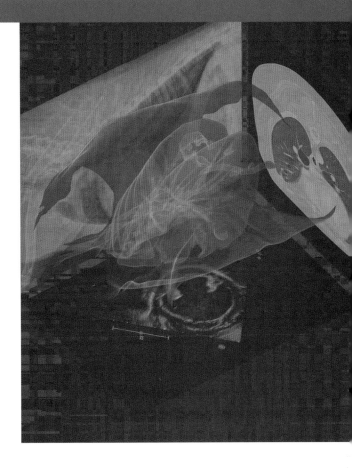

## Overview

The feline thorax is presented in this separate chapter because cats are not small dogs, and have their own set of idiosyncratic "rules of the road." All the rules and guidelines established for the dog do not fit for the cat and thereby normal anatomy, variants, and common thoracic abnormalities are presented in this chapter even though feline examples have been presented in the previous chapters.

## Feline Thorax Interpretation Paradigm

The same interpretation paradigm as set forth in the previous chapters will be used. The paradigm will still work from the outside in, providing the clinician and student with a framework to work through the extrathoracic structures, the pleural space, the pulmonary parenchyma and vasculature, and the mediastinum.

The overall shape of the feline thorax is narrower ventro-dorsally and more elongated (in a craniocaudal direction) compared with the dog, giving the feline thorax a more triangular appearance (Figure 19.1). The cardiac silhouette has a more acute angle relative to the sternum on lateral projections compared with the dog. Radiographs should be made on peak inspiration as noted for the dog (Figure 19.2).

## Extrathoracic Structures

Cranially, the thorax extends to the level of the thoracic inlet at the level of the manubrium ventrally, first ribs laterally, and cervicothoracic spinal junction dorsally. The diaphragm marks the caudal extension of the thorax. Ventrally, the diaphragmatic cupula extends cranially to the level of T8–T10. Dorsally,

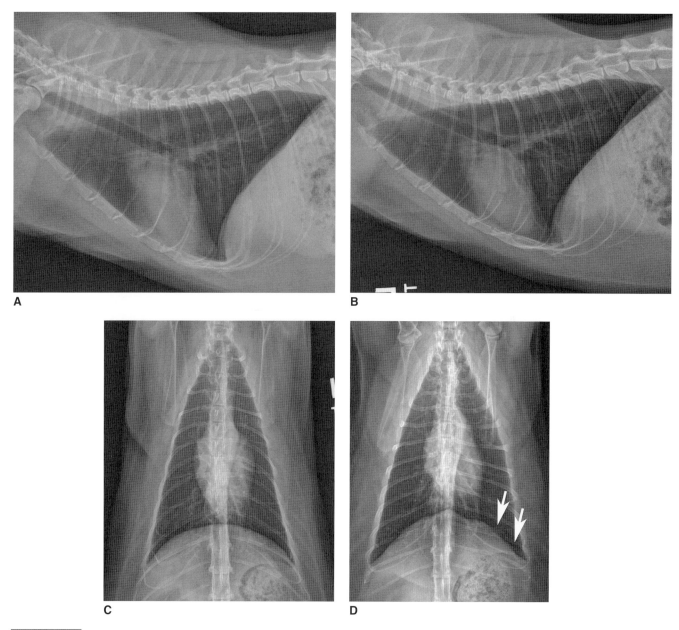

**FIGURE 19.1** Normal feline thorax including right lateral (**A**), left lateral (**B**), ventrodorsal (**C**), and dorsoventral (**D**) images. On the dorsoventral image, there is mild hyperinflation and diaphragmatic tenting (white arrows) noted on the left side.

the diaphragmatic crura extend to the level of T13–L1 on peak inspiration and attach to the ventral border of L3 and L4. On right versus left lateral radiographs, minimal separation of the right and left crura is noted, unlike that seen in the dog.

The 13 pairs of ribs protect the normal thoracic wall [1–3]. The first pair of ribs is attached to the manubrium whereas ribs 2 through 9 attach to the intersternebral disc spaces of the sternum. The costal portions of the ribs will mineralize in cats as in dogs; however, the mineralization is often multipartite and thin lined rather than solid and complete. Congenital anomalies of the sternebrae are common, often with fusion or decrease in number compared to the normal eight sternebrae (the manubrium is the first, xiphoid process is the eighth).

Pectus excavatum is an uncommon congenital sternal anomaly resulting in dorsal deviation of the caudal sternum and ventrodorsal narrowing of the thorax noted on lateral radiographs [4, 5] (Figure 19.3).

## Pleural Space

The pleural space is a potential space located between the parietal and visceral pleura, and is not visualized on normal thoracic radiographs. The pleural space is closed cranially and caudally, but there are mediastinal fenestrations connecting the right and left pleural spaces. The parietal pleura is a mesothelial

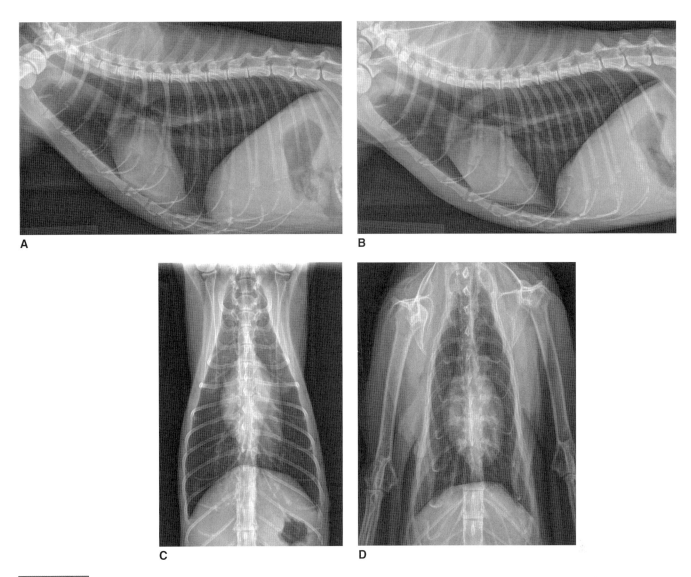

**FIGURE 19.2**   Right lateral (**A**), left lateral (**B**), and ventrodorsal (**C**) radiographs from a normal middle-aged cat taken on peak inspiration. A ventrodorsal "humanoid" radiograph where the thoracic limbs are pulled in a caudal direction is shown in (**D**). Note the ability to visualize the entire extent of the right and left cranial lung lobes without the superimposition of the scapulae in this image.

lining located along the thoracic wall, diaphragm, and mediastinum; the visceral pleura is a mesothelial lining around the pulmonary parenchyma. A small amount of lubricating fluid allows the visceral and parietal pleura to slide against each other during respiration.

The pleural space extends between lung lobes, creating pleural fissure lines between the right cranial and middle lung lobes, the right middle and caudal lung lobes, and the left cranial and caudal lung lobes (Figure 19.4). Occasionally, pleural fissure lines will be seen as linear opacities due to pleural thickening from fibrosis. The longus coli and hypaxial muscles are located ventral to the thoracic spine, creating a soft tissue opacity between the caudodorsal lungs and spine. This can be mistaken for pleural effusion on peak inspiration on lateral images (Figure 19.5).

# Pulmonary Parenchyma and Anatomy

There are six lung lobes present in the cat, as in the dog (Figure 19.4). The right lung is divided into right cranial, middle, caudal and accessory lung lobes. The left lung is divided into left cranial (cranial and caudal subsegments) and caudal lung lobes. The trachea terminates into the right and left principal bronchi. The right cranial lung lobe bronchus is the first branch off the right principal bronchus and extends cranially. The right middle lung lobe bronchus courses ventrally over the cardiac silhouette, best seen on the left lateral radiograph. The right caudal lobe bronchus continues caudal and dorsal.

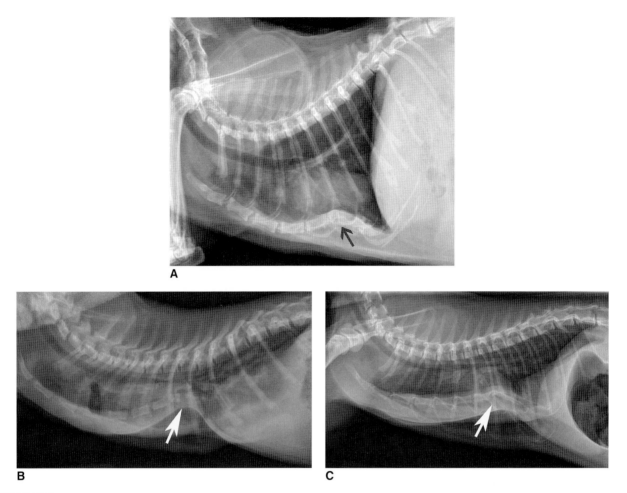

**FIGURE 19.3** Three right lateral radiographic images from different cats with a pectus excuvatum deformity of the sternum (white arrows).

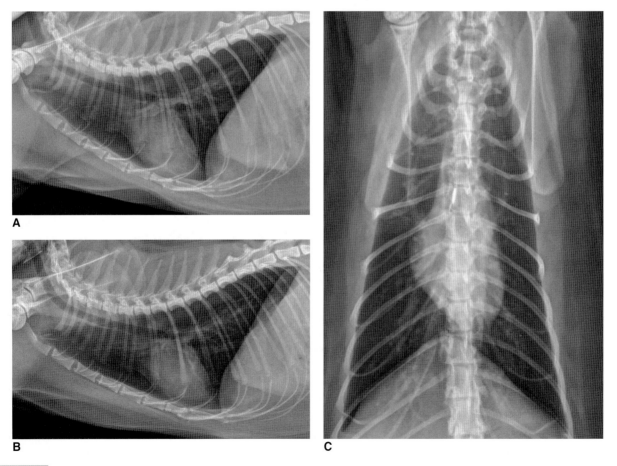

**FIGURE 19.4** Right lateral (**A**), left lateral (**B**), and ventrodorsal (**C**) images from a middle-aged cat. The radiographs are considered normal. The pulmonary parenchyma, cardiac silhouette, mediastinum, and pleural space are all normal.

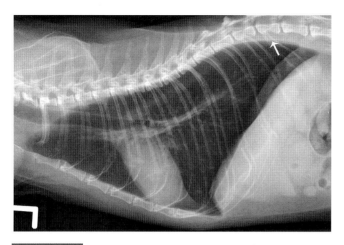

**FIGURE 19.5**   Peak inspiration, lateral radiograph from a normal cat. The caudodorsal soft tissue opacity (white arrow) is the ventral hypaxial musculature and should not be mistaken for pleural fluid.

The accessory lung lobe bronchus originates along the ventromedial aspect of the right caudal lung lobe bronchus. The left cranial lung lobe bronchus extends ventral and cranial away from the left principal bronchus. Within several millimeters of its origin, it bifurcates into cranial and caudal subsegment bronchi. The cranial subsegment bronchus extends cranially; the caudal subsegment bronchus extends ventrally. The left caudal bronchus extends caudal and dorsal into the left caudal lung lobe.

The pulmonary parenchyma consists of alveoli, interstitial tissue, bronchial walls, and pulmonary vasculature. Background opacity of the normal lung is primarily due to pulmonary arteries and veins, with the bronchi and interstitium contributing to a lesser extent. The small airways will not be visualized in the lung periphery although larger airways will be seen centrally. The fourth- and fifth-generation vessels (pulmonary arteries and veins) can be seen in the peripheral portions of the lungs. The descending thoracic aorta and the caudal vena cava are well visualized due to surrounding lung. The plica vena cava of the accessory lung lobe wraps around the caudal vena cava, which enters the right side of the diaphragm at the caval foramen. The descending thoracic aorta enters the abdomen at the level of the aortic hiatus in a central position between the right and left diaphragmatic crura (Figure 19.6).

The pulmonary arteries lie dorsal to the cranial bronchi on the lateral view, with the corresponding pulmonary veins located ventral to the bronchus (Figure 19.6). They should be approximately equal in size, and smaller than the diameter of the proximal third of the fourth rib [6]. On ventrodorsal or dorsoventral radiographs, the pulmonary artery is located lateral to the caudal bronchus with the corresponding pulmonary vein located medial. The pulmonary artery and vein are typically equal in size and the vessels are smaller than the right and left ninth ribs where they intersect on ventrodorsal/dorsoventral projections. Caudal lobar vessels are best seen on a dorsoventral projection when surrounded by more fully expanded caudal lung lobes and are magnified.

# Mediastinum

The mediastinum is a true open space between the right and left pleural cavities. The cranial mediastinum connects to the deep fascia of the neck, while the caudal mediastinum communicates with the retroperitoneum via the aortic hiatus. The mediastinum is incomplete in cats and dogs such that a transudate and modified transudate may pass through mediastinal fenestrations, and will present as a bilateral pleural effusion. In the case of exudative effusion, the pleural fluid may not cross the mediastinum easily, and may be unilateral.

The mediastinum can be divided into cranial, middle, and caudal portions. In the dorsal aspect of the cranial mediastinum are a collection of vessels, esophagus, nerves, and cranial mediastinal lymph nodes. The sternal lymph nodes and internal thoracic vessels are in the cranioventral mediastinal reflection between the ventral aspects of the left and right cranial lung lobes (Figure 19.7). The sternal lymph nodes (not normally visible) are located dorsal to the cranial aspect of the third sternebra, and drain the pericardium, cranial aspect of the diaphragm and the abdominal cavity [7, 8]. In young cats, the thymus is located in the ventral aspect of the cranial mediastinum. The thymus will enlarge until the age of maturity, then involutes and will be no longer visualized (Figure 19.8) [8, 9].

The trachea extends through the cervical region into the thoracic cavity at the thoracic inlet. The trachea does not deviate as dramatically from the thoracic spine as in dogs, but does angle ventrally to the base of the cardiac silhouette. The trachea terminates at the carina typically located at the fifth or sixth intercostal space. The normal thoracic tracheal diameter in the cat has been reported as 5.5 mm or 18% of the thoracic inlet (20% in normal Persian cats) [10]. The esophagus, vagus, and phrenic nerves, other cranial mediastinal vasculature (cranial vena cava, left subclavian, aortic arch, brachiocephalic trunk), and lymph nodes (cranial mediastinal dorsally and sternal ventrally) are not routinely visualized.

The descending thoracic aorta, esophagus, and tracheobronchial lymph nodes are located in the dorsal aspect of the middle mediastinum. The esophagus and tracheobronchial lymph nodes are not seen on normal thoracic radiographs. There are three primary tracheobronchial lymph nodes or lymphocenters. The right tracheobronchial lymph node is found medial to the right cranial lung lobe bronchus and lateral to the trachea. The left tracheobronchial lymph node is found medial to the cranial subsegment of the left cranial lung lobe bronchus and lateral to the trachea. The central tracheobronchial lymph node is found between the two caudal lobar bronchi just caudal to the bifurcation of the carina. These nodes are located slightly more cranial than those in the dog, and receive afferent lymphatics from the lungs [9].

The cardiac silhouette is located in the ventral middle mediastinum, and in the cat measures between 2 and 2.5 intercostal spaces on the lateral radiograph. It has an elongated, "almond" shape when compared with the dog. The vertebral heart scale can be used to assess cardiac size, and in the normal

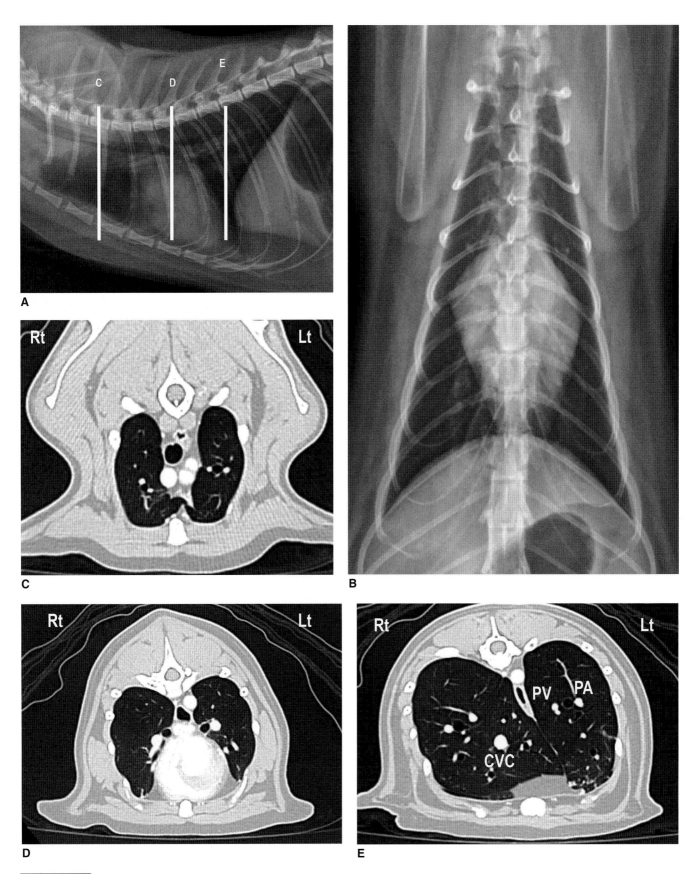

**FIGURE 19.6** Right lateral (**A**) and ventrodorsal (**B**) radiographs showing the relationship of the pulmonary vessels to the central bronchi. Image (**A**) shows the transverse slices for the three additional transverse CT slices (with contrast medium) showing anatomy of lungs relative to cranial, middle, and caudal thorax (**C–E**). The pulmonary veins are located ventral (lateral images) and central (dorsoventral or ventrodorsal image). The pulmonary arteries are located dorsal (lateral view) and lateral (ventrodorsal or dorsoventral views) relative to the principal bronchi. PA, pulmonary artery; PV, pulmonary vein; CVC, caudal vena cava; Rt, right side of the thorax; Lt, left side of the thorax.

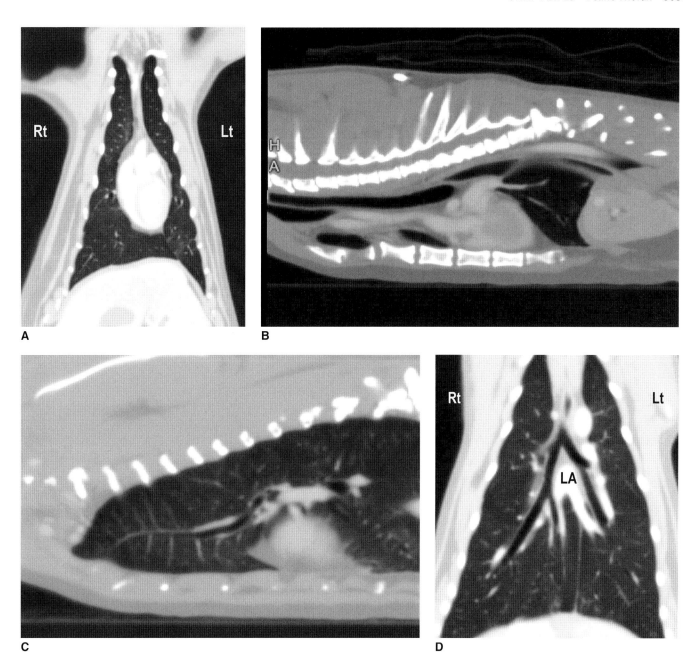

**FIGURE 19.7**   Four different CT images (post contrast administration) from a normal feline thorax. (**A**) Dorsal plane image showing the cranioventral mediastinum between the right and left cranial lung lobes as well as the caudoventral mediastinal reflection at the lateral-most aspect of the accessory lung lobe (extends from the apex of the heart to the diaphragm along the left caudal thorax). (**B**) Central sagittal plane reconstructed image documenting the sagittal structures of the mediastinum. Dorsal to the third sternebral segment is the internal thoracic vessels (cranial) and the sternal lymph node (caudal) seen as separate soft tissue attenuating structures. (**C**) Sagittal plane image of the right cranial lung lobe with the pulmonary artery being dorsal to the bronchus and the pulmonary vein (ventral and partially seen). (**D**) Dorsal plane image of the dorsal thorax at the heart base documenting the pulmonary veins entering the left atrium (LA). These vessels are central or medial relative to the principal bronchi and caudal bronchi. The accessory lung lobe bronchus is seen originating from right caudal lobe bronchus. The pulmonary arteries are lateral to the right and left caudal bronchi.

cat measures 7.5 ± 0.3 on the lateral image and 8.1v ± 0.45 on DV/VD projections (Figure 19.9) [11–13]. The apex of the cardiac silhouette is typically separated from the cupula on both lateral and ventrodorsal projections. On the ventrodorsal radiograph, the apex of the feline cardiac silhouette is typically to the left of the midline. In geriatric cats, the cardiac silhouette may align more horizontally along the sternum on the lateral projections.

In addition, the aortic arch may elongate and become tortuous, or "redundant" (Figure 19.10). This creates an aortic "knob" on the ventrodorsal image just to the left of the midline. The cause of these changes has not been determined. However, thickening of the tunica intima and media has been shown histologically in aged cats. It is hypothesized that these changes in the aortic arch and descending aorta will shift the base of the

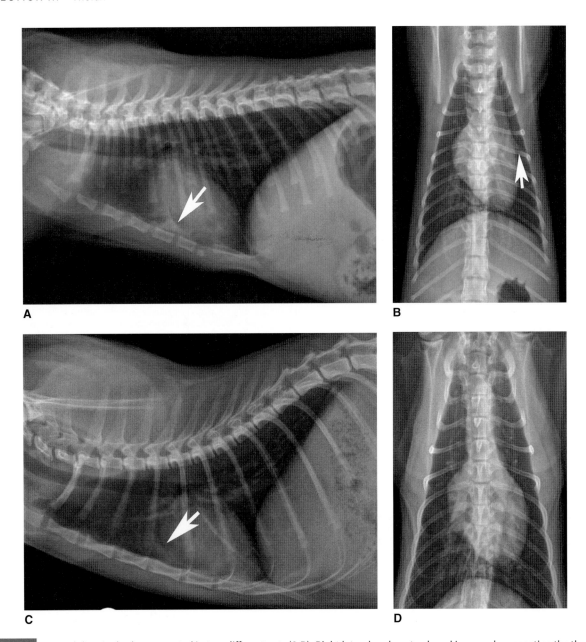

**A**

**B**

**C**

**D**

FIGURE 19.8 Normal thymic shadows as noted in two different cats (**A,B**). Right lateral and ventrodorsal images documenting the thymic soft tissue on both images (right lateral). More commonly, the thymus is seen in the cat on just the lateral view (right lateral more so than left lateral) as noted in the second cat (**C,D**; white arrow on the right lateral view).

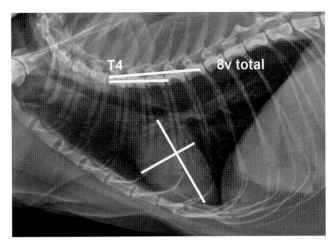

T4    8v total

FIGURE 19.9 The vertebral heart score is calculated on this thoracic radiograph (right lateral view). The short axis and long axis of the cardiac silhouette are drawn and measured against the thoracic vertebrae starting at T4. In this cat, the VHS = 8 vertebrae (normal).

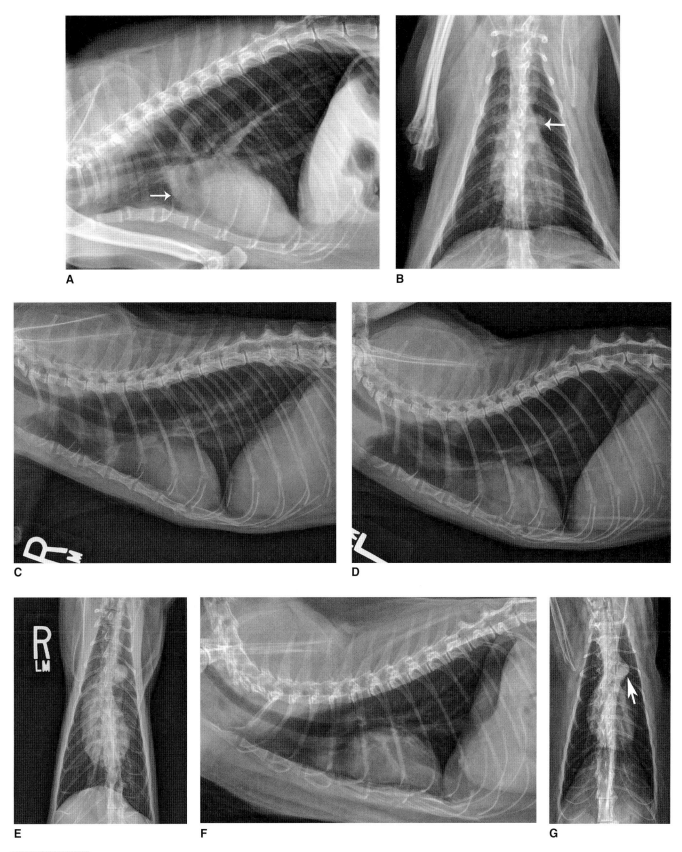

**FIGURE 19.10**   Four different aged cats documenting varying degrees of a geriatric thorax (cat 1 – **A,B**; cat 2 – **C–E**; cat 3 – **F,G**; cat 4 – **H,I**). There is cranioventral rotation of the cardiac silhouette ("lazy heart") and redundant aortic arch (white arrows) and descending thoracic aorta. Excessive aortic changes have been seen in cats with systemic hypertension in the authors' experience (**C–E**).

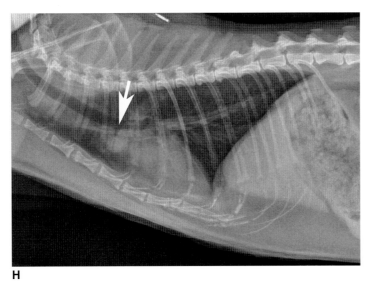

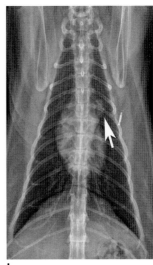

**FIGURE 19.10** (Continued)

cardiac silhouette into a more cranioventral position [14]. In obese cats, fat deposition around the pericardium creates the appearance of cardiomegaly, especially on ventrodorsal or dorsoventral images (Figure 19.11).

The descending thoracic aorta is seen in the dorsal aspect of the caudal mediastinum. The azygous vein and thoracic lymphatic ducts run adjacent to the aorta, but are too small to be seen. The esophagus enters the abdomen just to the left of the central diaphragm at the level of the esophageal hiatus. Ventrally, a mediastinal reflection between the accessory lung lobe and the left caudal lung lobe is present, extending from the apex of the heart to the left side of the diaphragm. This is best visualized on the ventrodorsal image but is less commonly seen in the cat (Figure 19.12).

# Extrathoracic Abnormalities

Rib fractures (most commonly due to trauma) are a common cause of extrathoracic abnormalities. The appearance will be variable [15]. A flail thorax is a condition where multiple contiguous segmental rib fractures are present (potentially along with sternal or thoracic vertebral anomalies, pleural effusion, pneumothorax, or pulmonary contusions). Paradoxical motion of the flail segment results in outward motion on expiration and inward motion on inspiration. Nontraumatic rib fractures can occur with chronic pleural, pulmonary or mediastinal diseases [15, 16]. This condition is called a *thoracic bellows effect* (Figure 19.13).

Rib tumors are rare in the cat [15, 17–19]. Expansile, proliferative, and lytic lesions often result in an extrapleural sign and/or a pleural effusion. The most common rib tumor in the cat is osteosarcoma. Metastatic lesions to the ribs have also been reported with pulmonary carcinomas and plasma cell tumors (multiple myeloma) (Figure 19.14).

The most common congenital diaphragmatic abnormality in the cat is a peritoneo-pericardial diaphragmatic hernia. In this condition, the central portion of the diaphragm (*septum transversum*) fails to fuse with the pleuroperitoneal and pleuropericardial folds, resulting in a cranioventral opening in the diaphragm [20–23]. The condition results in variable abdominal contents herniating cranially into the pericardial sac. Commonly this is an incidental finding. On lateral radiographs, a short curvilinear opacity between the caudal pericardium and the cranial diaphragm, called the *dorsal pericardial-peritoneal mesothelial remnant*, can be seen (Figure 19.15) [21]. The most common acquired diaphragmatic abnormality is diaphragmatic rupture secondary to trauma (Figure 19.16) [24–27]. Depending on the abdominal contents cranially displaced and size of diaphragm tear, the degree of contralateral mediastinal shift and pleural space changes will vary. Pleural effusion may be present with both acute and chronic hernias.

# Pleural Space Abnormalities

Pleural space abnormalities include pleural effusion and pneumothorax. Fluid in the pleural space results in a widened, radiopaque pleural space, retraction of the lung lobes from the thoracic wall (resulting in a scalloped appearance), and the presence of multiple pleural fissure lines. A mild pleural effusion will result in border effacement of the ventral aspect of the cardiac silhouette and cranioventral aspect of the diaphragm (Figure 19.17). With more severe effusion, there is an increase in the retraction of the lung lobes with fluid separation of parietal and visceral pleural surfaces on both lateral and VD/DV views. There is widening of the pleural fissure lines adjacent to the thoracic wall with a convex curvilinear soft tissue opacity extending toward the pulmonary

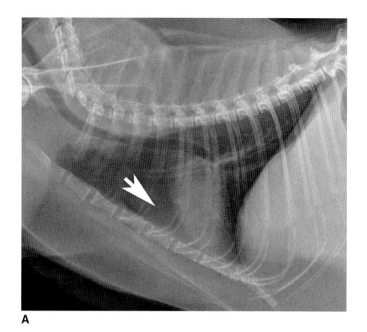

A

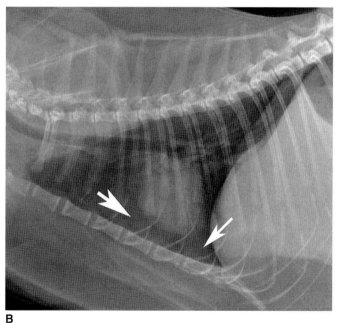

B

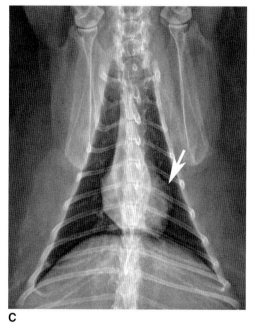

C

**FIGURE 19.11** Fat deposition around the cardiac silhouette (white arrows) in this three-view thorax (**A** – right lateral, **B** – left lateral, **C** – ventrodorsal) in an obese cat. On the ventrodorsal view, the arrow denotes the outer margin of the fat whereas the inner curved border represents the actual cardiac silhouette.

hilum. These fissure lines occur in the specific locations as noted previously.

The lungs take on a leaf-like or triangular shape as they become atelectatic. This will also result in an overall increased pulmonary opacity due to an unstructured interstitial pattern. In cats, as pleural fluid progresses, it is very common for lung lobes to collapse with only a single air bronchogram extending into the completely atelectatic lung lobe (Figure 19.18). The borders of the atelectatic lung lobe will not be visualized due to border effacement with the pleural fluid. Severe pleural effusion results in the cardiac silhouette and inflated lung lobes

appearing to "float in the fluid" on the lateral projections. The carina will still be located at the level of the fifth or sixth intercostal space, but the trachea may be elevated [28].

With the cat in dorsal recumbency (ventrodorsal view), the cardiac silhouette can be visualized as pleural fluid tends to accumulate dorsally in the paravertebral regions. When the cat is in ventral recumbency (dorsoventral view), the cardiac silhouette cannot be visualized due to border effacement with the ventrally distributed fluid. On lateral projections, a radiolucent line can sometimes be seen ventral to the cardiac silhouette representing subpericardial fat.

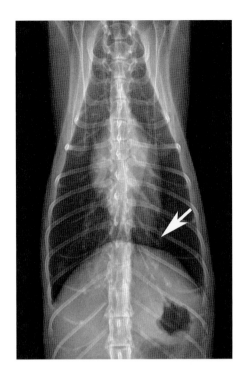

**FIGURE 19.12** Ventrodorsal image from a normal cat. The cranioventral mediastinal reflection is noted to be on the midline when compared with dogs (just to the left of midline). A thin radiopaque line represents the caudoventral mediastinal reflection (white arrow). This represents the leftward-most extent of the accessory lung lobe.

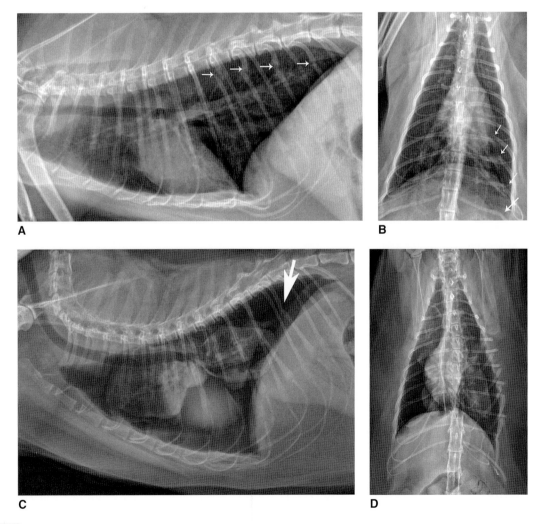

A

B

C

D

**FIGURE 19.13** Thoracic bellows effect noted in two different cats. The first cat (**A,B**) has chronic bronchial changes and rib fractures noted (white arrows). There is also sternal lymph node enlargement and mild cardiomegaly. The second cat (**C,D**) has a chronic chylothorax, restrictive pleuritis, moderate to severe pneumothorax, and multiple rib fractures (white arrow).

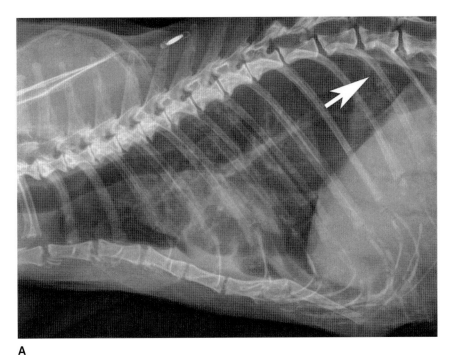

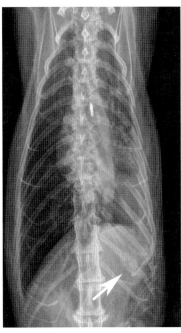

A

B

**FIGURE 19.14**    Multiple expansile lesions of the ribs are noted in this cat with metastatic urothelial carcinoma (white arrow). There is collapse of the left lung lobes with ill-defined masses consistent with pulmonary metastatic disease. In addition, pleural irregular margination is noted on the lateral radiograph consistent with pleural metastatic disease. All changes were confirmed at necropsy.

Unilateral pleural effusions are more common in cats than in dogs (Figure 19.19). The most common cause of a unilateral pleural effusion is pyothorax, most likely the result of a ventral pneumonia and transpleural localization of bacteria into the pleural space [29–31]. Other causes of exudative effusions include chylothorax, feline infectious peritonitis, hemorrhage or neoplastic effusions [28]. Chronic effusion can result in thickening of the visceral pleura surrounding lung lobes (*restrictive* or *fibrosing pleuritis*) [32–35]. This results in rounding of lung lobes and inability to fully inflate even after removal of pleural effusion. A pneumothorax may occur to fill in the empty space between incompletely inflated lung lobes and chest wall (Figure 19.20).

Pneumothorax results in radiolucent air between the visceral and parietal pleural surfaces so that the lung lobe appears radiopaque with surrounding radiolucent pleural space. Retraction and partial collapse of lung lobes and separation of the cardiac silhouette from the sternum can be seen. The more severe the pneumothorax, the more severe the lung lobe retraction will become (Figure 19.21), resulting in progressive atelectasis of the affected lobes. Pneumothorax is routinely bilateral. In the case of a tension pneumothorax, a progressive increase in the amount of pleural gas accumulates (one-way valve effect) as the cat breathes, resulting in a severe unilateral pneumothorax, contralateral mediastinal shift, flattening of the diaphragm on the affected side, and an increase in the diameter of the hemithorax involved (Figure 19.22). This condition is life-threatening and pleurocentesis/thoracic tube placement is required.

# Pulmonary Parenchymal Abnormalities

The pulmonary interpretation pattern has been previously reviewed in Chapter 16. A review of all the radiographic projections, and a determination of normal versus abnormal is still the first question. If abnormal, are the abnormalities radiolucent or radiopaque? Is the abnormality focal, multifocal, or generalized? If focal or multifocal, what lung lobes are involved and where in the lobe is the abnormality? The distribution of the abnormal opacity is essential in the differential diagnosis. A review of common diseases that cause or result in pulmonary changes will be described and illustrated.

A true generalized decrease in lung opacity in the cat is secondary to either hypovolemia or hyperinflation (Figure 19.23). Hyperinflation is usually associated with small airway disease such as feline asthma, where bronchoconstriction or thickening of the small airways restricts flow out of the alveoli and distal bronchioles. This results in progressive inflation of the lungs (up to a certain point) [36]. The diaphragmatic crura are displaced caudally to the level of L1–2 or beyond. On the ventrodorsal radiograph, diaphragmatic "tenting" (small diaphragmatic projections caused by pulling of the diaphragm against the costal attachment) may be visible (Figure 19.24).

Focal or multifocal areas of decreased opacity can be circular (oval) or lobar in appearance. Circular radiolucent focal or multifocal areas are commonly caused by bullae (secondary

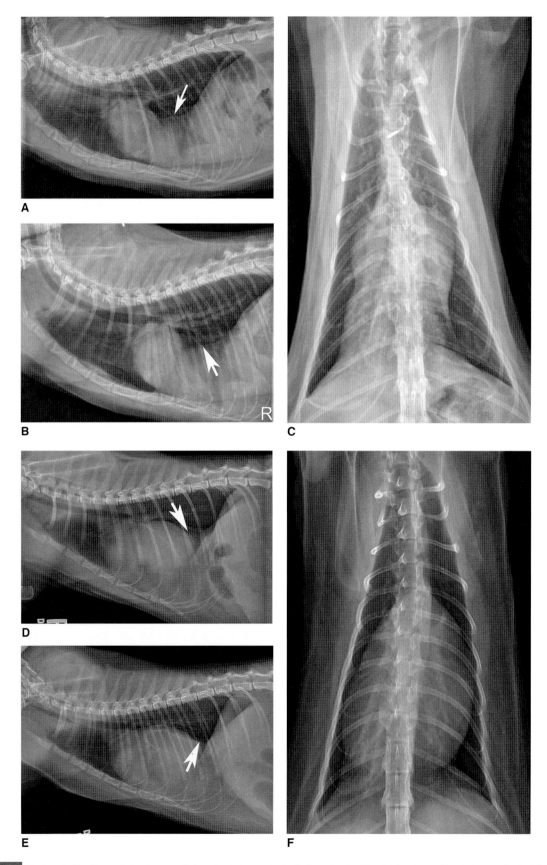

**FIGURE 19.15** Pericardial peritoneal diaphragmatic hernias in two cats, both found as incidental findings when being evaluated for metastatic disease. The first cat (**A** – right lateral, **B** – left lateral, **C** – ventrodorsal) has a soft tissue opaque structure noted caudal to the cardiac silhouette with cranial displacement of the cranial abdominal structures. A soft tissue opaque line is present ventral to the caudal vena cava that is called the dorsal peritoneopericardial mesothelial remnant (white arrow). In the second cat (**D** – right lateral, **E** – left lateral, **F** – ventrodorsal), the liver, gall bladder, and omentum are herniated cranially into the pericardial sac. The cardiac silhouette is markedly enlarged. The gastrointestinal tract is displaced cranially on all images. The dorsal peritoneopericardial mesothelial remnant is seen ventral to the caudal vena cava (white arrow) on the lateral images.

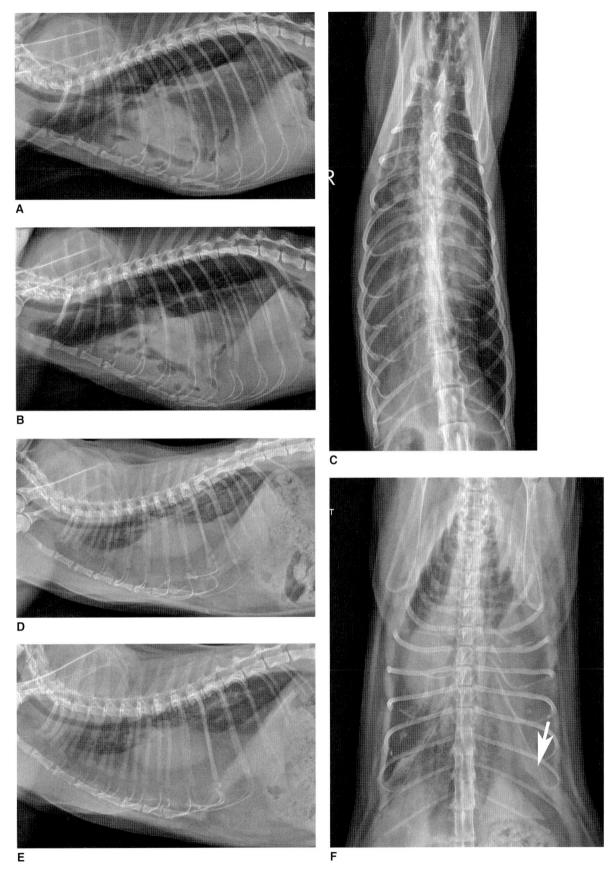

**FIGURE 19.16** Diaphragmatic rupture post trauma in two cats. In the first cat (**A** – right lateral, **B** – left lateral, **C** – ventrodorsal), there is a right-sided diaphragmatic rupture with leftward displacement of the cardiac silhouette and mediastinal structures. Small intestinal segments and soft tissue opaque structures are herniated into the right pleural space. In the second cat (**D** – right lateral, **E** – left lateral, **F** – ventrodorsal), there is a left-sided diaphragmatic rupture with cranial displacement of fat and soft tissue opaque structures including the spleen (white arrow). There is a rightward mediastinal shift of the cardiac silhouette and mediastinal structures. On the lateral images, there is primarily fat opacity noted (omentum) within the ventral thorax with dorsal displacement of the cardiac silhouette. There is a mild generalized unstructured pulmonary pattern consistent with atelectasis.

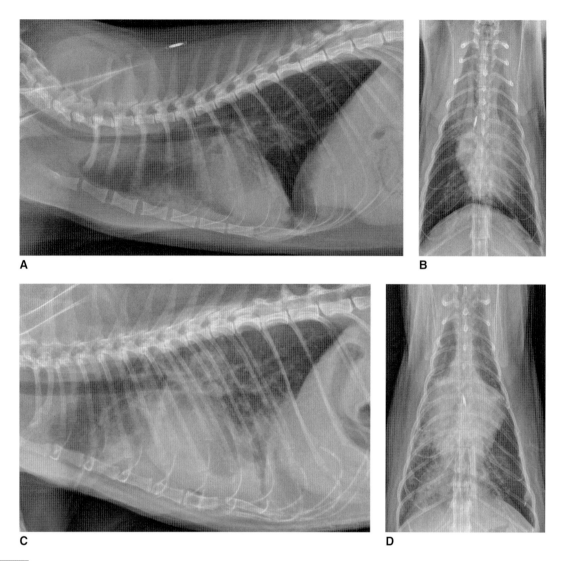

**FIGURE 19.17** Mild pleural effusion in two cats. In the first cat (**A** – right lateral, **B** – ventrodorsal), an increase in soft tissue opacity is noted cranial to the cardiac silhouette along the ventral cranial thorax on the right lateral. The cardiac silhouette is mildly enlarged and was determined to be a pleural effusion secondary to a primary cardiomyopathy. In the second cat (**C** – right lateral, **D** – ventrodorsal), there is border effacement of the cardiac silhouette noted on the lateral image. The cardiac silhouette is enlarged and there is an unstructured interstitial pulmonary pattern with a multifocal distribution. The trachea is elevated dorsally on the lateral radiograph. The radiographic changes were determined to be secondary to a primary cardiomyopathy.

to trauma), neoplasia, or parasitic granulomas (*Paragonimus kellicotti*; Figure 19.25). Lobar decreased opacity is usually secondary to pulmonary thromboembolism, although this is a rare finding in cats.

Atelectasis results in loss of normal lung volume and, depending on the degree of volume loss, can result in an unstructured interstitial (mild to moderate) or alveolar (severe) pulmonary pattern. Atelectasis may be secondary to pleural effusion/pneumothorax, prolonged recumbency, or bronchial obstruction. In the cat, the right middle lung lobe may collapse secondary to bronchial obstruction by a mucous plug, and is associated with asthma/bronchitis (Figure 19.26) [37, 38]. When totally collapsed, the right middle lobe appears as a curvilinear soft tissue opacity superimposed over the cardiac

silhouette on the left lateral radiograph. On the ventrodorsal radiograph, the collapsed right middle lung lobe appears as a small soft tissue opaque triangle that border effaces the right side of the cardiac silhouette.

Solitary pulmonary masses are a common radiographic presentation for primary lung tumors in cats, (Figure 19.27) [39–45]. Common primary lung lobe tumors include bronchogenic carcinoma, squamous cell carcinoma, and bronchoalveolar carcinoma [46]. Pulmonary masses can be cavitated secondary to central necrosis or invasion of a bronchus with replacement of the necrotic fluid with air. Ill-defined areas of multifocal mineralization may also be seen (Figure 19.27). Similar cavitated masses can occur with pulmonary abscess, but these are rare in the cat. Lobar atelectasis with an associated

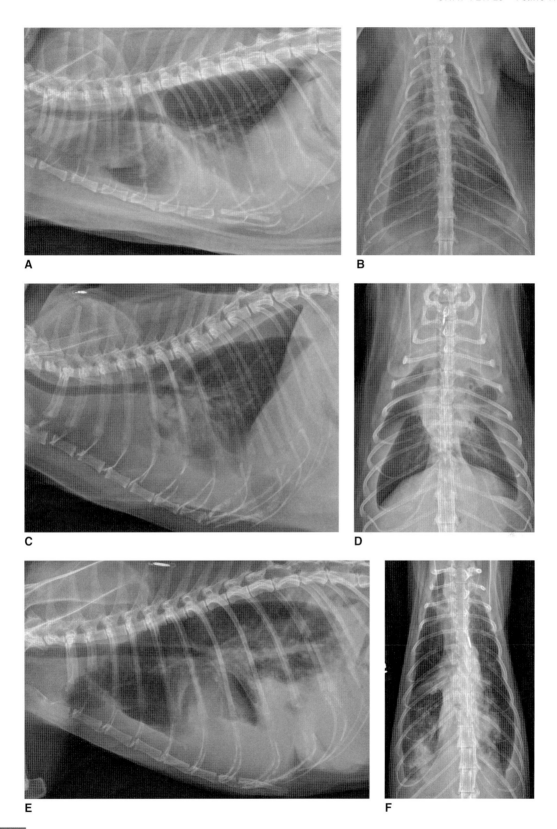

**FIGURE 19.18** Moderate to severe pleural effusion in three different cats. The first and third cats (**A** – right lateral, **B** – dorsoventral, **E** – right lateral, **F** – dorsoventral) have dorsoventral views that result in border effacement of the cardiac silhouette. The second cat (**C** – right lateral, **D** – ventrodorsal) has a ventrodorsal image so that the pleural fluid pools in the dorsal thoracic pleural space and the cardiac silhouette can be seen and is not border effaced. There is retraction of the lung lobes away from the thoracic walls and the presence of pleural fissure lines filled with soft tissue opacity. The pleural effusions were secondary to modified transudate – first cat with lymphoma, second cat with a cranial mediastinal mass, and metastatic carcinoma in the third cat.

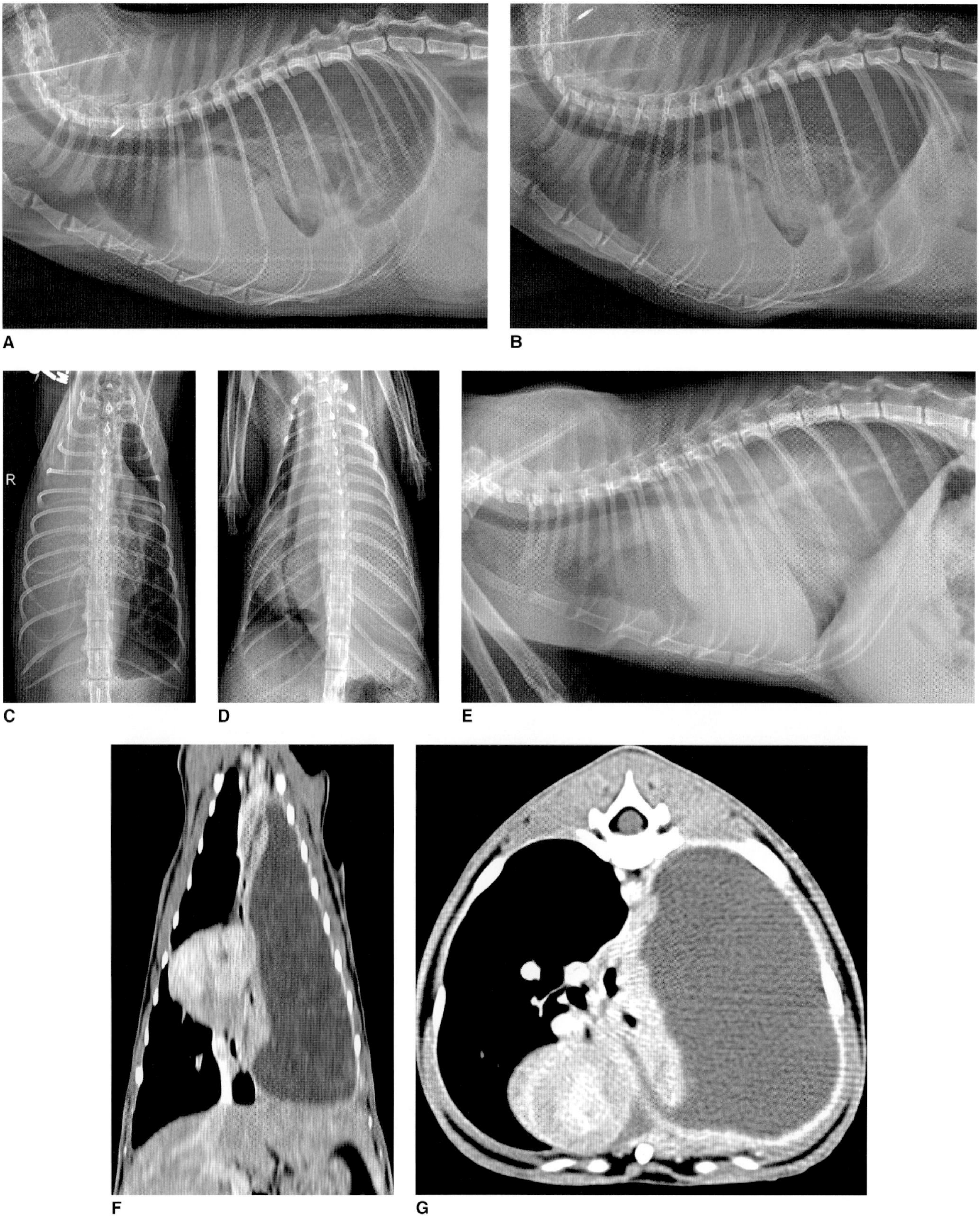

**FIGURE 19.19** Unilateral pleural effusion from two different cats both secondary to a pyothorax. In the first cat (**A** – right lateral, **B** – left lateral, **C** – ventrodorsal), the pyothorax was right-sided and there is a leftward contralateral mediastinal shift of the cardiac silhouette and right lung lobes (which are collapsed). In the second cat (**D** – right lateral, **E** – ventrodorsal), there is a severe left-sided pleural effusion/space-occupying mass effect with a contralateral rightward mediastinal shift and collapse of the left lung lobes. Follow-up CT images (**F** – reconstructed dorsal plane, **G** – transverse CT) document a soft tissue attenuating effusion with collapse of the left lung lobes and peripheral rim enhancement of the thickened parietal pleura secondary to the pyothorax.

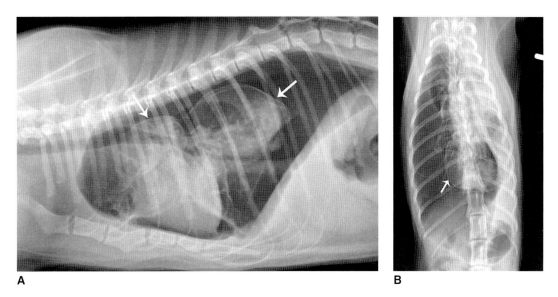

**FIGURE 19.20** Predominantly unilateral pneumothorax in a cat with a restrictive pleuritis secondary to a chronic pyothorax. There is rounding of the right caudal lung lobe (and cranial lung lobe) with thickening of the visceral pleura (white arrow on the right lateral and dorsoventral images) consistent with a restrictive pleuritis.

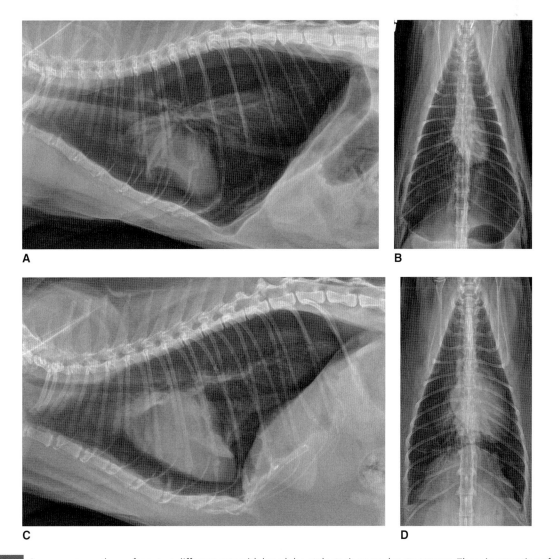

**FIGURE 19.21** Severe pneumothorax from two different cats with lung lobe atelectasis secondary to trauma. There is retraction of the lung lobes away from the thoracic wall and dorsal elevation of the cardiac silhouette away from the sternum in both cats (cat 1 **A** – right lateral, **B** – ventrodorsal; cat 2 **C** – right lateral, **D** – ventrodorsal).

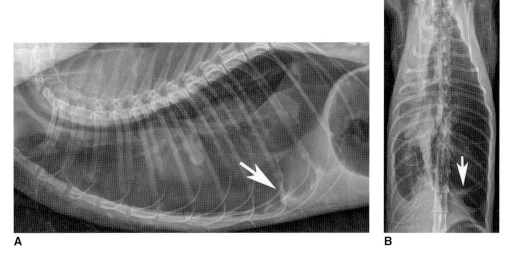

**FIGURE 19.22** Left-sided tension pneumothorax in a cat post trauma (**A** – right lateral, **B** – ventrodorsal). There is a severe contralateral mediastinal shift with collapse of multiple lung lobes, a severe left-sided pneumothorax with tenting of the diaphragm (white arrows) and severe expansion of the left pleural space.

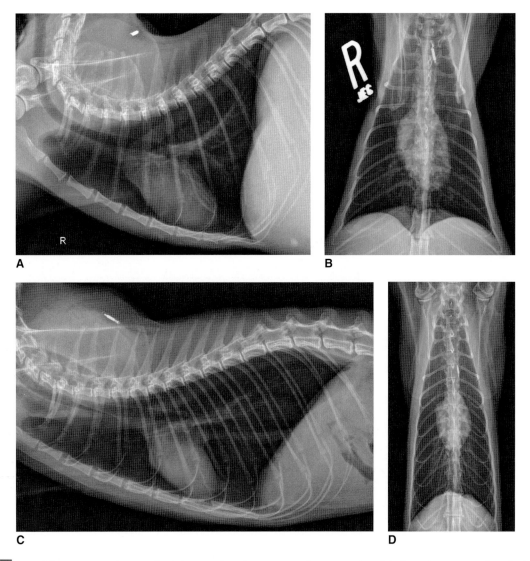

**FIGURE 19.23** Two different cats with generalized decrease in pulmonary opacity. In cat 1 (**A** – right lateral, **B** – ventrodorsal), there is generalized oligemia, particularly in the peripheral lung lobes. This decrease in pulmonary vascular size could be secondary to extreme hypovolemia or pulmonary thromboembolic disease. At necropsy, severe generalized thromboemboli were noted throughout the pulmonary arteries of all lung lobes. The exact etiology was not determined in this cat. In the second cat (**C** – right lateral, **D** – ventrodorsal), there is a generalized increase in lung volume resulting in an overall decrease in pulmonary opacity. This was secondary to hyperinflation in this cat related to feline hyperthyroidism and weight loss.

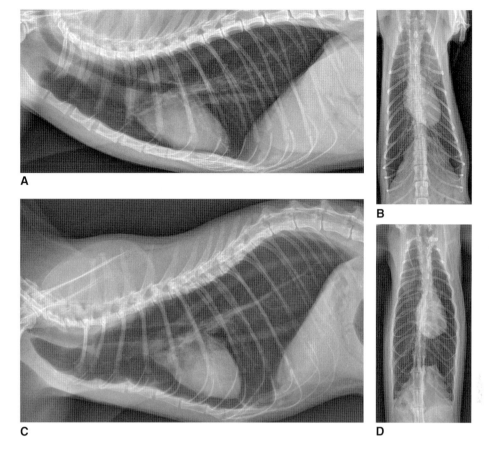

**FIGURE 19.24** Hyperinflation with diaphragmatic tenting in two cats that responded clinically to treatment for feline asthma (cat 1 – **A**, **B**; cat 2 – **C**, **D** with right lateral and ventrodorsal images presented respectively). Originally, the cats presented with a history of cough. There are triangular soft tissue opacities noted along the ventral diaphragm on the ventrodorsal images consistent with diaphragmatic tenting secondary to hyperinflation. On the right lateral from the second cat (**C**), there is dorsal elevation of the cardiac silhouette away from the sternum. This was caused by the hyperinflation and is not secondary to a pneumothorax.

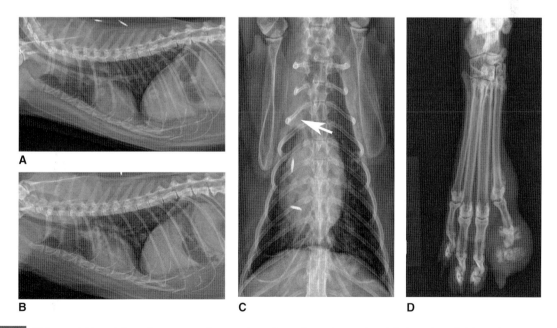

**FIGURE 19.25** Right cranial lung lobe collapse secondary to a bronchogenic carcinoma (**A** – right lateral, **B** – left lateral, **C** – ventrodorsal). On the ventrodorsal image (**C**), there is an ipsilateral rightward mediastinal shift. There are multiple cavitated nodules noted within the remainder of the lung lobes in this older cat. In image (**D**), there is a soft tissue mass associated with the fifth digit with underlying periosteal reaction of the distal fifth metacarpal bone and the proximal, middle, and distal phalanges. There is osteolysis of the ungual process of the distal phalanx of the fifth digit. This cat presented for lameness related to the pelvic limb digit. Thoracic radiographs documented the primary lung tumor with intrapulmonary and digital metastatic disease (lung–digit syndrome).

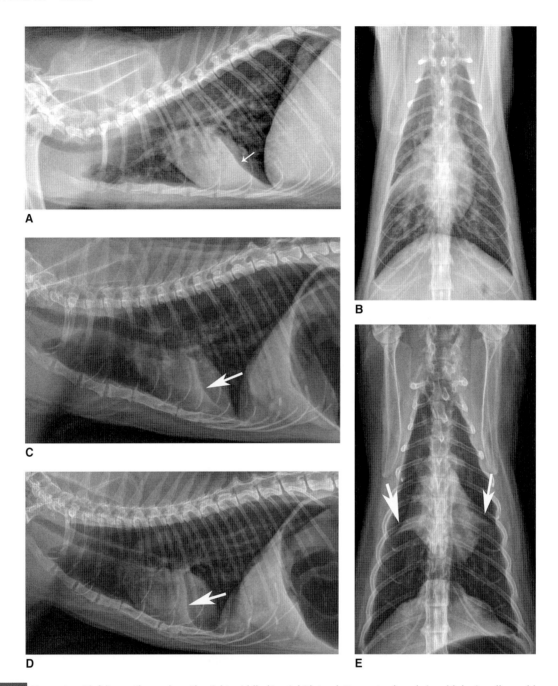

**FIGURE 19.26** Two cats with feline asthma where the right middle (**A** – right lateral, **B** – ventrodorsal views) lobe is collapsed (complete atelectasis) in the first cat. In the second cat (**C** – right lateral, **D** – left lateral, **E** – ventrodorsal), there is collapse of the right middle and caudal subsegments of the left cranial lung lobes. A mild to moderate bronchial pattern is present in both cats. These changes are consistent with lobar collapse secondary to mucous plugging from feline allergic lung disease or feline asthma.

mediastinal shift can occur when the associated bronchus is obstructed by tumor (Figure 19.25).

Primary lung lobe tumors can metastasize to the distal phalanges of any of the limbs, resulting in an aggressive, osteolytic lesion of that digit. This "lung–digit syndrome" is reported in cats (Figure 19.28) [47–49].

In addition to focal pulmonary masses, primary lung tumors in the cat can result in diffuse interstitial, bronchial, alveolar, or mixed patterns (Figure 19.29) [39–45]. Because of bronchial circulation, pulmonary metastasis can result from a

primary pulmonary tumor (Figure 19.25). Metastatic pulmonary disease from any distant site may present as a well-defined pulmonary nodular pattern, although a mixed appearance of poorly defined nodules, alveolar pattern, and/or unstructured interstitial patterns is more common [40, 45, 50]. Pleural effusion and cranial mediastinal or tracheobronchial lymph node enlargement are additional thoracic radiographic changes that have been reported with primary lung tumors in cats.

Fungal pneumonia (histoplasmosis, blastomycosis) most often results in a structured interstitial pattern, either nodular

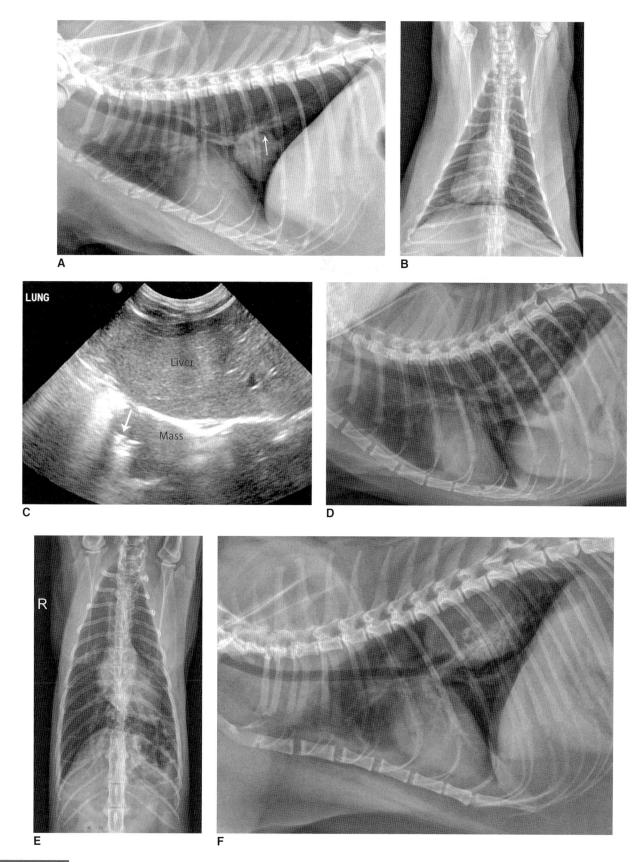

**FIGURE 19.27** Three different cats each with different patterns of a primary lung tumor (bronchoalveolar carcinoma in each cat). The first cat (**A** – right lateral, **B** – ventrodorsal, **C** – transabdominal ultrasound using the liver as a window), there is a right caudal pulmonary mass with a mild degree of cavitation (white arrow). In the second cat (**D** – right lateral, **E** – ventrodorsal), there is a large left caudal lung lobe mass that is severely cavitated. A mass becomes cavitated when the necrotic center drains into a bronchus and is replaced by air. Notice the internal margins of the mass are irregularly thickened (unlike a bulla with a simple thin wall). In the third cat (**F** – right lateral), there is a left caudal pulmonary mass with focal areas of mineralization. The mass is in the dorsal peripheral aspect of the left caudal lung lobe. There is retraction of the caudal aspect of the left lung lobe and increased soft tissue opacity along the ventral thorax consistent with pleural involvement and mild pleural effusion.

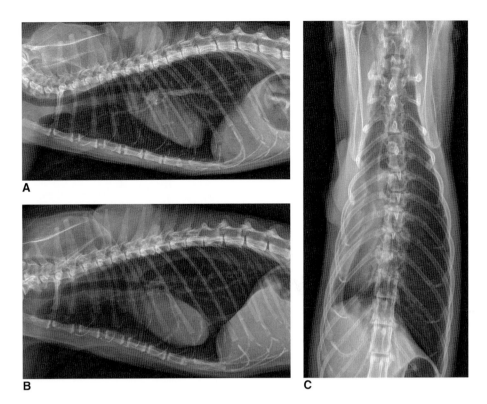

**FIGURE 19.28** Right middle and caudal lung lobe mass with complete collapse of those lobes and a significant ipsilateral mediastinal shift noted on all three projections (**A** – right lateral, **B** – left lateral, **C** – ventrodorsal). In addition, there is a subcutaneous mass noted adjacent to the right thoracic wall. The subcutaneous and pulmonary mass cytology was consistent with carcinoma (presumed primary lung in origin).

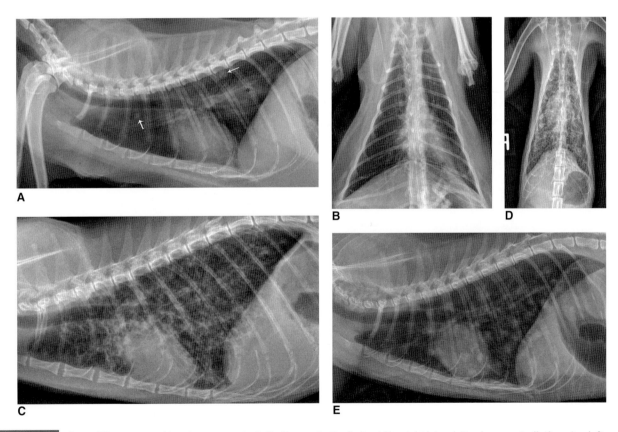

**FIGURE 19.29** Three different cats with pulmonary metastatic disease. In the first cat (**A** – right lateral, **B** – dorsoventral), there is a left caudal pulmonary mass (asterisk) with intrapulmonary nodules (white arrows). These metastatic lesions were secondary to a primary lung tumor in the left caudal lobe. In the second cat (**C** – right lateral, **D** – ventrodorsal), there is a diffuse bronchial pulmonary pattern with an underlying structured interstitial (miliary) pulmonary pattern. On cytology evaluation of the pulmonary parenchyma, carcinoma was identified. Other mass lesions were not present, so this was presumed to be a disseminated form of pulmonary carcinoma. In the third cat (**E** – right lateral), there are multiple small to varying sized soft tissue nodules noted throughout the pulmonary parenchyma consistent with metastatic disease. A soft tissue sarcoma was present in the left pelvic limb and was considered the primary source of the metastatic disease.

or miliary [51–57]. Pleural effusion and alveolar patterns can also be present.

A lung lobe torsion results when a lobe rotates along its axis at the pulmonary hilum [58–61]. This is often secondary to preexisting pleural effusion. The lung lobe becomes congested, resulting in edema, hemorrhage, and necrosis. The right middle and left and right cranial lung lobes are most commonly affected. Although this is rare in cats, it should be suspected when persistent consolidation is noted (post thoracocentesis), air bronchograms extend in an abnormal direction, or small gas lucencies are noted in the affected lung lobe.

Vascular changes (increased size) will result in increased opacity that is typically generalized. The caudal lobar pulmonary arteries can thicken as the cat ages where the arteries will become larger than the pulmonary veins, but the pulmonary arteries will not be tortuous as seen in feline heartworm disease (Figure 19.30) [14]. Enlargement of the pulmonary arteries and veins can be seen with volume overload and cats with left to right shunting cardiac congenital anomalies (Figure 19.31). Venous enlargement is often seen in dogs with left-sided congestive heart failure. In cats, however, pulmonary artery and vein enlargement is common [62]. As the vessels become enlarged, over time, they will become tortuous, particularly on the lateral views (Figure 19.31).

Feline bronchial disease is likely a combination of a variety of bronchial disorders including feline asthma, feline allergic lung disease, and chronic bronchitis [36–38, 63–69]. In feline asthma, eosinophilic airway inflammation and bronchoconstriction occur. A neutrophilic inflammation and increased mucus production are the hallmarks of chronic bronchitis. Thickened bronchial walls secondary to increased mucus production, cellular infiltrate, and bronchoconstriction result

in a bronchial pattern, with formation of prominent "rings and lines" in the periphery of the lung fields (Figure 19.32). Chronic airway inflammation will result in chronic obstructive pulmonary disease with overinflation or multifocal areas of hyperlucency (representing areas of emphysema) [36]. Hyperinflation of the lung lobes secondary to small airway trapping is a common finding in cats with feline asthma, and results in hyperlucency and diaphragmatic tenting. If lateral radiographs are made on both inspiration and expiration, persistent overexpansion will be noted due to the trapping of air in the lower airways (Figure 19.33).

Bronchiectasis can be an irreversible sequela of chronic airway disease, and results most often in cylindrical dilation of the bronchi (Figure 19.34) [64, 70, 71]. As described under the section on atelectasis, the right middle and/or caudal subsegment of the left cranial lung lobe can be collapsed secondary to mucous plugging and obstruction with resorption of air. Chronic lower airway disease can result in midbody rib fractures (typically ribs 9–11) [16]. This can also be seen in cats with chronic pleural effusions (thoracic bellows). In some cats, broncholithiasis (mineralized mucus plugs) can occur because of chronic lower airway inflammation resulting in multifocal mineral opaque structures in the alveoli and distal airways (Figure 19.35) [72, 73].

In the cat, radiographic changes of lower airway disease and clinical signs do not always correlate. Thoracic radiographs can be normal despite the presence of disease.

Multifocal and generalized unstructured interstitial and alveolar pulmonary changes can be caused by a number of different disease processes. It should be noted that these patterns form a continuum, and may represent different degrees of severity of the same disease process. Distribution

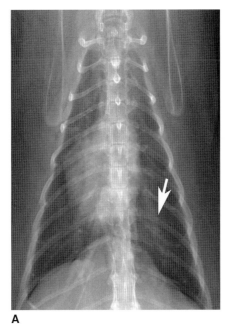 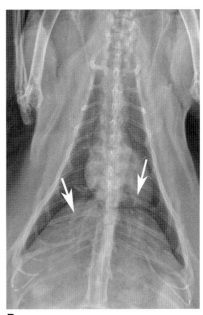

A        B

**FIGURE 19.30** Two different cats with pulmonary arterial enlargement (white arrows). In the first cat (**A**), the left caudal lobar pulmonary artery was enlarged. Heartworm disease was ruled out in this cat and pulmonary artery enlargement secondary to age related change was considered most likely. In comparison, the second cat (**B**) had enlargement of both left and right caudal pulmonary arteries.

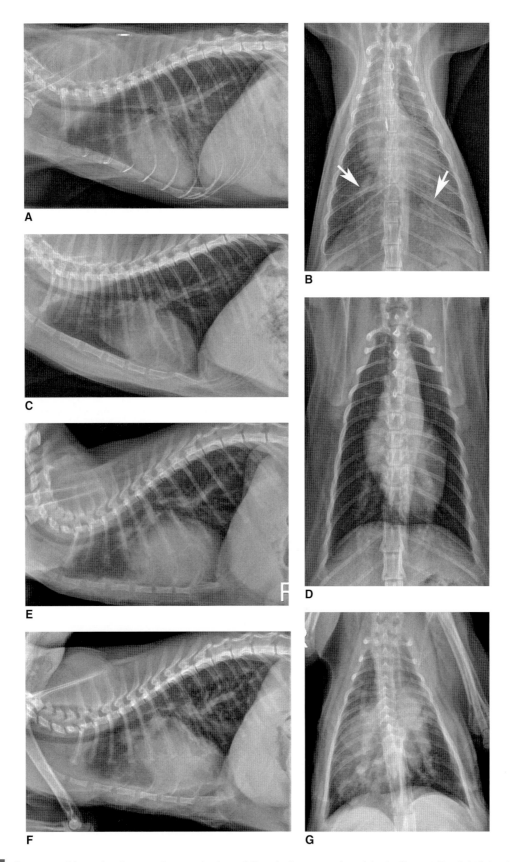

**FIGURE 19.31** Three cats with varying degrees of congestive heart failure (pulmonary edema). In the first cat (**A** – right lateral, **B** – dorsoventral), there is a moderate unstructured interstitial pulmonary pattern, primarily in a ventral distribution on the right lateral. The cardiac silhouette and pulmonary vessels are enlarged (white arrows). The echocardiographic diagnosis was hypertrophic cardiomyopathy with left atrial enlargement. In the second cat (**C** – right lateral, **D** – ventrodorsal), there is a moderate cardiac silhouette and pulmonary vessels are enlarged. The echocardiographic diagnosis was left to right shunting ventricular septal defect. In the third cat (**E** – right lateral, **F** – left lateral, **G** – dorsoventral), there is a generalized, mild, unstructured, interstitial pulmonary pattern. The cardiac silhouette and the pulmonary vessels are severely enlarged and there is enlargement of the descending thoracic aorta at the fourth intercostal space. The pulmonary vessels are not only enlarged but also tortuous in appearance. The echocardiographic diagnosis was left to right patent ductus arteriosus.

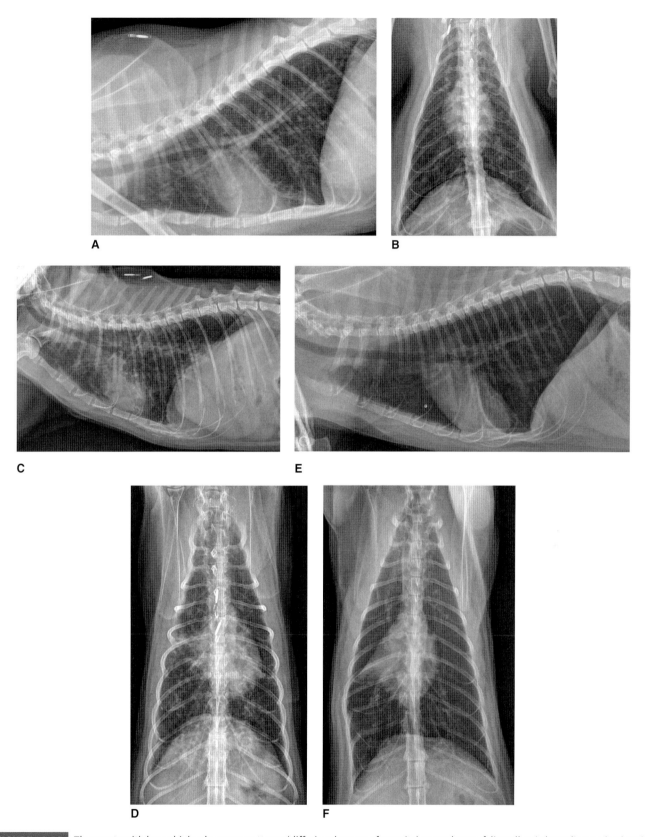

**FIGURE 19.32**  Three cats with bronchial pulmonary patterns (differing degrees of severity) secondary to feline allergic lung disease (asthma). In cat 1 (**A** – right lateral, **B** – ventrodorsal), there is a generalized bronchial pulmonary pattern with some degree of bronchiectasis. In cat 2 (**C** – right lateral, **D** – ventrodorsal) there is a generalized severe bronchial pulmonary pattern with areas of hyperlucency (pulmonary emphysema) and some bronchiectasis consistent with chronic obstructive pulmonary disease. In cat 3 (**E** – left lateral, **F** – ventrodorsal), there is a mild to moderate bronchial pattern. In addition, there is incomplete collapse of the right middle lung lobe with air bronchograms, uniform soft tissue opacity, border effacement of the small structures and a lobar sign (alveolar pulmonary pattern) and a rightward ipsilateral mediastinal shift.

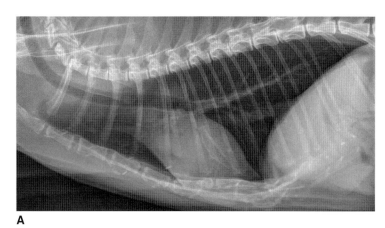
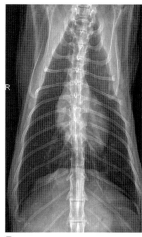

**A**                                                                                          **B**

**FIGURE 19.33**   Expiratory radiographs (**A** – right lateral, **B** – ventrodorsal images) from a cat with feline asthma. A difference between expiratory and inspiratory images was not seen consistent with air trapping secondary to peripheral bronchoconstriction.

of the pulmonary opacity is an important part of the diagnostic process.

Cardiogenic pulmonary edema in the cat usually has a multifocal mixed unstructured interstitial and alveolar pulmonary patterns, without a consistent distribution [74, 75]. Unlike the dog, cats with left-sided congestive heart failure often have accompanying pleural effusion [74, 76, 77]. While pulmonary veins are often enlarged in canine left-sided congestive heart failure, the pulmonary arteries and veins are more frequently distended in the cat (Figure 19.36) [62]. Noncardiogenic edema is also a mixed pattern and may be bilateral, primarily affecting the caudal and dorsal lung fields. Bacterial pneumonia (secondary to aspiration or inhalation of air-borne bacteria) is less common in the cat than the dog, but has a similar cranioventral distribution (Figure 19.37).

Multifocal mixed unstructured interstitial, bronchial, or alveolar pulmonary patterns are common with a number of different diseases. These include fungal disease (histoplasmosis, blastomycosis, cryptococcosis), parasitic disease (*Toxoplasma* and *Aelurostrongylus*), endogenous lipid pneumonia, cardiogenic pulmonary edema, feline infectious peritonitis (noneffusive form), and pulmonary fibrosis (Figures 19.38–19.40).

# Mediastinal Abnormalities

The mediastinum is a common site for feline thoracic abnormalities The mediastinum can be divided into thirds (cranial, middle, and caudal). Each division will be reviewed separately. Recognize that some diseases (esophageal) can result in the involvement of the entire mediastinum. The heart is included in the middle mediastinum, and acquired cardiac disease is a common abnormality that can result in mediastinal, pulmonary parenchymal, and pleural changes (considered to be multicompartmental disease).

The most common abnormality of the cranial mediastinum is a cranial mediastinal mass. Mediastinal masses are central in location on the ventrodorsal image and, depending on the size of the mass, will displace other mediastinal structures, such as the trachea. The cranial lung lobes are displaced laterally and caudally with larger masses. Elevation of the trachea and caudal displacement of the carina (caudal to the sixth intercostal space) may also occur. Cranial mediastinal masses, if large enough, will border efface the cranial aspect of the cardiac silhouette. Pleural effusion commonly accompanies cranial mediastinal masses (Figure 19.41).

In cats, the most common cranial mediastinal mass is lymphoma [78–80]. Other differentials include thymoma, ectopic thyroid adenoma or carcinoma, and a variety of cranial mediastinal cysts (Figure 19.42). A paraneoplastic syndrome has been described in cats with thymoma, in which a megaesophagus is present secondary to a myasthenia-like syndrome [81, 82]. Cranial mediastinal cysts can originate from a variety of different sources including ectopic parathyroid, thyroglossal ducts, and thymic branchial cysts [83–86]. In general, cranial mediastinal cysts are located more caudally than other cranial mediastinal masses, often in contact with the cardiac silhouette (Figure 19.43). A pleural effusion is not seen with these cysts.

Sternal lymph nodes are located just dorsal to the second and third sternebrae, and with enlargement, result in an ill-defined oval soft tissue opacity dorsal to this region (Figure 19.44). Enlargement of the sternal lymph node is primarily consistent with inflammatory or neoplastic disorders of the abdomen.

Middle mediastinal masses are much less common in the cat than in the dog (unrelated to the cardiac silhouette). Differentials for a soft tissue opaque mass over the cardiac silhouette would include tracheobronchial lymph node enlargement or an esophageal foreign body (Figure 19.45). The most common causes of tracheobronchial lymph node enlargement would include systemic fungal disease or round cell tumors such as lymphoma (although less common than in dogs).

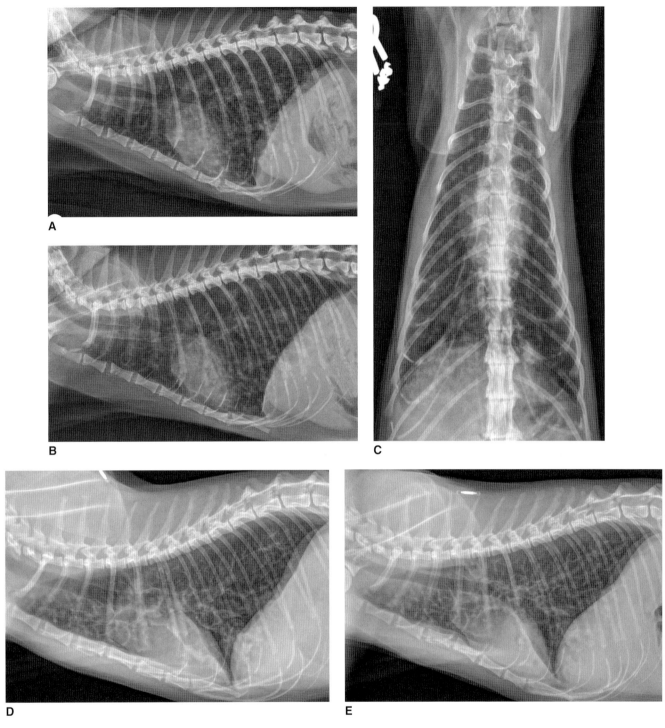

**FIGURE 19.34**   Bronchiectasis in two cats with chronic airway disease. In cat 1 (**A** – right lateral, **B** – left lateral, **C** – ventrodorsal), there is a generalized bronchial pulmonary pattern, severe, with some (moderate) degree of bronchial distension. In cat 2 (**D** – right lateral, **E** – left lateral, **F** – dorsoventral, **G** – ventrodorsal), there is a severe bronchial pulmonary pattern and severe bronchiectasis (combination of mostly saccular and some tubular bronchiectasis). Several of the airways are filled with soft tissue opaque material and there is marked bronchial wall thickening and dilation. There is collapse of the right middle lung lobe. A CT study was done in the same cat 2 (post IV contrast medium; **H** – dorsal plane reconstruction, **I** – transverse plane, **J** – sagittal plane reconstruction). Images are presented in an abdominal window (WW 450 and WL 80). Fluid-filled airways are also present on the transverse and sagittal plane images consistent with pus within the bronchiectatic airway secondary to lack of mucociliary clearance.

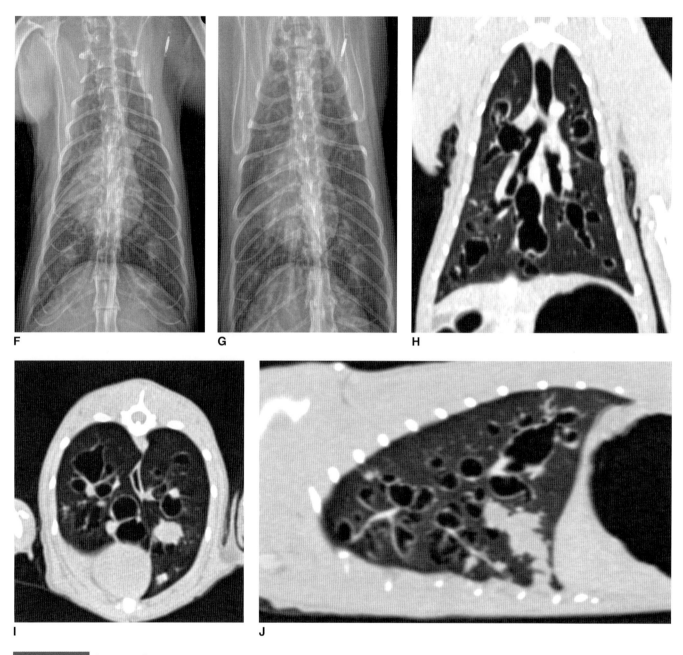

F

G

H

I

J

**FIGURE 19.34** (Continued)

Caudal mediastinal masses typically occur close to the diaphragm. The most common caudal mediastinal mass in the cat is a hiatal hernia, where a portion of the stomach (cardiac and/or fundus) herniates through the esophageal hiatus (Figure 19.46). This is usually dynamic and is seen on either a left lateral and/or ventrodorsal radiograph as a midline (VD/DV) rounded soft tissue opacity within the caudodorsal mediastinum. Other causes of esophageal enlargement (foreign body, neoplasia) should also be considered. A positive contrast esophagram will aid in differentiating these diseases. Other caudal mediastinal masses (soft tissue sarcomas) are rare.

Tracheal abnormalities are rare in the cat. Most commonly, tracheal disorders are acquired and related to trauma or iatrogenic trauma secondary to undue endotracheal cuff pressure [87–90]. Following endotracheal intubation and pressure-induced necrosis of the trachea induced by the cuff, fibrosis and stricture can occur. These strictures typically are seen at the thoracic inlet (Figure 19.47). External trauma, such as being hit by a car, can result in tracheal avulsion in the cranial thorax. A pneumomediastinum will result but the cat may continue to "breathe" the air in this gap between the cranial and caudal segments of the tracheal avulsion. Tracheal foreign bodies can be aspirated and may be

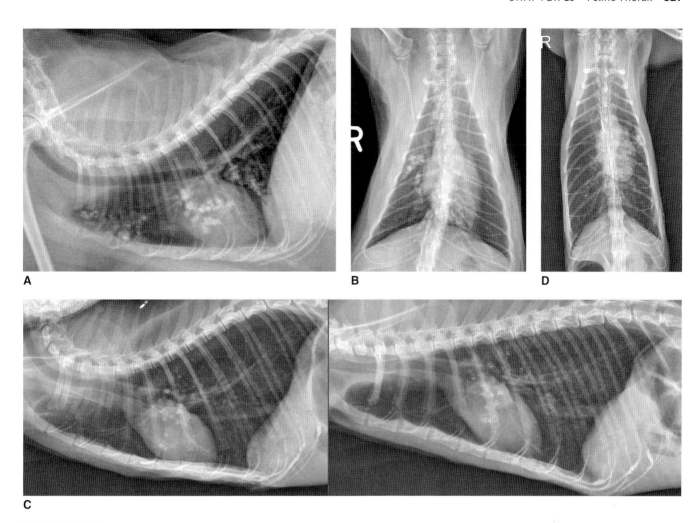

**FIGURE 19.35**   Broncholithiasis from two cats with chronic asthma. In cat 1 (**A** – left lateral, **B** – ventrodorsal), there are multifocal areas of mineralization noted within the airways of the right cranial, middle, and accessory lung lobes. In cat 2 (**C** – right and left lateral, **D** – ventrodorsal), there are multiple broncholiths noted with airway mineralization in the left cranial lung lobe. This cat is hyperinflated consistent with air trapping secondary to bronchoconstriction related to the feline allergic lung disease.

well visualized secondary to contrast with air in the trachea (Figure 19.48).

Disorders of the esophagus in the cat are similar to the dog. However, feline idiopathic congenital or acquired megaesophagus is rare. Megaesophagus can be seen secondary to distal esophageal stricture, myasthenia gravis (rare), and dysautonomia (Figure 19.49).

# Diseases of the Cardiac Silhouette

The normal Roentgen signs for the cardiac silhouette are described in an earlier chapter (Chapter 18).

The radiographic appearance of the feline heart differs slightly from that of the canine [91, 92]. On lateral radiographs,

the cardiac base is broad, tapering to a narrower apex (see Figures 19.1 and 19.2). The heart is located usually between the fourth and sixth intercostal spaces. On VD/DV projections, the apex is more variable than in the dog, usually located just to the left of the midline. Individual cardiac chambers are similar to the dog, with some unique features. The feline left atrium is located slightly more cranial than the dog, making it more difficult to identify on lateral views. On the VD/DV view, the feline main pulmonary artery is located more medially and cranially compared to the 1:00–2:00 position noted in the dog. Enlargement may not be identified radiographically. The appearance of the normal feline heart is less affected by breed and positioning compared to the dog although the Maine coon cat tends to have larger vertebral heart scores (VHS) than other domestic breeds.

Radiographic assessment of cardiomegaly in the cat is often challenging because of more subtle enlargement patterns [91–94]. Right heart enlargement in the cat can result

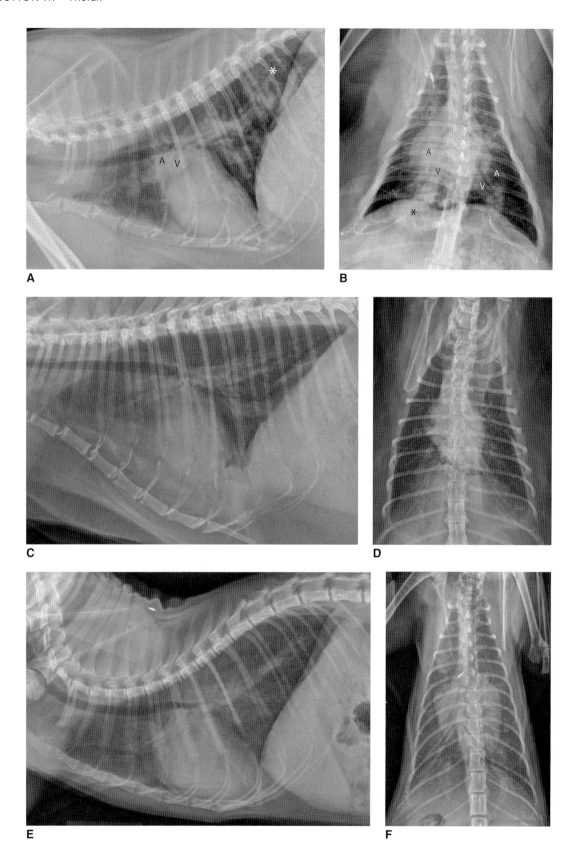

**FIGURE 19.36** Three cats with varying degrees of heart failure. In cat 1 (**A** – right lateral, **B** – ventrodorsal), there is a right caudal cavitated mass (asterisk). The cat also had primary hypertrophic cardiomyopathy with pulmonary vessel enlargement (A, pulmonary artery; V, pulmonary vein). In cat 2 (**C** – right lateral, **D** – ventrodorsal), there is pulmonary edema and pleural effusion secondary to a restrictive cardiomyopathy with mild to moderate pulmonary vessel enlargement. In cat 3 (**E** – right lateral, **F** – ventrodorsal), there is a moderate unstructured interstitial pulmonary pattern, cardiomegaly and pulmonary vascular enlargement consistent with hypertrophic cardiomyopathy and resultant pulmonary edema and vascular enlargement.

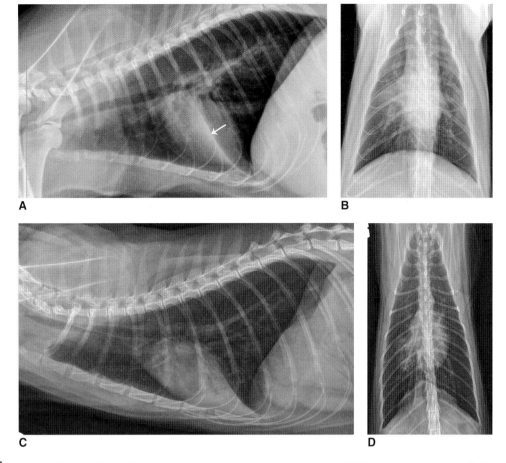

**FIGURE 19.37** Confirmed bacterial bronchopneumonia in two separate cats. In cat 1 (**A** – left lateral, **B** – ventrodorsal), there is a generalized bronchial pulmonary pattern, moderate in severity. There is an alveolar pulmonary pattern in the right middle lung lobe. A fluid-filled esophagus is noted. This cat had an esophagitis with aspiration pneumonia. In cat 2 (**C** – left lateral, **D** – ventrodorsal), there is an ill-defined unstructured interstitial to alveolar pulmonary pattern in the right middle lung lobe. The cat is hyperinflated with mild diaphragmatic tenting noted on the ventrodorsal image. Positive culture from a transtracheal wash was noted in the medical record. NOTE: Bronchopneumonia is relatively uncommon in the cat compared with the dog.

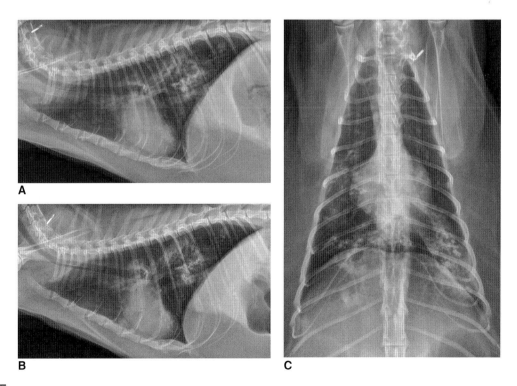

**FIGURE 19.38** Endogenous lipid pneumonia in a cat that presented for respiratory distress with a chronic cough noted for the past month (**A** – right lateral, **B** – left lateral, **C** – ventrodorsal). There are ill-defined unstructured interstitial and alveolar pulmonary changes with multifocal areas of mineralization. Biopsy confirmed the diagnosis of endogenous lipid pneumonia. This disease has not been described in the dog.

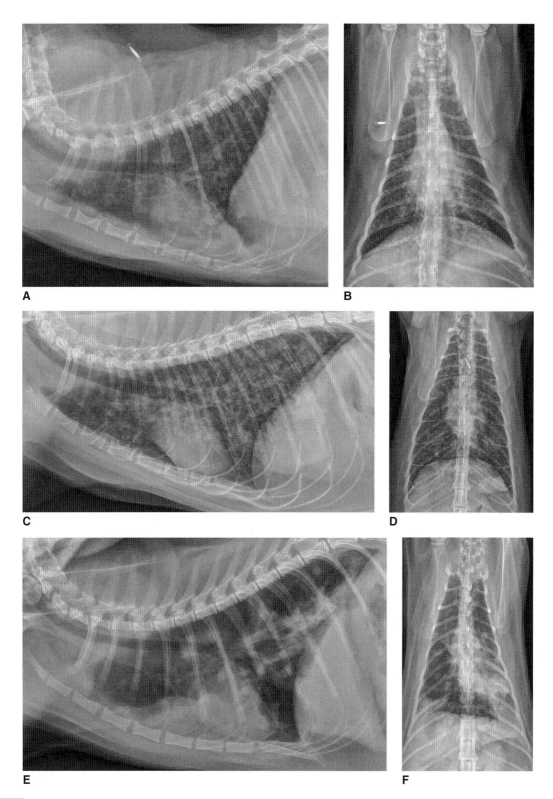

**FIGURE 19.39** Three separate cats with active inflammatory lung disease. These changes are relatively nonspecific. In cat 1 (**A** – right lateral, **B** – ventrodorsal), there is a generalized bronchial pulmonary pattern that is severe and a moderate unstructured interstitial pulmonary pattern. This cat was confirmed to have lungworm (*Aelurostrongylus abstrusus*) infestation and the radiographic changes cleared after adulticide anthelmintic therapy. In cat 2 (**C** – right lateral, **D** – ventrodorsal), there is a generalized bronchial pulmonary pattern and a structured, miliary, interstitial pulmonary pattern. This was determined to be secondary to histoplasmosis after fine needle aspirates of the lung under ultrasound guidance. In cat 3 (**E** – right lateral, **F** – ventrodorsal), there are multiple pulmonary nodules and masses with some pleural involvement (mild effusion and rounding of the caudal lung lobe borders). Ultrasound-guided fine needle aspirate documented *Mycobacterium* infection on cytology and culture.

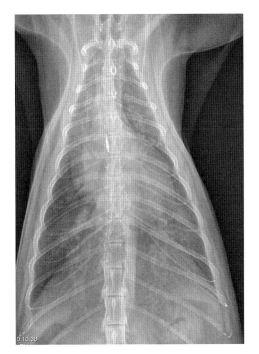 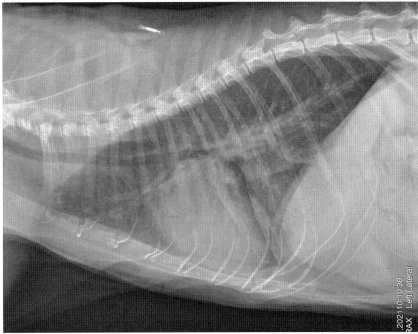

**FIGURE 19.40**   Cardiogenic pulmonary edema in a cat (ventrodorsal and left lateral images). There is cardiomegaly, pulmonary vessel enlargement and an unstructured interstitial pulmonary pattern (multifocal and ventral distribution). These changes were secondary to hypertrophic cardiomyopathy and left heart failure (pulmonary edema).

in widening of the cardiac silhouette, with dorsal deviation of the apex and elevation of the trachea on the lateral view (Figure 19.50). Left ventricular enlargement can cause subtle bulging of the caudal cardiac margin, elevation of the trachea, and increased length and width of the cardiac silhouette (Figure 19.51). Left atrial enlargement is a consistent feature of most forms of cardiomyopathy, but radiographic recognition is difficult. Rarely does the enlarged left atrium bulge dramatically dorsally as it does in the dog, although the overall cardiac length can be increased. On VD/DV views, the enlarged left atrium/left auricle creates a wider base cranially, without affecting the apex ("valentine"-shaped heart). Objective measurements of the heart using the VHS or the left atrium vertebral heart score (LA-VHS) can be performed, with VHS measurements of 8 and LA-VHS measurements of 1 considered normal [11–13]. However, there appears to be poor agreement between radiographic assessment (both subjective and objective) and echocardiographic values for left atrial enlargement [13].

# Tying It All Together (Compartmental and Multicompartmental Disease)

Each of the different areas of the thorax can be involved individually or in combination with other areas, making the disease process multicompartmental in nature. Using a systematic interpretation paradigm in your approach to the feline thorax is a critical piece of the puzzle once well positioned and appropriate technical quality radiographs have been obtained. Cats are *not* small dogs, and one should consider the species differences outlined in this chapter for radiographic interpretation.

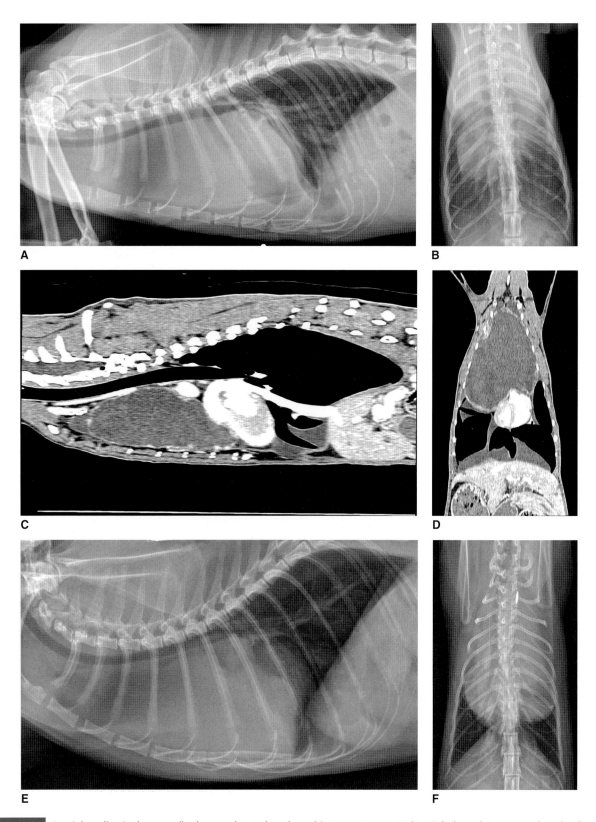

**FIGURE 19.41** Cranial mediastinal masses (both secondary to lymphoma) in two cats. In cat 1 (**A** – right lateral, **B** – ventrodorsal radiographs, **C** – sagittal reconstruction CT, **D**– dorsal plane reconstruction post contrast medium) there is mild pleural effusion. There is dorsal displacement of the thoracic trachea with caudal displacement of the carina (7th intercostal space) and the cardiac silhouette. The cranial border of the cardiac silhouette is border effaced with the mass. These changes are also seen on the CT of the thorax with mild to moderate contrast enhancement. In cat 2 (**E** – right lateral, **F** – ventrodorsal), there is a large cranial mediastinal mass with similar radiographic changes as described for cat 1. In both cats, on the ventrodorsal images there is relatively equal caudal displacement of the left and right cranial lung lobes.

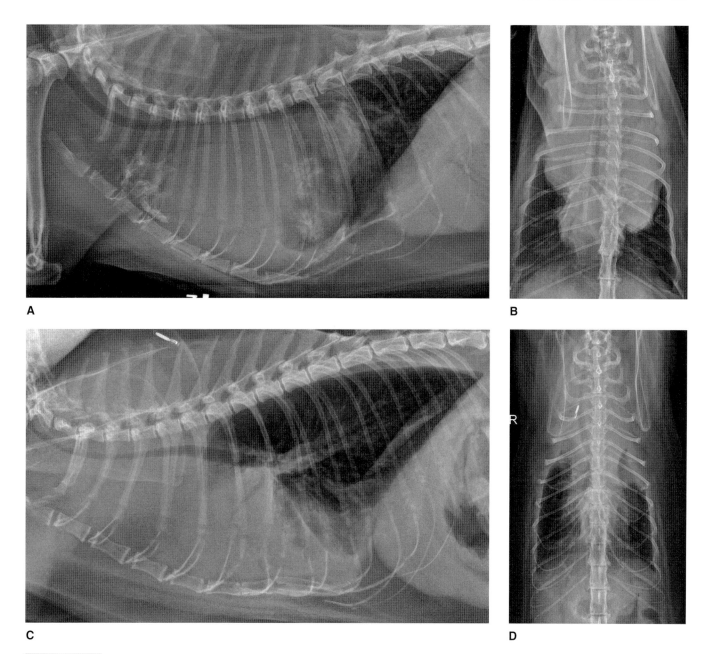

**A**

**B**

**C**

**D**

**FIGURE 19.42** Thymoma (cranial mediastinal masses) in two cats. In cat 1 (**A** – right lateral, **B** – ventrodorsal), there is dorsal and rightward deviation of the thoracic trachea. On the ventrodorsal image, there is caudal displacement of the left cranial lung lobe relative to the caudally displaced right cranial lobe. Other features as described for Figure 19.41 are present. Similar radiographic abnormalities are noted in cat 2 (**C** – right lateral, **D** – ventrodorsal).

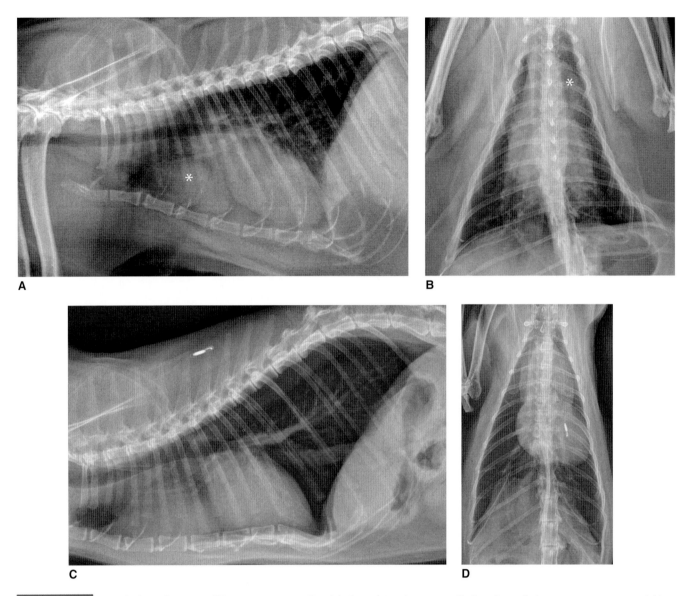

A

B

C

D

**FIGURE 19.43** Branchial cyst from two different cats. In cat 1 (**A** – right lateral, **B** – dorsoventral), there is a soft tissue opaque mass cranial to the cardiac silhouette (white asterisk). Unlike the cranial mediastinal mass presented in Figure 19.42, the trachea is in a normal position and the cranial mediastinal mass is in a ventral caudal position, but does not appear to border efface the cranial aspect of the cardiac silhouette. In cat 2 (**C** – right lateral, **D** – dorsoventral), the mass is in a similar position as noted in cat 1 in this figure. The trachea is mildly elevated dorsally and there is only partial border effacement with the cardiac silhouette, despite a more caudal position in the cranial mediastinum. On ultrasound of both cats, a thin-walled cystic structure was noted.

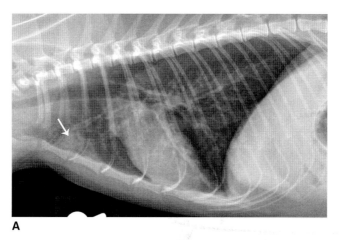

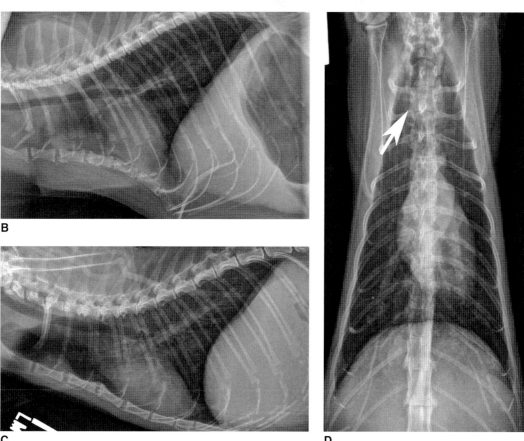

**FIGURE 19.44**   Three different cats with sternal lymph node enlargement. A white arrow is present in (**A**) to denote the enlarged sternal lymph node. In cat 2 (**B** – right lateral radiograph), there is a focal tissue opacity dorsal to the caudal second and cranial third sternebrae consistent with sternal lymph node enlargement. Hepatomegaly is also present. In cat 3 (**C** – right lateral, **D** – ventrodorsal), there is a soft tissue opaque structure in the cranioventral mediastinum (white arrow on the ventrodorsal image). In all three cats, the sternal lymph node enlargement was noted to be secondary to abdominal inflammatory or neoplastic diseases. In cats 1 and 3, there is a moderate generalized bronchial pulmonary pattern present.

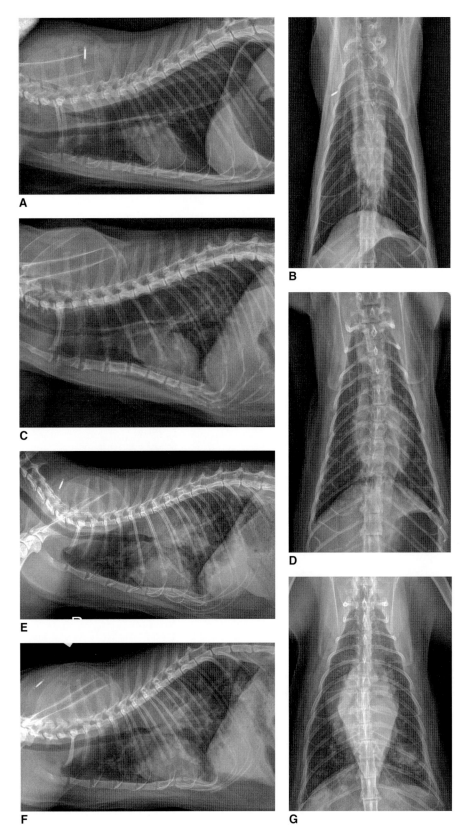

**FIGURE 19.45** Three different cats with dorsal mediastinal abnormalities. In cat 1 (**A** – right lateral, **B** – ventrodorsal), there is generalized gas distension of the esophagus. Additionally, there is a mixed soft tissue and gas opaque structure noted in the cranial esophagus at the thoracic inlet. A hairball was removed at endoscopy. In cat 2 (**C** – right lateral, **D** – ventrodorsal), there is an ill-defined soft opacity noted in the caudal thoracic esophagus. There is a structured, interstitial pulmonary pattern that is generalized. The remainder of the cranial thoracic esophagus was gas distended with ventral displacement of the trachea and cardiac silhouette. The esophageal mass was a squamous cell carcinoma with pulmonary metastatic nodules. In cat 3 (**E** – right lateral, **F** – left lateral, **G** – ventrodorsal), there is a large soft tissue mass noted dorsal to the cardiac silhouette. There is mild ventral deviation of the carina caudal bronchi. There are multiple ill-defined pulmonary nodules noted throughout the pulmonary parenchyma. This cat was determined to have severe central tracheobronchial lymph node enlargement and granulomatous pneumonia secondary to cryptococcosis. Mild sternal lymph node enlargement is also evident on the lateral images.

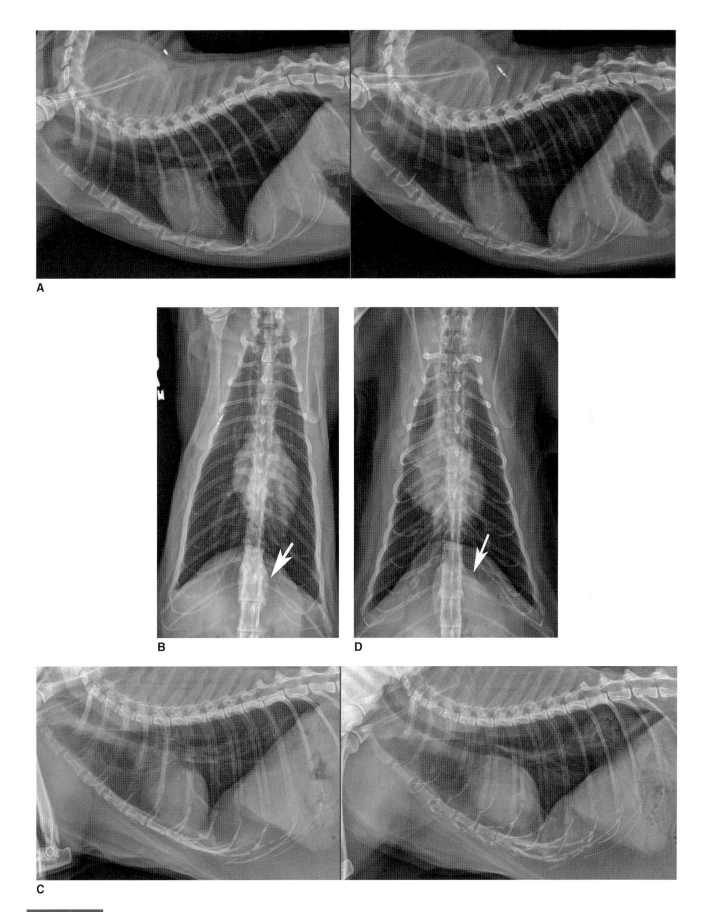

**FIGURE 19.46** Two different cats with a hiatal hernia. In cat 1 (**A** – right and left lateral, **B** – ventrodorsal), there is an ill-defined soft tissue opacity in the caudal dorsal mediastinum at the esophageal hiatus. This is better delineated on the ventrodorsal image (white arrow). In cat 2 (**C** – right and left lateral, **D** – ventrodorsal), there is a dynamic sliding hiatal hernia seen on the left lateral (right image of **C**) and the ventrodorsal image (**D** – white arrow). This is not seen on the right lateral image (left image of **C**). A rightward mediastinal shift of the cardiac silhouette is present on the ventrodorsal image consistent with an ipsilateral shift from partial volume loss in the right cranial and middle lung lobes.

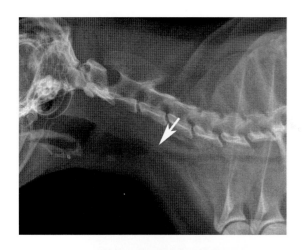

**FIGURE 19.47**  A right lateral radiograph of the neck from a cat with inspiratory stridor. There is focal narrowing of the cervical trachea (white arrow). This was an acquired stricture secondary to prior anesthesia and overinflation of the tracheal cuff.

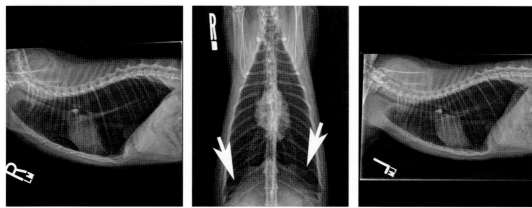

**FIGURE 19.48**  Tracheal foreign body (rock) in a cat with hyperinflation (right lateral – left image; ventrodorsal – middle image; left lateral – right image). There is hyperinflation as noted by flattening of the diaphragm on the lateral images and diaphragmatic tenting noted on the ventrodorsal image (white arrows).

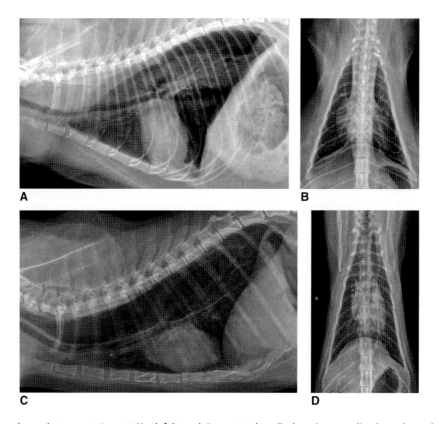

**FIGURE 19.49**  Megaesophagus in two cats. In cat 1 (**A** – left lateral, **B** – ventrodorsal), there is generalized esophageal dilation secondary to foreign material (as seen also in the stomach). There is ventral deviation of the trachea and increased soft tissue opacity of the left cranial lung lobe (caudal subsegment) consistent with an aspiration pneumonia. A cloth foreign body was removed at endoscopy. In cat 2 (**C** – left lateral, **D** – ventrodorsal), there is generalized gas distension of the esophagus with ventral displacement of the cardiac silhouette and trachea. A mild bronchial pulmonary pattern is also present. The megaesophagus was determined to be idiopathic.

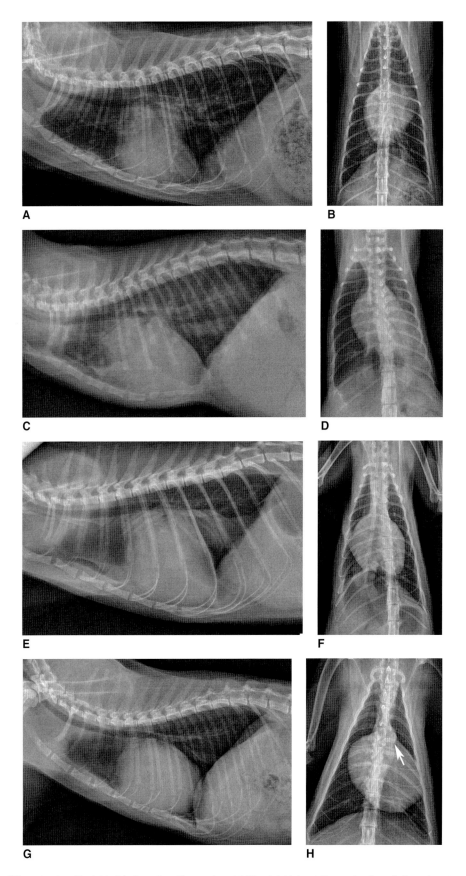

**FIGURE 19.50** Four different cats with right-sided cardiac disease. In cat 1 (**A** – right lateral, **B** – ventrodorsal), there is enlargement of the soft tissues of the heart base and enlargement and rounding of the right atrial/ventricular region on the right lateral view. Right ventricular cardiomyopathy was diagnosed in this cat and the dorsal cardiac changes were all attributed to enlargement of the right atrium. In cat 2 (**C** – right lateral, **D** – dorsoventral), there is enlargement of the cardiac silhouette. There is a moderate to severe unstructured interstitial pulmonary pattern in the left caudal lung lobe with enlargement of the pulmonary vasculature. This cat was determined to have tricuspid and mitral valve dysplasia with biatrial and ventricular enlargement and left caudal pulmonary edema. In cat 3 (**E** – right lateral, **F** – dorsoventral), there is severe enlargement of the right side of the cardiac silhouette and caudal vena cava. There is a mild pleural effusion present. Tricuspid dysplasia was diagnosed in this cat. In cat 4 (**G** – right lateral, **H** – dorsoventral), there is enlargement of the right side of the cardiac silhouette. There is a focal indentation noted in the descending thoracic aorta (white arrow on the dorsoventral). Tricuspid valve dysplasia and aortic coarctation were diagnosed in this cat.

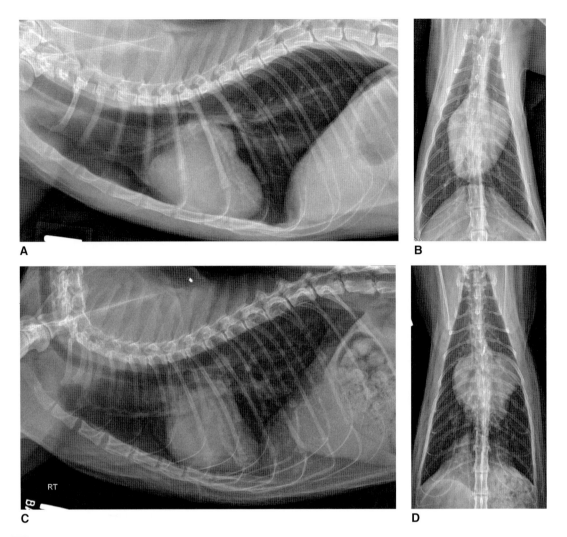

**FIGURE 19.51** Hypertrophic cardiomyopathy from two cats with a valentine heart appearance noted on the ventrodorsal images. In both cats, there is a shape change noted on the right laterals at the atrioventricular level along the caudal cardiac border. In cat 1 (**A** – right lateral, **B** – ventrodorsal), there is severe enlargement of the atria (determined to be left atrial on echocardiography). In cat 2 (**C** – right lateral, **D** – ventrodorsal), there is severe enlargement of the atria (again, determined to be left atrial enlargement on echocardiography).

# References

1. Hudson, L.C. and Hamilton, W.P. (1993). *Atlas of Feline Anatomy for Veterinarians*, 23–76. Philadelphia, PA: WB Saunders.
2. Done, S.H., Goody, P.C., Evans, S.A. et al. (1996). *Color Atlas of Veterinary Anatomy*, vol. 3, 10.2–10.33. London: Mosby-Wolfe.
3. Farrow, C.S., Green, R., and Shively, M. (1994). *Radiology of the Cat*, 45–130. London: Mosby-Wolfe.
4. Boudrieau, R.J., Fossum, T.W., Hartsfield, S.W. et al. (1990). Pectus excavatum in dogs and cats. *Compend. Cont. Educ. Small Anim. Pract.* 12: 341–355.
5. Hy, Y., Mann, F.A., and Jeong, S. (2008). Surgical correction of pectus excavatum in two cats. *J. Vet. Sci.* 9: 335–337.
6. Hayward, N.J., Baines, S.J., Baines, E.A., and Gerrtage, M.E. (2004). The radiographic appearance of the pulmonary vasculature in the cat. *Vet. Radiol. US* 45: 501–504.
7. Smith, K. and O'Brien, R. (2012). Radiographic characterization of enlarged sternal lymph nodes in 71 dogs and 13 cats. *J. Am. Anim. Hosp. Assoc.* 48: 176–181.
8. Tompkins, M. (1993). Lymphoid system. In: *Atlas of Feline Anatomy for Veterinarians* (ed. L. Hudson and W. Hamilton), 114–126. Philadelphia, PA: Saunders.
9. Baines, E. (2008). The mediastinum. In: *BSAVA Manual of Canine and Feline Thoracic Imaging* (ed. T. Schwarz and V. Johnson), 177–199. Gloucester, UK: British Small Animal Veterinary Association.
10. Hammond, G., Geary, M., Coleman, E. et al. (2011). Radiographic measurements of the trachea in domestic shorthair and Persian cats. *J. Feline Med. Surg.* 13: 881–884.

11. Lister, A.L. and Buchanan, J.W. (2000). Vertebral scale system to measure heart size on radiographs of cats. *J. Am. Vet. Med. Assoc.* 216: 210–214.

12. Ghadiri, A., Avizeh, R., Rasekh, A. et al. (2008). Radiographic measurement of vertebral heart score in healthy stray carts. *J. Feline Med. Surg.* 10: 61–65.

13. Guglielmini, C., Baron Toaldo, M., Poser, H. et al. (2014). Diagnostic accuracy of the vertebral heart score and other radiographic indices in the detection of cardiac enlargement in cats with different cardiac disorders. *J. Feline Med. Surg.* 16: 812–825.

14. Rogers, W.A., Bishop, S., and Rohousky, M. (1971). Pulmonary arterial medial hypertrophy and hyperplasia in conventional and specific pathogen free cats. *Am. J. Vet. Res.* 32: 767–774.

15. Adams, C., Streeter, E.M., King, R. et al. (2010). Cause and clinical characteristics of rib fractures in cats: 33 cases (2000–2009). *J. Vet. Emerg. Crit. Care* 20: 436–440.

16. Hardie, E.M., Ramirez, O., Clary, E.M. et al. (1998). Abnormalities of the thoracic bellows: stress fractures of the ribs and hiatal hernia. *J. Vet. Intern. Med.* 12: 279–287.

17. Ehrhart, N.P., Ryan, S.D., and Fan, T.M. (2013). Tumors of the skeletal system. In: *Small Animal Clinical Oncology*, 5e (ed. S.J. Withrow, D.M. Vail and R.L. Page), 463–503. St Louis, MO: Elsevier/Saunders.

18. Bitetto, W.V., Patnaik, A.K., Schrader, S.C. et al. (1987). Osteosarcoma in cats: 22 cases (1974–1984). *J. Am. Vet. Med. Assoc.* 190: 91–94.

19. Keenihan, E.K., Lynch, S., Priestnall, S.L. et al. (2013). Unusual rib metastasis in two cats with pulmonary carcinoma. *J. Feline Med. Surg.* 15: 1145–1148.

20. Evans, S.M. and Biery, D.N. (1980). Congenital peritoneopericardial diaphragmatic hernia in the dog and cat: a literature review and 17 additional case histories. *Vet. Radiol.* 21: 108–116.

21. Berry, C.R., Koblik, P.D., and Ticer, J.W. (1990). Dorsal peritoneopericardial mesothelial remnant as an aid to the diagnosis of feline congenital peritoneopericardial diaphragmatic hernia. *Vet. Radiol.* 31: 239–245.

22. Burns, C.G., Bergh, M.S., and McLoughlin, M.A. (2013). Surgical and nonsurgical treatment of peritoneopericardial diaphragmatic hernia in dogs and cats: 58 cases (1999–2008). *J. Am. Vet. Med. Assoc.* 242: 643–650.

23. Reimer, S.B., Kyles, A.E., Filipowicz, D.E. et al. (2004). Long-term outcome of cats treated conservatively of surgically for peritoneopericardial diaphragmatic hernia: 66 cases (1987–2002). *J. Am. Vet. Med. Assoc.* 224: 728–732.

24. Besalti, O., Pekcan, Z., Caaliskan, M. et al. (2011). A retrospective study on traumatic diaphragmatic hernias in cats. *Ankara. Univ. Fak. Derg.* 58: 175–179.

25. White, J.D., Tisdall, P.L.C., Norris, J.M. et al. (2003). Diaphragmatic hernia in a cat mimicking a pulmonary mass. *J. Feline Med. Surg.* 5: 197–201.

26. Voges, A.K., Bertrand, S., Hill, R.C. et al. (1997). True diaphragmatic hernia in a cat. *Vet. Radiol. Ultrasound* 2: 116–119.

27. Minihan, A.C., Berg, J., and Evans, K.L. (2004). Chronic diaphragmatic hernia in 34 dogs and 16 cats. *J. Am. Anim. Hosp. Assoc.* 40: 51–63.

28. Snyder, P.S., Sato, T., and Atkins, C.E. (1990). The utility of thoracic radiographic measurement for the detection of cardiomegaly in cats with pleural effusion. *Vet. Radiol.* 31: 89–91.

29. Davies, C. and Forrester, S.D. (1996). Pleural effusion in cats: 82 cases (1987–1995). *J. Small Anim. Pract.* 37: 217–224.

30. Waddell, L.S., Brady, C.A., and Drobatz, K.J. (2002). Risk factors, prognostic indicators, and outcome of pyothorax in cats: 80 cases (1986–1999). *J. Am. Vet. Med. Assoc.* 221: 819–824.

31. Barrs, V.R., Allan, G.S., Martin, P. et al. (2005). Feline pyothorax: a retrospective study of 27 cases in Australia. *J. Feline Med. Surg.* 7: 211–222.

32. Fossum, T.W. (2004). Chylothorax. In: *Textbook of Respiratory Disease in Dogs and Cats* (ed. L.G. King), 597–604. St Louis, MO: Saunders.

33. Fossum, T.W., Mertens, M.M., Miller, M.W. et al. (2004). Thoracic duct ligation and pericardectomy for treatment of idiopathic chylothorax. *J. Vet. Intern. Med.* 18: 307–310.

34. Fossum, T.W. (2001). Chylothorax in cats: is there a role for surgery? *J. Feline Med. Surg.* 3: 73–79.

35. Fossum, T.W., Evering, W.N., Miller, M.W. et al. (1992). Severe bilateral fibrosing pleuritis associated with chronic chylothorax in five cats and two dogs. *J. Am. Vet. Med. Assoc.* 201: 317–324.

36. Thrall, D.E. (2013). The canine and feline lung. In: *Textbook of Veterinary Diagnostic Radiology*, 6e (ed. D.E. Thrall). St Louis, MO: Elsevier Saunders.

37. Foster, S.F., Allan, G.S., Martin, P. et al. (2004). Twenty-five cases of feline bronchial disease (1995–2000). *J. Feline Med. Surg.* 6: 181–188.

38. Adamama-Moraitou, K.K., Patsikas, M.N., and Koutinas, A.F. (2004). Feline lower airway disase: a retrospective study of 22 naturally occurring cases from Greece. *J. Feline Med. Surg.* 6: 227–233.

39. Koblik, P.D. (1986). Radiographic appearance of primary lung tumors in cats. A review of 41 cases. *Vet. Radiol.* 27: 66–73.

40. Miles, K.G. (1988). A review of primary lung tumors in the dog and cat. *Vet. Radiol.* 29: 122–128.

41. Hahn, K.A. and McEntee, M.F. (1997). Primary lung tumors in cats: 86 cases (1979–1994). *J. Am. Vet. Med. Assoc.* 21: 1257–1260.

42. Ballegeer, E.A., Forrest, L.J., and Stepien, R.L. (2002). Radiographic appearance of broncholveolar carcinoma in nine cats. *Vet. Radiol. US* 43: 267–271.

43. Oliveira, C.R., Mitchell, M.A., and O'Brien, R.T. (2011). Thoracic computed tomography in feline patients without use of chemical restraint. *Vet. Radiol. US* 52: 368–376.

44. Sauvé, V., Drobatz, K.J., Shokek, A.B. et al. (2005). Clinical course, diagnostic findings and necropsy diagnosis in dyspneic cats with primary pulmonary parenchymal diseases: 15 cats (1996–2002). *J. Vet. Emerg. Crit. Care* 15: 38–47.

45. Suter, P.F., Carrig, C.V., O'Brien, T.R. et al. (1974). Radiographic recognition of primary and metastatic pulmonary neoplasms of dogs and cats. *J. Am. Vet. Rad. Soc.* 15: 3–25.

46. Rebhun, R.B. and Culp, W.T.N. (2013). Pulmonary neoplasia; section D, tumors of the respiratory system. In: *Withrow and MacEwen's Small Animal Clinical Oncology*, 5e (ed. S.J. Withrow, D.M. Vail and R.L. Page). St Louis, MO: Elsevier Saunders.

47. Goldfinch, N. and Argyle, D. (2012). Feline lung-digit syndrome. Unusual metastatic patterns of primary lung tumours in cats. *J. Feline Med. Surg.* 14: 201–208.

48. Gottfried, S.D., Popovitch, C.A., Goldschmidt, M.H. et al. (2000). Metastatic digital carcinoma in the cat: a retrospective study of 36 cats (1992–1998). *J. Am. Anim. Hosp. Assoc.* 36: 501–509.

49. Jacobs, T.M. and Tomlinson, M.J. (1997). The lung-digit syndrome in a cat. *Feline Practice* 25: 31–36.

50. Forrest, L.J. and Graybush, C.A. (1998). Radiographic patterns of pulmonary metastasis in 25 cats. *Vet. Radiol. US* 39: 4–8.

51. Lioret, A., Hartmann, K., Pennisi, M.G. et al. (2013). Rare systemic mycoses in cats: blastomycosis, histoplasmosis and coccidioidomycosis. ABCD guidelines on prevention and management. *J. Feline Med. Surg.* 15: 624–627.

52. Aulakh, H.K., Aulakh, K.S., and Troy, G.C. (2012). Feline histoplasmosis: a retrospective study of 22 cases (1998–2009). *J. Am. Anim. Hosp. Assoc.* 48: 182–187.

53. Gingerich, K. and Guptil, L. (2008). Canine and feline histoplasmosis: a review of a widespread fungus. *Vet. Med.* 103: 248–261.

54. Kerl, M.E. (2003). Update on canine and feline fungal diseases. *Vet. Clin. North Am. Small Anim. Pract.* 33: 721–747.

55. Brömel, C. and Sykes, J. (2005). Histoplasmosis in dogs and cats. *Clin. Tech. Small Anim. Pract.* 20: 227–232.

56. Brömel, C. and Sykes, J. (2005). Epidemiology, diagnosis, and treatment of blastomycosis in dogs and cats. *Clin. Tech. Small Anim. Pract.* 20: 233–239.

57. Davies, J.L., Epp, T., and Burgess, H.J. (2013). Prevalence and geographic distribution of canine and feline blastomycosis in the Canadian prairies. *Can. Vet. J.* 54: 753–760.

58. Brown, N. and Zontine, W.J. (1976). Lung lobe torsion in the cat. *J. Am. Vet. Rad. Soc.* 17: 219–223.

59. D'Anjou, M.A., Tidwell, A.S., and Hecht, S. (2005). Radiographic diagnosis of lung lobe torsion. *Vet. Radiol. US* 46: 478–484.

60. McLane, M.J. and Buote, N.J. (2011). Lung lobe torsion associated with chylothorax in a cat. *J. Feline Med. Surg.* 13: 135–138.

61. Dye, T.L., Teague, H.D., and Poundstone, M.L. (1998). Lung lobe torsion in a cat with chronic feline asthma. *J. Am. Anim. Hosp. Assoc.* 34: 493–495.

62. Schober, K.E., Wetli, E., and Drost, W.T. (2014). Radiographic and echocardiographic assessment of left atrial size in 100 cats with acute left-sided congestive heart failure. *Vet. Rad. US* 55: 359–367.

63. Nafe, L.A., Declue, A.E., Dee-Fowler, T.M. et al. (2010). Evaluation of biomarkers in bronchoalveolar lavage fluid for discrimination between asthma and chronic bronchitis in cats. *Am. J. Vet. Res.* 71: 583–591.

64. Venema, C. and Patterson, C. (2010). Feline asthma. What's new and where might clinical practice be heading? *J. Feline Med. Surg.* 12: 681–692.

65. Ettinger, S. (2010). Diseases of the trachea and upper airway. In: *Textbook of Veterinary Internal Medicine: Diseases of the Dog and Cat*, 7e (ed. S.J. Ettinger and E.C. Feldman). St Louis, MO: Saunders Elsevier.

66. Lin, C.H., Lee, J.J., and Liu, C.H. (2014). Functional assessment of expiratory flow pattern in feline lower airway disease. *J. Feline Med. Surg.* 16: 616–622.

67. Gadbois, J., d'Anjou, M.A., Dunn, M. et al. (2009). Radiographic abnormalities in cats with feline bronchial disease and intra- and interobserver variability in radiographic interpretation: 40 cases (1999–2006). *J. Am. Vet. Med. Assoc.* 234: 367–375.

68. Bay, J.D. and Johnson, L.R. (2004). Feline bronchial disease/asthma. In: *Textbook of Respiratory Disease in Dogs and Cats* (ed. L.G. King). St Louis, MO: Saunders.

69. Cooper, E.S., Syring, R.S., and King, L.G. (2003). Pneumothorax in cats with a clinical diagnosis of feline asthma: 5 cases (1990–2000). *J. Vet. Emerg. Crit. Care* 13: 95–101.

70. Robbins, S. (1989). The respiratory system. In: *Robbins' Pathologic Basis of Disease*, 4e. Philadelphia, PA: Saunders.

71. Norris, C.R. and Samii, V.F. (2000). Clinical, radiographic, and pathologic features of bronchiectasis in cats: 12 cases (1987–1999). *J. Am. Vet. Med. Assoc.* 216: 530–534.

72. Talavera, J., Fernandez del Palacio, M.J., and Bayon, A. (2008). Broncholithiasis in a cat: clinical findings, long-term evolution and histopathological features. *J. Feline Med. Surg.* 10: 95–101.

73. Seo, J.B., Song, K.S., and Lee, J.S. (2002). Broncholithiasis: review of the causes with radiologic-pathologic correlation. *Radiographics* 22: s199–s213.

74. Benigni, L., Morgan, N., and Lamb, C.R. (2009). Radiographic appearance of cardiogenic pulmonary oedema in 23 cats. *J. Small Anim. Pract.* 50: 9–14.

75. McKlveen, T.L. and Moon, M.L. (1999). Radiographic appearance of cardiogenic pulmonary edema in cats. *Vet. Radiol. Ultrasound* 40: 676.

76. Goutal, C.M., Keir, I., Kenney, S. et al. (2010). Evaluation of acute congestive heart failure in dogs and cats: 145 cases (2007–2008). *J. Vet. Emerg. Crit. Care* 20: 330–337.

77. Johns, S.M., Nelson, O.L., and Gay, J.M. (2012). Left atrial function in cats with left-sided cardiac disease and pleural effusion or pulmonary edema. *J. Vet. Intern. Med.* 26: 1134–1139.

78. Scherrer, W.E., Kyles, A.E., Samii, V.F. et al. (2008). Computed tomographic assessment of vascular invasion and resectability of mediastinal masses in dogs and a cat. *New Zealand Vet. J.* 56: 330–333.

79. Day, M.J. (1997). Review of thymic pathology in 30 cats and 36 dogs. *J. Small Anim. Pract.* 38: 393–403.

80. Thamm, D.H. (2013). Miscellaneous tumors. In: *Small Animal Clinical Oncology*, 5e (ed. S.J. Withrow, D.M. Vail and R.L. Page), 679–715. St Louis, MO: Elsevier/Saunders.

81. Shilo, Y., Pypendop, B.H., and Barter, L.S. (2011). Thymoma removal in a cat with acquired myasthenia gravis: a case report and literature review of anesthetic techniques. *Vet. Anaesth. Analg.* 38: 603–613.

82. Gores, B.R., Berg, J., Carpenter, J.L. et al. (1994). Surgical treatment of thymoma in cats: 12 cases (1987–1992). *J. Am. Vet. Med. Asssoc.* 204: 1782–1785.

83. Zekas, L.J. and Adams, W.M. (2002). Cranial mediastinal cysts in nine cats. *Vet. Radiol. US* 43: 413–418.

84. Ellison, G.W., Garner, M.M., and Ackerman, N. (1994). Idiopathic mediastinal cyst in a cat. *Vet. Radiol. US* 35: 347–349.

85. Swainson, S.W., Nelson, O.L., Niyo, Y. et al. (2000). Radiographic diagnosis: mediastinal parathyroid cyst in a cat. *Vet. Radiol. US* 41: 41–43.

86. Reichle, J.K. and Wisner, E.R. (2000). Non-cardiac thoracic ultrasound in 75 feline and canine patients. *Vet. Radiol. US* 41: 154–162.

87. Thomas, E.K. and Syring, R.S. (2013). Pneumomediastinum in cats: 45 cases (2000–2010). *J. Vet. Emerg. Crit. Care* 23: 429–435.

88. Mitchell, S.L., McCarthy, R., and Rudloff E, Pernell R (2000). Trachea rupture associated with intubation in cats: 20 cases (1996–1998). *J. Am. Vet. Med. Assoc.* 216: 1592–1595.

89. Zambelli, A.B. (2006). Pneumomediastinum, pneumothorax and pneumoretroperitoneum following endoscopic retrieval of a tracheal foreign body from a cat. *J. S. Afr. Vet. Assoc.* 77: 45–50.

90. Hardie, E.M., Spodnick, G.J., Gilson, S.D. et al. (1999). Tracheal rupture in cats: 16 cases (1983–1998). *J. Am. Vet. Med. Assoc.* 214: 508–512.

91. Guglielmini, C. and Diana, A. (2015). Thoracic radiography in the cat: identification of cardiomegaly and congestive heart failure. *J. Vet. Cardiol.* 17: S87–S101.

92. Lord, P.F. and Zontine, W.J. (1977). Radiological examination of the feline cardiovascular system. *Vet. Clin. North Am. Small Anim. Pract.* 7: 291–308.

93. Rishniw, M. (2000). Radiography of feline cardiac disease. *Vet. Clin. North Am. Small Anim. Pract.* 30: 395–425.

94. Suter, P.F. and Lord, P.F. (ed.) (1984). *Thoracic Radiography: A Text Atlas of Thoracic Diseases in the Dog and Cat*. Wettswill: Eigenverlag.

# Abdomen

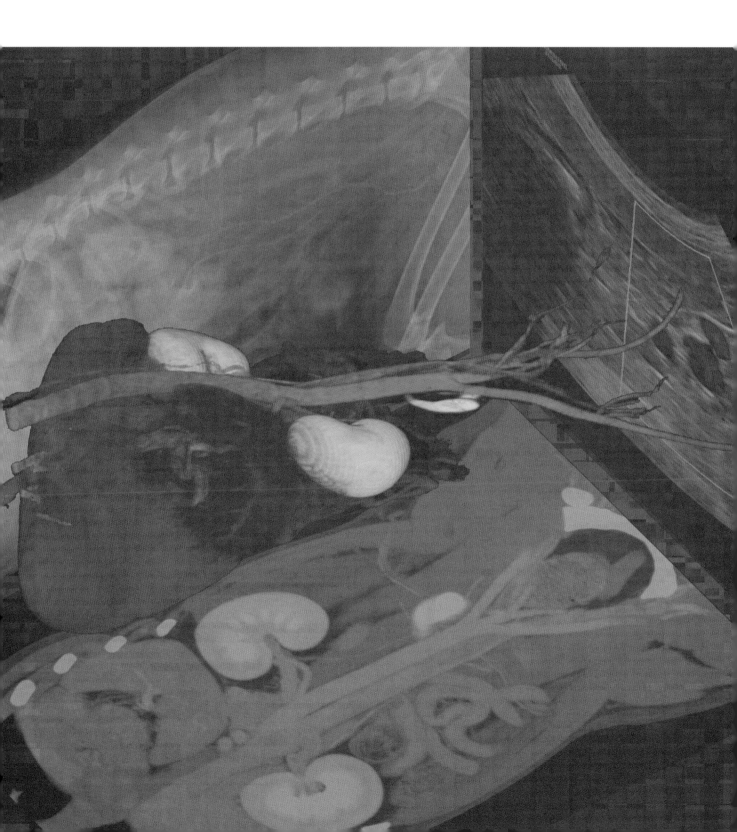

# CHAPTER 20

# Anatomy, Variants, and Interpretation Paradigm

**Elodie E. Huguet[1], Clifford R. Berry[2], and Robson Giglio[3]**

[1] Department of Small Animal Clinical Sciences, College of Veterinary Medicine, University of Florida, Gainesville, FL, USA
[2] Department of Molecular Biomedical Sciences, College of Veterinary Medicine, North Carolina State University, Raleigh, NC, USA
[3] College of Veterinary Medicine, University of Georgia, Athens, GA, USA

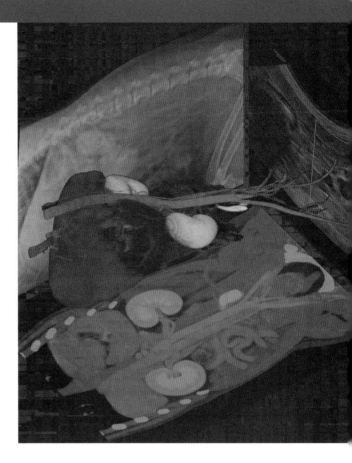

## Introduction

A wide range of normal variants are encountered when imaging the abdomen, and an understanding of the normal anatomy is important to recognize these variations. Various inherent and technical factors may influence interpretation of the normal anatomy, such as patient conformation, breed, and positioning. Some variations may mimic disease and should be interpreted with caution. To help guide image interpretation of the abdomen, an overview of the abdominal anatomy and commonly encountered variations are presented in this chapter (see also Appendix III).

## Diaphragm

The abdomen is bordered cranially by the diaphragm and caudally by the pelvic canal. The abdominal surface of the diaphragm is mostly border effaced by the liver on radiographs but increased intraperitoneal fat (falciform ligament in cats) or decreased size of the liver can improve delineation of the dorsal or ventral diaphragmatic margins (Figure 20.1). The normal margins of the diaphragm are smooth and continuous, with a convex contour extending cranially into the thoracic cavity (Figure 20.2). The diaphragmatic crura attach on the ventral aspects of the L3–L4 vertebral bodies; these margins will be ill defined compared to L2 and L5 (Figure 20.3). Between left and right lateral radiographs of the abdomen, variations in the position of the diaphragmatic crura are observed that will vary with species, patient breed and size, and x-ray beam centering. Due to gravitational displacement of the abdominal structures on lateral radiographs, increased intraabdominal pressure results in cranial displacement of the dependent diaphragmatic crus in relation to the contralateral nondependent diaphragmatic crus. On the right lateral projection, the diaphragmatic crura are parallel to each other, whereas on the left lateral projection, they are often tangentially oriented, diverging away from a central position, creating a V- or Y-shaped appearance (Figure 20.4). A similar variation should be taken into consideration when

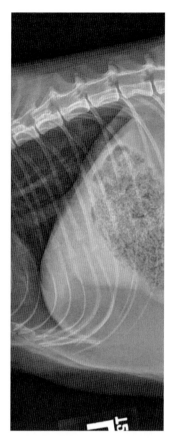

**FIGURE 20.1**   Increased delineation of the diaphragm on a left lateral radiograph associated with the presence of increased intraabdominal fat.

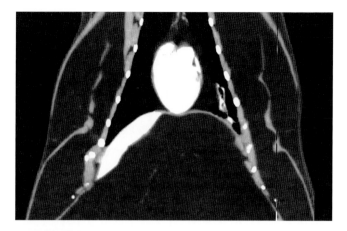

**FIGURE 20.2**   Computed tomographic image of the diaphragm in a dorsal plane.

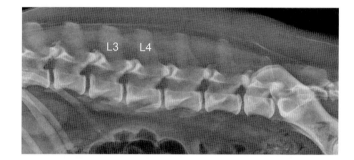

**FIGURE 20.3**   Radiograph of the diaphragmatic crura attachment on the ventral aspects of the L3–L4 vertebral bodies (note ill-defined ventral margin).

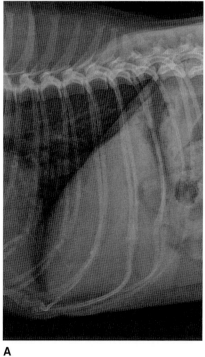

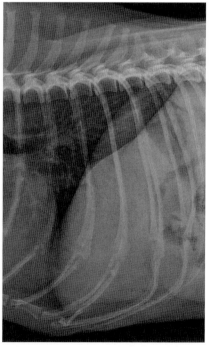

A                                                    B

**FIGURE 20.4**   Displacement of the diaphragmatic crura on right (**A**) and left lateral (**B**) radiographs, respectively.

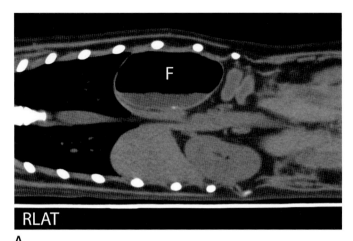

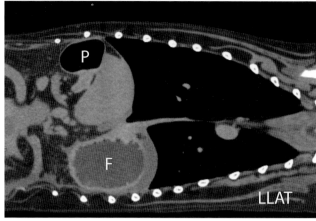

**A**          **B**

**FIGURE 20.5**   Computed tomographic images of the diaphragmatic crura in a dorsal plane, showing similar cranial extension of the diaphragmatic crura in right lateral recumbency (**A** - RLAT) where gas is present in the fundic portion (Label F) of the stomach. In (**B** LLAT) there is gas noted in the pylorus (P) and the left diaphragmatic crus is displaced cranially relative to the right. The fundus (F) of the stomach is filled with fluid.

imaging patients in lateral recumbency with other imaging modalities (Figure 20.5).

On ultrasound, the diaphragm cannot be isolated from the highly reflective hyperechoic interface of the lungs in the absence of pleural disease (Figure 20.6). The reflective interface of the lung–diaphragm usually causes a mirror image artifact, resulting in an image of abdominal structures (e.g. liver and gall bladder) noted on the thoracic side of the diaphragm (Figure 20.7).

# Abdominal cavity

The abdomen and pelvic cavities, as well as the scrotum in male patients, form a continuous peritoneal cavity. The wall of the peritoneal cavity is composed of the peritoneum, which has three parts (Figure 20.8).

1. *A parietal surface*: covers the inner surface of the abdominal and pelvic walls and the scrotum.

2. *A serosal surface*: covers the organs contained within those cavities.

3. *Connecting peritoneum*: forms various ligaments, mesentery, and omentum connecting the serosal peritoneum between organs or to parietal peritoneum. The mesentery more specifically connects the gastrointestinal tract to the dorsal abdominal wall.

The retroperitoneal space is a potential space between the dorsal parietal peritoneum and the hypaxial musculature. It extends from the diaphragm and extends into the pelvic cavity. Cranially, the retroperitoneal space and mediastinum communicate through the aortic hiatus, meaning that a pneumomediastinum can lead to a pneumoretroperitoneum. Contained within the retroperitoneal space are the kidneys, adrenal

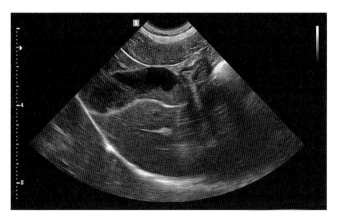

**FIGURE 20.6**   Indistinction of the diaphragm from the lung interface on ultrasound.

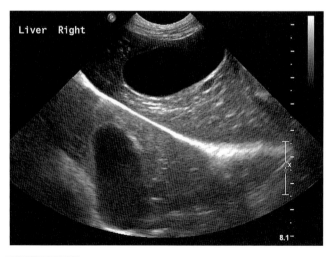

**FIGURE 20.7**   Mirror image artifact from the reflective interface of the lung–diaphragm on ultrasound.

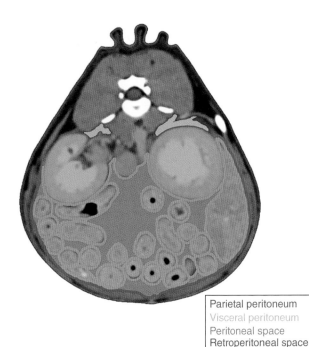

| | |
|---|---|
| Parietal peritoneum | |
| Visceral peritoneum | |
| Peritoneal space | |
| Retroperitoneal space | |

**FIGURE 20.8** Anatomic illustration of the peritoneum and associated spaces.

glands, ureters, cisterna chyli, major abdominal blood vessels, and parietal lymph nodes. In female dogs, the retroperitoneum includes part of the urinary bladder neck, unlike in male dogs where it extends more ventrally at the level of the pelvic inlet to include the ventral margin of the prostate.

The amount of fat present throughout the abdominal cavity depends on the patient's body condition. In obese patients, increased fat deposition may be observed predominantly around the falciform ligament and retroperitoneal space. The presence of fat in the peritoneal cavity aids with visualization of the serosal margins on abdominal radiographs (Figure 20.9). This is attributed to the lower density of fat in relation to fluid and/or

soft tissues within adjacent structures. Younger patients have a greater amount of brown fat with a higher water content and a mild amount of peritoneal effusion, both of which will result in an increase in soft tissue opacity throughout the abdominal cavity, thereby decreasing the overall serosal detail (Figure 20.10). Additionally, poor serosal detail is seen in emaciated patients due to the reduced presence of intrabdominal fat (Figure 20.11).

When evaluating the abdominal cavity with ultrasound, excess fat may partially attenuate the ultrasound beam, therefore limiting visualization of deeper abdominal structures, and can hinder the ultrasonographic evaluation of larger patients, making computed tomography a preferred modality (Figures 20.12 and 20.13). A scant amount of anechoic effusion within the peritoneal cavity represents a normal physiological variant, especially in young cats and dogs.

Within the peritoneal cavity, the fat may undergo focal necrosis and form a mobile intraabdominal mineralized body with a thin mineralized rim, called "Bates bodies," nodular fat necrosis or cholesterol inclusion cysts. These structures vary in size and location, and are of no clinical concern (Figure 20.14).

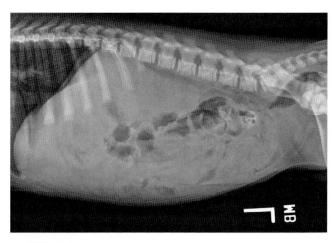

**FIGURE 20.10** Radiograph of a juvenile canine patient with poor serosal detail due to the presence of brown fat and mild amount of physiologic peritoneal effusion.

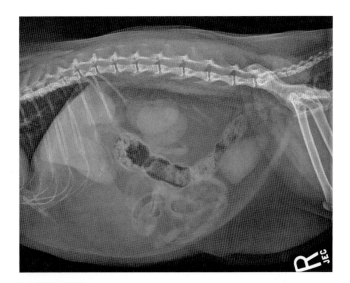

**FIGURE 20.9** Right lateral radiograph with good conspicuity of the serosal margins associated with the presence of a large amount of intraabdominal fat.

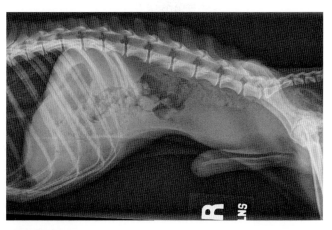

**FIGURE 20.11** Radiograph of an emaciated patient with poor serosal detail due to the reduced presence of intraabdominal fat.

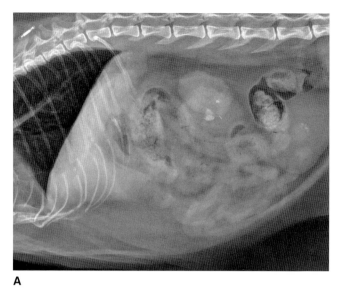

**A**

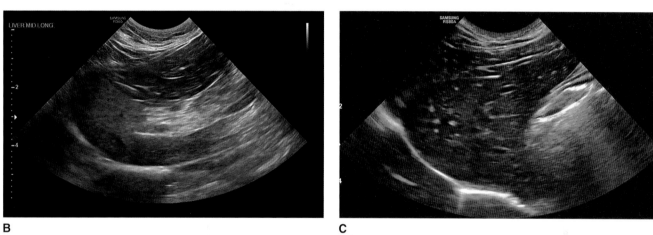

**B**

**C**

**FIGURE 20.12**   Radiograph (**A**) and ultrasound (**B**) images of the same cat with a large amount of falciform fat, causing attenuation of the ultrasound beam. Ultrasound image (**C**) of a normal feline liver for comparison.

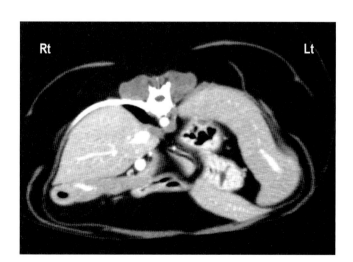

**FIGURE 20.13**   Improved assessment of the liver using computed tomography as opposed to ultrasound in obese patients.

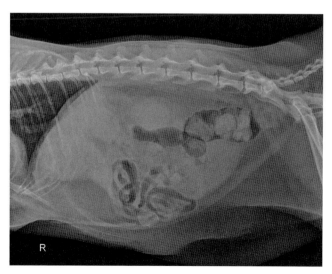

**FIGURE 20.14**   Right lateral radiograph of a feline patient with a ventrally located intraperitoneal mineralized structure, representing a Bates body.

# Gastrointestinal Tract

Radiographs are commonly used to assess the luminal contents of the gastrointestinal tract. The normal amount of gas within the gastrointestinal tract is variable. In normal fasted cats, small intestinal gas is rarely to mildly present, whereas in fasted dogs, approximately 30–60% of the small intestinal segments may be filled by gas under normal conditions. In nonfasted dogs and cats, the amount of intraluminal small intestinal gas may increase. The normal gastrointestinal wall cannot be reliably assessed due to border effacement with luminal contents or lack thereof and crowding with adjacent abdominal structures. Ultrasonography provides the best evaluation of the normal gastrointestinal wall; however, the presence of intraluminal gas may hinder visualization of the wall in the far field. The patient may need to be changed to a different recumbency for a more complete evaluation of the wall layers in such instances when doing an abdominal ultrasound.

## Stomach

The stomach has four regions: fundus, cardia, body, and pylorus (Figure 20.15). The craniodorsal and caudoventral surfaces of the stomach between the gastroesophageal and gastroduodenal junctions form the lesser and greater curvature, respectively. The stomach is located caudodorsal to the liver with the fundus/body centered in the left cranial abdomen. The pyloric antrum is ventrally located in relation to the fundus and extends to the right of midline in dogs (Figure 20.16). In comparison, it may be positioned along midline in cats (Figure 20.17). The stomach may contain a small amount of fluid and gas in fasted patients. Gas shifts within the nondependent aspect of the gastric lumen per recumbency as illustrated in Figure 20.18. Filling of the pyloric antrum with gas on the left lateral projection may aid with visualization of the gastroduodenal junction,

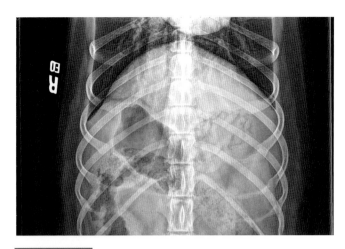

**FIGURE 20.16** Normal positioning of the stomach in dogs on a ventrodorsal radiograph.

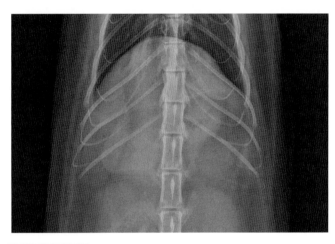

**FIGURE 20.17** Normal positioning of the stomach in cats on a ventrodorsal radiograph.

which may contain a small amount of gas tracking into the proximal duodenum under normal conditions (Figure 20.19). Gas within the gastric lumen in an underdistended stomach may contrast with rugal folds along the mucosal margins of the gastric wall, which are commonly most prominent in the gastric body and fundus (Figure 20.20). This finding is less commonly seen in cats. The size of the stomach varies based on the fasted state of the patient. In the absence of hepatomegaly, the caudal border of a relatively empty stomach should not extend beyond the last pair of ribs (Figure 20.21).

Ultrasound has the unique advantage of providing the best evaluation of the gastric wall layers, which are named and characterized as follows (from lumen to serosal surface, Figure 20.22).

1. Mucosal luminal interface: hyperechoic
2. Mucosa: hypoechoic and thickest
3. Submucosa: hyperechoic
4. Muscularis: hypoechoic
5. Serosal: hyperechoic and thinnest (not always identified)

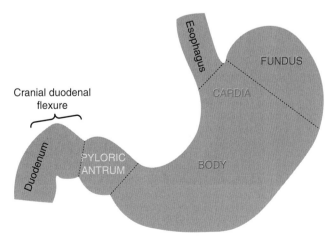

**FIGURE 20.15** Anatomic illustration of the canine and feline stomach.

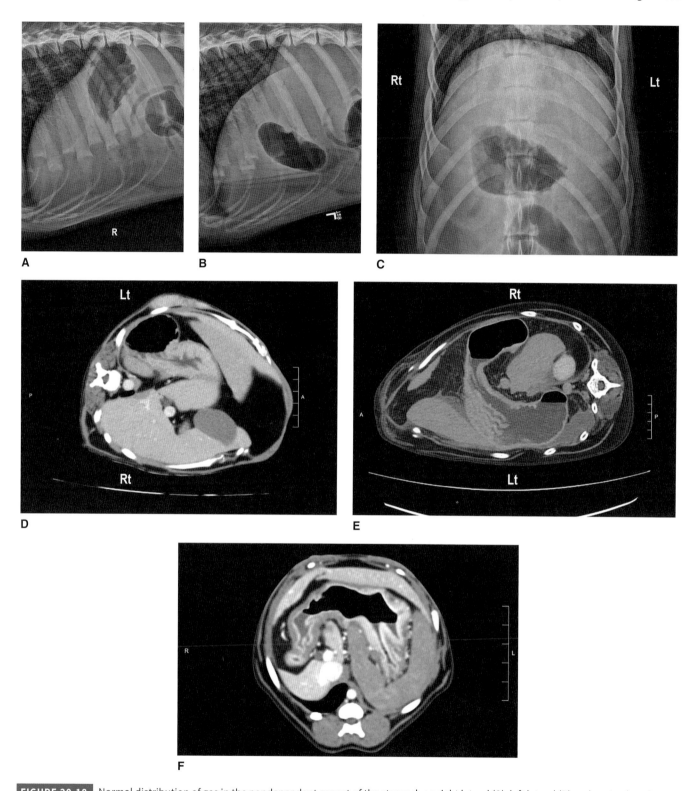

**FIGURE 20.18**   Normal distribution of gas in the nondependent aspect of the stomach on right lateral (**A**), left lateral (**B**) and ventrodorsal projections (**C**). CT images in the corresponding right recumbent (**D**), left recumbent (**E**), and dorsal recumbent (**F**) position show gas in different parts of the stomach depending on body position.

Measurements of the gastric wall thickness may be limited in the presence of an empty stomach and should be obtained with caution when only containing a small amount of ingesta as redundancy of the gastric wall may be falsely interpreted as gastric wall thickening (Figure 20.23). The overall thickness of the gastric wall should be measured between rugal folds and is <5 mm in dogs and <4 mm in cats [1]. The muscularis propria is thickest at the level of the pyloric sphincter and should not be misinterpreted as pathologic thickening.

While the gastric wall layers cannot be visualized on radiographs, cats have submucosal fat, which may be apparent on

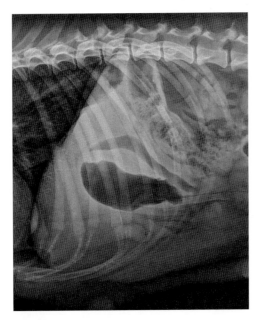

**FIGURE 20.19** Tracking of nondependent gas within the pyloric antrum, through the pyloroduodenal junction and into the descending duodenum on a left lateral radiographic projection.

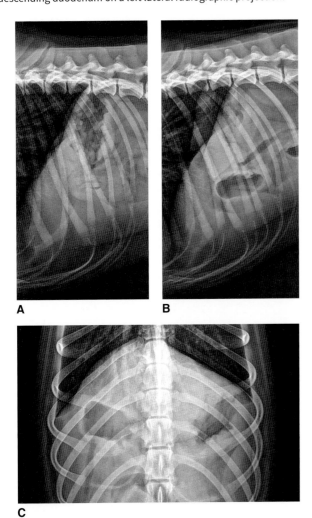

**A**      **B**

**C**

**FIGURE 20.20** Empty stomach with a small amount of intraluminal gas, highlighting normal rugal folds, on right lateral (**A**), left lateral (**B**) and ventrodorsal (**C**) radiographs.

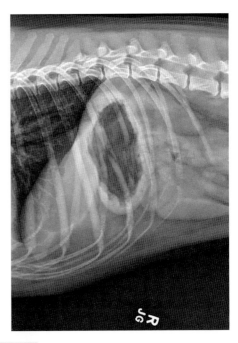

**FIGURE 20.21** Normal nondistended stomach on a right lateral radiograph (note how caudal margin of the stomach does not extend beyond the last pair of ribs).

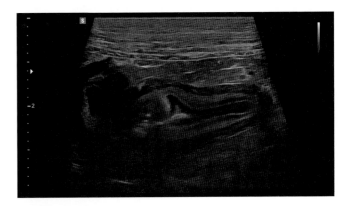

**FIGURE 20.22** Normal gastric wall layers on ultrasound.

ventrodorsal projections when the gastric body is empty and viewed enface (Figure 20.24) [2].

Computed tomography (CT) has the advantage of providing a three-dimensional image of the stomach without superimposition of other structures, permitting evaluation of the gastric wall despite the presence of intraluminal gas. CT may also improve evaluation of the stomach in large and/or deep-chested patients. While distinct wall layers are poorly recognized, the normal increased contrast enhancement of the gastric mucosa on images acquired during the arterial phase may help differentiate it from the other gastric wall layers (Figure 20.25).

## Small Intestine

The small intestine has three parts, which sequentially are the duodenum, jejunum, and ileum when traced in an aborad direction. The duodenum is divided into descending and

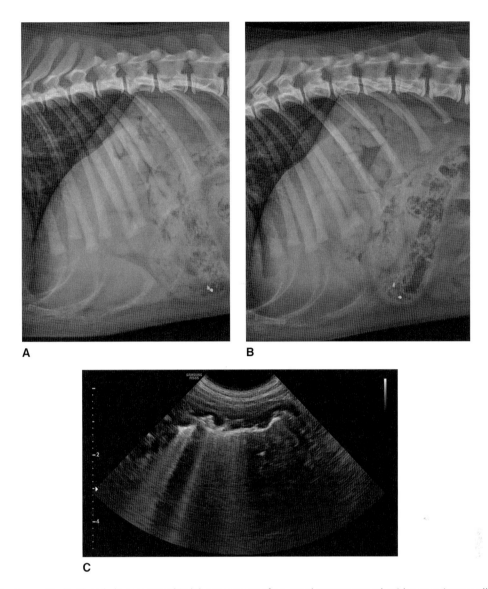

**FIGURE 20.23**   Radiographic (**A**, **B**) and ultrasonographic (**C**) appearance of a normal empty stomach with a prominent wall due to mural contraction and presence of rugal folds.

ascending parts. The descending duodenum extends caudally along the right lateral abdominal wall in the dog and then turns craniomedially at the caudal duodenal flexure before continuing for a short distance as the ascending duodenum. The ascending duodenum then joins with the jejunum in the mid to cranial abdominal region near midline. The jejunum makes up the majority of the small intestine and mostly occupies the mid abdomen. In cats, the pyloroduodenal junction is near midline so that the descending duodenum is in a more midline position compared with dogs. In cats with abundant fat and increased fecal material in the colon, most of the small intestine may be located to the right of midline. The ileum is the shortest small intestinal segment and cannot be differentiated from the jejunum on radiographs aside from localization at the ileocolic junction in dogs and the ileocecocolic junction in cats.

The small intestine has indistinguishable wall layers on radiographs with effaced mucosal margins in the absence of intraluminal gas. The overall thickness of the duodenum is often greater than the jejunum in dogs. The descending duodenum may contain a small amount of gas, especially on the left lateral projection due to extension of nondependent gas from the gastric lumen. Along the antimesenteric side of the duodenum, gas or positive contrast medium within the duodenal lumen may highlight small concave mucosal defects representing pseudoulcers secondary to gut-associated lymphoid tissue (GALT) or Peyer's patches (Figure 20.26). A similar finding may be observed with ultrasonography and CT (Figure 20.27). In cats, the small intestine may be evenly concentrically narrowed with a "string of pearls" appearance, representing peristalsis (Figure 20.28).

On ultrasound, the small intestine has well-defined wall layers, similar to the stomach, with normal wall layer thickness measurements listed in Table 20.1 [1]. The ileum may be differentiated from the jejunum due to its overall increased wall thickness and prominent submucosa and muscularis layers (Figure 20.29). In young patients, hyperechoic lines

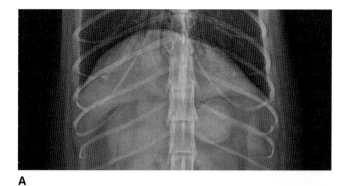

**A**

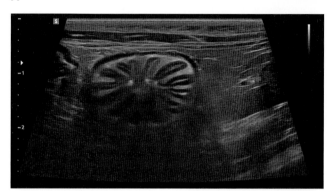

**B**

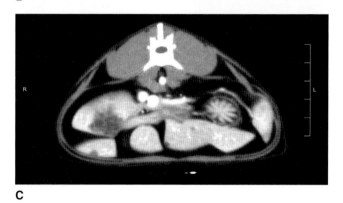

**C**

**FIGURE 20.24** Radiographic (**A**), ultrasonographic (**B**), and computed tomographic (**C**) appearance of the feline gastric wall with prominent submucosal fat (decreased opacity on radiographs, increased echogenicity on ultrasound and decreased attenuation on the CT study).

parallel to the submucosal may be observed within the outer aspect of the mucosa and may represent normal lymphoid tissues (Figure 20.29b). When viewing any portion of the small intestine in a short axis view, wedge-shaped hyperechoic regions are seen extending from opposing sides of the lumen into the mucosa and likely represent anisotropism due to tangential ultrasound beam alignment with the intestinal villi and intestinal crypts (Figure 20.30). Occasionally, hyperechoic striations along the luminal aspect of the mucosa may represent gas or ingesta within the intestinal crypts, most commonly seen in nonfasted patients, and may be indistinguishable from pathologic lymphangiectasia (Figure 20.31).

Similar to the stomach, the small intestinal wall layers cannot be differentiated on CT, with the exception of the mucosa following IV contrast due to normal increased contrast enhancement during the arterial phase (Figure 20.32).

## Colon

The colon is divided into ascending, transverse, and descending parts. The ileocecocolic (in cats) or ileocolic junction (in dogs) is commonly located in the right cranial to mid abdomen. At this level, the cecum represents a blind pouch which joins the ileocecocolic transition (in cats) or the ascending colon to form the cecocolic junction (in dogs). The ascending colon can be identified within the right cranial abdomen and traced cranially from the ileocolic junction to the right colic flexure, where it turns into the transverse colon. The transverse colon extends across midline into the left cranial abdomen before turning at the left caudal flexure and continuing caudally as the descending colon to the level of the pelvic inlet. The descending colon is more commonly located within the left abdomen but can be incidentally redundant and traced to the right of midline (Figure 20.33). The cecum and colon cannot always be differentiated on radiographs. When seen, the cecum often represents a lobular gas-filled structure in the right midabdominal region (Figure 20.34). Occasionally, fecal material may be identified within the cecum.

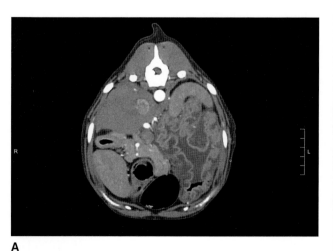

**A**

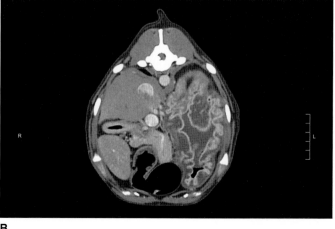

**B**

**FIGURE 20.25** Transverse computed tomographic images of the stomach acquired during the arterial (**A**) and venous (**B**) phases of contrast enhancement.

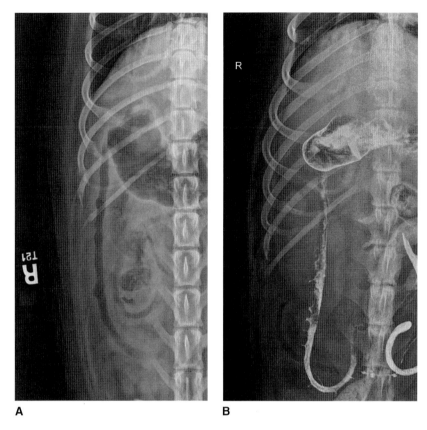

**A**        **B**

**FIGURE 20.26**   Radiographs of the stomach acquired before (**A**) and after (**B**) barium administration, highlighting small concave defects along the duodenal mucosa, most compatible with gut-associated lymphoid tissue or Peyer's patches.

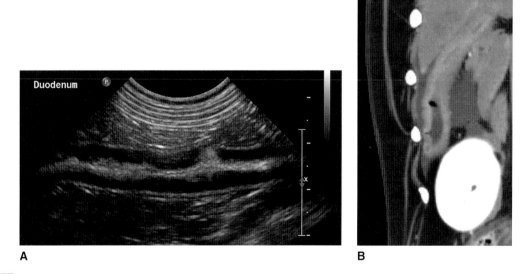

**A**        **B**

**FIGURE 20.27**   Ultrasonographic (**A**) and computed tomographic (**B**) images of the duodenum, showing the presence of small concave mucosal defects, representing gut-associated lymphoid tissue or Peyer's patches.

On radiographs, the cat cecum is not visualized. On ultrasound, the feline cecum may also be difficult to differentiate from the colon and represents a blind pouch continuous with the colon at the level of the ileocecocolic junction. When empty, the cecum in feline patients forms a lobular hypoechoic structure (Figure 20.35). The colonic contents can have a wide range of appearances and should be primarily heterogeneously soft tissue opaque.

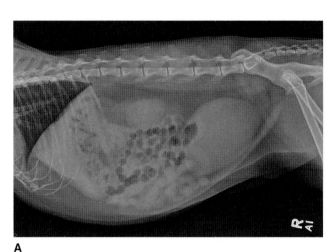

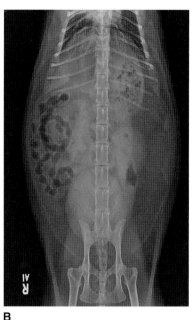

A

B

**FIGURE 20.28** Right lateral (**A**) and ventrodorsal (**B**) radiographs of normal small intestinal peristalsis in cats (e.g., "string of pearls" appearance).

| TABLE 20.1 | Normal wall layer thickness in dogs and cats. | | | |
|---|---|---|---|---|
| | | Duodenum (mm) | Jejunum (mm) | Ileum (mm) |
| Dog | <15 kg | 3.8 | 3.0 | 3.0 |
| | 15–30 kg | 4.1 | 3.5 | 3.5 |
| | >30 kg | 4.4 | 3.8 | 3.8 |
| Cat | | 2.2 | 2.2 | 2.8 |

There are no quantitative criteria establishing the normal colonic diameter in dogs on radiographs. In cats, a maximal colonic diameter to L5 vertebral length ratio of less than <1.28 is most representative of a normal colon [3]. When differentiation of the colon from the small intestine is limited, especially in the present of abnormal small intestinal dilation, a pneumocolonogram may be considered by rectally injecting the amounts of room air listed in Table 20.2 into the colon with a catheter tip syringe (Figure 20.36).

On ultrasound, the colon has a thin wall with similar wall layers as the remainder of the gastrointestinal tract, cumulatively measuring up to 1.5 mm in maximal thickness. Some variation in wall thickness may be observed in direct correlation with the amount of colonic distension present. Within the colonic submucosa in canine and feline patients, small, well-defined, rounded to ovoid and hypoechoic micronodules (1–3 mm in size) have been described to represent lymphoid follicles [4]. The clinical significance of these follicles remains unknown, representing an incidental finding or a reactive inflammatory/infectious response (Figure 20.37) [4].

# Pancreas

The pancreas is located just caudal to the stomach and is composed of left and right lobes situated along the greater curvature of the stomach and mesenteric side of the descending duodenum, respectively [5–8]. The body of the pancreas is centered between the two lobes at the level of the pylorus. It is contradictory among anatomists if a true pancreatic body is present in cats. In dogs, the normal pancreas cannot be visualized on radiographs. In contrast, the left pancreatic lobe in feline patients can occasionally be seen extending between the gastric fundus and splenic head/body, particularly with increased adiposity within the peritoneal cavity (Figure 20.38). The pancreas represents a thin, long and mildly lobular soft tissue opaque structure.

Using ultrasound, the right pancreatic lobe and body are readily identified in dogs and cats. In large patients or in the presence of gastric distension, the left pancreatic lobe may not be readily visualized in dogs. The entire pancreas is more reliably identified in cats. The pancreas should be relatively well demarcated with an echogenicity slightly less than the surrounding fat, but higher than the liver (Figure 20.39). The pancreas may be infiltrated with fat in obese patients and have an echogenicity similar to the mesenteric fat, rendering visualization more difficult (Figure 20.40). The mean normal thickness of the pancreas (dorsal to ventral dimension) is listed in Table 20.3 [9].

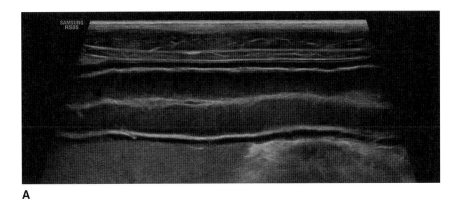

**A**

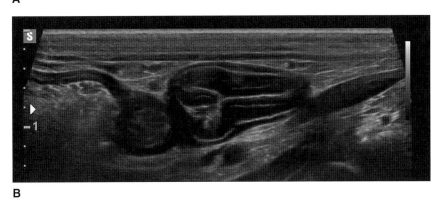

**B**

**FIGURE 20.29**   (**A**) Ultrasound image of normal jejunal wall layers in a dog. (**B**) Ultrasound image of normal ileal wall layers in a dog with the presence of a parallel hyperechoic mucosal line, representing normal lymphoid tissues.

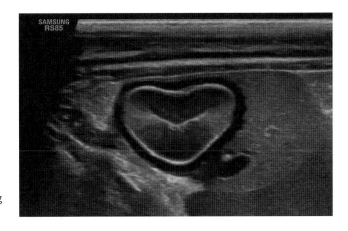

**FIGURE 20.30**   Transverse ultrasound image of the duodenum with artefactual bilateral regions of mucosal hyperechogenicity, representing anisotropy.

The use of ultrasound contrast agents may improve visualization of the pancreas in both canine and feline patients and can be used to evaluate normal perfusion [4, 5]. The limited availability and cost of ultrasound contrast agents currently limit the use of this technique in veterinary patients, but may be of future benefit to recognize pathological pancreatic changes.

Using ultrasound and CT, the pancreatic duct can occasionally be seen extending centrally within the left and right pancreatic lobes (Figure 20.41). In dogs, the extrahepatic bile duct and pancreatic duct separately enter the duodenum at the major duodenal papilla. In cats, the extrahepatic and pancreatic ducts join together just before entering the major duodenal papilla. The accessory pancreatic duct enters the duodenum at the minor duodenal papilla and is the main excretory duct in dogs. Normal upper reference ranges of <3 mm and <4 mm in diameter are reported in dogs and cats, respectively [9]. In older cats greater than 10 years of age, the normal pancreatic duct may be larger, measuring up to 5 mm in diameter (Figure 20.42) [10].

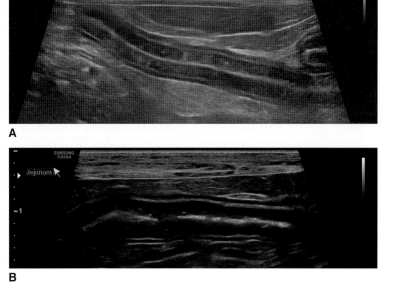

**FIGURE 20.31** Longitudinal ultrasound images of two small intestinal segments, containing mucosal hyperechoic striations (**A**), which represent gas or ingesta within the intestinal crypts, commonly seen in nonfasted dogs, and may be indistinguishable from pathologic lymphangiectasia. In (**B**), hyperechoic mucosal speckles are also present noted in a nonfasted dog.

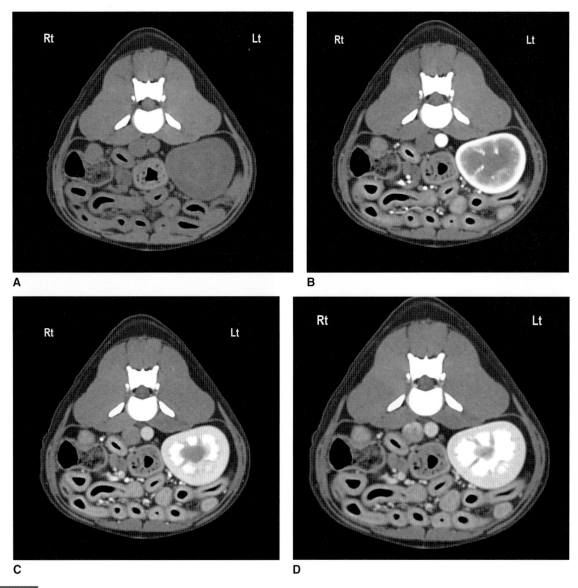

**FIGURE 20.32** Transverse computed tomographic images centered on the small intestine and acquired precontrast (**A**) and during the arterial (**B**), venous (**C**), and delayed (**D**) phases of contrast enhancement.

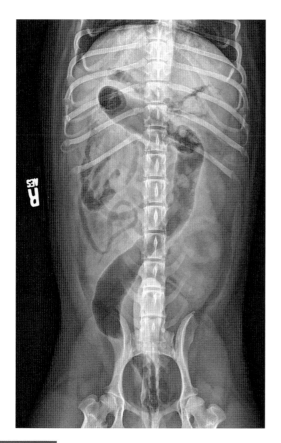

**FIGURE 20.33** Ventrodorsal radiographic projection of a redundant colon, as characterized by rightward deviation of the descending colon in the caudal abdomen.

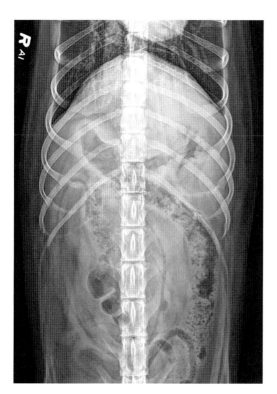

**FIGURE 20.34** Ventrodorsal radiograph showing a lobular and gas-filled bowel segment in the right midabdominal region, which represents a normal canine cecum.

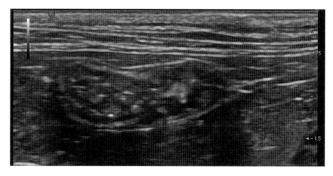

**FIGURE 20.35** Normal ultrasonographic appearance of the feline cecum.

| TABLE 20.2 | Recommended volumes of room air for pneumocolon negative contrast studies. |
|---|---|
| **Species** | **Volume (room air)** |
| Dog | 1–3 mL/kg |
| Cat | 20–30 mL |

On CT, the normal pancreas is soft tissue attenuating with a density lower than the liver and mean HU value of 61 in dogs and 48 in cats on precontrast images [7, 8]. Diffusely, the normal pancreas has heterogeneous arterial and homogenous venous contrast enhancement which remains slightly hypoattenuating to the liver during all phases of contrast enhancement. A peak attenuation value is observed during the venous phase in both cats and dogs with a mean HU value of 129 and 166, respectively (Figure 20.43) [7, 8].

# Biliary System

The gall bladder is a large saccular structure located within the gall bladder fossa of the liver, which is composed of the quadrate lobe of the liver medially and the right medial lobe laterally. The gall bladder communicates with the intrahepatic bile ducts via the cystic duct before continuing as the extrahepatic bile duct at the level of the porta hepatis. It continues caudally to the major duodenal papilla, that then enters the lumen of the proximal duodenum. While the normal gall bladder is routinely not identified on radiographs, it may occasionally represent a rounded focal soft tissue opaque bulge along the ventral margin of the liver in obese cats (Figure 20.44).

The size of the gall bladder is highly variable and may be quite voluminous in fasted or anorexic patients. Therefore, gall bladder size cannot be reliably used as an indicator of pathologic distension. In cats and dogs, the gall bladder is variable in size and shape and in normal cats it can be bilobed (Figure 20.45).

Ultrasound is the preferred modality to evaluate the gall bladder. The normal gall bladder contains anechoic bile and has

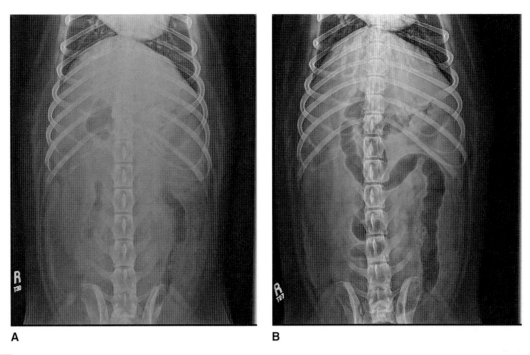

**A**                                    **B**

**FIGURE 20.36**   Ventrodorsal radiographs pre (**A**) and post (**B**) pneumocolon. Two mL/kg of room air was introduced into the colon and then an immediate exposure made for (**B**).

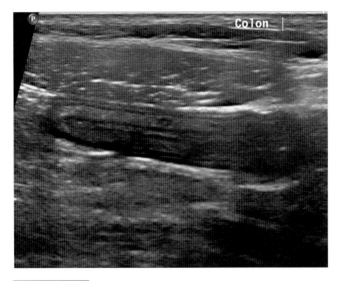

**FIGURE 20.37**   Feline colon US image (long axis) with a thickened mucosal layer and lymphoid follicles.

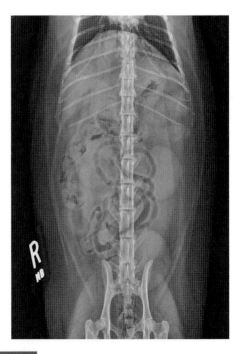

**FIGURE 20.38**   The tubular soft tissue opacity located between the spleen (craniolateral) and the left kidney (caudal) is the feline pancreas.

a thin and smoothly marginated hyperechoic wall, which measures less than 1 mm in thickness under normal conditions in cats and up to 2–3 mm in dogs [11, 12]. Contrast-enhanced ultrasonography has been reported as a way to increase the conspicuity of the gall bladder wall and may aid in the identification of wall defects due to necrosis or rupture [13]. Commonly, variable amounts of mobile, granular, echogenic and nonshadowing material, referred to as "sludge," may be identified incidentally within the gall bladder lumen in dogs (Figure 20.46) [14]. The clinical significance of this finding in cats is unclear and has been suggested as a sequela of cholestasis. Gall bladder sludge

may be recognized as more hyperattenuating nonmineralized material within the gall bladder lumen on CT (Figure 20.47).

Using ultrasound and CT, the cystic duct can be traced from the gall bladder and tapers before joining the intrahepatic bile ducts. The hepatic bile ducts represent thin branching tubular structures, which taper peripherally and can be differentiated

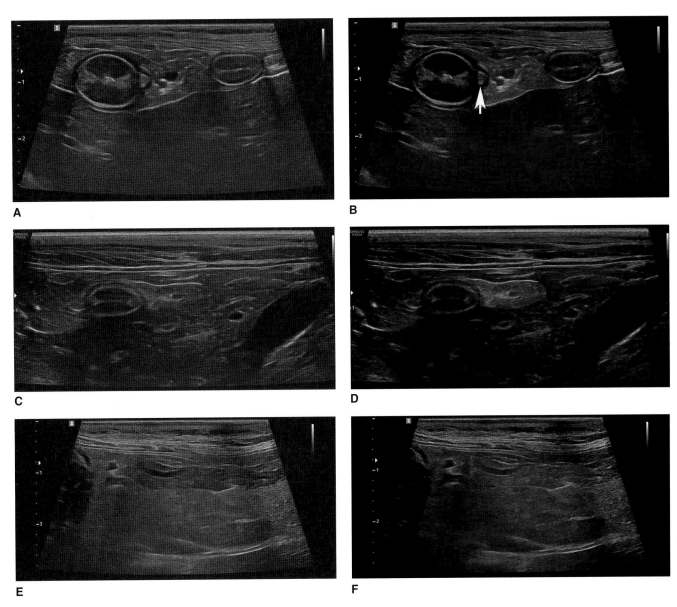

**FIGURE 20.39**   Three different ultrasound images without and with yellow highlights of the pancreas. (**A**) Short axis (transverse) view from the right cranial abdomen in a dog documenting the normal pancreas next to the duodenum. The duodenal papilla is partially visualized along the inside of the duodenum (medial margin, white arrow in (**B**)). Lateral is to the left. (**C**) Short axis (transverse) image from the right cranial abdomen in a normal cat. The right lobe of the pancreas extends toward the pancreatic body and the left lobe is noted (highlighted in yellow in (**D**)). Lateral is to the left. From the same cat (**E**), a transverse view documenting the left lobe of the pancreas (in long axis) as hypoechoic to the surrounding tissue (highlighted in yellow in (**F**)). Lateral is to the right of the image. In all images the pancreatic duct can be visualized.

from the hepatic vasculature using color or power Doppler. The extrahepatic bile duct is readily visualized, especially in cats, and should measure less than 5 mm in diameter in cats and 2 mm in dogs [15], although in dogs it is rarely seen under normal conditions.

# Liver

The liver is one of the largest intraabdominal organs and occupies the majority of the cranial abdominal cavity, with a larger portion extending to the right of midline. The liver is bordered cranially by the diaphragm and caudally by the stomach. Additionally, the caudate lobe of the liver conforms to the cranial pole of the right kidney to form the renal fossa (Figure 20.48). On radiographs, the liver is homogeneously soft tissue opaque with an angular caudoventral border, which as a general rule should not extend caudally beyond the costal arch in the absence of hepatomegaly (in expiratory radiographs) (Figure 20.49). Some variations may be seen in the presence of pulmonary hyperinflation, gastric distension or due to variability in body conformation.

The position of the gastric axis, representing a line drawn from the gastric fundus to the pylorus on lateral radiographic projections, may also be used to assess liver size.

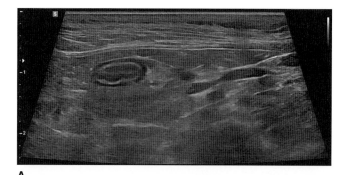

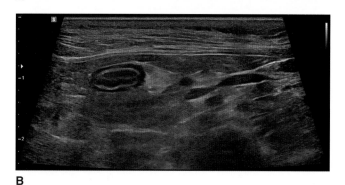

**FIGURE 20.40** (**A**) Short axis (transverse) view from the right cranial abdomen in a cat documenting a hyperechoic pancreatic right lobe next to the duodenum (highlighted in yellow in (**B**)). This is consistent with fatty infiltration. Lateral is to the left.

| TABLE 20.3 | Normal thickness of the pancreas in dogs and cats. | | |
|---|---|---|---|
| **Species** | **Right lobe** | **Body** | **Left lobe** |
| Dog | 8.1 mm | 6.3 mm | 6.5 mm |
| Cat | 4.4 mm | 6.2 mm | 5.8 mm |

Although some variations may exist, the gastric axis should be parallel to the long axis of the last ribs (Figure 20.50). Similar criteria are used to assess liver size in cats; however, the position of the pylorus tends to differ by being more medially positioned on ventrodorsal radiographic projections (Figure 20.51).

Liver size is difficult to assess with ultrasound. Under normal conditions, the liver should have a sharply marginated caudoventral border, which does not extend caudally beyond the gastric body (Figure 20.52).

The liver is composed of six lobes and two processes, characterized as follows: left lobe (divided into lateral and medial sublobes), quadrate lobe, right lobe (subdivided into lateral and medial sublobes), and caudate lobe with caudate and papillary processes (Figure 20.53). The caudate process of the caudate lobe can be recognized by the presence of the renal fossa, conformed to the cranial pole of the right kidney (Figure 20.54). Otherwise, these lobes cannot be differentiated

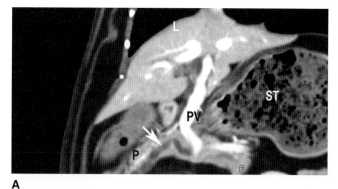

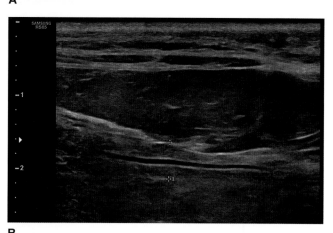

**FIGURE 20.41** Dorsal plane reconstruction CT (**A**) and transverse US image (**B**) from two normal cats. In (**A**) the portal vein (PV) is noted dorsal to the pancreas (P). A hypoattenuating tube is noted within the center of the pancreas representing pancreatic duct dilation (white arrow) which can be normal, particularly in older cats. L, liver; ST, stomach. In (**B**), the left lobe is seen in long axis for the pancreas deep to the spleen (marked by the green crosses for measurement). The pancreatic duct can be seen as the anechoic tube with echogenic walls within the center of the pancreas.

on ultrasound and CT, unless separated by a moderate to severe peritoneal effusion.

On ultrasound, the hepatic parenchyma is mildly hypoechoic to the spleen with a mildly coarser echotexture (Figure 20.55). The liver is hypoechoic to the falciform fat, which should not be mistaken to represent hepatic parenchyma, especially in obese patients (Figure 20.56). On CT, the liver parenchyma is homogeneously soft tissue attenuating. After contrast administration, there is strong and homogeneous enhancement of the parenchyma during the arterial phase, followed by progressive and homogeneous diffuse contrast enhancement of the parenchyma during the venous and delayed phases (Figure 20.57).

The hepatic vasculature may be assessed using ultrasound and CT angiography, and can be used to recognize individual hepatic lobes with a variable degree of certainty. Due to their small size, the hepatic arteries are not readily visible with ultrasound and are best visualized with CT during the arterial phase of contrast enhancement. In comparison, the hepatic and portal veins are easily recognized. On ultrasound, the portal veins have hyperechoic walls, which differentiate them from

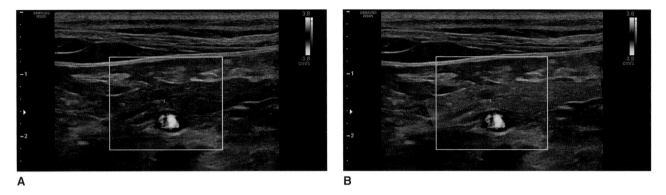

**FIGURE 20.42** (**A**) Body and left lobe of the feline pancreas with the portal vein in dorsal position (blue structure with color Doppler). The image is a transverse image with the left side of the image representing the cranial and right central portion of the cat abdomen. (**B**) Pancreas is highlighted in yellow. In both images, the pancreatic duct is measured between the green crosses and number 1 (2 mm).

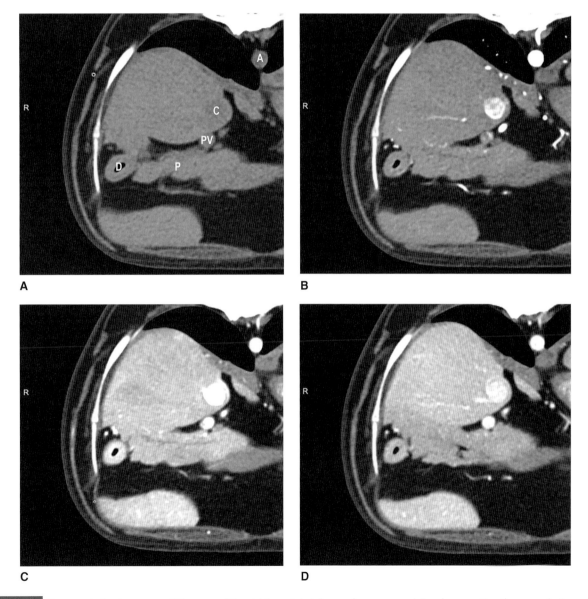

**FIGURE 20.43** Representative transverse CT images of the right cranial abdomen from a normal dog documenting the normal attenuation of the pancreas before (**A**) and after (**B–D**) contrast medium. (**B**) The arterial phase. (**C**) The portal venous phase. (**D**) The delayed venous phase studies. A, aorta; C, caudal vena cava (hepatic portion); PV, portal vein, P, pancreas; D, duodenum.

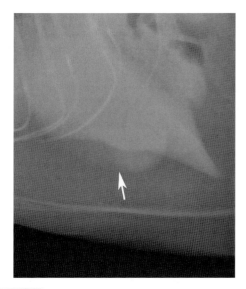

**FIGURE 20.44** Right lateral radiograph of the cranioventral abdomen from a cat. The gall bladder is distended and can be seen below the ventral hepatic margins (white arrow). The clinical significance of this finding needs to be correlated with a potential ultrasound and clinical findings associated with the cat. This has been seen in normal fasted cats without clinical relevance.

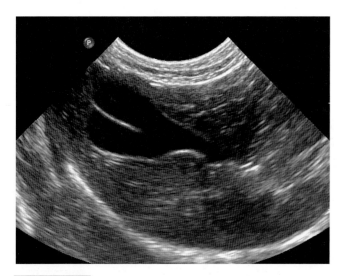

**FIGURE 20.45** Sagittal (long axis) ultrasound image of the cranial right abdomen in a cat with a bilobed gall bladder (normal variant).

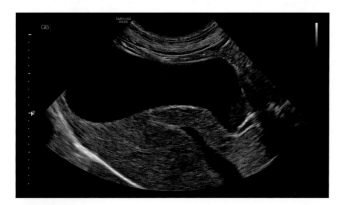

**FIGURE 20.46** Sagittal (long axis) ultrasound image of the cranial right abdomen in a dog with a small amount of echogenic material within the gall bladder lumen (normal variant).

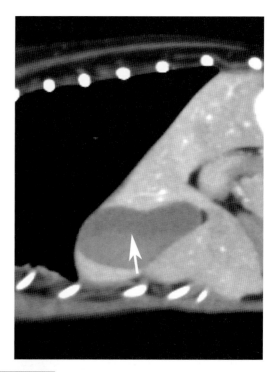

**FIGURE 20.47** Sagittal reconstructed CT image of the cranial right abdomen in a dog with a moderate amount of gravity-dependent hyperattenuating material within the gall bladder lumen (normal variant). The white arrow denotes the line between the biliary debris (ventral) and the normal bile (dorsal).

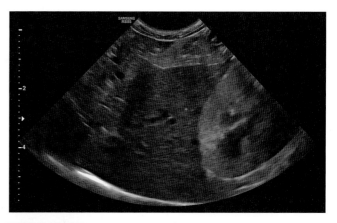

**FIGURE 20.48** Sagittal (long axis) ultrasound image of the cranial right abdomen in a dog documenting the difference in echogenicity between the caudate lobe of the liver and the cranial pole of the right kidney (hyperechoic cortex). The right kidney in the dog is usually fixed within the renal fossa of the caudate lobe of the liver whereas, in the cat, fat is often present between the liver and right kidney.

the hepatic veins (Figure 20.58). A more complete description of the abdominal vasculature is provided in a latter section of this chapter.

## Spleen

The spleen has three parts: head, body, and tail. The head of the spleen is located in the left midabdominal region and is

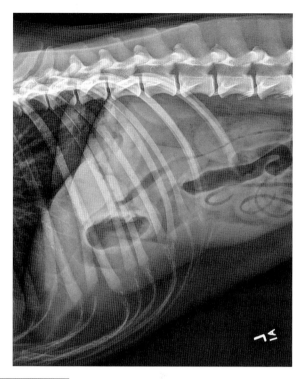

**FIGURE 20.49** Left lateral radiograph documenting normal hepatic size and gastric axis in a dog. The splenic margin is noted caudal to the hepatic silhouette. Gas is noted in the pylorus and the duodenum. The liver is contained within the costal arch; however, if the abdominal radiograph is made on peak inspiration, the liver margins will extend beyond the costal arch in a normal patient.

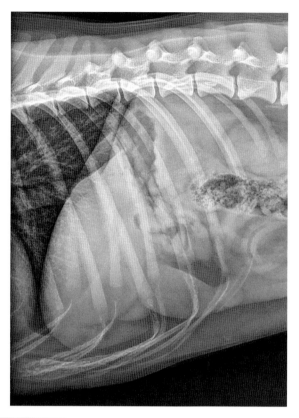

**FIGURE 20.50** Right lateral radiograph documenting normal hepatic size and gastric axis in a dog.

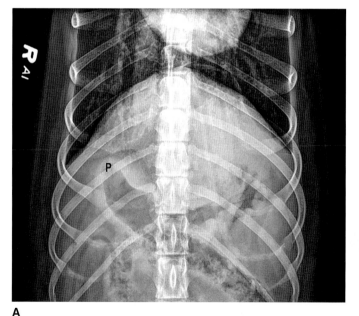

**A**

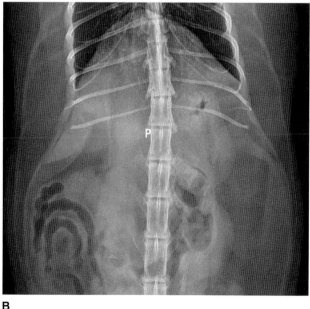

**B**

**FIGURE 20.51** Ventrodorsal radiographs from a dog (**A**) and a cat (**B**). Notice the position of the pylorus in the dog is near the right side of the abdomen (P) whereas the pylorus is in a more midline position for the cat (P).

routinely identified on lateral and ventrodorsal radiographic projections. The head of the spleen is relatively fixed due to its attachment to the stomach (fundic region) via the gastrosplenic ligament. The remainder of the spleen is mobile and may change in position between studies. The splenic tail may also be contained within the left abdominal cavity or extend ventrally across midline. The splenic tail is commonly visualized within the ventral abdominal cavity in dogs and rarely seen in cats under normal conditions. Some breed variations have been reported when evaluating the size of the spleen in

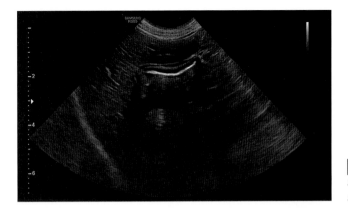

**FIGURE 20.52** Sagittal image (left side) from the cranial abdomen of a normal dog with normal liver size and positioning relative to the body and pyloric antrum of the stomach.

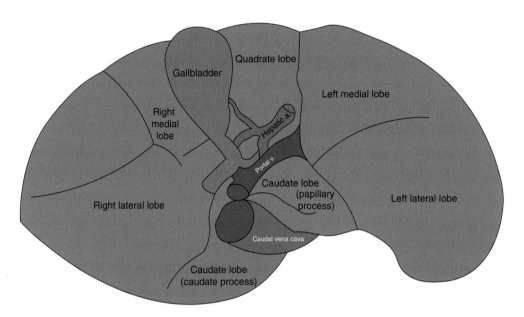

**FIGURE 20.53** Schematic of the normal liver lobes in a dog (caudal view).

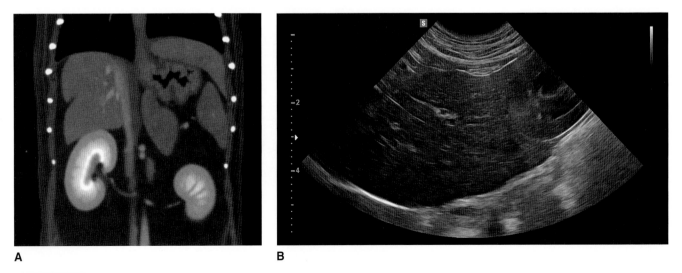

A

B

**FIGURE 20.54** (**A**) Dorsal plane reconstructed CT of the caudate lobe of the liver and position of the cranial pole of the right kidney adjacent to and in contact with the caudate lobe. The caudal vena cava is seen coursing through the hepatic parenchyma on the right side medial to the right kidney. (**B**) Sagittal plane ultrasound image of the caudate lobe of the liver and the right kidney. In this instance, the hepatic parenchyma and the kidney cortex are isoechoic to each other (compare with Figure 20.48).

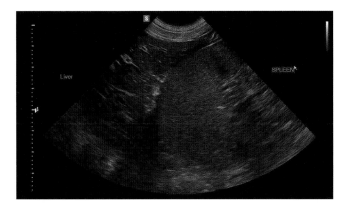

**FIGURE 20.55**   Left-sided sagittal image of an ultrasound from the cranial abdomen of a normal dog comparing the echogenicity and echotexture of the liver and the spleen. The spleen is noted to be hyperechoic and has a more tightly packed echotexture compared with the liver.

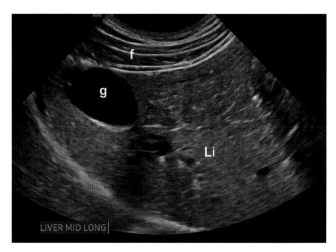

**FIGURE 20.56**   Normal sagittal ultrasound image from a cat on midline of the liver (Li). The gall bladder (G) in this cat is extending toward midline. There is some fat in the falciform ligament (F) noted in the near field of the image. As a cat deposits more fat in the falciform, the falciform can displace the liver dorsally away from the near field.

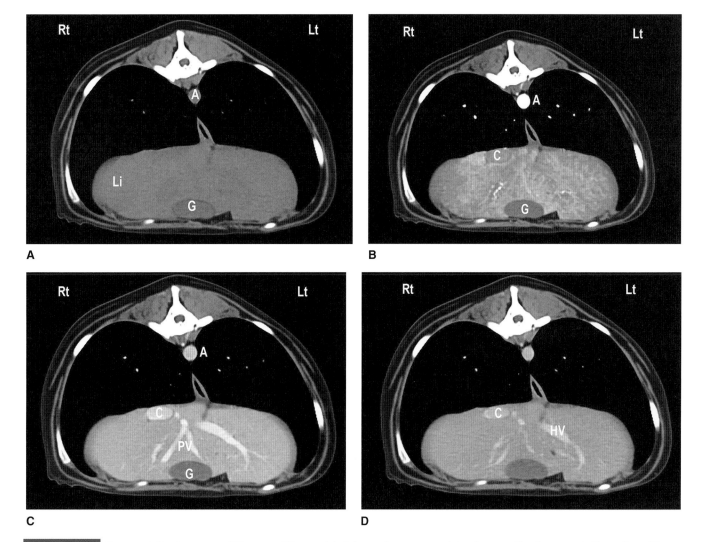

**FIGURE 20.57**   Representative transverse CT images of the cranial abdomen from a normal dog documenting the normal attenuation of the liver before (**A**) and after (**B–D**) intravenous contrast medium administration. (**B**) The arterial phase. (**C**) The portal venous phase. (**D**) Delayed venous phase studies. A, aorta; C, caudal vena cava; G, gall bladder; Li, liver; PV, portal vein contrast medium; HV, hepatic vein contrast medium.

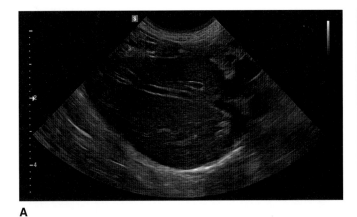

**A**

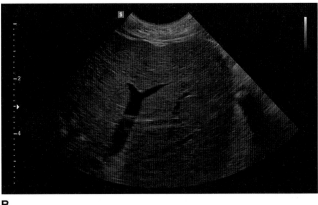

**B**

**FIGURE 20.58** Oblique imaging ultrasound planes of the liver from a dog documenting normal portal vein with echogenic walls (**A**) and hepatic veins (**B**). The portal veins should be traced back to the porta hepatis where they originate from the portal vein proper. The hepatic veins can be traced into the caudal vena cava.

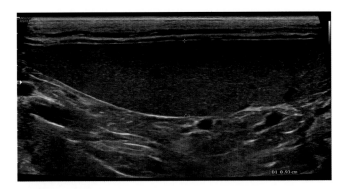

**FIGURE 20.59** Normal cat spleen measuring less than 10 mm in thickness at a central point.

dogs. For instance, German shepherd dogs and greyhounds tend to have a larger spleen than other dogs with a similar body weight. In larger dogs and especially deep-chested dogs, the splenic head may have a subcostal location and need to be visualized using an intercostal approach.

In the absence of objective criteria to evaluate the size of the canine spleen, a subjective assessment of the splenic volume and rounding of the splenic margins may indicate splenomegaly. A similar approach may be used to assess the size of the feline spleen. An objective measurement of the feline spleen is reported using ultrasound. At the level of the splenic hilus, the normal feline spleen should measure less than 1 cm in thickness (Figure 20.59) [16, 17]. Additionally, visualization of the splenic tail along the ventral abdominal cavity on abdominal radiographs, in the absence of splenomegaly, is very rare in cats.

The spleen is homogeneously soft tissue opaque on radiographs and may occasionally border efface with the caudoventral hepatic border at the level of the splenic tail on lateral radiographic projections and should not be misinterpreted as hepatomegaly (Figure 20.60). The splenic parenchyma has a homogeneous echogenicity that is most commonly hyperechoic to the liver and renal cortices with a fine (sandpaper-like) echotexture (Figure 20.61). The spleen is covered by a thin, strongly hyperechoic capsule, not seen on all other modalities. The splenic arteries and veins can be differentiated by assessing the direction of blood flow using color Doppler imaging or CT angiography (Figure 20.62). The splenic veins tend to be larger and more easily recognized. The spleen is homogeneously soft tissue attenuating on CT with strong inhomogeneous contrast enhancement during the arterial phase, especially in cats (Figure 20.63). On subsequent phases and especially in dogs, there is progressive diffuse contrast enhancement of the splenic parenchyma, occasionally persistently inhomogeneous in the absence of disease (see Figure 20.62). On the ventrodorsal radiograph, the "spaghetti sign" has been described where collateral vessels are noted adjacent to the body of the spleen in cats [18].

Using ultrasound and CT, ectopic splenic tissues vascularized by the splenic vasculature with an echogenicity/attenuation similar to the splenic parenchyma may be identified within the mesentery surrounding the spleen. These ectopic spleens are commonly referred as splenunculus, daughter or accessory spleen, and represent an incidental finding (Figure 20.64).

## Adrenal Glands

The adrenal glands are small paired structures identified craniomedial to the left and right kidneys. The left adrenal gland is located to the left of the aorta, cranial to the left renal artery and vein, and caudal to the celiac and cranial mesentery arteries. The right adrenal gland is more cranially located just to the right and slightly dorsal to the caudal vena cava, cranial to the celiac and cranial mesenteric arteries.

The left and right phrenicoabdominal veins lie along the ventral aspect of the adrenal glands and may be traced to the midportion of each corresponding ipsilateral adrenal gland. These vessels can be used as a landmark to identify the adrenal glands (Figure 20.65). The corresponding right and left

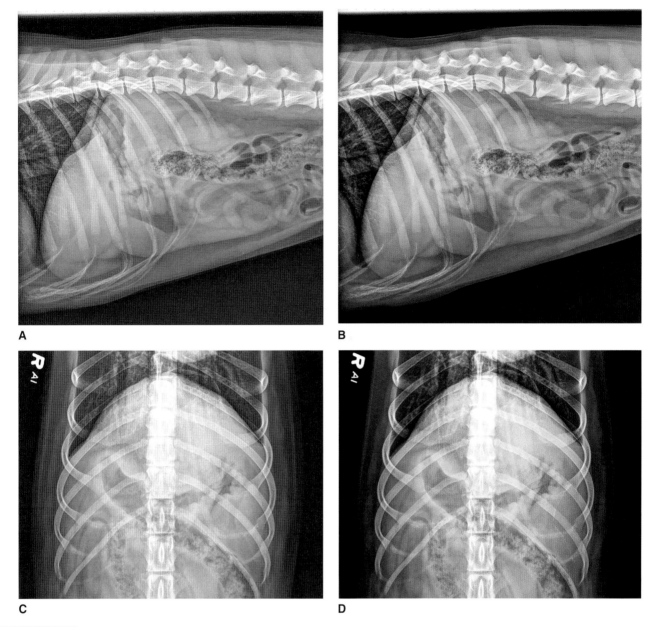

**FIGURE 20.60** Left lateral (**A**) and ventrodorsal (**C**) radiographs from a normal dog where the tail of the spleen is noted on the left lateral caudal to the liver and along the ventral abdomen. In addition, a portion of the head of the spleen is noted ventral to the T13–L1 intervertebral disc space (red highlights (**B**)). On the ventrodorsal image (**C**) the head of the spleen is lateral to the fundic portion of the stomach. This is highlighted in red (**D**).

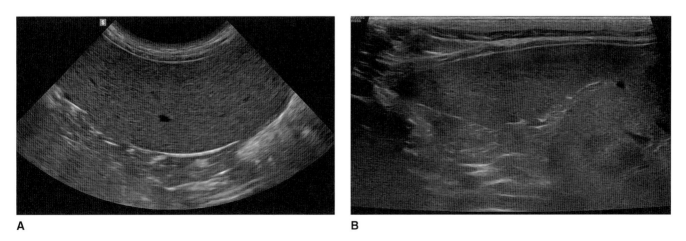

**FIGURE 20.61** Long axis images of the dog (**A**) and cat (**B**) spleen. The transducer is oriented in sagittal plane; however, the spleen is in transverse plane as it courses from left to right across the dog and cat abdomen.

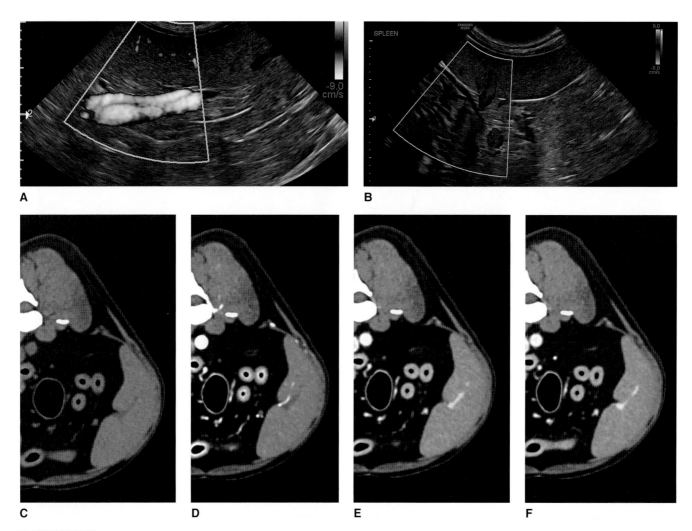

A   B

C   D   E   F

**FIGURE 20.62**   (**A,B**) Color Doppler images of the splenic arteries (red toward the transducer) and veins (blue away from the transducer). In addition, there are four transverse CT images of the left side of the abdomen from a dog pre (**C**) and post (**D-F**) intravenous contrast medium. There is homogeneous contrast attenuation throughout the splenic parenchyma on the arterial (**D**), portal vein (**E**), and delayed venous phases (**F**).

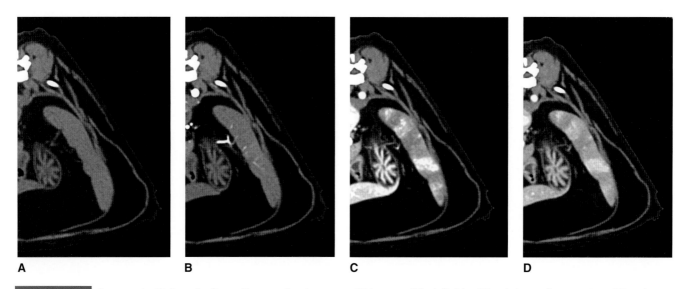

A   B   C   D

**FIGURE 20.63**   Compared with the prior figure, there are four transverse CT images of the left side of the abdomen from a cat pre (**A**) and post (**B-D**)intravenous contrast medium. There is heterogeneous contrast attenuation throughout the splenic parenchyma on the arterial (arteries present, **B**), portal vein (**C**), and delayed venous phases (**D**).

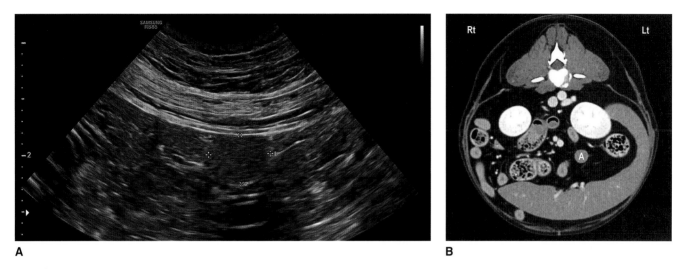

**FIGURE 20.64**   Focal accessory splenic tissue is noted in the ultrasound image (**A**) with markers denoting size and also within the central omentum on a transverse CT image post contrast administration (**B**). In the CT image, the accessory splenic tissue is marked with an A.

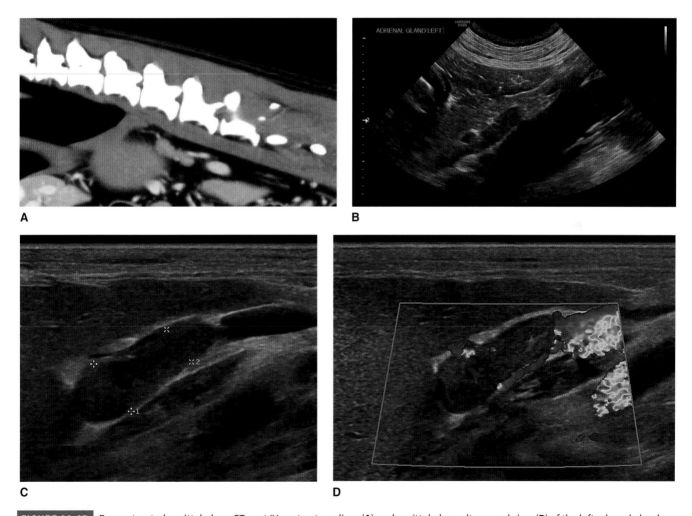

**FIGURE 20.65**   Reconstructed sagittal plane CT post IV contrast medium (**A**) and sagittal plane ultrasound view (**B**) of the left adrenal gland from a dog. On the CT scan, the phrenicoabdominal vessels are seen adjacent to the adrenal gland. On the US image (**B**), there is a hypoechoic oval along the ventral border of the adrenal gland consistent with the left phrenicoabdominal vein. In (**C**) and (**D**), sagittal images of the right adrenal gland from a normal cat are present. In (**C**), cranial and caudal poles are measured (4 and 3.8 mm, respectively). In (**D**), color Doppler has been engaged and the vessel along the ventral surface of the adrenal gland is the right phrenicoabdominal vein (blue and red due to the direction of blood flow relative to the transducer). There is blood flow caudal to the adrenal gland within the caudal vena cava with some color flow (mostly blue with some aliasing). Blood flow is noted within the abdominal aorta deep to the caudal vena cava (mostly red with some aliasing). The blood vessel along the dorsal aspect of the adrenal gland is the right phrenicoabdominal artery.

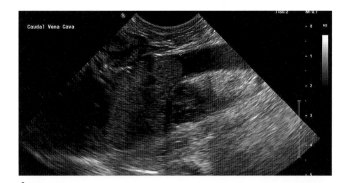

**A**

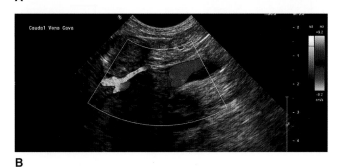

**B**

**FIGURE 20.66** Sagittal plane right cranial and dorsal abdominal ultrasound images from a dog with a right adrenal tumor that is invading the caudal vena cava. The tumor enters the caudal vena cava via a tumor thrombus extending through the phrenicoabdominal vein. (**A**) Gray-scale 2D image and (**B**) color Doppler image with blue flow in the caudal vena cava caudal to the tumor thrombus.

phrenicoabdominal arteries are noted to be dorsal to the midsection of each adrenal gland. Adrenal gland malignant neoplasms will invade the phrenicoabdominal veins and course into the caudal vena cava, resulting in tumor thrombosis of the caudal vena cava (Figure 20.66). The adrenal glands are bilobed with a cranial and caudal pole in canine patients. The left adrenal gland is most commonly peanut-shaped in small-breed dogs, whereas the right adrenal gland tends to be L- or

V-shaped (Figure 20.67). The adrenal glands are more elongated in large-breed dogs. While some cats may also have peanut-shaped adrenal gland, most commonly feline adrenal glands are ovoid in shape (Figure 20.68). The normal size reference ranges for canine and feline adrenal glands are shown in Table 20.4 [19].

Normal adrenal glands are not visualized on radiographs. Occasionally, feline adrenal glands may contain incidental dystrophic mineralization, which may be visualized on radiographs (Figure 20.69). Similar mineralization in canine adrenal glands may be associated with neoplasia and warrants further imaging when identified on radiographs.

Ultrasonography and CT are the modalities of choice to evaluate the adrenal glands in dogs and cats. On ultrasound, the adrenal glands are well demarcated and hypoechoic to the surrounding fat. The adrenal cortex can occasionally be differentiated from the medulla, representing a thick hypoechoic rim (Figure 20.70). Contrast-enhanced ultrasonography helps further differentiate the adrenal cortex from the medulla [20]. Following administration of an ultrasound contrast agent, adrenal gland enhancement is reported as homogeneous and centrifugal with rapid perfusion of the medulla followed by the cortex [20]. On CT, the adrenal glands are bilaterally homogeneously soft tissue attenuating and contrast enhancing (Figure 20.71).

# Kidneys

The kidneys are paired and bilaterally symmetrical structures surrounded by retroperitoneal fat. The renal parenchyma is divided into an outer cortex and inner medulla, which cannot be differentiated on standard radiographic projections. Under normal conditions, the kidneys have a homogeneous soft tissue opacity with the occasional exception of the renal hilus,

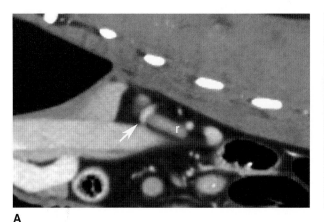

**A**

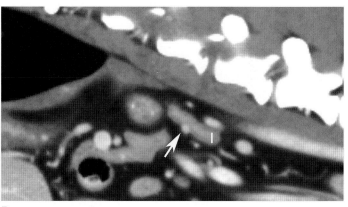

**B**

**FIGURE 20.67** Reconstructed sagittal plane images from a dog documenting the right (**A**) and left (**B**) adrenal glands. In (**A**), the right phrenicoabdominal vein (white arrow) can be seen exiting the caudal vena cava and coursing across the ventral aspect of the right adrenal gland (r). In (**B**), the left adrenal gland is noted in the retroperitoneal fat (l) with the left phrenicoabdominal vein (white arrow) coursing along the ventral aspect of the left adrenal gland.

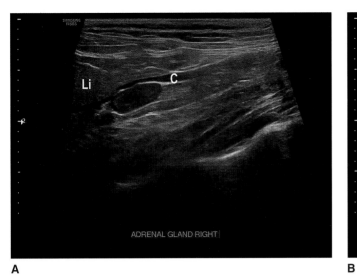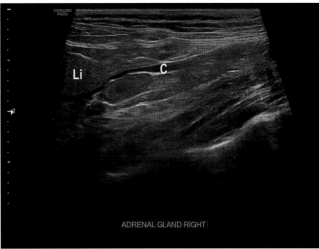

A

B

**FIGURE 20.68** Sagittal ultrasound image (**A**) of the normal right adrenal gland adjacent to the caudal vena cava (C) and caudal to the caudal lobe of the liver (Li). The adrenal gland is highlighted in green in (**B**). In (**A**), one can see the adrenal cortex and medulla.

| TABLE 20.4 | Normal adrenal gland size in dogs and cats. | |
|---|---|---|
| **Species** | **Weight** | **Size range of normal adrenal glands** |
| Dogs | <10 kg | 2.4–5.4 mm |
| | 10–30 kg | 3.1–6.8 mm |
| | >30 kg | 3.3–8.0 mm |
| Cats | | 3.5–4.5 mm |

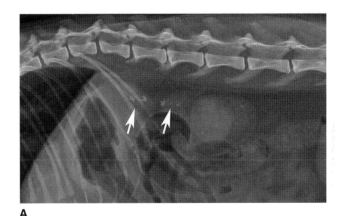

A

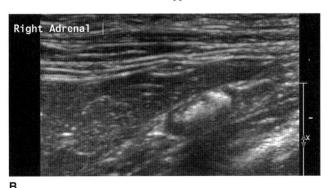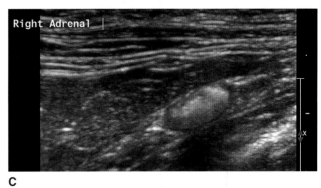

B

C

**FIGURE 20.69** (**A**) Close-up radiograph (right lateral) of a cat abdomen where there is dystrophic mineralization within the right and left adrenal glands (white arrows) and areas of renal dystrophic mineralization also present. (**B**) Sagittal ultrasound image of the right adrenal gland with areas of mineralization and distal shadowing. (**C**) Right adrenal highlighted in green from US image in (**B**).

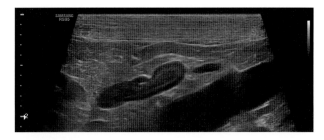

**FIGURE 20.70** Sagittal ultrasound image of the normal left adrenal gland in the dog adjacent to the abdominal aorta. The left phrenicoabdominal vein is noted on the ventral surface of the left adrenal gland and the large tubular anechoic structure deep to the left adrenal gland is the aorta.

which contains fat and may be recognized as a central region of decreased opacity (Figure 20.72). The right kidney often has more poorly defined margins than the left kidney on radiographs due to border effacement with the liver and superimposition with adjacent visceral structures. Normal ureters are not visualized on radiographs. Roughly located ventral to the fifth lumbar vertebra, the origin of the deep circumflex iliac arteries and veins may be seen end on and represents foci of increased opacity, which should not be misinterpreted as ureteroliths (Figure 20.73).

A more detailed evaluation of the renal anatomy and function is possible with an excretory urogram (EU). Positive contrast medium is administered intravenously and

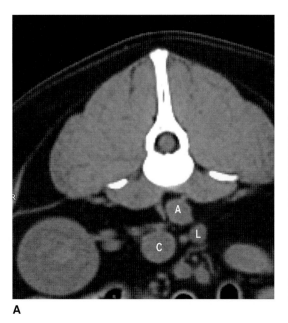

**A**

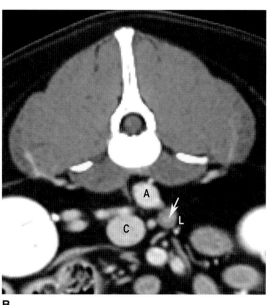

**B**

**FIGURE 20.71** Transverse CT images pre (**A**) and post (**B**) intravenous contrast medium administration. There is corticomedullary distinction noted on the postcontrast images (**B**) of the left adrenal gland with the medulla having increased attenuation (white arrow) relative to the outer cortex. A, aorta; C, caudal vena cava; L, left adrenal gland.

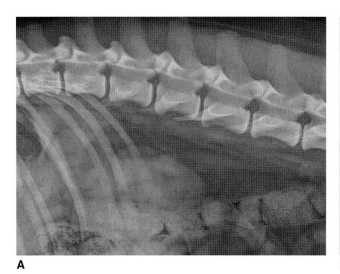

**A**

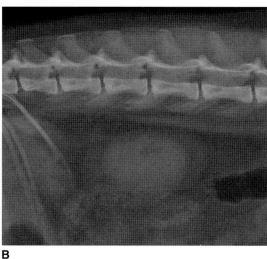

**B**

**FIGURE 20.72** Close-up lateral abdominal radiographs from a normal dog (**A**) and a normal cat (**B**). Fat (radiolucent) can be seen in the renal sinus in both the dog and cat kidneys. The tubular soft tissue opaque structure that courses over the dorsal aspect of the renal silhouettes is the caudal vena cava.

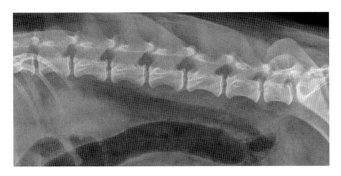

**FIGURE 20.73** The circular soft tissue opacities noted ventral to L6 represent end-on vessels within the retroperitoneal space in this lateral radiograph from a dog. These should not be mistaken for ureteroliths or lymph nodes.

radiographs are acquired at different time points to project the following phases of contrast enhancement (Figure 20.74, Table 20.5). Rarely, a small amount of gas may be identified within the renal veins due to inadvertent iatrogenic administration, most commonly using a saphenous intravenous catheter (Figure 20.75).

Ultrasound provides superior details of the renal anatomy. The renal cortex is hyperechoic to the medulla with good corticomedullary distinction (Figure 20.76). In obese cats, the renal cortices are occasionally more strongly hyperechoic due to increased cortical fat deposition (Figure 20.77). Angle-dependent regions of increased echogenicity at opposing ends of the kidneys are reported as artifact due to anisotropy and should not be misinterpreted as disease (Figure 20.78) [21]. The kidneys have smooth and well-defined margins with a thin hyperechoic rim, representing the renal capsule. The renal pelvis may contain a small amount of physiologic anechoic fluid, as a general rule measuring <2 mm in height centrally. Using a high-resolution transducer, the ureters are readily identified and traced to the vesicoureteral junction. The ureters should be <2 mm in diameter with a thin wall and intermittently may contain a minimal amount of anechoic fluid, indicating peristalsis.

Computed tomography provides good conspicuity of the kidneys with overall poorer parenchymal details in comparison to ultrasound. The renal parenchyma is soft issue attenuating with indistinct corticomedullary distinction. CT angiography/excretory urography results in similar phases of contrast enhancement as described above for radiography (Figure 20.79). Visualization of the ureters is best during the pyelogram phase (Figure 20.80).

On radiographs, the normal canine kidney is approximated to measure 2.5–3.5 times the length of L2 as measured on a ventrodorsal radiographic projection (Figure 20.81) [22, 23]. Some variation is reported between breeds of dogs, with mesaticephalic dogs have a higher ratio, occasionally measuring >3.5 on the ventrodorsal projection [16]. Additionally, higher ratios are observed in small-breed dogs [16]. Using a similar approach, the feline kidney has a normal ratio ranging between 2.4 and 3.0 times the length of L2 [22, 23].

Variations in renal size are present between some cat breeds [24]. In the authors' experience, similar size ratios may be applicable using CT to assess renal length in dogs and cats. Alternatively, subjective rounding and widening of the kidneys are suggestive of renomegaly. Using ultrasound, direct measurements of the canine kidney are limited in the absence of normal reference ranges considering variations in body weight and conformation between breeds. When feasible, especially in smaller patients, ratios of the renal length to aorta diameter or length of L5 or L6 may be used as normal reference ranges (Table 20.6). Given there are fewer variations in body size between cat breeds, the renal length is a relatively consistent means of measuring the normal feline kidney and ranges between 3.5 and 4.5 cm.

# Urinary Bladder

The urinary bladder extends cranially from the pelvic inlet to form a blind sac, which is homogeneously soft tissue opaque on radiographs (Figure 20.82). The size of the urinary bladder varies with the amount of urine it contains. Under normal conditions, the urinary bladder neck gradually tapers to the level of the vesicourethral junction. When volume underdistended, the urinary bladder may be partially intrapelvic in dogs. The feline urinary bladder has a more cranial position in comparison to dogs, especially when filled with urine (Figure 20.83). CT allows differentiation of fluid-attenuating urine from the normal soft tissue-attenuating urinary bladder wall (Figure 20.84). When distended, the urinary bladder wall is thin (<2 mm) with smooth margins. However, in the absence of luminal pressure to stretch the urinary bladder wall, it may recoil and be collapsed with an increased thickness and irregular margins (Figure 20.85). Radiographic evaluation of the urinary bladder wall is possible with a positive or double (positive and negative) contrast retrograde cystogram (Figure 20.86). The latter enhances visualization of the mucosal margin of the urinary bladder wall (Figure 20.87). Similar contrast studies are also possible using fluoroscopy or CT.

Ultrasonography is superior for evaluation of the urinary bladder wall and vesicoureteral junctions [27]. The urinary bladder wall has four layers, consisting of a hypoechoic mucosa, hyperechoic submucosa, hypoechoic muscularis, and hyperechoic serosa [27]. These layers may not be distinguishable when the urinary bladder is distended (Figure 20.88). The ureteral papillae are readily identified in the trigone region of the urinary bladder dorsally. The ureteral papillae represent focally thickened regions within the urinary bladder wall which slightly protrude along the luminal surface of the urinary bladder wall (Figure 20.89). Color and/or power Doppler ultrasonography aids with the identification of ureteral jets to assess ureteral patency, if present (Figure 20.90).

The urinary bladder should contain homogeneously anechoic or fluid-attenuating urine on ultrasound and CT, respectively. Using ultrasound, the urinary bladder lumen is

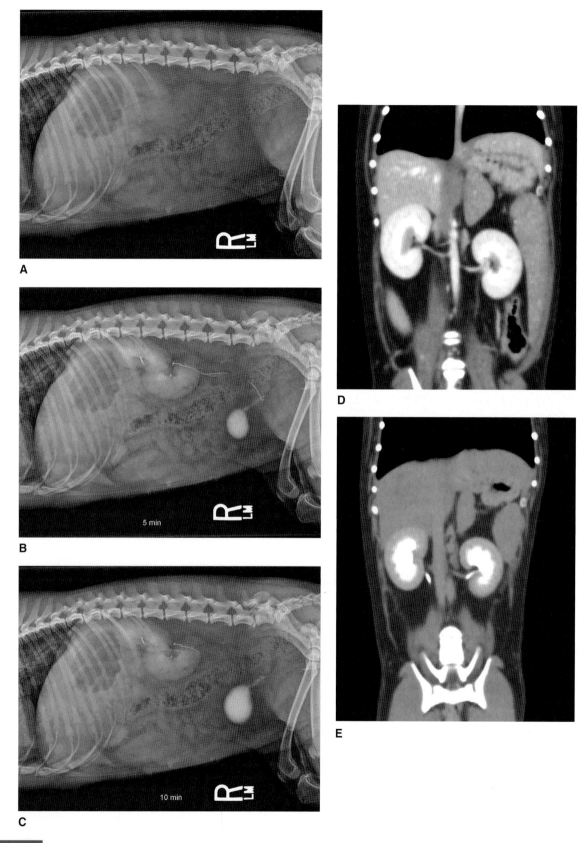

**FIGURE 20.74** Sequential right lateral radiographs obtained of a dog abdomen after being hit by a car, pre (**A**) and post intravenous contrast medium administration (**B** – 5 minutes, **C** – 10 minutes). On the initial set of images, there is a decrease in serosal detail within both the peritoneal and retroperitoneal spaces. There are caudal corner fractures associated with the caudoventral endplates of L5 and L6. There is a mild pneumothorax noted with dorsal elevation of the cardiac silhouette. On the 5- and 10-minute radiographs, there is a delay in renal opacification with the images appearing similar. The nephrogram phase delay is consistent with failure of normal renal excretion of the contrast medium. Progressive filling of the urinary bladder is not seen despite positive contrast medium being noted within the right and left ureters. Ureteral extravasation of contrast medium is not seen. From a different dog, dorsal plane reconstruction images of the kidneys is seen after contrast medium intravenous administration. In (**D**), there is an immediate blush and nephrogram phase with the positive contrast medium starting to collect in the medullary portion of the kidneys. In (**E**), there is progressive contrast medium accumulation within the renal medulla and pelves consistent with a normal pyelogram phase.

**TABLE 20.5**   Phases identified of a positive contrast excretory urogram (EU).

| | |
|---|---|
| Vascular phase | Immediate post IV contrast medium injection. Strong and rapid contrast enhancement of the vessels supplying the kidneys, particularly the renal cortices |
| Nephrogram phase (vascular + tubular) | Progressive homogeneous and uniform contrast enhancement of the renal parenchyma |
| Pyelogram phase | Progressive filling of the renal pelvis, diverticula, ureter, and urinary bladder. Progressive decrease in opacity of the renal parenchyma |

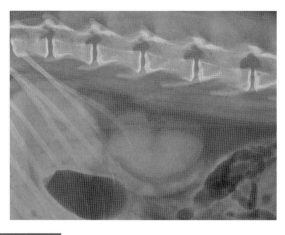

**FIGURE 20.75**   Close-up lateral radiograph from a cat that has a collection of gas bubbles within the renal veins after placement of a saphenous catheter. If enough air is injected, air emboli can result in the death of the patient.

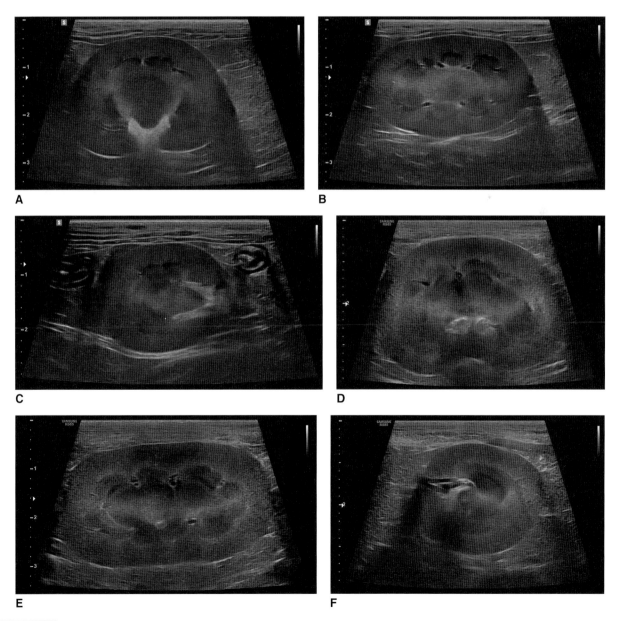

**FIGURE 20.76**   Normal dog and cat kidneys on ultrasound. Dorsal plane (**A**), sagittal plane (**B**), and transverse plane (**C**) images of the right kidney from a dog. Dorsal plane (**D**), sagittal plane (**E**), and transverse plane (**F**) images of the left kidney from a cat.

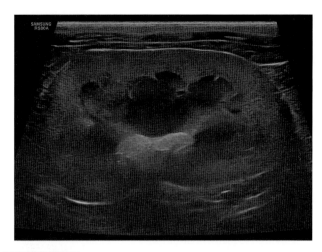

**FIGURE 20.77** Dorsal plane image from a cat of the left kidney. Notice the hyperechoic renal cortex relative to the renal medulla. Also, the bright echogenic material at the renal pelvis represents renal sinus fat.

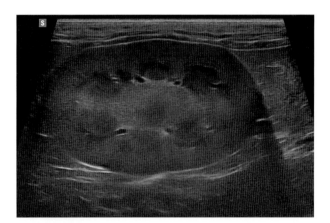

**FIGURE 20.78** Sagittal plane long axis image from the left kidney of a cat. There are several artifacts noted in this image. First, the cranial (left) and caudal (right) poles of the kidney are hyperechoic consistent with anisotropy and not disease. Second, there are edge refraction artifacts deep to the cranial and caudal curvature of the kidneys.

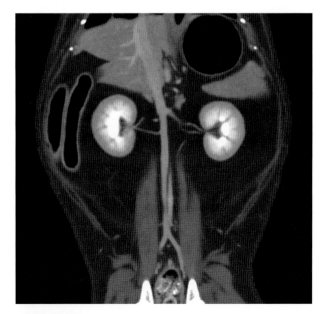

**FIGURE 20.79** Dorsal plane reconstructed view from a CT of a cat abdomen with normal contrast medium excretion within the renal cortices and medullary regions.

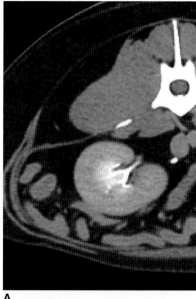

**A**

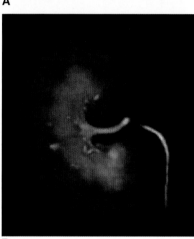

**B**

**FIGURE 20.80** Transverse CT image of the right kidney (**A**) in a cat with a normal pyelogram phase with positive contrast medium being present within the renal pelvis, renal diverticula, and right ureter (also noted adjacent to the caudal vena cava and exiting the renal sinus). (**B**) Three-dimensional rendering of the right kidney highlighting the relative amount of positive contrast medium within the cortex, medulla, renal pelvis, and ureter.

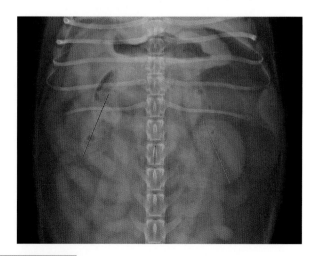

**FIGURE 20.81** Ventrodorsal radiograph from a normal dog where the lengths of the right and left renal silhouettes are compared against the length of L2. In this case the ratio of the renal length:L2 length is approximately 3.4:1.

**TABLE 20.6** Ratios for measurement of the canine kidney with ultrasonography.

| Ratios | Normal reference ranges |
| --- | --- |
| Renal length to aorta diameter[a] | 5.5–9.1 |
| Renal length to length of L5 or L6[b] | 1.3–2.7 |

[a] Mareschal et al. [25].
[b] Barella et al. [26].

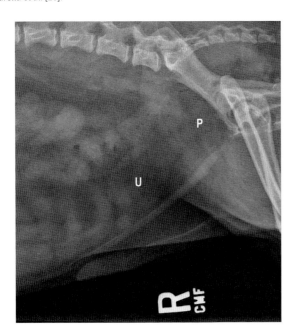

**FIGURE 20.82** Right lateral caudal abdomen from a neutered male dog where the urinary bladder is mildly volume distended. There is a normal fat opaque margin seen along the ventral aspect of the urinary bladder (U) and prostate gland. The prostate gland is noted to be small (P).

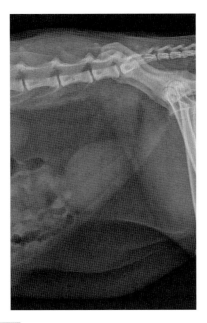

**FIGURE 20.83** Right lateral caudal abdomen from a neutered male cat where the urinary bladder is mildly to moderately volume distended. In the cat, the prostate gland is a histologic structure and not a distinct anatomic structure that can be visualized on radiographs unless abnormally enlarged secondary to neoplasia.

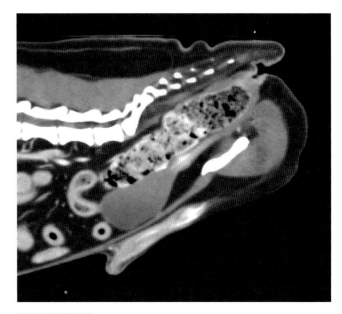

**FIGURE 20.84** Reconstructed sagittal image from a neutered male dog of the caudal abdomen presented in a soft tissue window. The urinary bladder can be seen with the small prostate gland just caudal to it. The colon and rectum with fecal material are noted to be dorsal to the urinary bladder, prostate, and urethra.

prone to side-lobe and grating-lobe artifacts which should not be misinterpreted as abnormal urinary bladder content (Figure 20.91).

# Urethra

The urethra in male dogs and cats is comprised of a pelvic and a penile part. The pelvic part includes preprostatic and prostatic portions. The distal penile urethra is contained within the urethral groove of the os penis in male dogs, and a lateral radiographic projection centered on the pelvis with the pelvis limb cranially retracted is recommended for a full evaluation of the urethral region in male canine patients. In contrast, the feline female urethra is diffusely equivalent to the preprostatic part of the pelvic urethra in the male. In cats, a longer portion of the urethra extends into the caudal abdominal cavity and may be recognized radiographically in cats with increased intraabdominal fat (Figure 20.92). The urethra is typically not visible on radiographs in dogs as it is effaced by the prostate in the caudal abdomen. While the outer margins of the urethra are better visualized on CT, evaluation of the urethral lumen on radiographs and CT is enhanced with positive retrograde or antegrade (cysto)urethrography (Figure 20.93).

In the presence of a full urinary bladder, the proximal portion of the urethra may be distended with a small amount of urine (Figure 20.94). While ultrasonography provides better detail resolution of the urethral wall, the pelvis and os penis partially obscure the visualization of the urethra, therefore limiting evaluation. In comparison, CT is advantageous in that the entire urethra can be visualized. The urethral wall has similar

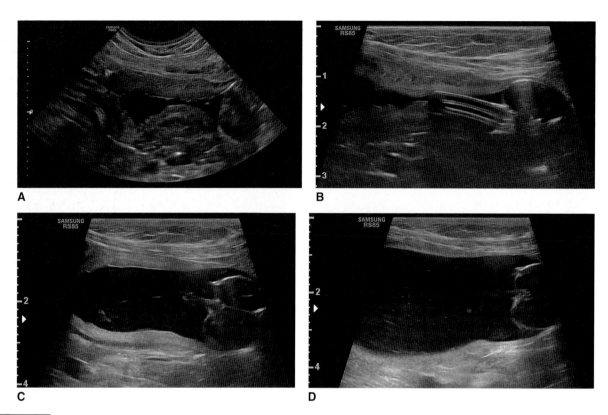

**FIGURE 20.85** (**A**) Empty urinary bladder and progressive filling of the urinary bladder with sterile saline (**B–D**) when visualized in sagittal plane on ultrasound images. The urinary bladder wall appears markedly thickened initially due to the lack of filling. On (**B–D**), progressive filling is noted and there is thinning of the urinary bladder wall. A balloon Foley catheter can be seen in these images within the lumen of the urinary bladder.

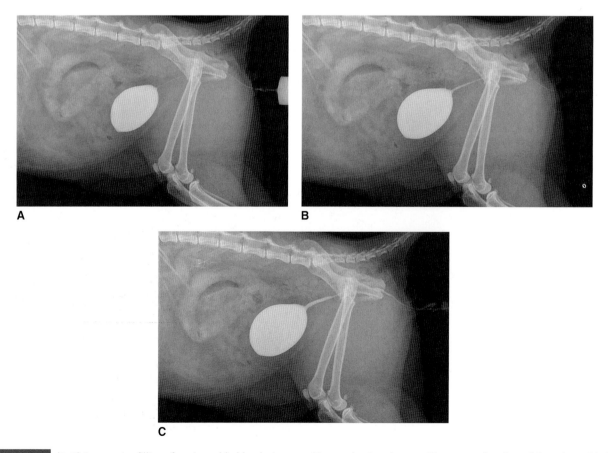

**FIGURE 20.86** (**A–C**) Progressive filling of a urinary bladder during a positive contrast cystogram. The mucosal surface of the urinary bladder wall is smooth; however, a small urachal remnant is noted in the cranioventral margin of the urinary bladder (most severe on **A**). On (**C**), vesicoureteral reflux is noted with positive contrast medium in the left ureter and renal pelvis.

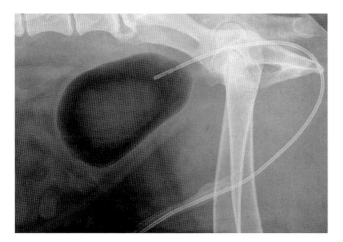

**FIGURE 20.87**  Double-contrast cystogram where a small amount of positive contrast medium is injected into the urinary bladder and then the remainder of the urinary bladder is filled with carbon dioxide (compared with room air). There is a focal area of positive and negative contrast medium within the cranioventral aspect of the urinary bladder consistent with a urachal remnant. The overall urinary bladder wall is thickened ventrally when compared with the dorsal wall, suggestive of a cystitis.

layers as the urinary bladder (see above description) and measures <2 mm in thickness under normal conditions.

The os penis in cats is small and variably faintly mineralized. If visualized, the os penis in feline patients should not be confounded to represent a urethral calculus (Figure 20.95). In dogs, the most distal portion of the os penis may also contain one or multiple ossification centers, which also should not be misinterpreted to represent urethral calculi (Figure 20.96).

# Prostate

The prostate gland in male dogs and cats surrounds the prostatic portion of the pelvic urethra. The normal prostate in castrated patients is not routinely visualized on radiographs. In intact patients, the normal prostate becomes hyperplastic and increases in size with age (Figure 20.97). On lateral radiographs, the height of the prostate should measure less than 70% of the height of the pelvic inlet (Figure 20.98). Regardless of its size, the normal prostate in intact dogs is a smoothly marginated and bilobed structure, which has homogeneous hyperechogenicity on ultrasound and soft tissue opacity and attenuation on radiographs and CT, respectively (Figure 20.99). Under normal conditions, the prostate should not contain any mineralization. In the presence of benign prostatic hyperplasia, the prostatic parenchyma may become heterogeneous and cystic (Figure 20.100).

# Ovaries

The ovaries are located in close proximity to the caudal poles of the kidneys and are ovoid in shape and small in size, measuring 1–2 cm in length [28]. Depending on the phase of the estrus cycle, the ovaries may increase in size and become rounded, as well as containing several capsule-deforming follicles (up to 10 follicles per ovary) [28]. While normal ovaries are not visible radiographically, ultrasound and CT are preferred modalities for the evaluation of the ovaries. On ultrasound, the ovaries have an inhomogeneous parenchyma which is hypoechoic to the surrounding

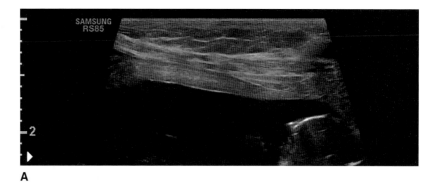

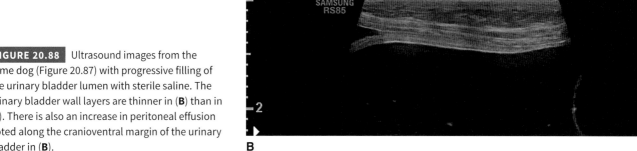

**FIGURE 20.88**  Ultrasound images from the same dog (Figure 20.87) with progressive filling of the urinary bladder lumen with sterile saline. The urinary bladder wall layers are thinner in (**B**) than in (**A**). There is also an increase in peritoneal effusion noted along the cranioventral margin of the urinary bladder in (**B**).

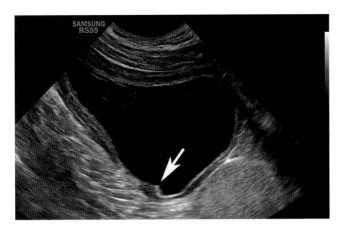

**FIGURE 20.89** Transverse ultrasound image from a dog documenting the ureteral papilla entrance into the urinary bladder (white arrow).

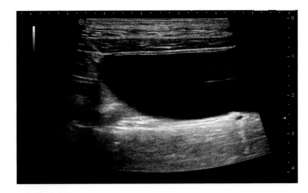

**FIGURE 20.91** Side-lobe artifacts within the urinary bladder (echogenic lines). This artifact should not be mistaken for urinary bladder debris, cells, etc.

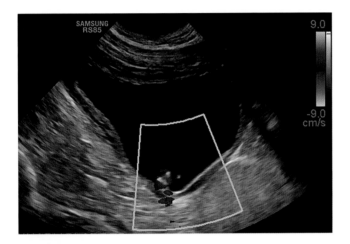

**FIGURE 20.90** Transverse ultrasound image from a dog documenting the ureteral jet entering the ureteral papilla using color Doppler.

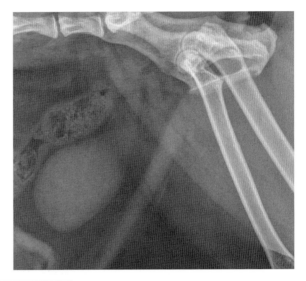

**FIGURE 20.92** Right lateral radiograph of the caudal abdomen from a cat documenting the urethra (soft tissue tubular structure) extending from the urinary bladder caudal margin.

fat (Figure 20.101). On CT, the ovaries are soft tissue attenuating with an inhomogeneous pattern of contrast enhancement, which may highlight noncontrast-enhancing cystic follicular structures (Figure 20.102). In spayed patients, metallic ligating implants or suture material are occasionally identified at the ovariectomy sites on any modality (Figure 20.103).

# Uterus

Dogs and cats have bicornuate uteri with two long horns, which unite to form the uterine body before joining the cervix. The left and right fallopian tubes connect the uterine horns to their corresponding ipsilateral ovary.

The appearance of the uterus is influenced by the different phases of estrus. The nongravid uterus is typically not seen on radiographs. Occasionally, it may be recognized as a tubular

structure extending cranially from the pelvic inlet between the descending colon and urinary bladder. Mild thickening of the uterus during proestrus, estrus, and metestrus, due to incomplete involution postpartum or from prior pregnancy, may increase its conspicuity on radiographs (Figure 20.104). In such cases, the uterus has a diameter measuring approximately equal to or less than the diameter of the small intestine under normal conditions.

The uterus lacks distinct wall layers but can be differentiated from the cervix by the overall thinner thickness of the uterine wall in comparison to the cervix on ultrasound and CT (Figure 20.105). In spayed female dogs and cats, the uterus is commonly removed to the level of the uterine body. The remaining portion of the uterine body and the cervix form the uterine stump, a blind-ended structure which may contain visible suture-like material (Figure 20.106). The uterine stump is most commonly identified using ultrasound, especially with the use of a high-resolution probe (Figure 20.107).

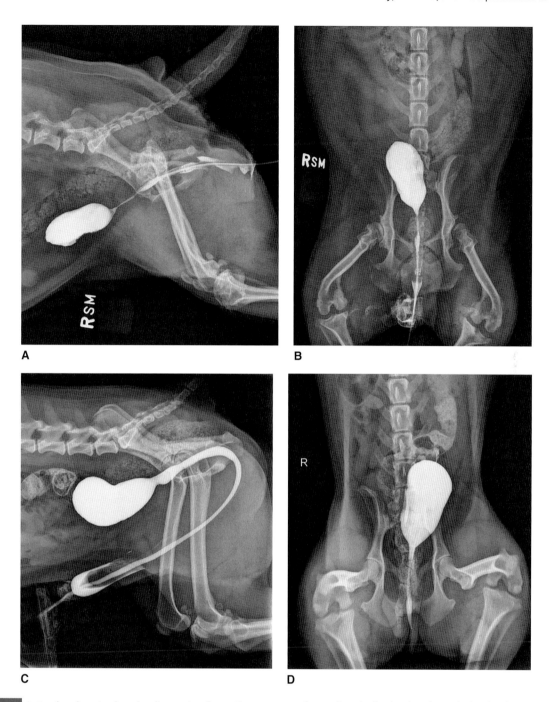

**FIGURE 20.93**   Lateral and ventrodorsal radiographs of a urethrocystogram from a female dog (**A,B**) and a male dog (**C,D**).

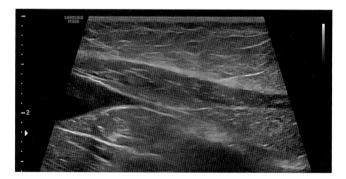

**FIGURE 20.94**   Sagittal ultrasound image of a normal urethra in a cat.

# Lymph Nodes

Abdominal lymph nodes are classified as either parietal or visceral. The parietal lymph nodes drain the abdominal and pelvic walls and include the lumbar, iliosacral, and iliofemoral lymph centers. The lumbar and iliosacral lymph nodes are located in the retroperitoneal space, whereas the iliofemoral lymph nodes are only occasionally present and located within the deep fascial planes in the distal part of the femoral triangle. The medial iliac lymph nodes represent the largest lymph nodes within the iliosacral lymph center and are routinely identified using ultrasound and CT (Figure 20.108).

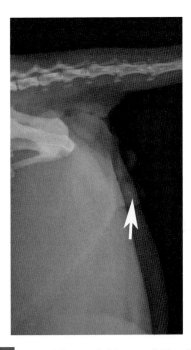

**FIGURE 20.95** Os penis in a cat (white arrow). This should not be mistaken for urethral calculi and is a normal anatomic variant.

The visceral lymph nodes drain particular organs after which they are named. These lymph nodes are grouped into celiac, cranial mesenteric, and caudal mesenteric lymph centers and include the following.

- Celiac: hepatic, splenic, gastric, and pancreaticoduodenal lymph nodes
- Cranial mesenteric: jejunal and colic lymph nodes
- Caudal mesenteric lymph nodes

Normal abdominal lymph nodes are not routinely identified on abdominal radiographs, with one exception. In obese cats, the colic lymph node may be occasionally identified on lateral projections (Figure 20.109). Ultrasonography and CT are the imaging modalities most commonly used for the evaluation of abdominal lymph nodes [29–32].

On ultrasound, abdominal lymph nodes can be well defined or ill defined if infiltrated with fat. Normal lymph nodes are fusiform in shape with a fatty hilus and parenchyma isoechoic to hypoechoic to the surrounding mesentery. Lymph nodes are best measured using their maximal short-axis dimension (Figure 20.110) [29–31]. Normal size reference ranges are most

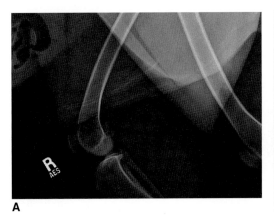

**A**

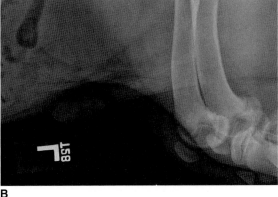

**B**

**FIGURE 20.96** Lateral radiographs (**A,B**) from two different dogs showing separate centers of ossification of the distal end of the os penis.

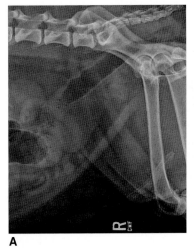

**A**

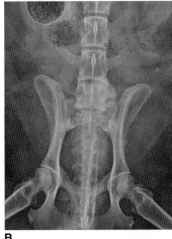

**B**

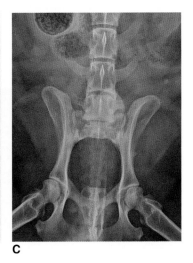

**C**

**FIGURE 20.97** Prostatic enlargement in an intact male dog. Based on the ultrasound evaluation, this was consistent with benign prostatic hyperplasia. Right lateral (**A**) and ventrodorsal (**B**) images of the caudal abdomen and pelvis. On the ventrodorsal image, the prostate gland takes up the entire pelvic opening (highlighted in blue, **C**).

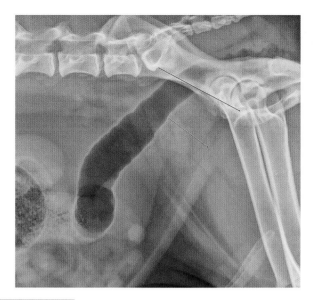

**FIGURE 20.98**  Right lateral radiograph of an intact male dog. The prostate is mildly enlarged and measures 54% of the pelvic opening (sacral promontory to the pubic bone eminence).

consistent in cats (Table 20.7), but vary in dogs given a greater size difference between breeds. Lymph node measurements should be used with caution and correlated with morphologic changes and alteration in the normal perinodal fat. Normal lymph nodes in young dogs and cats are inherently larger in size than those in older patients (Figure 20.111). Additionally, they may have a wide, peripheral and undulating to nodular hypoechoic rim (Figure 20.112).

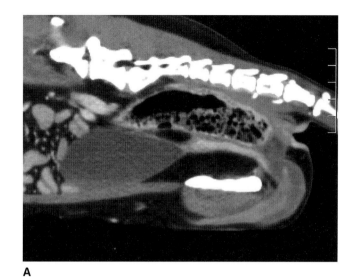

**A**

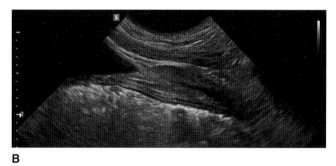

**B**

**FIGURE 20.99**  Normal sagittal CT (**A**) and US (**B**) of a prostate gland from a neutered male dog.

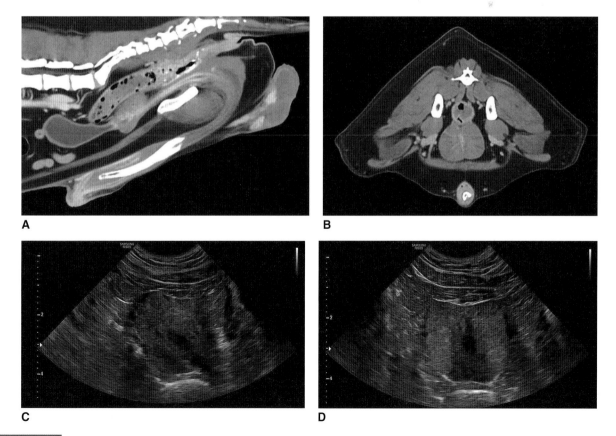

**A**                              **B**

**C**                              **D**

**FIGURE 20.100**  Benign prostatic hyperplasia from a sagittal and transverse CT (**A,B**) and from a sagittal and transverse US (**C,D**) from an intact male dog without urinary tract clinical signs.

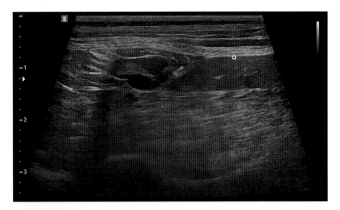

**FIGURE 20.101** Normal long axis (sagittal plane) image from an intact female cat documenting the left ovary with some follicular development.

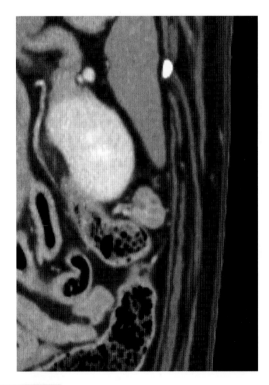

**FIGURE 20.102** Reconstructed dorsal plane image of the left ovary from an intact dog. There is normal follicular development.

The normal appearance of abdominal lymph nodes using CT has previously been described [29]. Visualization of the abdominal lymph nodes is improved in patients with increased intraabdominal fat. However, not all lymph nodes may be consistently identified, especially the colic lymph nodes. Most lymph nodes have an elongated contour and are homogeneously soft tissue attenuating and contrast enhancing (Figure 20.113). A distinct hypoattenuating hilus may occasionally be identified.

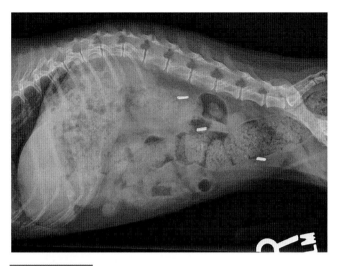

**FIGURE 20.103** Right lateral radiograph from a dog with prior ovariohysterectomy where metallic clamps have been used for the ovarian pedicles and the uterine stump.

# Abdominal Vasculature

In patients with increased intraabdominal fat, the caudal vena cava could be partially visible as a faintly tubular soft tissue opaque structure extending within the retroperitoneal space on lateral radiographic projections (Figures 20.114). The normal aorta and portal vein are not visible on radiographs. Evaluation of the abdominal vasculature on ultrasound requires increased operator experience. Color and power Doppler ultrasound identify flow within the vasculature to aid recognition of specific vascular structures within the abdominal cavity. Color Doppler is superior to power Doppler due to its ability to recognize the direction of blood flow (now also possible with power Doppler on newer ultrasound units). Recognizing the directionality of blood flow is important to characterize a normal vessel as arterial or venous in origin.

Along with ultrasound, CT angiography is one of the preferred methods for evaluation of the abdominal vasculature. CT provides a superior understanding of the vascular anatomy. As described in an earlier chapter, CT images are acquired at different phases of contrast enhancement to project images at peak arterial and venous uptake (Figure 20.115). The CT data can be reconstructed into three-dimensional images for surgical planning and three-dimensional printing.

## Aorta

The aorta is dorsally located, just to the left of midline, within the retroperitoneal space. It enters the abdominal cavity at the aortic hiatus and extends caudally. In the caudal sublumbar (L5–L6) region, the aorta divides into three branches (aortic

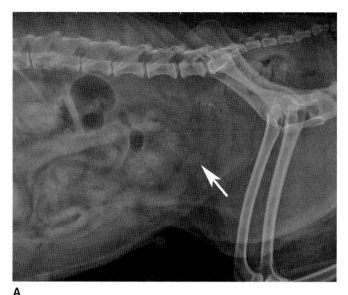

**A**

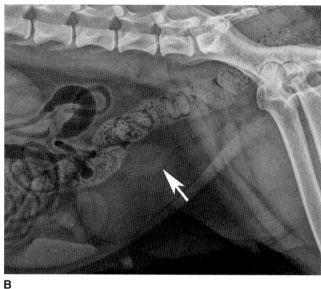

**B**

**FIGURE 20.104**   (**A,B**) Right lateral radiographs of the caudal abdomen from two different intact female dogs where the uterine shadow can be seen over the urinary bladder (white arrows) in the caudal abdomen.

trifurcation): the left and right external iliac arteries and the common internal iliac artery. This then branches into the right and left internal iliac arteries and median sacral artery. The normal anatomy of the aorta and its associated branches is illustrated in Figure 20.116.

The entire abdominal aorta is well visualized with ultrasound and CT angiography. The major branches of the aorta are readily identified with ultrasound, although visualization may be limited in larger patients. Color and power Doppler are essential for the identification of smaller branches. CT angiography provides an unobscured view of all arterial structures and smaller branches. Using pulsed wave Doppler, the aorta displays a triphasic laminar pattern. Peak aortic velocities are reached during ventricular systole and followed by a short rapid drop below baseline and immediate positive rebound, due to transient flow reversal from compliance of the aortic wall, called the Windkessel effect (Figure 20.117). The aorta has normal peak systolic velocities measuring up to 1.0–1.5 m/sec.

## Caudal Vena Cava

The caudal vena cava originates at the confluence of the left and right common iliac veins, dorsal to the aortic trifurcation (Figure 20.118). At the level of L6–L7, the caudal vena cava crosses the aorta to the right and continues ventral and parallel to the abdominal aorta before deviating ventrally at the level of L3. The caudal vena cava crosses the diaphragm

at the caval hiatus in a mid-dorsoventral position relative to the diaphragm as noted on a thoracic radiograph or a cranial abdominal radiograph. In patients with increased intraperitoneal fat, the caudal vena cava can be seen on lateral radiographs as it extends cranioventrally into the liver (Figure 20.114).

The location of the caudal vena cava bifurcation is variable, although most commonly identified at the level of the aortic trifurcation. Alternatively, five variations have been described [33] (Figure 20.119): caudal-partial split, partial duplication, complete duplication, left-sided location, and azygos continuation of the caudal vena cava

These variations are most easily identified using CT angiography, but may also be recognized with ultrasonography or on magnetic resonance imaging (MRI). Using pulsed-wave Doppler ultrasound, the caudal vena cava has a complex nonlaminar waveform influenced by cardiac and respiratory motions (Figure 20.120). Blood flow within the caudal vena cava has peak velocities ranging from 15 to 35 cm/sec.

## Portal Vein

The portal vein is located within the midaspect of the peritoneal cavity, dorsal to the pancreas, and enters the porta hepatis before dividing into the liver. The cranial and caudal mesenteric, splenic, and gastroduodenal veins join the portal venous system to form the portal vein proper, which enters the porta

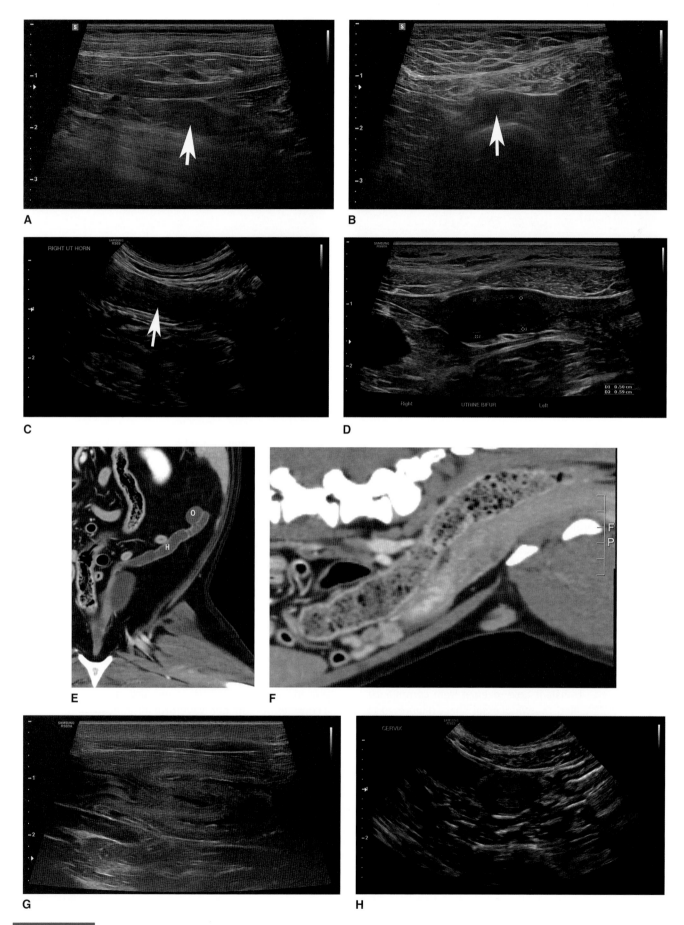

**FIGURE 20.105** Sagittal (**A**) and transverse (**B**) images of the uterine body from an intact female dog (white arrows). Right uterine horn in long axis (white arrow, **C**) and transverse image of the uterine division into the right and left uterine horns (demarcated by measurement tools, **D**). Dorsal plane (**E**) reconstructed CT image post IV contrast medium administration showing the uterine horn (H) and ovary (O). There is fluid noted in the uterine horn (cat was in estrus). Sagittal reconstructed CT (**F**) and US (**G**) images and transverse images (**H**) of the uterine body and cervix from an intact female dog in estrus.

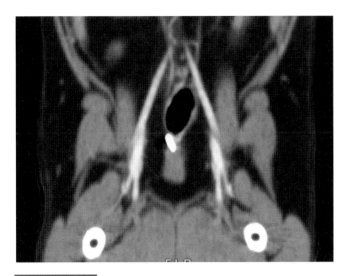

**FIGURE 20.106**  Dorsal plane reconstruction CT image post contrast medium documenting a metallic clip at the cranial aspect of the uterine body post ovariohysterectomy.

lobes) and continues on as the left divisional branch (left hepatic lobes).

The portal vein is not visualized on radiographs. Ultrasound and CT angiography are the modalities of choice for evaluation of the portal system. Although rarely performed, splenoportography is another reported technique for evaluating the anatomy of the portal vein and major tributaries and branches. With ultrasound guidance, positive contrast medium is injected within the splenic parenchyma and temporal uptake of contrast within the portal vein is imaged using radiography, CT, nuclear medicine (radionuclide injection), and/or fluoroscopy.

Ultrasound is superior in its ability to allow identification and characterization of blood flow within the portal vein. On pulsed-wave Doppler, blood flow is hepatopetal and nonlaminar with a flat waveform and positive velocities measuring between 10 and 25 cm/sec (Figure 20.120). The direction of blood flow within the portal vein may also be evaluated using color Doppler ultrasonography.

hepatis and divides into a slightly different branching pattern in dogs and cats, as follows.

- *Dogs*: small right divisional branch (caudate and right lateral liver lobes), small central branch and large left divisional branch (right medial, quadrate, and left hepatic lobes).
- *Cats*: right divisional branch (right liver lobes) and the central divisional branch (quadrate and central hepatic

# Summary

Abdominal variants and normal diagnostic imaging findings in the dog and cat have been reviewed in this chapter. These radiographic features should be considered when interpreting abdominal radiographs. The differences between dog and cat should also be considered when evaluating abdominal imaging.

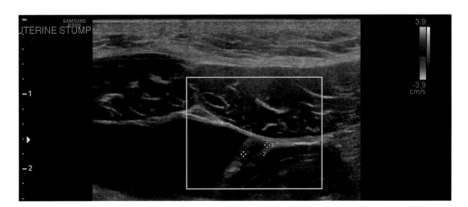

**FIGURE 20.107**  Transverse US image documenting a uterine stump adjacent to the urinary bladder (outlined by measurement tools). There is no flow noted on the this color Doppler image within the color box.

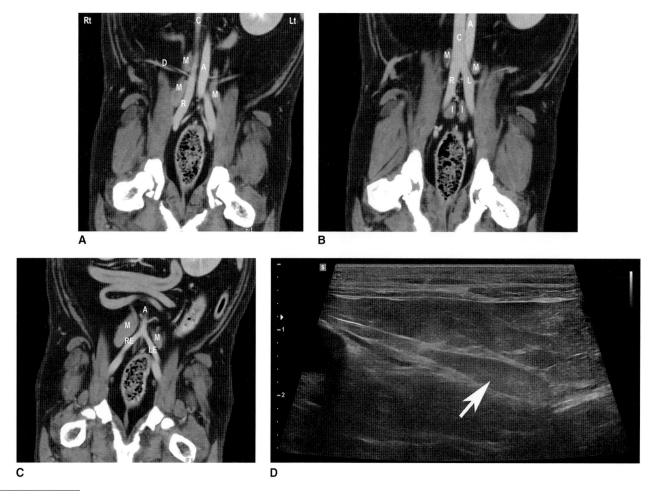

**FIGURE 20.108** Dorsal plane reconstructed CT images post contrast medium administration (**A–C**) and US image (**D**) from the caudal lumbar region in a normal dog. In (**A**), normal medial iliac lymph nodes (M) are noted adjacent to the caudal abdominal vasculature (a, aorta; r, right common iliac vein; c, caudal vena cava; d, right deep circumflex iliac vessels). In (**B**), the right (R) and left (L) common iliac veins are labeled. This slice is ventral to (**A**). Additional to the medial iliac lymph nodes (M), the internal iliac lymph nodes (I) are noted. In (**C**), the right (RE) and left (LE) external iliac arteries are labeled and the medial iliac lymph nodes (M) are noted just lateral to the trifurcation of the caudal abdominal aorta (a). In (**D**), the medial iliac lymph node (white arrow) is highlighted adjacent to the caudal abdominal aorta at the trifurcation (not shown in image) in the same dog.

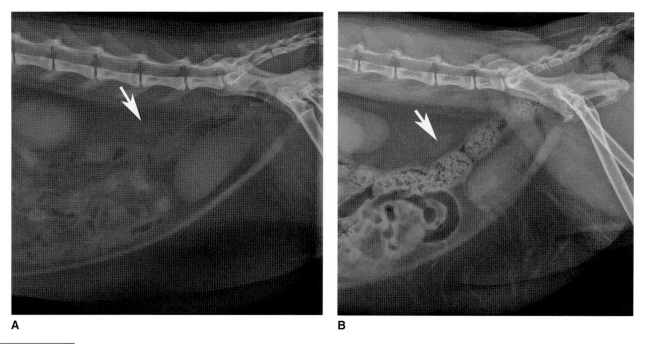

**FIGURE 20.109** Lateral abdominal radiographs from two different cats (**A,B**) documenting a mildly enlarged left colic lymph node (white arrow) within the fat just dorsal to the colon. In both cases, these were reactive lymph nodes and not metastatic disease.

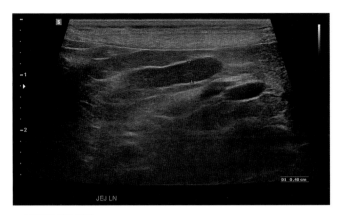

**FIGURE 20.110** Normal long axis image of a jejunal lymph node from a dog (between green crosses).

| TABLE 20.7 | Normal size of intraabdominal lymph nodes in dogs and cats using ultrasonography. | | |
|---|---|---|---|
| **Lymph node** | **Dogs (mm)** | **Cats (mm)** | **Figure 20.111** |
| Pancreaticoduo-denal | n/a | 4.6 (3.6–6.2)[c] | A |
| Ileocolic | n/a | 4.1 (2.7–4.8)[c] | B |
| Jejunal | 3.9 (1.6–8.2)[a] | 5.0 (2.8–7.2)[c] | C |
| Hepatic | n/a | 2.9 (2.5–3.6)[c] | D |
| Medial iliac | 4.6–4.8 (±0.18–0.20)[b] | 4.5 (1.3–14.0)[c] | E |

[a] Agthe et al. [30].
[b] Mayer et al. [31].
[c] Schreurs et al. [29].

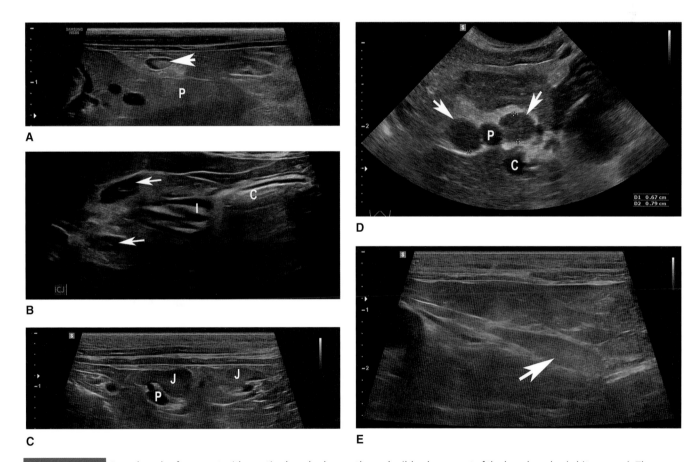

**FIGURE 20.111** Lymph nodes from a cat with reactive lymphadenopathy and mild enlargement of the lymph nodes (white arrows). These lymph nodes include (**A**) pancreatic-duodenal lymph node (P, pancreas); (**B**) ileocecocolic lymph nodes (I, ileum; C, colon); (**C**) jejunal lymph nodes (J) surrounding the portal vessels (P) and branches of the cranial mesenteric artery; (**D**) hepatic lymph nodes adjacent to the portal vein in the porta hepatis (P, portal vein; C, caudal vena cava); and (**E**) right medial iliac lymph node (white arrow).

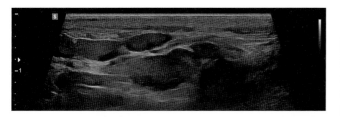

**FIGURE 20.112** Reactive lymph node enlargement can be seen in puppies and kittens up to 12 months of age. Long axis US image of reactive jejunal lymph nodes. Often there are hypoechoic nodules noted along the periphery of the lymph nodes, as seen in this image. These are presumed to represent reactive lymphoid tissue.

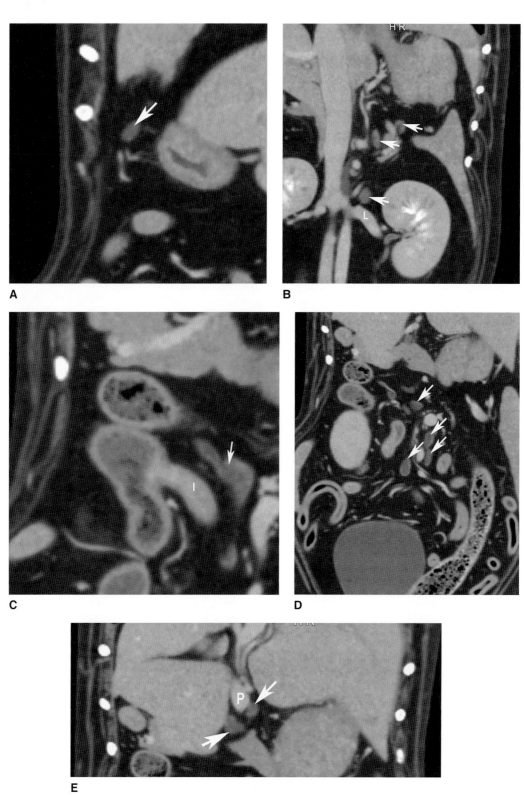

**FIGURE 20.113** Multiplanar reformats (dorsal plane) CT images post intravenous contrast medium documenting normal locations of various lymph nodes (white arrows) from a dog. These include (**A**) pancreatic-duodenal lymph node; (**B**) splenic lymph nodes and renal lymph nodes (adjacent to left renal vein (L)); (**C**) ileocolic lymph nodes (I, ileum); (**D**) jejunal lymph nodes; and (**E**) hepatic lymph nodes (P, portal vein).

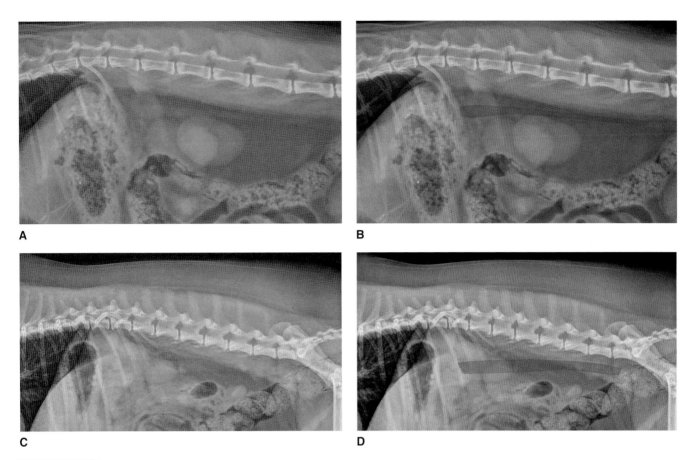

**FIGURE 20.114** Left lateral abdominal radiographs from a cat (**A**) and a dog (**C**). The caudal vena cava can be visualized in the dorsal retroperitoneal space and has been highlighted in blue (**B,D**).

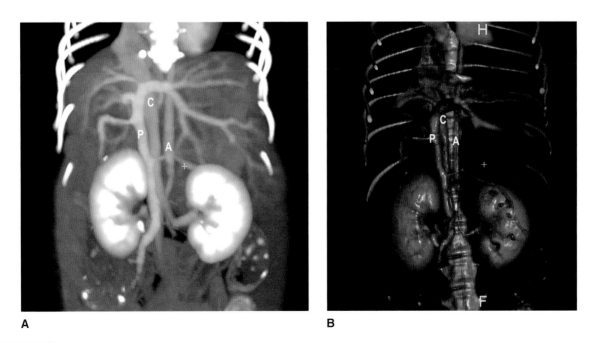

**FIGURE 20.115** Three-dimensional CT renderings of the abdominal vasculature including (**A**) MIP dorsal plane study and (**B**) 3D color rendering. P, portal vein; C, caudal vena cava; A, aorta. (Note that in **B**, H stands for head end of the patient.)

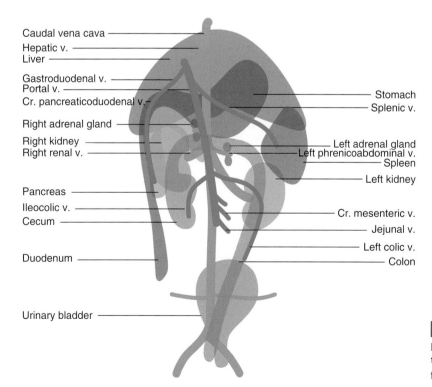

**FIGURE 20.116** Schematic representation of the abdominal aorta and its branches. Source: Reproduced with permission from *Today's Veterinary Practice*.

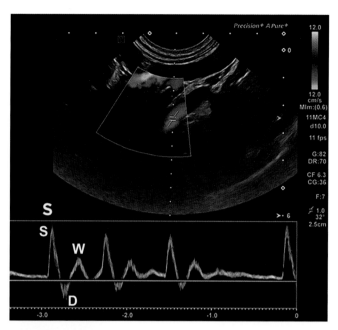

**FIGURE 20.117** Triplex imaging of the abdominal aorta. On the pulsed-wave Doppler tracing there are four systolic beats. The aorta has a triphasic recording with an initial upstroke for systole (S), then a rapid deceleration associated with the end of systole and a diastolic flow reversal (D), then another positive peak secondary to passive relaxation of the stretched aortic arch and ascending aorta from systolic stretch of the these vessels and the diastolic flow reversal (called the *Windkessel effect* [W]). In this example, flow is toward the transducer coded as red. The PW spectral wave form is also laminar with an outer echogenic envelope and no central signal.

**FIGURE 20.118** Schematic representation of the portal vein (green) and caudal vena cava (blue) and their branches. Source: Reproduced with permission from *Today's Veterinary Practice*.

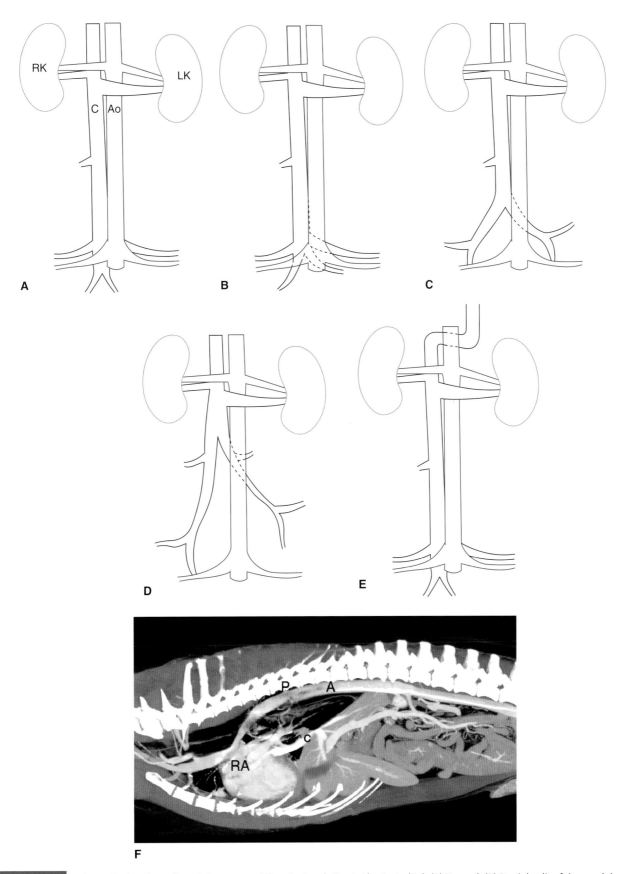

**FIGURE 20.119**   Schematic drawings of caudal vena cava (C) variants relative to the Aorta (Ao). (**A**) Normal. (**B**) Partial split of the caudal vena cava. (**C**) Partial duplication of the caudal vena cava. (**D**) Complete duplication of the caudal vena cava. (**E**) Azygos (A) continuation of the caudal vena cava. (**F**) Sagittal MIP showing azygos continuation of the abdominal caudal vena cava into the right atrium (RA). Drainage of hepatic veins is into a small caudal vena cava (C) that enters the right atrium.

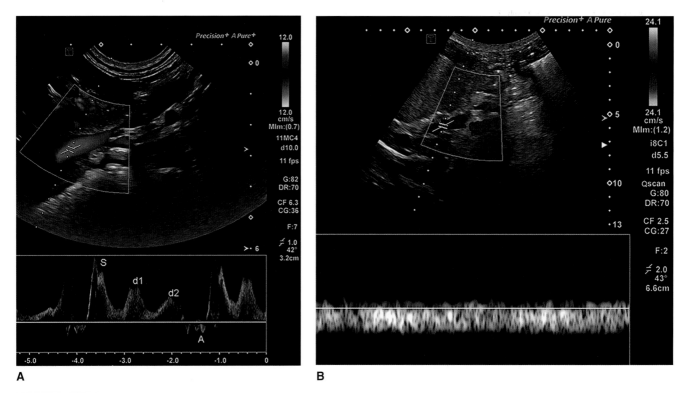

**A**  **B**

**FIGURE 20.120** Triplex imaging of the caudal vena cava (**A**) and portal vein (**B**). In the PW Doppler signal of the cauda vena cava (**A**), there are four components. S, ventricular systole where flow moves toward the ventricle after atrial systole. D1 and D2, diastolic filling once the tricuspid valve is open (occurring in two phases over time – d1 and d2). A, atrial systole where there is flow reversal. Note in this image the color coding and spectral mapping have been reversed so that red is away from the transducer and the positive deflections are away from the transducer. In (**B**), the portal vein velocity is approximately 12 cm/sec and it is away from the transducer (reads negative or below the baseline). The flow in (**B**) is also nonlaminar.

# References

1. Penninck, D. and d'Anjou, M.A. (2015). Gastrointestinal tract. In: *Atlas of Small Animal Ultrasonography*, 2e (ed. D. Penninck and M.A. d'Anjou). Hoboken, NJ: Wiley Blackwell.

2. Heng, H.G., Wrigley, R., Kraft, S., and Powers, B. (2005). Fat is responsible for an intramural radiolucent band in the feline stomach wall. *Vet. Radiol. Ultrasound* 46 (1): 54–56.

3. Trevail, T., Gunn-Moore, D., Carrera, I. et al. (2011). Radiographic diameter of the colon in normal and constipated cats and in cats with megacolon. *Vet. Radiol. Ultrasound* 52 (5): 516–520.

4. Citi, S., Chimenti, T., Marchetti, V. et al. (2013). Micronodular ultrasound lesions in the colonic submucosa of 42 dogs and 14 cats. *Vet. Radiol. Ultrasound* 54 (6): 646–651.

5. Johnson-Neitman J., O'Brien, R., and Wallace, J. (2012). Quantitative perfusion analysis of the pancreas and duodenum in healthy dogs by use of contrast-enhanced ultrasonography. *Am. J. Vet. Res.* 73 (3): 385–392.

6. Leinonen, M.R., Raekallio, M., Vainio, O. et al. (2010). Quantitative contrast-enhanced ultrasonographic analysis of perfusion in the kidneys, liver, pancreas, small intestine, and mesenteric lymph nodes in healthy cats. *Am. J. Vet. Res.* 71 (11): 1305–1311.

7. Cáceres, A.V., Zwingenberger, A., Hardam, E. et al. (2006). Helical computed tomographic angiography of the normal canine pancreas. *Vet. Radiol. Ultrasound* 47 (3): 270–278.

8. Secrest, S., Sharma, A., and Bugbee, A. (2018). Triple phase computed tomography of the pancreas in healthy cats. *Vet. Radiol. Ultrasound* 59 (2): 163–168.

9. Penninck, D. and d'Anjou, M.A. (2015). Pancreas. In: *Atlas of Small Animal Ultrasonography*, 2e (ed. D. Penninck and M.A. d'Anjou). Hoboken, NJ: Wiley Blackwell.

10. Larson, M.M., Panciera, D., Ward, D. et al. (2005). Age-related changes in the ultrasound appearance of the normal feline pancreas. *Vet. Radiol. Ultrasound* 46 (3): 238–242.

11. Hittmair, K.M., Vielgrader, H.D., and Loupal, G. (2001). Ultrasonographic evaluation of gallbladder wall thickness in cats. *Vet. Radiol. Ultrasound* 42 (2): 149–155.

12. Spaulding, K.A. (1993). Ultrasound corner: gallbladder wall thickness. *Vet. Radiol. Ultrasound I* 34: 270–272.

13. Bargellini, P., Orlandi, R., Palloni, C. et al. (2016). Evaluation of contrast-enhanced ultrasonography as a method for detecting gallbladder necrosis or rupture in dogs. *Vet. Radiol. Ultrasound* 57 (6): 611–620.

14. Brömel, C., Barthez, P., Léveillé, R., and Scrivani, P. (1998). Prevalence of gallbladder sludge in dogs as assessed by ultrasonography. *Vet. Radiol. Ultrasound* 39 (3): 206–221.

15. d'Anjou, M.A. and Penninck, D. (2015). Liver. In: *Atlas of Small Animal Ultrasonography*, 2e (ed. D. Penninck and M.A. d'Anjou). Hoboken, NJ: Wiley Blackwell.

16. Johnson, K.L., Porter, E.G., and Berry, C.R. (2017). Analysis of feline splenic radiographic measurements and their correlation to ultrasonographic measurements. *J. Feline Med. Surg.* 19 (10): 985–991.

17. Reese, S.L., Zekas, L., Iazbik, M. et al. (2013). Effect of sevoflurane anesthesia and blood donation on the sonographic appearance of the spleen in 60 healthy cats. *Vet. Radiol. Ultrasound* 54 (2): 168–175.

18. Specchi, S., Panopoulos, I., Adrian, A. et al. (2018). A "spaghetti sign" in feline abdominal radiographs predicts spleno-systemic collateral circulation. *Vet. Radiol. Ultrasound* 59 (1): 13–17.

19. Soulsby, S.N., Holland, M., Hudson, J., and Behrend, E. (2015). Ultrasonographic evaluation of adrenal gland size compared to body weight in normal dogs. *Vet. Radiol. Ultrasound* 56 (3): 317–326.

20. Pey, P., Rossi, F., Vignoli, M. et al. (2011). Contrast-enhanced ultrasonography of the normal canine adrenal gland. *Vet. Radiol. Ultrasound* 52 (5): 560–567.

21. Ruth, J.D., Heng, H., Miller, M., and Constable, P. (2013). Effect of anisotropy and spatial compound imaging on renal cortical echogenicity in dogs. *Vet. Radiol. Ultrasound* 54 (6): 659–665.

22. Lobacz, M.A., Sullivan, M., Mellor, D. et al. (2012). Effect of breed, age, weight and gender on radiographic renal size in the dog. *Vet. Radiol. Ultrasound* 53 (4): 437–441.

23. Finco, D.R., Stiles, N.S., Kneller, S.K. et al. (1971). Radiologic estimation of kidney size of the dog. *J. Am. Vet. Med. Assoc.* 159: 995–1002.

24. d'Anjou, M.A. and Penninck, D. (2015). Kidneys and ureters. In: *Atlas of Small Animal Ultrasonography*, 2e (ed. D. Penninck and M.A. d'Anjou). Hoboken, NJ: Wiley Blackwell.

25. Mareschal, A., d'Anjou, M.-A., Moreau, M. et al. (2007). Ultrasonographic measurement of kidney-to-aorta ratio as a method of estimating renal size in dogs. *Vet. Radiol. Ultrasound* 48 (5): 434–438.

26. Barella, G., Lodi, M., Sabbadin, L., and Faverzani, S. (2012). A new method for ultrasonographic measurement of kidney size in healthy dogs. *J. Ultrasound* 15 (3): 186–191.

27. Sutherland-Smith, K. and Penninck, D. (2015). Bladder and urethra. In: *Atlas of Small Animal Ultrasonography*, 2e (ed. D. Penninck and M.A. d'Anjou). Hoboken, NJ: Wiley Blackwell.

28. Pollard, R. and Hecht, S. (2015). Female reproductive tract. In: *Atlas of Small Animal Ultrasonography*, 2e (ed. D. Penninck and M.A. d'Anjou). Hoboken, NJ: Wiley Blackwell.

29. Schreurs, E., Vermote, K., Barberet, V. et al. (2008). Ultrasonographic anatomy of abdominal lymph nodes in the normal cat. *Vet. Radiol. Ultrasound* 49 (1): 68–72.

30. Agthe, P., Caine, A., Posch, B., and Herrtage, M. (2009). Ultrasonographic appearance of jejunal lymph nodes in dogs without clinical signs of gastrointestinal disease. *Vet. Radiol. Ultrasound* 50 (2): 195–200.

31. Mayer, M.N., Lawson, J., and Silver, T. (2010). Sonographic characteristics of presumptively normal canine medial iliac and superficial inguinal lymph nodes. *Vet. Radiol. Ultrasound* 51 (6): 638–641.

32. Beukers, M., Grosso, F.V., and Voorhout, G. (2013). Computed tomographic characteristics of presumed normal canine abdominal lymph nodes. *Vet. Radiol. Ultrasound* 54 (6): 610–617.

33. Ryu, C., Choi, S., Choi, H. et al. (2019). CT variants of the caudal vena cava in 121 small breed dogs. *Vet. Radiol. Ultrasound* 60 (6): 680–688.

# CHAPTER 21

# Extraabdominal Structures and the Abdominal Body Wall

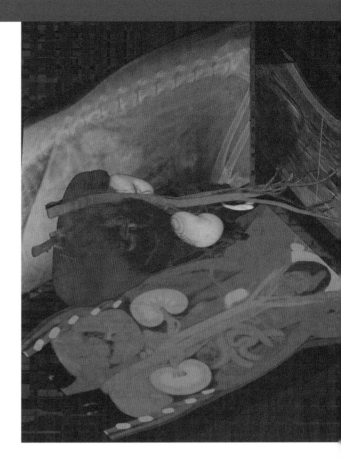

**Matthew D. Winter**

Department of Small Animal Clinical Sciences,
College of Veterinary Medicine, University of Florida,
Gainesville, FL, USA

## Introduction

The abdomen extends from the diaphragm to the pelvis. The extra abdominal structures consist of the body wall, the caudal thorax, the included portion of the vertebral column, and included portions of the pelvis and pelvic limbs. These structures are important to evaluate for alterations in body condition, body wall compromise, for osseous lesions that may reflect degenerative or aggressive diseases, and soft tissue or fat opaque masses. Evaluation of the osseous structures is covered in the musculoskeletal section. Evaluation of the diaphragm is covered in the thoracic section. The reader is referred to these respective sections for review of these components of the abdominal body wall assessment.

## Body Wall Anatomy

The cranial abdominal cavity is separated from the thoracic cavity by the diaphragm. The abdominal wall consists of the different abdominal muscles, fascia, and fat. The lateral and ventral margins of the abdominal body wall consist of the muscle, fascia, fat, and cutaneous tissues. Specifically, the musculature of the abdominal body wall includes the external abdominal oblique muscles, the internal abdominal oblique muscles, the rectus abdominis muscles, the transverse abdominal muscles, and the cutaneous trunci. These are also connected via various fascia and aponeuroses [1]. Fat is interspersed between these layers, within the fascial planes.

The cranial margin of the abdomen is the diaphragm, and the caudal margin is continuous with the pelvic canal at the pelvic inlet. The pelvic canal is bounded caudally by the pelvic diaphragm which consists of the coccygeus and levator ani muscles. Dorsally, the abdominal body wall includes the osseous components of the vertebral column and the paraspinal musculature.

Lymph nodes are also present in the inguinal region, and should be evaluated on imaging studies. The superficial inguinal lymph nodes are located in the furrow between the ventrolateral abdominal body wall and the muscles of the thigh. These lymph nodes drain the caudoventral abdominal body wall, including the caudal mammary glands in the female, and the prepuce and scrotum in the male [1]. These can occasionally be seen in the inguinal fat of feline and canine patients, even in normalcy, and may indeed be visible when enlarged.

Ventrally in the female, mammae and mammillae are present, and can enlarge during various stages of estrus and parturition in the intact dog and cat (Figure 21.1). These can also be the source of mass lesions, including neoplasia, infection, and abscessation.

# Hernias

Congenital hernias of the diaphragm are covered in the thoracic section. The most common congenital hernia of the abdominal wall is an umbilical hernia, where a small amount of fat/omentum is herniated into an opening at the umbilicus and extends into the subcutaneous tissues (Figure 21.2). A larger hernia at the umbilicus is called an *omphalocele*. In this congenital anomaly, there is intestinal tract or other abdominal organ herniation outside the abdominal wall at the umbilicus. Traumatic ruptures of the abdominal wall occur commonly post trauma with varying degrees of abdominal organ herniation (Figure 21.3). Herniation of organs into the inguinal canals can occur post trauma as well.

One of the features to evaluate radiographically is the presence of subcutaneous gas. This can be post trauma, postoperative surgical, secondary to abscess formation or fluid administration. The location and extent of the subcutaneous emphysema would be seen as a reflection of the location and degree of trauma. Ultrasound and CT can be useful to identify and characterize any herniated abdominal contents (Figure 21.4) and to better define abdominal body wall defects (Figure 21.5).

In intact male dogs, caudal perineal hernias can occur. Herniation of the urinary bladder, prostate gland or other intestinal segments can occur through the pelvic canal and into a perineal hernia due to the weakening of the perineal muscles by the testosterone levels in the male dog.

# Masses

Masses can originate from any of the tissues that comprise the abdominal body wall. Fat opaque masses associated with the abdominal body wall are common in dogs (Figure 21.6), but are rarely seen in cats. The most common of these are lipomas, a benign lipomatous mass that is typically characterized by well-differentiated adipocytes that occur within the subcutaneous tissues, muscles, and abdominal cavity. Other lipomatous masses are also recognized, including infiltrative lipomas, and angiolipomas, which are less common. Liposarcoma represents a malignant form of lipomatous mass that is also rare [2]. On CT, lipomas were characterized as round to oval, homogeneously fat-attenuating masses with well-defined margins. Infiltrative lipomas had similar, uniform fat attenuation, but had a more irregular shape. Liposarcomas were characterized by heterogeneous attenuation with ill-defined soft tissue components and a multinodular appearance [2].

Primary masses of mesenchymal origin can arise from the soft tissues of the abdominal body wall, often collectively termed soft tissue sarcomas (Figure 21.7). This can encompass tumors such as fibrosarcoma, perivascular wall tumors, liposarcoma, malignant fibrous histiocytoma, mesenchymoma, myxosarcoma, nonlexus-derived peripheral nerve sheath tumors, and undifferentiated sarcoma. Other abdominal wall masses include mammary gland adenocarcinomas and a variety of different types of soft tissue sarcomas (rhabdomyosarcoma, fibrosarcoma or undifferentiated sarcoma) [3]. Rhabdomyosarcoma, lymphangiosarcoma, and leiomyosarcoma are often excluded from this list of soft tissue sarcomas [3], but can also be the source of masses of the abdominal body wall.

Mammary gland tumors are the most common neoplasms in female dogs. These most often involve the caudal abdominal or inguinal mammary glands. It is speculated that this is due to their greater volume of glandular tissue. CT has been used successfully to stage disease in dogs (Figure 21.8). Injection of positive contrast media into the subareolar tissue of the mammary tissue has resulted in some sensitive and specific features to help identify sentinel lymph nodes, specifically hypoattenuating heterogeneity observed 1 minute post injection [4]. It is still challenging to differentiate between reactive and metastatic lymphadenomegaly. The size and shape of the lymph node were found to be less reliable.

# Summary

The abdominal wall consists of layered soft tissue and fat opaque regions that vary depending on the body condition of the dog or cat. Traumatic injuries to the body wall are common and herniations of different abdominal contents can occur. Imaging is helpful in identifying and characterizing contents. Masses also occur, and while lipomas are common and benign, it is important to be aware of more malignant masses that may occur.

The body wall and extraabdominal structures are a critical part of the interpretation paradigm.

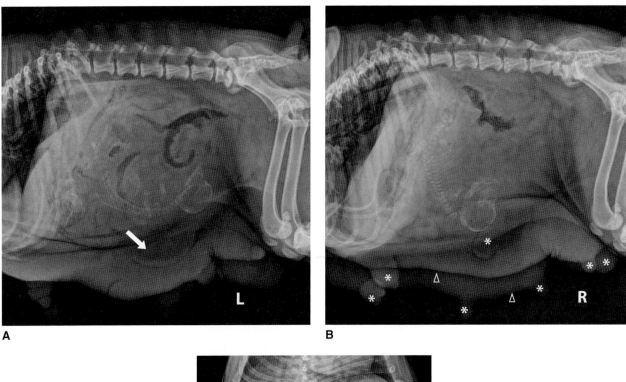

**FIGURE 21.1** Right lateral (**A**), left lateral (**B**), and ventrodorsal (**C**) projections of the abdomen of a pregnant bulldog. Note the thickened mammae (open arrowheads) and large mammillae (*). A single mineralized fetus is present. Also note the bonus lesion on the left lateral projection, a lipoma (white arrow).

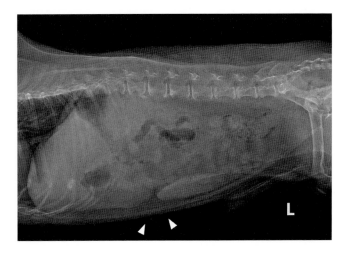

**FIGURE 21.2** Left lateral projection showing a small, ventrally located, well-defined, fat opaque mass in the subcutaneous tissues in the region of the umbilicus consistent with an umbilical hernia.

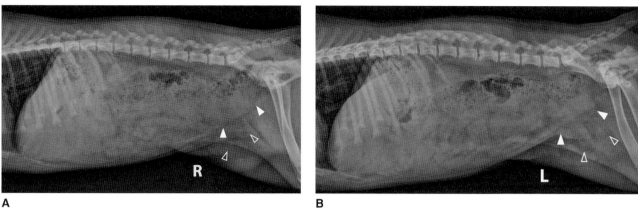

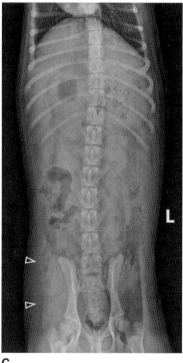

**FIGURE 21.3**   Right lateral (**A**), left lateral (**B**), and ventrodorsal (**C**) images of a dog with a history of recent trauma. Note the extent of the right inguinal body wall defect (white arrowheads) and the extension of tubular soft tissue structures within the subcutaneous tissues of the right inguinal region (open arrowheads).

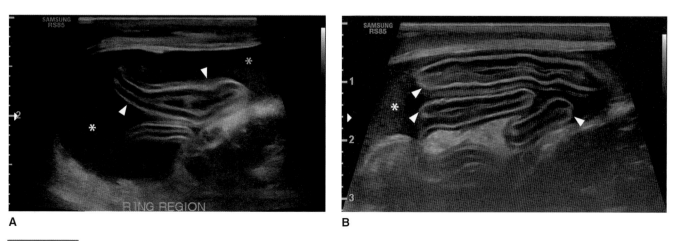

**FIGURE 21.4**   Ultrasound images (**A**,**B**) of the right inguinal region of the same dog as in Figure 21.2, showing the presence of small intestinal segments within the hernia (white arrowheads) and the presence of echogenic fluid (*).

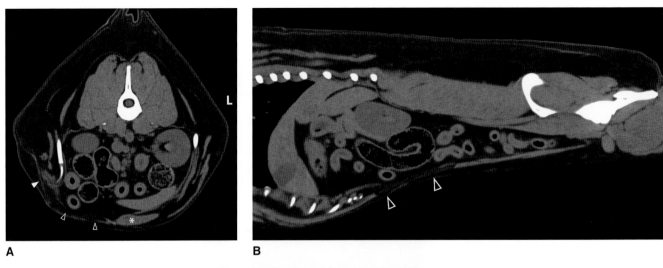

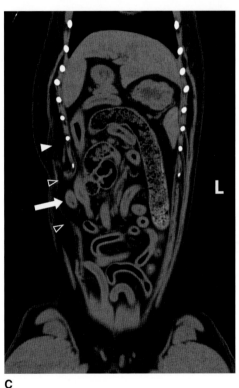

**FIGURE 21.5** Transverse (**A**) soft tissue reconstruction and sagittal (**B**) and dorsal plane (**C**) reformatted images showing a right ventral midabdominal body wall defect (open arrowheads) and increased fluid attenuation in the subcutaneous tissues cranial and dorsal to the defect (white arrowhead).

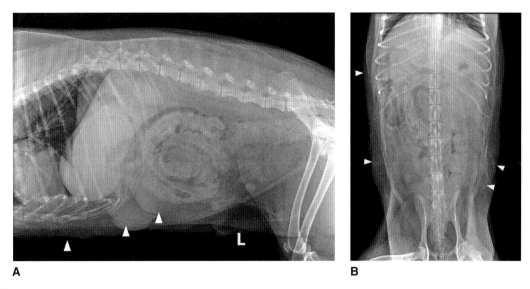

**FIGURE 21.6** Left lateral (**A**) and ventrodorsal (**B**) images of a dog with multiple subcutaneous fat opaque masses (white arrowheads) consistent with lipomas.

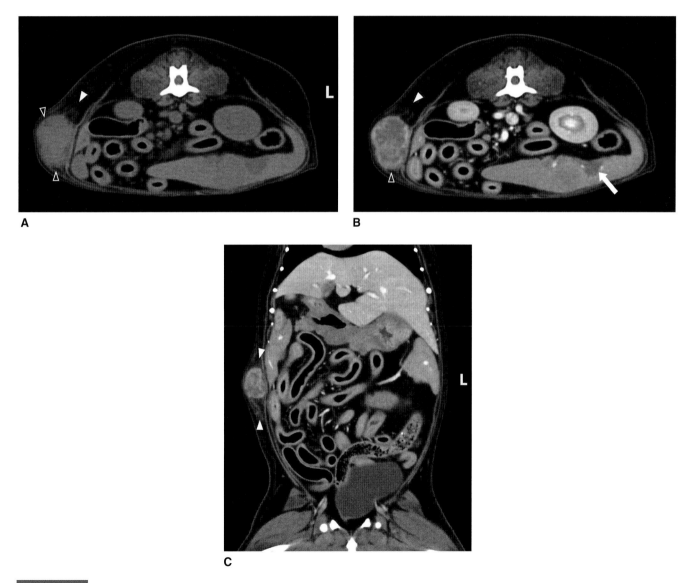

**FIGURE 21.7** Transverse precontrast (**A**) and postcontrast (**B**) as well as dorsal plane reformatted postcontrast (**C**) images of a dog with a subcutaneous soft tissue sarcoma. Note that the margins of the mass are relatively well defined, and contrast enhancement is heterogeneous (open arrowheads). Also note the contrast-enhancing, finger-like protrusions from the mass into the surrounding subcutaneous fat (white arrowheads) suggestive of extension of the mass into the surrounding body wall.

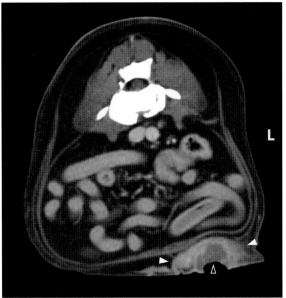
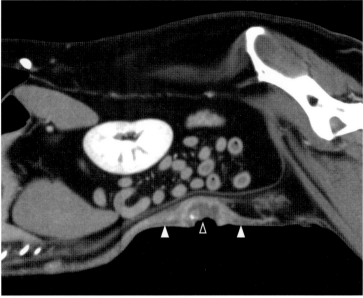

**A**                    **B**

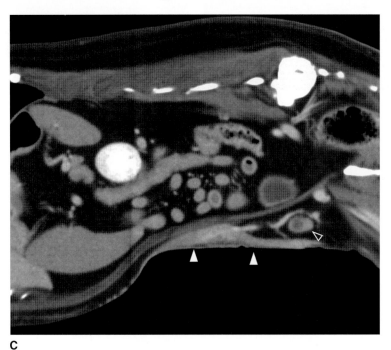

**C**

**FIGURE 21.8** Transverse reconstruction (**A**) and sagittal postcontrast reformatted images (**B,C**) of a dog with an ulcerated and necrotic mammary carcinoma. Note the heterogeneous contrast enhancement of the mammary mass (white arrowheads) with a central cavitation (open arrowhead) that has a fluid-attenuating component. In (**C**), note the enlargement of the superficial inguinal lymph node, which has a central hypoattenuating region with peripheral contrast enhancement.

# References

1. Evans, H. and de Lahunta, A. (2012). *Miller's Anatomy of the Dog*, 4e. St Louis, MO: Saunders.

2. Spoldi, E., Schwarz, T., Sabattini, S. et al. (2017). Comparisons among computed tomographic features of adipose masses in dogs and cats. *Vet. Radiol. Ultrasound* 58: 29–37.

3. Bray, J.P. (2016). Soft tissue sarcoma in the dog – part 1: a current review. *J. Small Anim. Prac.* 57: 510–519.

4. Soultani, C., Patsikas, M.N., Karayannopoulou, M. et al. (2017). Assessment of sentinel lymph node metastasis in canine mammary gland tumors using computed tomographic indirect lymphography. *Vet. Radiol. Ultrasound* 58: 186–196.

# CHAPTER 22

# The Peritoneal and Retroperitoneal Space

Matthew D. Winter

Department of Small Animal Clinical Sciences, College of Veterinary Medicine, University of Florida, Gainesville, FL, USA

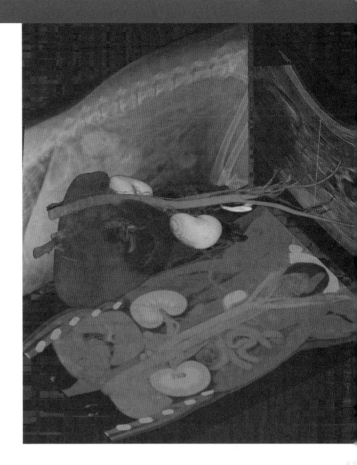

## Normal Anatomy

The peritoneum is a serous membrane that is primarily constructed of connective tissue and is broadly divided into the parietal and visceral peritoneum. The parietal peritoneum lines the abdominal cavity, pelvic cavity, and scrotum. The visceral peritoneum covers all or portions of the organs in the abdominal, pelvic, and scrotal cavities. Embryologically, organs descend ventrally into, or form within, the peritoneum, resulting in the creation of folds connecting peritoneum that are commonly referred to as the mesentery, omenta, or ligaments of these various organs. These resultant folds, spaces or cavities are also often the site of fat deposition [1]. The peritoneal space, then, is simply the potential space bounded by the peritoneal membranes that surround the abdominal organs.

The cavities described above created by this peritoneal investment are essentially closed cavities, with no organs actually existing within the peritoneal space itself. The exception is an opening of the cranial/abdominal margin of the uterine tube, which in theory connects the peritoneal cavity through the female genital tract to the outside world. Therefore, during ovulation, an ovum may be considered to be, briefly, peritoneal in location [1]. Otherwise, the peritoneal space contains only a small amount of lubricating fluid to reduce friction between adjacent organs as well as between organs and the abdominal body wall. This small amount of fluid is typically not visible when imaging normal patients.

The testes are covered with an investment of peritoneum, termed the *vaginal process*. The complex descension of the testes into the scrotum results in the creation of the cavity of the vaginal process. This cavity is continuous with the peritoneal space at the level of the vaginal ring. Similarly, the ovaries are covered with an investment of peritoneum, and are suspended in the peritoneal space via the mesovarium [1].

Organs that lie against the walls of the abdominal or pelvic cavities and have peritoneum covering only a single surface are considered retroperitoneal. The dorsal surface of the kidneys lacks a peritoneal covering, and may be separated from

*Atlas of Small Animal Diagnostic Imaging*, First Edition. Edited by Clifford R. Berry, Nathan C. Nelson, and Matthew D. Winter.
© 2023 John Wiley & Sons, Inc. Published 2023 by John Wiley & Sons, Inc.
Companion website: www.wiley.com/go/berry/atlas

the sublumbar musculature by fat. Ventrally and cranially, the kidneys have a peritoneal covering. The ureters course caudally from the renal pelvis, and are also retroperitoneal, bounded dorsally by the psoas musculature and ventrally by the peritoneum, before diving ventrally through the lateral ligament of the bladder (and the broad ligament in females) and entering the urinary bladder.

Finally, the adrenal glands are also considered retroperitoneal, contacting the retroperitoneal surfaces of the kidneys, renal hilus, and abdominal aorta. The right adrenal gland may be continuous with the adventitial lining of the caudal vena cava in dogs [1].

# Imaging Findings

## Serosal Margin Detail in the Normal Patient

In a normal patient, serosal margin detail, or the ability to define the margins of abdominal organs on the radiograph, is dependent on the amount of fat in the cavities created by the peritoneal folds, such as the omentum and mesentery. This fat becomes interspersed between abdominal organs, providing contrast between adjacent soft tissue structures.

On initial radiographic evaluation, serosal margin detail should be assessed. Specifically, evaluate the ability to visualize the serosal margins of the abdominal organs, and the amount of fat in the abdomen. Each patient should be treated individually, as there is significant variation in the amount of intraabdominal fat associated with body condition. Also, larger dogs produce more scatter radiation, reducing contrast resolution. In addition, brown fat in young patients does not provide the same degree of contrast as the yellow fat in more mature patients.

In mature patients with moderate peritoneal and retroperitoneal fat, the margins of abdominal organs should be easy to delineate (Figure 22.1). Thin patients will have poor serosal margin detail (Figure 22.2). Detecting free peritoneal fluid in these patients can be challenging. Be sure to also consider the contour of the abdominal body wall in these patients. If an emaciated patient with poor abdominal serosal detail has a rounded, distended abdominal body wall, consider the possibility of free peritoneal fluid.

## Causes of Altered Serosal Margin Detail

**Effusion**  Radiographically, the presence of fluid in the peritoneal space results in decreased serosal margin detail. The fluid in the peritoneal space will gradually border efface with the margins of abdominal organs, making them hard or impossible to see. With mild fluid, the margins of organs may look blurry or smudged rather than sharp and well defined.

Progressively, the margins of organs in the vicinity of larger volumes of fluid become obliterated entirely (Figure 22.3). Fat in the region of mild peritoneal fluid may look heterogeneous, with soft tissue streaks interspersed with fat in the mesentery, omentum, or retroperitoneal space. Occasionally, this is referred to as *fat stranding*.

Loss of detail can be focal or generalized, depending on the cause. Regional inflammation, such as that caused by pancreatitis, can be localized to the right cranial abdominal quadrant. The presence of large volumes of fluid, such as that seen with hypoproteinemia, severe uroabdomen, or severe hemorrhage, often creates generalized loss of serosal margin detail. If localized, often this may provide direction to a particular organ or organ system as the source of pathology.

Normal body cavity fluid, including peritoneal fluid, has low cell and protein concentrations, typically less than 3000 cells/µL and less than 2.3 g/dL respectively [2]. Effusions typically occur due to increases in the amount of fluid entering the cavity, or from decreased removal. The nature of the fluid varies with etiology. Peritoneal effusion may retain the characteristics of normal peritoneal fluid. Alternatively, it may have increased total nucleated cell count (TNCC), increased total protein, and may contain atypical cells. Identifying the type of fluid may help with differentials.

Traditionally, effusions have been classified as transudates or exudates based on alterations in cell count and protein, but parameters are variable. Transudates have been subdivided into pure transudates (1000–1500 cells/µL; <2.5 mg/dL protein) and modified transudates (TNCC 1000–5000 or 7000 cells/µL; >2.5 mg/dL protein). Exudates have been variably described as having a total protein >2.0, 2.5, or 3 g/dL and TNCC greater than 3000, 5000, or 7000. A simplified classification scheme has been proposed, with a cutoff between of 3000 cells/µL considered useful in the discrimination of transudates and exudates. Further, dividing transudates into low- and high-protein categories using a threshold of 2.5 g/dL was deemed more useful in determining differential diagnoses [2].

Radiography is insensitive to the underlying cause of effusions. The presence of an increased amount of fluid in the peritoneal and/or retroperitoneal spaces results in reduced serosal margin detail due to border effacement (Figure 22.4). Recall that fluid and soft tissue have the same opacity, and therefore the margins of structures in contact with the fluid will not be visible. The type or classification of the effusion cannot be distinguished radiographically. Still, generalized differentials for effusion identified radiographically are limited, and would include hemoabdomen, uroabdomen, septic abdomen, neoplastic/malignant effusion, or bile peritonitis. In some cases, localizing reduced serosal margin detail to a particular region of the abdomen may assist in prioritizing differentials. For example, focally reduced serosal margin detail in the right cranial abdomen may implicate the pancreas, gall bladder, right liver, stomach, or duodenum as potentially abnormal. When synthesized with patient information and other clinicopathologic data, differentials may be reprioritized.

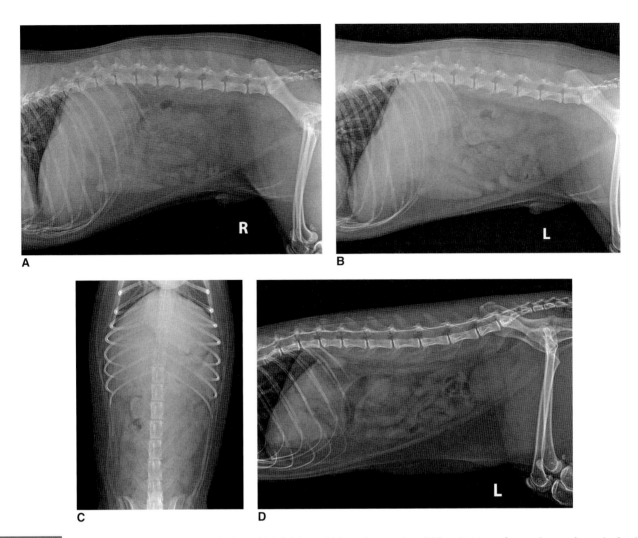

**FIGURE 22.1** Normal serosal margin detail. Right lateral (**A**), left lateral (**B**), and ventrodorsal (**C**) projections of normal serosal margin detail in a large-breed dog with good to increased body condition. Observe the normal margins of the liver, spleen, and intestinal loops. The left kidney is well visualized on the left lateral; the cranial pole of the right kidney is border effaced with the caudate process of the liver. On the ventrodorsal projection, it is more difficult to delineate specific organs, especially centrally, due to superimposition of more structures and thicker patient dimension. Left lateral projection (**D**) of a cat that has average body condition with normal serosal margin detail. Note the exquisite detail seen in cats, where most organs are surrounded by fat and easily defined.

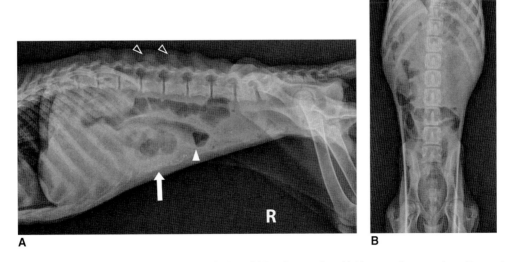

**FIGURE 22.2** Normal serosal margin detail in a thin patient. Right lateral (**A**) and ventrodorsal (**B**) images of a young dog with poor body condition. Note the protrusion of the spinous process resulting in an undulating cutaneous margin (open arrowheads), the lack of subcutaneous fat, and the absence of falciform and retroperitoneal fat. The ventral margin of the abdomen is not rounded, but is tucked and tapers to the pelvic canal (white arrow). As a result of poor body condition, it is difficult to delineate margins of intestinal segments (white arrowhead), or any other abdominal organs.

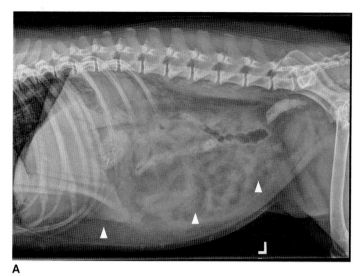
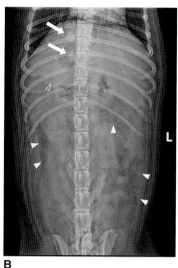

**FIGURE 22.3** Mild to moderate peritoneal effusion. Left lateral (**A**) and ventrodorsal (**B**) projections of a dog with mild to moderate peritoneal effusion. Note the blurred margins of the intestinal segments and the lateral abdominal body wall (white arrowheads) and the streaking in the region of the falciform fat. Note the rounded right liver and displacement of the pylorus, suggestive of a right-sided liver mass (open arrowhead). And note the pulmonary nodules (white arrows).

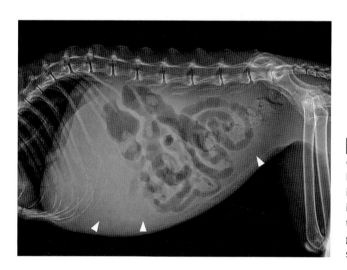

**FIGURE 22.4** Lateral projection of a geriatric cat with poor body condition and peritoneal effusion. While there is protrusion of the lumbar spinous processes as seen in Figure 22.2, note that the abdomen is distended, suggesting that there is enlargement of the abdomen, in this case due to the presence of fluid (white arrowheads). Also note that serosal margin detail is very poor. Delineating segments of the gastrointestinal tract is only possible due to the gas within the lumen of small intestinal segments and feces in the colon.

The sonographic appearance of peritoneal fluid varies, and echogenicity increases with cell count and protein (Figure 22.5). On computed tomography (CT), peritoneal effusion appears as fluid-attenuating material within the peritoneal space (Figure 22.6). The attenuation of peritoneal fluid as an aid to characterization of underlying etiology has limited utility in people. Attenuation values greater than 20 Hounsfield units (HU) are suggestive of infection versus ascites, although patients with malignancies were not included in this study population [3]. Further investigation on the utility of HU in the prediction of fluid types is required. However, in general, accuracy in predicting fluid types is increased with the consideration of additional imaging findings such as nodules and masses.

**Steatitis** Steatitis is the inflammation of fat, typically yellow fat, and is most commonly described in the mesenteric fat of the abdomen and seen in conjunction with peritonitis. This can result in saponification, necrosis, and mineralization [4, 5]. Radiographically, this can result in an increase in opacity of the peritoneal fat, which contributes to the loss of peritoneal serosal margin detail seen with peritoneal effusion [5]. Sonographically, inflamed fat shows an increase in echogenicity (Figure 22.7).

**Carcinomatosis** Neoplasms of abdominal organs can cause disruption of the peritoneal lining, thereby disseminating neoplastic cells throughout the peritoneal space. The result can be metastatic neoplastic nodules within the peritoneal space that occur concurrently with peritoneal effusion, often termed *carcinomatosis* [6]. The term carcinomatosis has been used generally to describe the presence of peritoneal nodules of neoplastic origin, regardless of tumor type. It has been suggested that the terms *lymphomatosis* and *sarcomatosis* are used to differentiate cell types associated with specific malignant nodules within the peritoneal space [7].

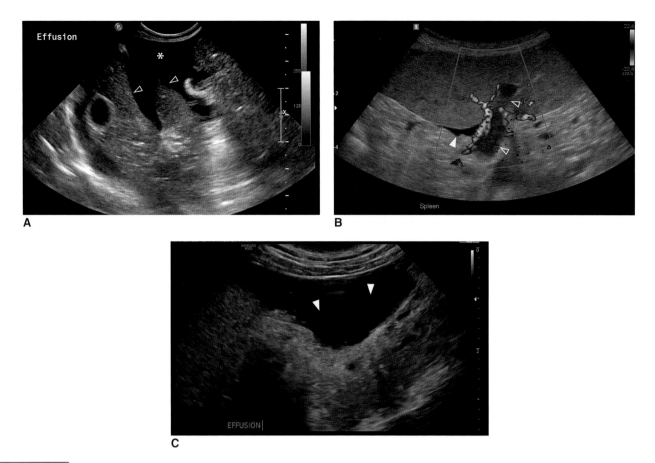

**FIGURE 22.5** Sonographic images of peritoneal effusion. In (**A**) note the fluid in the peritoneal space ventral to the liver (*) and how it outlines the margins of the liver lobes (open arrowheads). Image (**B**) shows a splenic vein thrombus (open arrowheads); note the small amount of fluid adjacent to the spleen (white arrowhead). In (**C**) note that the fluid contains an echogenic component (white arrowheads) suggesting the presence of cells and/or protein.

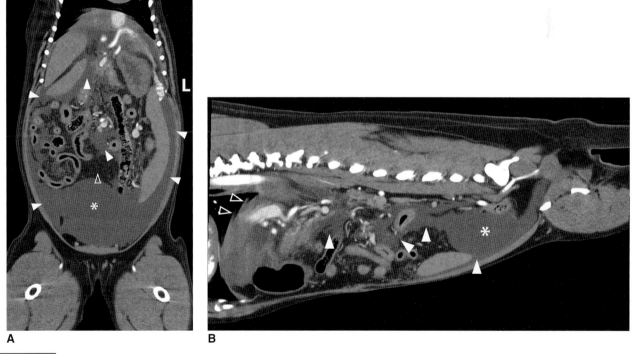

**FIGURE 22.6** Dorsal (**A**) and sagittal (**B**) reformatted, postcontrast CT images of a dog with multiple acquired shunts secondary to portal hypertension resulting from arterioportal fistula. Note the fluid in the peritoneal space surrounding the abdominal organs (white arrowheads). Even without contrast, the high contrast resolution of CT can allow fluid and soft tissue organs to be distinguished. The small intestines adjacent to the fluid can be distinguished. The (*) demarcates the urinary bladder. The urinary bladder contents have attenuation values of 4 HU, and the peritoneal effusion has attenuation values of 12 HU. This small difference in attenuation can be faintly distinguished visually on this soft tissue algorithm. Measuring HU can be helpful in characterizing effusions. The open arrowheads indicate motion artifact along the margin of the diaphragm associated with respiration.

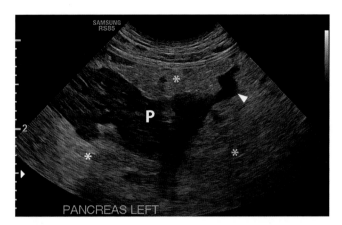

**FIGURE 22.7** Sonographic image of the pancreas in a dog with pancreatitis and regional steatitis. The pancreas (P) is thickened, hypoechoic and irregular, with regional effusion also present (white arrowhead). Note that the regional fat (*) is hyperechoic, consistent with inflammation.

Because the nodular changes associated with peritoneal metastasis often occur alongside peritoneal effusion, radiography can be an insensitive test. However, in the absence of large volumes of peritoneal effusion, the presence of nodular, ill-defined, irregular soft tissue opacities within the mesentery can be resolved [6]. These findings could be suggestive of carcinomatosis, sarcomatosis, or lymphomatosis. In addition, identification of a mass effect may help identify an organ of origin, which should influence the differential diagnosis (Figure 22.8).

The cross-sectional modalities of CT and US also benefit from improved contrast resolution, allowing for discrimination between effusion and peritoneal nodules. Sonographically, the imaging characteristics of peritoneal nodules associated with carcinomatosis, sarcomatosis, and lymphomatosis overlap, appearing as small, single or coalescing hypoechoic nodules or masses associated with the visceral or parietal peritoneum and/or connecting mesenteries (Figure 22.9) [7–9]. On CT images, irregular, soft tissue-attenuating nodules associated with the visceral peritoneum, parietal peritoneum, and/or mesenteries are highly suggestive of carcinomatosis, sarcomatosis, and lymphomatosis (Figure 22.10). It is not possible to distinguish between the different cell types. However, cross-sectional imaging modalities may provide greater accuracy in identifying and

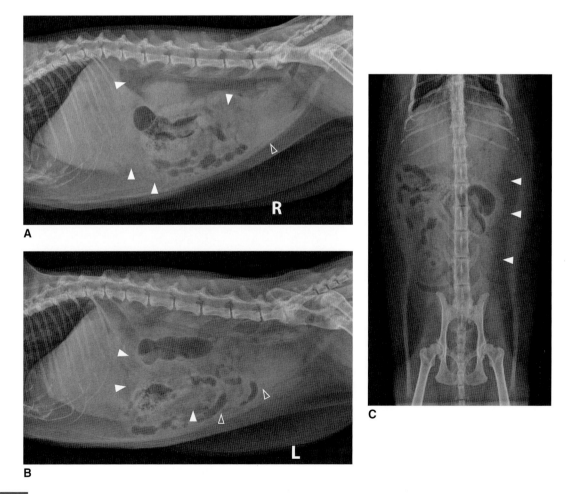

**FIGURE 22.8** Right lateral (**A**), left lateral (**B**), and ventrodorsal (**C**) radiographs of a cat with cholangiocarcinoma. Note the loss of serosal margin detail, which is most pronounced in the ventral abdomen on the lateral projections (open arrowheads) consistent with effusion. In addition, note the ill-defined nodular lesions in the abdominal fat (white arrowheads). These nodules are suggestive of mesenteric nodules, and would be consistent with carcinomatosis.

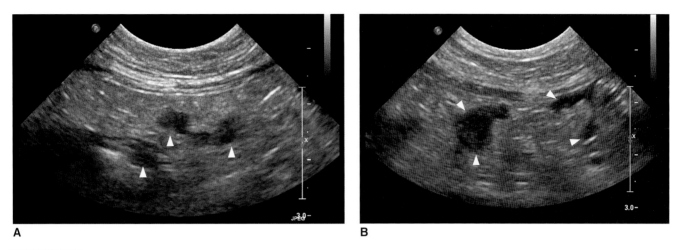

**FIGURE 22.9**   Sonographic images (**A**,**B**) of the same cat presented in Figure 22.8. Note the irregular, nodules within the mesenteric fat (white arrowheads) consistent with carcinomatosis. Also note that the fat is hyperechoic compatible with steatitis.

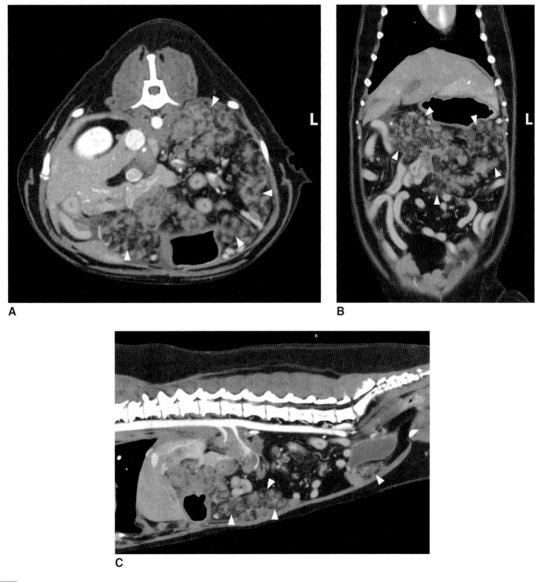

**FIGURE 22.10**   Transverse (**A**), dorsal (**B**), and sagittal (**C**) reformatted CT images of a 10-year-old mixed-breed dog with a history of rectal adenocarcinoma. Note the lobular and nodular mesentery (white arrowheads) consistent with carcinomatosis.

characterizing the primary neoplasm, which should aid in prioritization.

### Free Peritoneal Gas

Radiography can be an excellent test for the detection of free peritoneal gas. The identification of gas lucencies that cannot be reliably localized to the lumen of an intestinal segment is highly suggestive of free peritoneal gas (Figures 22.11 and 22.12). Additionally, the ability to visualize the peritoneal surface of the diaphragm, or the impression that serosal margin detail is increased in some areas, can further support a conclusion of free peritoneal gas. Barring recent abdominal surgery or full-thickness body wall trauma, the primary differential diagnosis for free peritoneal gas is a rupture in the gastrointestinal tract. This can be a complication of a chronic foreign body or mural lesion.

Ultrasound is also sensitive for the detection of free peritoneal gas. Recognition of comet tail artifacts in the near field and not associated with intestinal segments is possible. In one study, ultrasound detected free peritoneal gas more consistently than radiographs, although not all cases of intestinal perforation had evidence of free peritoneal gas on radiographs or ultrasound [10].

### Bates Bodies/Nodular Fat Necrosis

Bates bodies, also termed *nodular fat necrosis* or *nodular intraabdominal fat necrosis*, are thought to represent an extension of the same pathophysiology underlying steatitis: the inflammation of fat. Nodular intraabdominal fat necrosis has been reported in sheep, horses, pigs, dogs, and cats [5]. Hypothetically, these regions of nodular fat necrosis result from some form of ischemia due to pressure, trauma, regional inflammation, or other circulatory deficit within the regional fat typically relating to inflammation [11]. In one study [5], more of these were identified in cats than in dogs. This may be due to a lower incidence

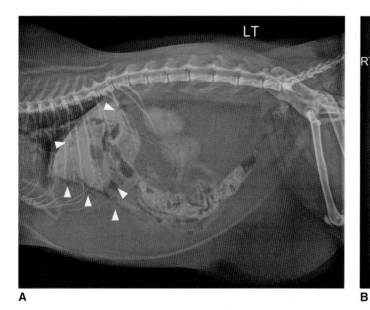
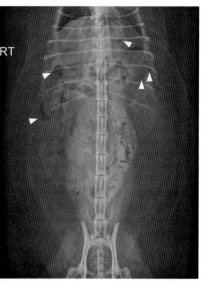

**A**  **B**

**FIGURE 22.11** Left lateral (**A**) and ventrodorsal (**B**) projections of the abdomen in a cat with free peritoneal gas. Note the regions of gas that track along organs like the liver, or are superimposed upon the liver (white arrowheads) and cannot be localized to intestinal segments.

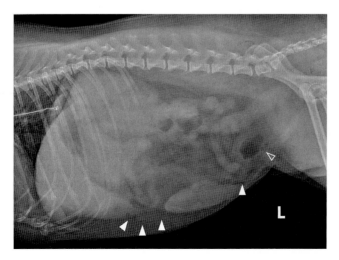

**FIGURE 22.12** Left lateral projection of the abdomen of a dog obtained postoperatively following cystotomy. Note the round, well-defined gas opacities in the peritoneal space superimposed on the caudoventral liver and the ventral intraabdominal fat, as well as along the caudal margin of the spleen (white arrowheads). The open arrowhead indicates gas in the urinary bladder and within or superimposed upon the urinary bladder wall.

in canine patients, or it may be that these are more frequently mineralized in feline patients, making them more easily identifiable radiographically. All lesions identified in feline patients were found in older, obese cats, and were considered to be incidental findings.

Radiographically, nodular fat necrosis is visible as a thin rim of mineral surrounding a fat to soft tissue opaque nodule or mass in the abdomen (Figure 22.13). Without the mineral component, these are difficult to identify radiographically (Figures 22.14 and 22.15). In instances in which the mineral has not yet formed, these may be visible on ultrasound or on CT (Figure 22.16).

**Masses**   Masses can also cause a reduction in serosal margin detail through compression of abdominal organs together, displacing the interspersed fat and eliminating contrast between soft tissue structures. Often, a mass is visible in these cases, and the focal loss of detail can be attributed to this. In some instances, this phenomenon can be caused by an extremely full urinary bladder or a distended stomach.

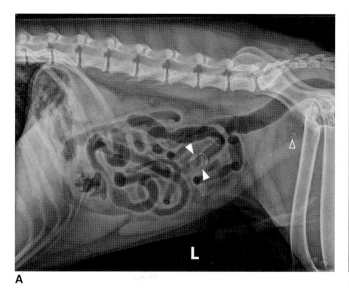
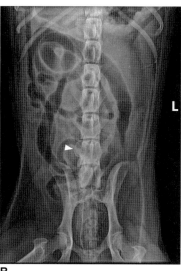

**FIGURE 22.13**   Left lateral (**A**) and ventrodorsal (**B**) projections of a dog with nodular fat necrosis. Note the focal thin, round rim of mineral in the caudal abdomen, just to the right of midline at the level of L6 (white arrowheads). On the lateral projection, mineral is seen ventral to the urinary bladder neck (open arrowhead), likely reflecting a suture granuloma from prior orchiectomy. Other small mineral foci are seen superimposed on intestinal segments, likely representing mineral ingesta.

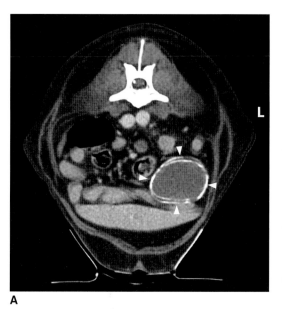
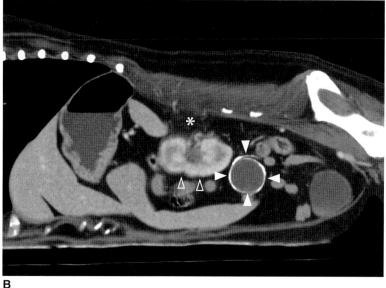

**FIGURE 22.14**   Transverse (**A**) and sagittal (**B**) images of a dog with nodular fat necrosis. Note the thin rim of mineral surrounding a central soft tissue-attenuating mass (white arrowheads). As the fat becomes inflamed, it does become hyperattenuating. Also note the irregular left kidney (open arrowheads) and the fluid located dorsal to the left kidney (*).

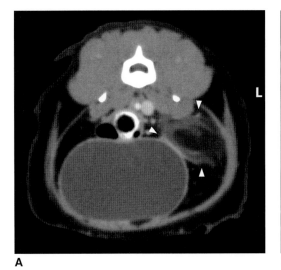

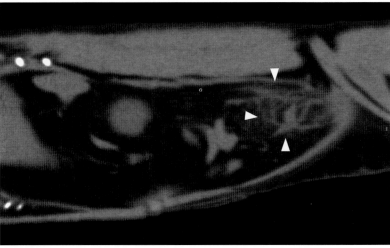

**A**      **B**

**FIGURE 22.15** Transverse (**A**) and sagittal reformatted (**B**) CT images of a dog with nodular fat necrosis. Note that there is no mineral currently surrounding the nodule (white arrowheads), and the increased attenuation is a heterogeneous mix of soft tissue and fat. The nodular structure is forming, but is ill defined.

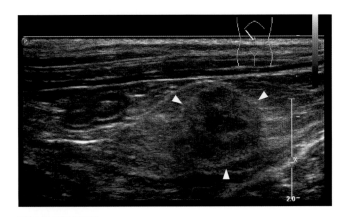

**FIGURE 22.16** Sonographic image of a forming region of nodular fat necrosis. The margins are well defined but not yet mineralized. The central region is heterogeneous (white arrowheads), with some areas containing fat with normal echogenicity centrally, and other regions showing hyperechoic fat suggestive of steatitis.

# Summary

The peritoneal space is a potential space. Serosal margin detail is primarily determined by the amount of fat deposited within the peritoneal folds that create the mesentery and omentum. Therefore, "normal" serosal margin detail can be quite variable depending on patient size and body condition.

Diseases that result in the deposition of soft tissue within the peritoneal space (effusion, nodules, etc.) reduce serosal margin detail on radiographs due to border effacement, which interferes with the ability to assess abdominal organs. The increase in the echogenicity of abdominal fat on ultrasound can also interfere with interrogation of abdominal organs.

Computed tomography can be a better option for evaluation of abdominal organs in cases where serosal margin detail is reduced.

Identification of free peritoneal gas in patients without recent abdominal surgery often constitutes an emergency. Be sure to spot the radiographic findings.

# References

1. Evans, H.E. and Miller, M.E. (2013). *Miller's Anatomy of the Dog*, 4e. St Louis, MO, Elsevier.
2. Bohn, A.A. (2017). Analysis of canine peritoneal fluid analysis. *Vet. Clin. North Am. Small Anim. Prac. Cytol.* 47: 123–133.
3. Allen, B.C., Barnhart, H., Bashir, M. et al. (2012). Diagnostic accuracy of intra-abdominal fluid collection characterization in the era of multidetector computed tomography. *Am. Surg.* 78: 185–189.
4. Komori, S., Nakagaki, K., Koyama, H. et al. (2002). Idiopathic mesenteric and omental steatitis in a dog. *J. Am. Vet. Med. Assoc.* 221: 1591–1593.
5. Schwarz, T., Morandi, F., Gnudi, G. et al. (2000). Nodular fat necrosis in the feline and canine abdomen. *Vet. Radiol. Ultrasound* 41: 335–339.
6. Root, C.R. and Lord, P.F. (1971). Peritoneal carcinomatosis in the dog and cat: its radiographic appearance1. *Vet. Radiol.* 12: 54–59.
7. Monteiro, C.B. and O'Brien, R.T. (2004). A retrospective study on the sonographic findings of abdominal carcinomatosis in 14 cats. *Vet. Radiol. Ultrasound* 45: 559–564.

8. Oetelaar, G.S., Lim, C.K., Heng, H.G. et al. (2020). Ultrasonographic features of colonic B-cell lymphoma with mesenteric lymphomatosis in a cat. *Vet. Radiol. Ultrasound* 61: E60–E63.

9. Paoloni, M.C., Penninck, D.G., and Moore, A.S. (2002). Ultrasonographic and clinicopathologic findings in 21 dogs with intestinal adenocarcinoma. *Vet. Radiol. Ultrasound* 43: 562–567.

10. Boysen, S.R., Tidwell, A.S., and Penninck, D.G. (2003). Ultrasonographic findings in dogs and cats with gastrointestinal perforation. *Vet. Radiol. Ultrasound* 44: 556–564.

11. Tharwat, M. and Buczinski, S. (2012). Diagnostic ultrasonography in cattle with abdominal fat necrosis. *Can. Vet. J.* 53: 41–46.

# CHAPTER 23

# Hepatobiliary Imaging

Matthew D. Winter

[1] Veterinary Consultants in Veterinary Medicine, Cambridge, UK
[2] Department of Small Animal Clinical Sciences, College of Veterinary Medicine, University of Florida, Gainesville, FL, USA

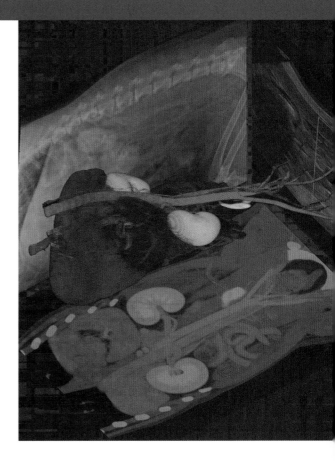

## Introduction

The liver can be a challenging organ to interpret on diagnostic imaging. The anatomy of the liver is complex, and many different pathologic mechanisms can create similar imaging features, which can complicate their interpretation, resulting in nonspecific findings.

## Normal Anatomy

The liver is an asymmetric organ that can be subdivided into left, central, and right divisions, each containing two lobes. The left division is subdivided into left lateral and left medial lobes. The central division is subdivided into quadrate and right medial lobes. The right division is divided into right lateral and caudate lobes. The caudate lobe is further subdivided into the caudate and papillary processes [1, 2]. Other references describe the liver as composed of four lobes, four sublobes, and two processes [3]. The right division is larger than the left; the hepatic lobes are separated by relatively deep fissures that are more pronounced in the left division. These fissures are difficult to visualize on imaging studies of normal dogs, and can complicate the location of hepatic lesions [4].

The primary blood supply to the liver is provided by the portal vein, which enters at the porta hepatis and provides 75–80% of normal hepatic blood flow [3]. The primary intrahepatic portal tributaries are the right, left, and central branches, which can also help to determine relative lobar anatomy. The hepatic artery also enters the liver at the porta hepatis and provides the remaining 20–25% of hepatic blood flow [3]. The liver is drained by the hepatic veins, which converge at the level of the diaphragm, slightly to the right of midline, to drain into the caudal vena cava. Special attention should be paid to the hepatic vasculature in cases of congenital or acquired portosystemic vascular anomalies.

The anatomy of the biliary system has been described [3]. Hepatocytes produce bile, which drains into bile canaliculi that ultimately form interlobular and lobar ducts, which are intrahepatic. The hepatic ducts represent the extrahepatic extension of the lobar ducts, and enter the excretory tree at the level of the cystic duct which is an extension of the gallbladder. The gallbladder is located ventrally between the quadrate lobe and the right medial lobe, with a fundus, body, and neck in the dog [3]. The neck is considered the beginning of the biliary duct system, extending from the gallbladder neck to the aforementioned junction of the hepatic ducts from the liver. The bile duct continues caudally to enter into the duodenum at the major duodenal papilla.

# Characterizing Hepatic Abnormalities

The characteristic features of hepatic disease are described using Roentgen signs, or modifications thereof, as mentioned in the introductory chapter. Once evaluation of the liver is performed, and conclusions are made, differentials should be listed and prioritized using your organizational scheme of choice (DAMN IT V or CITIMITV as mentioned in Chapter 1). While all Roentgen features are useful, an initial approach to evaluation of the liver often begins with assessment of size.

Deciding if the liver is enlarged or normal in size can be determined by comparison to adjacent structures, specifically the costal arch and the gastric axis (Figure 23.1). On radiographs, the caudoventral margin of the canine liver is generally described as ending at the level of the costal arch. However, this is dependent on the radiographs being expiratory and the breed of dog being evaluated. As a general principle, the observation of organ displacement is a window into the origin of masses in the abdomen. Specifically, then, the gastric axis can also be

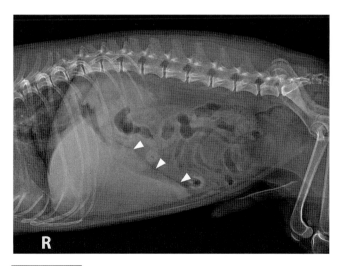

**FIGURE 23.1** Right lateral radiograph of a dog with generalized hepatomegaly. Note the extension of the hepatic margin beyond the costal arch, the rounded liver margins (white arrowheads) and the caudal displacement of the gastric axis relative to the thoracic spine.

used to evaluate hepatic size. The liver and stomach are loosely connected by a portion of the lesser omentum, the *hepatogastric ligament*. Therefore, caudal gastric displacement can serve as an indicator of hepatic enlargement. The *gastric axis* serves as an imaginary line that bisects the dorsal extent of the fundus and the ventral extent of the pylorus on a lateral projection. Generally, on a lateral abdominal radiograph, the gastric axis in the canine and feline patient is parallel to the ribs and perpendicular to the thoracic spine. On a ventrodorsal projection, the gastric axis can be represented as a line connecting the left lateral aspect of the gastric fundus to the right lateral aspect of the pylorus. These landmarks create a line that is typically located at the 10th to 12th intercostal space. The stomach itself is curvilinear, with the gastric body often curved caudally.

Relationship to the costal arch and alterations in the gastric axis can be effective tools to assess for changes in hepatic size. However, some breed and conformational variations exist. In deep-chested dogs, the caudal margin of the liver may be cranial to the costal arch and the gastric axis may be shifted cranially, resulting in an acute angle with the thoracic spine. In barrel-chested dogs, the normal liver may extend beyond the costal arch and the gastric axis may be slightly more caudal. In addition, differences in recumbency have been shown to create variation in these measurements, with right lateral recumbency resulting in larger relative measurements than left lateral recumbency in normal dogs and in dogs with hepatomegaly [5].

Similar anatomic guidelines can be used when assessing hepatic size on computed tomography (CT) examinations. Extension beyond the costal arch and gastric displacement can be good indicators of changes in hepatic size. Sonographically, changes in hepatic size relative to adjacent anatomy can be more subjective. Extension beyond the costal arch can be assessed during the examination, and displacement of the stomach can be evaluated with experience.

Fortunately, enlargement often also creates a shape change. Rounded hepatic margins may be the only feature of hepatic enlargement in some patients, and should be used as a strong indicator of hepatomegaly. Rounded hepatic margins can be identified on radiographs, CT, and ultrasound (US).

While many disease processes can overlap with regard to their imaging features, determining if hepatic enlargement is generalized, focal or multifocal can be a useful tool in narrowing the list of potential differentials. Making this distinction also involves assessment of hepatic margins. A focal rounded margin often suggests the presence of a mass, whereas a multifocal lobular or irregular margin may suggest many nodules, or multiple masses.

Some diseases result in a small liver (*microhepatia*) (Figure 23.2). As with enlargement, determination of hepatic size can generally be assessed by comparison to adjacent anatomy, specifically the costal arch and the gastric axis, with attention to breed variations. As with enlargement, evaluation of the shape and margins can help with generating differentials. Characterizing the margins as well defined and sharp versus lobular and irregular is valuable in differentiation of some congenital diseases from acquired diseases such as cirrhosis and nodular regeneration.

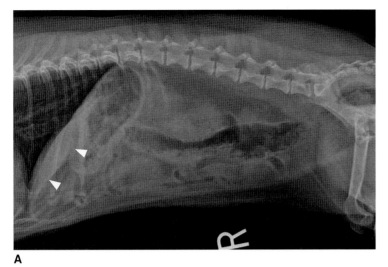
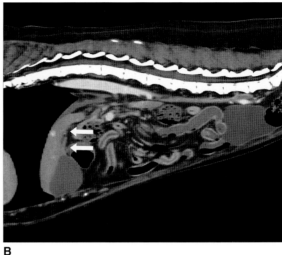

**A**  **B**

**FIGURE 23.2**  Right lateral radiograph (**A**) and sagittal reformatted image (**B**) of the abdomen of a dog with a congenital, extrahepatic portosystemic shunt. Note the caudal margins of the liver (white arrowheads) consistent with microhepatia.

The radiographic opacity of the liver is generally soft tissue. The liver is soft tissue attenuating on CT, and shows coarse but uniform echotexture on US. However, some diseases may change the opacity of the liver. Increases in opacity generally arise from the biliary tree rather than the hepatic parenchyma itself. Hepatolithiasis, or the presence of intrahepatic bile duct stones, can result in the identification of intrahepatic mineral. Because these stones are located in the arborized intrahepatic bile ducts, this mineral often can appear as curvilinear regions of mineral arranged in a branching pattern, depending on severity. Alternatively, these may be multifocal regions of mineral with no discernible pattern to their distribution.

Similarly, gas may contribute to decreased opacity of the liver. While not common, cases of gas identified within the portal vasculature have been reported, often in response to gastric pneumatosis, or in cases of gastric dilation and volvulus (Figure 23.3). This will also result in the impression of arborized, branching regions of gas within the hepatic parenchyma.

Focal accumulations of gas could also be present in the case of hepatic abscess, without arborization, but this has not been reported [6].

Ultrasound is an accessible tool for cross-sectional evaluation of the liver. While the conformation of some patients can preclude evaluation of the entire liver, ultrasound does provide information regarding the parenchyma, which can be characterized as normal, hypoechoic (darker than normal), hyperechoic (brighter than normal), and heterogeneous (nonuniform). These can be further combined to describe more complex changes to the hepatic parenchyma, with terms like heterogeneously hyperechoic used to reflect a nonuniform, coarse increase in hepatic echogenicity. In addition, ultrasound can be used to evaluate hepatic vasculature and the biliary tree.

Computed tomography affords nearly unparalleled ability to evaluate the entire liver, including vascular structures. Attenuation and contrast enhancement of the liver can be

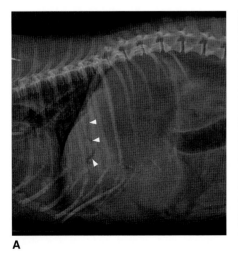
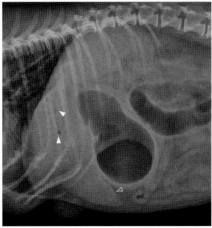
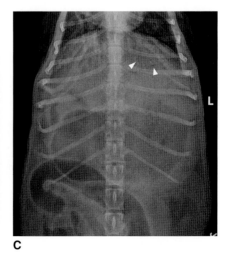

**A**  **B**  **C**

**FIGURE 23.3**  Right lateral (**A**), left lateral (**B**), and ventrodorsal (**C**) radiographs of a dog with intrahepatic gas localized to the portal venous system. Also note the cranioventral, fat opaque subcutaneous nodule, which is an incidental lipoma.

measured in Hounsfield units. Alterations in attenuation and enhancement patterns have been correlated with specific disease processes in some cases, though some features remain nonspecific. The evaluation of hepatic attenuation and contrast enhancement during dual- and triple-phase acquisitions can be useful in characterizing hepatic lesions and masses.

## Generalized Hepatomegaly

As mentioned above, while there are multiple tests for determination of hepatic size, in practice this determination is largely subjective. Generalized hepatomegaly is characterized on radiography, US, and CT often by a subjective assessment of the margin of the liver (rounded vs sharp); relationship with the costal arch, with careful consideration of breed and conformation; location of the gastric axis; and potential displacement of other abdominal organs (Figure 23.1).

Many diseases causing hepatopathy can result in generalized hepatomegaly, making this a relatively nonspecific finding that must be interpreted in the context of other data, including patient signalment, physical examination findings, clinicopathologic abnormalities, and additional diagnostic testing results. Table 23.1 lists some causes of generalized hepatomegaly categorized using the DAMN IT V system. It is evident that the observation/conclusion of generalized hepatomegaly without additional information is not particularly helpful in narrowing the list of differentials.

### Ultrasound Characteristics of Generalized Hepatomegaly
Sonographically, generalized hepatomegaly is similarly subjective and nonspecific. As a generalization,

inflammatory and infectious processes and toxicity may result in a generalized reduction in echogenicity. For example, leptospirosis and babesiosis often result in a generalized hepatic hypoechogenicity along with mild, generalized hepatomegaly. Toxins may cause acute hepatic necrosis, which may cause no sonographic abnormalities in the acute phase but have been reported to produce a mild reduction in hepatic echogenicity in the subacute phase.

Conversely, metabolic diseases such as diabetes mellitus and hyperadrenocorticism or exogenous corticosteroid administration result in glycogen storage and hepatic steatosis, which manifests as diffusely increased hepatic echogenicity.

Heterogeneous echogenicity can also be observed, and is often associated with nodular hyperplasia, extramedullary hematopoiesis, or metastatic neoplasia.

### CT Characteristics of Generalized Hepatomegaly
Attenuation refers to the relative reduction in x-rays as they pass through the patient. Attenuation is analogous to opacity on radiographs but CT has significantly greater contrast resolution, allowing for greater discrimination of tissue types. For example, fluid and soft tissue can be differentiated on CT, yet have the same opacity on radiographs. A full discussion of the physics of attenuation and calculation of attenuation coefficients is beyond the scope of this text, and the reader is directed to textbooks of medical physics.

Attenuation values in some organs can provide useful information when evaluating hepatic pathology. While generalized increases in hepatic attenuation have not been reported, a generalized reduction in hepatic attenuation has been reported in a case of a dog with hyperadrenocorticism [7]. In this case,

---

**TABLE 23.1** Summary of differentials for generalized hepatomegaly in the dog and cat.

| Category | Etiology |
|---|---|
| Degenerative/developmental | Nodular hyperplasia |
| | Storage disease (i.e., glycogen) |
| | Polycystic liver disease |
| Anomalous/autoimmune | |
| Metabolic | Vacuolar hepatopathy (diabetes mellitus, hyperadrenocorticism) |
| | Extramedullary hematopoiesis |
| Neoplastic/nutritional | Lymphoma |
| | Mast cell tumor Malignant histiocytosis |
| | Leukemia |
| | Diffuse metastasis |
| Inflammatory/infectious/iatrogenic/idiopathic | Acute hepatitis (i.e., leptospirosis, babesiosis) |
| | Fibrosis/early cirrhosis |
| Trauma/toxic | |
| Vascular | Congestion (right-sided congestive heart failure, Budd–Chiari syndrome) |

hepatic attenuation values were negative, and correlated with histopathologic analysis consistent with hepatic lipidosis [8]. Reductions in hepatic attenuation in cats have also been reported in cases of fasting-induced hepatic lipidosis, but negative attenuation values were not observed [8]. In addition, further evaluation of cats with naturally occuring hepatic lipidosis did not suggest great utility in the use of attenuation values as an aid to diagnosis.

Generalized hepatomegaly can also result from dissemination of hepatic nodules from either metastatic neoplasia or nodular hyperplasia. The discrimination of benign and malignant etiologies is challenging, and is discussed below.

## Focal Hepatomegaly

Recall that enlargement of an organ typically causes displacement of surrounding organs. This places further emphasis on the importance of normal radiographic anatomy and normal anatomic variants. Generalized enlargement tends to cause relatively uniform displacement of the gastric axis, while focal enlargements may result in focal displacement of the pylorus, fundus or possibly the gastric body (Figure 23.4a,b). In addition, focal enlargements involving the caudate lobe may result in caudal displacement of the right kidney. Therefore, it is critical to evaluate the location of all organs and identify any displacement. With regard to the liver specifically, reviewing imaging tests for focal displacement of the gastric fundus, body or pylorus can be helpful in identifying focal hepatic enlargement.

Focal masses can result from a multitude of etiologies. Table 23.2 summarizes some causes of focal hepatic enlargement. In general, primary hepatic neoplasms can be hepatocellular, biliary, neuroendocrine, or mesenchymal in origin [9]. The most common primary hepatic neoplasms in dogs are hepatocellular, whereas the most common primary hepatic neoplasms in cats are bile duct tumors [9]. Again, these would be prioritized based on additional information regarding patient signalment, physical examination findings, clinicopathologic abnormalities, and the results of other diagnostic testing.

### Ultrasound Characteristics of Nodules and Focal Hepatomegaly
The sonographic appearance of masses is variable, and discriminating between benign and malignant etiologies is challenging. In an investigation comparing the ability of US and CT to predict malignancy, the only significant sonographic feature that predicted malignancy was the presence of cavitation [10]. The presence of cavitation was proposed to reflect regions of necrosis often found in malignant neoplasm. However, CT was considered more accurate than US for predication of the nature of hepatic masses. Hypoattenuation with a threshold of 37 HU also helped predict malignancy, and was certainly influenced by the presence of cavitation. This further supports the concept that relative heterogeneity in both US and CT is suggestive of malignancy. In addition, larger masses were more often malignant, with an average diameter of approximately 8 cm compared to 4 cm in benign masses (Figure 23.5a-e).

Hepatic abscesses have features of focal hepatomegaly on both ultrasound and radiographs. Sonographically, hepatic abscesses are variable, and can appear hyperechoic, hypoechoic, or heterogeneous [6].

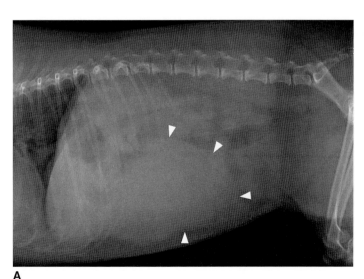
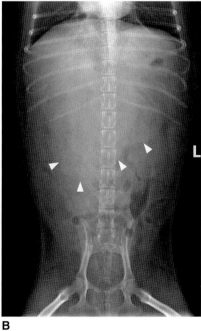

**FIGURE 23.4** Right lateral (**A**) and ventrodorsal (**B**) radiographs of a dog with focal hepatic enlargement. Note the right-sided distribution of the mass on the ventrodorsal projection, and the lobular margins (white arrowheads).

**TABLE 23.2** Summary of differentials for focal hepatomegaly.

| Category | Etiology | Comments/Notes |
|---|---|---|
| Degenerative/developmental | Nodular hyperplasia | Less likely to have capsular structure |
| | Cyst | Fluid attenuation on CT |
| Anomalous/autoimmune[a] | N/A | |
| Metabolic | N/A | |
| Neoplastic/nutritional | Adenoma | Diffuse enhancement similar to NH |
| | Hepatocellular carcinoma (dogs) | |
| | Hemangiosarcoma | |
| | Biliary carcinoma | |
| | Biliary adenoma | |
| Inflammatory/infectious/iatrogenic/idiopathic | Abscess | |
| Trauma/toxic | Liver lobe torsion | Dysplastic arteries shunt directly into portal veins |
| | Hematoma | |
| | Arterioportal fistula | |
| Vascular | High flow (Congenital) vascular malformations[a] | Early in the process, the arterialization of the portal vein may form a focal mass. Over time, this high-flow lesion results in congestion and ascites |

[a] Congenital anomalies of the portal venous system are described in the Vascular section.
CT, computed tomography; N/A, not applicable; NH, nodular hyperplasia.

Target lesions (Figure 23.6) can be helpful in the discrimination of benign versus malignant nodules. Target lesions appear as centrally hyper- to isoechoic, and are surrounded by a hypoechoic rim that is presumed to be a rim of compressed hepatocytes around the margins of a tumor [11]. These lesions were most commonly associated with primary or metastatic neoplasia. However, some of these lesions were associated with benign processes, further emphasizing the need for sampling in these situations.

## CT Characteristics of Nodules and Focal Hepatomegaly
Much has been published regarding the utility of CT in characterizing liver masses. Administration of iodinated, intravenous contrast with studies acquired during the arterial, portal, and venous phases of contrast enhancement can yield information regarding the vascular features of hepatic masses. Research in humans suggests that vascular features can help to characterize hepatic masses as benign or malignant, and even result in an accurate prediction of cellular diagnosis for some tumor types [12]. In general, neoplastic processes create leaky, poorly formed arterial supplies that should result in hyperenhancement during the arterial phase, isoenhancement during the portal phase, and hypoenhancement during the delayed venous phase. This premise has popularized research into the utility of dual- and triple-phase CT studies in veterinary patients (Figure 23.7).

The behavior of hepatic neoplasia on triple-phase contrast-enhanced CT has been studied [10, 13–16], and is variable, depending on tumor type. Commonalities in each study design include an evaluation of numerous CT characteristics, such as precontrast attenuation, enhancement intensity, size, and heterogeneity, to name a few. In addition, each study included both benign and malignant hepatic masses, with the malignant group consisting of multiple different cell types. Results of these investigations suggest that low attenuation values (<37 HU), heterogeneity, and mass size greater than 4.5 cm correlated positively with malignancy [10, 15] (Figure 23.8a–c). Further characterization of cell type is challenging based on this data due to the amalgamation of tumor types within each study population.

Characterizing fluid accumulations and cavitation in the liver can be helpful in narrowing the differential list, and would result in a reduction in overall attenuation. Fluid accumulations can indicate the presence of cysts and cyst-like regions or necrosis. Theoretical attenuation value thresholds have been reported to add information in the characterization of pathology, specifically in the differentiation of benign or malignant masses, although in practice, this is still challenging [10].

## Localizing Hepatic Masses
The accuracy of correctly locating hepatic masses has also been studied. Accurate location of hepatic masses is important in determining resectability [4]. In a study of 57 hepatic masses [1], the authors concluded that all imaging features of a hepatic mass should be used to accurately characterize the location of the mass, including its relationship to midline, to the portal vein, and to the gallbladder. In general, all masses located to the left of the midline were left divisional. Masses in the right division were located medial, dorsal, or lateral to the portal vein. Leftward displacement of the stomach resulted from a right divisional

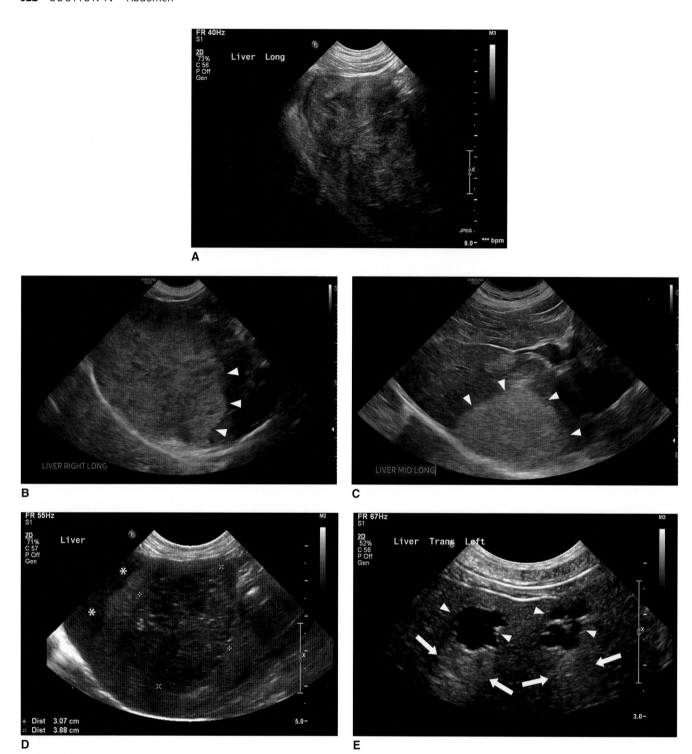

**FIGURE 23.5** Sonographic images of hepatic masses with variable echogenicities. (**A**) Focal, heterogeneous mass in the right liver of a dog (hepatocellular carcinoma). (**B**) Lobular and irregular, uniformly echogenic hepatic mass (hepatocellular carcinoma). (**C**) Uniformly hyperechoic mass with well-defined margins (nodular hyperplasia). (**D**) Heterogeneously hypoechoic, cavitated mass (calipers) in a cat with cholangiocarcinoma. Also note the effusion (asterisks). (**E**) Hepatic cysts in a cat (white arrowheads) with distal acoustic enhancement/through transmission artifact (white arrows).

mass. The identification of specific hepatic vein or portal branches was useful in accurately determining the division in which the mass originated.

In studies that compare the accuracy of CT and US in the accurate localization of masses, both imaging modalities have proven useful. In one study that reviewed the sensitivity, specificity, and positive predictive value of CT and US in the location of hepatic masses, CT was more sensitive than US for left divisional, central divisional, and right divisional masses. Specificity of CT was greater than that of US in all but central divisional masses, and therefore the positive predictive value of CT was also greater than US for correctly identifying right and left

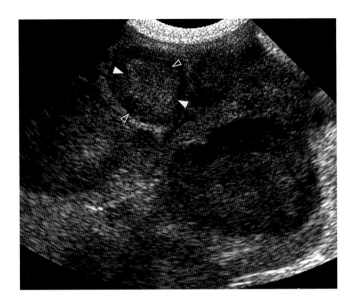

**FIGURE 23.6**   Target lesions in a dog. Note the central hyperechoic region (white arrowheads), surrounded by a peripheral hypoechoic rim (open arrowheads).

divisional masses, but not for central divisional masses [4]. In another study, US correctly identified the location of an hepatic mass in approximately half (51.8%) of all cases, with a sensitivity of 55% for the correct localization of left and right divisional masses [17]. For central divisional masses, sensitivity dropped to 29%. Specificity was relatively high for left divisional (98%), central divisional (87%), and right divisional (89%) masses. Correct localization was confounded by the presence of multifocal or diffuse hepatic disease.

## Microhepatia

Hepatic size can vary with breed and body conformation in normal canine patients, and is relatively consistent in feline patients. The diseases discussed thus far cause varying degrees of focal and generalized hepatic enlargement, but some diseases result in a small liver. Congenital anomalies, often involving vascular supply, are perhaps the most common causes of microhepatia in dogs and often (but not always) manifest in younger patients (Figure 23.2a,b). Chronic acquired diseases that result in progressive hepatic damage and fibrosis often terminate in cirrhosis. The imaging features of these two broad categories of microhepatia can be quite different.

**Vascular Malformations**   Congenital vascular malformations in the liver that may result in microhepatia include portosystemic shunts, hepatic microvascular dysplasia (HMD)/ primary portal hypoplasia, and portal vein atresia. Each of these abnormalities results in reduced portal blood flow through the liver, and reduced delivery of growth factors. Congenital macro portosystemic shunts may be characterized as intrahepatic or extrahepatic [18]. HMD, also known as portal atresia, may result in microshunting. These abnormalities are more common in dogs, but have also been reported in cats [19, 20].

**Extrahepatic Shunts**   The morphology of congenital extrahepatic portosystemic shunts has been extensively described using CT angiography and US examinations [18, 19, 21–28]. While US can be a very useful tool in the evaluation of portosystemic shunts, it is more operator dependent than CT, and CT images are often more useful for surgical planning. The classification scheme continues to evolve but there is a general lack of consensus regarding naming conventions.

   The continued study of anomalous vascular communications in portosystemic shunts and correlation with embryologic vascular development has provided insights to the classification scheme. Naming conventions help describe the relationship of normal and anomalous vasculature, but the utility and practicality of naming conventions can be questioned as it pertains to surgical intervention. A simplified approach suggests that the left gastric vein is nearly always involved in the morphology of an extrahepatic shunt at its origin, with variable

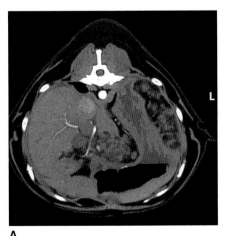

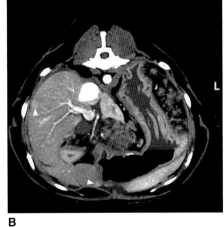

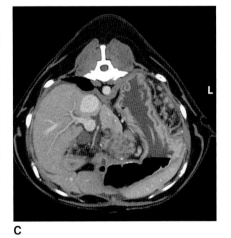

A                                    B                                    C

**FIGURE 23.7**   Identical slices of the liver in a dog obtained during arterial (**A**), portal (**B**), and venous (**C**) phases of contrast enhancement. Note the hyperattenuating nodules that are seen only on the portal phase (white arrowheads).

involvement of the right gastric vein, and with ultimate termi-nations in the prehepatic caudal vena cava at the level of either the epiploic foramen, the posthepatic cranial vena cava (occa-sionally via the phrenic vein), or the azygous vein (Figure 23.9). Table 23.3 summarizes some of the current naming conventions for extrahepatic portosystemic shunts.

**Intrahepatic Shunts** Traditionally, intrahepatic shunts have been broadly classified as left divisional, central

divisional, or right divisional but as with extrahepatic shunts, consensus is lacking. Left divisional intrahepatic shunts con-nect the left portal vein to the left hepatic vein and are often consistent with patent ductus venosus. Central divisional intrahepatic shunts often present with a window communica-tion directly between the portal vein and caudal vena cava. Right divisional intrahepatic shunts often have a long loop within the right lateral or caudate lobes and connect with the caudal vena cava [18].

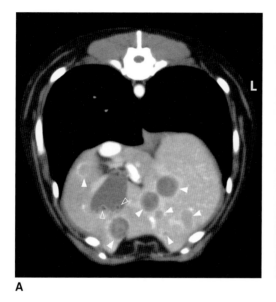
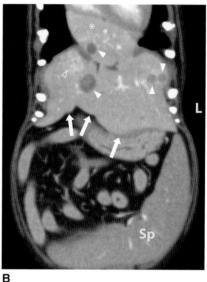

**A**  **B**

**FIGURE 23.8** (**A, B**) Hypoattenuating nodules in a dog with metastatic apocrine gland anal sac adenocarcinoma. Note the well-defined, heterogeneously enhancing nodules, with peripheral enhancement (white arrowheads). Also note the hypoattenuating gallbladder contents (open arrowheads) surrounded by mild hyperattenuating sludge. The white arrows indicate the rounded margins, an indicator of hepatic enlargement. Also note the bonus lesion (*), congenital peritoneal pericardial diaphragmatic hernia with herniation of the right medial liver lobe.

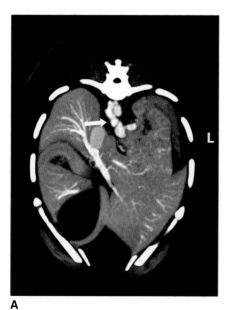
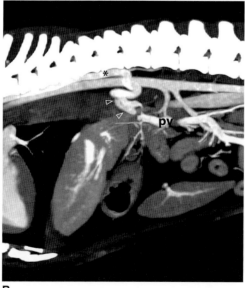
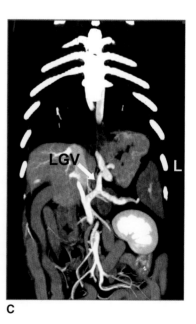

**A**  **B**  **C**

**FIGURE 23.9** Transverse (**A**), sagittal (**B**), and dorsal plane (**C**) images of a dog with an extrahepatic, congenital portosystemic shunt. This particular shunt is a left gastric-azygous. The anomalous vessel (white arrow) originates from the left gastric, and continues dorsally to the azygous vein (*), located to the right of the descending aorta. Note the tortuosity in the transverse and sagittal images (open arrowhead). PV, portal vein.

**TABLE 23.3** Summary of classification schemes for extrahepatic portosystemic shunts.

| Shunt origin | Shunt termination | White et al.[a] name/terminology | Nelson and Nelson[b] name/terminology |
|---|---|---|---|
| Left gastric vein | Posthepatic termination | Left gastrophrenic | Splenophrenic |
| | Left phrenic vein | Left gastrocaval | Splenophrenic |
| | Azygous vein | Left gastroazygous | Splenoazygous |
| | Posthepatic caudal vena cava (CVC) | | |
| | No normal gastrosplenic vein | RGV(i) | |
| | The splenic vein communicates normally with the portal vein | | Right gastric-caval |
| | The right gastric vein communicates with an anomalous left gastric vein | | |
| | The anomalous left gastric vein inserts into the prehepatic CVC | | |
| | Anomalous left gastric vein to CVC | RGV(ii) | Right gastric-caval with a caudal loop |
| | No normal gastrosplenic vein | | |
| | Anomalous communication between left gastric v. and splenic v. | RGV(iii) | Right gastric-caval |
| | No normal communication between the left gastric or the splenic v. with the CVC | | |
| Gastroduodenal v. | Terminates in azygous vein | | Right gastric-azygous with a caudal loop |

[a] Adapted from White et al. [27].
[b] Adapted from Nelson and Nelson [22].

Recently, a more detailed description of the anatomy of intrahepatic portosystemic shunts has been reported [29]. In this study, 44% of included intrahepatic shunts were right divisional, with the majority of these connecting the right portal vein branch with the right lateral hepatic vein (Figure 23.10). The remainder of the right divisional shunts in this study involved a connection between the right portal branch and the caudate hepatic artery. In the same study, 30% of dogs had a left divisional shunt. Approximately two-thirds of these had communication with the left hepatic vein, with the remaining left divisional shunts entering the left phrenic vein. Single central divisional shunts were less common, reported in 13% of dogs in this study. In half of these, communication between the left portal branch directly to the caudal vena cava was observed, suggesting that these were independent of the hepatic venous system. The remainder had variable communication with the quadrate hepatic vein, the central hepatic vein or the right medial hepatic vein.

An alternative classification scheme has also been proposed with four categories of intrahepatic shunts: patent/persistent ductus venosus; aneurysmal intrahepatic portosystemic shunt; one or more intrahepatic portosystemic shunts in one lobe; and multiple portosystemic shunts in multiple liver lobes. In this scheme, patent/persistent ductus

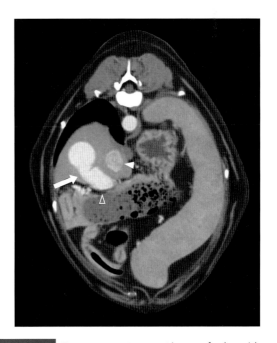

**FIGURE 23.10** Transverse postcontrast image of a dog with an intrahepatic shunt. The white arrow indicates the anomalous communication between the portal vein (open arrowhead) and the right hepatic vein. Note the mild enhancement of the caudal vena cava (white arrowhead).

| TABLE 23.4 | Summary of classification schemes for intrahepatic portosystemic shunts. | |
|---|---|---|
| **Category/location** | **Plested et al.[a]** | **Bertolini[b]** |
| Right divisional | Right lateral hepatic vein<br>Caudate hepatic vein | Persistent ductus venosus (right) |
| Left divisional | Left hepatic vein<br>Left phrenic vein | Persistent ductus venosus (left) |
| Central divisional | Quadrate hepatic vein<br>Central hepatic vein<br>Dorsal right medial hepatic vein<br>Ventral aspect of caudal vena cava | Persistent ductus venosus (central) |
| Multiple | Variable | One or more PSS in 1 liver lobe<br>Multiple PSS in several liver lobes |

[a] Plested et al. [29].
[b] Bertolini [30].
PSS, portosystemic shunt.

venosus can be categorized as left, central, or right divisional, but further discussion on characterization of definitive insertion was not included [1]. Table 23.4 summarizes the naming conventions used in characterizing extrahepatic shunts.

**Multiple Acquired Shunts** Multiple acquired shunts may result from any disease that causes an increase in portal venous resistance, including chronic fibrosis/cirrhosis, portal vein thrombus, arterioportal fistula, and portal hypoplasia, also called idiopathic portal hypertension (Figure 23.11a–d). Multiple acquired shunts are most often characterized by tortuous nests of vessels adjacent to the spleen, kidneys, urinary bladder, colon, or within the thoracic cavity (Figure 23.12a–c) [31].

Regardless of etiology, shunts can frequently result in reduced portal blood flow through the liver, which can be measured indirectly using imaging tools. Pulsed wave Doppler can be used to evaluate portal blood flow velocity (PBV) and direction [32]. Normal PBV has been described, and reductions in PBV have been correlated with shunting. Indeed, reversal of flow (hepatofugal flow) has been documented in some cases. In addition, portal vein diameter at the porta hepatis is frequently reduced compared to normal [33]. Relative portal vein diameter as a ratio to aortic diameter at the level of the porta hepatis has been reported to be sensitive and specific for both US and CT.

In some patients, a periportal hypoattenuating circumferential halo can be observed. This is described in people and is possibly associated with edema secondary to lymphatic obstruction and dilation resulting from a long list of potential etiologies for hepatobiliary disease, including viral hepatitis, blunt hepatic trauma, liver transplant (and rejection), tumors or malignant lymphadenopathy with compression of the lymphatics, congestive heart failure, kidney disease and aggressive fluid resuscitation [34]. In veterinary medicine, there has been a weak correlation with malignant hepatic lymphadenopathy and lymphatic obstruction, but this is not well established, and has been seen in dogs without hepatobiliary disease [34]. It is important to distinguish between a circumferential halo versus a focal hypoattenuating tube adjacent to the vasulature, which may indicate biliary dilation.

**Chronic Fibrosis/Cirrhosis** Hepatic fibrosis is commonly caused by chronic inflammation, and results from an imbalance in the synthesis and breakdown of extracellular matrix materials [35]. One of the most common causes of hepatic fibrosis is chronic hepatitis [36]. The underlying cause of chronic hepatitis is often unknown, though in a retrospective review up to 36% of cases were associated with underlying copper storage disease [37]. In the remaining patients, the pathogenesis is poorly understood. In many cases, there are few to no imaging abnormalities in cases of chronic hepatitis.

Cirrhosis is considered to be the endstage of fibrosis, resulting in the conversion of normal hepatic architecture into micro- or macronodules. At imaging, this can manifest as a small liver with irregular margins, although the liver may also appear completely normal. The abnormal hepatic parenchymal architecture also often results in increased portal pressure (portal hypertension) which subsequently creates various degrees of peritoneal effusion depending on severity.

On ultrasound, endstage cirrhosis may appear irregular and lobular, with heterogeneous to increased echogenicity and echotexture. Peritoneal effusion may be present, and the regional fat may be hyperechoic (Figure 23.13a,b). On Doppler interrogation, PBV may be reduced, and reversal of portal blood flow may be noted if acquired shunts are present.

# Biliary Abnormalities

Biliary pathology has been extensively described in the veterinary literature, although the majority of the knowledge base involves ultrasound [38]. The gallbladder wall cannot be assessed radiographically, although in some cases an enlarged gallbladder can be seen on lateral radiographs, ventral to the liver, especially in cats.

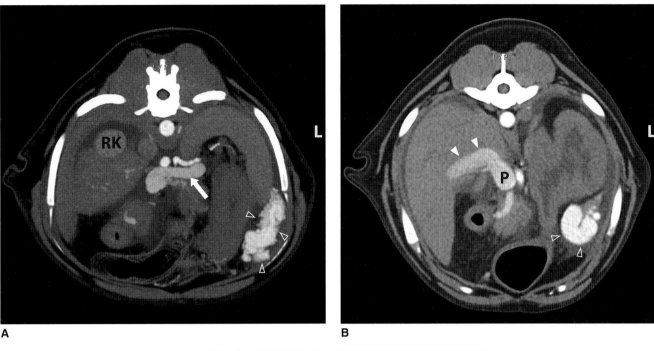

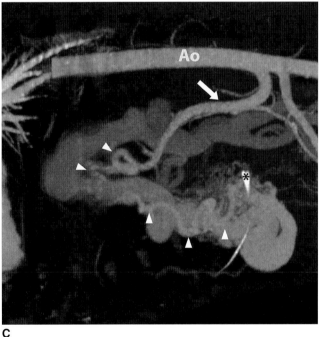

**FIGURE 23.11**   Transverse images (**A**, **B**) and volume-rendered image (**C**) of an arterial-phase acquisition in a dog with an arterioportal fistula. In (**A**) notice the enhancement of the portal vein and the splenic vein (white arrow) with subjective enlargement of the splenic vein. This is unusual during the arterial phase. In (**B**) note the congestion of the right portal branch (white arrowheads). The portal vein (P) is larger than the aorta. In (**C**) note the celiac artery (white arrow) and the tortuous splenic artery (white arrowheads) that courses cranioventral, then caudal within the spleen, to connect directly with the portal system.

Sonographic evaluation of the gallbladder wall allows for assessment of wall thickness as well as any irregularity of the mucosa. In cats, gallbladder wall thickness greater than 1 mm correlated with histopathologic abnormalities of the gallbladder wall [39]. Abnormal gallbladder contents can be recognized radiographically as mineral opaque structures that are often gravity dependent. US and CT can also be useful in identifying abnormal contents, especially those that are nonmineralized, which cannot be resolved on radiographs (Figure 23.14a,b).

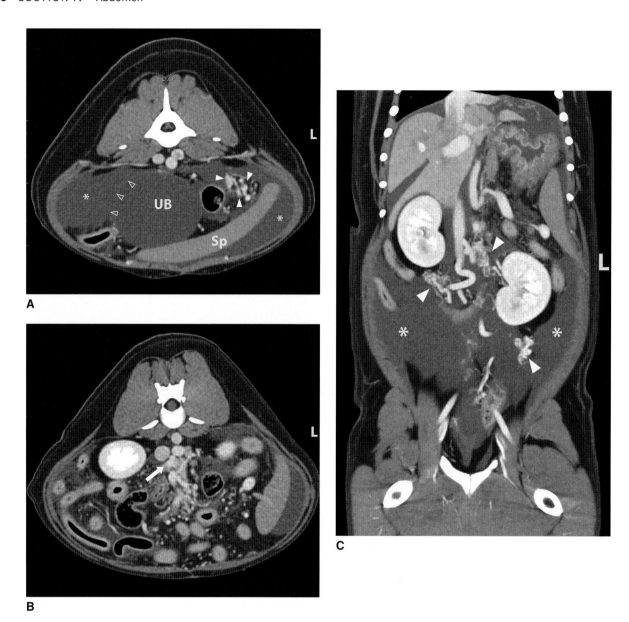

**FIGURE 23.12** Transverse (**A**, **B**) and dorsal plane (**C**) images of a dog with portal hypertension that has developed severe peritoneal effusion and multiple acquired shunts. (**A**) Note the plexus of vessels adjacent to the spleen (white arrows), the large volume of peritoneal fluid (*) and the margin of the urinary bladder adjacent to the peritoneal fluid (open arrowheads). (**B**) Note the plexus of vessels ventral to the aorta, caudal vena cava and renal veins, adjacent to the portal tributaries. (**C**) Note the plexus of vessels located caudal to each kidney and between the kidneys (white arrowheads) and the large volume of peritoneal fluid (*).

## Gallbladder sludge

It has been suggested that the presence of gallbladder sludge in some dogs is incidental [40]. More recently, dogs with >25% sludge as a function of total gallbladder volume were found to be more likely to have hyperadrenocorticism or hypothyroidism. Dogs with gallbladder sludge were older, and had greater gallbladder volume, suggesting that gallbladder sludge could reflect alterations in gallbladder function or contractility [41]. In cats, the presence of gallbladder sludge may be predictive of increased liver enzymes. In one study, gallbladder sludge was identified in 14% of the study population. When compared to a control group, the cats with gallbladder sludge had

a statistically significant increase in alanine aminotransferase, alkaline phosphatase, and total bilirubin [42].

## Gallbladder mucoceles

Gall bladder mucoceles are poorly understood and the pathogenesis is unknown. The disease is characterized by increased secretion of mucin by the gallbladder epithelium which can result in abnormally thick mucus that can culminate in obstruction of the bile duct and possibly rupture of the gallbladder [43]. The sonographic appearance of gallbladder mucoceles has classically been described as a stellate pattern of nonmotile

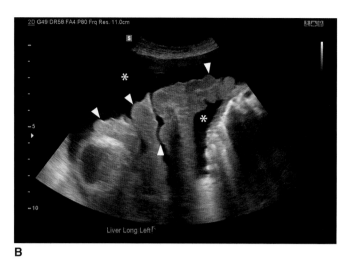

**FIGURE 23.13**   Sonographic images of a dog obtained during the subacute (**A**) and chronic (**B**) phases of hepatic fibrosis, with progression to cirrhosis. In (**A**) note the hypoechogenicity of the liver parenchyma and the lobular hepatic margins (white arrowheads). In the follow-up image obtained 2 months later, note how much smaller and more irregular the liver has become, with an overall increase in echogenicity (white arrowheads). Also note the development of anechoic peritoneal effusion.

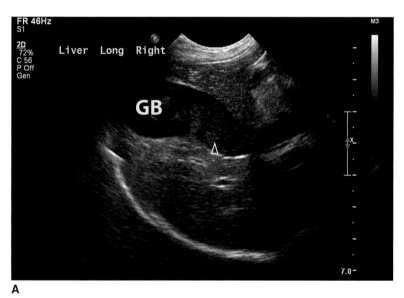
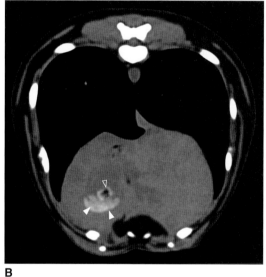

**FIGURE 23.14**   Sagittal sonographic image (**A**) and transverse CT image (**B**) of two different dogs with abnormal gallbladder contents. In (**A**) note the accumulation of gravity-dependent, nonshadowing material in the gallbladder (open arrowhead). This material was mobile on real-time imaging, and it can be important to note the gravity dependency. (**B**) Note the mineral-attenuating, gravity-dependent material in the ventral aspect of the gallbladder (white arrowheads), with a focal, fat-attenuating component (open arrowhead).

sludge, although some variations have been documented [44, 45] (Figure 23.15a–c). Gallbladder rupture is a common sequela to this disease, and can be recognized by features of wall discontinuity, regional effusion, and hyperechoic fat [44].

Evaluation of gallbladder pathology with CT has been more recently described, and the utility of precontrast CT in the diagnosis of gallbladder mucocele has been reported (Figure 23.16) [46]. The presence of centrally hyperattenuating bile with HU greater than 48.6 was suggestive of a gallbladder mucocele. More importantly, all dogs with centrally located gallbladder mineral had a gallbladder mucocele.

## Biliary Obstruction

Enlargement of the gallbladder may result from dysfunction, as mentioned above, but also from obstruction. Biliary obstruction is not visible radiographically, but on CT and US marked dilation of the bile duct (intra- and extrahepatic) can be identified (Figure 23.17). Sonographic features of biliary obstruction in cats and dogs have been reported. In cats, common bile duct diameter of greater than 5 mm was correlated with biliary obstruction [47].

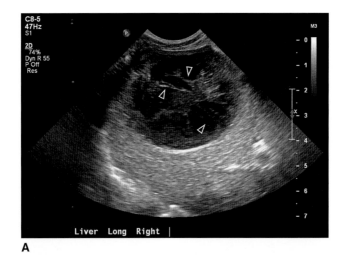

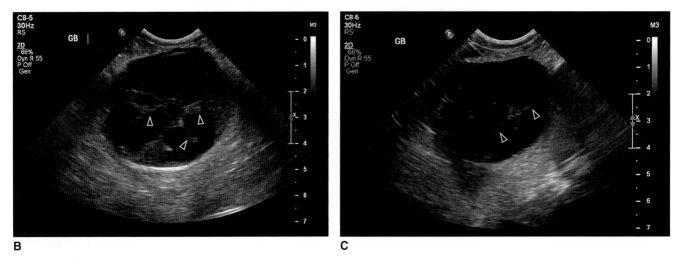

**FIGURE 23.15** Sonographic images (**A–C**) of dogs with gallbladder mucocele. Note the central location of the gallbladder material, with a stellate pattern that emanates from the center of the gallbladder toward the periphery (open arrowheads). In (**C**) note the hyperattenuating fat peripheral to the gallbladder, suggesting regional inflammation. This gallbladder had ruptured.

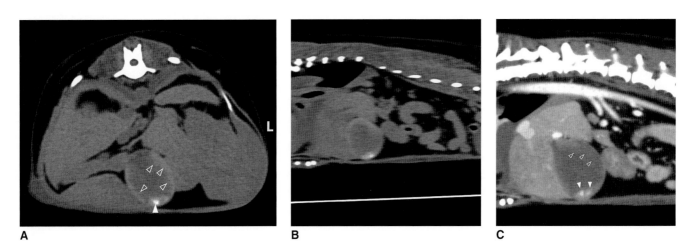

**FIGURE 23.16** Transverse and sagittal reformatted precontrast (**A,B**) and sagittal reformatted postcontrast (**C**) images of a dog with peripherally accumulated hyperattenuating gallbladder contents (open arrowheads) suggestive of gallbladder mucocele. A focus of mineral is seen in a gravity-dependent position (white arrowhead). In (**C**) there is no enhancement of this material, and the mineral material persists (white arrowheads).

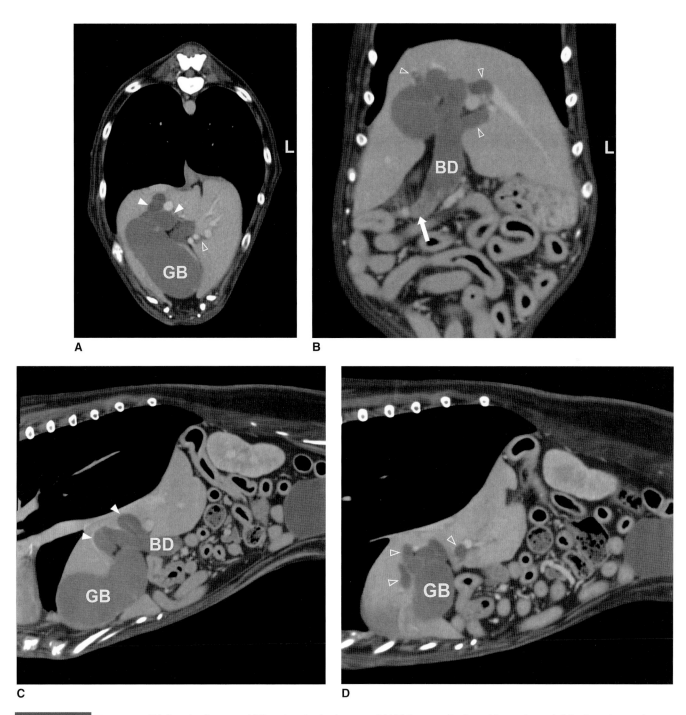

**FIGURE 23.17**   Transverse (**A**) dorsal reformatted (**B**) and sagittal reformatted (**C,D**) images of a dog with extrahepatic bile duct obstruction. Note the enlargement of the gallbladder (GB) and the bile duct (BD), with dilation of the intrahepatic bile ducts (open arrowheads). Note how tortuous the bile duct is (white arrowheads) due to dilation and congestion. On the dorsal image (**B**), the white arrow indicates the mildly contrast-enhancing mass responsible for the obstruction (biliary carcinoma).

## Summary

The hepatobiliary system is complex, and this is reflected in the imaging challenges presented herein. In general, determination of focal versus generalized enlargement can significantly narrow the list of differential diagnoses. Prediction of benign versus malignant disease is challenging, and work continues on this front. Progressive heterogeneity of masses on ultrasound and computed tomography generally correlate with malignancy, though this is not always true.

Vascular diseases of the liver are also complex, and a significant body of work has been compiled in the pursuit of consensus in describing and naming congenital shunts as well as acquired vascular diseases.

# References

1. Lamb, C.R., Steel, R., and Lipscomb, V.J. (2018). Determining the anatomical origin of canine hepatic masses by CT: CT of hepatic masses. *J. Small Anim. Pract.* 59: 752–757.

2. Covey, J.L., Degner, D.A., Jackson, A.H. et al. (2009). Hilar liver resection in dogs. *Vet. Surg.* 38: 104–111.

3. Evans, H. and de Lahunta, A. (2012). *Miller's Anatomy of the Dog*, vol. 4. St Louis, MO: Saunders.

4. Cheney, D.M., Coleman, M.C., Voges, A.K. et al. (2019). Ultrasonographic and CT accuracy in localising surgical- or necropsy-confirmed solitary hepatic masses in dogs. *J. Small Anim. Pract.* 60: 274–279.

5. Kim, S., Yoon, Y., Hwang, T. et al. (2018). Comparison for radiographic measurements of canine liver size by left and right recumbency. *J. Vet. Clin.* 35: 13–16.

6. Farrar, E.T., Washabau, R.J., and Saunders, H.M. (1996). Hepatic abscesses in dogs: 14 cases (1982–1994). *J. Am. Vet. Med. Assoc.* 208: 243–247.

7. Carloni, A., Paninarova, M., Cavina, D. et al. (2019). Negative hepatic computed tomographic attenuation pattern in a dog with vacuolar hepatopathy and hepatic fat accumulation secondary to cushing's syndrome. *Vet. Radiol. Ultrasound* 60: E54–E57.

8. Nakamura, M., Chen, H.-M., Momoi, Y. et al. (2005). Clinical application of computed tomography for the diagnosis of feline hepatic lipidosis. *J. Vet. Med. Sci.* 67: 1163–1165.

9. Selmic, L.E. (2017). Hepatobiliary neoplasia. Vet. *Clin. North Am. Small Anim. Pract. Hepatol.* 47: 725–735.

10. Griebie, E.R., David, F.H., Ober, C.P. et al. (2017). Evaluation of canine hepatic masses by use of triphasic computed tomography and B-mode, color flow, power, and pulsed-wave Doppler ultrasonography and correlation with histopathologic classification. *Am. J. Vet. Res.* 78: 1273–1283.

11. Cuccovillo, A. and Lamb, C.R. (2002). Cellular features of sonographic target lesions of the liver and spleen in 21 dogs and a cat. *Vet. Radiol. Ultrasound* 43: 275–278.

12. Blachar, A., Federle, M.P., Ferris, J.V. et al. (2002). Radiologists' performance in the diagnosis of liver tumors with central scars by using specific CT criteria. *Radiology* 223: 532–539.

13. Fukushima, K., Kanemoto, H., Ohno, K. et al. (2012). CT characteristics of primary hepatic mass lesions in dogs. *Vet. Radiol. Ultrasound* 53: 252–257.

14. Jones, I.D., Lamb, C.R., Drees, R. et al. (2016). Associations between dual-phase computed tomography features and histopathologic diagnoses in 52 dogs with hepatic or splenic masses. *Vet. Radiol. Ultrasound* 57: 144–153.

15. Leela-Arporn, R., Ohta, H., Shimbo, G. et al. (2019). Computed tomographic features for differentiating benign from malignant liver lesions in dogs. *J. Vet. Med. Sci.* 81: 1697–1704.

16. Shaker, R., Wilke, C., Ober, C. et al. (2021). Machine learning model development for quantitative analysis of CT heterogeneity in canine hepatic masses may predict histologic malignancy. *Vet. Radiol. Ultrasound* 62: 711–719.

17. Wormser, C., Reetz, J.A., and Giuffrida, M.A. (2016). Diagnostic accuracy of ultrasound to predict the location of solitary hepatic masses in dogs. *Vet. Surg.* 45: 208–213.

18. Lamb, C.R. and White, R.N. (1998). Morphology of congenital intrahepatic portacaval shunts in dogs and cats. *Vet. Rec.* 142: 55–60.

19. Lamb, C.R., Forster-van Hijfte, M.A., White, R.N. et al. (1996). Ultrasonographic diagnosis of congenital portosystemic shunt in 14 cats. *J. Small Anim. Pract.* 37: 205–209.

20. Sugimoto, S., Maeda, S., Tsuboi, M. et al. (2018). Multiple acquired portosystemic shunts secondary to primary hypoplasia of the portal vein in a cat. *J. Vet. Med. Sci.* 80: 874–877.

21. Frank, P., Mahaffey, M., Egger, C. et al. (2003). Helical computed tomographic portography in ten normal dogs and ten dogs with a portosystemic shunt. *Vet. Radiol. Ultrasound* 44: 392–400.

22. Nelson, N.C. and Nelson, L.L. (2011). Anatomy of extrahepatic portosystemic shunts in dogs as determined by computed tomography angiography. *Vet. Radiol. Ultrasound* 52: 498–506.

23. Parry, A.T. and White, R.N. (2015). Portal vein anatomy in the dog: comparison between computed tomographic angiography (CTA) and intraoperative mesenteric portovenography (IOMP): comparison between CTA and IOMP. *J. Small Anim. Pract.* 56: 657–661.

24. White, R.N. and Parry, A.T. (2016). Morphology of splenocaval congenital portosystemic shunts in dogs and cats: portosystenic shunts involving the splenic vein. *J. Small Anim. Pract.* 57: 28–32.

25. White, R.N. and Parry, A.T. (2015). Morphology of congenital portosystemic shunts involving the right gastric vein in dogs. *J. Small Anim. Pract.* 56: 430–440.

26. White, R.N. and Parry, A.T. (2013). Morphology of congenital portosystemic shunts emanating from the left gastric vein in dogsand cats. *J. Small Anim. Pract.* 54: 459–467.

27. White, R.N., Warren-Smith, C., Shales, C. et al. (2020). Classification of portosystemic shunts entering the caudal vena cava at the omental foramen in dogs. *J. Small Anim. Pract.* 61: 659–668.

28. Zwingenberger, A.L., Schwarz, T., and Saunders, H.M. (2005). Helical computed tomographic angiography of canine portosystemic shunts. *Vet. Radiol. Ultrasound* 46: 27–32.

29. Plested, M.J., Zwingenberger, A.L., Brockman, D.J. et al. (2020). Canine intrahepatic portosystemic shunt insertion into the systemic circulation is commonly through primary hepatic veins as assessed with CT angiography. *Vet. Radiol. Ultrasound* 61: 519–530.

30. Bertolini, G. (2019). Anomalies of the portal venous system in dogs and cats as seen on multidetector-row computed tomography: an overview and systematization proposal. *Vet. Sci.* 6: 10.

31. Bertolini, G. (2010). Acquired portal collateral circulation in the dog and cat. *Vet. Radiol. Ultrasound* 51: 25–33.

32. Szatmári, V., Sótonyi, P., and Vörös, K. (2001). Normal duplex Doppler waveforms of major abdominal blood vessels in dogs: a review. *Vet. Radiol. Ultrasound* 42: 93–107.

33. d'Anjou, M.-A., Penninck, D., Cornejo, L. et al. (2004). Ultrasonographic diagnosis of portosystemic shunting in dogs and cats. *Vet. Radiol. Ultrasound* 45: 424–437.

34. Glăvan, C. (2021). CT periportal halo sign in dogs – comparasion with human medicine. *Sci. Papers J.* 64 (2): 44–48.

35. Favier, R.P. (2009). Idiopathic hepatitis and cirrhosis in dogs. *Vet. Clin. North Am. Small Anim. Pract. Hepatol.* 39: 481–488.

36. Eulenberg, V.M. and Lidbury, J.A. (2018). Hepatic fibrosis in dogs. *J. Vet. Intern. Med.* 32: 26–41.

37. Poldervaart, J.H., Favier, R.P., Penning, L.C. et al. (2009). Primary hepatitis in dogs: a retrospective review (2002–2006). *J. Vet. Intern. Med.* 23: 72–80.

38. Brand, E.M., Lim, C.K., Heng, H.G. et al. (2020). Computed tomographic features of confirmed gallbladder pathology in 34 dogs. *Vet. Radiol. Ultrasound* 61: 667–679.

39. Hittmair, K.M., Vielgrader, H.D., and Loupal, G. (2001). Ultrasonographic evaluation of gallbladder wall thickness in cats. *Vet. Radiol. Ultrasound* 42: 149–155.

40. Brömel, C., Barthez, P.Y., Léveillé, R. et al. (1998). Prevalence of gallbladder sludge in dogs as assessed by ultrasonography. *Vet. Radiol. Ultrasound* 39: 206–210.

41. Cook, A.K., Jambhekar, A.V., and Dylewski, A.M. (2016). Gallbladder sludge in dogs: ultrasonographic and clinical findings in 200 patients. *J. Am. Anim. Hosp. Assoc.* 52: 125–131.

42. Harran, N., d'Anjou, M.-A., Dunn, M. et al. (2011). Gallbladder sludge on ultrasound is predictive of increased liver enzymes and total bilirubin in cats. *Can. Vet. J.* 52: 999–1003.

43. Aicher, K.M., Cullen, J.M., Seiler, G.S. et al. (2019). Investigation of adrenal and thyroid gland dysfunction in dogs with ultrasonographic diagnosis of gallbladder mucocele formation. *PLoS One* 14: e0212638.

44. Besso, J., Wrigley, R., Gliatto, J. et al. (2000). Ultrasonographic appearance and clinical findings in 14 dogs with gallbladder mucocele. *Vet. Radiol. Ultrasound* 41: 261–271.

45. Choi, J., Kim, A., Keh, S. et al. (2014). Comparison between ultrasonographic and clinical findings in 43 dogs with gallbladder mucoceles. *Vet. Radiol. Ultrasound* 55: 202–207.

46. Fuerst, J.A. and Hostnik, E.T. (2019). CT attenuation values and mineral distribution can be used to differentiate dogs with and without gallbladder mucoceles. *Vet. Radiol. Ultrasound* 60: 689–695.

47. Gaillot, H.A., Penninck, D.G., Webster, C.R.L. et al. (2007). Ultrasonographic features of extrahepatic biliary obstruction in 30 cats. *Vet. Radiol. Ultrasound* 48: 439–447.

# CHAPTER 24

# Spleen

**Cintia R. Oliveira**

VetsChoice Radiology, Madison, WI, USA

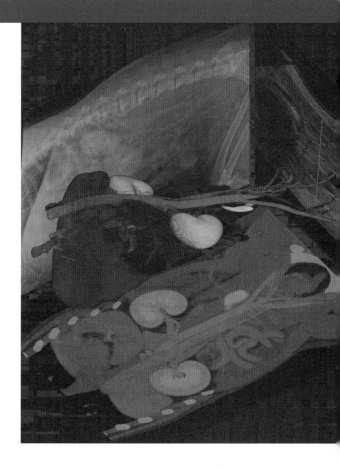

## Introduction

In small animals, the spleen is a mobile organ, with only its proximal extremity or head being fixed to the stomach by the gastrosplenic ligament, in the left craniodorsal aspect of the abdomen. The body and distal extremity, or tail of the spleen, are not fixed and therefore variable in position.

On lateral radiographic views in dogs, the tail of the spleen is seen as a triangular soft tissue opacity caudal and slightly ventral to the liver and pylorus (Figure 24.1). Occasionally, the head of the spleen may be seen in dogs or cats on lateral views in the dorsal and cranial abdomen just caudal to the stomach and dorsal to the right kidney margins (Figure 24.1). On ventro-dorsal views, the body of the spleen is seen as a triangular soft tissue opacity in the cranial and left aspects of the abdomen, caudolateral to the stomach and craniolateral to the left kidney in both dogs and cats (Figures 24.1 and 24.2). If the spleen is positioned alongside the left body wall, it may not be visible on lateral radiographs but may be visible entirely on the ventrodorsal view.

The feline spleen differs from the canine spleen in that it is smaller and thinner, and less variable in size and position (Figure 24.2). The body and tail of the feline spleen are not usually seen on lateral views in normal cats. The head may be visible on lateral views as a small triangular soft tissue opacity caudal and dorsal to the stomach. Like the dog, on the ventro-dorsal view the head of the spleen can be seen in the left cranial abdomen caudolateral to the stomach and craniolateral to the left kidney. Frequently, the entire feline spleen is visible on ventrodorsal views since its tail extends caudally along the left lateral abdominal wall (Figure 24.2). The normal thickness of the feline spleen is 1 cm as measured on radiographs and ultrasound [1].

On ultrasound (US), the canine spleen is identified on the left side caudal and lateral to the stomach. Since its body and distal extremity are movable, they often extend into the caudal

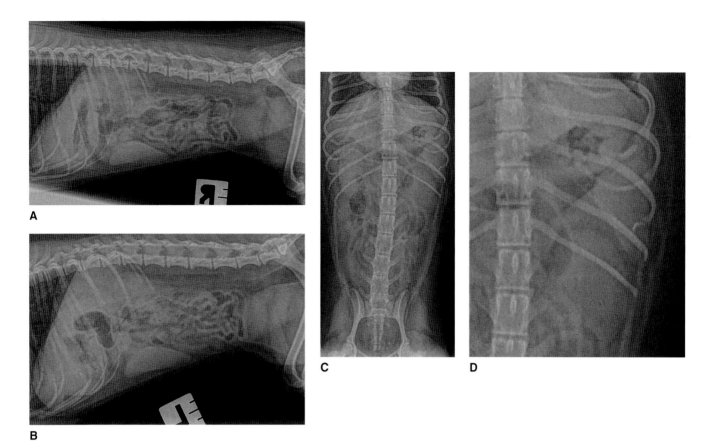

**FIGURE 24.1**   Right lateral (**A**), left lateral (**B**), and ventrodorsal (**C**) radiographs from a dog with a normal spleen for size, position, shape, and margination. On the lateral images, the tail of the spleen is located caudal and ventral to the stomach and caudal to the liver. On the ventrodorsal radiographs (**C** and close-up **D**), the splenic head is located in the left cranial abdomen, lateral to the fundic portion of the stomach, and has a variable position relative to the caudal ribs on the left. The renal silhouette is located caudal and medial to the splenic head.

abdomen and across midline to the right side and the spleen often appears folded on itself (Figures 24.3 and 24.4) [1]. The feline spleen may be difficult to find ultrasonographically in some cats because of its small size (Figure 24.5). Intercostal windows may be necessary with the transducer placed in a more dorsal and cranial position than expected [1]. As opposed to dogs, the feline spleen rarely folds on itself unless enlarged. Sonographically, when enlarged, the spleen may extend more caudally, being visible next to the urinary bladder, and the splenic margins become rounded or blunted, as opposed to the normal sharp appearance [1, 2].

Ectopic spleen has been reported in dogs and cats. It has been described ultrasonographically as round to triangular homogeneous structures isoechoic to spleen in the perisplenic region and with computed tomography (CT) as multiple heterogeneous intraabdominal and intrahepatic masses resembling hepatic tumor with abdominal metastasis [3, 4].

Splenic thickness greater than 1 cm in cats is suggestive of splenomegaly. A recent study found a weak correlation between radiographic and ultrasonographic measurement of splenic size in cats. In that study, the feline spleen measured ultrasonographically had a mean of $8.0 \pm 1.6$ mm, similar to previous reports [5]. In dogs, there is no absolute normal size for the spleen. Suspect splenomegaly on ultrasound can be confirmed with radiographs or palpation, but radiographic assessment of splenic size is subjective because the spleen varies in size in normal dogs and cats.

Radiography and ultrasound are still the primary imaging methods used to evaluate the spleen, in part due to their noninvasive nature and the ease with which evaluation and sampling can be carried out with US. Contrast-enhanced US can be used for further characterization of focal and diffuse splenic lesions although the accuracy of contrast-enhanced US in differentiating between benign and malignant splenic lesions is conflicting [3, 6–10]. A study evaluating the assessment of feeding vessels with contrast-enhanced US found that echogenicity and persistent hypoperfusion cannot be used alone to distinguish between malignant and benign focal splenic lesions but the presence of tortuous and persistent feeding vessels may be helpful in distinguishing malignancy since no benign lesions in the study had such a characteristic [11]. Contrast enhancement parameters for normal spleen have been published using different contrast agents [8].

The use of CT to evaluate the spleen is usually reserved for specific disease processes such as trauma, vascular disorders, staging of neoplasia or in acute abdomen cases (Figure 24.3). However, CT has been used with increasing frequency to evaluate splenic disease and its use is paramount for complete

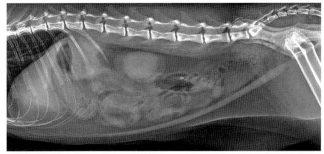

A

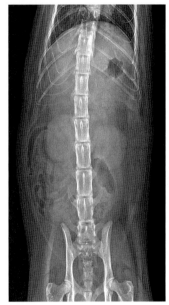

B

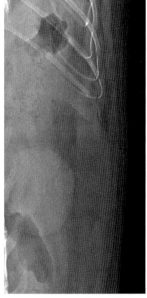

C

**FIGURE 24.2** Right lateral (**A**) and ventrodorsal (**B**) radiographs from a cat with a normal spleen for size, position, shape, and margination. On the lateral images, the tail of the spleen is routinely not visualized. On the ventrodorsal radiograph, the splenic head is in the left cranial abdomen, lateral to the fundic portion of the stomach. (**C**) Ventrodorsal radiograph of a normal cat spleen where the length of the spleen is seen along the left lateral abdominal wall.

detection and evaluation of vascular disorders. A recent study described the presence of collateral circulation using CT angiography in a dog with splenic vein obstruction and presumed splenic vein hypertension [12].

Magnetic resonance imaging (MRI) is not used routinely to evaluate the spleen since US and CT are faster and allow for immediate sampling of lesions. Studies describing the normal MRI appearance of the canine and feline spleen are available as well as studies evaluating splenic disease (Figure 24.3). Elastography (ultrasound technique for determining stiffness of the spleen) of the normal spleen has also been reported but currently its use is still reserved for research.

The imaging features of the normal spleen in four imaging modalities are listed in Table 24.1. A recent study evaluated the US appearance of the spleen in nine normal puppies from 4 to 60 weeks using a high-frequency linear transducer and found that the splenic parenchymal patterns changed with age from a granular appearance at 4 weeks of age to a reticulonodular

pattern characterized by well-defined hypoechoic nodules which was most marked at 28–36 weeks of age, which then gradually changed into a more homogeneous granular pattern at 60 weeks [13]. Care must be taken during ultrasound examination of very young dogs since some of these patterns resemble disease, including neoplasia.

# Focal Splenic Changes

## Primary and Secondary Neoplasia

Splenic neoplasia has a high prevalence in dogs, with a high frequency of malignant tumors, and in the presence of hemoabdomen, a splenic mass is more likely to be neoplasia [14, 15]. Hemangiosarcoma is the most prevalent malignant neoplasia of the spleen in dogs (Figures 24.6–24.9) [15]. Other malignant tumors of the spleen in dogs include sarcoma, lymphoma, carcinoma, mast cell tumor, and metastasis (Figures 24.10–24.18) [16–19].

In a study of 455 cats with splenic disease, primary and metastatic neoplasia accounted for 37% of cases [20]. Most cats had mastocytoma followed by lymphoma, myeloproliferative disease, and hemangiosarcoma. A much smaller percentage of benign lesions was found, including accessory spleen (4%), hyperplastic nodules and/or hematomas (4%), splenitis (2%), and thromboembolism with infarction (1%) [20].

Splenic nodules are a common nonspecific finding in dogs for which differentials include nodular hyperplasia, extramedullary hematopoiesis (EMH), hematoma, or neoplastic or infectious lesions [21]. These nodules can be of variable size and echogenicity and no ultrasound criteria can be confidently applied to differentiate benign from malignant nodules. Nodular hyperplasia and EMH are a common finding in older dogs and they should not be regarded as metastatic lesions in the presence of a primary neoplasia elsewhere without sampling [20, 22].

Splenic masses are usually vascular, and bleeding often occurs if the masses rupture. Bleeding of splenic hemangiosarcoma is one of the most common causes of canine hemoabdomen [23]. In some dogs with hemoabdomen, a "sentinel clot sign" may be detected in proximity to the bleeding source. The sentinel clot sign is the highest attenuation hematoma adjacent to a bleeding organ or mass [24]. Active bleeding can be detected on postcontrast CT images by the presence of a serpiginous or amorphous, highly attenuating area originating from an organ parenchyma which would be consistent with extravasation of contrast medium into the peritoneal space [24].

With radiography, neoplasia can be seen as a distinct mass or changes to the splenic contour/margins (Figure 24.8). A variety of changes can be seen with US and CT and there are no specific findings to differentiate between benign or malignant disease or between specific types of neoplasia [17, 21, 25].

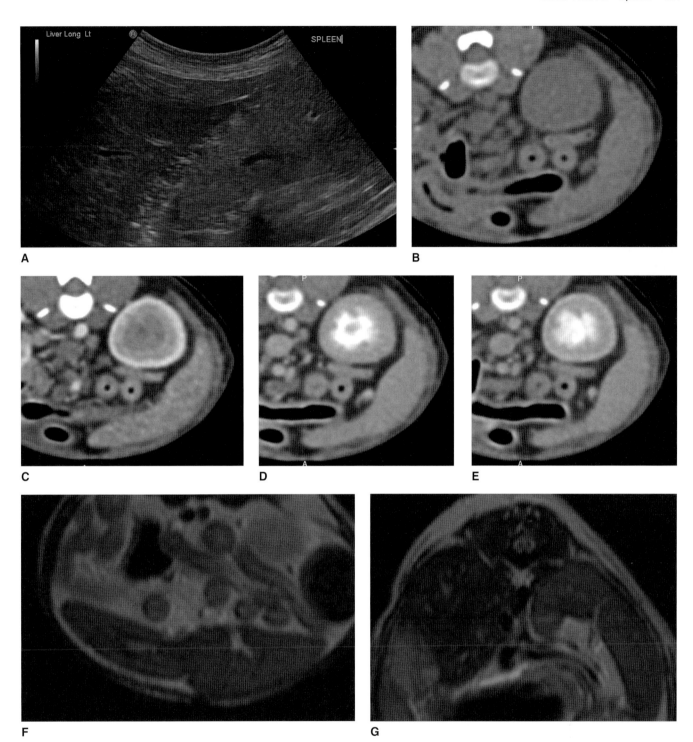

**FIGURE 24.3** (**A**) Sagittal (long axis) ultrasound image from a dog of the left side of the liver (left side of the image) and the spleen (right side of the image). Note the differences in echogenicity and echotexture. Transverse plane precontrast (**B**) and postcontrast arterial (**C**), portal (**D**), and venous (**E**) phases. The spleen has a heterogeneous patchy enhancement on the arterial phase. On portal and venous phase, the enhancement is homogeneous. Transverse plane T2 (**F,G**), T1 precontrast (**H**) and T1 postcontrast (**I**) images. Liver/spleen comparison (**G**). The spleen is hyperintense compared to the liver on T2-weighted images (**F,G**). On T1 precontrast image (**H**) the spleen is hypointense compared to liver and has homogeneous contrast enhancement (**I**). Splenic veins are apparent as hypoechoic structures within the spleen and along its hilar margin (**J, K**).

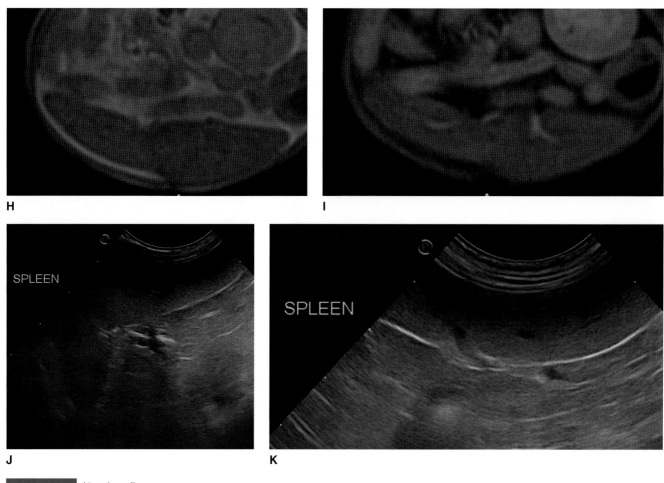

H

I

J

K

**FIGURE 24.3**  (Continued)

**TABLE 24.1**  **Imaging characteristics of normal canine and feline spleen.**

|  | **Radiographs** | **US** | **CT** | **MRI** |
|---|---|---|---|---|
| Dog | Soft tissue opaque | Finely textured, hyperechoic compared to liver and renal cortex | Splenomegaly is common since patients usually under general anesthesia<br><br>Precontrast: homogeneous soft tissue attenuation<br><br>Postcontrast:<br><br>Arterial: heterogeneous enhancement<br><br>Venous: homogeneous enhancement<br><br>Delayed: homogeneous enhancement | T2W: hyperintense compared to liver<br><br>T1W precontrast: hypointense compared to liver<br><br>T1W postcontrast: homogeneously contrast enhancing, slightly hypointense compared to liver<br><br>STIR: hypointense compared to liver |
| Cat | Soft tissue opaque | Finely textured, hyperechoic compared to renal cortex | Splenomegaly is common since patients usually under general anesthesia<br><br>Postcontrast:<br><br>Arterial: patchy heterogeneous enhancement<br><br>Venous: patchy heterogeneous or homogeneous enhancement<br><br>Delayed: homogeneous enhancement | T2W: hyperintense compared to liver<br><br>T1W precontrast: hypointense compared to liver<br><br>T1W postcontrast: markedly enhancing, first 60 seconds heterogeneous pattern of high and low signal intensity, after 60 seconds homogeneous enhancement |

CT, computed tomography; MRI, magnetic resonance imaging; STIR, short tau inversion recovery; T1W, T1 weighted; T2W, T2 weighted; US, ultrasound.

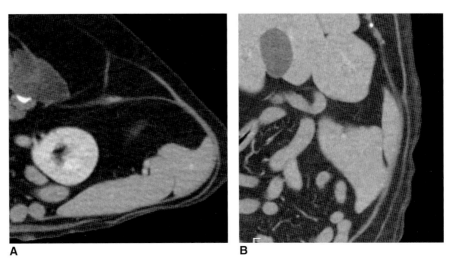

**FIGURE 24.4** Eleven-year-old mixed-breed Labrador with history of shortness of breath. CT transverse plane postcontrast (**A**) and dorsal plane postcontrast (**B**) CT images. The spleen is moderately enlarged and folding upon itself. This is likely congestion because of general anesthesia.

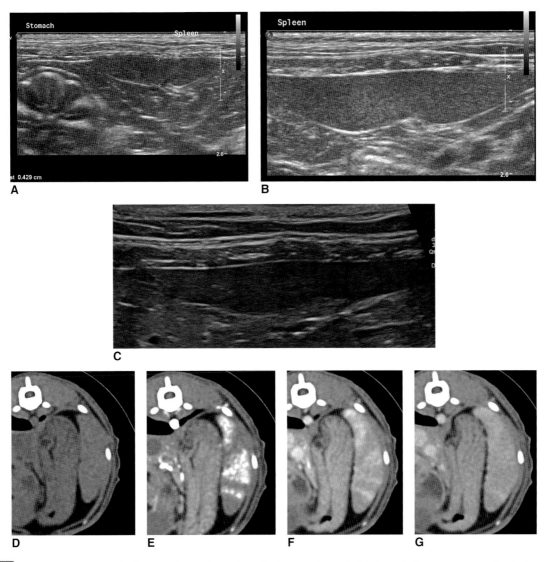

**FIGURE 24.5** Ultrasound image (**A,B**) of a normal cat spleen. The splenic parenchyma is tightly packed in echotexture, slightly hypoechoic relative to the surrounding mesenteric fat, and outlined by a hyperechoic capsule. The spleen measures 0.43 cm in thickness. The fundic portion of the feline stomach is seen in the left of the image (**A**) with a hyperechoic serosal outer border and a hyperechoic submucosal fat layer and an inner hyperechoic mucosal luminal interface. (**B**) Close-up of the spleen of the same cat. (**C**) Ultrasound image from a different cat with a close-up of the spleen. The spleen has a tightly packed echotexture, is relatively isoechoic to the surrounding mesentery and lacks the portal splenic vascular markings more commonly seen in the dog. Transverse plane precontrast (**D**) and postcontrast arterial (**E**), venous (**F**), and delayed (**G**) phases of the spleen of another cat. The spleen has a heterogeneous patchy enhancement on the arterial and venous phases. On the delayed phase, the enhancement is starting to be more homogeneous.

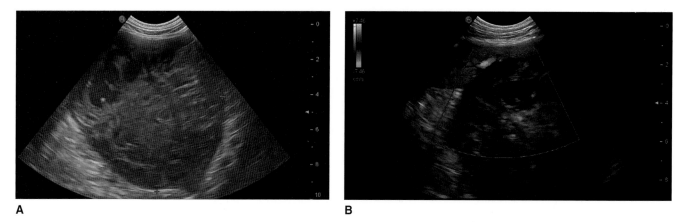

**A**     **B**

**FIGURE 24.6**   (**A**) Sagittal (long axis) ultrasound image of a 11-year-old golden retriever presented with a 2-month history of lethargy and decreased appetite. A large round complex cavitated mass is present in association with the spleen. Upon color Doppler evaluation, multiple regions of the mass had no blood flow (**B**). Not demonstrated in the images was a mild amount of peritoneal effusion. Fine needle aspiration of the mass was performed, and sarcoma was confirmed on cytology.

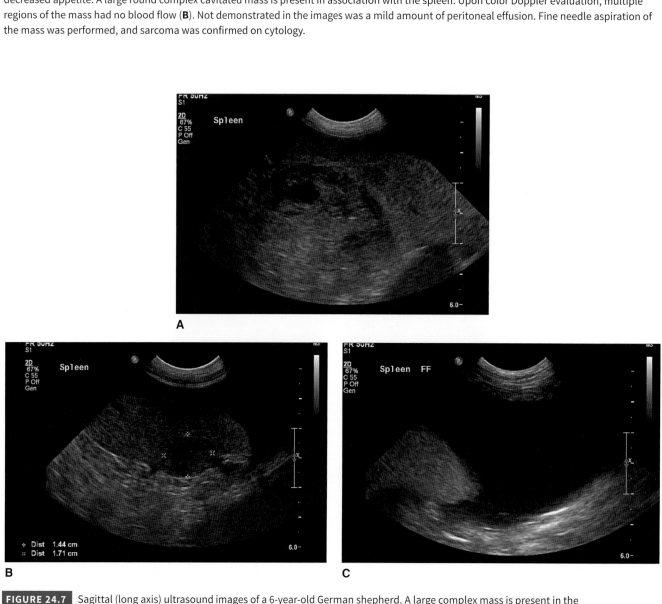

**A**

**B**     **C**

**FIGURE 24.7**   Sagittal (long axis) ultrasound images of a 6-year-old German shepherd. A large complex mass is present in the spleen (**A**). Multiple hypoechoic nodules are present throughout the spleen (**B**). A marked amount of anechoic peritoneal effusion was also present (**C**). Sarcoma and hemorrhage were diagnosed on cytology based on fine needle aspiration of the splenic nodules and effusion respectively.

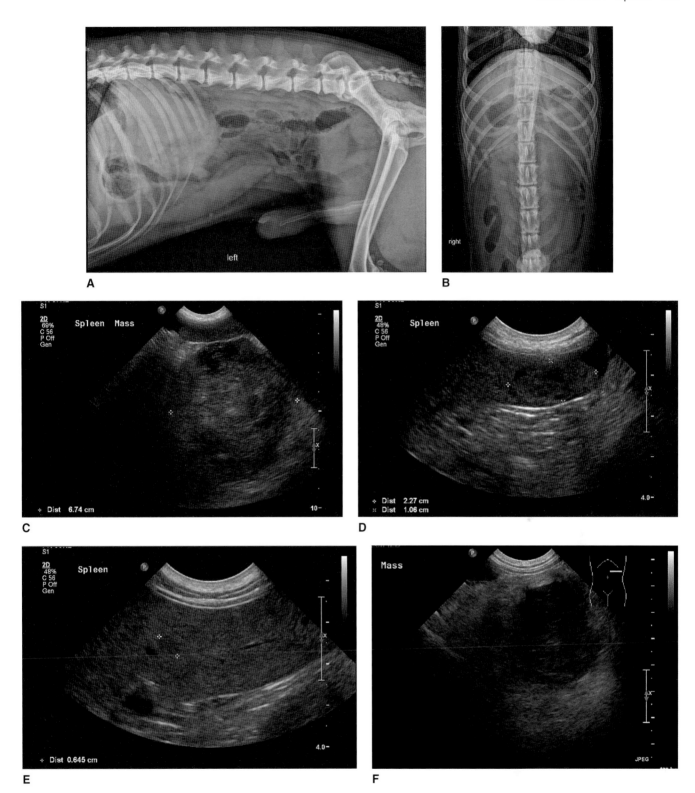

**FIGURE 24.8** Ten-year-old dog presented with vomiting, regurgitation, anorexia, fever, and tense abdomen. (**A,B**) Left lateral and ventrodorsal radiographs of the abdomen. A well-defined large soft tissue opaque mass with irregular margins is present in the craniodorsal abdomen (**A**). The mass is causing ventral and caudal displacement of the colon and small intestines (**A,B**). The spleen is enlarged with rounded margins. There is generalized decreased serosal detail. (**C–F**) Sagittal (long axis) ultrasound images. A large heterogeneous mass is present within the head of the spleen (**C**) along with multiple hyper- and hypoechoic nodules (**D,E**). The mesentery was hyperechoic adjacent to the splenic mass (**F**). A mild amount of peritoneal effusion was present (not shown). Sarcoma was diagnosed on cytology based on fine needle aspiration of the splenic mass.

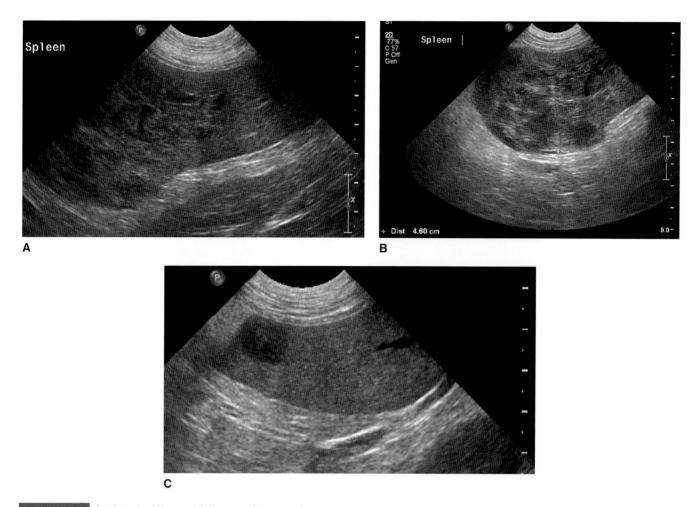

**FIGURE 24.9** (A-C) Sagittal (long axis) ultrasound images of a 9-year-old dog presented with anorexia and panting. A large heterogeneous mass with multiple anechoic areas within and ill-defined margins is seen within the spleen (**A,B**). The mass causes deformation of the splenic border. A well-defined smoothly marginated hypoechoic nodule is present in the splenic parenchyma (**C**). A moderate amount of peritoneal effusion was present (not shown). Sarcoma was diagnosed on cytology of fine needle aspirate of the mass and confirmed later with histopathology.

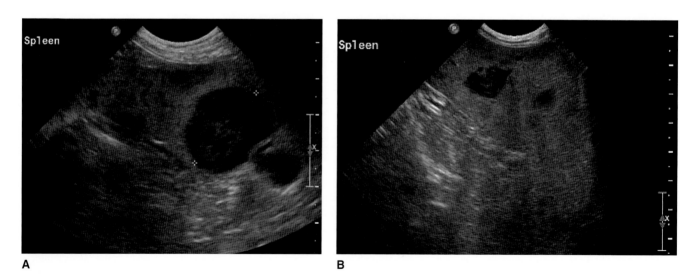

**FIGURE 24.10** (A,B) Sagittal (long axis) ultrasound images of a 12-year-old mixed-breed dog with enlarged mandibular lymph nodes. The spleen is moderately enlarged. Multiple hyper- and hypoechoic nodules and masses are present in the spleen, some of them bulging the splenic capsule. Other US findings included an enlarged and diffusely hyperechoic liver and multiple enlarged and hypoechoic lymph nodes. The dog also had a cranial mediastinal mass on thoracic radiographs. Cytology from fine needle aspirate of the liver and spleen confirmed lymphoma.

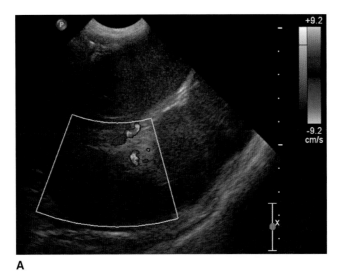

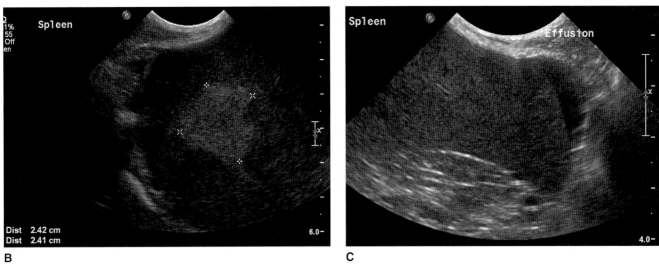

**FIGURE 24.11** Sagittal (long axis) ultrasound images of a 5-year-old dachshund presented with inappetence and lethargy. The spleen is severely enlarged, lobular and folding (**A**). Multiple iso-, hyper-, and hypoechoic nodules are present, some causing bulging of the splenic capsule (**B**). Mild amount of peritoneal effusion was present (**C**). Cytology from fine needle aspirate of the splenic parenchyma and splenic nodules confirmed lymphoma.

**FIGURE 24.12** Sagittal (long axis) ultrasound image of a 9-year-old Catahoula Leopard Hog dog presented for further workup of lymphoma. The spleen is moderately enlarged with a Swiss cheese appearance seen as multiple small hypoechoic nodules throughout the parenchyma. Multiple abdominal lymph nodes were severely enlarged and hypoechoic. The liver was normal, but cytology based on fine needle aspiration of the liver confirmed lymphoma. Cytology of the spleen also confirmed lymphoma.

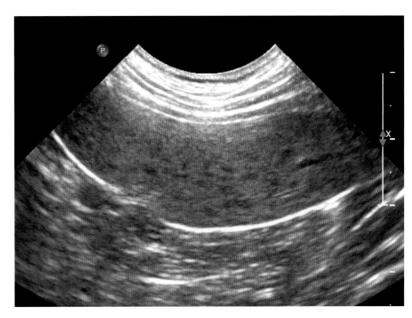

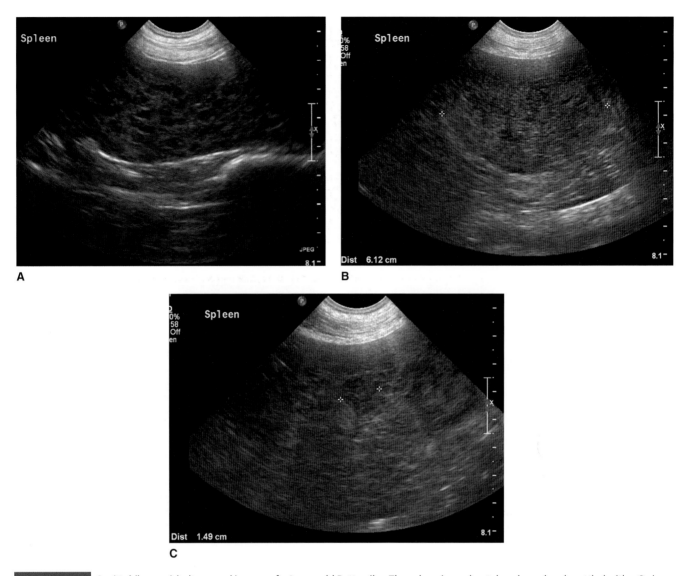

**FIGURE 24.13** Sagittal (long axis) ultrasound images of a 9-year-old Rottweiler. The spleen is moderately enlarged and mottled with a Swiss cheese appearance (**A**). A large heterogeneous mass as well as a few larger hypoechoic nodules were also present in the spleen (**B,C**). Multiple abdominal lymph nodes were severely enlarged and hypoechoic. Cytology based on fine needle aspirates of the spleen confirmed lymphoma.

On US, neoplasia commonly manifests as poorly margin-ated nodules or masses that are anechoic or hypoechoic, with or without target-like lesions, or are complex in appearance and may distort the splenic contour [17, 21, 26–28]. With CT, a multitude of characteristics have been reported with overlap between benign and malignant masses [25, 29, 30]. Malignant masses may be precontrast hypoattenuating and enhance less than the splenic parenchyma on postcontrast images, or they can have mild or strong heterogeneous enhancement [25, 30]. Less commonly, neoplastic lesions may be hyperechoic or hyperattenuating on US and CT respectively [25, 30].

Hemangiosarcomas can appear as a mass of variable size, may be solid or cavitated, isoechoic, hypo- or hyperechoic compared to the splenic parenchyma, or have mixed echo-genicity [31]. Ultrasonographically, they are indistinguishable from hematomas, abscesses, EMH or benign neoplasia such as hemangioma [26, 31–33]. With CT, they have been found to

have marked generalized enhancement in early-phase images that persisted in delayed images, or homogeneous poor enhancement on all phases. In one study, 77% of the heman-giosarcomas and all hematomas had contrast accumulation compatible with active hemorrhage [34, 35].

Other malignant neoplasia that have similar US appear-ance include other sarcomas such as histiocytic sarcoma, lym-phoma, and metastatic disease [18, 28]. In a CT study comparing malignant and nonmalignant splenic masses in dogs, malig-nant masses had significant lower attenuation values (Houn-sfield units, HU) on both pre- and postcontrast images and the authors recommend a cutoff value of less than 55 HU as being suggestive of a malignant mass [34]. A study comparing CT with histopathologic diagnosis of dogs with hepatic or splenic masses found a large overlap between pre- and postcontrast CT features of malignant and nonmalignant masses and con-cluded that dual-phase CT provides limited specific diagnostic

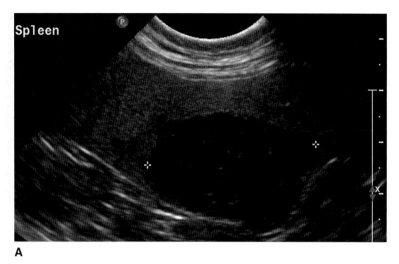

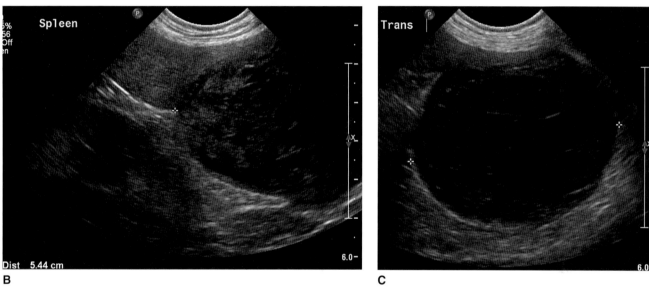

**FIGURE 24.14**   Sagittal (long axis) (**A,B**) and (**C**) transverse (short axis) ultrasound images of a 11-year-old German shepherd presented with T13–L1 myelopathy. Abdominal US was performed to rule out concurrent disease prior to decompressive spinal surgery. The spleen is moderately enlarged and contains multiple round well-circumscribed heterogeneously hypoechoic nodules and masses measuring up to 6.2 cm, many of which are distorting the splenic capsule. Cytology based on fine needle aspiration of the largest splenic mass confirmed lymphoma.

information in these patients [35]. A more recent study found that precontrast lesion attenuation was significantly different between splenic malignant and benign tumors, with malignant tumors having a mean and standard deviation lesion attenuation of 40.3 ± 5.9 HU, and benign tumors 52.8 ± 6.8 HU [36].

Target-like lesions seen on US, nodules with a hyperechoic center surrounded by a hypoechoic rim resembling a bull's eye target, have been associated with malignant lesions in both humans and dogs, although these lesions can also be seen with a variety of benign diseases (Figures 24.17, 24.18, and 24.32) [27]. Sampling of any splenic lesion is necessary for a final diagnosis.

## Nodular Hyperplasia

Nodular hyperplasia and hematoma are among the most common splenic lesions in dogs [1]. These lesions are a particularly common finding in ultrasound examinations of older dogs and should not be regarded as malignant lesions without sampling. In a study evaluating 1480 dogs with splenic disease, nodular hyperplasia and hematoma made up the majority of the cases [20]. In a study evaluating 105 dogs presented with incidentally found nonruptured splenic masses, 70.5% had a benign lesion, of which 50% had nodular hyperplasia. In a similar study in cats, however, these lesions comprised only 4% of the cases [20]. This suggests that splenic nodules or masses in cats are less likely to be benign compared to dogs and therefore more aggressive sampling may be indicated.

With US, these benign lesions have a variable appearance and therefore cannot be distinguished from malignant nodules (Figures 24.19–24.22). With CT, these lesions tend to be hyperattenuating on precontrast images and remain so on postcontrast images or be isoattenuating on precontrast images and hyperattenuating on postcontrast images (Figures 24.23 and 24.24) [25, 34]. Another differential for such lesions is EMH.

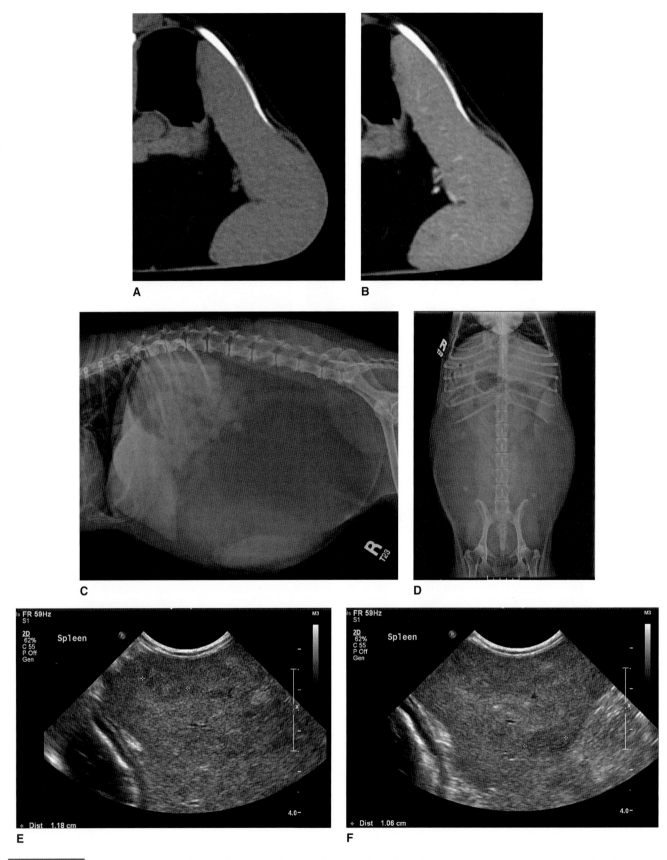

**FIGURE 24.15** Thirteen-year-old miniature schnauzer with decreasing appetite and vomiting. Transverse plane precontrast (**A**) and postcontrast (**B**) CT images of the spleen. Multiple precontrast isoattenuating and postcontrast hypoattenuating nodules are present on the spleen on CT. The spleen is moderately enlarged. (**C,D**) Right lateral and ventrodorsal views of the abdomen. The spleen is moderately enlarged with rounded lobulated margins. A large intraabdominal lipoma is also present. (**E,F**) Sagittal (long axis) ultrasound images. The spleen is moderately enlarged with multiple hyperechoic (**E**) and hypoechoic (**F**) nodules. Cytology confirmed mast cell tumor.

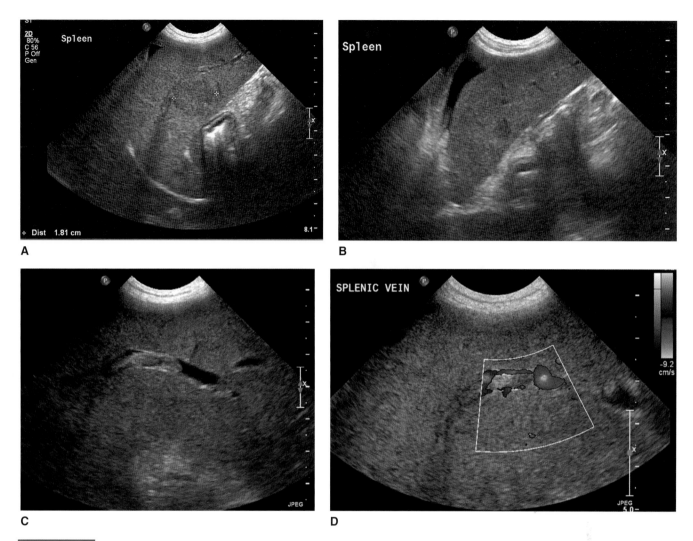

**FIGURE 24.16** Sagittal (long axis) ultrasound images of a 9-year-old pit bull terrier with 2 weeks of lethargy, anorexia, and weight loss. The spleen is moderately enlarged with multiple hyper- and hypoechoic nodules (**A,B**). A large hyperechoic structure is present in the lumen of the splenic vein representing a thrombus. (**C**). On color Doppler evaluation, partial flow is present around this structure (**D**). Other US findings included enlarged and diffusely hyperechoic liver, multiple enlarged and hypoechoic lymph nodes and mild peritoneal effusion. Cytology from fine needle aspiration of the liver, splenic parenchyma, and lymph nodes confirmed mast cell tumor.

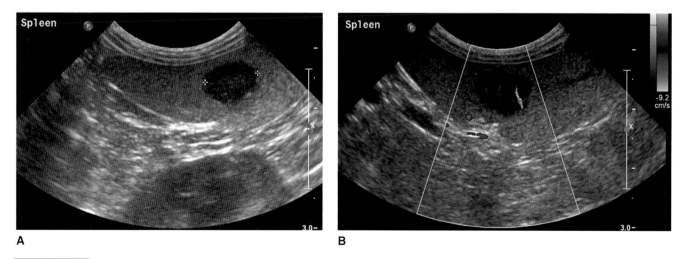

**FIGURE 24.17** Sagittal (long axis) ultrasound images of a 13-year-old German pinscher presented for front limb lameness, lethargy, and weakness. A solitary well-circumscribed round hypoechoic nodule with a target appearance (hyperechoic center) is present in the splenic body (**A**). Multiple similar-looking nodules were present in the liver. Upon color Doppler evaluation of the splenic nodule, a large feeding vessel can be seen at the periphery and entering the nodule (**B**). Cytology from fine needle aspiration of the hepatic and splenic nodules diagnosed hepatocellular carcinoma.

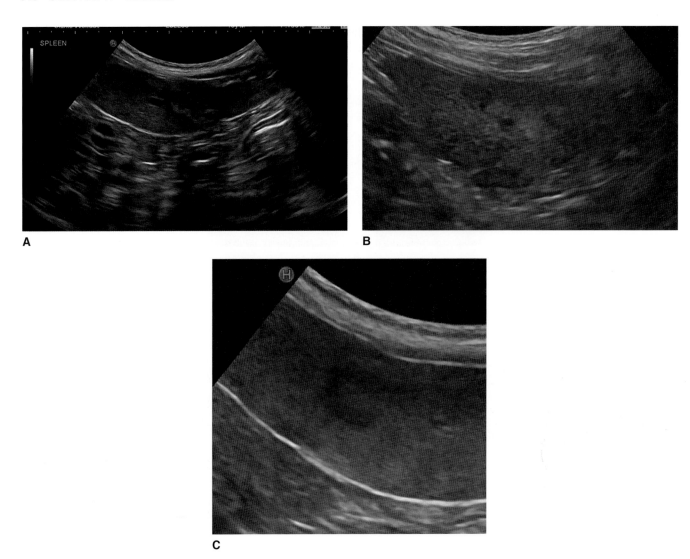

**FIGURE 24.18** Sagittal (long axis) ultrasound images of a 14-year-old dachshund with squamous cell carcinoma. Multiple heterogeneous hyperechoic masses are present in the spleen (**A**). In addition, multiple ill-defined hypoechoic nodules, some with a target appearance, are also present in the spleen (**B,C**). Cytology from fine needle aspiration of the splenic nodules diagnosed metastasis from tonsillar squamous cell carcinoma.

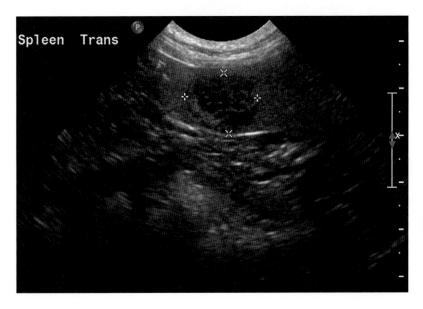

**FIGURE 24.19** Sagittal (long axis) ultrasound image of a 10-year-old boxer. A round well-circumscribed hypoechoic nodule is present in the spleen. Cytology from fine needle aspiration of the nodules diagnosed nodular hyperplasia.

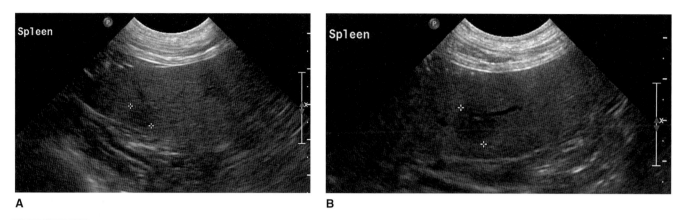

**FIGURE 24.20** (**A,B**) Sagittal (long axis) ultrasound images of a 8-year-old boxer diagnosed with mast cell tumor in the left thigh. Multiple round well-circumscribed hypoechoic nodules are present in the spleen. Cytology from fine needle aspiration of the nodules diagnosed nodular hyperplasia.

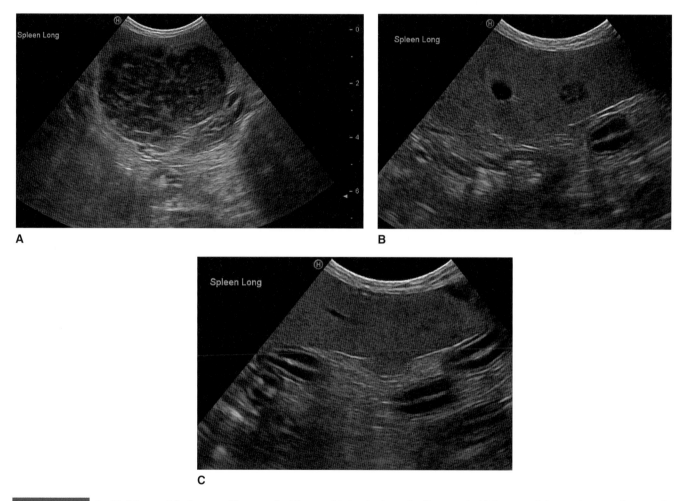

**FIGURE 24.21** Sagittal (long axis) ultrasound images of a 11-year-old standard poodle diagnosed with hepatocellular carcinoma. A large well-circumscribed cavitated mass is present in the spleen (**A**). In addition, multiple hypoechoic and isoechoic nodules are present throughout the splenic parenchyma (**B,C**), some bulging the capsule (**C**). Cytology from fine needle aspiration of the nodules diagnosed nodular hyperplasia.

## Hematoma

Splenic hematomas may occur because of trauma, spontaneously, or secondary to lymphoma or hemangiosarcoma. The appearance of hematomas varies with time and hemoglobin content. Radiographically, a well-defined soft tissue opaque mass may be seen with poor peritoneal detail in cases of hemorrhage [1, 2, 26]. On US, they are seen as focal lesions possibly with distortion of the parenchyma. These can be ill defined, well defined or encapsulated and anechoic, hypoechoic or

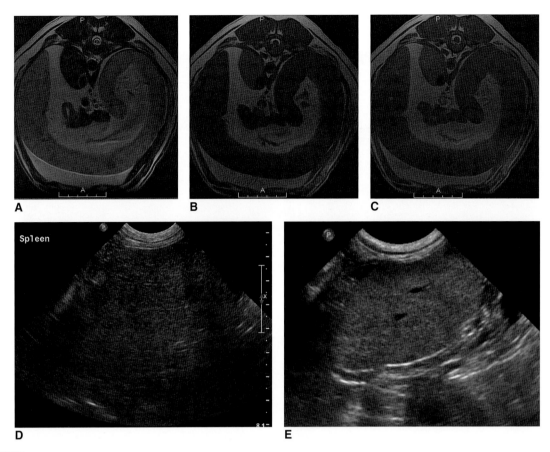

**FIGURE 24.22**  Ten-year-old mixed-breed dog with progressive pelvic limb weakness. Transverse T2 (**A**), T1 precontrast (**B**), and T1 postcontrast (**C**) MRI images. Multiple T2 and T1 hypointense nodules are present throughout the spleen (**A,B**). Some of the nodules show mild contrast enhancement (**C**). (**D,E**) Sagittal (long axis) ultrasound images. The spleen is diffusely mottled with multiple hyperechoic nodules. A mild amount of peritoneal effusion was present. Cytology from fine needle aspiration of the splenic nodules diagnosed nodular hyperplasia.

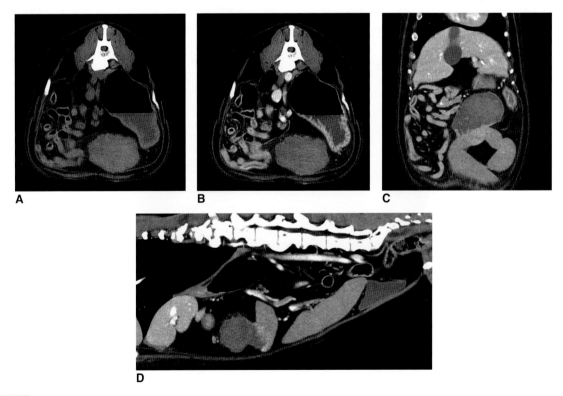

**FIGURE 24.23**  Eleven-year-old Great Dane presented with anorexia and palpable organomegaly. Transverse plane precontrast (**A**) and postcontrast (**B**), dorsal (**C**), and sagittal (**D**) plane postcontrast CT images. An irregular marginated well-circumscribed round soft tissue-attenuating rim-enhancing mass extends from the cranial margin of the spleen. Surrounding the mass are areas of increased fluid attenuation suggestive of effusion. Cytology from fine needle aspiration of the mass diagnosed nodular hyperplasia and extramedullary hematopoiesis.

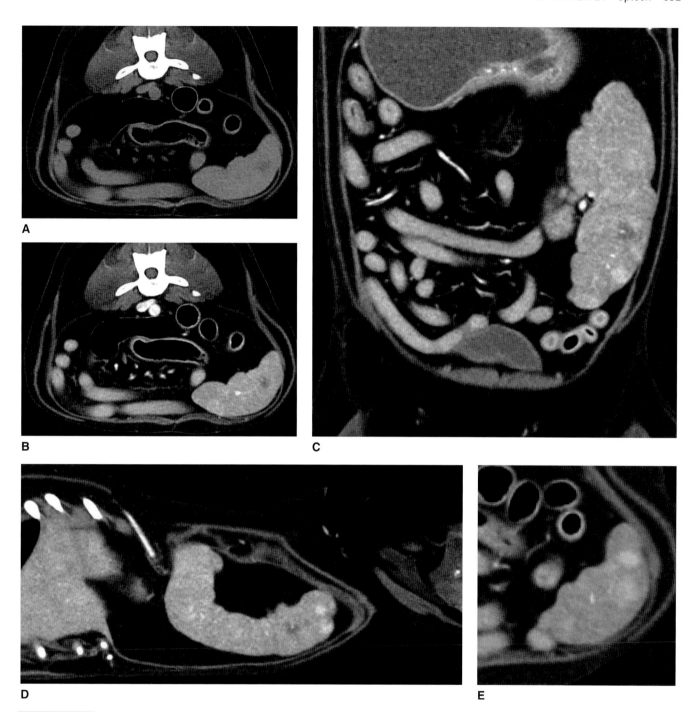

**FIGURE 24.24** Ten-year-old Rottweiler with pain on opening the mouth and firm nonmobile mass on top of the head. Transverse plane precontrast (**A**) and postcontrast (**B**), dorsal (**C**), and sagittal (**D**) plane postcontrast CT images. Close-up image of the spleen (**E**). The spleen has irregular margins and multiple well-circumscribed round nodules measuring up to 1 cm in diameter that are isoattenuating to spleen on precontrast images and strongly contrast enhancing on postcontrast images. A few ill-defined hypoattenuating nodules were also present on postcontrast images. Cytology from fine needle aspiration of the nodules diagnosed nodular hyperplasia.

hyperechoic compared to surrounding splenic parenchyma, depending on chronicity (Figures 24.25 and 24.26) [1, 2, 26].

In a study evaluating 71 dogs with a splenic mass presenting with hemoabdomen and requiring a blood transfusion, a hematoma was present in seven of the 17 dogs that had a benign mass. The other 10 dogs with a benign mass had nodular hyperplasia, with a total of 23.9% (17/71) of the dogs having a benign mass [14]. In the study, 54 of the dogs (76.1%) had

a malignant mass, with 92.6% having hemangiosarcoma [14]. In cats, the spleen may be enlarged, mottled, and irregular [26]. A study evaluating prognostic factors in 35 dogs with splenic hematomas found a median survival time of 674 days, which is much higher than that of dogs with hemangiosarcoma [37].

On CT, acute hematomas are isoattenuating to splenic parenchyma. They become hypoattenuating over time as the hemoglobin content decreases and the water content

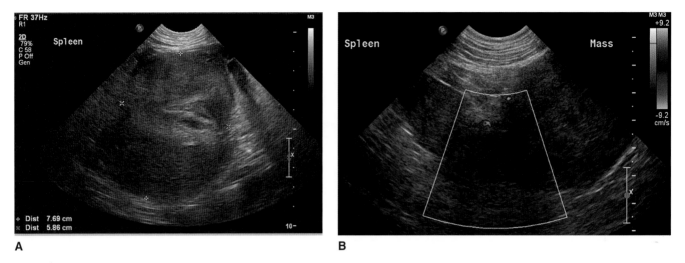

**FIGURE 24.25** Sagittal (long axis) ultrasound images of a 11-year-old German shepherd with palpable abdominal mass. A large lobulated heterogeneous mass with multiple anechoic thin-walled regions is present in the splenic tail (**A**). On color Doppler evaluation of the mass, there was evidence of minimal blood supply within the mass (**B**). A moderate amount of peritoneal effusion was present. Histopathology of the mass confirmed hematoma. The peritoneal effusion was hemorrhagic.

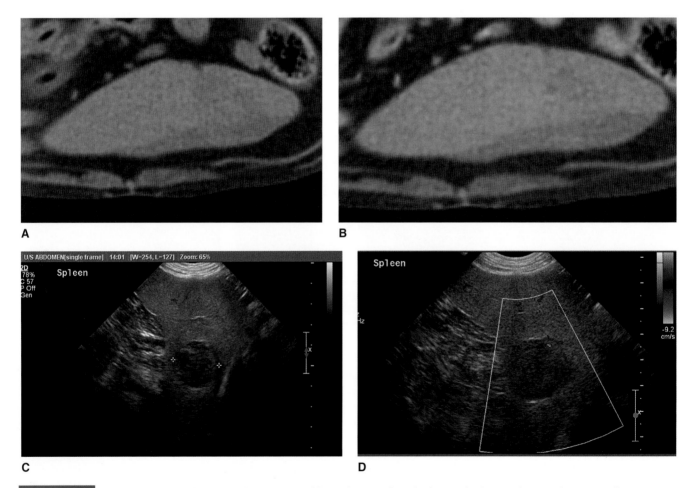

**FIGURE 24.26** Seven-year-old Rhodesian ridgeback presented for evaluation of a right thoracic limb mass diagnosed as mast cell tumor. Transverse plane precontrast (**A**) and postcontrast (**B**) CT images of the spleen. A 3 cm ill-defined hypoattenuating noncontrast-enhancing mass is present in the tail of the spleen (**A,B**). The mass becomes slightly more conspicuous on postcontrast images where it is seen against the contrast-enhancing splenic parenchyma (**B**). The mass is predominantly rounded and becomes linear shaped as it extends to the periphery of the spleen. (**C,D**) Sagittal (long axis) ultrasound images. A 3 cm rounded well-circumscribed hyperechoic mass was present (**C**). Upon color Doppler evaluation, there was no evidence of blood flow within the mass (**D**). On gross evaluation, the capsule of the spleen was lifted from normal splenic parenchyma by a large focus of massive hemorrhage.

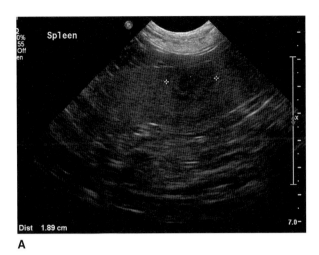

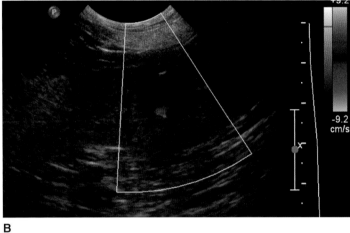

**A**                                           **B**

**FIGURE 24.27**   Sagittal (long axis) ultrasound images of a 9-year-old golden retriever presented with seizure. A round well-circumscribed heterogeneous hypoechoic nodule is present in the splenic body (**A**). Upon color Doppler evaluation, a mild amount of blood flow is present (**B**). Cytology from fine needle aspiration of the nodule diagnosed extramedullary hematopoiesis.

increases. On postcontrast images they appear as noncontrast-enhancing masses and are therefore easier to identify post contrast administration (Figure 24.26) [25].

## Extramedullary Hematopoiesis

Extramedullary hematopoiesis, the formation of blood cells outside the bone marrow, occurs frequently in the spleen in dogs and can manifest as nodules or masses and have similar variable US and CT findings as nodular hyperplasia or malignant lesions (Figures 24.27–24.32) [26]. A recent study evaluating the multiphase CT appearance of cytologically confirmed EMH found that the most common appearance of these lesions was multiple nodules that were hyperattenuating to the spleen in the arterial and portal phases, with approximately half (45%) of those lesions being hyperattenuating in the interstitial (venous) phase and the other half isoattenuating (Figure 24.32). Other appearances included multifocal nodular aspect, a mass, diffuse heterogeneous parenchyma, and normal spleen [22]. Diffuse or focal changes may be present and there is usually splenomegaly. As with nodular hyperplasia, these are common lesions in dogs so focal splenic lesions in dogs should not be assumed to be malignant based on imaging alone.

## Abscess

Splenic abscesses are very uncommon. Radiographically, there may be ill-defined or irregular accumulations of gas within the spleen with or without a visible mass, splenomegaly or a mass associated with the spleen in combination with peritoneal effusion without the presence of gas [38–40]. They have been associated with *Clostridium* spp., *Klebsiella pneumoniae*, *Enterococcus* spp., and *Staphylococcus* infection [39]. On US, abscesses can appear as poorly marginated hypoechoic or hyperechoic lesions

or complex masses of mixed echogenicity (Figure 24.33) [38, 40]. If gas is present, multiple small hyperechoic foci associated with reverberation will be seen [38]. On CT, abscesses appear as focal well-circumscribed rim-enhancing masses with multiple gas-attenuating regions within. Pneumoperitoneum and fat stranding have been reported in association with a splenic abscess in a dog with widespread hemangiosarcoma metastasis [29].

## Splenic Thrombosis

Splenic vein thrombosis is often found as an incidental finding without associated clinical signs or any other splenic changes. However, a variety of conditions have been associated with splenic vein thrombosis including neoplasia, corticosteroid administration, systemic inflammatory response, disseminated intravascular

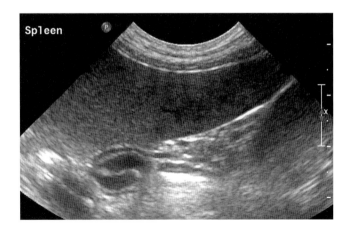

**FIGURE 24.28**   Sagittal (long axis) ultrasound image of a 9-year-old bulldog with history of multiple low to intermediate grade mast cell tumors. Multiple ill-defined hypoechoic nodules are present in the spleen. Cytology from fine needle aspiration of the nodules diagnosed extramedullary hematopoiesis.

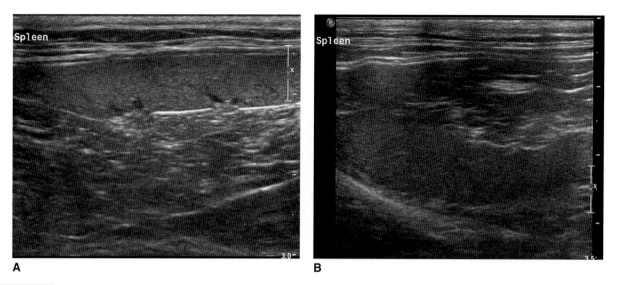

**FIGURE 24.29** (**A,B**) Sagittal (long axis) ultrasound images of a 10-year-old domestic shorthair presented with a mass in the cranial abdomen. The spleen is moderately enlarged with rounded margins and normal echogenicity and texture. Cytology from fine needle aspiration of the spleen diagnosed extramedullary hematopoiesis.

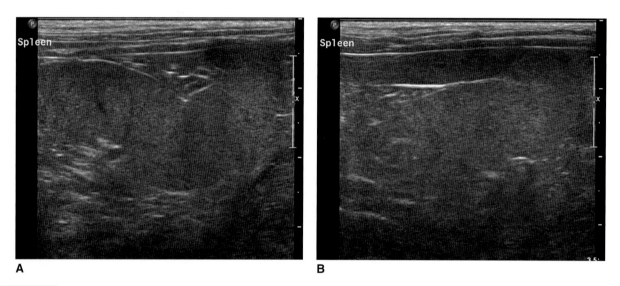

**FIGURE 24.30** (**A,B**) Sagittal (long axis) ultrasound images of a 9-year-old domestic shorthair presented for suspect lymphoma. The spleen is moderately enlarged with rounded margins and normal echogenicity and texture and folding upon itself. Cytology from fine needle aspiration of the spleen diagnosed extramedullary hematopoiesis.

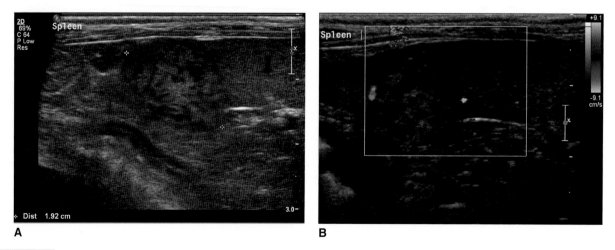

**FIGURE 24.31** Sagittal (long axis) ultrasound images of a 7-year-old Pomeranian. A large heterogeneous mass with multiple anechoic regions within is present in the head of the spleen, causing bulging of the splenic capsule (**A**). Upon color Doppler evaluation, there is no blood flow within the mass (**B**). Cytology from fine needle aspiration of the splenic mass diagnosed extramedullary hematopoiesis and lymphoid hyperplasia.

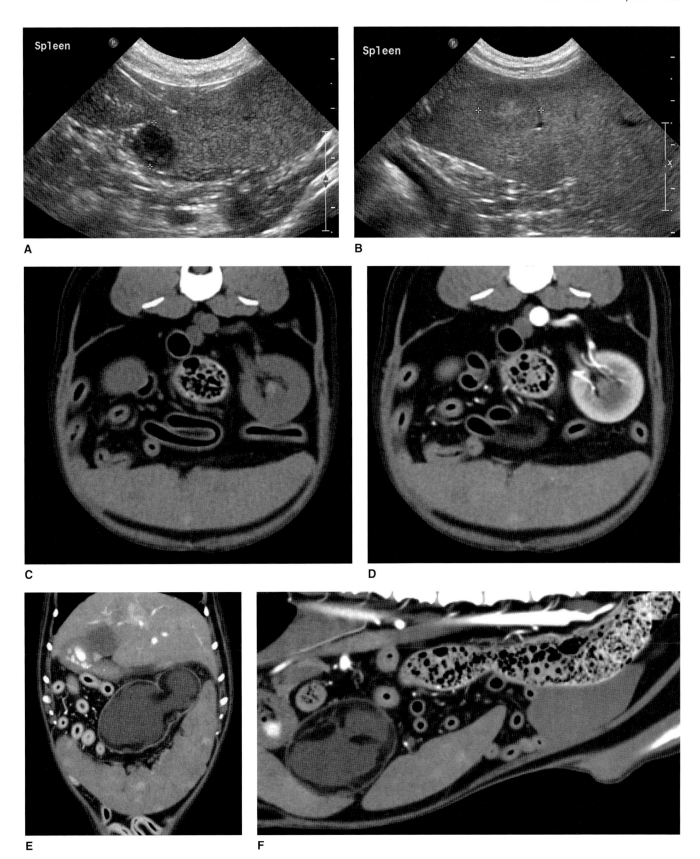

**FIGURE 24.32** Sagittal (long axis) ultrasound images of a 9-year-old Labrador with several weeks onset of lethargy. Multiple hypoechoic and hyperechoic nodules are present throughout the spleen (**A,B**), one of which has a target appearance with a hyperechoic center surrounded by a hypoechoic region (**B**). Transverse plane precontrast (**C**) and postcontrast (**D**), dorsal (**E**), and sagittal (**F**) plane postcontrast CT images. Multiple isoattenuating and hyperattenuating (compared to splenic parenchyma) nodules are present on precontrast images (**C**), some with mild contrast enhancement (**D–F**). The spleen is diffusely enlarged, likely secondary to general anesthesia. In addition, the patient had a fat- and fluid-attenuating mass in the cranial abdomen and multiple gastric and duodenal foreign material. Cytology from fine needle aspiration of the target-appearing splenic nodule diagnosed extramedullary hematopoiesis.

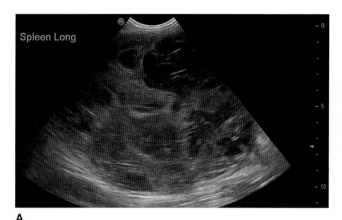

A

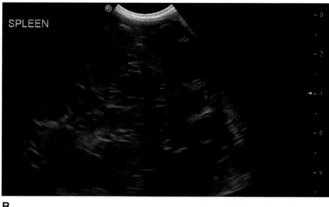

B

**FIGURE 24.33** (**A,B**) Sagittal (long axis) ultrasound images of a 12-year-old mixed-breed Labrador retriever presented with lethargy and fever. A large intraabdominal mass was palpated at the rDVM. A large complex cavitated mass with multiple anechoic regions and hyperechoic septa is present in the body and tail of the spleen. On color Doppler evaluation, the mass was highly vascular with multiple blood vessels being traced between the mass and splenic parenchyma. A marked amount of peritoneal effusion was present. Multiple cavitated masses were present in the liver and left kidney. On cytology based on fine needle aspiration of the splenic mass, suppurative inflammation with bacterial sepsis was diagnosed, consistent with an abscess. The patient was suspected to have underlying multicentric neoplasia.

coagulation, pancreatitis, and immune-mediated diseases [41, 42]. In a study evaluating 80 dogs with splenic vein thrombosis, the majority had neoplasia as a concurrent disease process from which lymphoma was the most common tumor. The most common immune-mediated disease was immune-mediated hemolytic anemia. Concurrent splenic infarcts were present in 33% of dogs in the study [41]. It is important therefore to check for underlying disease in dogs with splenic vein thrombosis.

On US, splenic vein thrombosis will appear as a nonmovable hyperechoic focus within the lumen of the splenic vein (Figures 24.16, 24.34, and 24.35) [43]. Doppler US should be used to differentiate slow turbulent echogenic blood flow from true thrombosis [42]. On CT, splenic thrombosis would be expected to appear as a round intraluminal filling defect [44].

## Infarction

Splenic infarct can occur secondary to thrombosis, embolism, torsion or systemic disease. Multiple concurrent diseases is common, including hypercoagulable diseases, neoplasia or thrombosis secondary to cardiac disease [45]. On US, affected areas commonly appear as a wedge-shaped or triangular, sharply demarcated region of hypoechogenicity (Figure 24.36). Most commonly, the ventral extremity of the spleen is affected [45]. These areas will demonstrate reduced or absent blood flow upon color Doppler evaluation. On CT, infarcted spleen can be iso- or hypoattenuating and lacking enhancement on postcontrast images.

## Myelolipomas

These are strongly hyperechoic nodules in the mesenteric border of the spleen, commonly seen adjacent to the splenic vein on US examinations (Figures 24.37 and 24.38). They may have acoustic shadowing and can be solitary or encompass the entire splenic parenchyma [1, 46]. These lesions are benign and common,

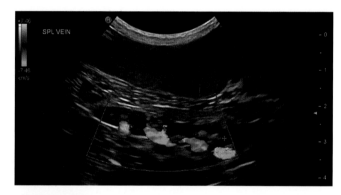

**FIGURE 24.34** Sagittal (long axis) ultrasound image of a 8-year-old miniature schnauzer diagnosed with multicentric lymphoma stage IVb. Multiple well-defined hyperechoic structures are present in the lumen of the splenic vein, partially occluding the blood flow, representing thrombi.

especially in older dogs and cats. Due to their characteristic US appearance, sampling of these lesions is usually not undertaken.

## Mineralization

Mineralization of the splenic parenchyma may be seen representing dystrophic calcification in association with metabolic conditions such as Cushing' disease or chronic hepatitis, abscesses, hematomas or neoplastic masses (Figure 24.39) [1].

# Diffuse Splenic Changes

## Splenomegaly

Splenomegaly can be caused by a variety of factors, including inflammatory changes, infectious or infiltrative disease,

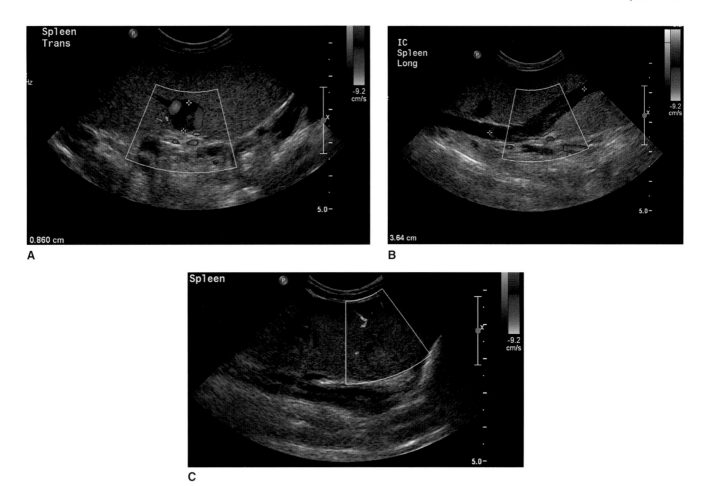

**FIGURE 24.35** Ultrasound images of a 13-year-old greyhound presented with ataxia and weight loss. A large hyperechoic structure is present in the lumen of an intraparenchymal splenic vessel occupying almost approximately 80% of the diameter of the lumen (**A,B**). Upon color Doppler evaluation, this structure is confirmed to be nonmobile. Blood flow is present in the splenic parenchyma adjacent to the affected vessel (**C**). In addition, the spleen is moderately enlarged with a mottled parenchyma. Multiple small ill-defined hypoechoic and hyperechoic nodules are present (not shown). Necropsy confirmed intraparenchymal splenic arterial thrombosis. Multiple other small splenic arteries had thrombus within. Histopathologically, the most significant findings in this patient were a pituitary adenoma and parathyroid carcinoma.

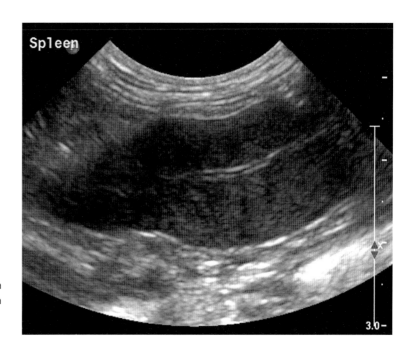

**FIGURE 24.36** Sagittal (long axis) ultrasound image of a 14-year-old mixed-breed dog presented with pancytopenia and lethargy. A focal well-demarcated wedge-shaped hypoechoic region is present in the spleen.

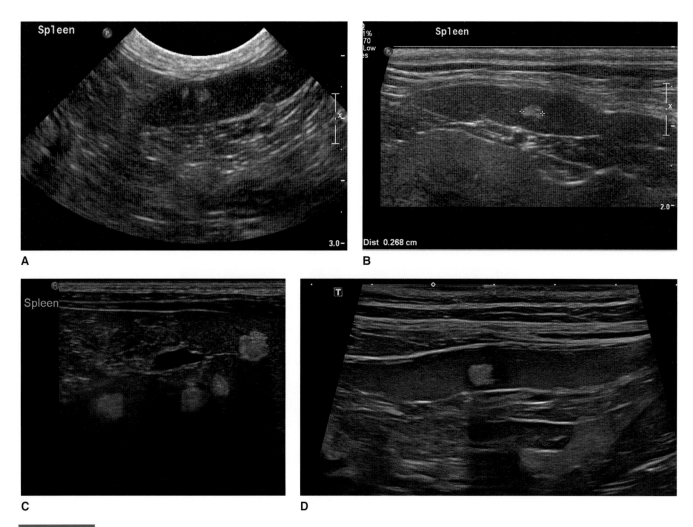

**FIGURE 24.37** Sagittal (long axis) ultrasound images of four cats presented for conditions unrelated to the spleen. Round well-circumscribed hyperechoic nodules are present in the spleen (**A–D**). Some of the nodules have an associated acoustic shadowing (**C,D**). This appearance is characteristic of myelolipomas, an incidental finding. In cat **C** there is also splenomegaly and folding of the spleen.

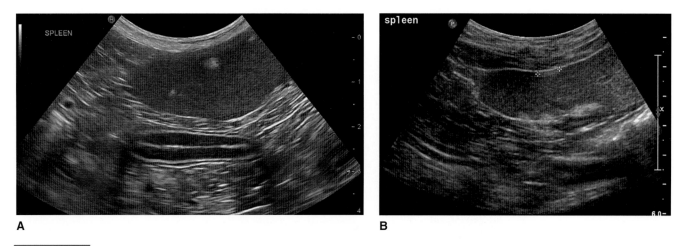

**FIGURE 24.38** (**A,B**) Sagittal (long axis) ultrasound images of two dogs presented for conditions unrelated to the spleen. Multiple well-circumscribed variably shaped hyperechoic nodules are present in the spleen of each dog, characteristic of myelolipomas, an incidental finding.

splenic torsion, and congestion secondary to anesthesia/sedation, portal hypertension or congestive heart failure. It is a subjective assessment with radiographs, ultrasound, and computed tomography. In general, splenomegaly results in dorsal and caudal displacement of the small intestines on lateral radiographic views along with rounded, thickened margins of the spleen. On ventrodorsal views, the small intestines may be displaced to the right or left if the body and/or tail are enlarged,

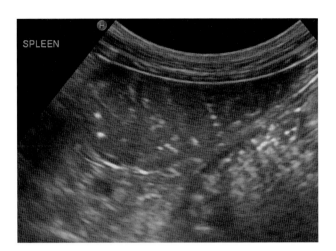

**FIGURE 24.39**   Sagittal (long axis) ultrasound image of a 15-year-old rat terrier presented with a caudal ventral abdominal wall abscess. The patient has unregulated diabetes mellitus. Multiple hyperechoic linear shaped structures are present in the spleen representing mineralization compatible with chronic endocrinopathy.

and cranial displacement of the stomach may occur if the head of the spleen is enlarged (Figure 24.40). The margins remain smooth but the thickness increases and the borders become rounded. In cats, splenomegaly is presumed if the body and tail are seen on the lateral view (Figure 24.41) [2].

A variety of anesthetic drugs are known to cause splenic congestion, including acepromazine and thiopental [47]. Propofol was shown to not cause splenic enlargement in a group of healthy beagles [47]. The effects of butorphanol and dexmedetomidine during contrast-enhanced US of the spleen were evaluated in six healthy beagles [48]. Dexmedetomidine was found to reduce the splenic enhancement causing diffuse parenchymal hypoechogenicity during the entire exam whereas butorphanol did not affect the perfusion of the spleen; therefore the use of butorphanol was recommended if sedation is necessary for splenic contrast ultrasound [48].

Sevofluorane anesthesia and blood donation did not subjectively change the splenic size, echogenicity or echotexture on ultrasonographic evaluation of the spleen in 60 healthy

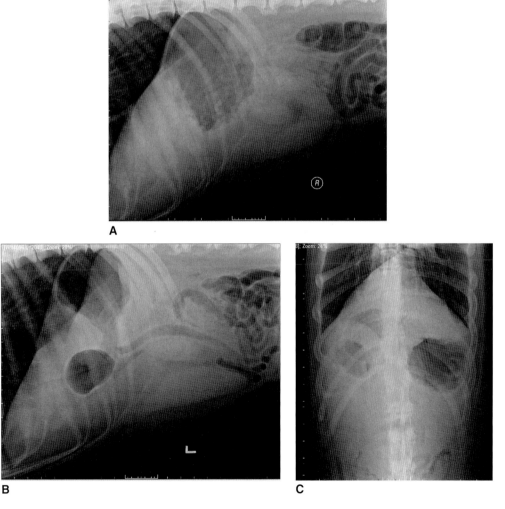

**A**

**B**

**C**

**FIGURE 24.40**   Right (**A**), left (**B**), and ventrodorsal (**C**) radiographs of a 6-year-old Great Dane sedated with acepromazine. The spleen is rounded and moderately enlarged, causing cranial displacement of the stomach and caudal displacement of the small intestines. On the VD view, a large portion of the spleen can be seen in the right cranial abdomen caudal to the pylorus, creating a mass effect. The patient was suspected to have splenic torsion based on radiographic and clinical findings.

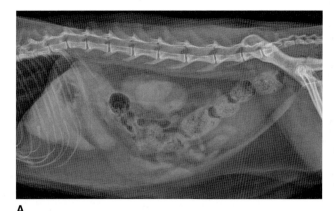

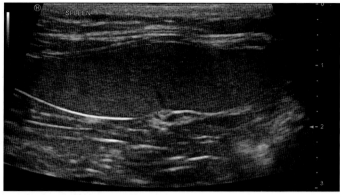

**A**

**B**

**FIGURE 24.41** Right lateral view and sagittal (long axis) ultrasound image of a 9-year-old Ragdoll. The spleen has rounded margins and is visible on the lateral view (**A**). On US, the spleen is subjectively moderately enlarged with normal echotexture and measured 1.1 cm in thickness (**B**). Fine needle aspiration of the spleen yielded normal spleen.

cats [49]. A recent study evaluated the radiographic and ultrasonographic splenic size in 15 healthy cats following five sedative drugs or drug combinations: acepromazine alone, dexmedetomidine alone, butorphanol alone, a combination of dexmedetomidine, butorphanol and ketamine, and a combination of midazolam and butorphanol, and found that acepromazine resulted in a significant increase in splenic size in both radiographs and ultrasound for up to three hours post sedation [50]. With butorphanol alone, there was no significant change in splenic size and with dexmedetomidine and the two combinations of drugs there was a trend toward splenic enlargement [50].

A study evaluated the effects of multiple anesthetic drugs on canine splenic volume using CT [51]. In this study, acepromazine, thiopental, and propofol resulted in splenomegaly, dexmedetomidine did not alter splenic volume, and hydromorphone slightly decreased splenic volume [51]. A similar study evaluated the effect of alfaxalone on spleen volume in dogs using CT and found that splenic volume was significantly increased at 15 minutes and 30 minutes after alfaxalone administration [52].

## Torsion

Torsion is typically seen in large- or giant-breed dogs, particularly German shepherd or Great Dane, and is commonly associated with gastric dilatation-volvulus. The spleen is usually severely enlarged and commonly there is peritoneal effusion [44, 53–56]. Radiographic signs include increased thickness and rounding of splenic margins and, most importantly, abnormal position of the spleen with loss of visualization of the body of the spleen in the left cranial abdomen on the ventrodorsal view [57]. A large reverse C-shaped soft tissue opaque midabdominal mass may be seen on both lateral and ventrodorsal views (Figures 24.42 and 24.43). If necrosis or gas-producing bacteria are present, regions of gas may be seen within the parenchyma [54, 57]. With US, besides enlargement, the spleen usually has a characteristic coarse lacy appearance. Use of Doppler is of paramount

importance to confirm lack of blood flow within the splenic vessels (Figures 24.42–24.44). Echogenic thrombi may also be detected within the splenic vessels [54, 58]. It is important to consider that these findings can also be seen in cases of lymphoma with malignant thrombosis. A hyperechoic triangular perivenous sign may be seen with torsion corresponding to invagination of mesenteric tissue. Care must be taken not to confuse this sign with myelolipomas [59].

In a case report of isolated splenic torsion evaluated with CT, the spleen was enlarged and less attenuating than the liver on precontrast images. The rotated pedicle was seen as a whirled focus of soft tissue-containing vessels in the midabdomen. Following contrast administration, the spleen did not enhance [55]. In a more recent study, the CT appearance of splenic torsion was described in eight dogs that had surgical confirmation of torsion [44]. The CT characteristics included enlarged folded C-shaped spleen (8/8), rounded spleen (7/8) with subjectively no parenchymal or vascular enhancement (6/8) and peritoneal effusion (6/8). A whirl sign, as described in the previously mentioned study, was seen in 7/8 cases but in this more recent study the whirl sign was noted to have a strong hyperattenuating center on precontrast images in 5/7 cases, all of which had complete torsion. This hyperattenuating center was attributed to represent hyperattenuation of vessels due to arterial or venous thrombosis (Figure 24.45) [44].

A recent study described chronic splenic torsion in a dog with an accessory spleen. In the study, the abnormal accessory spleen was misdiagnosed as a liver torsion. The study highlights that a normal spleen does not rule out splenic torsion in a dog [60]. Another recent study described the use of US and CT to diagnose complete splenic duplication, torsion and splenic vein hypertension [61].

## Primary and Secondary Neoplasia

Tumors that can cause diffuse splenic changes include lymphoma, mast cell tumor, histiocytic sarcoma, hemangioma,

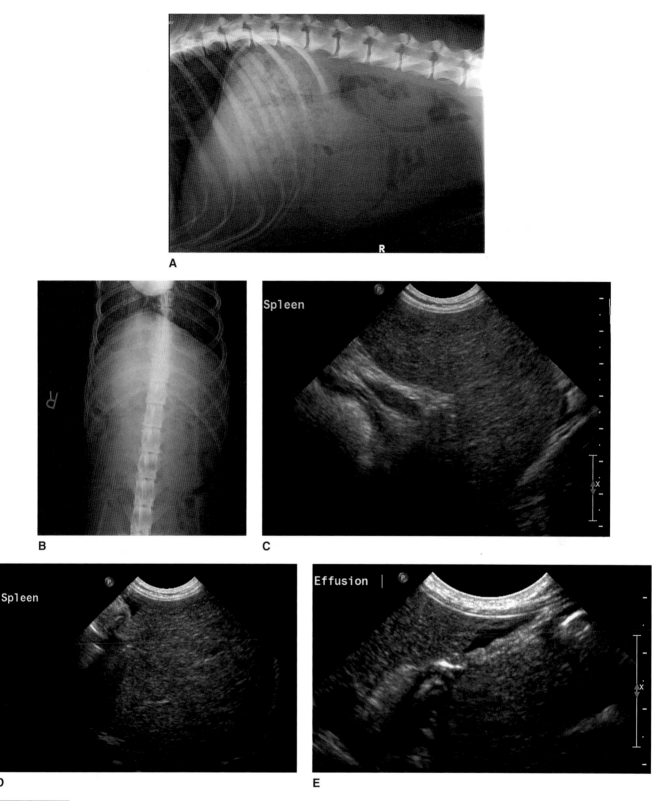

**FIGURE 24.42** Right and ventrodorsal radiographs of a 5-year-old German shepherd presented with history of weight loss, lethargy, and abnormal behavior. The spleen is severely enlarged, appearing as a reversed C-shaped mass on the right lateral view (**A**) and as a midabdominal soft tissue opaque mass on the VD view (**B**). The spleen is causing caudal and dorsal displacement of the small intestines. There is generalized poor peritoneal detail. (**C–E**) Sagittal (long axis) ultrasound images. The spleen is enlarged with rounded lobular margins and has a classic lacy appearance with multiple hypoechoic areas interspersed with linear shaped hyperechoic foci (**C,D**). A mild volume of peritoneal effusion was present (**D, E**). Not demonstrated in the images but present were multiple triangular-shaped hyperechoic regions in the splenic hilus in close proximity to the splenic vein. Splenic torsion was confirmed on histopathology.

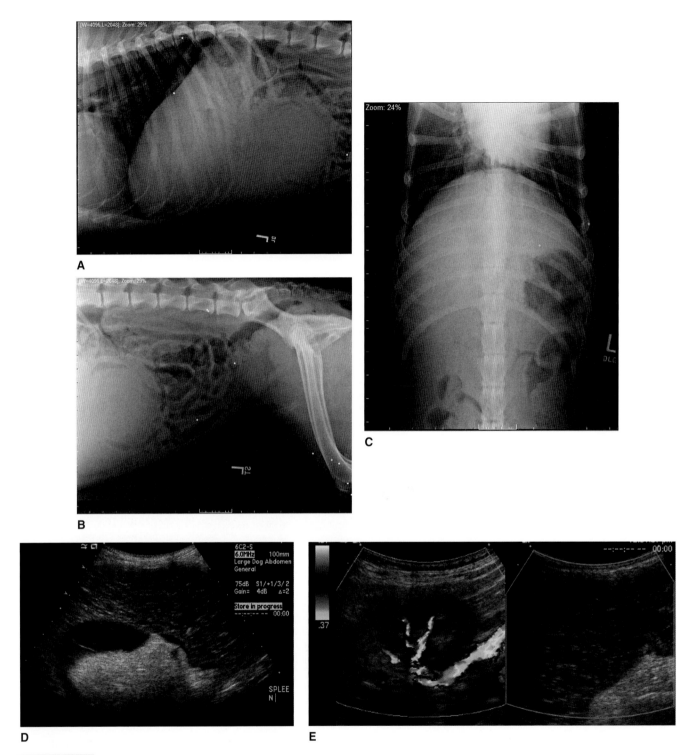

**FIGURE 24.43** Left and ventrodorsal radiographs of a 5-year-old German shepherd presented with decreased appetite and weight loss. A large rounded well-defined soft tissue opaque mass resembling a reversed C-shape is present in the cranial abdomen (**A–C**). The mass causes dorsal and left displacement of the gastric axis and caudal displacement of the small intestines. There is generalized poor peritoneal detail. (**D,E**) Sagittal (long axis) ultrasound images. The spleen is markedly enlarged and diffusely hypoechoic with a classic lacy appearance. A large focus of hyperechoic fat adjacent to a hypoechoic fusiform-shaped area is present near to the spleen, presumed to be the site of torsion (**D**). Upon color Doppler interrogation, no flow was detected in the splenic parenchyma or vessels in the hilar region (**E**, right image; left image is the left kidney to demonstrate color Doppler flow). No peritoneal effusion was present. On surgery, the spleen was large with torsion in an upside down "u" shape spanning the whole width of the abdomen. Splenic torsion was confirmed on histopathology.

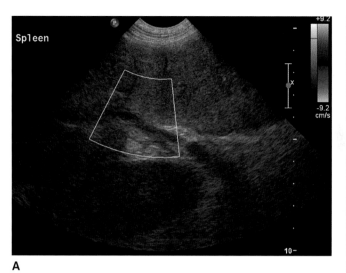

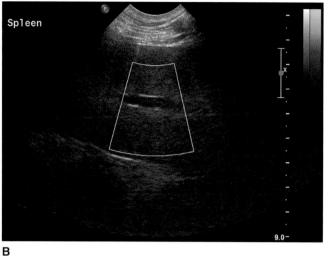

**A** **B**

**FIGURE 24.44** Sagittal (long axis) ultrasound images of a 5-year-old mastiff presented with history of vomiting, uncomfortable abdomen, and anorexia. The spleen is enlarged with rounded margins and folding upon itself and diffusely mottled. Upon color (**A**) and power (**B**) Doppler evaluation, there was no evidence of blood flow within the splenic vein or throughout the splenic parenchyma. A moderate amount of peritoneal effusion was present, not depicted in the images. On histopathology, diffuse severe congestion of the spleen consistent with occlusion of vascular drainage resulting from splenic torsion was found.

and hemangiosarcoma (diffuse nodular changes). Radiographically, the spleen will be enlarged and may have changes in its contour/margins. Lymphoma has a large range of ultrasonographic changes, including a normal appearance, multiple variably sized hypoechoic nodules, diffuse hypoechogenicity or hyperechogenicity or focal or multifocal complex masses (see Figures 24.10–24.14) [62].

The classic US appearance of splenic lymphoma in dogs has been described as a Swiss cheese or honeycomb pattern characterized by the presence of diffuse small hypoechoic nodules [31]. Mast cell tumor likewise can result in no US changes or a variable range of changes in both dogs and cats (see Figures 24.15 and 24.16) [16, 26]. The sensitivity of US to detect mast cell tumor in the spleen of dogs was low, at 43%, in one study and the authors recommend performing splenic aspiration regardless of the US appearance in dogs with aggressive mast cell tumor [19].

A study evaluating the use of CT for staging mast cell tumor in the liver and spleen in dogs found that four out of five dogs with liver or splenic metastasis had an abnormal spleen, with two having focal hypoattenuating nodular changes, two having a diffusely heterogeneous splenic parenchyma, and one of the dogs having a normal spleen [30]. In the same study, four out of those five dogs had a normal hepatic parenchyma and the authors concluded that sampling of the liver and spleen should be performed in the absence of CT findings in these organs during the staging of mast cell tumors.

Another study evaluating the sensitivity and specificity of US to detect hepatic and splenic abnormalities for the diagnosis of lymphoma found 100% sensitivity of US for detecting lymphoma in the spleen. Therefore the authors recommended performing fine needle aspirates of the spleen only if the organ is abnormal on US, whereas they suggest fine needle aspiration of the liver should be performed regardless of ultrasonographic characteristics, even if the liver is normal on US [18].

## Immune-Mediated Disease

Immune-mediated hemolytic anemia and immune-mediated thrombocytopenia can cause generalized splenomegaly with US or CT. splenic vein thrombosis may be seen [41].

## Extramedullary Hematopoiesis

Extramedullary hematopoiesis can cause focal or diffuse lesions with a variable range of US and CT patterns (see section on focal changes).

## Bacterial, Fungal or Parasitic Infection

Infections may cause secondary splenomegaly with normal or reduced echogenicity on US. Histoplasmosis in cats often causes splenomegaly and a hypoechoic spleen. Discrete nodules can also be seen [63]. With feline infectious peritonitis, the spleen may have normal echogenicity or be hypoechoic and enlarged, and peritoneal effusion is usually present [26]. A spleen with normal echogenicity was more common in a study evaluating 16 cats. *Bartonella henselae* has been reported to cause splenic vasculitis, thrombosis, and infarction with a hypoechoic splenic parenchyma in a dog [64].

Infectious processes that can cause splenic changes are many and include babesiosis, erlichiosis, leishmaniasis, toxoplasmosis, granulomatous disease, and hepatozoonosis, among others [65].

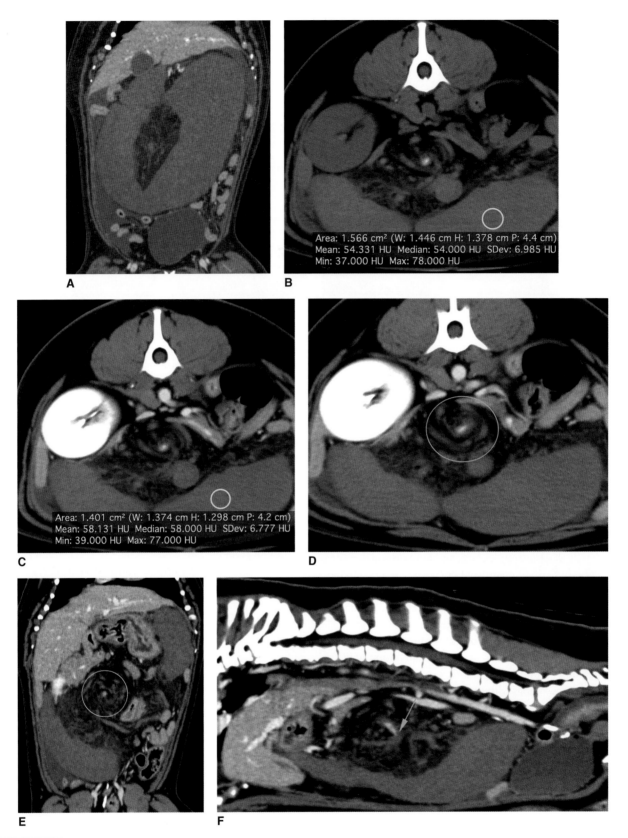

**FIGURE 24.45** Two-year-old English bulldog presented for progressive worsening lethargy and anemia. On A-FAST ultrasound (no images available), there was moderate peritoneal free fluid that was aspirated and resembled blood. A mass-like structure resembling the spleen was also seen on A-FAST. Dorsal plane postcontrast CT images (**A,E**); transverse plane precontrast (**B**) and postcontrast (**C**) CT images; transverse plane postcontrast CT image (**D**); sagittal plane postcontrast CT image (**F**). The spleen is severely enlarged and C-shaped (**A**) with negligible enhancement (HU precontrast = 54, HU postcontrast = 58) and generalized homogeneous parenchyma (**B,C**). A "whirl sign" is present as multiple vessels and soft tissue structures travel around a rotated pedicle, creating a "mass-like" structure with a strongly hyperattenuating center representing the splenic artery (circle, **D,E**). There is abrupt occlusion of the contrast medium in the splenic artery as it travels toward the spleen (arrow, **F**). A moderate amount of peritoneal effusion is present as well as multiple strands of fluid surrounding the spleen (all figures). The patient had exploratory laparotomy confirming a splenic torsion. On histopathology, there was diffuse marked splenic congestion with siderotic plaques and multifocal marked acute hemorrhage of the omentum.

# Summary

The most common splenic abnormalities and their imaging appearance have been described. As a rule of thumb, splenic masses and nodules cannot be finally diagnosed with imaging alone and sampling is needed. These lesions are very common in old dogs and care must be taken not to condemn those patients without sampling or identifying the presence of other imaging abnormalities suggestive of malignancy. Some disease processes can be more confidently diagnosed with imaging, such as myelolipomas, infarct, thrombosis, and torsion. Ultrasound-guided fine needle aspiration of the spleen is performed routinely and the incidence of complications is extremely low. The reader is encouraged to refer to the referenced literature for additional information.

# References

1. Nyland, T.G. and Mattoon, J.S. (2015). Spleen. In: *Small Animal Diagnostic Ultrasound*, 3e (ed. J.S. Mattoon and T.G. Nyland). St Louis, MO: Elsevier.

2. Armbrust, L. (2009). The spleen. In: *BSAVA Manual of Canine and Feline Abdominal Imaging* (ed. R. O'Brien and F. Barr). Quedgeley, UK: British Small Animal Veterinary Association.

3. Rossi, F., Leone, V.F., Vignoli, M. et al. (2008). Use of contrast-enhanced ultrasound for characterization of focal splenic lesions. *Vet. Radiol. Ultrasound* 49: 154–164.

4. Kutara, K., Seki, M., Ishigaki, K. et al. (2017). Triple-phase helical computed tomography in dogs with solid splenic masses. *J. Vet. Med. Sci.* 79 (11): 1870–1877.

5. Johnson, K.L., Porter, E.G., and Berry, C.R. (2017). Analysis of feline splenic radiographic measurements and their correlation to ultrasonographic measurements. *J. Feline Med. Surg.* 19 (10): 985–991.

6. Ivancic, M., Long, F., and Seiler, G.S. (2009). Contrast harmonic ultrasonography of splenic masses and associated liver nodules in dogs. *J. Am. Vet. Med. Assoc.* 234: 88–94.

7. Nakamura, K., Sasaki, N., Murakami, M. et al. (2010). Contrast-enhanced ultrasonography for characterization of focal splenic lesions in dogs. *J. Vet. Intern. Med.* 24: 1290–1297.

8. Ohlerth, S., Dennler, M., Rüefli, E. et al. (2008). Contrast harmonic imaging characterization of canine splenic lesions. *J. Vet. Intern. Med.* 22 (5): 1095–1102.

9. Ohlerth, S., Rüefli, E., Poirier, V. et al. (2007). Contrast harmonic imaging of the normal canine spleen. *Vet. Radiol. Ultrasound* 48 (5): 451–456.

10. Rossi, F., Fina, C., Stock, E. et al. (2016). Effect of sedation on contrast-enhanced ultrasonography of the spleen in healthy dogs. *Vet. Radiol. Ultrasound* 57 (3): 276–281.

11. Taeymans, O. and Penninck, D.G. (2011). Contrast enhanced sonographic assessment of feeding vessels as a discriminator between malignant vs. benign focal splenic lesions. *Vet. Radiol. Ultrasound* 52: 457–461.

12. Specchi, S. and Bertolini, G. (2020). CT angiography identifies collaterals in dogs with splenic vein obstruction and presumed regional splenic vein hypertension. *Vet. Radiol. Ultrasound* 61: 636–640.

13. Hwang, Y., Noh, D., Choi, S. et al. (2020). Changes of ultrasonographic pattern of the spleen examined with a high-frequency linear transducer during growth in puppies. *Vet. Radiol. Ultrasound* 1–6.

14. Hammond, T.N. and Pesillo-Crosby, S.A. (2008). Prevalence of hemangiosarcoma in anemic dogs with a splenic mass and hemoperitoneum requiring a transfusion: 71 cases (2003–2005). *J. Am. Vet. Med. Assoc.* 232 (4): 553–558.

15. Eberle, N., von Babo, V., Nolte, I. et al. (2012). Splenic masses in dogs. Part 1: epidemiologic, clinical characteristics as well as histopathologic diagnosis in 249 cases (2000–2011). *Tierarztl Prax Ausg K Kleintiere Heimtiere* 40 (4): 250–260.

16. Sato, A.F. and Solano, M. (2004). Ultrasonographic findings in abdominal mast cell disease: a retrospective study of 19 patients. *Vet. Radiol. Ultrasound* 45: 51–57.

17. Cruz-Arámbulo, R., Wrigley, R., and Powers, B. (2004). Sonographic features of histiocytic neoplasms in the canine abdomen. *Vet. Radiol. Ultrasound* 45: 554.

18. Crabtree, A.C., Spangler, E., Beard, D., and Smith, A. (2010). Diagnostic accuracy of gray-scale ultrasonography for the detection of hepatic and splenic lymphoma in dogs. *Vet. Radiol. Ultrasound* 51 (6): 661–664.

19. Book, A.P., Fidel, J., Wills, T. et al. (2011). Correlation of ultrasound findings, liver and spleen cytology, and prognosis in the clinical staging of high metastatic risk canine mast cell tumors. *Vet. Radiol. Ultrasound* 52 (5): 548–554.

20. Spangler, W.L. and Culbertson, M.R. (1992). Prevalence, type, and importance of splenic diseases in dogs: 1,480 cases (1985–1989). *J. Am. Vet. Med. Assoc.* 200 (6): 829–834.

21. Ramirez, S., Douglass, J.P., and Robertson, I.D. (2002). Ultrasonographic features of canine abdominal malignant histiocytosis. *Vet. Radiol. Ultrasound* 43: 167–170.

22. Cordella, A., Caldin, M., and Bertolini, G. (2020). Splenic extramedullary hematopoiesis in dogs is frequently detected on multiphase multidetector-row CT as hypervascular nodules. *Vet. Radiol. Ultrasound* 61: 1–7.

23. Pintar, J., Breitschwerdt, E.B., Hardie, E.M., and Spaulding, K.A. (2003). Acute non-traumatic hemoabdomen in the dog: a retrospective analysis of 39 cases (1987–2001). *J. Am. Anim. Hosp. Assoc.* 39: 518–522.

24. Specchi, S., Auriemma, E., Morabito, S. et al. (2017). Evaluation of the computed tomographic "Sentinel Clot Sign" to dentify bleeding abdominal organs in dogs with hemoabdomen. *Vet. Radiol. Ultrasound* 58 (1): 18–22.

25. Kutara, K., Konno, T., Kondo, H. et al. (2017). Imaging diagnosis – ectopic spleen mimicking hepatic tumor with intra-abdominal metastases investigated via triple-phase helical computed tomography in a dog. *Vet. Radiol. Ultrasound* 58 (3): 26–30.

26. Hanson, J.A., Papageorges, M., Girard, E. et al. (2001). Ultrasonographic appearance of splenic disease in 101 cats. *Vet. Radiol. Ultrasound* 42: 441–445.

27. Cuccovillo, A. and Lamb, C.R. (2002). Cellular features of sonographic target lesions of the liver and spleen in 21 dogs and a cat. *Vet. Radiol. Ultrasound* 43: 275–278.

28. Ballegeer, E.A., Forres, L.J., Dickinson, R.M. et al. (2007). Correlation of ultrasonographic appearance of lesions and cytologic and histologic diagnoses in splenic aspirates from dogs and cats: 32 cases (2002–2005). *J. Am. Vet. Med. Assoc.* 230: 690–696.

29. Shanaman, M.M., Schwarz, T., Gal, A., and O'Brien, R.T. (2013). Comparison between survey radiography, B-mode ultrasonography, contrast-enhanced ultrasonography and contrast-enhanced multi-detector computed tomography findings in dogs with acute abdominal signs. *Vet. Radiol. Ultrasound* 54 (6): 591–604.

30. Hughes, J.R., Szladovits, B., and Drees, R. (2019). Abdominal CT evaluation of the liver and spleen for staging mast cell tumors in dogs yields nonspecific results. *Vet. Radiol. Ultrasound* 60: 306–315.

31. Wrigley, R.H., Konde, L.J., Park, R.D., and Lebel, J.L. (1988). Ultrasonographic features of splenic lymphosarcoma in dogs: 12 cases (1980–1986). *J. Am. Vet. Med. Assoc.* 193: 1565–1568.

32. Wrigley, R.H., Park, R.D., Konde, L.J. et al. (1988). Ultrasonographic features of splenic hemangiosarcoma in dogs: 18 cases (1980–1986). *J. Am. Vet. Med. Assoc.* 192: 1113.

33. Wrigley, R.H., Konde, L.J., Park, R.D. et al. (1989). Clinical features and diagnosis of splenic hematomas in dogs: 10 cases (1980–1987). *J. Am. Anim. Hosp. Assoc.* 25: 371.

34. Fife, W.D., Samii, V.F., Drost, W.T. et al. (2004). Comparison between malignant and nonmalignant splenic masses in dogs using contrast-enhanced computed tomography. *Vet. Radiol. Ultrasound* 45: 289–297.

35. Jones, I.D., Lamb, C.R., Drees, R. et al. (2016). Associations between dual-phase computed tomography features and histopathologic diagnosis in 52 dogs with hepatic or splenic masses. *Vet. Radiol. Ultrasound* 57 (2): 144–153.

36. Lee, M., Park, J., Choi, H. et al. (2018). Presurgical assessment of splenic tumors in dogs: a retrospective study of 57 cases (2012–2017). *J. Vet. Sci.* 19 (6): 827–834.

37. Patten, S.G., Boston, S.E., and Monteith, G.J. (2016). Outcome and prognostic factors for dogs with a histological diagnosis of splenic hematoma following splenectomy: 35 cases (2001–2013). *Can. Vet. J.* 57 (8): 842–846.

38. Ginel, P.J., Lucena, R., Arola, J. et al. (2001). Diffuse splenomegaly caused by splenic abscessation in a dog. *Vet. Rec.* 149 (11): 327–329.

39. Gaschen, L., Kircher, P., Venzin, C. et al. (2003). Imaging diagnosis: the abdominal air-vasculogram in a dog with splenic torsion and clostridial infection. *Vet. Radiol. Ultrasound* 44: 553–555.

40. Abdellatif, A., Gunther, C., Pepler, C., and Kramer, M. (2014). A rare case of splenic abscess with septic peritonitis in a German shepherd dog. *BMC Vet. Res.* 10: 201.

41. Laurenson, M.P., Hopper, K., Herrera, M.A., and Johnson, E.G. (2010). Concurrent diseases and conditions in dogs with splenic vein thrombosis. *J. Vet. Intern. Med.* 24 (6): 1298–1304.

42. Jaehwan, K. (2019). A case of acute splenic vein thrombosis in a dog. *J. Vet. Med. Sci.* 81 (10): 1492–1495.

43. Lamb, C.R., Wrigley, R.H., Simpson, K.W. et al. (1996). Ultrasonographic diagnosis of portal vein thrombosis in four dogs. *Vet. Radiol. Ultrasound* 37 (2): 121–129.

44. Hughes, J.R., Johnson, V.S., and Genain, M.-A. (2020). CT characteristics of primary splenic torsion in eight dogs. *Vet. Radiol. Ultrasound* 61: 261–268.

45. Hardie, E.M., Vaden, S.L., Spaulding, K., and Malarkey, D.E. (1995). Splenic infarction in 16 dogs: a retrospective study. *J. Vet. Intern. Med.* 9: 141–148.

46. Schwarz, L.A., Penninck, D.G., and Gliatto, J. (2001). Canine splenic myelolipomas. *Vet. Radiol. Ultrasound* 42: 347–348.

47. O'Brien, R.T., Waller, K.R., and Osgood, T.L. (2004). Sonographic features of drug-induced splenic congestion. *Vet. Radiol. Ultrasound* 45: 225–227.

48. Rossi, F., Rabba, S., Vignoli, M. et al. (2010). B-mode and contrast-enhanced sonographic assessment of accessory spleen in the dog. *Vet. Radiol. Ultrasound* 51 (2): 173–177.

49. Reese, S.L., Zekas, L.J., Iazbik, M.C. et al. (2013). Effect of sevoflurane anesthesia and blood donation on the sonographic appearance of the spleen in 60 healthy cats. *Vet. Radiol. Ultrasound* 54 (2): 168–175.

50. Auger, M., Fazio, C., de Swarte, M. et al. (2019). Administration of certain sedative drugs is associated with variation in sonographic and radiographic splenic size in healthy cats. *Vet. Radiol. Ultrasound* 60: 717–728.

51. Baldo, C.F., Garcia-Pereira, F.L., Nelson, N.C. et al. (2012). Effects of anesthetic drugs on canine splenic volume determined via computed tomography. *Am. J. Vet. Res.* 73 (11): 1715–1719.

52. Hasiuk, M.M.M., Garcia-Pereira, F.L., Berry, C.R., and Ellison, G.W. (2018). Effects of a single intravenous bolus injection of alfaxalone on canine splenic volume as determined by computed tomography. *Can. J. Vet. Res.* 82 (3): 203–207.

53. Neath, P.J., Brockman, D.J., and Saunders, H.M. (1997). Retrospective analysis of 19 cases of isolated torsion of the splenic pedicle in dogs. *J. Small Anim. Pract.* 38 (9): 387–392.

54. Konde, L.J., Wrigley, R.H., Lebel, J.L. et al. (1989). Sonographic and radiographic changes associated with splenic torsion in the dog. *Vet. Radiol. Ultrasound* 30: 41.

55. Patsikas, M.N., Rallis, T., Kladakis, S.E., and Dessiris, A.K. (2001). Computed tomography of isolated splenic torsion in a dog. *Vet. Radiol. Ultrasound* 42: 235–237.

56. DeGroot, W., Giuffrida, M.A., Rubin, J. et al. (2016). Primary splenic torsion in dogs: 102 cases (1992–2014). *J. Am. Vet. Med. Assoc.* 248 (6): 661–668.

57. Stickle, R.L. (1989). Radiographic signs of isolated splenic torsion in dogs: eight cases (1980–1987). *J. Am. Vet. Med. Assoc.* 194 (1): 103–106.

58. Saunders, H.M., Neath, P.I., and Brockman, D.J. (1998). B-mode and Doppler ultrasound imaging of the spleen with canine splenic torsion: a retrospective evaluation. *Vet. Radiol. Ultrasound* 39: 349–353.

59. Mai, W. (2006). The hilar perivenous hyperechoic triangle as a sign of acute splenic torsion in dogs. *Vet. Radiol. Ultrasound* 47: 487–491.

60. Mergl, J.C., Hanselman, B., and Kirsch, M. (2022). Chronic splenic torsion in a dog with an accessory spleen. *Can. Vet. J.* 63 (2): 147–151.

61. Battiato, P., Salgüero, R., Specchi, S., and Longo, M. (2022). Ultrasonographic and CT diagnosis of a complete splenic duplication with right splenic torsion and presumed regional splenic vein hypertension in a dog. *Vet. Radiol. Ultrasound* 63: E1–E5.

62. Lamb, C.R., Hartzband, L.E., Tidwell, A.S., and Pearson, S.H. (1991). Ultrasonographic findings in hepatic and splenic lymphosarcoma in dogs and cats. *Vet. Radiol. Ultrasound* 32: 117–120.

63. Atiee, G., Kvitko-White, H., Spaulding, K., and Johnson, M. (2014). Ultrasonographic appearance of histoplasmosis identified in the spleen in 15 cats. *Vet. Radiol. Ultrasound* 55 (3): 310–314.

64. Friedenberg, S.G., Balakrishnan, N., Guillaumin, J. et al. (2015). Splenic vasculitis, thrombosis, and infarction in a febrile dog infected with Bartonella henselae. *J. Vet. Emerg. Crit. Care* 25 (6): 789–794.

65. Ferri, F., Zini, E., Auriemma, E. et al. (2017). Splenitis in 33 dogs. *Vet. Pathol.* 54 (1): 147–154.

# CHAPTER 25

# Gastrointestinal Tract

**Seamus Hoey**

School of Veterinary Medicine, University College Dublin, Veterinary Science Centre, Dublin, Ireland

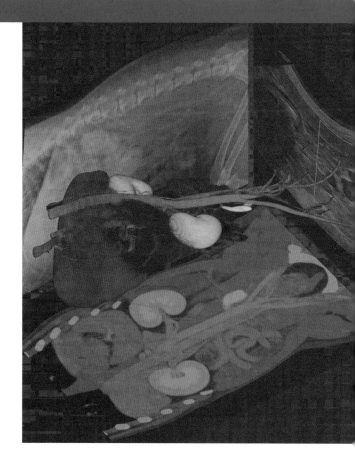

## Introduction

The gastrointestinal system is one of the most evaluated systems in small animal veterinary practice. A thorough clinical history and physical examination are critical in attempting to narrow down the area to be evaluated in these patients. The complexity of the anatomy and the varied complex disease processes involved in the patient's clinical problem can make assessment difficult. Radiography is an excellent survey tool for evaluating the gastrointestinal tract. With the addition of contrast medium, one can evaluate the gastrointestinal tract in a more comprehensive manner.

## Diagnostic Imaging Modalities

Radiography is routinely used in evaluating the gastrointestinal tract. Unfortunately, the fluid contents of the gastrointestinal lumen are soft tissue opaque, the same as the soft tissue opaque gastrointestinal wall. To improve our assessment of the gastrointestinal tract, we can use contrast radiography, whereby material of a different opacity is introduced into the gastrointestinal lumen. Gas opaque negative contrast medium (such as room air or carbon dioxide gas) can be introduced via tube into the esophagus, stomach, or colon. Mineral to metal opaque positive contrast medium (such as barium or iodine-based solutions) can be administered to assess function in real time via fluoroscopy or radiography, as well as the morphology of the lumen of the entire gastrointestinal tract. The risk of aspiration of positive contrast medium must be mentioned, as aspiration of barium may act as a physical barrier to gas exchange (Figure 25.1) whereas iodine may be associated with pneumonitis.

Ultrasonographic evaluation of the gastrointestinal tract is commonly done, replacing abdominal radiography in many institutions. However, the two imaging modalities are complementary and initial survey abdominal radiographs can help in dictating the course of the ultrasound examination.

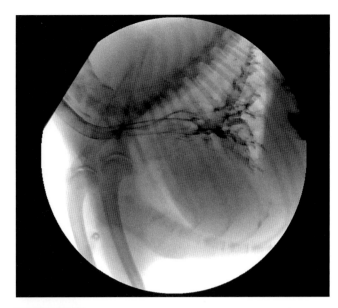

**FIGURE 25.1** Fluoroscopic image of the cranial thorax of a 6-year-old male pug, with difficulty swallowing and a history of cough. Barium contrast medium has been aspirated, coating the tracheal mucosal surface and extending into the proximal primary and secondary bronchi.

The wall of the esophagus, stomach, small and large intestines is composed of four layers: inner mucosa, submucosa, muscularis, and serosa. The high spatial resolution of ultrasound allows assessment of wall thickness, and the integrity of the wall layers.

Computed tomography (CT), with its speed of image acquisition and ability to image larger patients, is increasingly being employed in the workup of gastrointestinal cases, with and without the administration of intravenous or luminal contrast medium.

# Stomach

The stomach is a large tubular organ which extends between the caudal esophageal sphincter and the pyloric sphincter. It is located caudal to the liver and cranial to the colon, pancreas, spleen, and kidneys. The stomach is divided into fundus, body, and pylorus. The pyloric antrum continues to the pyloric sphincter and proximal duodenum.

The stomach is routinely evaluated using radiography and ultrasonography, radiography acting as a screening test for gastric disease and ultrasound yielding further information about mural and intraluminal changes. CT is being used more and more as an adjunct to these modalities in complicated or equivocal cases. In human radiology, magnetic resonance imaging (MRI) is being increasingly used for gastrointestinal imaging but is not routinely used in veterinary medicine.

Ultrasonographically, the gastric wall is composed of four layers, like the rest of the gastrointestinal tract: inner mucosa, submucosa, muscularis and serosal layers. The mucosal

surface is corrugated by indentations called *rugal folds* within the gastric fundus and orad gastric body but not within the pylorus. Due to the indentation of the mucosal rugal folds, the wall thickness must be measured at the thinnest point, which would be at the base of the rugal fold. The normal wall thickness should be 2–5 mm in the dog and 2–4 mm in the cat; however, it must be remembered that stomach filling will affect wall thickness. A limitation of ultrasound is the effect of gas dilation of the stomach leading to inability of ultrasound beam penetration.

Radiographically, normally the empty stomach is soft tissue opaque, and border effaces with the hepatic silhouette. With gas in the stomach, the gastric location can be better determined. In left lateral recumbency, gas moves freely into the gastric pylorus, pyloric antrum, and proximal duodenum. In right lateral recumbency, gas moves into the gastric fundus. In dorsal recumbency, gas moves into the gastric body. Lastly, in sternal recumbency, gas moves into the gastric body and pylorus. As such, each component of the stomach lumen can be evaluated if a moderate amount of gas is present in the gastric lumen.

The gastric axis is a line drawn from the gastric fundus to the gastric pylorus. On lateral view, this line should be within an angle parallel with the 10th ribs, or perpendicular to the long axis of the L2 vertebral body. On ventrodorsal or dorsoventral views, the gastric axis should be perpendicular to the vertebral column in the dog. In the cat, the stomach forms more of a "J-shape," with the pylorus located in a more caudal position relative to the fundus. Additionally, the pyloroduodenal junction is located close to midline in a cat and not along the right lateral body wall, as noted in a dog.

Contrast gastrography can be done using negative and/or positive contrast medium. As such, pneumogastrography can be done using an orogastric or nasogastric tube with the introduction of gas into the gastric lumen (2–20 mL/kg; Figure 25.2) [1].

Alternatively, positive contrast medium gastrography, either alone or as part of an upper gastrointestinal study, can be performed whereby in dogs <20 kg, 8–12 mL/kg of 30–60% w/v barium sulfate solution can be administered and in dogs >20 kg, 5–7 mL/kg of 30–60%w/v barium sulfate can be administered either by syringe or via orogastric tube [2]. Liquid barium contrast should progress through the stomach so that there is gastric emptying in the normal dog by 3 hours and in the normal cat by 1 hour [3].

Computed tomography is useful in investigation of the stomach in that superimposition is avoided and the differences between soft tissue- and fluid-attenuating material can be appreciated, especially post intravascular contrast administration with enhancement of the gastric wall.

## Gastric Dilation

Gastric dilation can be identified radiographically as a gas- or soft tissue opacity-filled stomach which extends caudal to the costal arch. The gastric fundus, recognized by the rugal folds

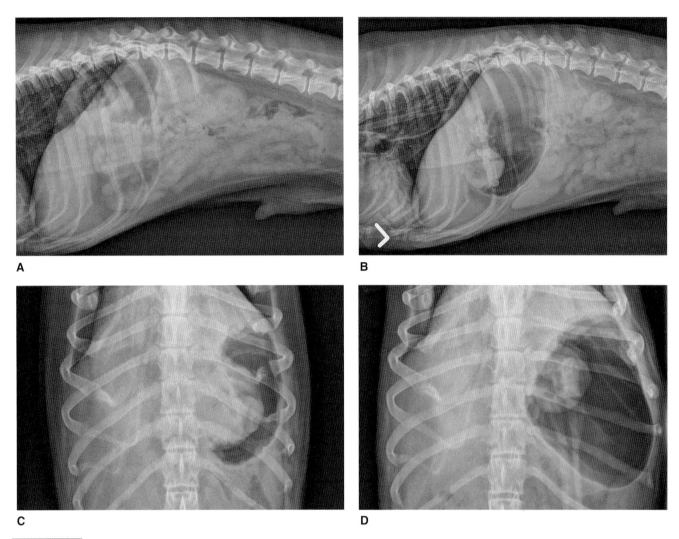

**FIGURE 25.2**   Left lateral and ventrodorsal views of the cranial abdomen of a 10-year-old male castrated dachshund with acute onset vomiting over the last 24 hours. The images are before (**A,C**) and after (**B,D**) nasogastric tube placement and gastric gas administration. A poorly defined soft tissue opaque rounded structure is within the gastric body, better highlighted after gas administration (pneumogastrography). This was retrieved and was a piece of blanket.

extending into the gastric lumen, remains in a normal position within the left dorsal abdomen. Gas distension of the stomach can be secondary to aerophagia secondary to anesthesia or sedation. The stomach can be filled with mixed soft tissue and gas opaque material, or well-defined ovoid-shaped soft tissue opaque material corresponding to food engorgement, or due to gastric outflow obstruction secondary to pyloric hypertrophy, gastritis, pyloric neoplasia or foreign bodies [4] (Figures 25.3 and 25.4).

## Gastric Dilation and Volvulus

Gastric dilation and volvulus (GDV) is an emergency condition in which the stomach is markedly gas dilated and subsequently rotates about its own axis. The pylorus and fundus are in an abnormal position, with the most common GDV being a 180° rotation whereby the fundus is displaced to the right and ventral, and the pylorus is displaced to the left and dorsal. The best

view to document this volvulus is the right lateral where the gas extends into the abnormally positioned pylorus and the fluid extends into the abnormally displaced fundus. The pylorus is narrower and has a smoother mucosal surface than the fundus, with an absence of rugal folds. The interface between the pylorus and the fundus on right lateral view is a linear soft tissue opacity, causing "compartmentalization" of the gas-filled stomach. This shows a characteristic "double bubble" appearance (Figures 25.5 and 25.6). It is important to note any gas within the gastric wall or portal vasculature.

## Foreign Bodies

Gas-filled, mineral or metal opaque foreign bodies are easier to identify within the gastric lumen on routine radiography (Figures 25.7 and 25.8). Frequently, patients with gastric foreign bodies are presented with a history of vomiting or regurgitation. As such, clinical signs and radiographic features of aspiration

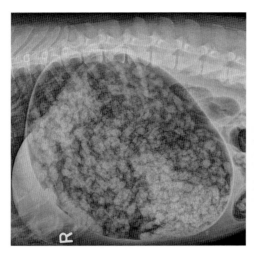
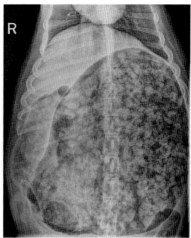

**FIGURE 25.3** Right lateral and ventrodorsal views of the cranial abdomen of an 8-year-old female spayed Weimaraner with acute abdominal bloat an hour after eating. The stomach is markedly dilated with gas (from the level of T8 to L5) and multiple small rounded mixed soft tissue and gas opaque material.

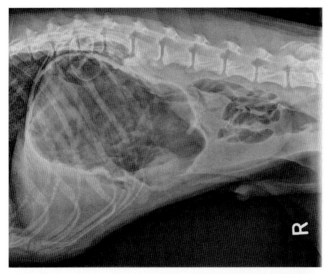

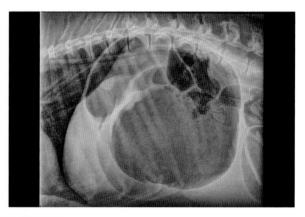

**FIGURE 25.5** Right lateral view of the cranial abdomen of a 7-year-old, female spayed Great Dane who was presented with acute bloat. Marked gastric gas dilation, with dorsal displacement of the gastric pylorus and ventral displacement of the fundus and an interposed compartmentalization, consistent with gastric dilation and volvulus.

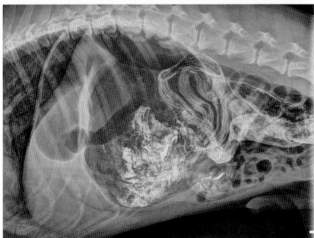

**FIGURE 25.4** Right lateral views of the cranial abdomen before and after oral positive contrast medium administration. The stomach is markedly gas dilated on the initial image, from the level of T10 to L4. There is a small amount of gas within the craniodorsal peritoneal cavity, caudal to the diaphragm, consistent with pneumoperitoneum secondary to ruptured gastric ulcer.

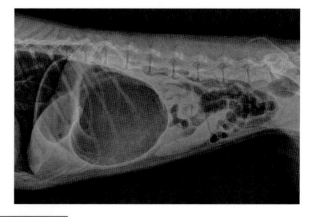

**FIGURE 25.6** Right lateral abdominal view of a 7-year-old female spayed mixed-breed dog with acute abdominal bloating. The gas-filled stomach shows dorsal displacement of the pylorus and ventral displacement of the fundus with a soft tissue band interposed (compartmentalization), consistent with gastric dilation and volvulus.

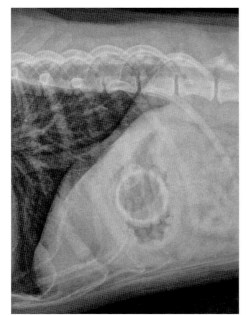
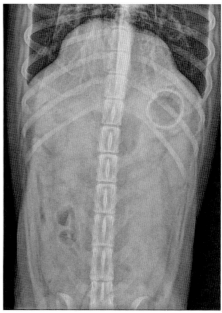

**FIGURE 25.7**   Right lateral and ventrodorsal views of the cranial abdomen of a 3-year-old male castrated Swiss mountain dog. A rounded gas opaque structure with a thick, soft tissue to mineral opaque rim is within the gastric fundus on ventrodorsal view and the gastric body on right lateral view, consistent with recent ingestion of a tennis ball.

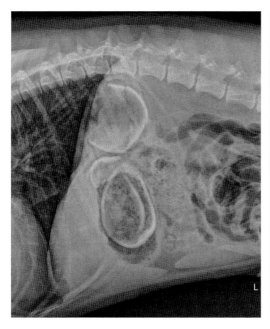
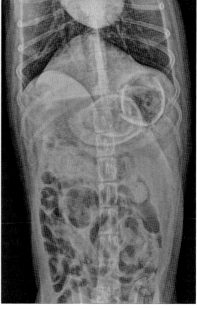

**FIGURE 25.8**   Left lateral and ventrodorsal abdominal views of a 7-year-old male castrated golden retriever, presented for acute dullness and vomiting. Multiple rounded gas opaque structures with incomplete thick, soft tissue to mineral opaque rims are within the gastric lumen. These were portions of tennis balls recently ingested.

pneumonia must be considered. Gastric foreign bodies which are soft tissue opaque can be difficult to see if surrounded by soft tissue opaque stomach wall and luminal contents. They are easier to identify with gas surrounding the foreign body (Figure 25.9). Positive contrast gastrography can also be useful in highlighting soft tissue opaque foreign bodies (Figure 25.10).

Given that the variable opacities of gastric foreign bodies and the gastric ingesta may be similar, it is frequently difficult to determine the difference between normal ingesta and a clinically significant obstructive foreign body. Screening radiographs may show suspicion of gastric outflow obstruction with/without gastric dilation, however, if the patient has been vomiting secondary to gastric outflow obstruction. In such cases, ultrasound is useful in the assessment of the gastric wall and contents, taking the limitation of gas hindering penetration of the ultrasound beam into account (Figure 25.11).

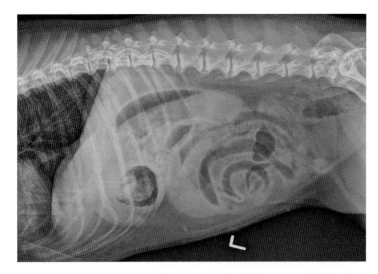

**FIGURE 25.9** Left lateral abdominal view of a 13-year-old female spayed pit bull terrier, with a 1-month history of diarrhea and a 1-day history of lethargy and vomiting. There are several gas-filled small intestinal loops. The gastric body-pylorus contains a mild amount of gas with a central heterogeneous soft tissue opacity. A long soft tissue opaque structure with a linear pattern is within a markedly dilated proximal duodenum. A sock was retrieved on surgical exploration.

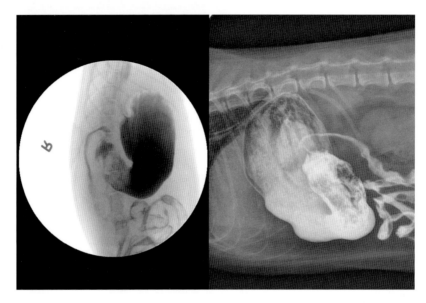

**FIGURE 25.10** Oblique ventrodorsal fluoroscopic image and a right lateral view of the cranial abdomen post oral contrast administration of an 8-month-old male castrated domestic shorthair cat. A rounded defect is within the gastric pylorus, with filling of the remainder of the stomach and the proximal duodenum, consistent with a pyloric textile foreign body.

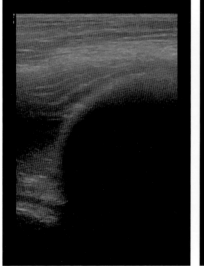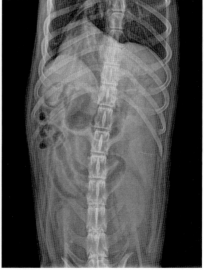

**FIGURE 25.11** A longitudinal ultrasonographic examination of the gastric pylorus, and a ventrodorsal view of the cranial abdomen of a 9-year-old male castrated German shepherd dog with a history of anorexia and vomiting. A smoothly marginated curvilinear hyperechoic structure is within the gastric pyloric lumen, with distal acoustic shadowing. An ovoid gas opacity is within the gastric pylorus with poorly defined soft tissue rim, consistent with a pyloric foreign body (a ball).

# Gastric Neoplasia

Gastric neoplasia includes gastric carcinoma, lymphoma, and leiomyomas. Gastric adenocarcinoma accounts for up to 80% of gastric neoplasia in the dog. Gastric neoplasia may be associated with intraluminal extension of the mass and can be easily confused with gastric foreign bodies. Pneumogastrography or positive contrast gastrography can identify a soft tissue opaque nodule or mass confluent with the gastric wall.

Gastric ultrasound is useful in characterizing the nature of the gastric wall thickening, to differentiate gastric neoplasia, gastric polyps, and foreign bodies.

In more complex cases and in areas where ultrasound is unable to penetrate to image the stomach due to gastric, intestinal, or even free peritoneal gas, CT can be used to assess the gastric wall (Figures 25.12–25.14).

# Gastritis and Ulceration

Gastritis can be caused by ingestion of a chemical or physical irritant, or as a side-effect of drugs. Radiographically, the stomach often has a normal appearance, in the absence of the identification of foreign bodies. Ultrasonography can be useful to assess gastric wall thickness in cases of gastritis, and in more severe cases aid in the detection of gastric wall ulceration. Gastric ulcers are erosions of the gastric mucosa, whereby gastric contents can penetrate the wall of the stomach. Ultrasonographically, mobile echogenic fluid or gas can be identified in defects within the

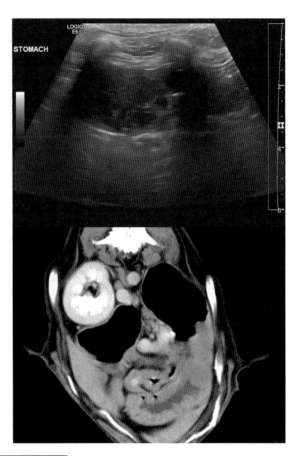

**FIGURE 25.13**   Transverse ultrasound image of the gastric fundus wall (top image) and transverse post contrast CT image of the cranial abdomen (bottom image) in soft tissue window of an 11-year-old male castrated German shepherd. There is marked lobular thickening of the greater curvature wall of the gastric wall. The thickening is heterogeneously hyperechoic with loss of wall layering. On CT, the thickening mass is homogeneously hypoattenuating and homogeneously contrast enhancement. Biopsy revealed histiocytic sarcoma.

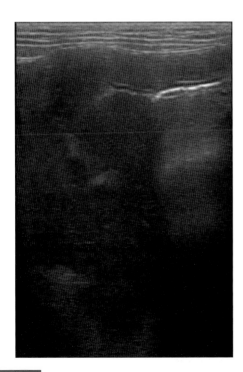

**FIGURE 25.12**   Longitudinal ultrasound image of the gastric pylorus of a 5-year-old male castrated domestic shorthair cat, vomiting for 6 months. Marked thickening of the pyloric wall, with loss of wall layering, diagnosed as adenocarcinoma on cytology.

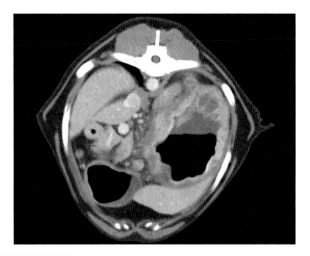

**FIGURE 25.14**   Transverse postcontrast image of the cranial abdomen in soft tissue window of a 7-year-old female spayed Labrador retriever, with a 3-month history of weight loss. There is a large hypoattenuating, centrally poorly enhancing and peripherally strongly contrast-enhancing mass at the dorsolateral aspect of the gastric fundus, diagnosed as gastric adenocarcinoma.

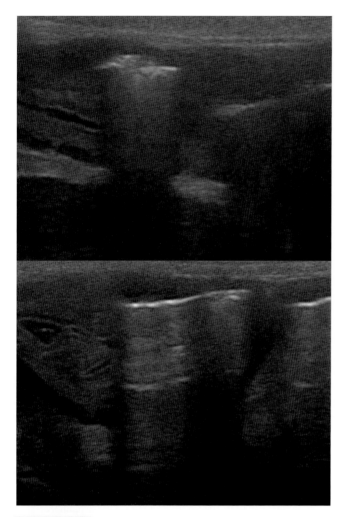

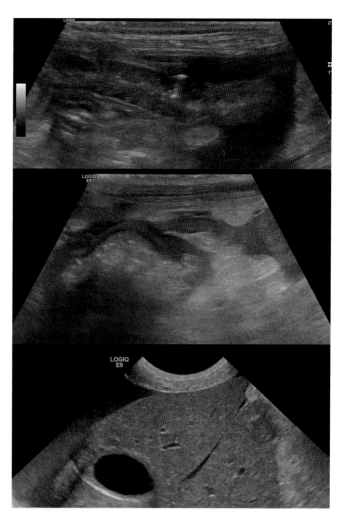

**FIGURE 25.15**  Longitudinal ultrasound images of the gastric pyloric wall of a 10-year-old female spayed shih tzu, presented with trembling and lethargy. Hyperechoic material is within the gastric wall, with distal reverberation artifact and loss of wall layering, consistent with gastric ulceration and gas tracking into the wall.

**FIGURE 25.16**  Ultrasound images of the jejunum (top and middle) and the liver and gall bladder (bottom), of a 12-year-old male neutered German shorthaired pointer with a 3-year history of intermittent diarrhea. A linear hyperechogenicity extends from the jejunal mucosa to the serosal margin, surrounded by a hypoechoic region within the adjacent wall. Heterogeneous echogenic material is within the peritoneal space, with hyperechoic fat. A full jejunal ulcer with septic peritoneal effusion, consistent with intestinal perforation, was noted.

gastric mucosa (Figure 25.15). Gastric ulcers may also extend through the entire gastric wall, resulting in gastric perforation.

## Gastric Perforation

Gastric perforation can occur in a variety of cases such as gastric ulceration, GDV, penetrating foreign body, and gastric neoplasia. With gastric perforation, the gastric contents enter the peritoneal space. As such, a chemical peritonitis can occur with peritoneal effusion, as well as the escape of gas into the peritoneum, leading to pneumoperitoneum.

Radiographically, due to the loss of normal peritoneal fat between peritoneal organs, and the peritoneal effusion causing border effacement with the organs, there is a loss of peritoneal serosal detail. Free gas is frequently identified within the peritoneal cavity adjacent to the stomach within the inflamed peritoneal fat as well at the most dependent part of the abdomen, which is generally at the level of the diaphragm (Figures 25.4 and 25.16).

## Small and Large Intestines

The small intestinal tract is divided into duodenum, jejunum, and ileum. In summary, the duodenum is confluent with the pyloric sphincter, making a cranial duodenal flexure at the level of the sphincter before coursing caudally along the right abdominal body wall as the descending duodenal loop. The descending duodenum turns to form a caudal duodenal flexure, becoming the ascending duodenum and continuing cranially before transitioning to the jejunum. The jejunal loops then course throughout the peritoneal cavity before becoming the short ileum which interfaces with the ascending colon at the ileocolic sphincter.

The cecum is a blind-ended diverticulum of the proximal colon, which opens into the ascending colon adjacent to the ileocolic opening in the dog or the ileocecocolic junction in the cat. The cecum is generally located to the right of midline within the dorsal peritoneal cavity. From the cecum, the ascending colon courses cranially to a point just caudal to the stomach, where at the right colic flexure the transverse colon turns medially to cross midline. At the left colic flexure, the transverse colon meets the descending colon which runs caudally through the pelvic inlet to the rectum. The mesentery contains the arteries, intestinal lymphatics and nerve plexus supplying the intestinal loops.

When assessing the small intestinal loops radiographically, they are generally of soft tissue opacity. In dogs, a mild amount of intraluminal gas is normal, whereas in the cat only a very minimal amount of gas is considered normal. Radiographically, small intestinal loops should be of a similar diameter, with the diameter of no loop measuring greater than twice the diameter of another. In the dog, small intestinal loop diameter should not measure greater than 1.6 times the height of the midbody of L5. In cats, no small intestinal loop should measure greater than 12 mm in diameter.

Contrast radiography can be used in the assessment of the small intestinal lumen, as well as function. An upper gastrointestinal study (upper GI) can be done. As stated above in gastrography, in dogs <20 kg, 8–12 mL/kg of 30–60% w/v barium sulfate solution can be administered and in dogs >20 kg, 5–7 mL/kg of 30–60% w/v barium sulfate can be administered either by syringe or via orogastric tube [2]. The barium contrast medium coats the walls of the small intestine during transit, as well as foreign material within the tract. It must be noted that within the small intestine, there may be normal outpouchings of intraluminal contrast medium into the Peyer's patches lymphoid tissue, which can appear like intestinal ulcers (Figure 25.17).

Ultrasonographically, small intestinal loops are similar in composition. The wall is like the stomach and esophagus, composed of four layers; mucosa, submucosa, muscularis, and serosa. The mucosa is the thickest layer owing to the presence of intestinal villi, glands, and lymph nodules. Intestinal wall layers should be distinguishable from each other during ultrasonographic assessment. The intestinal wall thickness can be measured ultrasonographically. Multiple sources of normal wall thickness in the dog and cat are available (Table 25.1).

Radiographically, in the dog, the cecum can often be visible due to intraluminal gas, whereas in the cat the cecum is rarely identified on survey radiographs. The colon can be filled with gas, heterogeneous gas, and soft tissue opaque or purely soft tissue to mineral opaque fecal material. The colon should measure less than the length of the seventh lumbar vertebra in the dog. In the cat, it is reported that the colon should not exceed 2.8 times the length of the height of the endplate of the second lumbar vertebra (L2) or 1.3 times the length of the fifth lumbar vertebra (L5) [5, 6].

A limitation of ultrasound is intraluminal gas within the intestinal loops, with the associated reverberation artifacts preventing ultrasonographic evaluation of the deeper structures.

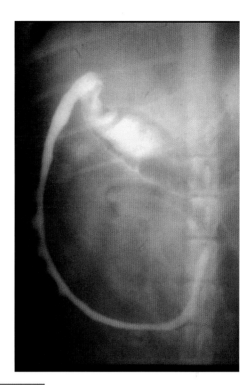

**FIGURE 25.17** Ventrodorsal image of the cranial-left abdomen with positive contrast filling the duodenum. Multiple areas of contrast extend into the lateral margin of the duodenum, consistent with "pseudoulcers" from Peyer's patches lymphoid tissue.

| TABLE 25.1 | Maximal small intestinal wall thickness measurements (mm) for the dog and cat with references. | |
| --- | --- | --- |

| Site | Maximal wall thickness measurements in mm | |
| --- | --- | --- |
| Species | Dog | Cat |
| Duodenum | 6 | 2.2 |
| Jejunum | 4.7 | 2.2 |
| Ileum | 3.8 | 2.8 |

Delaney et al. (2003) Ultrasound evaluation of small bowel thickness compared to weight in normal dogs. VRUS 44(5):577–580; Di Donato et al. (2014) Ultrasonographic measurement of the relative thickness of intestinal wall thickness of intestinal wall layers in clinically healthy cats. J. Feline Med. Surg. 16(4):333–339; Gladwin et al. (2014) Ultrasonographic evaluation of the thickness of the wall layers in the intestinal tract of dogs. Am. J. Vet. Res. 75:349–352; Winter et al. (2014) Ultrasonic evaluation of relative gastrointestinal layer thickness in cats without clinical evidence of gastrointestinal tract disease. J. Feline Med. Surg. 16(2):118–124.

Computed tomographic examination of the small intestinal loops is increasingly being performed. With CT, intraluminal gas does not prevent evaluation of the loop. Similarly, the different attenuation values of fluid and soft tissues help differentiate intestinal wall from intestinal contents. However, the spatial resolution of CT is less than that of ultrasound so distinct intestinal wall layers are often not discernible, with improved layer conspicuity after administration of intravenous contrast (up to 77% in late phase) [7].

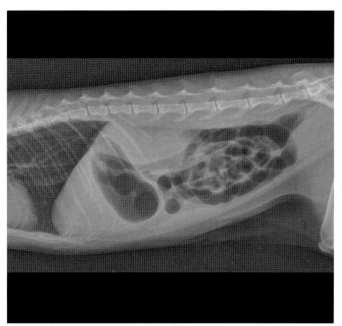
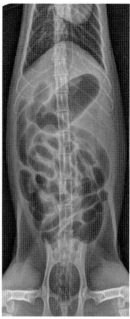

**FIGURE 25.18**   Right lateral and ventrodorsal views of the abdomen of a 7-year-old female spayed domestic shorthair cat presented for vomiting. The stomach and small intestinal tract contain a moderate amount of gas, with all loops of small intestine similar in diameter, consistent with functional ileus.

## Functional Ileus

Ileus is the absence of or reduction in intestinal motility. This can be functional in the absence of a mechanical obstruction, seen in postoperative patients, chronic enteropathies, and a variety of metabolic and toxic conditions [8]. In functional ileus, all loops of intestine can be dilated, measuring greater than normal (>1.6× midbody of L5 in dogs or >12 mm in cats), making a single population of dilated small intestinal loops (Figures 25.18 and 25.19).

## Mechanical Obstruction

Mechanical obstruction, also known as *mechanical ileus*, is frequently due to intraluminal foreign body. Mechanical obstruction can also be due to extraluminal or mural lesions causing obstruction of the gastric or small intestinal lumen. The radiographic diagnosis of mechanical obstruction is made by identifying "two populations of small intestinal loops." This is where there are several normal-sized loops of small intestine, and others which measure greater than normal (>1.6× midbody of L5 in dogs or >12 mm in cats), or one loop of intestine is greater than twice the diameter of another loop (Figures 25.20 and 25.21). It has been reported that patients with intestinal diameter ≥2.4×L5; ≥3.4×the diameter of the smallest loop; or ≥1.9×the average diameter of the small intestinal loops are likely obstructed and could be sent directly to surgery if ultrasound is not available or declined [9].

Although CT has been shown to be more sensitive and specific for the detection of mechanical obstruction in the dog, it is

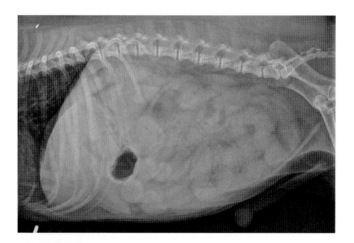

**FIGURE 25.19**   Left lateral view of the abdomen of a 10-year-old male castrated Welsh terrier with a history of vomiting and diarrhea. All small intestinal loops are distended and soft tissue opaque, consistent with functional ileus.

reported that for experienced radiologists recommending surgery, the sensitivity and specificity were higher for radiography [10].

In some cases, a single loop of intestine is identified, which is distended and measuring greater than twice the diameter of another loop. In the absence of a distinct colon, the question of whether the loop is a distended small intestinal loop or a normal colonic loop is of the utmost importance. In this instance, a pneumocolon can be performed by inserting a flexible tube or catheter-tipped syringe into the descending colon/ rectum and administering room air at a dose of 1–3 mL/kg in the dog, and a total of 20–30 mL of room air in the cat. The goal

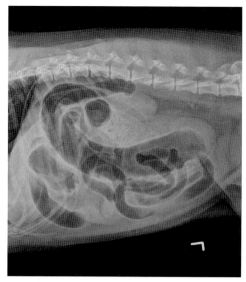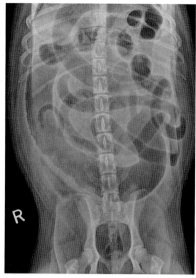

**FIGURE 25.20** Left lateral and ventrodorsal views of the abdomen of a 6-year-old female spayed Labrador retriever, presented for vomiting and dullness. A gas-filled loop of small intestine is markedly dilated, measuring twice the diameter of the other small intestinal loops. Heterogeneous soft tissue and gas opaque material superimpose the distended loop dorsally, consistent with mechanical obstruction.

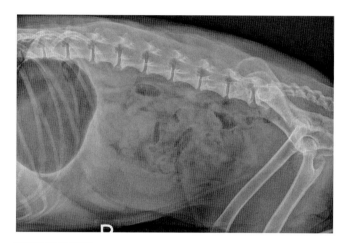

**FIGURE 25.21** A right lateral view of the abdomen of an 11-year-old female spayed Border collie, presented for vomiting. A markedly soft tissue distended small intestinal loop is within the ventral abdomen, confirmed as mechanical obstruction caused by mural adenocarcinoma.

is to fill the colon with gas to allow differentiation from small intestinal loops (Figure 25.22). Ultrasound is more accurate and provides a high level of diagnostic confidence in the diagnosis of mechanical obstruction in vomiting dogs [11].

## Foreign Bodies

Small intestinal foreign bodies are the most common cause of mechanical obstruction. In some cases, the foreign bodies can be mineral or metal opaque, but frequently they are soft tissue opaque or mixed soft tissue and gas opaque like normal adjacent ingesta. In cases of foreign bodies causing a mechanical obstruction, a soft tissue opaque or mixed gas and soft tissue opaque distended portion of the small intestinal

tract abruptly interfaces with a smaller, usually empty portion of small intestinal loop. The obstructive foreign material is located at the interface between the distended and normal intestinal segments (Figures 25.23 and 25.24). In equivocal cases, ultrasound can be used to assess the intestinal contents.

Foreign bodies can be of various sizes, shapes, and echogenicity. A hyperechoic interface with distal shadowing is highly suggestive of a foreign body [12]. Mechanical obstruction secondary to the foreign body can be identified as distension of the orad intestinal loop (Figure 25.25).

Linear foreign bodies such as string or twine can be difficult to identify. Linear foreign bodies become anchored at a point and the peristaltic waves of the intestinal tract cause plication (bunching) of intestinal loops within the peritoneal cavity. Perforation must be assessed concurrently. It is of paramount importance to evaluate the base of the tongue for a site of attachment. Radiographically, small "comma-shaped" gas bubbles can be identified within small intestinal loops due to plication. Perforation pneumoperitoneum is identified as free gas bubbles within the peritoneum, especially at the level of the diaphragm. Concurrent peritonitis can be identified as poor peritoneal serosal detail (Figure 25.26). Ultrasonographically, linear foreign bodies are identified as linear echogenicity extending within the lumen across corrugated loops of small intestine (Figure 25.27).

## Intestinal Neoplasia

Intestinal neoplasia is common in older dogs and cats. Lymphoma is the most common neoplasm of the cat and one of the most common in the dog. Lymphoma can be identified affecting the entire gastrointestinal tract or one segment. Adenocarcinoma is the second most common intestinal

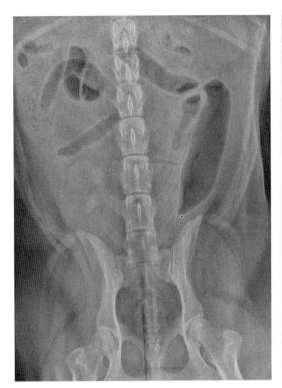
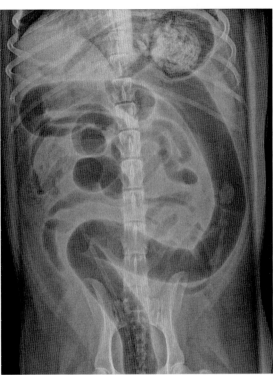

**FIGURE 25.22**   Ventrodorsal views of the abdomen of a 7-year-old female spayed Labrador retriever with a history of vomiting overnight. Images are before and after pneumocolon (with a tube superimposing the descending colon). A heterogeneous gas and soft tissue opaque filled intestinal loop is identified on the initial image, which measures greater than twice the diameter of another small intestinal loop. Pneumocolon is performed to fill the colon, thereby identifying the initial loop as distinct from the colon and confirming a distended small intestinal loop in small intestinal mechanical obstruction.

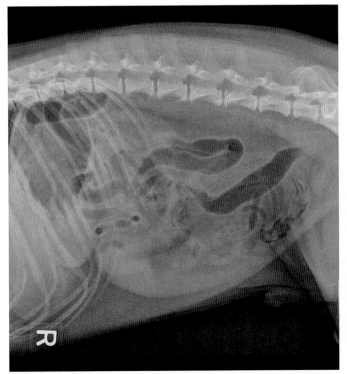
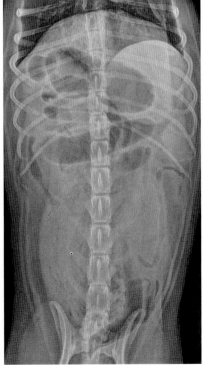

**FIGURE 25.23**   Right lateral and ventrodorsal abdominal views of a 4-year-old male castrated mixed-breed dog, presented for vomiting. There is a dilated soft tissue loop within the caudal right abdomen, containing multiple linear gas opacities centrally, consistent with a textile foreign body.

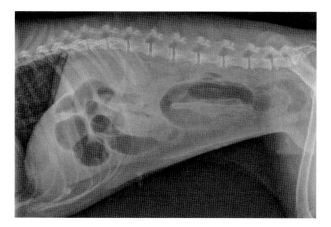

**FIGURE 25.24** Left lateral abdominal view of a 1-year-old female Vizsla, with a history of vomiting. There are multiple gas-filled small intestinal loops which are greater than twice the diameter of other small intestinal loops, and measuring greater than normal (>1.6 × midbody height of L5), consistent with mechanical obstruction.

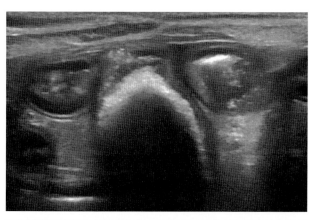

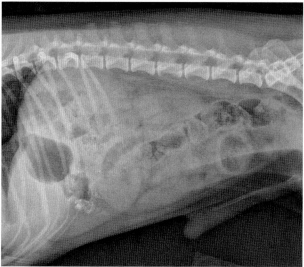

**FIGURE 25.25** Ultrasound image (top image) of the jejunum and right lateral view of the abdomen of an 8-year-old male castrated Chihuahua, with a 3-day history of vomiting. The jejunal lumen is dilated with a moderate amount of hyperechoic material showing distal acoustic shadowing. On radiography (bottom image), there are multiple mineral opacities within the gastric pyloric lumen. Multiple gas bubbles are within a distended small intestinal loop caudal to the region of the pylorus, consistent with gastric and jejunal textile foreign material.

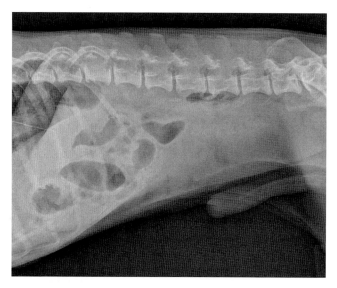

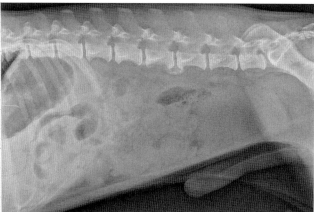

**FIGURE 25.26** Left (top) and right (bottom) lateral views of the abdomen of a 10-year-old male castrated springer spaniel, with pain on abdominal palpation. Multiple small intestinal loops are bunched within the ventral and cranial abdomen. Some irregularly shaped gas bubbles are within the intestinal lumen on the left lateral view. A linear foreign body was removed at surgery.

neoplasm of the cat and one of the most common in the dog. Carcinomas generally develop as solitary masses. Other neoplasms such as leiomyomas or leiomyosarcomas are less common.

Radiographically, intestinal neoplasia may show mechanical obstruction, signs of concurrent disease such as hepatic or splenic enlargement or may show no changes (Figure 25.28). Ultrasonographically, intestinal neoplasia is associated with hypoechoic thickening of the intestinal wall, frequently with loss of wall layering. Concurrent regional lymphadenopathy is common. In some feline alimentary lymphoma cases, the muscularis layer can be thickened where the muscularis may be the same thickness as the mucosa (Figures 25.29 and 25.30). In adenocarcinoma, the ultrasonographic changes are like those of lymphoma, although adenocarcinomas tend to affect a shorter length of intestine and are more likely to be associated with mechanical obstruction than lymphoma (Figure 25.31).

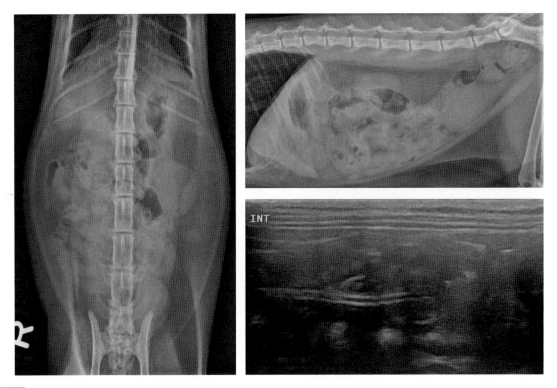

**FIGURE 25.27** Ventrodorsal and right lateral views of the abdomen, and ultrasound image of the jejunum of a 2-year-old male castrated domestic shorthair cat with a 2-day history of vomiting. There is bunching of the small intestinal loops within the ventral abdomen, with comma-shaped gas bubbles within the intestinal lumen. A linear hyperechoic structure is identified within the jejunal lumen, confirming a linear foreign body within the jejunum.

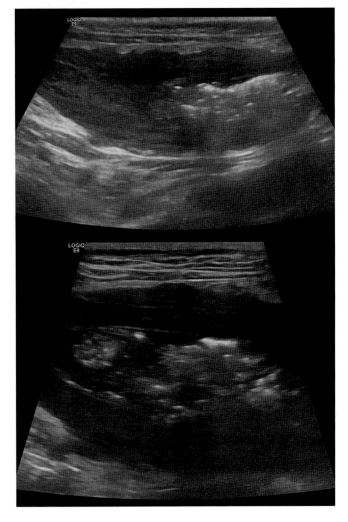

**FIGURE 25.28** Longitudinal ultrasound images of the jejunum of an 11-year-old female spayed Siamese cat with a 3-day history of anorexia and lethargy. There is marked circumferential thickening of the jejunal walls, with loss of wall layering, confirmed as intestinal lymphoma.

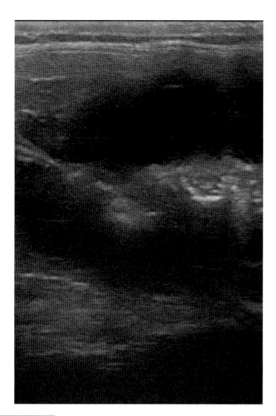

**FIGURE 25.29** Longitudinal ultrasound image of the jejunum of a 6-year-old female spayed domestic shorthair cat, presented for vomiting and lethargy. There is circumferential hypoechoic thickening of the wall of the jejunum, with loss of wall layering, confirmed as intestinal lymphoma.

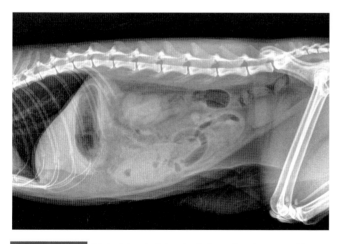

**FIGURE 25.30** Right lateral abdominal view of an 11-year-old female spayed Siamese cat with a history of anorexia and lethargy. There is a rounded soft tissue opacity within the ventral abdomen, with multifocal soft tissue opaque material within the adjacent peritoneal fat and associated decreased serosal detail. Peritoneal effusion with a cytology confirmed diagnosis of intestinal lymphoma.

Computed tomography can be used to evaluate the small intestinal loops, and postcontrast images can show thickening of the intestinal walls and concurrent changes such as regional lymphadenopathy, splenomegaly, or hepatomegaly (Figure 25.32).

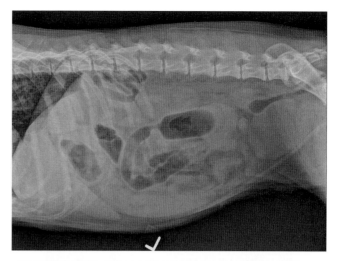

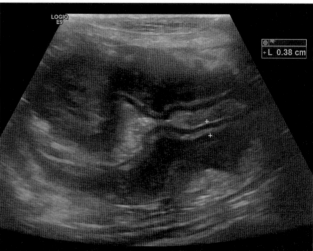

**FIGURE 25.31** Left lateral abdominal radiograph and longitudinal ultrasound image of the jejunum of an 8-year-old female spayed Australian shepherd with a week-long history of diarrhea. On radiographs, there is a gas-distended small intestinal loop cranial to a larger rounded soft tissue opaque mass cranial to the urinary bladder. Ultrasound shows an asymmetric circumferential thickening of the intestinal wall, with loss of wall layering, consistent with intestinal lymphoma.

## Chronic Enteropathy/Inflammatory Bowel Disease

Chronic enteropathy (CE), also known as inflammatory bowel disease (IBD), is frequently identified as a cause of gastroenteritis in dogs and cats. This is a complex disease process, and discussion of CE/IBD pathophysiology is beyond the scope of this text [13]. Changes in wall thickness can be identified, but wall thickness measurements are not sensitive or specific for diagnosing CE in dogs as the wall thickness can be normal to mild thickening. Loss of wall layering has been shown as an important finding differentiating inflammatory lesions from neoplastic and granulomatous lesions where layering is lost. The majority of patients with CE have normal intact wall layering [14, 15].

In some cases, multiple hyperechoic parallel lines can be identified within the mucosa, perpendicular to the lumen.

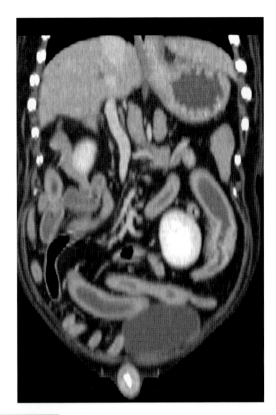

**FIGURE 25.32** A dorsal reconstructed CT study post intravenous contrast medium image of the abdomen displayed in soft tissue window of a 6-year-old male castrated bulldog cross presented with chronic vomiting and anorexia. There is a focal area of asymmetric circumferential thickening of the jejunal wall and a small area of soft tissue-attenuating material within the adjacent peritoneal fat. Jejunal adenocarcinoma was diagnosed on cytology.

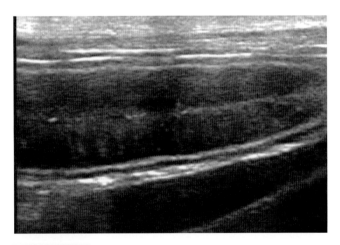

**FIGURE 25.33** Longitudinal ultrasound image of the jejunum of a 7-year-old female spayed pug, with a chronic history of diarrhea and weight loss. Multiple parallel hyperechoic lines within the mucosal layer, consistent with lymphangiectasia.

These have been shown to represent lymphangiectasia (Figure 25.33). These striations have been identified in patients with protein-losing enteropathy including CE and intestinal neoplasia such as lymphoma. Lymphangiectasia is also identified physiologically in cases of a recent meal.

## Intestinal Ulceration

Intestinal ulceration is like gastric ulceration, whereby a defect forms in the mucosal surface of the small intestinal loop and intestinal contents and gas can dissect into the wall. Ulceration can occur in cases of enteritis or intestinal neoplasia. In extreme cases, the ulcer can perforate and intestinal contents can enter the peritoneal cavity, with resultant peritonitis and pneumoperitoneum (Figure 25.34).

## Intussusception

Intussusception is an invagination of one portion (intussusceptum) of the gastrointestinal tract into the lumen of an adjoining segment (intussuscepiens), along with the adjacent mesentery, lymph nodes, and vasculature. The condition is common

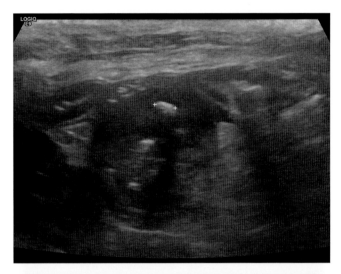

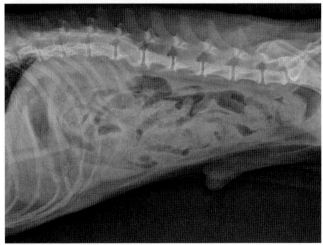

**FIGURE 25.34** Ultrasonographic examination of the jejunum and right lateral radiographic view of the abdomen of a 12-year-old male castrated cocker spaniel with chronic vomiting. There is marked asymmetric hypoechoic thickening of the jejunal wall, with a hyperechoic structure (calipers) within the superficial wall. On radiography, there is poor cranial peritoneal serosal detail. There are several gas-filled small intestinal loops. A jejunal adenocarcinoma with ulceration and associated peritoneal effusion was diagnosed.

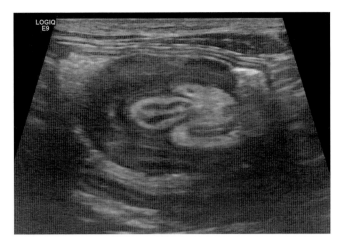

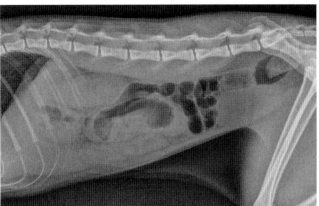

in young dogs and most often ileocolic in location. The intussusception can cause partial obstruction or obstruction and ischemia or infarction of the intussusceptum and localized peritonitis [16]. Radiographic findings can show a soft tissue opaque mass within the midabdomen, or may be nonspecific. Ultrasound shows "a loop within a loop": concentric rings in transverse images or parallel lines reflecting the multiple layers of intestinal walls (Figures 25.35 and 25.36).

## Intestinal and Colonic Volvulus

Intestinal torsion is the twisting of an intestinal segment around its long axis. Intestinal or mesenteric volvulus is a rotation of intestine around the mesenteric axis. Radiographically, colonic volvulus is seen as gaseous distension of a loop of intestine within the right cranial and mid/abdomen, leftward displacement of the cecum, and generalized increased small intestinal gas (Figure 25.37) [17].

Colonic torsion is a life-threatening emergency, as is intestinal volvulus. The radiographic findings associated with a group of 14 dogs included severe, segmental distension of the colon, focal narrowing of the colon, displacement of the cecum and descending colon, and mild to no small intestinal abnormal distension (Figure 25.37) [18]. In some dogs, a barium enema was done, and there was a focal narrowing of the colon and longitudinal striations arranged in a spiral pattern that was described as the "torsion sign" [18].

## Megacolon

The colon can become impacted with feces in constipation, obstipation, and megacolon. Megacolon can be due to chronic

**FIGURE 25.35**   Ultrasound image of the ileum and left lateral radiographic view of a 3-year-old male castrated domestic longhair cat with a history of inappetence. At the level of the ileum, the ileocolic junction is surrounded by an additional intestinal loop (loop within a loop). On radiography, there is a soft tissue opaque rounded mass, ventral to the renal silhouettes, consistent with ileocolic intussusception.

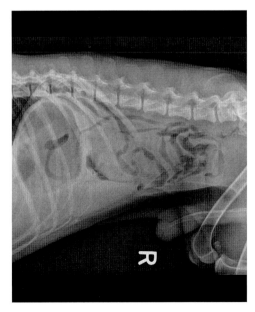
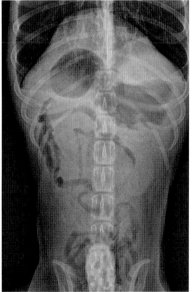

**FIGURE 25.36**   Right lateral and ventrodorsal views of the abdomen of a 3-year-old male shar pei, with a history of diarrhea. There is a rounded soft tissue opaque mass within the right cranial abdomen, with several gas-filled jejunal loops which are normal in diameter. A jejunojejunal intussusception was diagnosed at surgery.

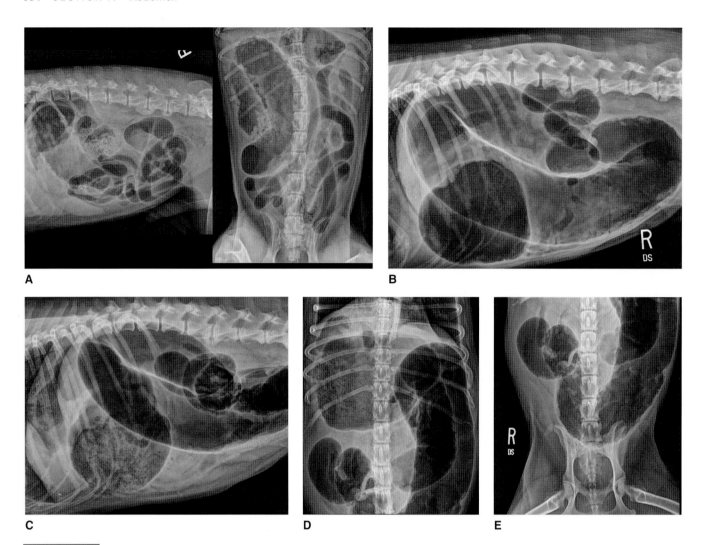

**FIGURE 25.37** (**A**) Right lateral and ventrodorsal abdominal views of a 14-year-old male castrated mixed-breed dog, with acute-onset vomiting. The colon is markedly gas filled and displaced to the right, consistent with colonic torsion. The jejunal loops are gas filled, with all measuring similar in diameter. (**B–E**) Right lateral, left lateral, and ventrodorsal images from a 10-year-old FN bassett hound. The colon is severely gas distended and displaced to the left and ventrally. The stomach is moderately gas distended. The cecum is dorsally and caudally displaced. These changes were consistent with a colonic torsion that was confirmed at surgery.

constipation and obstipation or neurologic, metabolic, or anatomic anomalies. One example is mechanical obstruction of the colon due to malunion fracture healing causing pelvic narrowing or pelvic masses such as prostatic or uterine masses as well as sarcomas. Intraluminal colonic masses can also cause colonic obstruction. In cats, megacolon is associated with a colonic diameter to length of L5 ratio of >1.5 (Figure 25.38).

## Colonic Neoplasia

In cats, lymphoma is the most common colonic neoplasm with concentric, eccentric wall thickening or diffuse wall thickening [19]. In dogs, adenocarcinoma is the most common colonic neoplasm. Differential diagnosis would include pythium infestation in dogs (Figure 25.39). Adenocarcinomas can be solitary masses or form concentric strictures.

# Summary

Abdominal radiographs play an important role when surveying the gastrointestinal tract. Although abdominal ultrasound and computed tomography provide additional important information, the screening test should still be abdominal radiography. This will help dictate the type of secondary imaging study and help the practitioner develop specific questions to answer related to the original abdominal radiography. It cannot be overemphasized that the routine abdominal radiographic study should include right lateral, left lateral and ventrodorsal images. They should be obtained on peak expiration and should be straight for appropriate interpretation. Obliqued lateral abdominal radiographs can be nondiagnostic, particularly if there are multiple equivocal changes present on the radiographs.

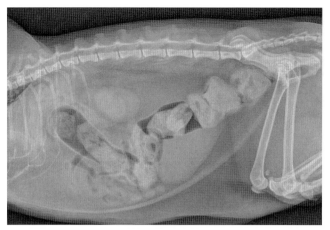

**FIGURE 25.38** Right lateral abdominal view of an 8-year-old male castrated domestic shorthair cat, presented with constipation. The moderately distended descending colon contains mineral opaque, rounded to rectangular structures and gas, consistent with desiccated feces.

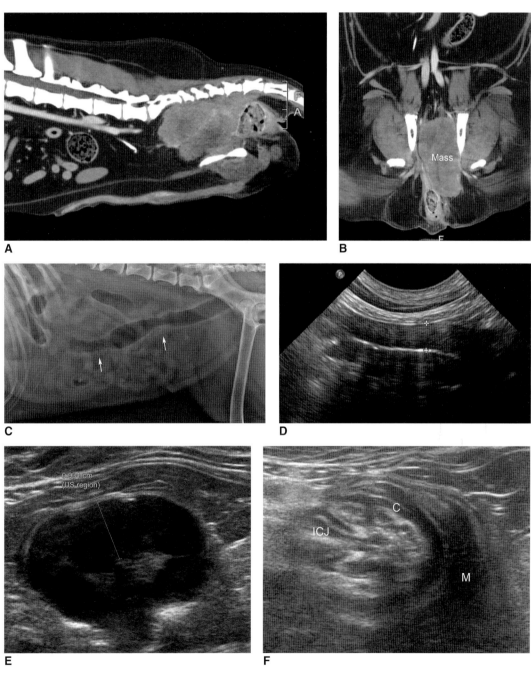

**FIGURE 25.39** Sagittal (**A**) and dorsal plane (**B**) reconstructions from a dog with an eccentric rectal mass (post intravenous contrast medium administration). On histology, this mass was an adenocarcinoma. (**C**) Right lateral radiograph documenting thickening of the colonic wall (white arrows) that was persistent on multiple views. Fine needle aspirates under US guidance documented carcinoma. Multiple cystic and ureteral calculi are also noted. (**D–F**) Ultrasound images from a dog with pythium documenting colonic wall thickening, mass, and loss of wall layering. Fungal hyphae were evident on ultrasound-guided fine needle aspirates of the mass.

One of the most common questions that is being asked of the interpretation of the abdominal radiographs is whether the case is a surgical case (GDV, obstruction, etc.) or a case to manage medically? The important concepts reviewed in this chapter include an understanding of the normal radiographic anatomy of the gastrointestinal tract and the common abnormalities of size, shape, margin, and opacity being recognized as many of the Roentgen changes seen in gastrointestinal tract abnormalities.

# References

1. Muhlbauer, M. and Kneller, S. (2013). *Radiography of the Dog and Cat: Guide to Making and Interpreting Radiographs.* Ames, IA: Wiley.
2. Wallack, S. (2003). *The Handbook of Veterinary Contrast Radiography.* San Diego, CA: San Diego Veterinary Imaging.
3. Miyabayashi, T. and Morgan, J.P. (1984). Gastric emptying in the dog – a contrast radiographic technique. *Vet. Radiol.* 25: 187.
4. Smart, L., Reese, S., and Hosgood, G. (2017). Food engorgement in 35 dogs (2009–2013) compared with 36 dogs with gastric dilation and volvulus. *Vet. Rec.* 181: 563.
5. Adams, W.M., Sisterman, L.A., Klauer, J.M. et al. (2010). Association of intestinal disorders in cats with findings of abdominal radiography. *J. Am. Vet. Med. Assoc.* 236: 880.
6. Trevail, T., Gunn-Moore, D., Carrera, I. et al. (2011). Radiographic diameter of the colon in normal and constipated cats and in cats with megacolon. *Vet. Radiol. Ultrasound* 52: 516.
7. Fitzgerald, E. (2017). Improving conspicuity of the canine gastrointestinal wall using dual phase contrast-enhanced computed tomography: a retrospective cross-sectional study. *Vet. Radiol. Ultrasound* 58 (2): 151–162.
8. Whitehead, K., Cortes, Y., and Eirmann, L. (2016). Gastrointestinal dysmotility disorders in critically ill dogs and cats. *J. Vet. Emerg. Crit. Care* 26 (2): 234–253.
9. Finck, C., d'Anjou, M.-A., Alexander, K. et al. (2014). Radiographic diagnosis of mechanical obstruction in dogs based on relative small intestinal external diameters. *Vet. Radiol. Ultrasound* 55 (5): 472–479.
10. Drost, W., Green, E., Zekas, L. et al. (2016). Comparison of computed tomography and abdominal radiography for detection of canine mechanical intestinal obstruction. *Vet. Radiol. Ultrasound* 57 (4): 366–375.
11. Sharma, A., Thompson, M., Scrivani, P. et al. (2011). Comparison of radiography and ultrasonography for diagnosing small intestinal mechanical obstruction in vomiting dogs. *Vet. Radiol. Ultrasound* 52 (3): 248–255.
12. Tidwell, A. and Penninck, D. Ultrasonography of gastrointestinal foreign bodies. *Vet. Radiol. Ultrasound* 33: 160–169.
13. Dandrieux, J. (2016). Inflammatory bowel disease versus chronic enteropathy in dogs: are they one and the same? *J. Small Anim. Pract.* 57 (11): 589–599.
14. Penninck, D., Smyers, B., Webster, C.R. et al. (2003). Diagnostic value of ultrasonography in differentiating enteritis from intestinal neoplasia in dogs. *Vet. Radiol. Ultrasound* 44 (5): 570–575.
15. Rudorf, H., van Schaik, G., O'Brien, R.T. et al. (2005). Ultrasonographic evaluation of the thickness of the small intestinal wall in dogs with inflammatory bowel disease. *J. Small Anim. Pract.* 46 (7): 322–326.
16. Lamb, C. and Mantis, P. (1998). Ultrasonographic features of intestinal intussusception in 10 dogs. *J. Small Anim. Pract.* 39: 437–441.
17. Nemzek, J., Walshaw, R., and Hauptman, J. (1993). Mesenteric volvulus in the dog: a retrospective study. *J. Am. Anim. Hosp. Assess.* 29: 357–362.
18. Gremillion, C.L., Savage, M., and Cohen, E.B. (2018). Radiographic findings and clinical factors in dogs with surgically confirmed or presumed colonic torsion. *Vet. Radiol. Ultrasound* 59 (3): 272–278.
19. Schwarz, T. (2018). Large bowel. In: *Textbook of Veterinary Diagnostic Radiology*, 7e (ed. D.E. Thrall). St Louis, MO: Elsevier.

# CHAPTER 26

# Pancreas

## Cintia R. Oliveira[1] and Nathan C. Nelson[2]

[1] VetsChoice Radiology, Madison, Wisconsin, USA
[2] Department of Molecular Biomedical Sciences, College of Veterinary Medicine, North Carolina State University, Raleigh, NC, USA

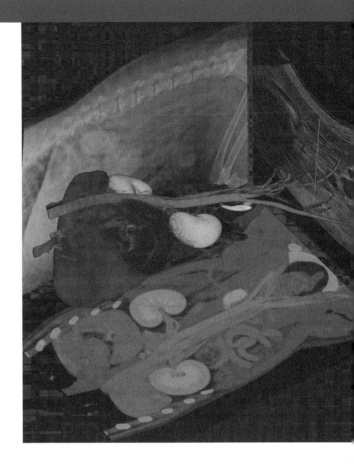

## Anatomy

The pancreas consists of two lobes and a body, and is located in close apposition to a number of adjacent organs which efface its margins on radiographs (Figure 26.1). The left lobe is located caudal to the body and fundus of the stomach in the dog. In the cat, the left lobe extends further laterally, toward the hilus of the spleen. It is surrounded by fat and not in contact with other organs, and as a result is routinely seen on abdominal radiographs in cats (Figure 26.2). The remainder of the pancreas is not seen radiographically in cats or dogs when normal.

The pancreas is more readily identified on ultrasound. The body of the pancreas is immediately caudal to the proximal descending duodenum in the dog and cat. The right lobe extends caudally to the medial or dorsal aspect of the duodenum. The right lobe is proportionally longer in the dog compared to the cat, and is reliably seen adjacent to the duodenum on ultrasound, particularly when using a dorsal right intercostal approach (Figure 26.3). The echogenicity of the pancreas is similar to normal liver, and may contact the liver cranially, partially obscuring its margins on ultrasound. In the dog, the pancreaticoduodenal vein may be seen within the right lobe of the pancreas, aiding identification. The left lobe of the pancreas is not often seen in dogs, as gas within the adjacent fundus obscures it. In the cat, the left lobe is readily seen, particularly laterally by the splenic hilus (Figure 26.4). The pancreatic duct is often most evident in the left lobe and usually less than 2 mm diameter, though this diameter increases with age.

The entire pancreas is readily seen on CT images of the dog (Figure 26.5) and cat (Figure 26.6). Given its small size, thin slices (2 mm or less) aid in identification of the pancreas, particularly cranially where it contacts the stomach, colon, and liver. Its attenuation values are similar to the liver and other soft tissue structures.

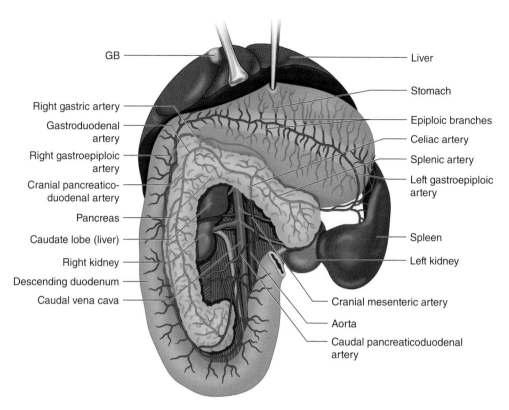

GB

Right gastric artery

Gastroduodenal artery

Right gastroepiploic artery

Cranial pancreatico- duodenal artery

Pancreas

Caudate lobe (liver)

Right kidney

Descending duodenum

Caudal vena cava

Liver

Stomach

Epiploic branches

Celiac artery

Splenic artery

Left gastroepiploic artery

Spleen

Left kidney

Cranial mesenteric artery

Aorta

Caudal pancreaticoduodenal artery

**FIGURE 26.1** Diagram of normal pancreatic anatomy showing proximity of the duodenum to the right lobe and the body and the fundus and splenic vein to the left lobe.

# Pancreatitis in Dogs and Cats

Pancreatitis refers to inflammation of the exocrine pancreas and is the most common exocrine pancreatic disorder in dogs and cats, being divided into acute or acute necrotizing, and chronic [1–5]. The differences between acute and chronic pancreatitis are histologic and not necessarily clinical.

Acute pancreatitis is associated with varying degrees of inflammation, necrosis, and edema, whereas chronic pancreatitis histologically demonstrates irreversible and progressive fibrosis and acinar loss [2–5]. Although several causes have been reported, in most cases it is considered idiopathic [2–4]. Histopathology is the gold-standard method of diagnosing pancreatitis but is not commonly performed due to its invasive nature. A presumptive diagnosis is usually made by a combination of clinical signs and clinicopathologic and diagnostic imaging findings. Pancreatitis has been reported to be one of the most common causes of portal vein thrombosis in dogs and CT angiography is the gold-standard method for the diagnosis of portal vein thrombosis [6, 7].

The major radiographic sign of pancreatitis is loss of peritoneal detail with increased soft tissue opacity in the right cranial abdomen which is a result of focal peritonitis (Figure 26.7). Other signs include a mass effect in the right cranial abdomen and a persistent gas-filled proximal descending duodenum, termed a "sentinel loop sign." The proximal duodenum may also be displaced ventrally or laterally, appearing to have a broader curvature, and the pylorus of the stomach may be displaced toward the left. However, none of these signs are specific for pancreatitis and radiographs may appear normal.

Ultrasound is usually the imaging modality of choice to diagnose pancreatitis in dogs and cats, but CT has been performed more often recently. Ultrasound findings in acute pancreatitis include an enlarged, possibly mass-like pancreas with hypoechoic parenchyma, adjacent hyperechoic mesentery, and peritoneal effusion [1, 8–10] (Figures 26.8–26.15). With pancreatic necrosis, there may be irregular hypoechoic and hyperechoic areas and nonenhanced pancreatic tissue [11] (Figure 26.16). The hypoechoic areas within the pancreas are usually caused by inflammation, hemorrhage, necrosis or edema, and the hyperechoic areas are usually caused by fibrosis [2]. Other ultrasound findings include cystic-like or cavitated lesions, dilation of the pancreatic duct, especially in cats, duodenal or gastric thickening with or without loss of layering and corrugation of the duodenum, and extrahepatic biliary obstruction [1, 9, 10] (Figure 26.10). It is important to remember that dilation of the pancreatic duct in cats can also be associated with aging [12, 13]. Ultrasound may also be normal in cats and dogs and may be normal in the initial stages in dogs [9, 10].

A study evaluating ultrasonographic monitoring in 38 dogs with clinically suspected pancreatitis found that approximately one-third of the dogs did not have ultrasound findings of acute pancreatitis at the first ultrasound but did on the second examination performed 40–52 hours later [14]. The authors suggested waiting at least 52 hours after admission to perform ultrasound on a dog suspected of having acute pancreatitis [14]. In a study

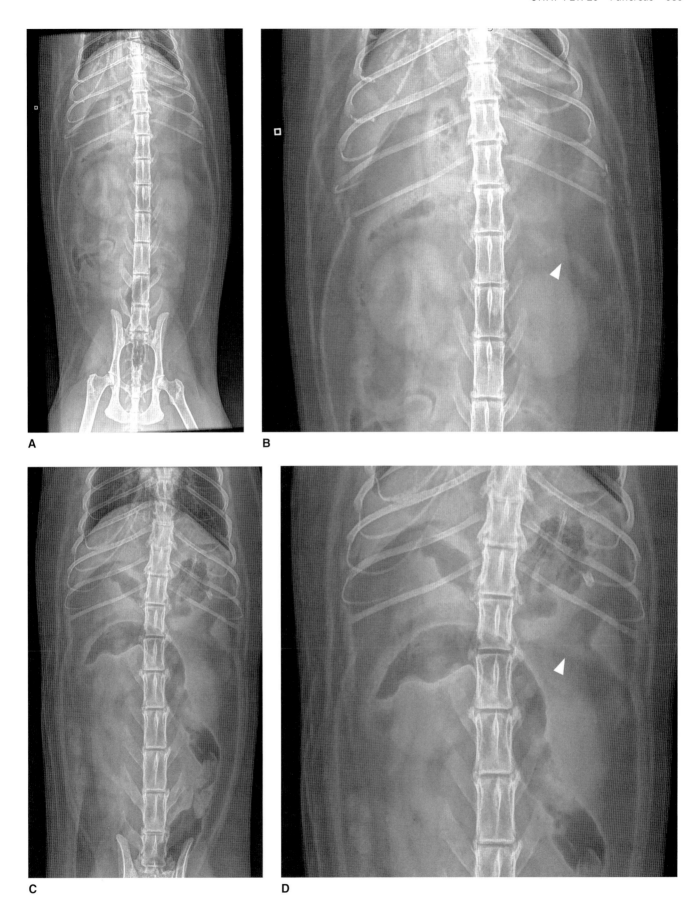

**FIGURE 26.2** Ventrodorsal views of the abdomen (**A,C**) and close-up images (**B,D**) of the normal pancreas in two different cats. The pancreas can be seen as a fusiform soft tissue opaque structure in the left cranial abdomen between the fundus of the stomach, the spleen, and the left kidney (arrowheads).

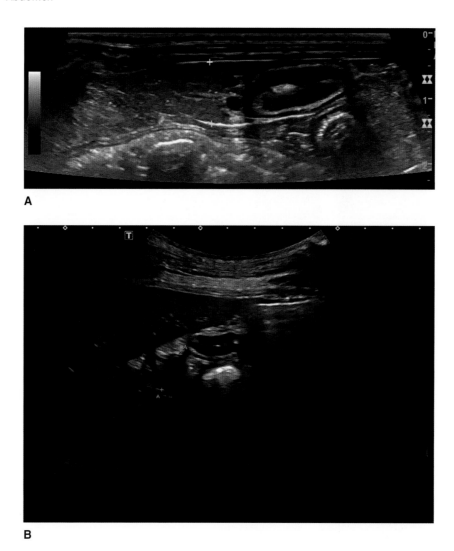

**FIGURE 26.3** Transverse (short axis) ultrasound images of dogs with a normal pancreas (between the calipers). (**A**) Using a linear transducer in a small-breed dog. (**B**) A large-breed dog imaged with a macroconvex transducer. The right lobe of the pancreas can be seen as an isoechoic to slightly hypoechoic structure medial or dorsomedial to the descending duodenum. The pancreaticoduodenal vein is seen as a round anechoic structure in the center of the pancreas. In dogs, the right lobe is easier to identify than the left lobe.

evaluating 25 cats with B-mode and contrast-enhanced power and color Doppler ultrasonography of the pancreas, vascularity and blood volume for all Doppler methods were significantly higher in cats with pancreatic disease compared to normal cats [15]. B-mode ultrasound findings in the diseased cats included hypoechogenicity of the pancreas compared to the liver, irregular contour, presence of masses, nodules or cysts within the pancreas, inhomogeneous pancreas, hyperechoic mesentery, and free fluid. Eight cats in the study had pancreatitis, four had nodular hyperplasia and four had neoplasia. Also in this study, significantly higher values were found with postcontrast compared to precontrast color or power Doppler ultrasound [15].

In a study evaluating contrast-enhanced ultrasound (CEUS) of the pancreas in healthy dogs and dogs with acute pancreatitis, the mean pixel and peak intensity of the pancreatic parenchyma in dogs with pancreatitis was significantly higher than that of dogs with normal pancreas,

suggesting CEUS can be useful for diagnosing canine pancreatitis and pancreatic necrosis [16]. In a similar study evaluating CEUS in 23 dogs with naturally occurring pancreatitis and 12 normal dogs, of all the parameters evaluated, a significant difference was found only for peak time, with dogs with pancreatitis having a prolonged peak time compared to control dogs [17]. The study suggests CEUS can be used in dogs for the detection of pancreatic perfusion changes as a possible sign of pancreatitis.

Computed tomographic findings are similar, including an enlarged pancreas with ill-defined borders and homogeneous or heterogeneous enhancement, adjacent peritoneal effusion possibly with fat stranding, thickening of the adjacent duodenum and/or gastric wall, dilated gall bladder and biliary tract due to compression and obstruction by the enlarged pancreas [8, 10, 18] (Figures 26.14–26.17). In a study evaluating the use of CT angiography in sedated dogs with suspected pancreatitis, an enlarged homogeneously or

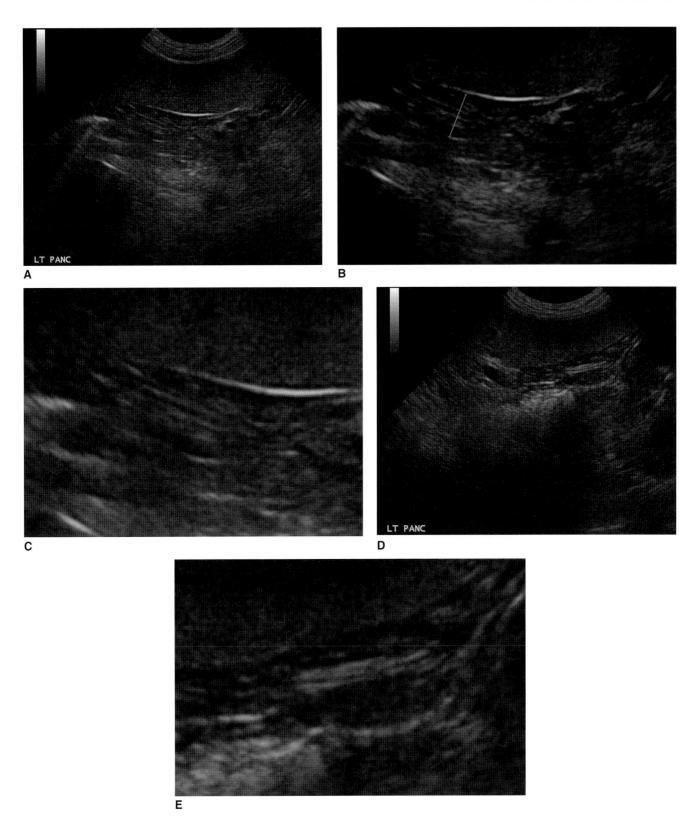

**FIGURE 26.4** Sagittal (long axis) ultrasound images of a cat with normal pancreas. (**B**) is a close-up of (**A**), (**E**) is a close-up of (**D**). The left lobe of the pancreas (**A–E**) can be seen as a fusiform isoechoic to slightly hypoechoic structure medial or dorsomedial to the spleen (on (**B**) the green line indicates the pancreas diameter). It is also caudal to the stomach and cranial to the transverse colon. In cats, the left lobe and body of the pancreas are easier to identify than the right lobe.

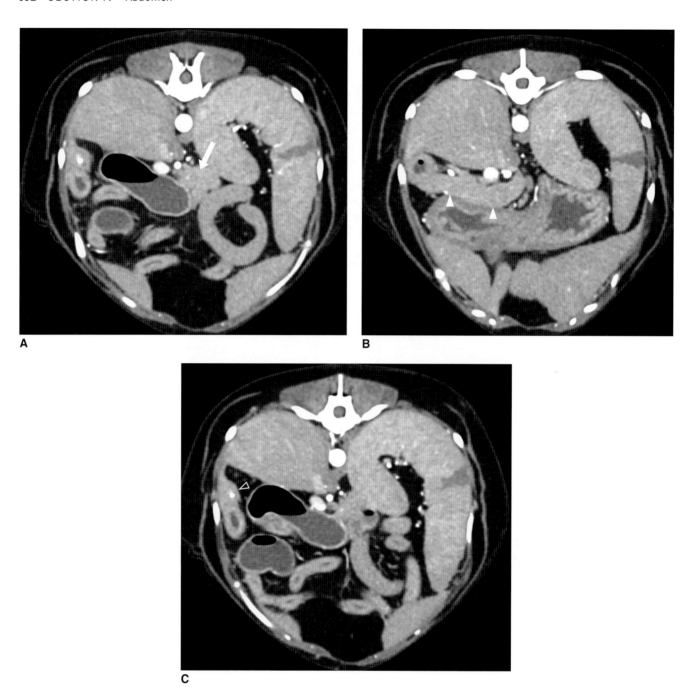

**FIGURE 26.5** Transverse plane postcontrast CT images of the abdomen of a 10-year-old poodle with a normal pancreas. (**A**) Left lobe of the pancreas (arrow). (**B**) Body of the pancreas (closed arrowheads). (**C**) Right lobe of the pancreas (open arrowhead).

heterogeneously enhancing pancreas with ill-defined margins were the main findings [18]. In addition to these findings, three out of 10 dogs had portal vein thrombi. Not surprisingly, the portal vein thrombi seen with CT was not found on US on any of the dogs (given the challenge of examining the portal vein with US in dogs). The authors also found that three out of four dogs with heterogeneous enhancement had overall poorer outcome compared to the dogs with homogeneous enhancement, concluding that the heterogeneous enhancement may correspond to necrotic or fibrotic nonenhancing regions in the pancreas. However, the overall number of dogs with heterogeneous enhancement is very small and a larger number of

cases would need to be studied for meaningful conclusion of this finding [18].

Another study compared the use of computed tomography angiography (CTA) with ultrasound in the diagnosis of acute pancreatitis in dogs and concluded that CTA did not significantly identify pancreatitis better than ultrasound. However, it allowed visualization of the entire pancreas and detected portal vein thrombosis and biliary mineralization significantly better than ultrasound [10].

Acute pancreatitis has been associated with pulmonary complications in dogs [19, 20]. A study evaluated 26 dogs presenting with acute pancreatitis and found 21 of the 26 had

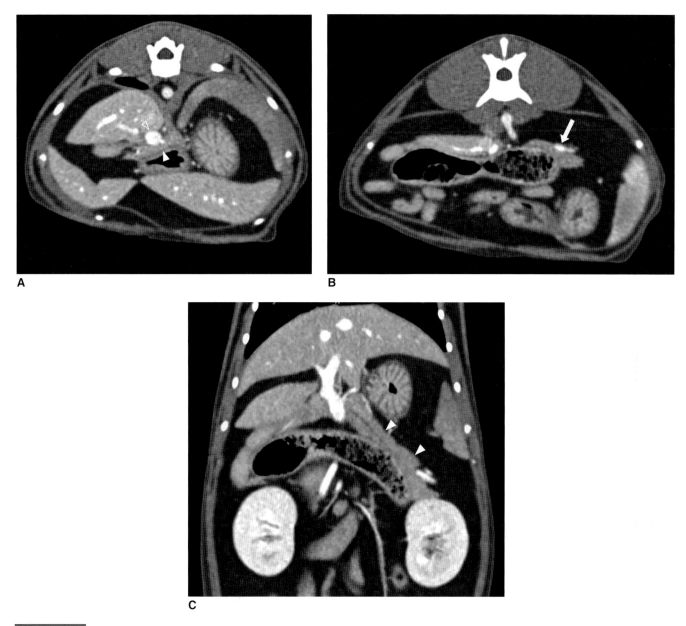

**FIGURE 26.6** Tranverse CT image of the body (**A**), left lobe (**B**), and dorsal image of the left lobe (**C**) of a normal pancreas in a cat. The pancreas is indicated by closed arrowheads. The body of the pancreas is ventral to the portal vein (open arrowhead). The left lobe extends immediately cranial to the colon and caudal to the stomach, and is ventral to the splenic vein (arrow). The pancreatic duct is seen in the left lobe.

clinical and radiographic signs of pulmonary disease, including alveolar and interstitial pattern, indicative of acute lung injury or pneumonia [20]. In a study evaluating the accuracy of CT for the diagnosis of feline pancreatitis, only two of the 10 cats had CT changes consistent with pancreatitis, which were described as enlarged pancreas and reduced contrast in the surrounding fat in one of the cats [21]. In this study, visualization of the pancreas was considered difficult on CT and not possible without intravenous contrast administration. In a recent study evaluating 21 cats with pancreatitis, the pancreas was seen on CT in 18 out of 19 cats, but differences in pancreatic dimensions were not seen in cats with pancreatitis compared to normal cats. Measurements included diameter, contour, enhancement, and pre- and postcontrast density [8]. These two studies

suggest lack of support for the use of CT in the diagnosis of pancreatitis in cats [8, 21].

There are very few reports on the use of magnetic resonance imaging (MRI) for evaluation of the pancreas. With MRI, the pancreas is assessed by evaluating the intensity changes on T1- and T2-weighted sequences, the contrast enhancement, the presence of pancreatic and common bile duct dilation, and by evaluating the surrounding soft tissues for the presence of fluid and inflammation indicating peritonitis. Magnetic resonance cholangiopancreatography has been used to image the biliary tract and pancreatic duct in normal cats and in cats with cholangitis and pancreatitis [22]. MRI findings in cats with pancreatitis included enlargement, pronounced signal intensity abnormalities with T1 precontrast hypointense and T2

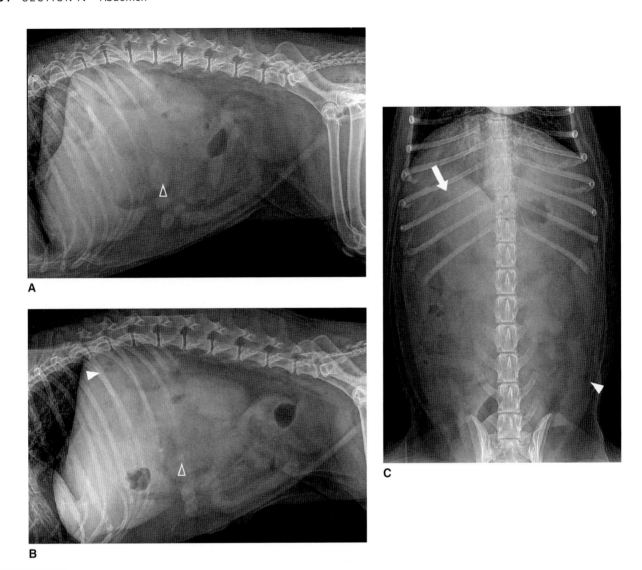

**FIGURE 26.7** Right lateral (**A**), left lateral (**B**), and ventrodorsal (**C**) views of the abdomen of a 10-year-old mixed-breed dog. The owners found it laterally recumbent. Septic peritonitis was diagnosed by ER service via abdominocentesis. There is generalized poor peritoneal detail with multiple small free gas bubbles (closed arrowheads). A large, poorly defined soft tissue opaque mass is present caudal to the stomach on the lateral views ((**A,B**) open arrowheads), and there is increased soft tissue opacity on the right cranial abdomen on the VD view ((**C**) arrow). Differentials include neoplasia, abscess, or granuloma possibly from spleen, pancreas, or liver. An abdominal exploratory surgery revealed an approximately 5 × 4 cm mass with purulent exudate effacing the left lobe of the pancreas and extending into the root of the mesentery with a focal area of necrosis. There was generalized peritonitis and large amounts of serosanguinous fluid. The primary differential diagnosis was necrotizing pancreatitis. The patient was euthanized, and a final histologic diagnosis was not obtained.

hyperintense pancreatic parenchyma (normal pancreas in cats is T1 hyperintense and T2 hypointense), contrast enhancement, and dilated pancreatic duct [22].

The diagnosis of chronic pancreatitis is very challenging, and the differentiation of acute and chronic pancreatitis may also be challenging [1-4]. With chronic pancreatitis, radiographs are usually normal. With ultrasound, the pancreas may be normal or decreased in size, with mixed echogenicity, nodular lesions and hyperechoic shadowing lesions corresponding to fibrosis and/or mineralization [1, 9, 10]. In cats, enlargement or irregularity of the pancreatic ducts may be seen as well as dilated common bile duct if there is partial or complete

common bile duct obstruction. Pancreatitis in cats may be seen associated with hepatic lipidosis, cholangitis, diabetes mellitus or inflammatory bowel disease [3, 4].

Concurrent pancreatitis, inflammatory bowel disease, and hepatic lipidosis is a medical condition in cats called *triaditis* [3, 4]. Ultrasound signs associated with triaditis in addition to those seen with pancreatitis include diffuse hyperechoic liver and changes in the small intestine layering and/or thickness (see Triaditis below).

Pancreatitis cannot be reliably differentiated from pancreatic neoplasia based on imaging alone and sampling is needed for definitive diagnosis.

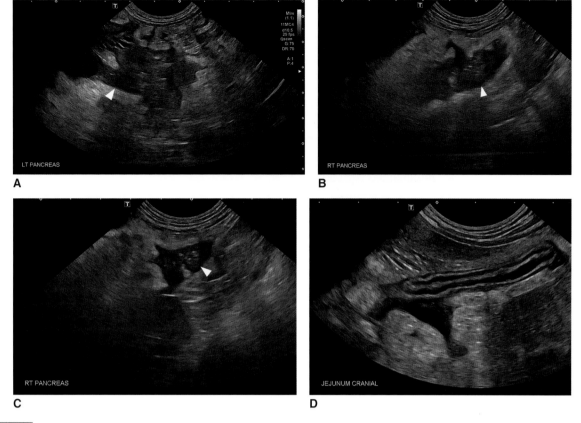

**FIGURE 26.8** Transverse (short axis (**A–C**)) ultrasound images of a 4-year-old cockapoo presented for inappetence, vomiting, and lethargy. The left and right lobes of the pancreas are severely enlarged and hypoechoic (arrowheads (**A,B**)). Multiple hyperechoic regions are also present in the pancreas (**C**). There is a large amount of anechoic free fluid in the abdomen and the mesentery is hyperechoic (**D**). A fine needle aspiration of the pancreas was performed. The cytologic diagnosis was pancreatitis.

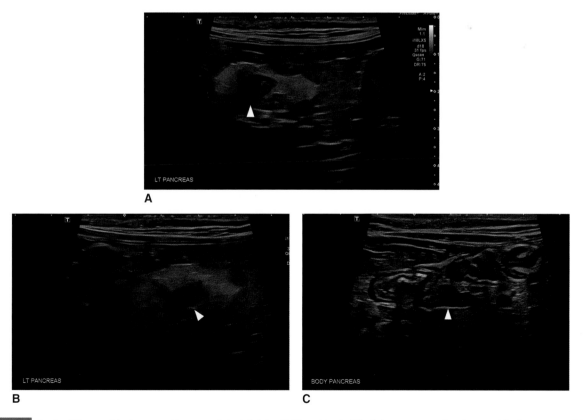

**FIGURE 26.9** Sagittal (long axis) ultrasound images of the left lobe (**A,B**) and body (**C**) of the pancreas of a 12-year-old DSH presented for further workup of chronic vomiting. Blood work showed abnormal fPLI. The left lobe and body of the pancreas (arrowheads) are hypoechoic and enlarged with surrounding hyperechoic mesentery. A small amount of free fluid was present. The findings are suggestive of acute pancreatitis.

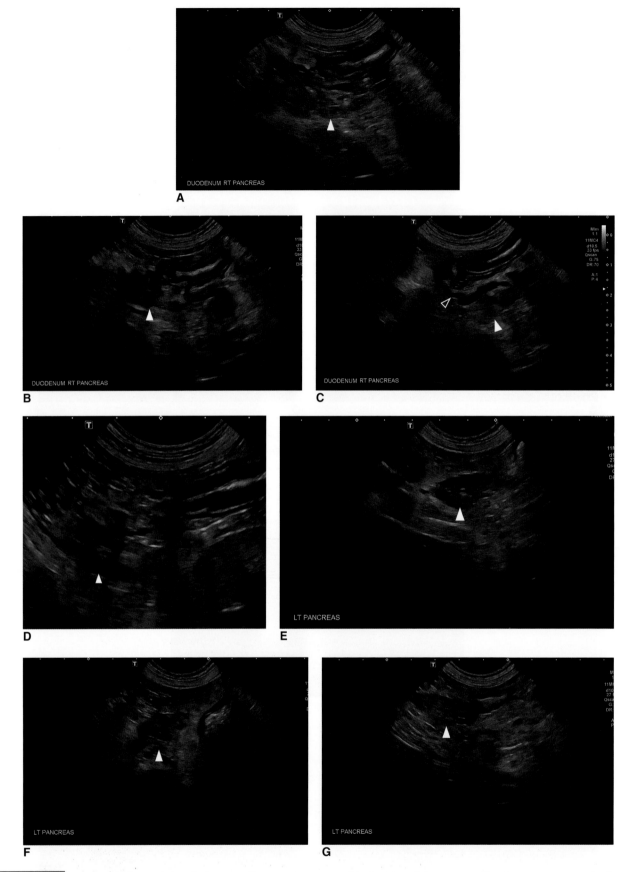

**FIGURE 26.10** Transverse (short axis (**A–G**)) ultrasound images of a 11-year-old mixed-breed dog presented to the emergency service for lethargy, weight loss, inappetence, and a distended abdomen. The right (**A–C**) and left (**D–G**) lobes of the pancreas are enlarged and hypoechoic (arrowheads). A small amount of free fluid is present, and the surrounding mesentery is hyperechoic. The pancreatic duct is mildly dilated, measuring 0.3 cm in diameter ((**C**) open arrowhead). The patient underwent exploratory surgery for biopsies due to severely elevated liver enzymes. On surgery, the pancreas was enlarged and the liver was fibrotic with multiple nodules. Histopathology of the pancreas revealed subacute pancreatitis with necrosis, edema, hemorrhage, and evidence of chronic pancreatitis with pancreatic acinar fibrosis and degeneration. No infectious organisms or neoplastic cells were visualized in the pancreas. The patient was also diagnosed with cirrhosis and Cushing disease.

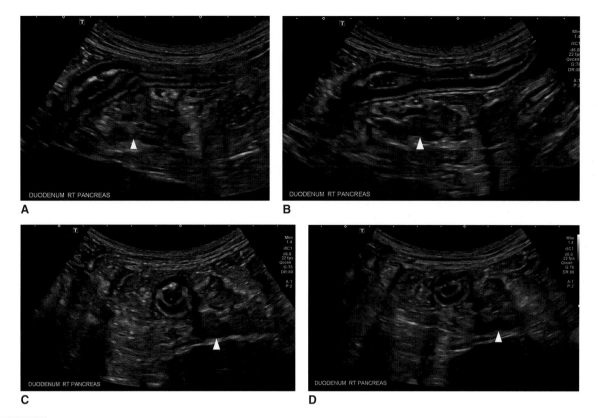

**FIGURE 26.11** Transverse (short axis (**A**–**C**)) and longitudinal (long axis (**D**)) ultrasound images of a 11-year-old goldendoodle presented for acute onset of vomiting, anorexia, and extreme lethargy. The right lobe of the pancreas is enlarged and heterogeneously hypoechoic (arrowheads) with some hyperechoic regions. A small amount of free fluid is present, and the mesentery is hyperechoic. The findings are suggestive of acute pancreatitis, possibly with a component of chronic pancreatitis. Pancreatic neoplasia cannot be ruled out.

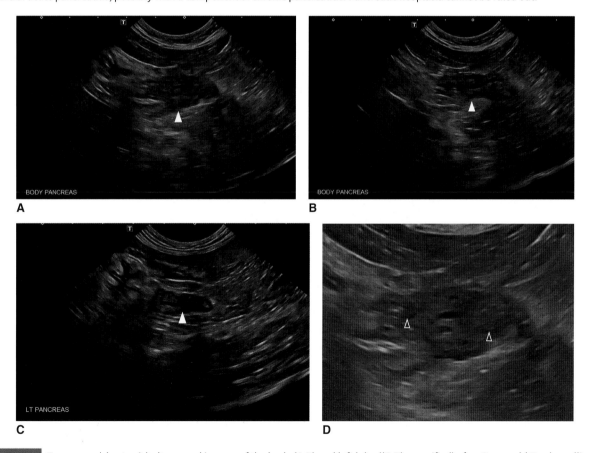

**FIGURE 26.12** Transverse (short axis) ultrasound images of the body (**A,B**) and left lobe ((**C,D**) magnified) of an 8-year-old Border collie presented for persistent hypercalcemia and suspect lymphoma. The pancreas is mildly enlarged and hypoechoic (closed arrowheads) with multiple ill-defined hypoechoic nodules (open arrowheads). The findings are suggestive of acute pancreatitis with concurrent nodular hyperplasia or neoplasia. A final diagnosis was not obtained.

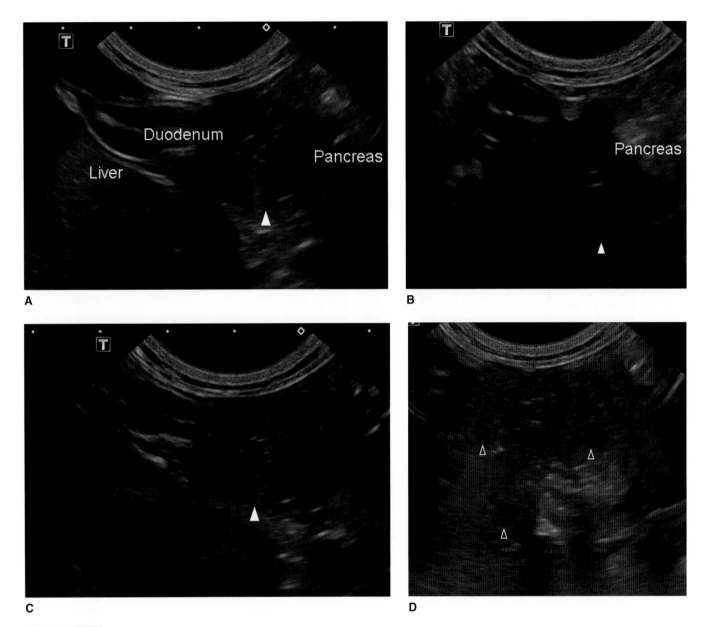

**FIGURE 26.13** Transverse (short axis (**A–D**)) ultrasound images of a 7-year-old mixed-breed dog presented with vomiting. The right lobe of the pancreas is diffusely and moderately enlarged and hypoechoic (closed arrowheads). Some hypoechoic nodules are present ((**D**) open arrowheads). The surrounding mesentery is hyperechoic. The findings are suggestive of acute pancreatitis with nodular hyperplasia and steatites. Pancreatic neoplasia cannot be completely ruled out.

# Triaditis

Triaditis refers to feline inflammatory gastrointestinal disease due to concurrent inflammation of the small intestines, pancreas and hepatobiliary system, and has been reported in 50–56% of cats with pancreatitis [3, 4, 23, 24]. Clinical signs include anorexia, weight loss, diarrhea, vomiting, pyrexia, and dyspnea, and hematologic and biochemical abnormalities consistent with liver disease, pancreatitis, and inflammatory bowel disease or lymphoma may be present.

Ultrasound findings may include those consistent with pancreatitis, hepatopathy, and small intestinal inflammation such as enlarged and hypoechoic pancreas, pancreatic duct dilation and choleliths, hyperechoic mesentery, peritoneal effusion, enlarged and hyperechoic liver, intrahepatic or extrahepatic bile duct enlargement, choleliths, gall bladder wall abnormalities, thickened small intestines, muscularis hypertrophy, and mesenteric lymphadenopathy (Figures 26.18 and 26.19). Common comorbidities include hepatic lipidosis, inflammatory liver disease, bile duct obstruction, diabetes

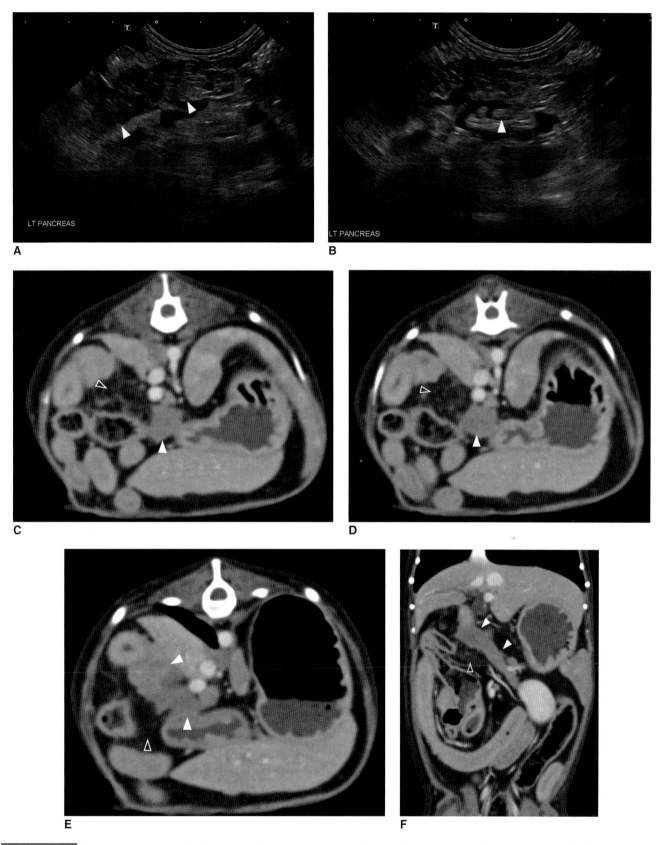

**FIGURE 26.14** Transverse (short axis (**A,B**)) ultrasound images of a 10-year-old goldendoodle presented for inappetence and lethargy. Blood work revealed hypoalbuminemia and elevated liver enzymes. The pancreas is moderately enlarged and hypoechoic (closed arrowheads). There is a mild amount of anechoic free fluid surrounding the pancreas and the surrounding mesentery is hyperechoic. Transverse (**C–E,G,H**), sagittal (**I**), and dorsal plane (**F**) postcontrast CT images. A mild amount of fluid attenuating material is present within the peritoneal cavity, predominantly surrounding the pancreas with a fat stranding appearance (open arrowheads). The pancreas (closed arrowheads) is enlarged, rounded, and lobulated with multiple noncontrast-enhancing regions. The liver and gall bladder are enlarged and the common bile duct is distended, measuring up to 0.7 cm ((**G**) arrow). Some of the intrahepatic ducts are also distended ((**H**) arrow). The duodenum (asterisk) and jejunum are diffusely mildly thickened and with poor contrast enhancement (**I**). The US and CT diagnosis was acute pancreatitis and steatitis suspect causing common bile duct obstruction. Pancreatic neoplasia cannot be completely ruled out. Cytology of liver demonstrated cholestasis and suppurative inflammation.

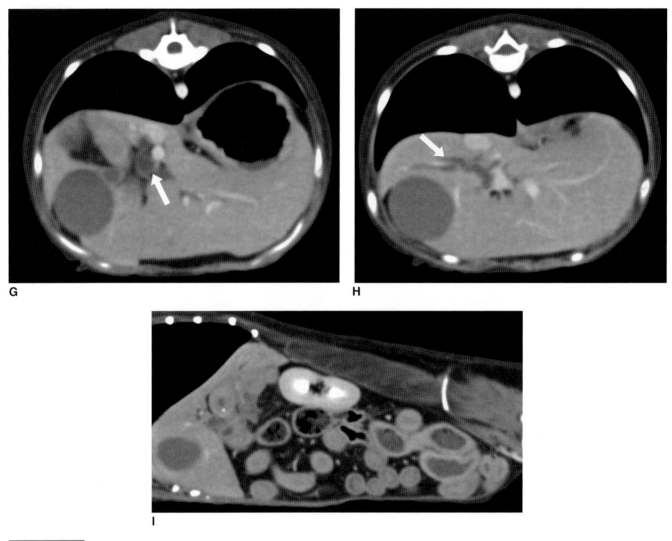

G

H

I

**FIGURE 26.14** (Continued)

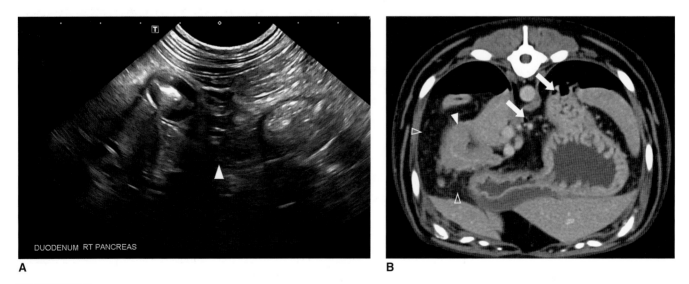

A

B

**FIGURE 26.15** Transverse (short axis (**A**)) ultrasound image of a 9-year-old Labrador retriever presented for inappetence and vomiting. The pancreas is mildly enlarged and hypoechoic (closed arrowhead) and there is anechoic free fluid in the abdomen. Transverse plane postcontrast CT image (**B**) of the same patient. Fluid-attenuating material (open arrowhead) and gas (arrows) are present within the peritoneal cavity with a fat stranding appearance. The pancreas is mildly enlarged and rounded (closed arrowhead). The patient has other abnormalities on the CT not described here. The findings are suggestive of pancreatitis. The patient had exploratory surgery due to septic abdomen and a duodenal perforation was diagnosed.

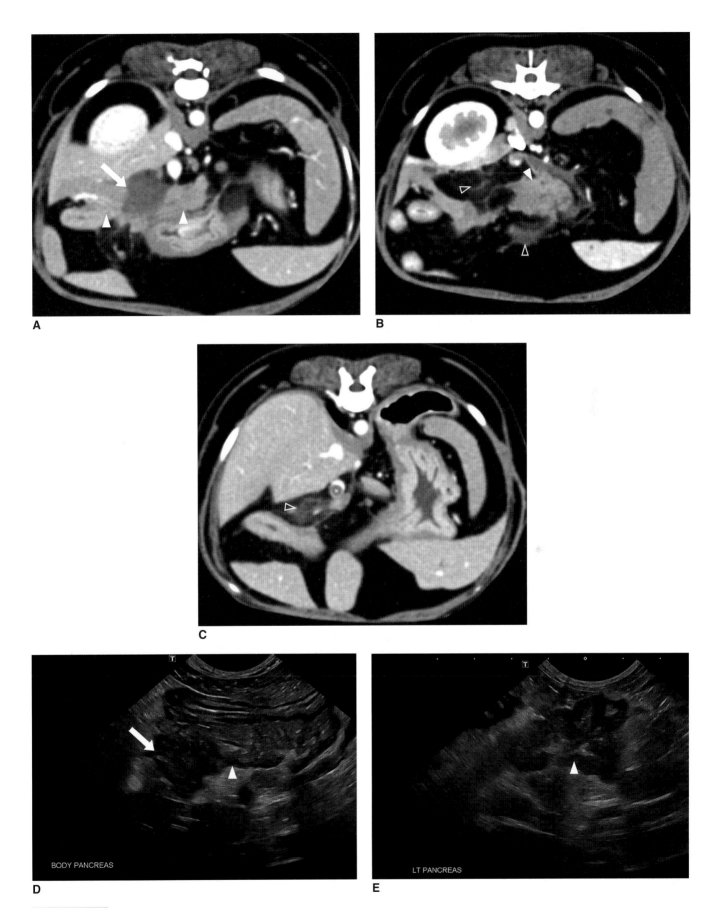

**FIGURE 26.16** Transverse postcontrast CT images (**A**–**C**) and sagittal (long axis) ultrasound images (**D,E**) of a 6-year-old shih tzu presented for vomiting and lethargy. The cPLI was abnormal. A large hypoattenuating nonenhancing lesion is present in the body of the pancreas (arrow (**A,D**)). The pancreas is diffusely enlarged (arrowheads). There is a small amount of peripancreatic free fluid with fat stranding (open arrowheads). A thrombus is present in the portal vein (asterisk (**C**)). The dog went to surgery and was diagnosed with acute necrotizing pancreatitis, confirmed on histopathology.

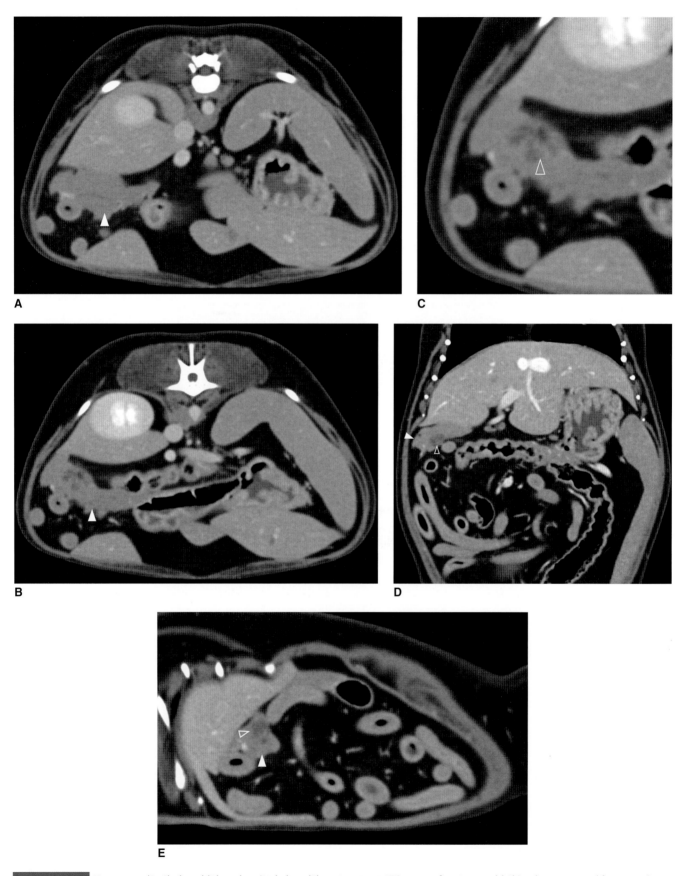

**FIGURE 26.17** Transverse (**A–C**), dorsal (**D**), and sagittal plane (**E**) postcontrast CT images of an 8-year-old Akita dog presented for anorexia, vomiting, and lethargy. The cPLI was abnormal. (**C**) is a close-up image of (**B**). The pancreas is mildly enlarged (closed arrowhead); a postcontrast hypoattenuating region is present in the right pancreatic lobe (open arrowheads). A small hypoattenuating nodule is present in the right pancreatic lobe (arrow). There was a small amount of peripancreatic fat stranding. The patient had other abnormalities on the CT not described here. The CT diagnosis was acute pancreatitis with focal necrotic regions.

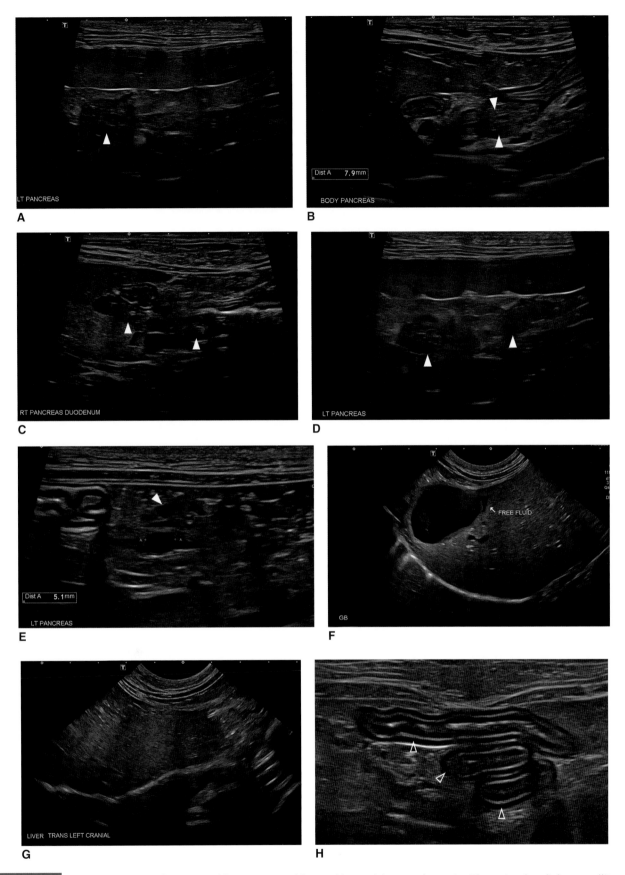

**FIGURE 26.18** Ultrasound images of a 14-year-old DSH presented for vomiting and decreased appetite. The patient has diabetes mellitus. (**A-D**) The left and right lobe and body of the pancreas are hypoechoic and moderately enlarged (arrowheads) with surrounding hyperechoic mesentery. A large hypoechoic nodule is present in the left lobe measuring 0.5 cm ((**E**) between calipers). A small amount of free fluid is present in the abdomen, adjacent to the gall bladder (**F**). The liver is diffusely enlarged and hyperechoic (**F,G**). Multiple loops of jejunum are mildly thickened with matching of the mucosal and muscularis layers ((**H**) open arrowhead indicates the thickened muscularis layer). The ultrasound and clinical diagnosis were acute pancreatitis with triaditis. The hypoechoic nodule in the pancreas is suspected to correspond to nodular hyperplasia. Neoplasia cannot be completely ruled out.

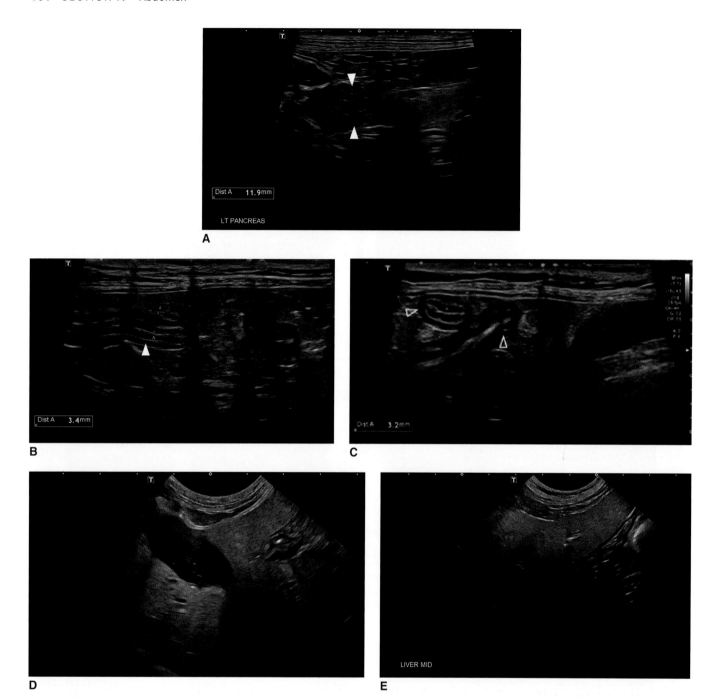

**FIGURE 26.19** Transverse (short axis) ultrasound images of a 10-year-old DSH presented for anorexia and vomiting with suspect diabetic ketoacidosis. The left lobe of the pancreas is hypoechoic and enlarged, measuring 1.2 cm ((**A**) closed arrowhead). Loops of jejunum are diffusely thickened with matching of the mucosal and muscularis layers (calipers indicate wall thickness, open arrowhead indicates the muscularis layer (**B,C**)). The liver is diffusely enlarged and hyperechoic (**D,E**). The findings are consistent with acute pancreatitis with triaditis. Pancreatic neoplasia cannot be completely ruled out.

mellitus, inflammatory bowel disease, and intestinal lymphoma, among other diseases [3]. Ultrasound-guided fine needle aspiration of hepatic parenchyma and bile may be helpful in confirming active bacterial infection [24].

A definitive diagnosis of triaditis requires integration of patient history, clinical examination findings, laboratory and diagnostic imaging findings, and histopathologic evaluation of the pancreas, liver, and small intestines [3, 24]. Bacterial, infectious, immune-mediated, and idiopathic mechanisms are considered as possible causes of inflammation in the pancreas, liver, and small intestines that could cause the development of triaditis [3].

# Pancreatic Nodular Hyperplasia

Pancreatic exocrine nodular hyperplasia is a benign condition that is commonly identified in older dogs and cats. It is not associated with inflammatory or other conditions, and is considered an incidental finding [25]. Nodular hyperplasia is most commonly identified on ultrasound examination, where there are multiple small (usually 0.3–1.0 cm diameter) hypoechoic nodules that can result in mild pancreatic enlargement [26] (Figure 26.20). Given their small size, they are less commonly recognized on CT, but will cause subtle, contrast-enhancing nodules when present (Figure 26.21).

Although nodular hyperplasia does not cause clinical signs, it has some imaging features that overlap with malignant neoplasia (e.g., diffuse nodules, increase in pancreatic size) which complicates diagnosis and may require aspiration/cytology for definitive diagnosis.

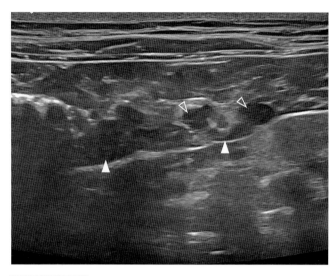

**FIGURE 26.20** Longitudinal image of the left pancreas in a cat. Pancreas is indicated by closed arrowheads. There are multiple hypoechoic nodules in the pancreas, consistent with nodular hyperplasia (open arrowheads). The cat was asymptomatic.

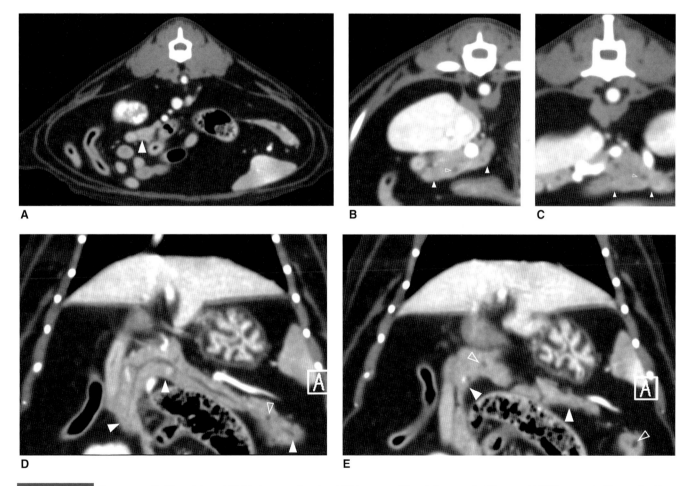

**FIGURE 26.21** Transverse (**A–C**) and dorsal (**D,E**) plane postcontrast CT images of the abdomen of a 19-year-old DHS presented for evaluation of an oral mass. A thoracic CT was performed for metastasis check. (**B,C**) Close-up views of the pancreas. The pancreas (arrowheads) is normal in size with a few well-circumscribed postcontrast hypoattenuating nodules (open arrowheads) measuring up to 0.2 cm in diameter. The nodules are presumed to be benign and correspond to nodular hyperplasia but malignant neoplasia cannot be completely ruled out.

# Pancreatic Cysts and Pseudocysts

Cysts and pseudocysts have been infrequently reported in cats and dogs. In both, the most common clinical sign associated with pancreatic cysts, pseudocysts, and abscesses is vomiting with or without anorexia, and these lesions are often associated with acute or chronic pancreatitis and diabetes mellitus [27].

Ultrasound or CT are the imaging modalities of choice to diagnose cystic lesions in the pancreas. On ultrasound, they appear as an anechoic mass with distal acoustic enhancement associated with the pancreas. On CT, they appear as a round or oval lesion containing fluid-attenuating material with a thin soft tissue-attenuating wall and rim enhancement on postcontrast images. Differentials for such lesions include pancreatic cyst, pseudocyst, abscess, neoplasia or loculated effusion. Ultrasound can be used to guide aspiration of these lesions which serves to collapse them as well as for cytologic evaluation, bacterial culture, and determination of amylase and lipase activities [26, 27].

True cysts are defined as an enclosed structure surrounded by a capsule internally coated with cuboidal epithelium and filled with liquid or semi-solid component. In contrast to inflammatory pseudocysts, true cysts do not contain exudate. True pancreatic cysts are rare in dogs and cats and few sporadic reports are available. One report described a 5-year-old cat with a history of vomiting. On ultrasound, a cystic pedunculated mass was attached to the body of the pancreas. Exploratory surgery was performed, and the mass confirmed to be a cyst [28]. A 15-year-old cat presented with chronic vomiting and azotemia had an abdominal ultrasound performed, which demonstrated a well-defined multilobulated cystic structure cranial and medial to the left kidney measuring up to 2.8 cm in diameter [27]. A laparoscopy was performed and a cystic structure approximately 7 cm in length was present between the spleen and left kidney, appearing to originate from the left pancreatic lobe. Brown fluid was aspirated from the lesion. Laparoscopic omentalization was performed. On histopathology, the lesion had an irregular wall consisting of cuboid epithelium with apical secretory vesicles and the diagnosis was pancreatic cyst [27].

Another report describes an 11-month-old cat presented for recurring vomiting. Abdominal US revealed the presence of a cystic anechoic structure with well-defined edges with close contact with the duodenum and pancreas. An exploratory surgery was performed showing a cystic structure approximately 3 cm in diameter in the pancreas. The lesion was completely removed and submitted for histopathology. The structure contained brown liquid and was diagnosed as a pancreatic cyst [29].

Multiple recurrent pancreatic cysts were described in a cat with pancreatic inflammation, atrophy, and diabetes mellitus [30]. On ultrasound, compartmentalized anechoic structures were present within the pancreas connecting to a peritoneal mass which was multilobulated and hypoechoic with intralesional hyperechoic strands. On CT, a fluid-filled mass was present within the left pancreatic lobe. The mass had a thin wall with moderate contrast enhancement and internal septations. Exploratory surgery and histopathology confirmed the lesion as being a true cyst [30].

Pancreatic pseudocysts are enzyme-rich fluid collections that lack an epithelial layer and may contain exudate, pancreatic secretions, and necrotic debris [31]. In humans, they are the most common cystic lesion of the pancreas and may complicate acute pancreatitis, chronic pancreatitis or pancreatic trauma. The pathogenesis is not well understood. One possibility is premature activation of digestive enzymes by pancreatitis causing inflammation and necrosis of the pancreatic parenchyma and resulting in the formation of a cystic structure [32]. Pseudocysts are also rare in dogs and cats and only reported sporadically but are more common than true cysts [32–34].

In one study, pancreatic pseudocysts were diagnosed in four dogs and two cats [32]. Ultrasound revealed anechoic to slightly echoic cyst-like lesions in the pancreatic region. Distal acoustic enhancement was observed in all lesions. Multiple pseudocysts were seen in one cat. In all patients, the pancreatic parenchyma was hypoechoic and the surrounding omental and peritoneal fat were hyperechoic, suggesting acute pancreatitis. Cytologically, the pseudocyst fluid was aseptic in all patients and had low numbers of inflammatory cells in five of the six patients. All had high lipase activity in the pseudocyst fluid and in two dogs and one cat, the lipase activity fluid was greater than that in the serum [32].

# Pancreatic Abscess

Pancreatic abscesses are rare in dogs and cats, but most commonly occur as sequelae to pancreatitis in dogs [35]. Radiographs do not readily identify pancreatic abscesses as they occur concurrently with pancreatitis, and both result in pancreatic enlargement and loss of regional detail. A mass effect could be present in the case of a very large abscess, but differentiation of enlargement from pancreatitis alone is not possible.

Ultrasound is more sensitive in detecting pancreatic abscesses, revealing an accumulation of fluid within the pancreatic parenchyma (Figure 26.22). The fluid is typically highly echogenic, reflecting the high cellular/protein content of the fluid. Gas is not usually seen within the abscess. Regional inflammation and fluid reflective of pancreatitis are expected. Pancreatic neoplasms can develop secondary abscessation, so identification of an abscess on ultrasound still requires cytologic or histopathologic examination to rule out concurrent neoplasia.

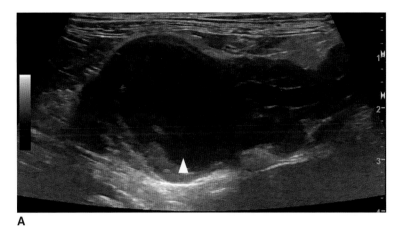

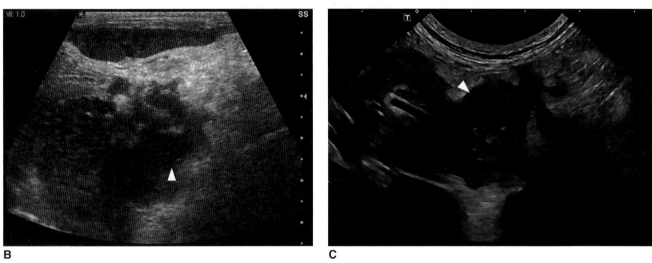

**FIGURE 26.22** Ultrasound images of a cat (**A**), small-breed dog (**B**), and large-breed dog (**C**) with pancreatic abscesses. There is a large fluid-filled, echogenic mass within each pancreas (arrowheads) consistent with a pancreatic abscess. Purulent fluid was aspirated from each under ultrasound guidance.

# Pancreatic Carcinoma

Exocrine pancreatic tumors are rare in dogs and cats, with pancreatic adenocarcinoma being the most common type. The diagnosis is challenging because clinical signs and hematologic results are nonspecific or may be normal [26, 36, 37]. Possible radiographic findings in dogs and cats with pancreatic tumor are a mass effect and effusion. Ultrasonographic findings include the presence of an enlarged and hypoechoic pancreas with or without nodules and masses, abdominal effusion, enlarged regional lymph nodes, and extrahepatic biliary obstruction [26, 38] (Figures 26.23–26.26).

In a study evaluating 30 cats with extrahepatic biliary obstruction, 12 cats had neoplasia as the cause of the obstruction, with three being carcinoma [38]. In a study evaluating 19 cats with pancreatic neoplasia and nodular hyperplasia, 14 cats had neoplasia, of which 11 had adenocarcinoma [26]. The remaining tumors were composed of one each of lymphoma, squamous cell carcinoma, and lymphangiosarcoma.

The most common ultrasonographic findings for neoplasia in general were focal pancreatic mass or nodule (8/14), lymphadenopathy (7/14), and abdominal effusion (7/14) [26]. Cats with nodular hyperplasia (5/19) had multiple hypoechoic nodules that were mostly small, ranging from 0.3 to 1.0 cm. Although overlap in the size between neoplasia and nodular hyperplasia was present, the presence of a single pancreatic nodule/mass larger than 2.0 cm was unique to pancreatic neoplasia in this study [26].

In a study evaluating the ultrasonographic findings in 14 cats with histology- or cytology-proven carcinomatosis, three cats had pancreatic tumor as the primary tumor site, two with carcinoma and one with adenocarcinoma. Peritoneal effusion and masses in the connecting peritoneum described as small, separate to confluent, hypoechoic, round to oval were found in all cats [39].

A recent study described the CT and ultrasound features of canine and feline carcinomatosis and sarcomatosis in 31 patients [40]. In this study, two dogs and six cats had pancreatic

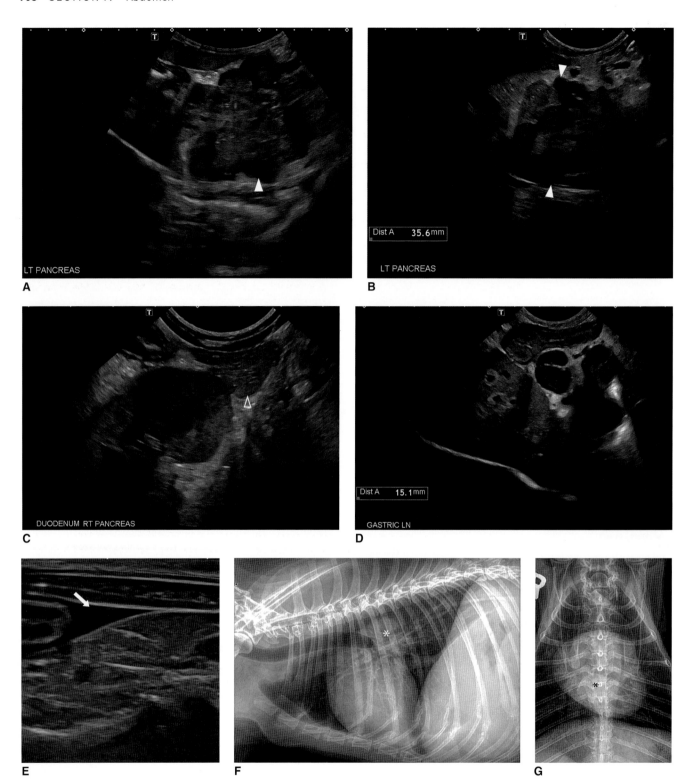

**FIGURE 26.23** Transverse (short axis) ultrasound images of a 12-year-old poodle presented with chronic pancreatitis and inappetence. cPLI was severely increased. There is a large, lobulated heterogeneous hypoechoic mass associated with the left pancreatic lobe ((**A,B**) arrowheads). The right lobe of the pancreas is enlarged and mildly hypoechoic ((**C**) open arrowhead). Multiple mesenteric lymph nodes are severely enlarged and hypoechoic ((**D**) between calipers). There is a moderate amount of free fluid, and the mesentery is hyperechoic ((**E**) arrow). In addition, there was severe thickening of the stomach and multiple hepatic nodules. Right lateral (**F**) and ventrodorsal (**G**) views of the thorax. A large, poorly demarcated soft tissue opaque mass is present in the hilar region (asterisk) causing ventral displacement of the trachea consistent with severe tracheal bronchial lymphadenopathy. The findings are suggestive of multicentric neoplasia. Cytology of a mesenteric lymph node was diagnostic for histiocytic sarcoma.

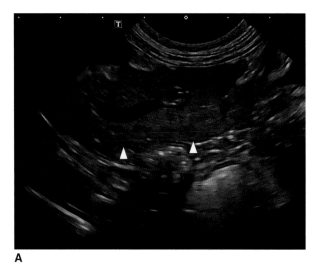

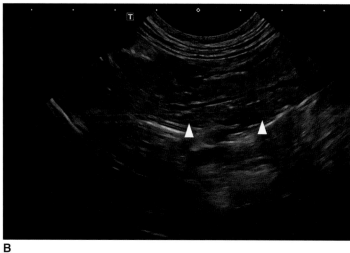

A                                                                                          B

**FIGURE 26.24** Sagittal (long axis) ultrasound images of a 12-year-old Labrador presented for a trial for multiple myeloma. Doing well at home with no clinical signs. The pancreas is moderately enlarged ((**A,B**) arrowhead) with a mild hypoechoic texture and heterogeneous. The differentials included neoplasia such as multiple myeloma, carcinoma or pancreatitis.

carcinoma as the primary tumor type. On ultrasound and CT, multiple pleural and peritoneal lesions were commonly seen (10/14 cases) as opposed to solitary lesions (4/14 cases). Nodules were present remote to the primary tumor in all cases, and less frequently observed close to the primary tumor (8/14 cases) [40].

In a study reviewing 34 cases of feline pancreatic carcinoma, the most common presenting signs were weight loss, decreased appetite, vomiting, palpable abdominal mass, and diarrhea. Metastatic disease was confirmed in 11 cats and the median survival time was 97 days [41]. Ultrasonographic findings in this study demonstrated nodular changes to the pancreas in all cats. Additional ultrasound findings included abdominal effusion in 16 cats, liver abnormalities in 12 cats, splenic nodules in two, abdominal lymphadenopathy in 11, nodular appearance to adipose tissue in three cats and bile duct and pancreatic duct dilation in two cats each [41].

In a study reviewing 23 cases of canine pancreatic carcinoma, the most common clinical signs included anorexia, lethargy, vomiting, and abdominal pain [37]. Ultrasound findings included masses along the left, right or body of the pancreas that were described as heterogeneous with well-defined borders and occasional cavitation. Out of eight patients with diffuse carcinoma histologically, two had grossly normal pancreas on ultrasound. Metastatic disease was detected in 78% (18/23) of the dogs at the time of diagnosis, with the most common sites being the liver (12/23) or regional lymph nodes (10/23) [37].

Recently, a study described a case of suspected needle tract seeding in a cat undergoing fine needle aspiration of a pancreatic nodule that was histologically diagnosed as pancreatic adenocarcinoma [42]. Studies specifically describing the CT appearance of feline and canine pancreatic neoplasia are lacking in the veterinary literature. Expected findings are a mass on the pancreas or pancreatic enlargement, peritoneal

effusion, regional lymphadenopathy and presence of metastasis in other organs such as liver and spleen (Figure 26.27).

# Endocrine Tumors

Insulinomas are neuroendocrine tumors primarily composed of abnormal beta cells, and cause clinical signs due to their inappropriate, excessive production of insulin. They are well characterized in dogs and very rare in cats [43]. The most accurate clinical criteria for diagnosis are paired blood glucose and insulin levels, with hypoglycemia occurring in the face of normal or elevated insulin level.

Imaging is used to stage the patient prior to surgical intervention. Ideally, the primary tumor is identified within the pancreas, and the absence of apparent metastatic lesions provides a more favorable prognosis for surgical cure.

CT examination is the most sensitive method in detecting insulinomas and screening a patient for metastasis [44]. It provides evaluation of the entire pancreas, without the limitations of ultrasound when gas from adjacent gastrointestinal structures may limit complete pancreatic evaluation. Triple-phase angiography should be performed, as insulinomas are often more apparent in early-phase arterial imaging (Figure 26.28) compared to the adjacent pancreatic parenchyma [45]. Later venous or delayed phases may still demonstrate the primary tumor (Figure 26.29). CT also provides a more complete evaluation of the liver for metastasis as well as regional lymph nodes compared to ultrasound. Hepatic lymph nodes are common sites of metastasis (Figure 26.28), though the pancreaticoduodenal lymph node (Figure 26.29) and regional mesenteric lymph nodes should also be evaluated for evidence of metastasis (Figure 26.30).

If not obscured by gas in the gastrointestinal tract, insulinomas can be identified on ultrasound and typically are iso- to hypoechoic nodules or masses within the pancreatic parenchyma

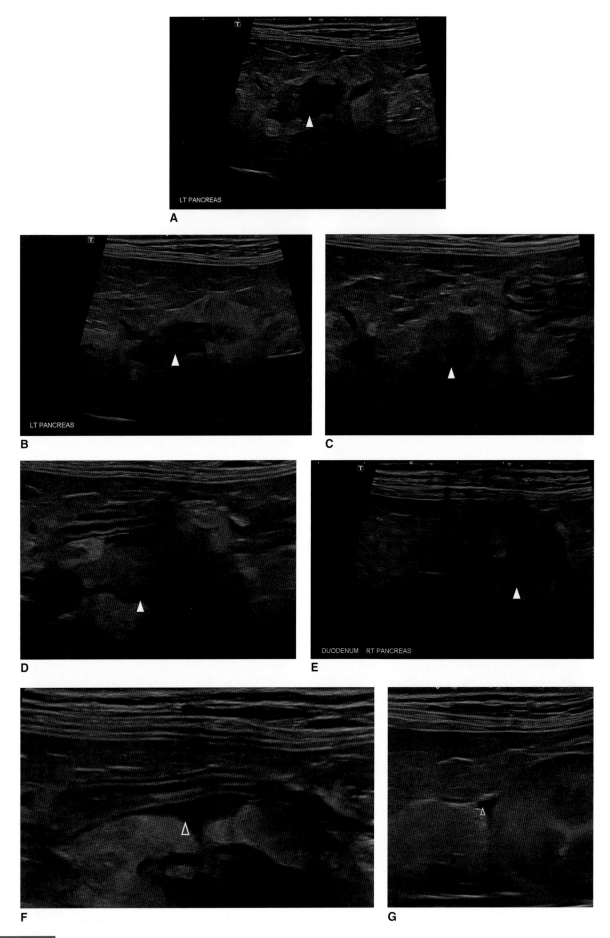

**FIGURE 26.25** Sagittal (long axis) ultrasound images of a 12-year-old DSH presented for intermittent anorexia and vomiting. The pancreas is diffusely moderately enlarged, irregular and hypoechoic with surrounded hyperechoic mesentery ((**A–E**) arrowhead). Free fluid is present ((**F,G**) open arrowhead). The findings are suggestive of pancreatitis or pancreatic neoplasia. Cytology of the pancreas diagnosed carcinoma.

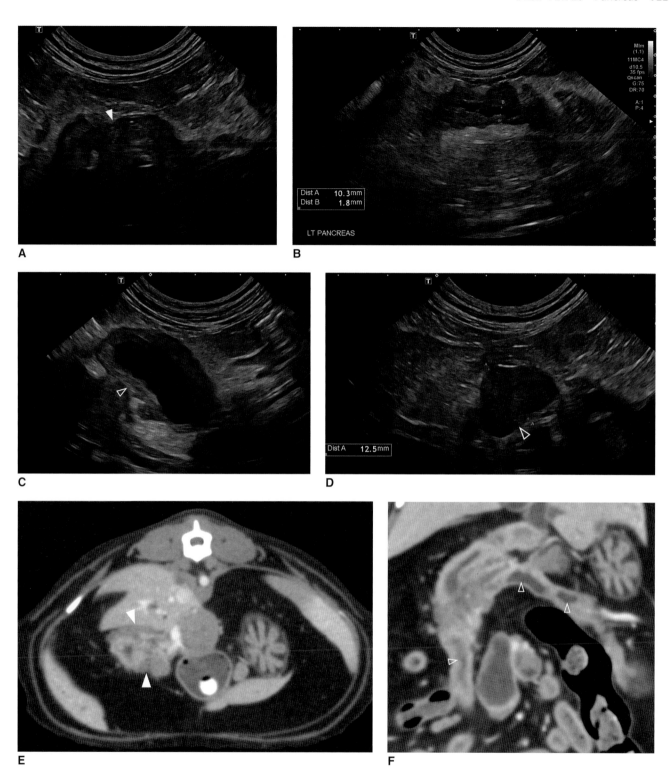

**FIGURE 26.26** Sagittal (long axis) ultrasound images of a 6-year-old DSH presented for icterus, inappetence, and elevated liver values. The right lobe of the pancreas is moderately enlarged, mass-like, and hypoechoic with surrounded hyperechoic mesentery ((**A**) arrowhead). The left lobe is mildly enlarged ((**B**) between calipers; calipers also indicate the pancreatic duct). Regional lymph nodes are severely enlarged and cavitated ((**C,D**) open arrowheads). Free fluid is present. Transverse (**E,G–I,K**) and dorsal (**F,J**) plane postcontrast CT images of the abdomen. The pancreas (arrowheads) is enlarged and heterogeneous with ill-defined nodules and masses (**E**). The pancreatic duct is diffusely dilated, measuring up to 0.5 cm in diameter ((**F**) open arrowheads). Regional lymph nodes are severely enlarged and cavitated and some can be connected to the pancreas ((**G**) arrow). The gall bladder is moderately distended (**H**). The intrahepatic ducts are diffusely dilated and there is diffuse dilation of the cystic and common bile duct ((**H–J**) asterisk). Multiple soft tissue-attenuating nodules are present throughout the peritoneal cavity, some strongly contrast enhancing ((**K,L**) within circles). A mild amount of fluid is present in the peritoneal cavity. The findings are consistent with pancreatic malignant neoplasia such as carcinoma with severe metastatic lymphadenopathy, biliary tract obstruction, and carcinomatosis. Cytology of the hepatic lymph node was consistent with carcinoma.

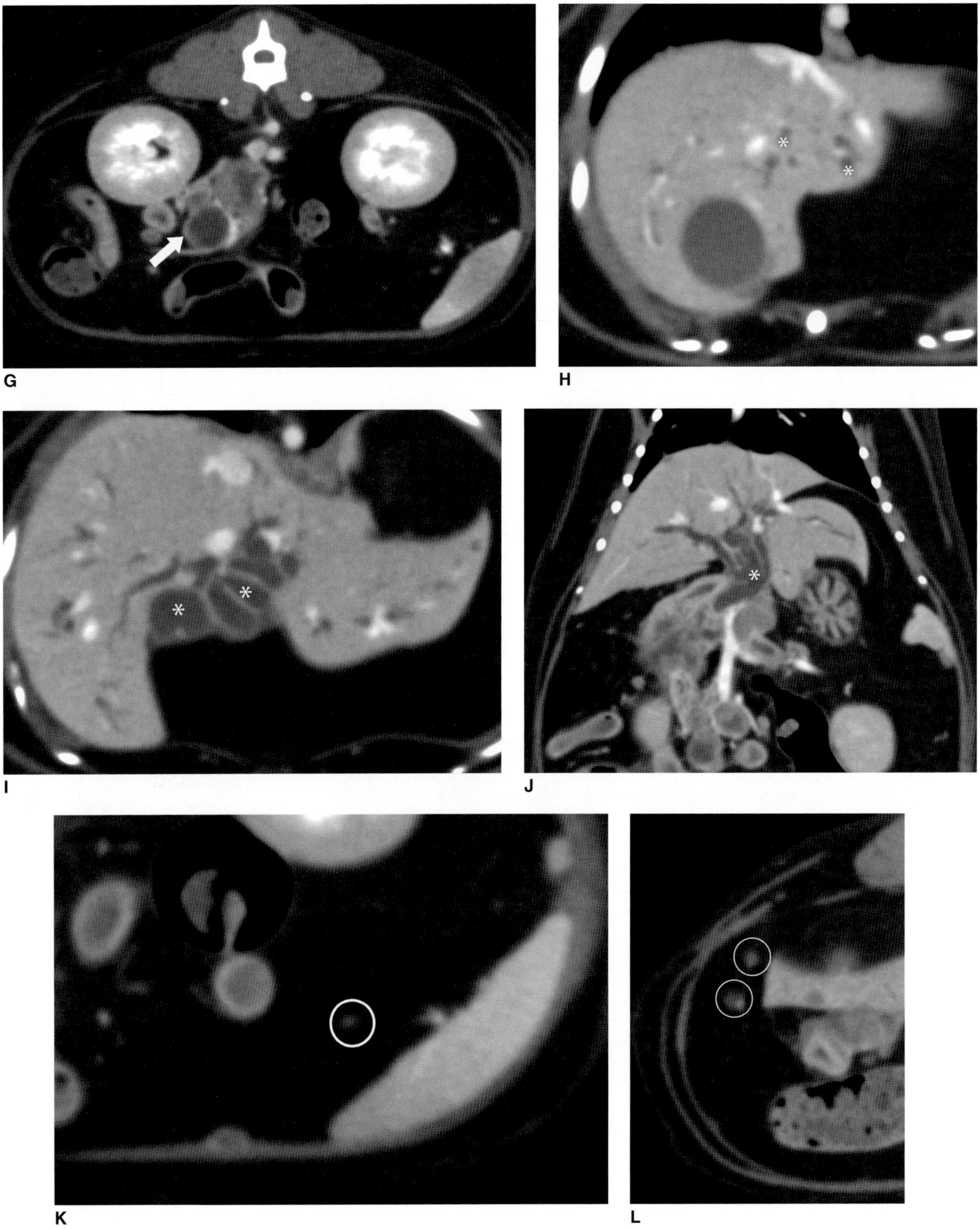

G

H

I

J

K

L

**FIGURE 26.26** (Continued)

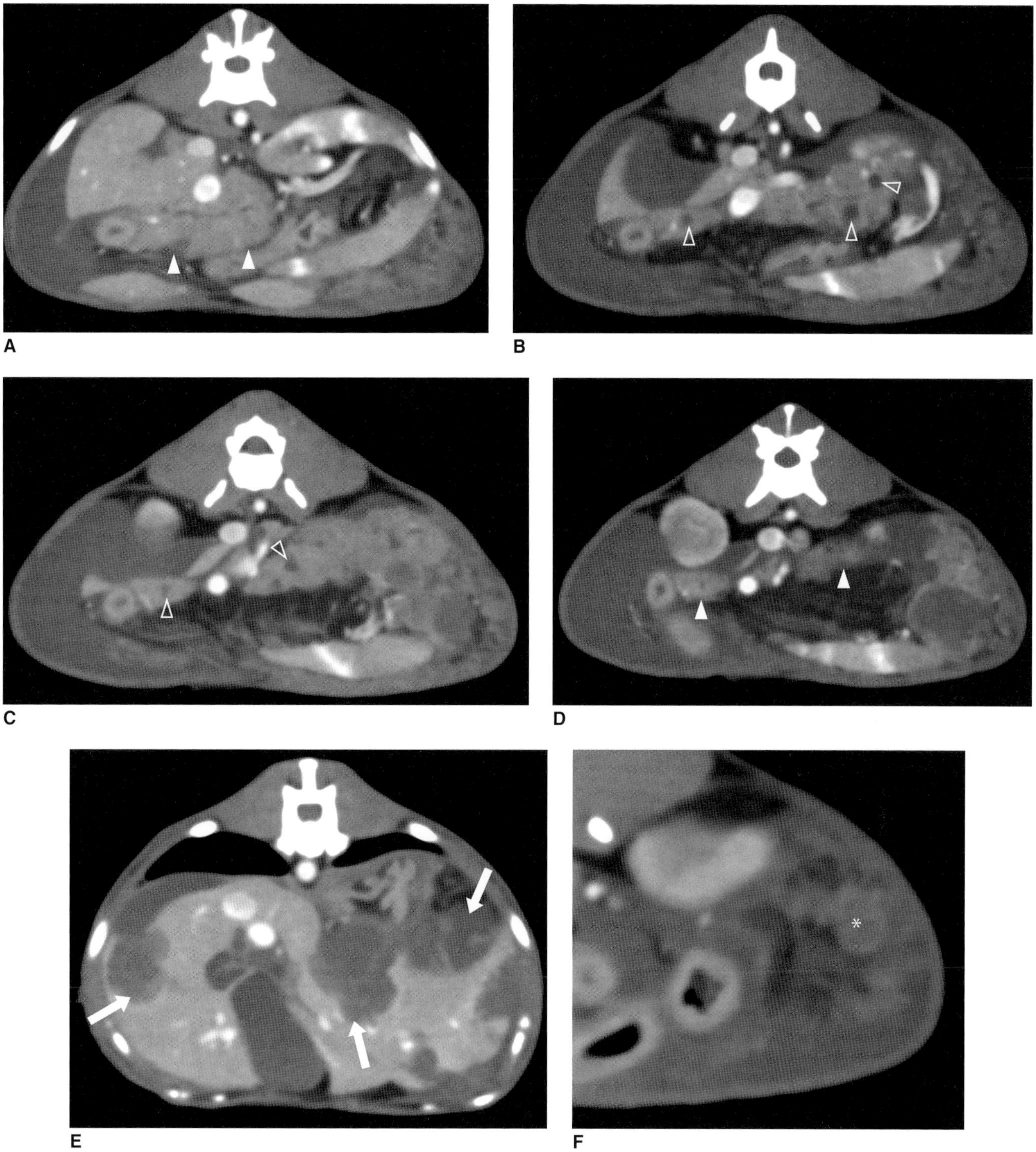

**FIGURE 26.27** Transverse plane postcontrast CT images of a 13-year-old DSH presented for lethargy and not doing well. A hemoabdomen was diagnosed during presentation. The pancreas is severely diffusely enlarged with a large cavitated mass (arrowhead) measuring approximately 3 cm in diameter and multiple hypoattenuating nodules (open arrowheads) (**A–D**). Multiple large hypoattenuating cavitated masses and nodules are present throughout the liver ((**E**) arrows). A severe amount of fluid-attenuating material is present in the abdomen. Multiple ill-defined contrast-enhancing nodules are present in the mesentery, predominantly adjacent to the spleen and pancreas ((**F**) asterisk). The CT findings are suggestive of malignant neoplasia with carcinomatosis. The primary tumor could be pancreatic or hepatic in origin. A final diagnosis was not obtained.

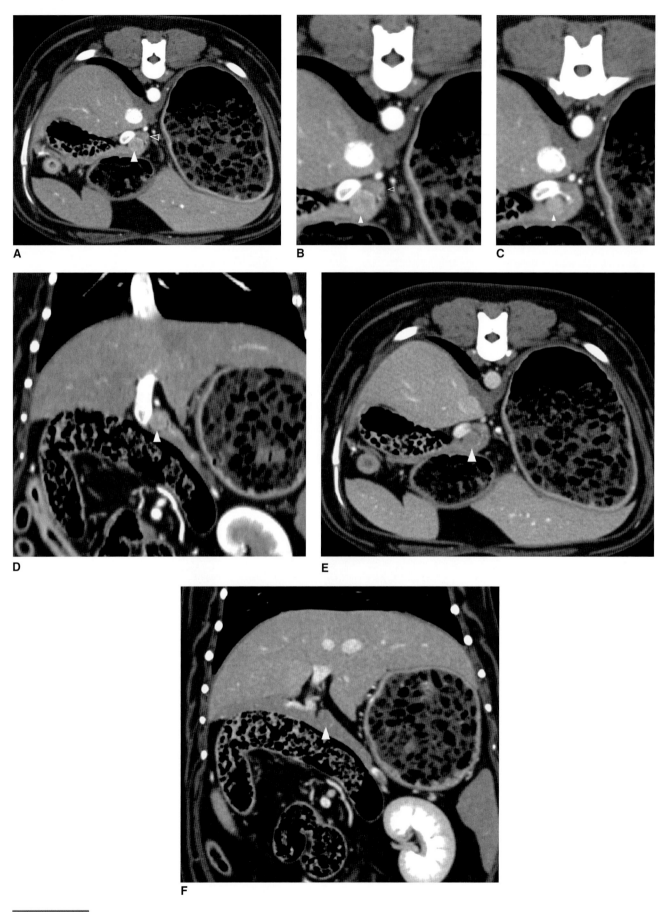

**FIGURE 26.28** Transverse (**A**–**C**,**E**) and dorsal (**D**,**F**) plane postcontrast CT images of the abdomen of a 6-year-old pit bull presented for decreased appetite and energy, with hypoglycemia. Figures (**A**–**D**) are late arterial phase, (**E**) and (**F**) are venous phase images. (**B**) is a close-up of (**A**). A round, relatively well-circumscribed soft tissue-attenuating strong contrast-enhancing mass (arrowheads) is present in the left lobe of the pancreas, seen ventral to the portal vein measuring approximately 1.5 cm in diameter. The mass is more enhancing on the late arterial phase (**A**–**D**) compared to the venous phase images (**E**,**F**). The left hepatic lymph node is mildly enlarged and heterogeneously enhancing and confluent with the mass (open arrowhead). The findings are consistent with an insulinoma with metastatic lymphadenopathy.

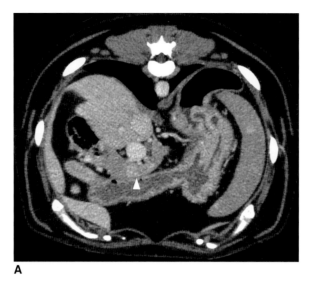

**A**

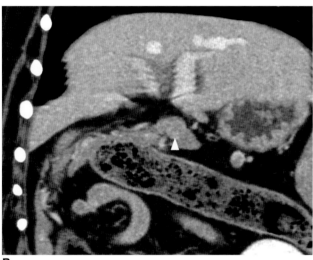

**B**

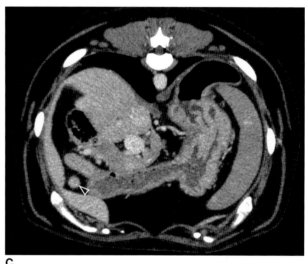

**C**

**FIGURE 26.29**   Transverse (**A,C**) and dorsal (**B**) plane postcontrast CT images of the abdomen of a 11-year-old mixed-breed dog presented for workup of hypoglycemia. A poorly defined soft tissue-attenuating contrast-enhancing mass (arrowheads) is present in the body and left lobe of the pancreas seen ventral and to the left of the portal vein, measuring approximately 2.6 × 1.5 cm (**A,B**). The pancreaticoduodenal lymph node is enlarged ((**C**) open arrowhead). The findings are consistent with an insulinoma. On surgery, a mass was present in the left lobe of the pancreas. The histologic diagnosis was islet cell neoplasia with metastatic pancreaticoduodenal lymph node.

(Figure 26.31). As they can be small or obscured by adjacent anatomy, inability to identify a primary pancreatic nodule on US or CT examination does not preclude a diagnosis of insulinoma and may ultimately require surgical exploratory and biopsy for definitive diagnosis. Identification of nodules within the liver in a patient with insulinoma is not definitive for metastasis, as there is overlap in benign and other causes of nodules in the liver.

Tumors may arise from other islet neuroendocrine cells in the pancreas and result in glucagonomas, gastrinomas, or somatostatinomas, depending on the hormone secreted by the neoplasm. These are rare tumors in dogs and cats and poorly characterized, but have a similar appearance to insulinomas.

# Pancreatic Edema

Pancreatic edema in the absence of acute pancreatitis is characterized by fluid in the interlobular septa of the pancreas. On ultrasound, it appears as multiple linear anechoic areas that divide the gland and give it a characteristic "tiger stripe" appearance [46] (Figures 26.32 and 26.33). It has been associated with hypoalbuminemia or portal hypertension in dogs in conditions such as anaphylaxis, portosystemic shunt, and iatrogenic overhydration, among other causes [46]. Pancreatic edema is usually an incidental finding.

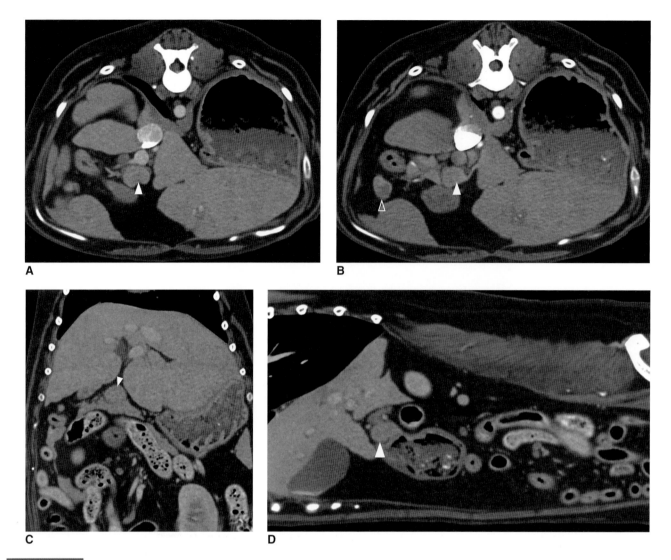

**FIGURE 26.30** Transverse (**A** and **B**), dorsal (**C**), and sagittal (**D**) plane postcontrast CT images of the abdomen of an 8-year-old Alaskan malamute presented for anorexia and lethargy. Blood work showed hypoglycemia. A soft tissue-attenuating contrast-enhancing nodule is present within the body of the pancreas (closed arrowheads). Multiple mesenteric lymph nodes were moderately enlarged and heterogeneously enhancing ((**B**) pancreaticoduodenal lymph node; open arrowhead). The findings are consistent with an insulinoma with suspect metastatic lymphadenopathy. Typically insulinomas will enhance on the arterial phase of a CT study (three phase not obtained in this dog).

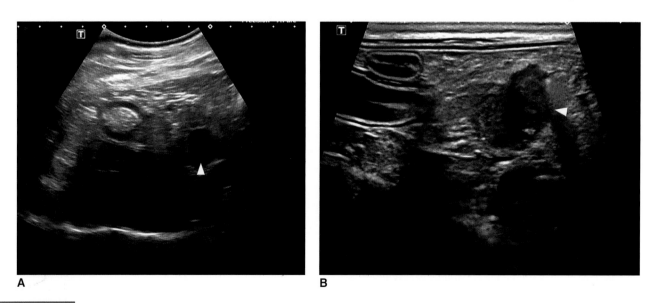

**FIGURE 26.31** Transverse (short axis) images of two dogs with insulinoma in the right lobe (arrowheads). In the dog in (**A**), the insulinoma is nearly anechoic, whereas in (**B**) the insulinoma is only slightly different in echogenicity from adjacent pancreatic parenchyma.

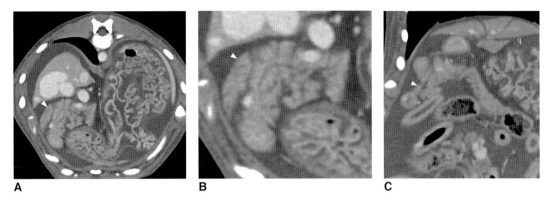

**FIGURE 26.32** Transverse (**A,B**) and dorsal (**C**) plane postcontrast CT images of the abdomen of a 6-month-old boxer presented for further evaluation of an intrahepatic shunt. Blood work showed severe hypoalbuminemia. (**B**) is a close-up image of (**A**). The pancreas (closed arrowheads) has a typical "tiger stripe" appearance, being diffusely enlarged with multiple striated hypoattenuating regions throughout the parenchyma (**A–C**). There is also severe peritoneal effusion and gastric wall edema (open arrowhead) among other findings. The CT findings for the pancreas are consisting with edema likely secondary to hypoalbuminemia and/or portal hypertension.

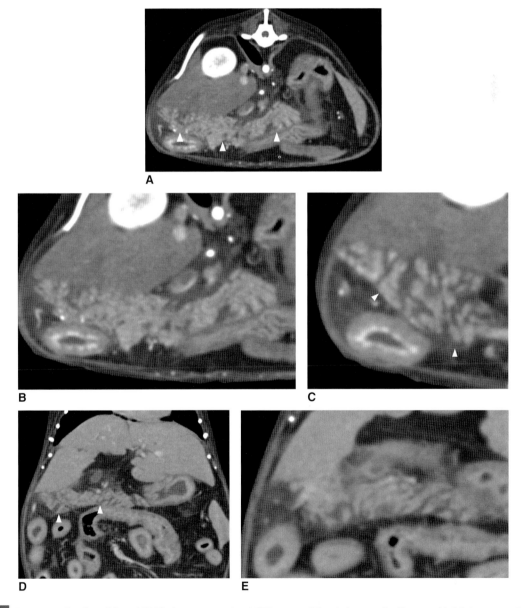

**FIGURE 26.33** Transverse (**A–C**) and dorsal (**D,E**) plane postcontrast CT images of the abdomen of a 12-year-old shih tzu presented with acute onset of anemia and diabetes, being managed for protein-losing enteropathy. Blood work showed marked hypoalbuminemia. (**B**) is a close-up image of (**A**), (**E**) is a close-up image of (**D**). The pancreas (arrowheads) has a typical "tiger stripe" appearance, being diffusely enlarged with multiple striated hypoattenuating regions throughout the parenchyma. There is peritoneal effusion, the liver is enlarged, and heterogeneous and multiple loops of jejunum are mildly thickened. The CT findings for the pancreas are consistent with edema secondary to hypoalbuminemia.

# References

1. Xenoulis, P.G. (2015). Diagnosis of pancreatitis in dogs and cats. *J. Small Anim. Pract.* 56 (1): 13–26.

2. Watson, P. (2015). Pancreatitis in dogs and cats: definitions and pathophysiology. *J. Small Anim. Pract.* 56 (1): 3–12.

3. Simpson, K.W. (2015). Pancreatitis and triaditis in cats: causes and treatment. *J. Small Anim. Pract.* 56 (1): 40–49.

4. Cerna, P., Kilpatrick, S., and Gunn-Moore, D.A. (2020). Feline comorbidities: what do we really know about feline triaditis? *J. Feline Med. Surg.* 22 (11): 1047–1067.

5. Forman, M.A., Steiner, J.M., Armstrong, P.J. et al. (2021). ACVIM consensus statement on pancreatitis in cats. *J. Vet. Intern. Med.* 35 (2): 703–723.

6. Sato, K., Sakamoto, Y., Sakai, M. et al. (2020). Diagnostic utility of computed tomographic angiography in dogs with portal vein thrombosis. *J. Vet. Med. Sci.* 82 (10): 1421–1427.

7. von Stade, L.E., Shropshire, S.B., Rao, S. et al. (2021). Prevalence of portal vein thrombosis detected by computed tomography angiography in dogs. *J. Small Anim. Pract.* 62 (7): 562–569.

8. Forman, M.A., Marks, S.L., De Cock, H.E. et al. (2004). Evaluation of serum feline pancreatic lipase immunoreactivity and helical computed tomography versus conventional testing for the diagnosis of feline pancreatitis. *J. Vet. Intern. Med.* 18 (6): 807–815.

9. Hecht, S. and Henry, G. (2007). Sonographic evaluation of the normal and abnormal pancreas. *Clin. Tech. Small Anim. Pract.* 22 (3): 115–121.

10. French, J.M., Twedt, D.C., Rao, S., and Marolf, A.J. (2019). Computed tomographic angiography and ultrasonography in the diagnosis and evaluation of acute pancreatitis in dogs. *J. Vet. Intern. Med.* 33 (1): 79–88.

11. Jaeger, J.Q., Mattoon, J.S., Bateman, S.W., and Morandi, F. (2003). Combined use of ultrasonography and contrast enhanced computed tomography to evaluate acute necrotizing pancreatitis in two dogs. *Vet. Radiol. Ultrasound* 44 (1): 72–79.

12. Larson, M.M., Panciera, D.L., Ward, D.L. et al. (2005). Age-related changes in the ultrasound appearance of the normal feline pancreas. *Vet. Radiol. Ultrasound* 46 (3): 238–242.

13. Hecht, S., Penninck, D.G., Mahony, O.M. et al. (2006). Relationship of pancreatic duct dilation to age and clinical findings in cats. *Vet. Radiol. Ultrasound* 47 (3): 287–294.

14. Leoni, F., Pelligra, T., Citi, S. et al. (2020). Ultrasonographic monitoring in 38 dogs with clinically suspected acute pancreatitis. *Vet. Sci.* 7: 180.

15. Rademacher, N., Ohlerth, S., Scharf, G. et al. (2008). Contrast-enhanced power and color Doppler ultrasonography of the pancreas in healthy and diseased cats. *J. Vet. Intern. Med.* 22 (6): 1310–1316.

16. Rademacher, N., Schur, D., Gaschen, F. et al. (2016). Contrast-enhanced ultrasonography of the pancreas in healthy dogs and in dogs with acute pancreatitis. *Vet. Radiol. Ultrasound* 57 (1): 58–64.

17. Lim, S.Y., Nakamura, K., Morishita, K. et al. (2015). Quantitative contrast-enhanced ultrasonographic assessment of naturally occurring pancreatitis in dogs. *J. Vet. Intern. Med.* 29 (1): 71–78.

18. Adrian, A.M., Twedt, D.C., Kraft, S.L., and Marolf, A.J. (2015). Computed tomographic angiography under sedation in the diagnosis of suspected canine pancreatitis: a pilot study. *J. Vet. Intern. Med.* 29 (1): 97–103.

19. Vrolyk, V., Wobeser, B.K., Al-Dissi, A.N. et al. (2017). Lung inflammation associated with clinical acute necrotizing pancreatitis in dogs. *Vet. Pathol.* 54 (1): 129–140.

20. Gori, E., Pierini, A., Ceccherini, G. et al. (2020). Pulmonary complications in dogs with acute presentation of pancreatitis. *BMC Vet. Res.* 16 (1): 209.

21. Gerhardt, A., Steiner, J.M., Williams, D.A. et al. (2001). Comparison of the sensitivity of different diagnostic tests for pancreatitis in cats. *J. Vet. Intern. Med.* 15 (4): 329–333.

22. Marolf, A.J., Kraft, S.L., Dunphy, T.R., and Twedt, D.C. (2013). Magnetic resonance (MR) imaging and MR cholangiopancreatography findings in cats with cholangitis and pancreatitis. *J. Feline Med. Surg.* 15 (4): 285–294.

23. Fragkou, F.C., Adamama-Moraitou, K.K., Poutahidis, T. et al. (2016). Prevalence and clinicopathological features of triaditis in a prospective case series of symptomatic and asymptomatic cats. *J. Vet. Intern. Med.* 30 (4): 1031–1045.

24. Lidbury, J.A., Mooyottu, S., and Jergens, A.E. (2020). Triaditis: truth and consequences. *Vet. Clin. North Am. Small Anim. Pract.* 50 (5): 1135–1156.

25. Newman, S.J., Steiner, J.M., Woosley, K. et al. (2005). Correlation of age and incidence of pancreatic exocrine nodular hyperplasia in the dog. *Vet. Pathol.* 42 (4): 510–513.

26. Hecht, S., Penninck, D.G., and Keating, J.H. (2007). Imaging findings in pancreatic neoplasia and nodular hyperplasia in 19 cats. *Vet. Radiol. Ultrasound* 48 (1): 45–50.

27. Bruckner, M. (2019). Laparoscopic omentalization of a pancreatic cyst in a cat. *J. Am. Vet. Med. Assoc.* 255 (2): 213–218.

28. Coleman, M.G., Robson, M.C., and Harvey, C. (2005). Pancreatic cyst in a cat. *N. Z. Vet. J.* 53 (2): 157–159.

29. Cavalcanti, E.B.O., Cerqueira, A.C.F., Kaiser, B.B. et al. (2021). Pancreatic cyst in a cat. *Ciencia Rura, Santa Maria* 51 (11): www.scielo.br/j/cr/a/Bp9H7ZvhHprWfqpNQQpqDpq/.

30. Branter, E.M. and Viviano, K.R. (2010). Multiple recurrent pancreatic cysts with associated pancreatic inflammation and atrophy in a cat. *J. Feline Med. Surg.* 12 (10): 822–827.

31. Rabie, M.E., El Hakeem, I., Al Skaini, M.S. et al. (2014). Pancreatic pseudocyst or a cystic tumor of the pancreas? *Chin. J. Cancer* 33 (2): 87–95.

32. VanEnkevort, B.A., O'Brien, R.T., and Young, K.M. (1999). Pancreatic pseudocysts in 4 dogs and 2 cats: ultrasonographic and clinicopathologic findings. *J. Vet. Intern. Med.* 13 (4): 309–313.

33. Hines, B.L., Salisbury, S.K., Jakovljevic, S., and DeNicola, D.B. (1996). Pancreatic pseudocyst associated with chronic-active necrotizing pancreatitis in a cat. *J. Am. Anim. Hosp. Assoc.* 32 (2): 147–152.

34. Smith, S.A. and Biller, D.S. (1998). Resolution of a pancreatic pseudocyst in a dog following percutaneous ultrasonographic-guided drainage. *J. Am. Anim. Hosp. Assoc.* 34 (6): 515–522.

35. Anderson, J.R., Cornell, K.K., Parnell, N.K., and Salisbury, S.K. (2008). Pancreatic abscess in 36 dogs: a retrospective analysis of prognostic indicators. *J. Am. Anim. Hosp. Assoc.* 44 (4): 171–179.

36. Bennett, P.F., Hahn, K.A., Toal, R.L., and Legendre, A.M. (2001). Ultrasonographic and cytopathological diagnosis of exocrine pancreatic carcinoma in the dog and cat. *J. Am. Anim. Hosp. Assoc.* 37 (5): 466–473.

37. Pinard, C.J., Hocker, S.E., and Weishaar, K.M. (2021). Clinical outcome in 23 dogs with exocrine pancreatic carcinoma. *Vet. Comp. Oncol.* 19 (1): 109–114.

38. Gaillot, H.A., Penninck, D.G., Webster, C.R., and Crawford, S. (2007). Ultrasonographic features of extrahepatic biliary obstruction in 30 cats. *Vet. Radiol. Ultrasound* 48 (5): 439–447.

39. Monteiro, C.B. and O'Brien, R.T. (2004). A retrospective study on the sonographic findings of abdominal carcinomatosis in 14 cats. *Vet. Radiol. Ultrasound* 45 (6): 559–564.

40. Weston, P.J., Baines, S.J., Finotello, R., and Mortier, J.R. (2021). Clinical, CT, and ultrasonographic features of canine and feline pleural and peritoneal carcinomatosis and sarcomatosis. *Vet. Radiol. Ultrasound* 62 (3): 331–341.

41. Linderman, M.J., Brodsky, E.M., de Lorimier, L.P. et al. (2013). Feline exocrine pancreatic carcinoma: a retrospective study of 34 cases. *Vet. Comp. Oncol.* 11 (3): 208–218.

42. Jegatheeson, S., Dandrieux, J.R., and Cannon, C.M. (2020). Suspected pancreatic carcinoma needle tract seeding in a cat. *JFMS Open Rep.* 6 (1): 2055116920918161.

43. Gifford, C., Morris, A., Kenney, K., and Estep, J. (2020). Diagnosis of insulinoma in a Maine Coon cat. *J. Feline Med. Surg. Open Rep.* 6 (1): 2055116919894782.

44. Robben, J.H., Pollak, Y.W., Kirpensteijn, J. et al. (2005). Comparison of ultrasonography, computed tomography, and single-photon emission computed tomography for the detection and localization of canine insulinoma. *J. Vet. Intern. Med.* 19 (1): 15–22.

45. Fukushima, K., Fujiwara, R., Yamamoto, K. et al. (2016). Characterization of triple-phase computed tomography in dogs with pancreatic insulinoma. *J. Vet. Med. Sci.* 77 (12): 1549–1553.

46. Lamb, C.R. (1999). Pancreatic edema in dogs with hypoalbuminemia or portal hypertension. *J. Vet. Intern. Med.* 13 (5): 498–500. Figure 26.18    (Continued)

# CHAPTER 27

# Urogenital Tract

**Elizabeth Huynh**

VCA West Coast Specialty and Emergency Animal Hospital, Fountain Valley, CA, USA

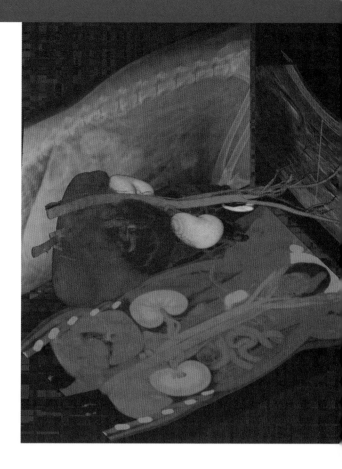

## Kidneys

### Normal Imaging Findings

See Chapter 20.

### Abnormal Imaging Findings

**Size**   Normal renal size does not rule out renal disease. Renal parenchymal diseases such as toxicity, amyloidosis, glomerulonephritis, acute nephritis, and pyelonephritis may be present without changes in renal size.

**Large Kidney(s)**   Renomegaly (>3.5 times the length of L2 in dogs; >3.0 times the length of L2 in cats) can be diagnosed using abdominal radiographs. Severe unilateral or bilateral renomegaly causes peripheral displacement of adjacent

abdominal contents. Renomegaly may be associated with parenchymal, capsular, or renal pelvic abnormalities. Usually, additional studies, using intravenous contrast medium or ultrasound, are needed to further assess the underlying cause of renomegaly.

Differentials for smoothly marginated renomegaly include hydronephrosis, perinephric pseudocyst (Figure 27.1), lymphomsa (may be bilateral) (Figure 27.2), amyloidosis (usually mild renomegaly), compensatory hypertrophy (Figure 27.3), renal hypertrophy secondary to portosystemic shunts (usually mild and more often seen in dogs than cats) (Figure 27.4), acromegaly, acute nephritis, toxicity, or acute renal failure (mild renomegaly).

Differentials for irregularly marginated renomegaly include neoplasia (primary or metastatic) (Figure 27.5), focal renal cyst, polycystic kidney disease (Figure 27.6), feline infectious peritonitis, abscess (Figure 27.7), or hematoma.

Excretory urography is used to diagnose parenchymal and ureteral changes of the kidneys as well as providing information

*Atlas of Small Animal Diagnostic Imaging*, First Edition. Edited by Clifford R. Berry, Nathan C. Nelson, and Matthew D. Winter.
© 2023 John Wiley & Sons, Inc. Published 2023 by John Wiley & Sons, Inc.
Companion website: www.wiley.com/go/berry/atlas

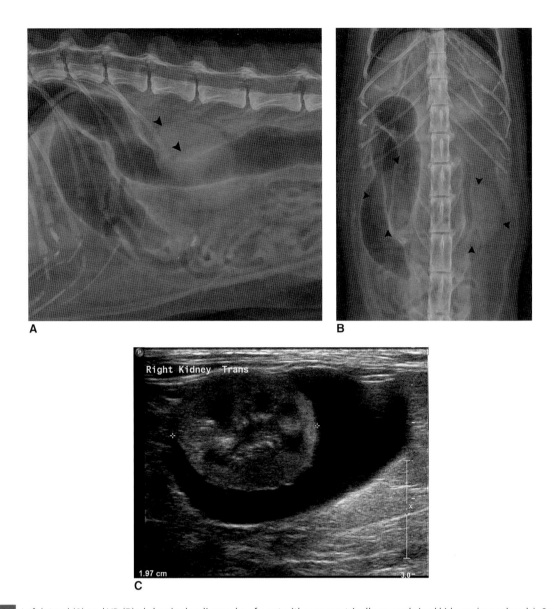

**FIGURE 27.1** Left lateral (**A**) and VD (**B**) abdominal radiographs of a cat with asymmetrically normal sized kidneys (arrowheads). Sagittal plane ultrasound image (**C**) of a small right kidney in the same cat with a large perinephric pseudocyst.

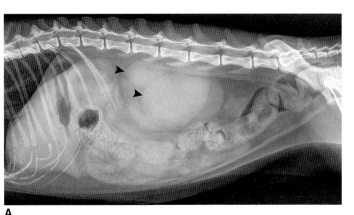
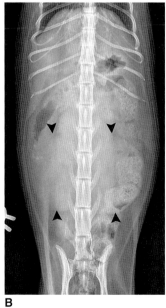

**FIGURE 27.2** Right lateral (**A**) and VD (**B**) abdominal radiographs of a cat with bilateral renomegaly (arrowheads), diagnosed with renal lymphoma.

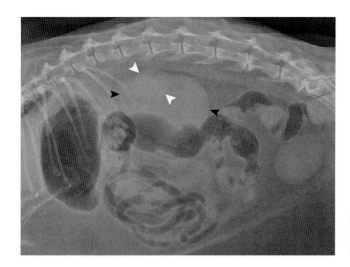

**FIGURE 27.3** Right lateral abdominal radiograph of a cat with a small right kidney (white arrowheads) and left renomegaly (black arrowheads), consistent with compensatory hypertrophy.

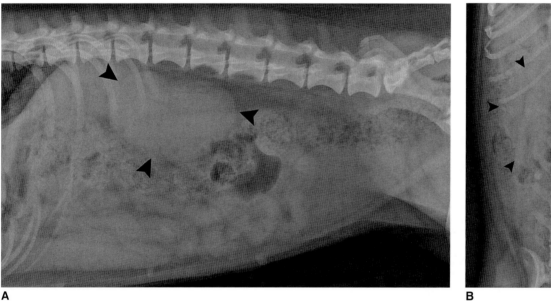

**A**

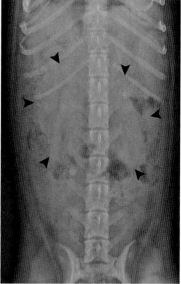

**B**

**FIGURE 27.4** Right lateral (**A**) and VD (**B**) abdominal radiographs of a dog with bilateral renomegaly (arrowheads), consistent with renal hypertrophy secondary to a congenital extrahepatic portosystemic shunt. Note the microhepatia and cranial displacement of the gastric axis on the right lateral radiograph.

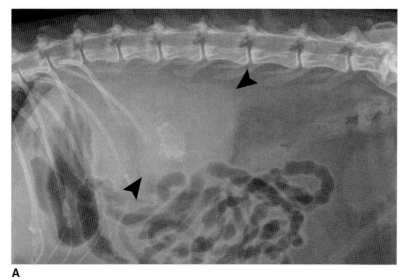

**A**

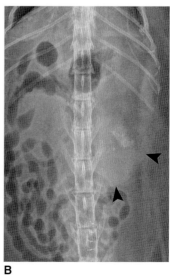

**B**

**FIGURE 27.5** Right lateral (**A**) and VD (**B**) abdominal radiographs of a dog with unilateral irregularly marginated renomegaly (arrowheads), consistent with primary malignant carcinoma.

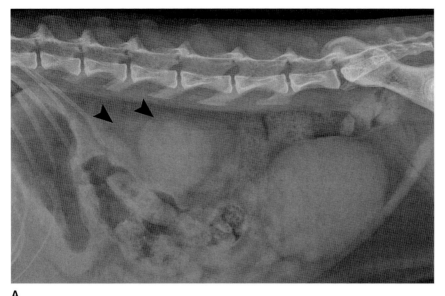
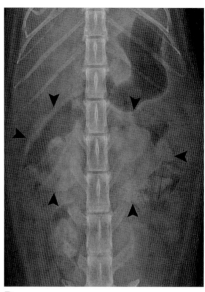

**A**                                                                 **B**

**FIGURE 27.6**   Right lateral (**A**) and VD (**B**) abdominal radiographs of a cat with bilateral irregularly marginated renomegaly (arrowheads), consistent with polycystic kidney disease.

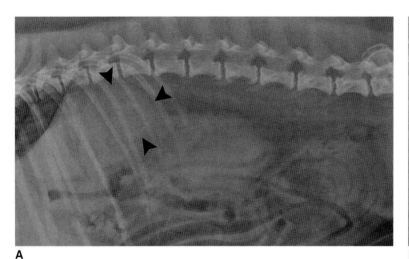
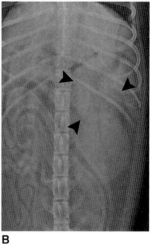

**A**                                                                 **B**

**FIGURE 27.7**   Left lateral (**A**) and VD (**B**) abdominal radiographs of a dog with unilateral irregularly marginated soft tissue opaque mass effect contiguous with the cranial pole of the left kidney (arrowheads), consistent with a renal abscess.

regarding renal function. Diffuse and focal renal parenchymal diseases cause variable changes in the nephrogram and pyelogram phases. The contrast study may be normal if renal function is sufficient with minimal architectural changes. If renal function is poor, there may be decreased opacification of the nephrogram and/or pyelogram phase. Differentials for enlarged, unopacified kidneys include hydronephrosis, neoplasia, inflammation, severe cystic disease, renal trauma, and renal vein thrombosis. Neoplasia, cysts, abscesses, infarctions (Figure 27.8), and hematoma may result in focal or multifocal unopacified disruptions of the nephrogram phase.

Nonspecific changes associated with renomegaly can be seen as diffuse renal cortical hyperechogenicity on ultrasound. Considerations for these changes include glomerulonephritis, interstitial nephritis, acute tubular necrosis, endstage renal disease, lymphoma, feline infectious peritonitis, hypercalcemic nephropathy, pyelonephritis, congenital renal dysplasia, and renal diverticular mineralization. In more progressive renal disease, decreased or loss of renal corticomedullary distinction (Figure 27.9) is noted and is caused by increased medullary and cortical echogenicity. A medullary rim sign is a thin hyperechoic band of the outer renal medulla (Figure 27.10), which can be seen in both normal and diseased kidneys (i.e., hypercalcemic nephropathy, chronic interstitial nephritis, and acute tubular necrosis) [1–5].

Acute renal failure associated with ethylene glycol toxicity usually results in severely hyperechoic renal cortices with or without hyperechoic renal medullae [5]. Renal hypertrophy from the loss of contralateral renal function or congenital portosystemic shunts should appear normal in echogenicity and

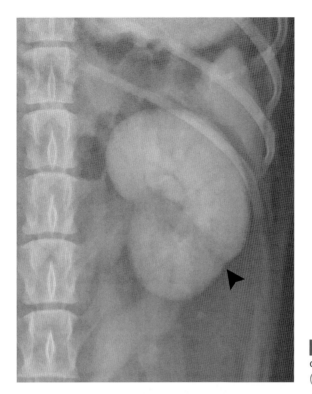

**FIGURE 27.8** Excretory urogram. Collimated VD abdominal radiograph of a dog with a triangular-shaped, unopacified disruption of the nephrogram phase (arrowhead), consistent with a renal cortical infarction.

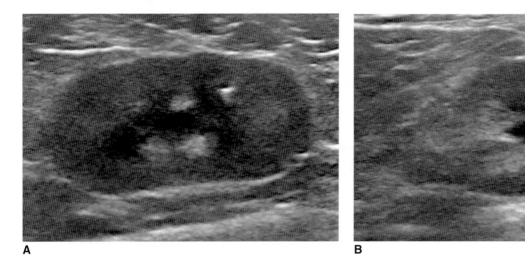

A

B

**FIGURE 27.9** Sagittal (**A**) and transverse (**B**) plane ultrasound images of a small left kidney of a cat with chronic renal disease, further characterized by loss of corticomedullary distinction, mild pyelectasia seen on the transverse plane image (between the calipers), and a small renal diverticular mineralization seen on the sagittal plane image (between the calipers).

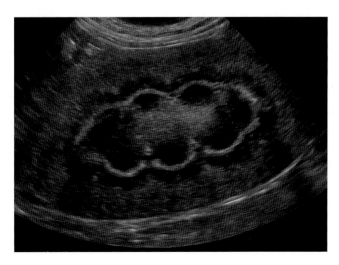

**FIGURE 27.10** Sagittal plane ultrasound image of the left kidney of a dog with a medullary rim sign with no renal dysfunction.

architecture. More severe generalized renomegaly can occur with diffuse infiltrative neoplasia, such as lymphoma, or feline infectious peritonitis. Lymphoma often results in bilateral renal changes, pyelectasia, loss of corticomedullary distinction, renomegaly, renal deformity, hypoechoic lesions, and, rarely, hyperechoic lesions [6]. In cats, hypoechoic subcapsular thickening is associated with renal lymphoma [7] (Figure 27.11); this may represent neoplastic infiltration into the subcapsular region. Subcapsular thickening is also seen with renal carcinoma and feline infectious peritonitis [8].

Renal cysts, abscesses, hematomas, or neoplasia causes irregular renomegaly. Polycystic kidney disease is a genetic disorder where normal renal tissue is displaced by multiple cysts (Figure 27.12). This is typically seen in Persian cats or Persian mixed-breed cats and has been reported in cairn and bull terrier

dogs [9–12]. Cystadenocarcinomas (Figure 27.13) in German shepherd dogs are associated with dermatofibrosis. On ultrasound, they may appear as cavitated, complex masses [13, 14]. A few cysts are usually incidental, benign, round, variably sized, anechoic lesions with distal acoustic enhancement on ultrasound.

Renal abscesses and hematomas are rare but result in focal renal changes. Abscesses may occur secondary to regional infection or hematogenous spread of bacteria. Renal abscesses (Figure 27.14) have variable ultrasonographic appearances but are often seen as cavitated lesions with thick, irregular walls. Intralesional hyperechoic shadowing gas or reverberation artifact can be seen, secondary to gas-producing bacteria. Parenchymal (Figure 27.15) or subcapsular hematomas may be caused by trauma, coagulopathy, or renal biopsy. Hematomas

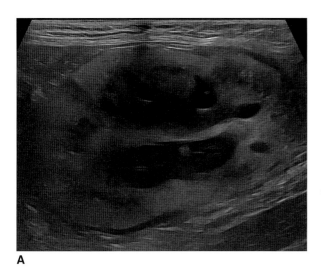
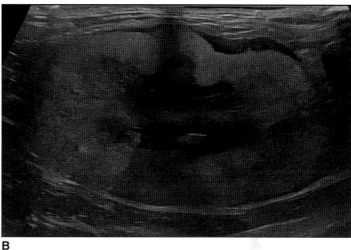

**A**    **B**

**FIGURE 27.11** Sagittal plane ultrasound images of the left (**A**) and right (**B**) kidneys of a cat with renal lymphoma. Note the enlarged, irregularly marginated kidneys with hyperechoic renal cortices, decreased corticomedullary distinction, multifocal hypoechoic nodules, and hypoechoic subcapsular thickening.

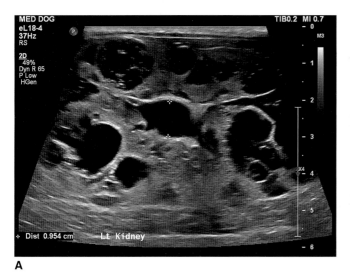
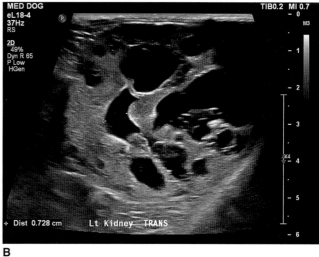

**A**    **B**

**FIGURE 27.12** Sagittal (**A**) and transverse (**B**) plane ultrasound images of the left kidney of a cat with polycystic kidney disease. The left kidney is enlarged and there are numerous, amorphous and round, anechoic renal cortical cysts, and severely dilated renal pelvis (between the calipers).

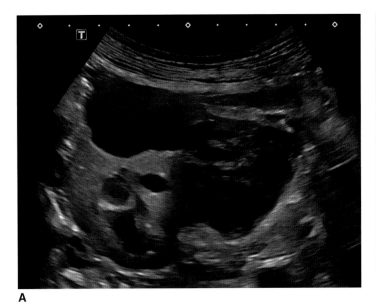

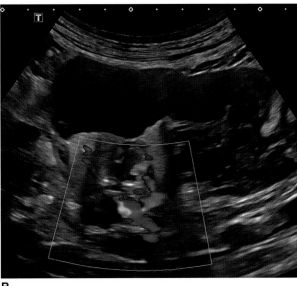

A

B

**FIGURE 27.13** Sagittal plane ultrasound image without color Doppler (**A**) and with color Doppler (**B**) of the kidney of a German shepherd with a cystadenocarcinoma.

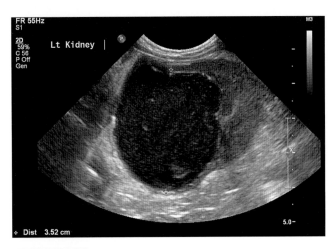

**FIGURE 27.14** Sagittal plane ultrasound image of the kidney of a dog with a renal abscess. Note the cavitated lesion with a thick irregular wall and echogenic intraluminal material.

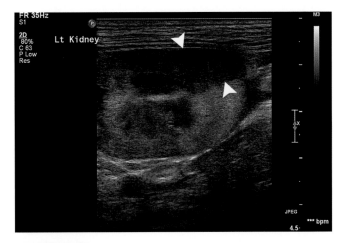

**FIGURE 27.15** Transverse plane ultrasound image of the kidney of a dog with a well-defined, hypoechoic, renal hematoma (arrowheads).

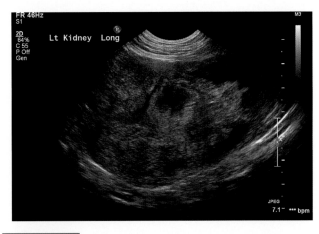

**FIGURE 27.16** Sagittal plane ultrasound image of the kidney of a dog with renal carcinoma. There is a large, poorly delineated, heterogeneous mass of the left kidney and no normal renal architecture is appreciated.

can also occur within the renal pelvis, resulting in obstructive hydronephrosis. Abscesses and hematomas may have identical ultrasonographic appearances to renal neoplasia.

Although neoplasia (i.e., lymphoma) may cause generalized renomegaly, it can also cause focal or multifocal enlargement. Epithelial neoplasms, such as carcinomas, are the most common primary renal neoplasm in the dog; a mass can be seen at either the cranial or caudal pole of the kidney. While these are usually unilateral, both kidneys can be affected. On ultrasound, renal carcinoma (Figure 27.16) may be hypoechoic, hyperechoic, or complex, completely obliterating the normal renal architecture [15]. Renal metastatic lesions cause hyperechoic, hypoechoic, or isoechoic masses. Hemangiosarcoma, osteosarcoma, melanoma, mast cell tumor, pulmonary carcinoma, mammary gland, and gastrointestinal tract have all been reported to metastasize to the kidneys.

Subcapsular or perirenal disease usually causes smoothly marginated generalized renomegaly or, less commonly, irregularly marginated renomegaly. Perinephric pseudocysts (Figure 27.17) have been reported most often in cats and result in focal fluid accumulation around one or both kidneys [16]. The development of these cysts is unknown. On ultrasound, the kidney is surrounded by a thin, round, anechoic fluid-filled structure. Renal hyperechogenicity may be artifactual secondary to acoustic enhancement from the fluid or secondary to diffuse nephropathy.

### Small Kidney(s)

Small renal sizes (<2.5 times the length of L2 in dogs; <2 times the length of L2 in cats) can usually be

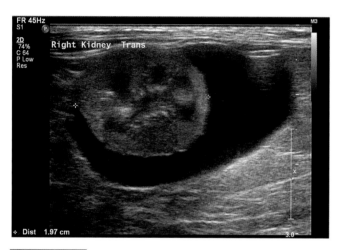

**FIGURE 27.17**   Sagittal plane ultrasound image of the kidney with a perinephric pseudocyst in a cat.

diagnosed using abdominal radiography. Differential diagnoses for small, smoothly marginated kidneys include renal hypoplasia, amyloidosis, and endstage renal disease. Differential diagnoses for small, irregularly marginated kidneys include chronic or endstage renal disease (Figure 27.18).

Small kidneys may be caused by congenital renal disease (which is present at birth), familial renal disease (which may result in chronic renal failure at a young age), or acquired chronic renal disease. Small kidneys secondary to chronic renal disease may be irregular in margination due to cortical infarctions. Ultrasound of the affected kidney typically shows a small, irregular, hyperechoic kidney with decreased corticomedullary distinction. Chronic renal cortical infarctions (Figure 27.19) appear as hyperechoic, wedge-shaped, cortical lesions [17].

# Ureters

## Excretory Urography

To assess the ureters and further assess the urinary tract using radiography, excretory urography may be helpful. Indications for excretory urography include trauma to the urinary tract, hematuria, suspicion for ectopic ureters, retroperitoneal mass effect, or decreased retroperitoneal serosal detail. Excretory urography uses intravenous positive contrast medium, in the form of nonionic iodinated contrast medium, to opacify the urinary tract. Uncommon adverse effects to intravenous iodinated

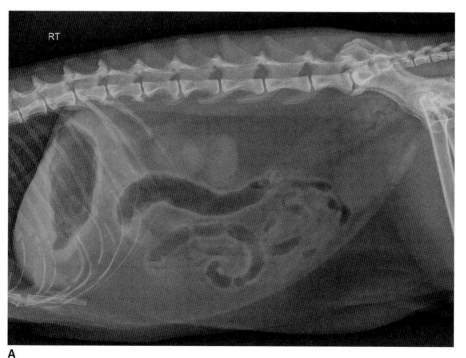
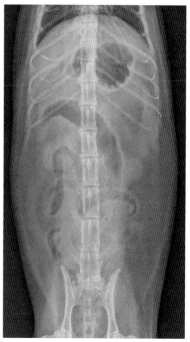

A                                    B

**FIGURE 27.18**   Right lateral (**A**) and VD (**B**) abdominal radiographs of a cat with bilaterally small and irregular kidneys, representing chronic kidney disease.

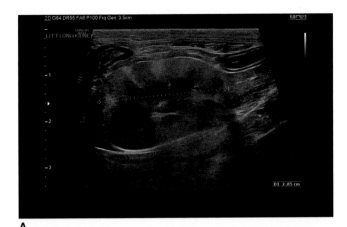

**A**

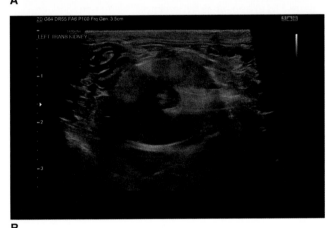

**B**

**FIGURE 27.19** Sagittal (**A**) and transverse (**B**) plane ultrasound images of the chronic kidney disease of a cat. There are well-defined, hyperechoic, triangular-shaped, chronic renal cortical infarctions. The left kidney is also small and exhibits decreased corticomedullary distinction.

contrast medium include nausea, vomiting, hives, hypotension, and contrast medium-induced anuric renal failure. Contraindications for excretory urography include azotemia, anuric renal failure, dehydration, hypotension, or known hypersensitivity reactions to iodinated contrast medium.

In preparation for a diagnostic excretory urogram, the patient should be fasted for at least 12 hours before the study. An enema should be performed to avoid additional superimposition of colonic feces over the urinary tract. Baseline bloodwork should also be performed to ensure that the patient has adequate renal function. Survey collimated abdominal radiographs are recommended prior to excretory urogram to ensure adequate radiographic exposure and efficacy of the enema.

An intravenous catheter should be placed. Sedation or general anesthesia is recommended. Iodinated contrast medium is administered intravenously as a bolus injection at 600–700 mgI/kg of body weight. Ventrodorsal (VD) and right lateral radiographs should be performed immediately after contrast medium administration. Oblique radiographs to further assess the ureters can also be performed. Radiographs should be repeated after 5, 20, and 40 minutes or until a diagnosis is reached. To evaluate the renal arteries, VD radiographs should be taken 5–7 seconds after the bolus injection of contrast medium.

**Normal Excretory Urography** At 5–7 seconds after contrast medium administration, the renal arteries are opacified. Excretory urogram can be divided into three phases: (i) nephrogram phase, (ii) pyelogram phase, and (iii) cystogram phase.

The *nephrogram phase* (Figure 27.20) begins after 10 seconds and lasts up to 2 minutes, with peak opacity

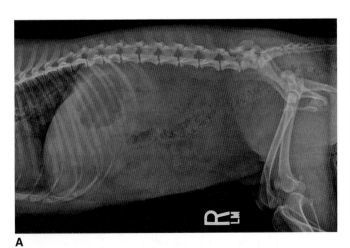

**A**

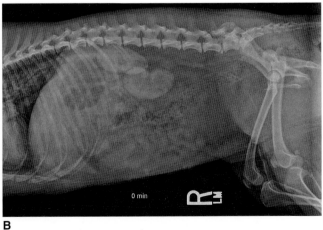

**B**

**FIGURE 27.20** Excretory urography. Survey right lateral abdominal radiograph (**A**) and right lateral abdominal radiograph at the time of intravenous administration of contrast medium (**B**) denoting a normal nephrogram phase of a dog. Note the contrast medium uptake in the renal cortex when compared to the survey abdominal radiograph. This patient sustained a vehicular trauma. There is decreased retroperitoneal and peritoneal serosal detail, prompting this study to rule out uroperitoneum and uroretroperitoneum. In addition, there is also mild pneumothorax, pelvic fractures, right coxal luxation, and multiple caudal lumbar vertebral fractures.

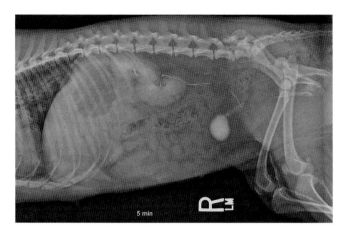

**FIGURE 27.21** Excretory urography. Right lateral abdominal radiograph taken 5 minutes after intravenous administration of contrast medium in the same dog denoting a normal pyelogram phase. Note the decreased renal cortical contrast enhancement and increased renal medullary contrast enhancement in addition to renal pelvic and ureteral contrast filling. There is also mild contrast filling within the urinary bladder, representing part of the cystogram phase.

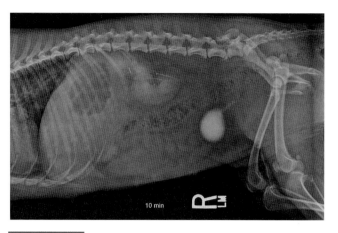

**FIGURE 27.22** Excretory urography. Right lateral abdominal radiograph taken 10 minutes after intravenous administration of contrast medium in the same dog denoting a normal cystogram phase.

at 10–30 seconds. This phase occurs when the contrast medium arrives in the glomerular vessels and filters into the nephron, leading to uniform opacification of the renal parenchyma. Initially, the renal cortex can be more opaque than the medulla. The intensity and duration of the opacity of the kidneys in this phase depend on the dose of contrast medium, renal perfusion, glomerular filtration of the contrast medium, tubular resorption of water, and patency of the renal outflow tract. The renal parenchymal opacity should continue to decrease over time, but approximately 25% of normal dogs still have a detectable nephrogram 2 hours after the initial time of the study. As the nephrogram phase fades, the pyelogram phase begins.

The *pyelogram phase* (Figure 27.21) occurs when contrast medium collects in the collecting system as the nephrogram phase fades. The pyelogram phase can last for ≥2 hours after contrast medium injection. If renal function is normal, the collecting system is persistently more opaque than the renal parenchyma. The normal renal pelvis is curvilinear in shape, measuring ≤2 mm in width. The renal diverticula may be seen in some dogs and cats and are thin, sharply marginated, spikes radiating from the pelvis, measuring ≤1 mm in width. In some dogs, the renal diverticula are not well defined. The diverticula in cats are usually more prominent. During this phase, contrast medium fills the ureters. The normal ureteral diameter is variable in size due to intermittent ureteral peristalsis, but should not measure >3 mm in width. The caudal aspect of the ureters course in a cranial direction before entering the urinary bladder at the cranial aspect of the trigone.

The *cystogram phase* (Figure 27.22) occurs when a variable volume of contrast medium accumulates in the urinary bladder. An excretory urogram provides a crude assessment of renal function, although only 5% of renal function is needed for excretion of iodinated contrast media.

**Abnormal Excretory Urography** The lack of nephrogram and pyelogram phases with a history of trauma indicates renal avulsion (Figure 27.23). A poor initial nephrogram that fades immediately is usually due to an insufficient dose of contrast medium or primary anuric renal failure. A poor initial nephrogram followed by persistent opacity may represent severe generalized renal disease. A poor initial nephrogram followed by increasing opacity may be caused by prior systemic hypotension, acute extrarenal obstruction, or renal ischemia. A good initial nephrogram followed by persistent or increasing opacity may indicate systemic hypotension or contrast-induced renal failure, acute renal tubular necrosis, or acute renal obstruction. The opacity of the pyelogram phase may be decreased in the face of renal failure, because of increased urine volume and decreased concentrating ability.

## Percutaneous Antegrade Positive-Contrast Pyelography

Percutaneous positive-contrast pyelography introduces positive contrast directly into the renal pelvis, avoiding any potential adverse systemic reactions. This technique does not allow assessment of the renal parenchyma but rather assessment of the renal pelvic and ureteral size, shape, diameter, and patency. Indications for this procedure include unilateral hydronephrosis and hydroureter (Figure 27.24) to determine the degree and location of any ureteral obstruction.

In preparation for a diagnostic percutaneous positive-contrast pyelography, the patient should be fasted for at least 12 hours before the study. An enema should be performed to avoid additional superimposition of colonic feces over the urinary tract. Survey collimated abdominal radiographs are recommended to ensure the adequate radiographic exposure and efficacy of the enema.

An intravenous catheter should be placed. Sedation or general anesthesia is recommended. A 25 gauge spinal needle is inserted through a thin portion of the renal cortex into the

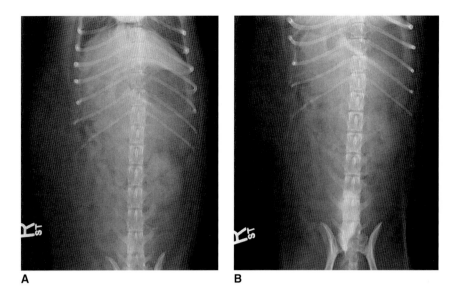

**A**   **B**

**FIGURE 27.23** Excretory urography. Ventrodorsal abdominal radiograph of a dog with a traumatic abdominal wall hernia and herniation of small intestine within the subcutaneous tissues. There is a normal nephrogram phase of the left kidney (**A**) and normal pyelogram phase of the left kidney (**B**). There is no normal nephrogram or pyelogram phase of the right kidney, representing right renal avulsion.

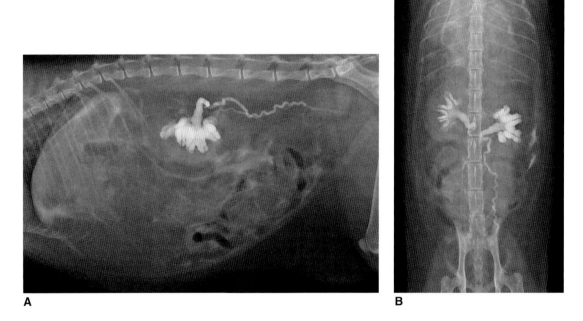

**A**   **B**

**FIGURE 27.24** Right lateral (**A**) and VD (**B**) radiographs after percutaneous antegrade positive-contrast pyelogram of a cat with bilateral hydronephrosis and hydroureter. There is mild iatrogenic retroperitoneal and peritoneal contrast medium extravasation.

dilated pelvis under ultrasound guidance. The large hilar and interlobar vessels should be avoided. A volume of urine is removed, depending on the degree of hydronephrosis, and an equivalent of one-half of the removed volume of nonionic iodinated contrast medium is slowly administered. Renal pelvic and ureteral filling can be visualized using fluoroscopy, if available, followed by VD and lateral abdominal radiographs.

The most common complications are leakage of contrast medium from the renal pelvis secondary to inadvertent needle puncture, and capsular leakage at the site of needle insertion.

Subcapsular hemorrhage and renal pelvic hemorrhage can be a serious complication.

## Abnormalities of the Collecting System

Abnormalities of the collecting system can occur secondary to pyelonephritis or hydronephrosis. The abnormalities are best visualized with intravenous contrast medium studies or ultrasonography.

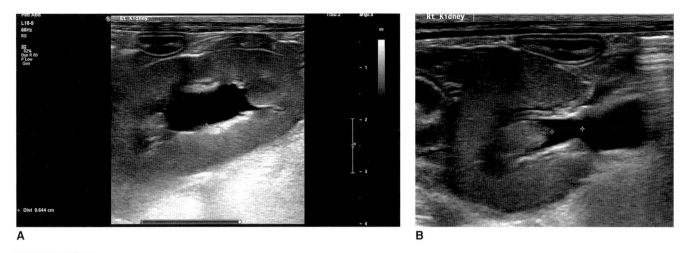

**A**                    **B**

**FIGURE 27.25** Sagittal (**A**) and transverse (**B**) plane ultrasound images of the right kidney of a cat with pyelonephritis. Note the distended renal pelvis with anechoic fluid (between the calipers).

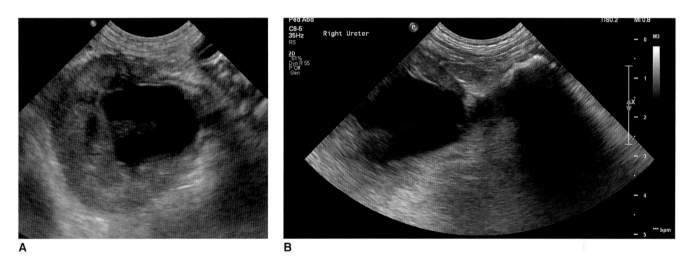

**A**          **B**

**FIGURE 27.26** Transverse plane ultrasound image of a kidney at the level of the kidney (**A**) and proximal ureter (**B**) of a dog with obstructive hydronephrosis secondary to hyperechoic shadowing proximal ureteral calculi.

Pyelonephritis (Figure 27.25) can result in pyelectasia (up to >3 mm is considered abnormal) [18] and mild proximal ureteral dilation. Ultrasound characteristics of pyelonephritis include hyperechoic renal cortices, decreased corticomedullary distinction, along with renal pelvic and proximal ureteral distension [19].

Hydronephrosis results in smoothly marginated, unilateral or bilateral renomegaly on abdominal radiographs. Depending on renal function, intravenous contrast medium administration usually causes contrast medium-dilated renal pelvis and diverticula. In severe hydronephrosis, there may be only a small rim of cortical tissue surrounding the markedly dilated renal pelvis. Ultrasonography provides excellent visualization of hydronephrosis (Figure 27.26). If the ureter is also dilated, it should be followed caudally to determine the cause of obstruction. Common causes of obstructive hydronephrosis include ureteral calculi, urinary bladder trigone neoplasia, ureteral stricture secondary to trauma or chronic ureteritis, blood clots following renal biopsy, or a combination of these.

Common causes of mineralization of the kidneys include renal diverticular mineralization and nephrolithiasis (renal

pelvic calculi) (Figure 27.27) that may extend into the proximal ureter. Only mineral opaque calculi (i.e., phosphates or oxalates) are visible on abdominal radiographs. Ultrasonography

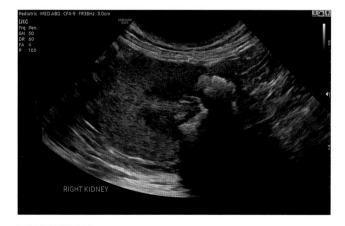

**FIGURE 27.27** Transverse plane ultrasound image of a kidney of a cat with nephrolithiasis. Note the hyperechoic shadowing calculus in the renal pelvis.

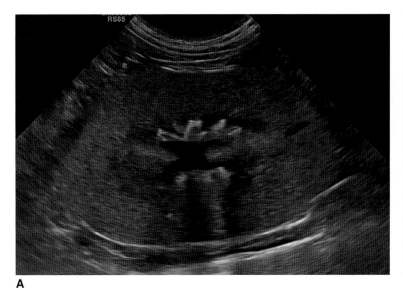

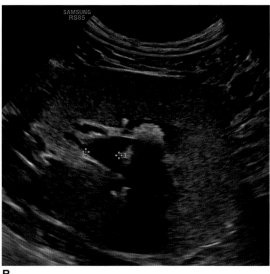

**A**  **B**

**FIGURE 27.28** Sagittal (**A**) and transverse (**B**) plane ultrasound images of the left kidney of a cat with hyperechoic shadowing, renal diverticular mineralization, decreased corticomedullary distinction, and pyelectasia.

can detect both radiolucent and radiopaque calculi both appearing hyperechoic with or without distal acoustic shadowing. If obstructive ureteral calculi are present, anechoic fluid dilation of the cranial ureter can be seen.

Renal diverticular mineralization (Figure 27.28) is characterized by dystrophic parenchymal mineralization and may be difficult to differentiate from nephrolithiasis on radiography or ultrasonography. Both conditions cause mineral opacities on radiographs and hyperechoic foci on ultrasound. Unless there is urine dilation of the affected ureteral segment, differentiation between renal diverticular mineralization and small nephrolithiasis may not be possible. Other causes of dystrophic mineralization include hematomas, cysts, abscesses, granulomas, and neoplasms.

Acute renal failure may result in perirenal retroperitoneal fluid (Figure 27.29). This is often subtle on radiographs. Ultrasonographically, the volume of fluid may only be mild to moderate. The fluid may accumulate adjacent to a failing kidney with unilateral ureteral obstruction, or in a patient without systemic signs of renal failure (azotemia). The amount of fluid does not correlate with the severity of renal failure. Often the fluid extends into the peritoneal space. The pathogenesis may involve excess hydrostatic pressure or vasculitis of capsular vessels in the affected kidney.

Renal secondary hyperparathyroidism, now known as chronic kidney disease-mineral and bone disease (CKD-MBD) [20], is a common complication of chronic kidney disease in dogs and cats and can manifest in the skeletal system with visible radiographic changes [21]. The skull and mandible show the earliest and most dramatic changes, with marked demineralization (Figure 27.30). The teeth may be increased in mineral opacity when compared to the other cranial osseous structure because of severe mineral loss in the lamina dura [22]. The changes are most marked and occur most rapidly in the immature patient. Metastatic calcification is a sequela of chronic renal disease and occurs when there is an elevated calcium:phosphate ratio. Mineralization is most prominent in the stomach (uremic gastropathy) (Figure 27.31), arteries, joints, and kidneys, although mineral opacities can also be seen in the myocardium, lungs, and liver.

## Abnormalities of the Ureters

Mineral opaque ureteral calculi can often be visualized on abdominal radiographs. Calcium oxalate calculi are the most common type of ureteral calculi in cats, with both calcium oxalate and struvite occurring in dogs. Both types are routinely mineral opaque and well visualized. However, additional studies may be needed if ureteral mineral opacities are seen, to determine whether they are real. Mineral opacities in the colon superimposed on the kidneys or ureters, as well as the end-on deep circumflex iliac vessels, can be mistaken for ureteral calculi (Figure 27.32). Mineral

**FIGURE 27.29** Sagittal plane ultrasound image of a kidney of a cat with acute renal failure. There is generalized renomegaly, loss of corticomedullary distinction, and mild anechoic perirenal effusion.

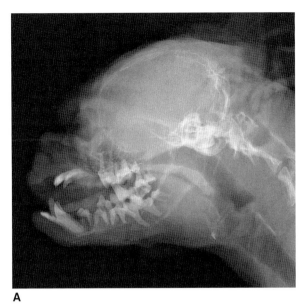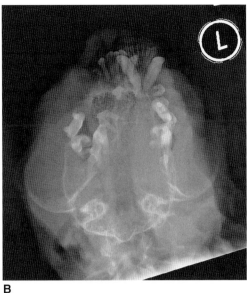

**A** **B**

**FIGURE 27.30** Lateral (**A**) and DV (**B**) skull radiographs of a young dog with renal secondary hyperparathyroidism. Note the diffuse decrease in mineral opacity of the skull and the appearance of "floating teeth."

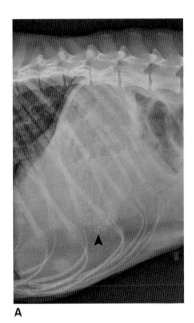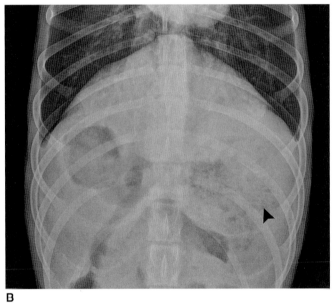

**A** **B**

**FIGURE 27.31** Right lateral (**A**) and VD (**B**) abdominal radiographs of a dog with uremic gastropathy. The gastric wall is mineralized and conforms to the rugal folds (arrowheads).

opaque ureteral calculi are most easily visualized as a discrete round or ovoid mineral opacity within the retroperitoneum on lateral abdominal radiographs. Superimposition of gas and feces on the VD projection may obscure the visualization of calculi.

Additional imaging studies are often needed to confirm the presence of ureteral calculi, especially nonmineral opaque calculi. On excretory urography, any calculi should cause a filling defect within the contrast medium-filled ureteral lumen. In addition, it may be possible to visualize the renal pelvis. It is important not to mistake transient ureteral peristalsis for a true filling defect. Serial radiographs should be done to help differentiate between peristalsis and a true filling defect.

Ureteral dilation usually occurs secondary to obstruction. Other causes of ureteral dilation include atony and ureteritis. A mass in the urinary bladder trigone can cause dilation of both ureters. Other causes of ureteral dilation include strictures, ureteral calculi (Figure 27.33), ureteral rupture, ectopic ureters, and luminal or extraluminal masses. Inadvertent ligation of a ureter during abdominal surgery is also a consideration. Calculi, strictures, and mural mass lesions should cause a filling defect within the affected segment with proximal dilation. Smooth filling defects are consistent with calculi, strictures, and extrinsic masses. Irregular filling defects may indicate neoplasia, inflammation, or fibrosis.

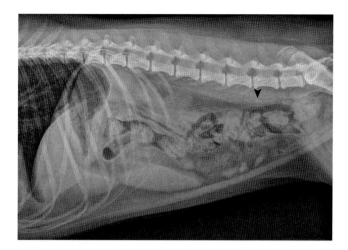

**FIGURE 27.32** Normal right lateral abdominal radiograph of a dog. Note the round, soft tissue to mineral opacity in the caudal retroperitoneal space, representing normal end-on deep circumflex iliac vessels (arrowhead), commonly mistaken for ureteral calculi.

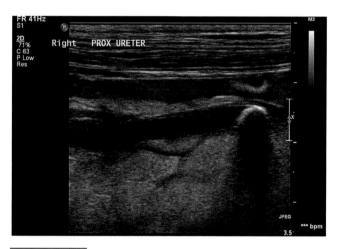

**FIGURE 27.33** Sagittal plane ultrasound image of a dilated right ureter with a large, round, hyperechoic shadowing, ureteral calculus.

Pyelonephritis commonly causes proximal ureteral dilation and mild pyelectasia.

Ectopic ureter is a congenital disorder of one or both ureters where the ureteral termination is located distal to the urinary bladder trigone. Excretory urography can be very helpful in the diagnosis of ectopic ureter(s), although additional imaging studies may be needed. The most common termination sites for ectopic ureters are the urinary bladder neck and urethra, although vaginal termination can also occur. The affected ureter is often dilated and tortuous, but can appear normal, on excretory urography. The ureters are best visualized at 5, 10, and 20 minutes following contrast medium injection, and oblique VD views taken at this time are helpful in visualizing the ureteral termination site without superimposition of the vertebral spine. Moderate distension of the urinary bladder with negative contrast medium prior to administration of positive contrast medium is helpful to visualize ureteral termination.

Even with these procedures, location of ureteral termination may not be possible because of superimposition of

the pelvis. Ureters with abnormal termination sites close to the urinary bladder trigone are particularly difficult to diagnose, especially if the ureter is not dilated. Intramural ectopic ureters appear externally to enter the urinary bladder at the normal location, but tunnel below the mucosa and open at an abnormal caudal site. If ureteral evaluation is incomplete on excretory urography, positive-contrast vaginography and urethrography can be performed. Computed tomography (CT) also has good success in the diagnosis of ectopic ureters and may be the imaging modality of choice for this condition [23].

Ureteroceles are cystic dilations of the intravesicular submucosal portion of the distal ureter near the termination site and may accompany ectopic ureters. They can be within the urinary bladder (i.e., intravesical or orthotopic) or in an abnormal position in association with an ectopic ureter (i.e., ectopic ureterocele) [24]. Orthotopic ureteroceles are contained entirely within the urinary bladder and have an opening in the region of the ureteral orifice. Ectopic ureteroceles have an abnormal location and may originate from the urinary bladder neck or urethral in association with an ectopic ureter. After excretory urography, the contrast medium-filled dilation is visible within the urinary bladder (especially if prefilled with negative contrast medium) or urethra. On ultrasound, it is round, thin walled, and fluid filled, and can be located within the urinary bladder lumen (Figure 27.34).

Ureteral rupture typically results in fluid accumulation in the retroperitoneal space, causing loss of serosal detail on radiographs. This is most often seen after abdominal trauma. This diagnosis is made best with contrast radiography. After contrast medium administration, the proximal aspect of the affected ureter is dilated and somewhat tortuous with contrast medium leakage at the rupture site. A ruptured ureter may be difficult to identify with ultrasound.

The ureters are not seen in normal dogs and cats on ultrasound, except for intermittent visualization of urine jets when it enters the urinary bladder at the ureterovesicular junction or trigone. However, with dilation the ureter becomes apparent as

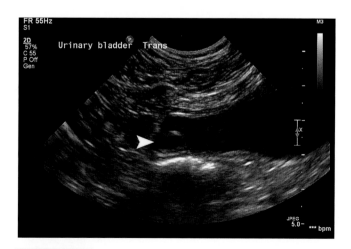

**FIGURE 27.34** Transverse plane ultrasound image of the urinary bladder with a ureterocele (arrowhead) in a dog diagnosed with ectopic ureters.

a distended tubular structure with anechoic luminal fluid. The dilated ureter should be followed to try to rule out an obstructive lesion. Ureteral calculi are a common cause and are seen as hyperechoic foci with distal acoustic shadowing within a dilated, tortuous, fluid-filled ureter. Ureteral dilation occurs in the proximal aspect initially despite the site of obstruction. Large trigonal masses usually cause bilateral ureteral obstruction.

Proximal ureteral dilation may occur with pyelonephritis. A dilated, tortuous ureter may be visualized on ultrasound, along with retroperitoneal effusion in cases of ureteral rupture. However, the most reliable diagnosis is made with excretory urography or antegrade pyelography.

Ultrasound may be used as an alternative imaging modality for diagnosis of ectopic ureters. Although not visible in every patient, the ureterovesicular junction can often be seen as a small "bump" projecting into the lumen of the caudodorsal urinary bladder wall (Figure 27.35). Urine jets can be seen intermittently at these sites, especially with Doppler ultrasonography and intravenous administration of a diuretic. The absence of a jet, and visualization of a ureter extending caudal to the urinary bladder trigone, are consistent with ectopic ureter. Ureteral dilation and ipsilateral hydronephrosis are often seen with concurrent ureteritis and stricture formation.

# Urinary Bladder and Urethra

## Normal Imaging Findings

See Chapter 20.

## Contrast Radiography

Although radiographs and ultrasound can be obtained with a cooperative conscious patient, most contrast examinations require the patient to be heavily sedated or anesthetized. General anesthesia for these purposes allows for better patient positioning, improves patient safety, and avoids artifacts arising from muscle spasm during contrast medium administration or catheterization.

In addition to the normal aspects of patient preparation for anesthesia, the descending colon and rectum should be evacuated prior to imaging. This is most appropriately achieved in dogs by administering an enema and providing the opportunity for defecation before premedication. Phosphate enemas are contraindicated in cats; instead low-volume lubricant or warm water enemas are preferred.

Survey radiographs should always be taken and assessed prior to performing a contrast study. This ensures that exposure factors are appropriate, enemas have been effective, and contrast studies are not needed if lesions are visible on survey images.

## Cystography

**Pneumocystography**   Pneumocystography (negative-contrast cystography) has some limitations and is rarely used as the sole imaging examination (Figure 27.36). The procedure is as follows.

- The patient is placed in left lateral recumbency.
- A cuffed urinary catheter (to avoid gas escape) is placed and the urinary bladder is emptied.
- The urinary bladder is then filled with room air or carbon dioxide and concurrently gently palpated to ensure proper filling. The volume needed to fill the urinary bladder is patient specific. When room air is used, there is a small risk of air embolism from the technique. If carbon dioxide

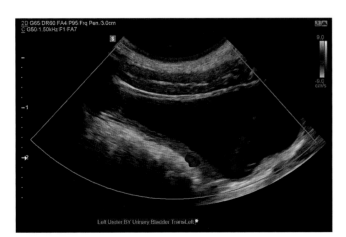

**FIGURE 27.35**   Sagittal plane ultrasound image of a normal ureterovesicular junction in a dog. Color Doppler is used to interrogate the urine jet entering the urinary bladder from the ureterovesicular junction.

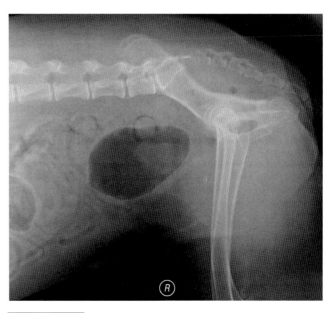

**FIGURE 27.36**   Pneumocystography of a dog with a large, soft tissue opaque, lobular trigonal mass.

is utilized, administration directly from the pressurized source must be avoided.

- The urinary catheter is removed, and the radiographs are obtained.

Pneumocystography may provide information on urinary bladder size, identification of urinary cystic calculi, anad verification of the location of the urinary bladder.

**Positive-Contrast Cystography** Positive-contrast cystography (Figure 27.37) is performed in a similar way to pneumocystography, except that a water-soluble iodine-based contrast agent is used. Contrast medium with a concentration of 120–400 mgI/mL is adequate. The main indication for positive-contrast cystography is suspected bladder wall rupture. A second indication is to provide appropriate backpressure for uniform urethral dilation for a retrograde urethrogram.

**Double-Contrast Cystography**  This technique has many advantages over negative- and positive-contrast cystography alone. The combination of urinary bladder distension with negative- and positive-contrast medium is the preferred technique for diagnosing most intraluminal and mural urinary bladder lesions.

In double-contrast cystography (Figure 27.38), the urinary bladder is distended with negative contrast medium and a small volume of centrally located, dependent, positive contrast medium. Intraluminal urinary bladder contents such as calculi and blood clots fall into the contrast medium pool and create a filling defect. Masses of the urinary bladder wall are nonmobile and may cause filling defects within the contrast medium pool or be outlined by gas with positive contrast medium.

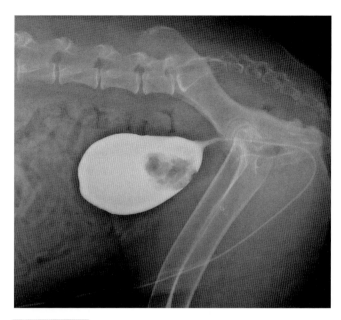

**FIGURE 27.38**  Double-contrast cystography of a dog with a large, lobular, trigonal mass, causing a positive-contrast defect.

Typically, the first phase of the study is a pneumocystogram. Once the urinary bladder is adequately full, a small volume of undiluted positive contrast medium is administered to create a small puddle to help identify small luminal lesions. In cats, 1 mL of contrast medium is usually adequate. A gradual scale of increasing volume of positive contrast medium is added to larger dogs, not exceeding 5 mL. Rotating the patient is helpful to coat the urinary bladder wall with contrast medium, encourage intraluminal lesions into the dependent contrast medium pool, and may result in bubble formation. Bubble formation may be confused with true intraluminal urinary bladder lesions. To avoid bubble formation, the urinary bladder should be emptied, and positive contrast medium is administered before air.

## Urethrography

Urethrography is useful to investigate urethral disease. For all procedures, nonionic iodinated positive contrast is used at a concentration of 120–400 mgI/mL.

**Normograde Urethrography** Normograde urethrography is occasionally indicated when retrograde studies have been unsuccessful, usually because of a failure of urethral catheterization. However, it is difficult to achieve good images because of variable urethral filling. To obtain a normograde urethrogram, the patient must be anesthetized. The urinary bladder is filled with positive-contrast medium percutaneously, urinary catheter, or intravenous urogram, and then expressed by applying pressure with a wooden paddle to fill the urethra at the time of radiographic exposure.

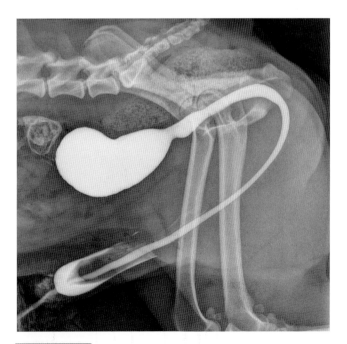

**FIGURE 27.37**  Retrograde positive-contrast urethrography and cystography in a male dog.

**Retrograde Urethrography**    The urethra is most readily evaluated with retrograde positive-contrast studies. Urethral relaxation is needed in this procedure to allow adequate filling without artifactual narrowing due to muscle spasm. A urinary catheter is prefilled with positive-contrast medium to avoid air bubbles in the urethra, which may mimic urinary calculi. This urinary catheter is then placed. The urethra is occluded around the catheter and the contrast medium injected. Radiographs are taken during the injection of contrast medium to obtain adequate urethral distension. Radiation safety, including proper protective equipment and avoiding the primary x-ray beam, is important.

In the male dog, the best catheter for injection is a Foley (balloon-tipped) catheter. In almost all adult dogs, an 8 Fr (or larger) catheter can be used. The tip is placed into the penile urethra and the balloon gently inflated with saline sufficiently to anchor it within the distal urethra. The pelvic limbs should be flexed cranially to obtain an unobstructed view of the tip of the penis. A single injection using a dosage of 1 mLI/kg of positive-contrast medium in the dog is needed to evaluate the entire urethra. When the urinary bladder is empty or incompletely filled, separate exposures may be necessary to evaluate the prostatic, membranous, and penile urethra.

In the male cat, a narrow-gauge urethral catheter (3–4 Fr) is used, ideally with an end-hole. To secure this and maintain distension during injection, atraumatic clips are placed above the catheter across the prepuce, not the penis. A volume of volume of 2–4 mL total of positive-contrast medium is needed.

**Vaginourethrography**    Because urethrography using a catheter obscures the urethra in females, a vaginourethrography is preferred. In the female dog, the tip of an 8 Fr Foley catheter is placed in the vulva, with the balloon inflated just inside the vulval lips, which are closed around it with atraumatic clips. A urethral catheter is used in the cat. Approximately 1 mLI/kg of positive-contrast medium is injected to fill the vagina and then overflow into the urethra as the radiographic exposure is obtained.

# Urinary Bladder Diseases

## Distension

Urinary bladder distension is usually subjective and the history of the patient should be taken into consideration (Figure 27.39).

## Rupture and Diverticula

Most animals with urinary bladder rupture present with collapse and abdominal distension. The primary finding on abdominal radiographs is loss of abdominal serosal detail secondary to uroperitoneum. Additional imaging is required to distinguish rupture of the ureter, bladder, or urethra. The urinary bladder may be ruptured and remain partially full. A visible urinary bladder on an abdominal radiograph does not rule out rupture. The preferred imaging procedure for confirmation of urinary bladder rupture is positive-contrast cystography where positive-contrast medium can be seen in the peritoneum adjace to the urinary bladder (Figure 27.40). As urethral rupture is an important differential diagnosis in these cases, a retrograde urethrogram should be performed first.

Urinary bladder diverticula are most often seen in cats, in the position of the urachal origin at the apex of the bladder (Figure 27.41). The presence of a diverticulum may be incidental. Incidental, secondary, diverticulum seen in some cats with a history of urethral obstruction will resolve following resolution of the obstruction and prolonged periods of urinary bladder decompression.

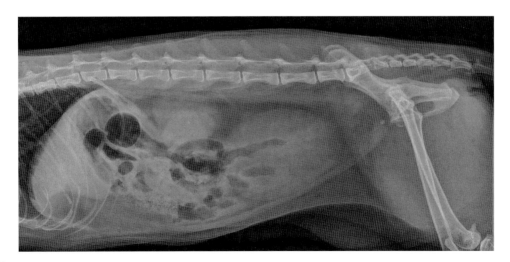

**FIGURE 27.39**    Left lateral abdominal radiograph of a cat with a severely dilated urinary bladder secondary to urethral obstruction. There is decreased peritoneal serosal detail associated with the urethral obstruction. In the caudoventral abdomen, there is a well-defined, round, mineral opaque calculus in the region of the urethra, likely the cause of the urethral obstruction.

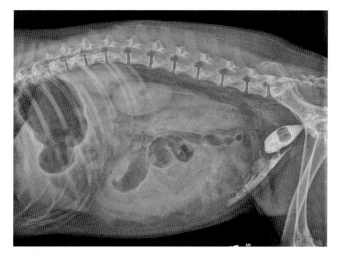

**FIGURE 27.40**  Lateral abdominal radiograph of a dog with a urinary bladder rupture, confirmed via positive-contrast cystography. Note the extravasated positive-contrast medium into the peritoneal space adjacent to the urinary bladder. Prior to positive-contrast cystography, an excretory urogram was performed, hence the diffuse extravasation of positive-contrast medium within the peritoneal space as well as faint nephrogram and pyelogram phases of the kidneys.

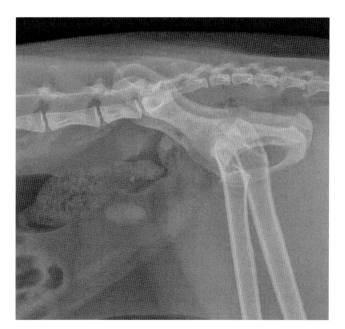

**FIGURE 27.41**  Caudally collimated right lateral abdominal radiograph of a cat with a focal outpouching of the apex of the urinary bladder. There is also a single, large, mineral opaque, urinary cystic calculus.

## Mineralization

Differential diagnoses for mineral opaque material in the urinary bladder include calculi, sand, dystrophic mineralization of soft tissues, or a foreign body. The opacity of uroliths varies with chemical composition. Calcium oxalate and struvite uroliths are generally mineral opaque, but 1.7–5.2% of these uroliths are not apparent on abdominal radiographs [25]. Urate, cystine, and calcium phosphate uroliths are variably mineral opaque and are not detected in approximately 25% of radiographs in patients with these uroliths [25]. Sand and all calculi are echogenic on ultrasonography, regardless of their mineral composition [26].

## Calculi

Mineral opaque calculi are typically visible on abdominal radiographs. The calculi shape varies according to their composition. Struvite uroliths (Figure 27.42) tend to be smooth with blunted margins. Rectangular-shaped calculi are typically silicate, and oxalates (Figure 27.43) tend to be grape-like clusters.

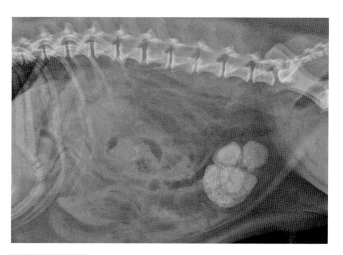

**FIGURE 27.42**  Lateral abdominal radiograph of a dog with severe struvite urinary calculi. Note the smooth and blunted edges of the urinary cystic calculi. There is also decreased retroperitoneal serosal detail, left renomegaly, and left nephrolithiasis, consistent with uroretroperitoneum and left obstructive hydronephrosis.

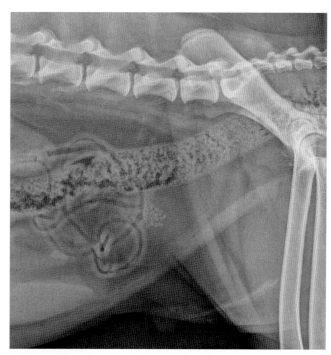

**FIGURE 27.43**  Caudally collimated abdominal radiograph of a dog with calcium oxalate calculi. Note the grape-like clusters.

Soft tissue opaque calculi are not visible on abdominal radiographs as they are border effaced by soft tissue opaque urine. Pneumocystography will cause them to appear soft tissue opaque within the negative-contrast medium, but double-contrast cystography is often more useful. Double-contrast cystography shows all types of calculi as well-defined filling defects in the contrast medium pool (Figure 27.44), similar to gas bubbles. Bubbles usually adhere to one another and accumulate at the peripheral margin of the contrast medium (Figure 27.45), whereas calculi fall into the central part of the contrast medium.

## Sand

Urine sand is not discrete on radiographs but appears as diffuse and irregular increases in opacity within the bladder lumen (Figure 27.46) on radiographs. On ultrasound, they are gravity dependent, granular, hyperechoic, and shadowing.

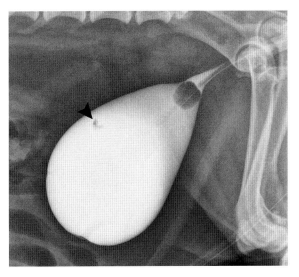

**FIGURE 27.44** Double-contrast cystography showing filling defects in the contrast medium pool, representing urinary cystic calculi (arrowhead).

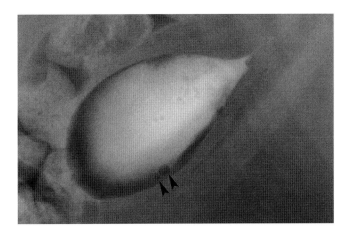

**FIGURE 27.45** Double-contrast cystography in a cat showing filling defects at the margin of the contrast medium pool, representing gas bubbles (arrowheads).

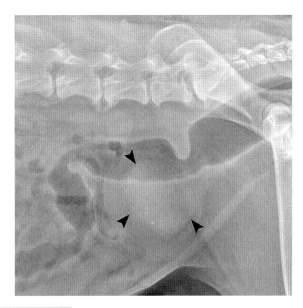

**FIGURE 27.46** Lateral abdominal radiograph of a dog with increased urinary bladder opacity, representing sand (arrowheads). There are also a few, small, solid, mineral opaque calculi.

## Urinary Bladder Wall

Mineralization of the bladder wall is a nonspecific finding, generally indicating dystrophic mineralization. It is uncommon and seen secondary to chronic inflammation, urinary bladder neoplasms such as transitional cell carcinoma, and cyclophosphamide-induced urinary cystitis. Mineral opaque urolithiasis can be confused with mural calcification and can be discerned using double-contrast cystography, positional radiography, and ultrasonography.

## Masses

Ultrasonography can be important in determining which layer of the urinary bladder wall is involved when a mass is present (Figure 27.47). Most urinary bladder masses are neoplastic, but polyps may have a similar appearance.

## Neoplasms

The most common urinary bladder neoplasm is transitional cell carcinoma (or urothelial carcinoma), representing >90% of all cases. This is typically a disease of older animals. It has a predilection for the trigone of the urinary bladder. The masses are usually focal, but satellite lesions may be present.

Contrast studies and abdominal ultrasonography are needed to detect urinary bladder wall neoplasms as they are undetectable on plain radiographs. On contrast study, there is irregularity of the urinary bladder margin, urinary bladder wall thickening, or large filling defects in the contrast medium pool (Figure 27.48). On ultrasound (Figure 27.47), these masses are irregularly marginated, variable in size, homogeneous or

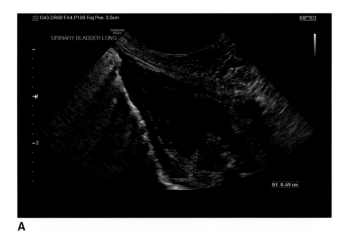

A

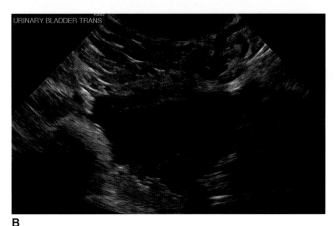

B

**FIGURE 27.47** Sagittal (**A**) and transverse (**B**) plane ultrasound images of a lobular, echogenic, urinary bladder trigone mass (between the calipers), consistent with a transitional cell carcinoma.

heterogeneous, and may involve one or multiple layers of the urinary bladder. On ultrasonography, penetration beyond the muscularis layer, heterogeneity, and trigonal location are characteristics that are significantly associated with shorter survival times in dogs diagnosed with transitional cell carcinoma [27].

Less common urinary bladder neoplasms are soft tissue sarcomas, including leiomyosarcoma and rhabdomyosarcoma. Rhabodmyosarcomas often affect younger animals (<1 year of age). Sarcomas arise from the muscular layers of the urinary bladder wall with no epithelial involvement. In animals with suspected urinary bladder neoplasia, thoracic radiography and ultrasonography of the sublumbar lymph nodes are recommended for staging.

## Polypoid Urinary Cystitis

Polypoid urinary cystitis is an important differential diagnosis for urinary bladder epithelial lesions. In contrast to transitional cell carcinoma, polyps are often multiple and tend to be centered on the cranioventral region of the urinary bladder rather than the trigone. Double-contrast cystography reveals multiple soft tissue lesions arising from the urothelium. On ultrasound, there is urinary bladder wall thickening, single or multiple, isoechoic, pedunculated, and irregular lesions (Figure 27.49) [28].

## Other Soft Tissue Masses

An important differential diagnosis for intraluminal soft tissue lesions is blood clots. These appear similar to multiple

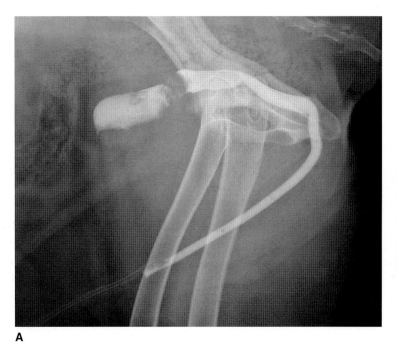

A

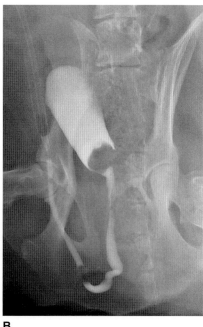

B

**FIGURE 27.48** Caudally collimated right lateral (**A**) and oblique VD (**B**) abdominal radiographs of a contrast cystogram in a dog with a large contrast filling defect of the trigone of the urinary bladder, representing a transitional cell carcinoma.

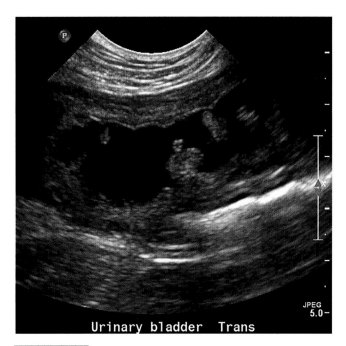

**FIGURE 27.49** Transverse plane ultrasound image of a dog with a thickened urinary bladder wall and multifocal, pedunculated, echogenic mucosal margin lesions, representing polypoid urinary cystitis.

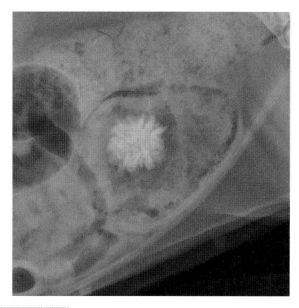

**FIGURE 27.51** Left lateral abdominal radiograph of a dog with a single, large, spiculated, mineral opaque urinary cystic calculus and irregular gas opacities conforming to the urinary bladder wall margin, consistent with emphysematous cystitis.

## Mural Gas

Intramural gas is strongly suggestive of emphysematous cystitis; this is due to the presence of gas-forming bacteria proliferating in the urinary bladder and depositing gas within the wall. Most commonly, emphysematous cystitis is associated with diabetes mellitus [29]. On radiographs, the urinary bladder wall has multifocal gas opacities in a thickened urinary bladder wall [30] (Figure 27.51).

# Abnormal Position

## Intrapelvic Urinary Bladder

In both female and male dogs, the urinary bladder is typically located entirely intraabdominal in position when distended. Some dogs have an intrapelvic bladder neck. This may be associated with urinary incontinence, but it is also a common finding in normal animals [31].

## Hernia or Rupture

Urinary bladder displacement can occur with defects in the abdominal body wall or perineum (i.e., perineal ruptures, inguinal hernias, and ventral abdominal body wall ruptures), causing urethral obstruction and subsequent urinary bladder distension. When this happens, the distended urinary bladder forms a soft tissue swelling over the affected area. If there is suspicion for urinary bladder displacement, ultrasonography

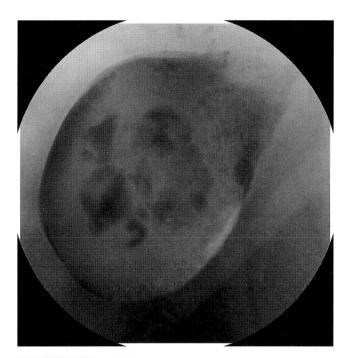

**FIGURE 27.50** Double-contrast cystography with centralized irregular filling defects within the contrast medium pool, representing blood clots. The variably sized, coalescing round, faint contrast filling defects represent gas bubbles. The slightly lobular caudoventrally located contrast filling defect represents a urinary bladder neoplasm. This patient was diagnosed with transitional cell carcinoma.

polyps on double-contrast cystography, producing irregular filling defects within the contrast medium pool (Figure 27.50). Ultrasound using color and power Doppler may be helpful to distinguish between the two.

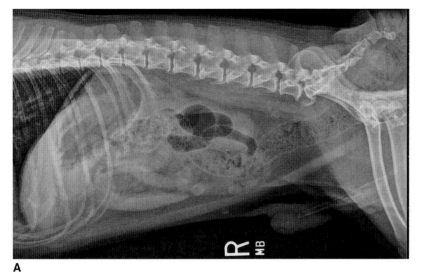
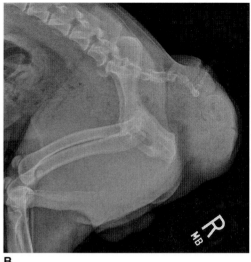

**A**   **B**

**FIGURE 27.52**   Right lateral (**A**) and caudally collimated right lateral (**B**) abdominal radiographs of a dog with a perineal urinary bladder hernia. Note the urinary bladder is not seen in the caudoventral abdomen on the right lateral projection.

or retrograde urethrography can be performed to delineate the urethra and urinary bladder. Prior to retrograde urethrography, urocystocentesis should be performed to alleviate the pressure within the urinary bladder.

In perineal hernias, the urethra is displaced laterally or dorsally and the apex of the bladder is retroverted into the perineum (Figure 27.52). The prostate is often concurrently herniated. Perineal ruptures are most commonly seen in intact male dogs.

Inguinal hernias of the urinary bladder may occur in males and females, although they are most commonly seen in middle-aged intact female dogs. Inguinal herniation is rare in cats. In this case, the urethra is ventrally deviated and the urinary bladder is displaced into the caudoventral subcutaneous tissues of the abdominal body wall (Figure 27.53).

# Urethral Diseases

## Calculi

Most urethral calculi are mineral opaque and can be seen on radiographs. Urate calculi, which are seen in Dalmatians and dogs with portosystemic shunts, are an exception. In the male dog, common sites of obstruction are the penile urethra in the region of the perineum (Figure 27.54) and immediately proximal to the os penis (Figure 27.55). Urethral obstruction is common in male cats. The region of obstruction is most often at the level of the penile urethra and the obstructive calculi or plugs are often not large enough or mineral opaque enough to visualize on radiographs. Urethral calculi are rare in female dogs and cats.

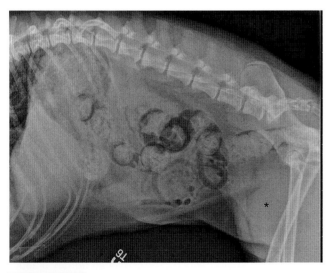

**FIGURE 27.53**   Right lateral abdominal radiograph of a dog with an inguinal urinary bladder hernia (*).

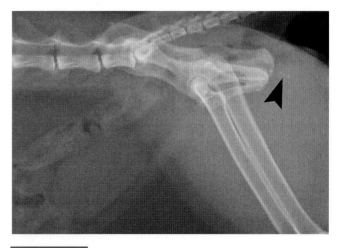

**FIGURE 27.54**   Left lateral radiograph of a cat with numerous mineral opaque caudal urethral calculi over the perineum (arrowhead).

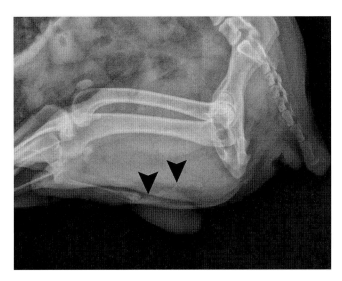

**FIGURE 27.55**   Caudally collimated, flex pelvic limb, right lateral perineal radiograph of a dog with numerous mineral opaque penile urethral calculi (arrowheads) immediately proximal to the os penis.

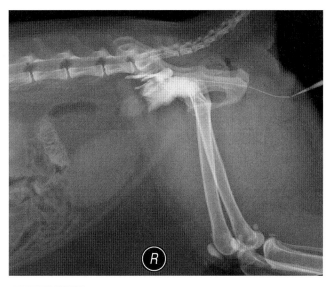

**FIGURE 27.56**   Caudally collimated right lateral abdominal radiographs with retrograde urethrogram of a cat with a urethral rupture. Note the contrast extravasation into the caudodorsal retroperitoneal space. No positive-contrast medium is seen in the urinary bladder lumen. The route of entry of positive-contrast medium cannot be determined.

Many cases of urethral calculi obstruction are managed by retrograde urohydropropulsion. Radiographs are taken during and after attempts at flushing to ensure that all calculi have been retropulsed into the urinary bladder.

## Rupture

Urethral rupture is usually associated with a history of trauma. The trauma may be iatrogenic, following difficult catheterization in male cats. Other findings seen with urethral rupture include perineal, inguinal, or inner thigh region bruising, swelling, cutaneous necrosis of the perineum and prepuce, ascites, and dysuria/anuria.

Urinary bladder rupture will cause urine to accumulate in the peritoneal cavity; however, more caudal urethral ruptures will cause urine to accumulate in the pelvic canal, perineum prepuce, or thigh. To diagnose the location of the urethral rupture and extent of injury, retrograde urethrography is more helpful than ultrasound. A finding on retrograde urethrography includes leakage of contrast medium into the periurethral soft tissues (Figure 27.56).

## Neoplasia

Urethral neoplasia is most seen in geriatric female dogs. It is less common in male dogs and in cats. Stranguria and hematuria may be present. Radiographs of the urinary bladder are usually unremarkable. Sublumbar lymphadenopathy and pulmonary metastasis may be seen.

Retrograde urethrography reveals distortion of the urethral lumen. Typically, there is evidence both of narrowing and irregular margination with an "apple core" appearance (Figure 27.57). On ultrasonography, there is diffuse urethral

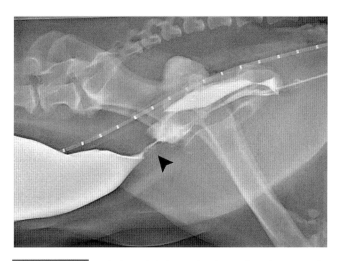

**FIGURE 27.57**   Right lateral abdominal radiograph with retrograde vaginocystourethrogram of a dog with a proximal urethral neoplasm. Note the "apple core" lesion (arrowhead). A callibration marker is present dorsal to the urethra, within the rectum.

wall thickening with a mass effect, hypoechogenicity, and hyperechoic regional fat. The appearance of urethral neoplasia is similar to severe inflammatory urethral disease, so histopathologic analysis, using urethroscopy or catheter suction technique, is required for a definitive diagnosis.

## Inflammation

Urethritis is less common than urethral neoplasia but is an important differential diagnosis for animals with supportive clinical signs. This cannot be seen radiographically. On ultrasound, there is thickening of the urethral wall.

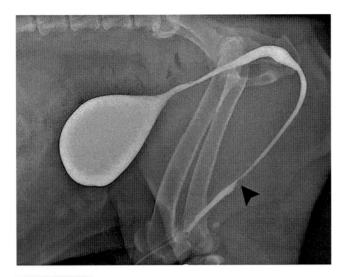

**FIGURE 27.58** Retrograde urethrogram of a dog with a penile urethral stricture (arrowhead) immediately caudal to the os penis.

## Stricture

Urethral stricture may be seen with neoplasia, urethritis, or prior trauma and is difficult to evaluate on abdominal radiographs as the only change seen may be urinary bladder distension. Given the location and extent of the urethra in dogs and cats, ultrasonography is limited to viewing the proximal portion of the urethra. Positive-contrast normograde or retrograde urethrogram of strictures secondary to neoplasia or urethritis causes an irregularly marginated mucosal surface, but with prior trauma, the urethral mucosal surface will be smooth (Figure 27.58).

# Developmental Disease

## Ureteral Ectopia

Ectopic ureter cannot be diagnosed on plain abdominal radiographs in dogs and cats. Retrograde urethrography and occasionally ultrasound are needed for diagnosis (Figure 27.59). In most dogs, the affected ureters are intramural where the ureter enters the urinary bladder in a normal position but tunnels through the wall and urethral walls prior to termination. In cats, ectopic ureters are typically extramural and are distinctly separate from the urinary bladder neck. Although most ectopic ureters are dilated in the intraabdominal portion, this is not often apparent in the distal part associated with the urethra. The typical termination of ectopic ureters in female dogs and cats is the intrapelvic urethra, although they can pass as far distally as the urethral orifice and open alongside the vestibulovaginal junction. Less common sites of opening are the vagina and uterus. In male dogs and cats, which are less commonly affected than females, the ureters typically enter in the region of the prostatic urethra (Figure 27.60). However, it is often difficult to localize the opening site definitively, because of overlying bones of the pelvis.

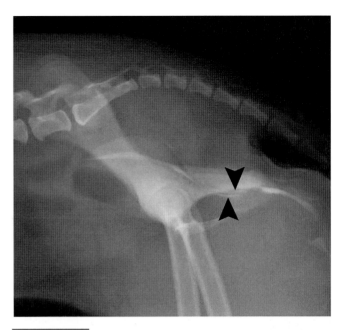

**FIGURE 27.59** Caudally collimated right lateral abdominal radiograph with retrograde urethrogram of a female dog with bilateral ectopic ureters (arrowheads).

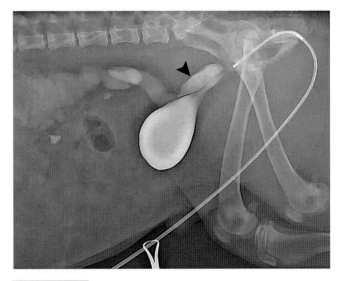

**FIGURE 27.60** Caudally collimated right lateral abdominal radiograph with retrograde urethrogram of a male dog with unilateral ectopic ureter and hydronephrosis and hydroureter.

## Ureterocele

Ureteroceles are cystic dilations of the intravesicular submucosal portion of the distal ureter. They can be entirely within the urinary bladder (intravesical or orthotopic) or in an abnormal position in association with an ectopic ureter (ectopic ureterocele) [32, 33]. These may be incidental findings during investigation of urinary incontinence or occasionally dysuria. Retrograde positive-contrast cystourethrogram studies may show contrast medium within a cystic dilation at the bladder neck (Figure 27.61), further characterized by a filling defect at

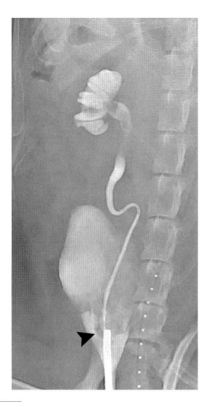

**FIGURE 27.61**   Caudally collimated VD abdominal radiographs with retrograde urethrogram of a female dog with a contrast filling defect at the caudal aspect of the urinary bladder, representing a ureterocele (arrowhead).

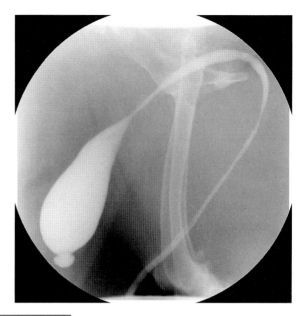

**FIGURE 27.62**   Lateral abdominal radiograph of a dog with a urinary bladder diverticulum, confirmed via positive-contrast cystography. Note the outpouching of the positive-contrast medium at the apex.

the dorsal urinary bladder lumen, separated from the urinary bladder lumen by a thin septum of urothelium.

## Diverticulum

Urethral diverticula are a rare cause of urinary incontinence and dysuria. Most diverticula are congenital but can be acquired. They may not be apparent on abdominal radiographs. On ultrasound and retrograde urethrocystogram, they are seen as discrete, smooth outpouchings of the urethral lumen (Figure 27.62) [34, 35].

# Female Reproductive Tract

## Anatomy

See Chapter 20.

## Normal Pregnancy

Radiographs and ultrasound are used to assess normal gestation in dogs and cats. The benefit of these imaging modalities varies depending on the stage of gestation.

**Radiography**   In dogs, uteromegaly can be detected on day 30 following ovulation on radiographs. The individual fetal sacs become apparent between 30 and 40 days post ovulation. The uterine horns become more tubular in shape between days 38 and 45 post ovulation. Fetal skeletal mineralization is the definitive sign of pregnancy and may be seen from day 41 post ovulation; visualization of fetal bone structures will be optimal after day 45.

Prior to the development of fetal mineralization, other considerations for uteromegaly include pyometra, mucometra, hydrometra, and hemometra. Due to the long potential life span of canine sperm in the uterus (up to 7 days), the exact date of fertilization and hence exact stage of fetal development are often not known. Therefore, it is possible to have a radiograph taken at 45 days post mating in a pregnant patient that shows no evidence of fetal mineralization. In these cases, ultrasound is needed.

Once fetal mineralization is visible, it progresses quickly and can be seen within 5 days; a radiograph taken at 45 days post mating that shows no evidence of mineralization could be repeated 7–10 days later. In the female cat, radiographically detectable uteromegaly has been reported as early as day 19 of pregnancy, although day 25–35 is usually a more reliable guide; fetal mineralization develops between days 35 and 45.

In both dogs and cats, the uterus is midventral and caudoventrally located in the abdomen as gestation progresses. Once the fetal skeleton is visible, radiography is a good method for assessing fetal numbers; the number of skulls attached to vertebral columns can be counted (Figure 27.63). The use of ionizing radiation in diagnostic radiography does present a potential risk to the fetus.

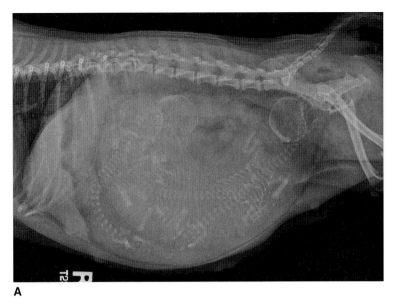

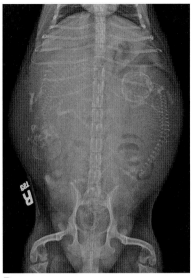

**A**          **B**

**FIGURE 27.63**   Right lateral (**A**) and VD (**B**) abdominal radiographs of a gravid female with three large mineralized feti.

**Ultrasonography**   For earlier detection of pregnancy, ultrasound is needed. Imaging of the gestational sac has been reported as early as day 10 of pregnancy in the female dog and day 11 in the female cat, and detection is most accurate between days 21 and 35. The fetal heartbeat is usually seen by day 21. Ultrasound may be less accurate at determining fetal numbers than radiographs. Uteromegaly may be seen after 7 days in the female dog and 4 days in the female cat. Early detection of pregnancy may be further restricted by interference from intraluminal gastrointestinal material.

**Postpartum Uterus**   Involution of the postpartum uterus is normally complete within 4 weeks in dogs and cats. The uterine wall is initially thick and irregular, with some intraluminal, variably echogenic material (Figure 27.64). As time progresses, the walls become thinner and the amount of intraluminal material decreases.

## Female Reproductive System Diseases

### Ovary

**Normal Imaging Appearance**   See Chapter 20.

**Uterus**   If the uterus is distended adequately, it may be seen on abdominal radiographs. Mild uterine body distension is located between the descending colon and urinary bladder but may be confused with segments of small intestine (Figure 27.65). Greater distension will lead to radiographically visible uterine horns on the VD radiograph; this is further

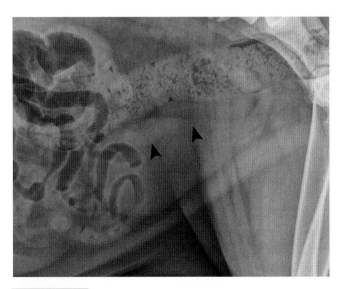

**FIGURE 27.65**   Caudally collimated right lateral abdominal radiograph of a mildly distended uterine body (arrowheads) in a dog appearing similar to the adjacent mildly gas-filled small intestinal segments.

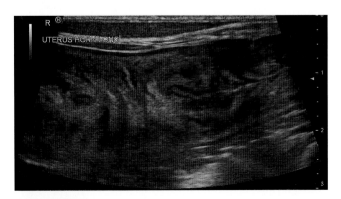

**FIGURE 27.64**   Sagittal plane ultrasound image of a thickened postpartum uterus in a dog.

characterized by large, tortuous, soft tissue tubular structures cranial to the urinary bladder and cranially displacing the small intestine (Figure 27.66). Rarely, an emphysematous pyometra develops and is seen on radiographs as tubular structures containing gas or mixed soft tissue and gas opacities (Figure 27.67). This has been associated with *Clostridium perfringens* and *Pseudomonas aeruginosa* infection and may be linked with metritis or fetal death [36, 37].

**Endometrial Disease**   Canine endometrial hyperplasia-pyometra complex is common and results from an abnormal response to chronic and repeated progesterone exposure and

subsequent infection leading to pyometra. In older patients (>6 years), cystic endometrial hyperplasia usually precedes pyometra. In younger female dogs, pyometra may develop without underlying endometrial disease.

**Ultrasonography**   Ultrasound is optimal for diagnosing cystic endometrial hyperplasia and pyometra. On ultrasound, cystic endometrial hyperplasia causes diffuse uterine wall thickening with multifocal anechoic cysts (Figure 27.68). As bilateral or unilateral pyometra develops, hypoechoic, anechoic, or echogenic fluid accumulates in the uterine horn(s). It is important to check for uterine distension on both sides

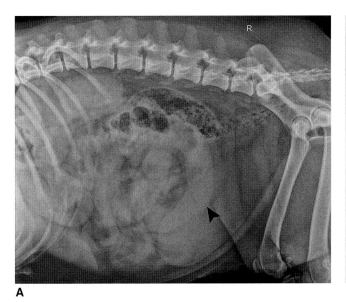
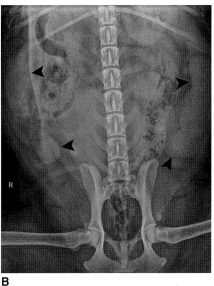

**A**

**B**

**FIGURE 27.66**   Right lateral (**A**) and VD (**B**) abdominal radiographs of a dog with bilateral uterine horn distension (arrowheads). This dog was diagnosed with pyometra.

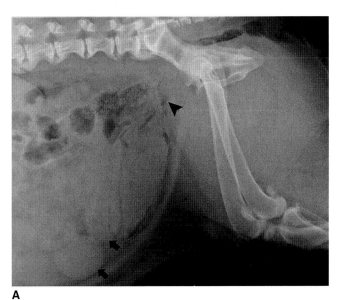
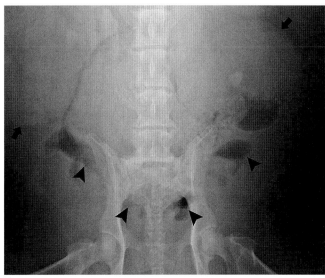

**A**

**B**

**FIGURE 27.67**   Caudally collimated right lateral (**A**) and VD (**B**) abdominal radiographs of a large-breed dog with emphysematous pyometra and emphysematous cystitis. Note the gas-filled uterine body and caudal uterine horns (arrowheads). Some portions of the uterine horns are markedly fluid filled (arrows).

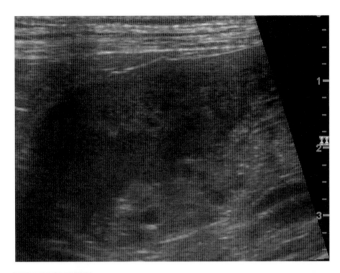

**FIGURE 27.68**  Sagittal plane ultrasound image of a dog with a thickened, cystic uterine wall with mild intraluminal echogenic fluid accumulation, consistent with cystic endometrial hyperplasia.

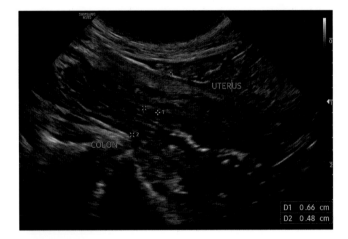

**FIGURE 27.69**  Sagittal plane ultrasound image of a minimally distended uterine body in a dog appearing similar to that of the adjacent empty colon.

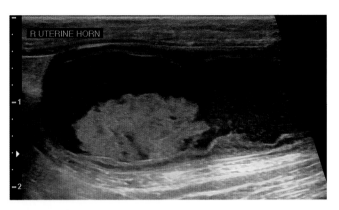

**FIGURE 27.70**  Sagittal plane ultrasound image of a markedly dilated uterine horn with echogenic fluid, inspissated hyperechoic material, and markedly thinned walls, consistent with pyometra.

of the abdomen. If mildly dilated, the uterine horns can be similar in size to the small intestine (Figure 27.69). Ultrasound will help differentiate a layered small intestinal segment from an indistinguishable layered uterine horn. When the uterus is markedly dilated, the uterine wall will become very thin (Figure 27.70).

**Uterine Stump Pyometra**  Uterine stump granuloma or stump pyometra can be difficult to diagnose on radiographs. On radiographs, there can be a soft tissue mass effect between the urinary bladder and descending colon with regional loss of serosal detail. Ultrasound is typically needed for this diagnosis. Typically, ultrasound shows a heterogeneous mass lesion between the urinary bladder and descending colon, immediately cranial to the pelvic inlet; small lesions may be difficult to identify (Figure 27.71).

**Focal Uteromegaly**  Focal uteromegaly may be seen on ultrasound or radiographs. Differential diagnoses include early

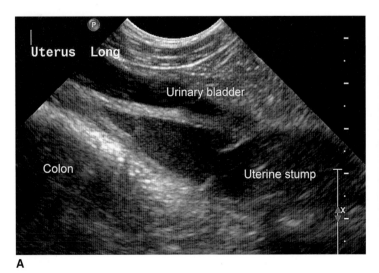

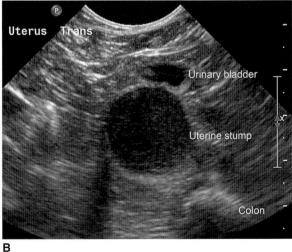

**FIGURE 27.71**  Sagittal (**A**) and transverse (**B**) plane ultrasound images of a dog with a dilated, centrally echogenic fluid-filled uterine stump pyometra.

pregnancy with a small litter size, focal pyometra, abscess, granuloma, and uterine neoplasia. Ultrasonography is most useful in confirming the involvement of the uterus and diagnosing the cause of enlargement.

Uterine neoplasms are uncommon in both the female dog and female cat (0.3–0.4% of all neoplasms in the female dog, 0.2–1.5% in the female cat) [38, 39]. Most canine uterine neoplasms are mesenchymal (leiomyomas, 85–90%; leiomyosarcomas, 10%) [39], but adenomas/adenocarcinomas, fibromas/fibrosarcomas, and lipomas can also occur [40, 41]. Most feline uterine neoplasms are adenocarcinomas, but leiomyomas/leiomyosarcomas, fibromas/fibrosarcomas, lipomas, and lymphoma have also been reported [41].

**Abnormal Findings during Pregnancy**   Radiographs and ultrasound are helpful in the investigation of abnormalities during gestation, including fetal distress, fetal death, fetal mummification, and dystocia.

**Fetal Distress**   This is only assessed on ultrasound by measuring the fetal heart rate. Normal fetal heart rate is twice that of the gravid female but may be reduced by fetal hypoxia secondary to dystocia.

**Fetal Death**   Fetal death may be determined using ultrasound or radiographs. Ultrasound assessment of fetal viability is based on the presence or absence of cardiac activity. Ultrasonography is generally more reliable than radiography for detecting early fetal death.

Radiographic evidence of fetal death is apparent after skeletal mineralization has occurred. Signs may include gas surrounding or within the fetus [42, 43], fetal anatomy disorganization, demineralization of fetal bones, overlapping of the calvarial bones ("Spalding sign"), or fetal malpositioning (i.e., hyperextension) [44]. Superimposed intestinal gas may mimic these changes.

**Fetal Mummification**   Mummification may happen after a fetus dies where compaction of the skeletal structures and increased mineral opacity occur (Figure 27.72). This may be seen with ectopic pregnancies, as the fetus appears in an abnormal location [45]. In these cases, there is often peritoneal effusion, making it difficult to differentiate fetal mummification from an acute uterine rupture.

Fetal death before 25 days probably results in resorption of the fetus, whereas after 35 days abortion is more likely. An aborted fetus quickly loses the normal ultrasonographic appearance and is usually expelled within a few days [46].

**Dystocia**   Dystocia is best assessed on radiographs. Radiographic findings include fetal malpresentation and fetal oversize, pelvic canal narrowing secondary to prior pelvic fractures, and uterine inertia where the fetuses fail to approach the pelvic inlet. Radiographs should be done if there is concern for retained fetuses.

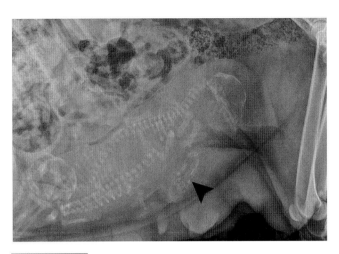

**FIGURE 27.72**   Right lateral abdominal radiograph of a gravid female dog with two mineralized feti and one mummified fetus (arrowhead).

**Cervix**   The cervix is usually poorly identified with diagnostic imaging and is likely to present an obviously abnormal appearance only when a large mass is present.

**Vagina and Vestibule**   The vagina and vestibule are best examined directly or via vaginoscopy; diagnostic imaging is usually unnecessary. To investigate vaginal and vulvar pathology, contrast radiography (vaginography or vaginourethrography) can be done, but CT is the imaging modality of choice due to the location of this portion of the anatomy.

Severe vaginal stenosis has been suspected in recurrent lower urinary or genital tract infections due to the retention of pooled urine in the vagina proximal to the stenosis [47–49]. Vaginal aplasia is a failure of development of the vagina. On vaginography, there is lack of vaginal contrast medium filling [50].

Vaginitis can occur in intact or spayed female dogs, and less commonly in female cats, and may result from bacterial (*Brucella canis* or *Mycoplasma* spp.) or viral (canine herpes virus) infections and chemical or mechanical irritation, generally presenting with a vulval discharge [51–53]. Vaginitis is usually diagnosed via cytology and vaginoscopy. However, on positive-contrast vaginography, vaginitis causes irregular mucosal margination. On CT, the vaginal wall is irregular in margination, thickened, and contrast enhancing.

Vaginal hypertrophy commonly occurs in younger female dogs. Brachycephalic breed dogs (boxer, but also bull mastiff and bulldog) are predisposed [54]. It results in a thickening and corrugation of the lining of the vagina.

Vaginal or uterine prolapse is congenital and results from a weakness of the supporting tissues. Hyperestrogenism due to cystic ovaries has also been implicated as the cause of this condition [55]. Uterine prolapse may be a complication before, during, immediately after, or up to 48 hours after parturition.

Vaginal or vestibular neoplasms include leiomyomas, fibromas, polyps, and leiomyosarcomas; most (~70%) are benign [56]. Caudally located masses are easily evaluated with visual inspection, but CT or contrast radiographs help delineate the more cranially located masses. On contrast vaginogram, vaginal masses usually appear as filling defects and are generally smoothly marginated.

## Miscellaneous Conditions

Uncommon conditions of the female reproductive system are often congenital and include intersexuality. These patients may have clitoral hypertrophy and radiography of the perineal area may show an os clitoris [57].

## Mammary Glands

There are usually five pairs of mammary glands in the female dog and four pairs in the female cat, although some variation is possible. The axillary and sternal lymph nodes drain the cranial mammary glands and the inguinal lymph nodes drain the caudal mammary glands [58]. The normal mammary gland cannot be distinguished from the surrounding fascial planes and cutaneous structures on radiographs. The use of ultrasonography to assess mammary glands has been reported [59–61]. The normal mammary gland has a homogeneous appearance on ultrasonography around the time of parturition.

### Mammary Gland Diseases

**Mammary Neoplasia**  Mammary neoplasia is very common in the female dog. The incidence of neoplasia is significantly reduced by ovariohysterectomy. The risk of malignant neoplasms is 0.05% if the animal is spayed prior to the first estrus, 8% if spayed after the first season, and 26% if spayed later than the second season [62]. Spaying at any age reduces the risk of benign neoplasms [63]. In dogs, approximately 50% of mammary neoplasms are benign and 50% are malignant [64]. The majority of the malignant canine mammary neoplasms are carcinomas, but sarcomas (i.e., fibrosarcomas, osteosarcomas) may occasionally occur. Benign neoplasms are most often fibroadenomas, but adenomas and benign mixed neoplasms may also occur [65].

Mammary neoplasia in the female cat is much more likely (~90%) to be malignant but occurs at less than half the frequency of the female dog [64]. Siamese cats seem to show an increased risk of mammary neoplasia. There is an effect of early spaying, with a sevenfold reduction in incidence reported when ovariohysterectomy is performed at 6 months of age [63]. Most feline mammary neoplasms are adenocarcinomas.

Radiographs do not play a huge role in the assessment of primary mammary neoplasia; palpation and histopathology are better methods of assessment. However, radiography is indicated if there is a risk of pulmonary metastatic disease or metastatic lymphadenopathy (i.e., sternal or sublumbar lymph nodes) [66]. Three-view thoracic radiographs should be evaluated for metastasis. In the female cat, metastatic spread to the

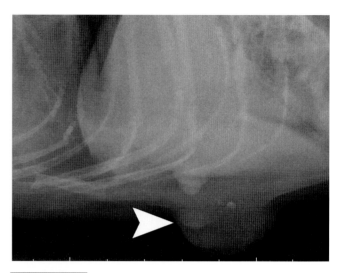

**FIGURE 27.73**  Left lateral thoracic radiograph of a dog with a mineralized mammary mass (arrowhead).

pleura has been reported [67]. To evaluate sublumbar metastatic lymphadenopathy, ultrasonography is the modality of choice when compared to radiography.

Mineralized mammary lesions have been reported and are more often associated with benign lesions than with malignant disease [68]. Mineralization may be seen on survey radiographs along the ventral body wall (Figure 27.73) and seen as distal acoustic shadowing on ultrasonography. Ultrasonographic assessment of sternal lymphadenopathy is more sensitive and specific than radiography.

**Mastitis**  On ultrasonography, mastitis will appear thickened, heterogeneous (i.e., echogenic lines and anechoic regions), and irregular in echotexture [69]. In severe cases, gas bubbles may be seen, and abscessation has been reported.

# Male Reproductive Tract

## Prostate Gland

### Normal Imaging Appearance  See Chapter 20.

### Positive-Contrast Retrograde Urethrography  The prostatic urethra and many diseases of the prostate can be evaluated using positive-contrast retrograde urethrography. The normal prostatic urethra should be uniformly distended and smoothly marginated with no filling defects. A normal tiny filling defect is sometimes visible in the dorsal wall of the urethra at the center of the prostate, representing the colliculus seminalis (where the vas deferens and prostatic ducts enter the urethra). The urethra may appear slightly wider in the center of the prostate and may taper a little at the cranial and caudal margins of the prostate. The extent of central dilation may vary depending on the pressure applied during contrast medium

injection, and a degree of normal variation from animal to animal is to be expected. The urinary bladder neck should be smoothly tapering.

Occasionally, intraprostatic reflux of contrast medium can occur in a normal dog. The reflux should only outline normal prostatic ducts. Abnormal reflux is a nonspecific finding and may occur with prostatitis, abscesses, cysts, or neoplasia.

## Prostatic Diseases

### Change in Size

**Increase in Size**    Generalized prostatomegaly (Figure 27.74) causes cranioventral deviation of the urinary bladder and dorsolateral deviation of the colon. The colonic lumen may narrow if the prostatomegaly is severe. Severe prostatomegaly may cause cranial displacement of the abdominal contents.

Asymmetrical prostatomegaly (e.g., cysts, abscess, neoplasia) may cause variations in the displacement pattern of the urinary bladder. A cyst or abscess extending dorsally may compress the urinary bladder ventrally. A lesion causing ventral prostatomegaly may dorsally deviate the urinary bladder from the ventral abdominal body wall.

Conditions such as acute prostatitis and neoplasia do not usually cause severe prostatomegaly. Severe prostatomegaly is much more likely to be seen with benign prostatic hyperplasia, cysts, or abscesses. Even in severe prostatomegaly, the margins of the prostate usually remain sharp. Indistinct prostatic margins in the presence of caudal intraabdominal fat is suggestive of prostatitis or prostatic neoplasia. Abscesses generally have sharp margins, but may result in decreased peritoneal serosal detail representing peritonitis.

**Decrease in Size**    Atrophy is common after neutering. The rate of prostate size change after neutering and the final size are not consistent. A neutered male is likely to have a very small prostate and may be difficult to identify if the animal was neutered at a very young age. Atrophy may also occur secondary to Sertoli cell neoplasia or estrogen therapy. Atrophy is also seen as a degenerative change associated with old age. On radiographs, the prostate gland will be small or indiscernible.

### Change in Opacity

**Increased Opacity**    The normal prostate is soft tissue opaque and mildly enlarged. As enlargement becomes more severe, the opacity of the prostate may become heterogeneous. Mineralization within the prostate is an unusual finding and warrants further investigation with ultrasonography and histopathologic analysis. Mineralization of the prostate is predictive of prostatic neoplasia in neutered male dogs with an overall sensitivity of 84% and specificity of 100% [70]. However, in intact male dogs, mineralization can occur with prostatic neoplasia, paraprostatic cysts, benign prostatic hyperplasia, or prostatitis.

**Decreased Opacity**    Gas opacities within the prostate are suggestive of severe infection from gas- producing bacteria.

**Metastases**    The most common malignant neoplasms of the prostate are adenocarcinoma and transitional cell carcinoma [71]. These commonly metastasize to regional lymph nodes (i.e., medial iliac and internal iliac lymph nodes) and adjacent osseous structures [72]. Metastatic osseous lesions are usually osteoproliferative, seen most often on the ventral surfaces of the caudal lumbar and sacral vertebral bodies, iliac

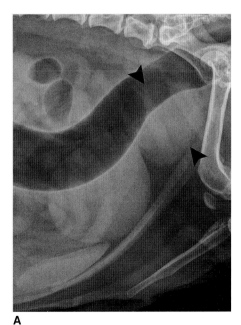
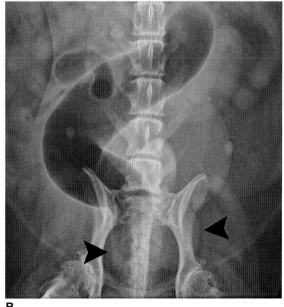

A                                                    B

**FIGURE 27.74**    Right lateral (**A**) and VD (**B**) abdominal radiographs of a dog with generalized prostatomegaly (arrowheads), cranially displacing the urinary bladder.

wings, and femoral diaphysis and other long bones. Prostatic carcinoma has been reported in conjunction with hypertrophic osteopathy [73, 74]. Thoracic metastasis occurs in the later stages of the disease.

### Benign Prostatic Hyperplasia

Benign prostatic hyperplasia is the most common finding in normal intact male dogs. It is a presumptive diagnosis in all middle-aged to older intact male dogs. Histologically, it has been shown to be present in 95% of intact dogs >9 years old [75]. Many dogs will never show clinical signs associated with prostatomegaly.

Benign prostatic hyperplasia commonly results secondary to symmetric glandular hyperplasia. On ultrasound, there is variable prostatic enlargement, heterogeneous echotexture, and hyperechogenicity. Mineralization is not usually seen unless concurrent disease is present. Parenchymal cysts of varying size and number may also be present (Figure 27.75).

Differentiation between benign prostatic hyperplasia, prostatitis, and neoplasia is difficult on ultrasound examination. Frequently, prostatic hyperplasia, neoplasia, and prostatitis coexist in the same prostate in older dogs. Histopathologic analysis is required for definitive diagnosis and complete staging.

### Cysts

#### Parenchymal Cysts

Parenchymal cysts may occur with benign prostatic hyperplasia. These cysts may occur secondary to dilated acini and ducts and can be acquired or congenital. They may also be seen with prostatitis and neoplasia. True cysts are smooth, anechoic, with distal acoustic enhancement. True cysts may become infected. If irregularly marginated structures with echogenic material are seen, abscess or hemorrhage should be considered. Cytologic analysis and culture and sensitivity are required for a definitive diagnosis.

### Paraprostatic Cysts

Paraprostatic cyst are large cystic structures that develop between the prostate and urinary bladder. They are derived from remnants of the uterus masculinus, vestigial Mullerian ducts, or subsequent to prostatic hematoma [76]. They usually arise from the craniodorsal aspect of the prostate and extend cranially. It can be difficult to determine which structure is the urinary bladder if the cyst is very large. Careful evaluation of the bladder neck and prostate position can help differentiate the urinary bladder from a cyst, but a cystogram or retrograde urethrogram may be necessary to positively identify the urinary bladder. Sometimes the walls of paraprostatic cysts are mineralized, creating an "eggshell" appearance on radiographs.

Typically, on ultrasound a paraprostatic cyst is a fluid-filled, anechoic to mildly echogenic structure with variable wall thickness. Where the walls are mineralized, they appear markedly hyperechoic. Septations may also be present. The cysts are variable in size but can be very large, occupying the majority of the caudal abdomen, extending into the pelvic cavity causing perineal hernias. Paraprostatic cysts may become infected, resulting in echogenic intralesional material. Occasionally, paraprostatic cysts may be solid, but have a mixed echogenicity.

### Prostatitis

Bacterial prostatitis in intact male dogs is common. Concurrent urinary tract infection is a predisposition to prostatitis; it can be an extension of testicular or epididymal disease. Fungal prostatitis is very rare.

On ultrasound, prostatitis may be asymmetrically or symmetrically enlarged, heterogeneous in echotexture, and contain multifocal anechoic cysts (Figure 27.76). Some cysts may have echogenic intralesional material. If one or multiple large cyst-like structures with irregularly thickened walls and echogenic material are seen, they may represent an abscess. Small

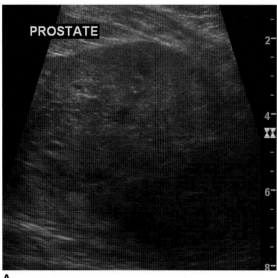
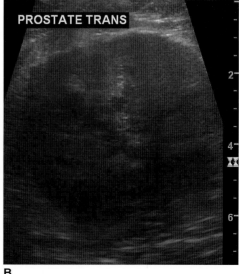

**FIGURE 27.75**   Sagittal plane (**A**) and transverse plane (**B**) ultrasound images of a cystic benign prostatic hyperplasia in a normal intact male dog.

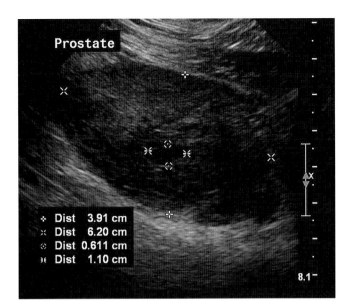

**FIGURE 27.76** Sagittal plane ultrasound image of a neutered male dog with prostatomegaly, heterogeneity, and slightly irregular margins, consistent with bacterial prostatitis.

foci of mineralization may be present with chronic prostatitis, but this finding is seen more commonly with neoplasia.

Caudal abdominal effusion may be present. Regional lymphadenopathy may also be present, although this is unusual and generally only mild. Serial ultrasounds after neutering may show resolution of prostatomegaly. The testes should also be examined as infection of the testes may be the primary cause or have secondary effects from prostatitis. Occasionally, prostatitis may resemble benign prostatic hyperplasia and have a homogeneous appearance. Definitive diagnosis often requires fine needle aspiration and culture and sensitivity.

**Abscesses**   Abscesses (Figure 27.77) may form as a result of acute or chronic prostatitis. Infection of benign prostatic cysts is common. The entire prostate can become abscessed.

**Neoplasia**   Prostatic neoplasia is uncommon in the dog and extremely rare in the cat. Prostatic carcinoma is seen in middle-aged to old, medium- to large-breed, intact and neutered dogs. Prostatomegaly in a neutered animal, especially with evidence of mineralization, is suggestive of neoplasia. Adenocarcinomas and transitional cell carcinomas are common. These tumor types may be difficult to differentiate histologically and are not distinguishable ultrasonographically. Lymphoma is very uncommon.

Ultrasonographically, the prostate is typically asymmetrically enlarged and heterogeneous. There may be multiple hyperechoic foci, some of which may be associated with distal acoustic shadowing, indicating mineralization (Figure 27.78). Cavitary lesions may be present, appearing similar to that seen with prostatitis. Biopsy of the prostate or lymph nodes is required to confirm the diagnosis.

**Atrophy**   The prostatic parenchyma usually appears uniformly hypoechoic on ultrasound.

## Testes and Scrotum

Radiographic examination of the testes and scrotum adds little when compared to a thorough clinical examination. Ultrasonography allows more detailed assessment of this area, in particular the testes. Indications for ultrasonography of the testes and scrotum include prostatic disease, feminization syndrome, infertility, a palpable mass, testicular asymmetry,

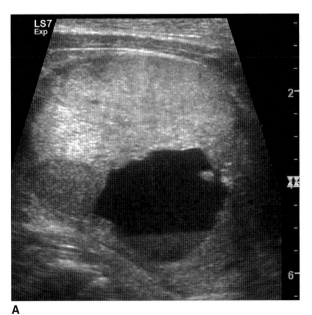

**A**

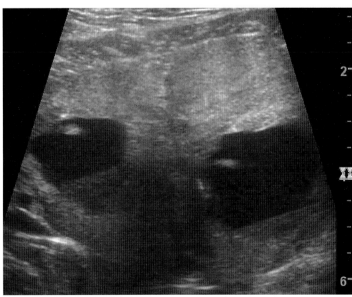

**B**

**FIGURE 27.77** Sagittal plane (**A**) and transverse plane (**B**) ultrasound images of a dog with prostatomegaly and a large, irregular cavitated structure with mild to moderate dependent echogenic material, consistent with a prostatic abscess.

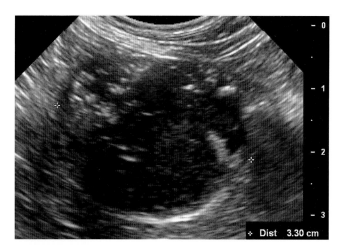

Transverse plane ultrasound image of a dog with prostatomegaly, diffuse hypoechogenicity, and multifocal hyperechoic foci, consistent with mineralized prostatic carcinoma.

testicular atrophy, pyrexia of unknown origin, scrotal swelling, and retained testicles. A 10–15 MHz linear probe is commonly used to evaluate the testes. The probe should be placed directly on each testicle.

## Normal Ultrasonographic Appearance

The paired testes are contained within the scrotum separated by the median septum. They are covered by connective tissue, which radiates septa centrally to join the median raphe where the testes are further divided into lobules. The epididymis comprises a head, body, and tail. The head lies at the cranial pole of the testis, the body is located along the lateral and dorsal aspect of the testis, and the tail is positioned caudally.

The normal testis is moderately echogenic with a homogeneous echotexture (Figure 27.79). The median raphe is a central hyperechoic linear structure in the midsagittal plane and a focal hyperechoic structure in the transverse plane. The head and body of the epididymis are nearly isoechoic with the testicle, and the tail is hypoechoic to anechoic and has a coarse echotexture. The head is cranially located, the body can be followed caudally, and the tail is located caudal to both the head and body.

## Testicular Diseases

**Neoplasia** Neoplasia of the testes is the second most common tumor in male dogs and considered rare in cats. Most neoplasms are benign, and of these, interstitial (Leydig) cell tumors are the most common; on ultrasound, they contain multifocal to coalescing, small, hypoechoic nodules. Bilateral interstitial cell tumors commonly occur. Other neoplasms include seminomas and Sertoli cell tumors. Seminomas (Figure 27.80) are often large and solitary, causing testicular enlargement; on ultrasound, they are hypoechoic relative to normal testicular echogenicity, but this is not always the case. Seminomas tend to be unilateral. Sertoli cell tumors may cause testicular enlargement with atrophy of the contralateral testicle if the tumor is producing estrogen. They tend to have a mixed echogenicity.

Cryptorchid animals are reported to be at 13 times greater risk of developing a Sertoli cell tumor or seminoma and may develop these neoplasms at a relatively young age [77]. Multiple concurrent neoplasms may also occur. Many Sertoli cell tumors are functional and often metastasize to the regional lymph nodes, liver, and lungs.

**Orchitis** Orchitis is often seen concurrently with epididymitis and may be secondary to retrograde infection from the ductus deferens. Less commonly, penetrating wounds may also cause orchitis. Secondary abscessation is common. Ultrasonographically, there is enlarged testicle and epididymis, variably thickened testicular walls, variable echogenicity [78], and a diffusely heterogeneous parenchyma. Chronic infection may result in a small testicle of mixed echogenicity. Orchitis may appear very similar to a neoplasm, but localized fluid accumulation is much less common in neoplasia.

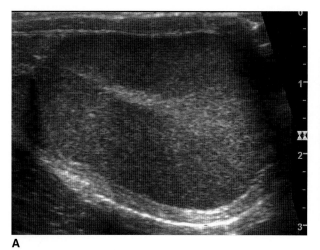

**A**

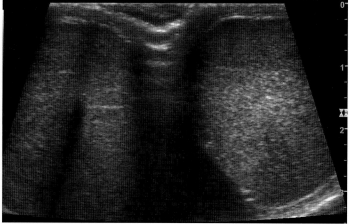

**B**

Sagittal plane (**A**) and transverse plane (**B**) ultrasound images of a normal testicle.

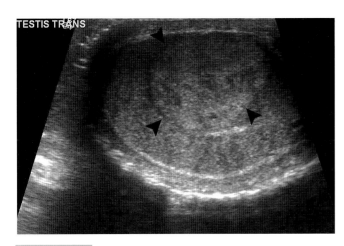

**FIGURE 27.80**  Sagittal plane ultrasound image of a testicular seminoma (arrowheads).

**Testicular Torsion**  Testicular torsion can occur in enlarged, intraabdominal, neoplastic testes. The characteristic appearance is of a diffuse increase in echogenicity with capsular thickening, epididymal and spermatic cord enlargement, and scrotal thickening. Differentiation between testicular torsion and orchitis is difficult.

**Atrophy**  The testicle is small in size and normal in echogenicity or hypoechoic on ultrasound. Atrophy may be secondary to age-related changes, may occur in one testicle from a Sertoli cell tumor in the contralateral testicle, or may occur with a retained testicle. Nonneoplastic retained testicles are usually very small and difficult to identify; they may be located anywhere from just caudal to the kidneys to the inguinal canal [79].

## Scrotal Diseases

**Hernia**  Scrotal herniation of the small intestine may be confirmed by seeing the gas-filled segments of intestine in the scrotal sac on radiographs. Ultrasonographically, the intestines may be identified by the distinctive layered appearance and peristalsis. Hyperechoic peritoneal fat also may herniate into the scrotum. Any herniated organ may become strangulated or necrotic, leading to local inflammation or fluid accumulation.

## Penis

**Radiography**  The only part of the penis identifiable on plain radiographs is the os penis which lies on the caudoventral aspect of the abdomen. In some dogs, the tip of the os penis may be discontinuous, representing a secondary center of ossification (Figure 27.81) which is often confused with a urethral calculus. On a properly positioned VD view, the prepuce overlies the vertebrae and is difficult to identify. Oblique VD views demonstrate the structure more clearly.

Radiography of the penis is of little value compared with a thorough clinical examination, with the exception of penile urethral calculi.

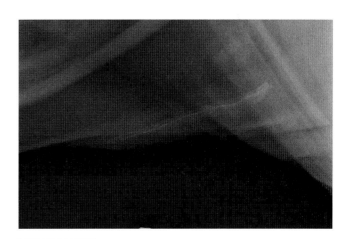

**FIGURE 27.81**  Collimated right lateral abdominal radiograph of a dog with a normal, rectangular-shaped mineral opacity cranial to the os penis, representing a secondary center of ossification of the os penis.

# References

1. Ferreira, A., Marwood, R., Batchelor, D. et al. (2020). Prevalence and clinical significance of the medullary rim sign identified on ultrasound of feline kidneys. *Vet. Rec.* 186: 533.
2. Biller, D.S., Bradley, G.A., and Partington, B.P. (1992). Renal medullary rim sign: ultrasonographic evidence of renal disease. *Vet. Radiol. Ultrasound* 33: 286–290.
3. Hart, D.V., Winter, M.D., Conway, J., and Berry, C.R. (2013). Ultrasound appearance of the outer medulla in dogs without renal dysfunction. *Vet. Radiol. Ultrasound* 54: 652–658.
4. Barr, F.J., Patteson, M.W., Lucke, V.M., and Gibbs, C. (1989). Hypercalcemic nephropathy in three dogs: sonographic appearance. *Vet. Radiol.* 30: 169–173.
5. Adams, W.H., Toal, R.L., Walker, M.A. et al. (1989). Early renal ultrasonographic findings in dogs with experimentally induced ethylene glycol nephrosis. *Am. J. Vet. Res.* 50: 1370–1376.
6. Taylor, A.J., Lara-Garcia, A., and Benigni, L. (2014). Ultrasonograhpic characteristics of canine renal lymphoma. *Vet. Radiol. Ultrasound* 55: 441–446.
7. Valdes-Martinez, A., Cianciolo, R., and Mai, W. (2007). Association between renal hypoechoic subcapsular thickening and lymphosarcoma in cats. *Vet. Radiol. Ultrasound* 48: 357–360.
8. Lewis, K.M. and O'Brien, R.T. (2010). Abdominal ultrasonographic findings associated with feline infectious peritonitis: a retrospective review of 16 cases. *J. Am. Anim. Hosp. Assoc.* 46: 152–160.

9. McKenna, S.C. and Carpenter, J.L. (1980). Polycystic disease of the kidney and liver in the cairn terrier. *Vet. Pathol.* 17: 436–442.

10. Biller, D.S., Chew, D.J., and DiBartola, S.P. (1990). Polycystic kidney disease in a family of Persian cats. *J. Am. Vet. Med. Assoc.* 196: 1288–1290.

11. O'Leary, C.A., Mackay, B.M., Malik, R. et al. (1999). Polycystic kidney disease in bull terrier: an autosomal dominant inherited disorder. *Aus. Vet. J.* 77: 361–366.

12. Beck, C. and Lavelle, R.B. (2001). Feline polycystic kidney disease in Persian and other cats: a prospective study using ultrasonography. *Aust. Vet. J.* 79: 181–184.

13. Lium, B. and Moe, L. (1985). Hereditary multifocal renal cystadenocarcinomas and nodular dermatofibrosis in the German shepherd dog: macroscopic and histopathologic changes. *Vet. Pathol.* 22: 447–455.

14. Moe, L. and Lium, B. (1997). Hereditary multifocal renal cystadenocarcinomas and nodular dermatofibrosis in 51 German shepherd dogs. *J. Small Anim. Pract.* 38: 498–505.

15. Bryan, J.N., Henry, C.J., Turnquist, S.E. et al. (2006). Primary renal neoplasia of dogs. *J. Vet. Intern. Med.* 20: 1155–1160.

16. Ochoa, V.B., Dibartola, S.P., Chew, D.J. et al. (1999). Perinephric pseudocysts in the cat: a retrospective study and review of the literature. *J. Vet. Intern. Med.* 13: 47–55.

17. Debruyn, K., Haers, H., Combes, A. et al. (2012). Ultrasonography of the feline kidney: technique, anatomy and changes associated with disease. *J. Feline Med. Surg.* 14: 794–803.

18. D'Anjou, M.A., Bedard, A., and Dunn, M.E. (2011). Clinical significance of renal pelvic dilatation on ultrasound in dogs and cats. *Vet. Radiol. Ultrasound* 52: 88–94.

19. Bouillon, J., Snead, E., Caswell, J. et al. (2018). Pyelonephritis in dogs: retrospective study of 47 histologically diagnosed cases (2005–2015). *J. Vet. Intern. Med.* 32: 249–259.

20. Foster, J.D. (2016). Update on mineral and bone disorders in chronic kidney disease. *Vet. Clin. North Am. Small Anim. Pract.* 46: 1131–1149.

21. Stillion, J.R. and Ritt, M.G. (2009). Renal secondary hyperparathyroidism in dogs. *Compend. Contin. Educ. Vet.* 31: E8.

22. Davis, E.M. (2015). Oral manifestations of chronic kidney disease and renal secondary hyperparathyroidism: a comparative review. *J. Vet. Dent.* 32: 87–98.

23. Schwarz, T., Bommer, N., Parys, M. et al. (2021). Four-dimensional CT excretory urography is an accurate technique for diagnosis of canine ureteral ectopia. *Vet. Radiol. Ultrasound* 62: 190–198.

24. Glassberg, K.I., Braren, V., Duckett, J.W. et al. (1984). Suggested terminology for duplex systems, ectopic ureters and ureteroceles. *J. Urol.* 132: 1153–1154.

25. Weichselbaum, R.C., Feeney, D.A., Jessen, C.R. et al. (1999). Urocystolith detection: comparison of survey, contrast radiographic and ultrasonographic techniques in an in vitro bladder phantom. *Vet. Radiol. Ultrasound* 40: 386–400.

26. Weichselbaum, R.C., Feeney, D.A., Jessen, C.R. et al. (2000). Relevance of sonographic artifacts observed during in vitro characterization of urocystolith mineral composition. *Vet. Radiol. Ultrasound* 41: 438–446.

27. Hanazono, K., Fukumoto, S., Endo, Y. et al. (2014). Ultrasonographic findings related to prognosis in canine transitional cell carcinoma. *Vet. Radiol. Ultrasound* 55: 79–84.

28. Takiguchi, M. and Inaba, M. (2005). Diagnostic ultrasound of polypoid cystitis in dogs. *J. Vet. Intern. Med. Sci.* 67: 57–61.

29. Fumeo, M., Manfredi, S., and Volta, A. (2019). Emphysematous cystitis: review of current literature, diagnosis and management challenges. *Vet. Med.* 10: 77–83.

30. Petite, A., Busoni, V., Heinen, M.P. et al. (2006). Radiographic and ultrasonographic findings of emphysematous cystitis in four nondiabetic female dogs. *Vet. Radiol. Ultrasound* 47: 90–93.

31. Adams, W.M. and DiBartola, S.P. (1983). Radiographic and clinical features of pelvic bladder in the dog. *J. Am. Vet. Med. Assoc.* 182: 1212–1217.

32. Stiffler, K.S., Stevenson, M.A., Mahaffey, M.B. et al. (2002). Intravesical ureterocele with concurrent renal dysfunction in a dog: a case report and proposed classification system. *J. Am. Anim. Hosp. Assoc.* 38: 33–39.

33. Lautzenhiser, S.J. and Bjorling, D.E. (2002). Urinary incontinence in a dog with an ectopic ureterocele. *J. Am. Anim. Hosp. Assoc.* 38: 29–32.

34. Remedios, A.M., Middleton, D.M., Myers, S.L. et al. (1994). Diverticula of the urinary bladder in a juvenile dog. *Can. Vet. J.* 35: 648–650.

35. Scheepens, E.T. and L'Eplattenier, H. (2005). Acquired urinary bladder diverticulum in a dog. *J. Small Anim. Pract.* 46: 578–581.

36. Hernandez, J.L., Besso, J.G., Rault, D.N. et al. (2003). Emphysematous pyometra in a dog. *Vet. Radiol. Ultrasound* 44: 196–198.

37. Mattei, C., Fabbi, M., and Hansson, K. (2018). Radiographic and ultrasonographic findings in a dog with emphysematous pyometra. *Acta Vet. Scand.* 60: 67.

38. Miller, M.A., Ramos-Vara, J.A., Dickerson, M.F. et al. (2003). Uterine neoplasia in 13 cats. *J. Vet. Diagn. Invest.* 15: 515–522.

39. Percival, A., Singh, A., Zur Linden, R.A. et al. (2018). Massive uterine lipoleiomyoma and leiomyoma in a miniature poodle bitch. *Can. Vet. J.* 59: 845–850.

40. Patsikas, M., Papazoglou, L.G., Jakovljevic, S. et al. (2014). Radiographic and ultrasonographic findings of uterine neoplasms in nine dogs. *J. Am. Anim. Hosp. Assoc.* 50: 330–337.

41. Vail, D.M., Thamm, D.H., and Liptak, J. (2013). *Withrow and MacEwen's Small Animal Clinical Oncology*. St Louis, MO: Elsevier.

42. Wicklund, H. (1957). The presence of free gas in the fetal circulatory system as a pathognomonic sign of intrauterine death. *Acta Soc. Med. Ups.* 62: 104–112.

43. Baharmast, J. and Rad, M.A. (1977). Diagnosis of emphysematous fetuses in dogs and cats. *Mod. Vet. Pract.* 58: 349–350.

44. Farrow, C., Morgan, J., and Story, E. (1976). Late term fetal death in the dog: early radiographic diagnosis. *Vet. Radiol.* 17: 11–17.

45. Lederer, H.A. and Fisher, L.E. (1960). Ectopic pregnancy in a dog. *J. Am. Vet. Med. Assoc.* 137: 61.

46. Lamm, C.G. and Njaa, B.L. (2012). Clinical approach to abortion, stillbirth, and neonatal death in dogs and cats. *Vet. Clin. North Am. Small Anim. Pract.* 42: 501–513, vi.

47. Kyles, A.E., Vaden, S., Hardie, E.M., and Stone, E.A. (1996). Vestibulovaginal stenosis in dogs: 18 cases (1987–1995). *J. Am. Vet. Med. Assoc.* 209: 1889–1893.

48. Crawford, J.T. and Adams, W.M. (2002). Influence of vestibulovaginal stenosis, pelvic bladder, and recessed vulva on response to treatment for clinical signs of lower urinary tract disease in dogs: 38 cases (1990–1999). *J. Am. Vet. Med. Assoc.* 221: 995–999.

49. Kieves, N.R., Novo, R.E., and Martin, R.B. (2011). Vaginal resection and anastomosis for treatment of vestibulovaginal stenosis in 4 dogs with recurrent urinary tract infections. *J. Am. Vet. Med. Assoc.* 239: 972–980.

50. Souther, S., Baik, N.J., Clapp, K. et al. (2019). A case of segmental aplasia of the uterus, cervix, and cranial vagina in a cat. *Front. Vet. Sci.* 6: 145.

51. Johnston, S. and Kustritz, M. (2001). Disorders of the canine vagina, vestibule, and vulva. In: *Canine and Feline Theriogenology*

(ed. S. Johnston, M. Kustritz and P. Olson), 235–237. Philadelphia: WB Saunders.

52. Beverly, J. (2003). Vaginal disorders. In: *Small Animal Theriogenology* (ed. M. Kustritz and S. Messonnier), 395–419. Waltham: Butterworth-Heinemann.

53. Soderberg, S.F. (1986). Vaginal disorders. *Vet. Clin. North Am. Small Anim. Pract.* 16: 543–559.

54. Post, K., Van Haaften, B., and Okkens, A.C. (1991). Vaginal hyperplasia in the bitch: literature review and commentary. *Can. Vet. J.* 32: 35–37.

55. Zedda, M.T., Bogliolo, L., Ariu, F. et al. (2016). Vaginal fold prolapse in a dog with pyometra and ovarian papillary cystadenocarcinoma. *J. Am. Vet. Med. Assoc.* 248: 822–826.

56. Thacher, C. and Bradley, R.L. (1983). Vulvar and vaginal tumors in the dog: a retrospective study. *J. Am. Vet. Med. Assoc.* 183: 690–692.

57. Sumner, S.M., Grimes, J.A., Wallace, M.L., and Schmiedt, C.W. (2018). Os clitoris in dogs: 17 cases (2009–2017). *Can. Vet. J.* 59: 606–610.

58. Evans, H.E. and de Lahunta, A. (2013). *Miller's Anatomy of the Dog*. St Louis, MO: Elsevier Saunders.

59. Vannozzi, I., Tesi, M., Zangheri, M. et al. (2018). B-mode ultrasound examination of canine mammary gland neoplastic lesions of small size (diameter < 2 cm). *Vet. Res. Commun.* 42: 137–143.

60. Soler, M., Dominguez, E., Lucas, X. et al. (2016). Comparison between ultrasonographic findings of benign and malignant canine mammary gland tumours using B-mode, colour Doppler, power Doppler and spectral Doppler. *Res. Vet. Sci.* 107: 141–146.

61. Moraes, N.S. and Borges, N.C. (2021). Sonographic assessment of the normal and abnormal feline mammary glands and axillary and inguinal lymph nodes. *Vet. Med. Int.* 2021: 9998025.

62. Sorenmo, K.U., Shofer, F.S., and Goldschmidt, M.H. (2000). Effect of spaying and timing of spaying on survival of dogs with mammary carcinoma. *J. Vet. Intern. Med.* 14: 266–270.

63. Overley, B., Shofer, F.S., Goldschmidt, M.H. et al. (2005). Association between ovariohysterectomy and feline mammary carcinoma. *J. Vet. Intern. Med.* 19: 560–563.

64. Bostock, D.E. (1986). Canine and feline mammary neoplasms. *Br. Vet. J.* 142: 506–515.

65. Tavasoly, A., Golshahi, H., Rezaie, A., and Farhadi, M. (2013). Classification and grading of canine malignant mammary tumors. *Vet. Res. Forum* 4: 25–30.

66. Misdorp, W. and Hart, A.A. (1979). Canine mammary cancer. II. Therapy and causes of death. *J. Small Anim. Pract.* 20: 395–404.

67. Zappulli, V., Rasotto, R., Caliari, D. et al. (2015). Prognostic evaluation of feline mammary carcinomas: a review of the literature. *Vet. Pathol.* 52: 46–60.

68. Cassali, G., Ferreira, E., Lavalle, G. et al. (2014). Consensus for the diagnosis, prognosis and treatment of canine mammary tumors. *Brazil. J. Vet. Pathol.* 7: 38–69.

69. Trasch, K., Wehrend, A., and Bostedt, H. (2007). Ultrasonographic description of canine mastitis. *Vet. Radiol. Ultrasound* 48: 580–584.

70. Bradbury, C.A., Westropp, J.L., and Pollard, R.E. (2009). Relationship between prostatomegaly, prostatic mineralization, and cytologic diagnosis. *Vet. Radiol. Ultrasound* 50: 167–171.

71. Packeiser, E.M., Hewicker-Trautwein, M., Thiemeyer, H. et al. (2020). Characterization of six canine prostate adenocarcinoma and three transitional cell carcinoma cell lines derived from primary tumor tissues as well as metastasis. *PLoS One* 15: e0230272.

72. Axiak, S.M. and Bigio, A. (2012). Canine prostatic carcinoma. *Compend. Contin. Educ. Vet.* 34: E1–E5.

73. Jennings, K. and Watts, J. (2018). Hypertrophic osteopathy in a castrated dog with prostatic carcinoma and prostatitis. *J. Small Anim. Pract.* 59: 719.

74. Withers, S.S., Johnson, E.G., Culp, W.T. et al. (2015). Paraneoplastic hypertrophic osteopathy in 30 dogs. *Vet. Comp. Oncol.* 13: 157–165.

75. Cunto, M., Mariani, E., Anicito Guido, E. et al. (2019). Clinical approach to prostatic diseases in the dog. *Reprod. Domest. Anim.* 54: 815–822.

76. Kyllar, M. and Čížek, P. (2020). An unusual case of infected uterus masculinus in a dog. *BMC Vet. Res.* 16: 194.

77. Hayes, H.M., Wilson, G.P., Pendergrass, T.W., and Cox, V.S. (1985). Canine cryptorchism and subsequent testicular neoplasia: case-control study with epidemiologic update. *Teratology* 32: 51–56.

78. Ober, C.P., Spaulding, K., Breitschwerdt, E.B. et al. (2004). Orchitis in two dogs with Rocky Mountain spotted fever. *Vet. Radiol. Ultrasound* 45: 458–465.

79. Felumlee, A.E., Reichle, J.K., Hecht, S. et al. (2012). Use of ultrasound to locate retained testes in dogs and cats. *Vet. Radiol. Ultrasound* 53: 581–585.

# CHAPTER 28

# Adrenal Glands and Lymph Nodes

Elizabeth Huynh

VCA West Coast Specialty and Emergency Animal Hospital, Fountain Valley, CA, USA

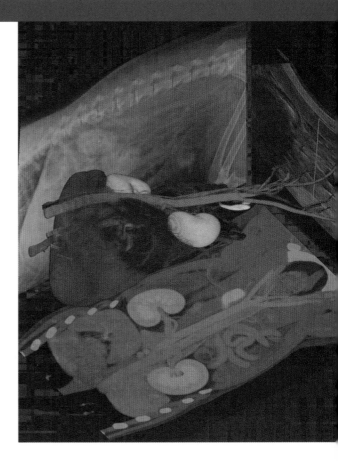

## Overview of Adrenal Glands

The left and right adrenal glands are located in the cranial retroperitoneal space, ventral to T13 through L2 vertebrae, and are closely associated with their respective kidneys, aorta, and caudal vena cava [1]. The left adrenal gland is made up of cranial and caudal poles and the right adrenal gland is made up of cranial and caudal aspects. The phrenicoabdominal vein splits the adrenal glands into cranial and caudal halves. The left adrenal gland is located craniomedial to the cranial pole of the left kidney, lateral to the aorta, caudal to the celiac and cranial mesenteric arteries, dorsal to the phrenicoabdominal vein, and ventral to the phrenicoabdominal artery. The right adrenal gland is located further cranial than the left, craniomedial to the cranial pole of the right kidney, lateral to the caudal vena cava, dorsal to the phrenicoabdominal vein, and ventral to the phrenicoabdominal artery. In cats, the right adrenal gland can be found within the renal fossa of the caudate process of the caudate lobe of the liver [1].

Normal adrenal glands cannot be visualized on radiographs in dogs and cats. Ultrasonography and computed tomography are preferred modalities to evaluate the adrenal glands. Magnetic resonance imaging is another modality less commonly used to evaluate the adrenal glands.

## Imaging Appearance of Normal Adrenal Glands

**Radiography** Radiographically, normal adrenal glands in dogs and cats cannot be visualized unless they are associated with a mass effect and/or mineralized. In some geriatric cats, incidental, likely clinically insignificant, adrenal gland mineralization (Figure 28.1) can be seen. Normal adrenal glands are soft tissue opaque and, therefore, are border effaced with the adjacent liver, surrounding musculature, and any other superimposed soft tissue structures.

*Atlas of Small Animal Diagnostic Imaging*, First Edition. Edited by Clifford R. Berry, Nathan C. Nelson, and Matthew D. Winter.
© 2023 John Wiley & Sons, Inc. Published 2023 by John Wiley & Sons, Inc.
Companion website: www.wiley.com/go/berry/atlas

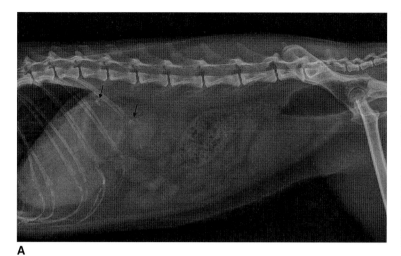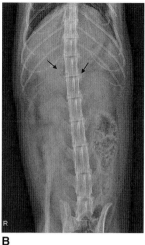

**A**  **B**

**FIGURE 28.1**  Left lateral (**A**) and ventrodorsal (**B**) abdominal radiographs of a geriatric cat with incidental adrenal gland mineralization (arrows).

**Ultrasonography**  Ultrasonography is a preferred method of assessing the adrenal glands and entails real-time scanning in parasagittal, dorsal, or oblique and transverse plane to depict the long and short axes of the gland. The highest frequency transducer that allows adequate penetration should be used. A 5 MHz transducer is usually required for larger dogs, although compression of the ventral abdominal wall with the transducer may allow use of a 7.5 MHz probe in compliant patients. Most animals are scanned in dorsal recumbency, after the hair is clipped and the skin is moistened with alcohol and acoustic coupling gel. A ventral abdominal or flank approach may be used.

The left adrenal gland is identified by first locating the cranial pole of the left kidney in the parasagittal long-axis plane, then sliding the transducer medially until the aorta is found. The left adrenal gland lies ventrolateral to the aorta, caudal to the celiac and cranial mesenteric arteries that branch from the aorta, and cranial to the renal artery that also branches from the aorta. The right adrenal gland is identified by locating the cranial pole of the right kidney in the parasagittal long-axis plane, then sliding the transducer medially until the caudal vena cava and portal vein are found. The right adrenal gland is closely associated with the caudal vena cava and can be mistaken as a venous branch of the caudal vena cava. The right adrenal gland is located within the renal fossa of the caudate process of the caudate lobe of the liver and can be easily mistaken as a hepatic nodule (Figure 28.2). Color and power Doppler can assist in differentiating the right adrenal gland from the surrounding vasculature.

The normal left adrenal glands (Figure 28.3a) in dogs are biconcave or oblong in shape and the right adrenal glands (Figure 28.3b) in dogs are biconcave, oblong, or triangular shaped. In cats, the adrenal glands are oval or bean shaped (Figure 28.4). The width and length of the adrenal glands are variable. Adrenal glands are hypoechoic to the surrounding

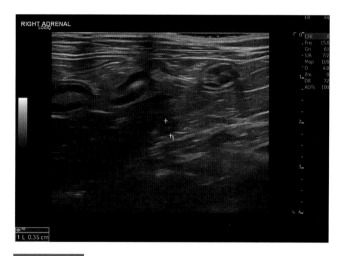

**FIGURE 28.2**  Ultrasound image of the right adrenal gland (between the calipers) in a normal adult cat, closely located to the caudate process of the caudate lobe of the liver.

retroperitoneal fat. In some instances, the corticomedullary distinction is well defined.

In dogs, the normal adrenal gland length and width are variable; however, the caudal pole width should measure between 6.0 and 7.4 mm [2–5]. Recent literature has suggested that the thickness of the caudal pole of the adrenal gland in the sagittal plane is correlated to body size: ≤5.4 mm for dogs <10 kg, ≤6.8 mm for dogs 10–30 kg, and ≤8.0 mm for dogs >30 kg [6]. Adrenal gland length has not been correlated with the age or size of dogs. Therefore, the caudal pole measurement is key to determining enlargement of the adrenal glands in dogs.

In normal cats, the cranial height of the adrenal glands ranges between 3.0 and 4.8 mm and the caudal height of the adrenal glands ranges between 3.0 and 4.5 mm [7]. The adrenal gland height in cats weighing ≤4 kg ranges between 2.2 and 4.1 mm and in cats weighing >4 kg ranges between 2.4 and 5.1 mm [8].

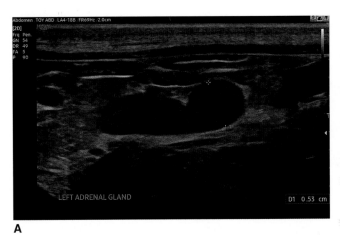

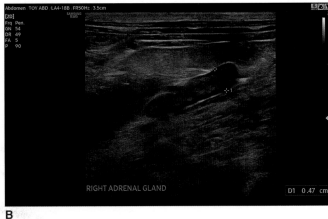

**FIGURE 28.3** Ultrasound images of the left (**A**) and right (**B**) adrenal glands (between the calipers) in a normal adult dog. Note the normal distinction of the cortex and the medulla of the adrenal glands.

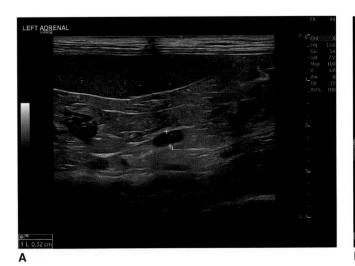

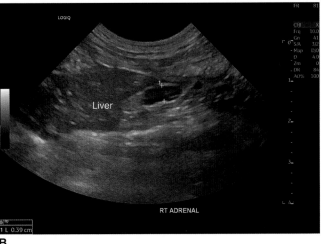

**FIGURE 28.4** Ultrasound images of the left (**A**) and right (**B**) adrenal glands in a normal adult cat. Note the anatomic landmarks around the left adrenal gland and the proximity of the caudate lobe of the liver to the right adrenal gland.

**Computed Tomography** Visualization of the adrenal glands with computed tomography (CT) is not restricted by patient size or gas in the overlying gastrointestinal tract. Typically, 3–5 mm thick transverse CT images of the abdomen in the region of the adrenal glands are obtained. Nonionic iodinated positive-contrast medium may be administered intravenously to help distinguish vessels from the adrenal glands. A bolus injection of 400–800 mgI/kg of body weight may be given and the adrenal gland scan repeated immediately. The left adrenal gland is ventrolateral to the aorta and psoas minor muscle and medial to the cranial pole of the left kidney (Figure 28.5a). The right adrenal gland is located dorsolateral to the caudal vena cava, ventral to the right diaphragmatic crus, and medial to the cranial pole of the right kidney (Figure 28.5b). The adrenal glands are oval, triangular, or round soft tissue-attenuating structures. Portions of the right adrenal gland may appear bipartite.

Orientation of each gland within the transverse plane also affects their measured width and thickness; therefore, these dimensions may not be comparable to those obtained with ultrasonography. The ventrolateral-to-dorsomedial dimension provides an estimation of the short axis of the gland. In a study of 10 healthy dogs, the maximum ventrolateral-to-dorsomedial dimension was 11.1 mm for the right gland and 14.6 mm for the left gland. In a study with 48 normal adult dogs, the mean CT volume of the left adrenal gland was 0.60 cm³ and the right adrenal gland was 0.55 cm³ [9].

## Imaging Abnormalities of Adrenal Glands

Radiographically, marked adrenomegaly secondary to neoplasia may cause a soft tissue opaque mass effect in the craniodorsal retroperitoneal space, caudolaterally displacing the kidneys (Figure 28.6) [10, 11]. Diffuse retroperitoneal change may also be present. Right adrenomegaly is more difficult to assess due to its proximity to the caudate process of the

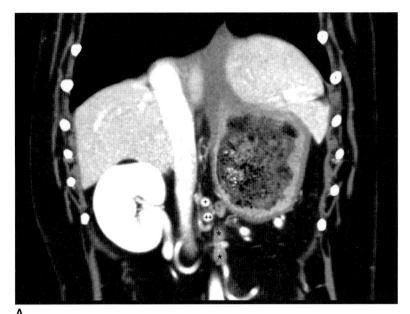
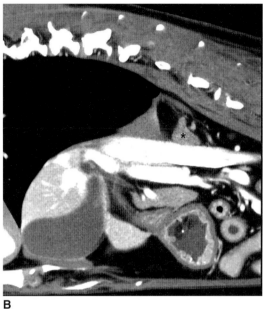

**A**    **B**

**FIGURE 28.5**  Computed tomographic angiogram (CTA) image of the normal left adrenal gland (*) in a dog in the dorsal plane (**A**), soft tissue window (window width 400, window level 40) of the cranial abdomen during the portal phase of contrast; note the normal regional anatomy including the celiac (+) and cranial mesenteric (++) arteries. Computed tomographic image of the normal right adrenal gland in a dog in the parasagittal plane (**B**), soft tissue window (window width 400, window level 40) of the cranial abdomen; note the normal triangular to V-shaped appearance of the adrenal gland.

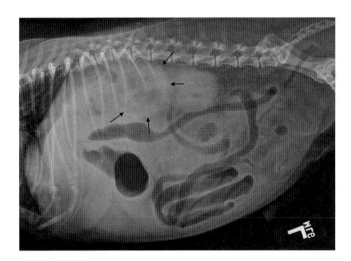

**FIGURE 28.6**  Left lateral abdominal radiograph of a geriatric dog with a large, partially mineralized right adrenal gland mass (arrows). This mass causes caudal displacement of the right kidney.

caudate lobe of the liver, border effacing the adrenal gland mass with the liver.

Although radiographs are not considered the ideal modality to diagnose adrenal gland abnormalities, they are essential to diagnose metastatic disease in the thorax in addition to secondary signs of adrenal gland disease (i.e., pendulous abdomen, hepatomegaly, bronchial and pulmonary mineralization, calcinosis cutis, abdominal soft tissue mineralization, and osteopenia) as seen in adrenal adenomatous cortical hyperplasia. Occasionally, adrenal gland calcification can be seen radiographically in dogs with adrenal adenoma or carcinoma [10].

Differentials for adrenal gland masses include adenocarcinoma (cortical involvement), pheochromocytoma (medulla involvement), metastasis, hyperplasia, and rarely neuroblastoma, ganglioblastoma, myelolipoma, hemorrhage, inflammation or infection, or cyst.

Adrenomegaly, adrenal gland nodules, and adrenal gland masses are better assessed on abdominal ultrasonography. Ultrasonography to detect adrenal lesions has high specificity (100%), but low sensitivity (63.7%) [12]. Differentials for adrenomegaly include hyperplasia or neoplasia such as adenocarcinoma, pheochromocytoma, metastatic disease, adenoma, or, less commonly seen, adrenalitis. An ultrasonographically normal-appearing adrenal gland does not preclude disease. Small adrenal glands on ultrasonography, on the other hand, may also be seen. Considerations for small adrenal gland include unilateral adrenal gland atrophy secondary to functional contralateral adrenal tumor, exogenous corticosteroid administration, or hypoadrenocorticism.

Adrenal carcinoma is the most common type of adrenal primary neoplasia and is generally seen unilaterally. Single or multiple nodules can be seen. The majority of adrenal carcinomas measure >10 mm in diameter. The echotexture is usually heterogeneous with small regions of mineralization (Figure 28.7); the echogenicity of these lesions may be hypo- to hyperechoic when compared to the renal cortex. Occasionally, vascular invasion of phrenicoabdominal veins can be seen in 23.5% of dogs with right-sided adrenal gland tumors, given the proximity to the caudal vena cava [12]. If extensive vascular invasion is seen, CT may be helpful for further investigation. Vascular invasion on CT is a

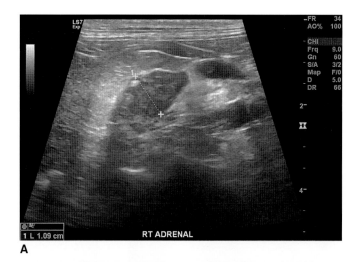

**A**

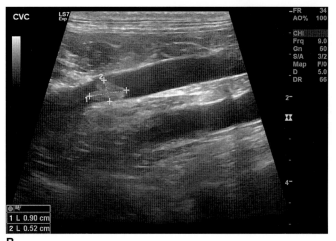

**B**

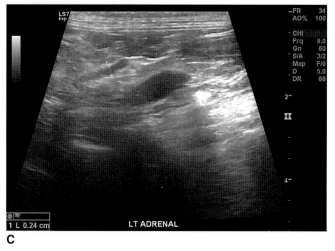

**C**

**FIGURE 28.7** Abdominal ultrasound images of a geriatric dog with a heterogeneous right adrenal gland mass (**A**) with focal intraluminal infiltration into the adjacent caudal vena cava (**B**) and a small left adrenal gland (**C**). Histopathologic diagnosis is consistent with a functional right adrenocortical carcinoma with secondary left adrenal gland atrophy.

hypoattenuating contrast filling defect on the venous phase of contrast.

Pheochromocytoma is the second most frequent primary adrenal gland neoplasia. It is usually large, amorphous, and irregular in margination with loss of internal architecture. Pheochromocytomas are usually >10 mm in diameter. They are variable in echogenicity. Vascular invasion extending into the phrenicoabdominal vein and caudal vena cava (Figure 28.8) can be seen in 40% of dogs diagnosed with pheochromocytoma [12].

Adrenal cortical adenomas are rare adrenal primary neoplasms. They are solitary (Figure 28.9) or exhibit multifocal nodules and can affect both adrenal glands. The echogenicity and echotexture may be heterogeneous. There may be small regions of calcification.

Adrenal adenomatous cortical hyperplasia occurs in approximately 32% of dogs with adrenal gland lesions [12] and are secondary to pituitary disease. Adrenal cortical hyperplasia is smaller and more numerous than adrenocortical adenomas. Hyperplasia of both adrenal glands can be seen in 91% of dogs diagnosed with adrenal cortical hyperplasia and is often more

hypoechoic [12]. The shape and margination of adrenal glands with hyperplasia are unaffected. This lesion usually affects the entire glandular parenchyma of the adrenal gland (Figure 28.9). Hyperplasia can also exhibit focal nodules that range from 3.1 to 10 mm in diameter [12].

Adrenal gland metastatic disease is usually bilaterally affected. There are usually multifocal, heterogeneous nodules, with irregular margins. Neoplasms that metastasize to adrenal glands include splenic hemangiosarcoma and pulmonary carcinoma. Lesions may measure up to 10 mm in diameter.

## Overview of Lymph Nodes

The lymphatic system is a complex system of cellular and vascular components which is responsible for the immune response of the body. The component of the lymphatic system commonly assessed on computed tomography (CT) and ultrasonography are the lymph nodes. Special procedures using positive contrast medium can help assess the lymphatic ducts via

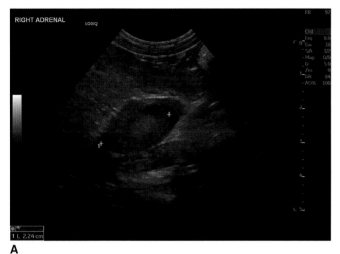

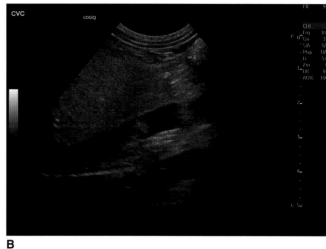

**A**  **B**

**FIGURE 28.8** Abdominal ultrasound images of a geriatric dog with a heterogeneous right adrenal gland mass (**A**) with focal intraluminal infiltration into the adjacent caudal vena cava (**B**). Histopathologic diagnosis is consistent with a right pheochromocytoma.

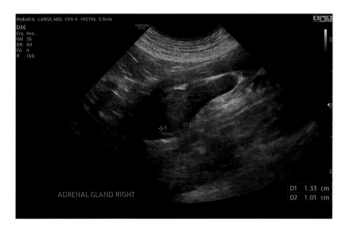

**FIGURE 28.9** Abdominal ultrasound image of a geriatric dog with a well-defined, round, homogeneously hyperechoic nodule (between the calipers) of the cranial aspect of the right adrenal gland. Considerations include adenoma or hyperplasia. No confirmed histopathologic diagnosis was made.

lymphangiogram, which can be imaged on radiography or CT. On survey radiography, lymph nodes are difficult to assess as they are normally small and tend to border efface adjacent soft tissue structures. Anatomical localization of the lymph nodes is essential to understand abnormalities of the lymphatic system.

## Imaging Characteristics of Normal Lymph Nodes

### Head and Cervical Region
Radiographic assessment of the lymph nodes of the skull and cervical region includes the mandibular and medial retropharyngeal lymph nodes, but these are border effaced by the surrounding soft tissue structures. Ultrasonography or CT are better modalities to assess these lymph nodes.

Mandibular lymph nodes form a group of two or three nodes that lie dorsal to the linguofacial vein in the region of the ramus of the mandible, best appreciated on lateral radiographs (Figure 28.10). Afferent lymph vessels to the mandibular lymph nodes come from most parts of the head [1]. On ultrasound (Figure 28.11), the mandibular lymph nodes in dogs and cats are superficial/subcutaneous, oval, and predominantly hypoechoic [13]. Mandibular lymph nodes on ultrasound are considered enlarged with a length >2 cm, width >1.5 cm, and height >0.5 cm [13]. On CT (Figure 28.12), normal mandibular lymph nodes are oval, usually paired into lateral and medial portions, homogeneously soft tissue attenuating, and measure 10–25 mm in length [14].

The medial retropharyngeal lymph node (Figure 28.10) is the largest node found in the head and neck. It lies ventral to the wing of the atlas and dorsal to the pharynx and larynx. Afferent lymph vessels to the medial retropharyngeal lymph nodes come from the deep structures of the head such as the tongue, walls of the oral, nasal, and pharyngeal region, salivary glands, and deep parts of the external ear, larynx, and esophagus [1]. On ultrasonography (Figure 28.13), the medial retropharyngeal lymph nodes are oblong and predominantly isoechoic to the adjacent mandibular salivary glands. Normal medial retropharyngeal lymph nodes can be moderately heterogeneous in echotexture in cats [15]. The size of these lymph nodes is increased with higher body weight and younger age in dogs and decreases in size with increased age [13, 16, 17]. In dogs, medial retropharyngeal lymph nodes are considered enlarged on ultrasound with a length >3 cm, width >2 cm, and height >1 cm [13]. In cats, normal medial retropharyngeal lymph nodes on ultrasound measure 20.7 (L) × 12.4 (W) × 3.7 (H) mm [15].

On CT (Figure 28.14), the medial retropharyngeal lymph node is seen within a fatty triangular space, defined by the wing of the atlas dorsomedially, the mandibular salivary gland ventrolaterally, and the common carotid artery medially. These lymph nodes are homogeneous and irregular in shape or flattened in dogs, bilaterally symmetric, and are mildly heterogeneous in cats [15]. In dogs,

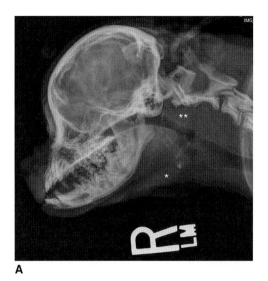

A

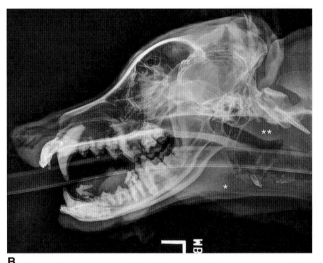

B

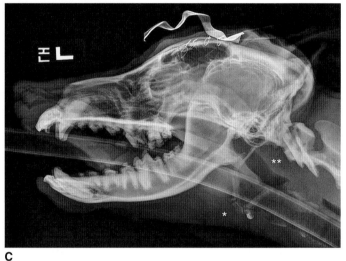

C

**FIGURE 28.10**   Lateral skull radiographs of a normal middle-aged brachycephalic dog (**A**), mesaticephalic dog (**B**), and dolichocephalic dog (**C**); note the regions of the mandibular (*) and medial retropharyngeal (**) lymph nodes.

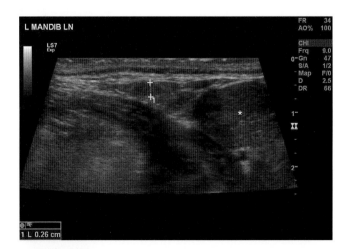

**FIGURE 28.11**   Transverse plane ultrasound image of a normal mandibular lymph node (between the calipers) in a middle-aged dog. Note the lateral location of the mandibular salivary gland (*) in relation to the mandibular lymph node.

normal medial retropharyngeal lymph nodes on CT measure 30–70 (L) × 10 (W) × 5–10 (H) mm [14] or 2.5–5.0 (L) × 1.0–2.0 (W) × 0.5–1.0 (H) cm [16].

In recent studies including 161 presumed normal dogs, the median short-axis transverse diameter of medial retropharyngeal lymph nodes measured 5.2 and 5.4 mm [18]. In cats, normal medial retropharyngeal lymph nodes on CT measured 20.7 (L) × 13.1 (W) × 4.7 (H) mm [15].

**Thorax**   Radiographic assessment of thoracic lymph nodes includes sternal, cranial mediastinal, and bronchial lymph nodes (Figure 28.15). The sternal lymph node is usually a single node on each side in the dog and a single node in the cat. In the dog, there is occasionally only a single medial node. The sternal lymph node is located in the cranioventral aspect of the mediastinum, immediately cranial to the transversus thoracis muscle, and medial to the second costal cartilage or second interchondral space. On lateral radiographs, the sternal

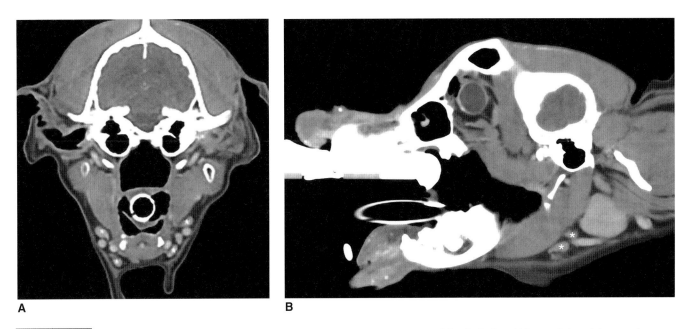

**FIGURE 28.12** Transverse (**A**) and parasagittal (**B**) plane, soft tissue window, CTA images of the skull of a middle-aged dog with normal mandibular lymph nodes (*).

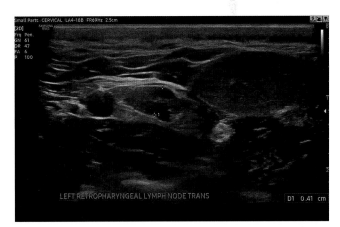

**FIGURE 28.13** Transverse ultrasound image of a normal medial retropharyngeal lymph node (between the calipers) in a dog. Note the mandibular salivary gland ventrolateral to the medial retropharyngeal lymph node and the anechoic external carotid artery adjacent to the medial retropharyngeal lymph node.

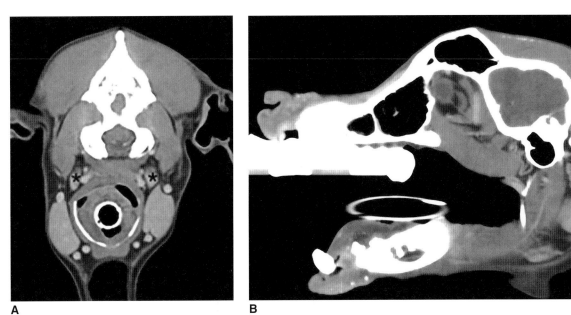

**FIGURE 28.14** Transverse (**A**) and parasagittal (**B**) plane, soft tissue window, CTA images of the skull of a normal middle-aged dog depicting normal medial retropharyngeal lymph nodes (*).

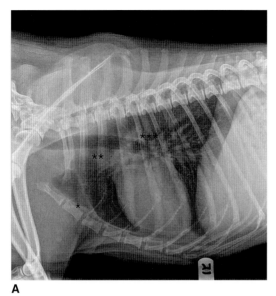

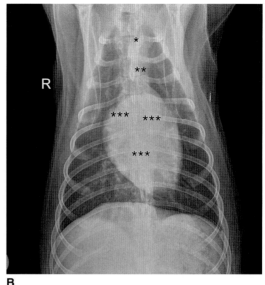

**FIGURE 28.15**    Right lateral (**A**) and ventrodorsal (**B**) thoracic radiographs of a normal middle-aged, medium-sized dog. Note the region of the sternal lymph nodes (*), cranial mediastinal lymph nodes (**), and tracheobronchial lymph nodes (***).

lymph node is located dorsal to the second sternebra in dogs and dorsal to the third sternebra in cats. Additionally, sternal lymph nodes can be evaluated on the ventrodorsal thoracic radiograph, over the cranial mediastinal reflection. The sternal lymph nodes drain a broad region of the thorax and abdomen, such as the ribs, sternum, thoracic and abdominal walls, thymus, abdominal and pelvic cavities, and cranial and caudal thoracic mammary glands [1, 19, 20]. Sternal lymph nodes, like other lymph nodes, are normally oval to round, isoechoic to slightly hypoechoic and can vary in size on ultrasound (Figure 28.16).

No reported normal sternal lymph node size on ultrasound has been reported in the literature. Sternal lymph nodes on CT are similar to those seen on ultrasound, where they are

paired, oval, soft tissue attenuating, homogeneously contrast enhancing, and located dorsal to the second sternebra in dogs (Figure 28.17); normal sternal lymph node size on CT can be measured using the ratio of the short-axis dimension of the sternal lymph nodes to the thickness of the second sternebrae; the mean ratio is 0.457 (95% prediction interval ranging from 0.317 to 0.596), or 3.16 ± 1.09 mm in width and 5.15 ± 1.89 mm in height [21]. In cats, normal sternal lymph node size on CT measures 3.93 ± 0.74 mm [22].

Similar to sternal lymph nodes, cranial mediastinal lymph nodes are also located over the cranial mediastinal reflection on the VD or DV thoracic radiograph and are adjacent to the great vessels of the cranial mediastinum (i.e., cranial vena cava, brachiocephalic trunk, left subclavian artery), and ventral to the trachea. However, on lateral thoracic radiographs, the cranial mediastinal lymph nodes are located within the craniodorsal mediastinum, ventral to the trachea (Figure 28.15). As such, cranial mediastinal lymphadenopathy usually causes dorsal deviation of the trachea on the lateral radiograph and rightward deviation of the trachea on the VD or DV radiograph (Figure 28.18).

Given the superimposition of the cranial mediastinum over the lungs, differentiation of cranial mediastinal and pulmonary masses can be challenging on radiographs, and can be confirmed on thoracic CT [23]. Many lung masses can be distinguished from mediastinal masses because the lung mass is lateral to the mediastinum and is therefore more sharply marginated because of the surrounding air-filled lung. Some mediastinal masses, however, may protrude laterally, or be in a thin portion of the mediastinum, and surrounded by air, making them sharply marginated and easily mistaken for a lung mass.

Cranial mediastinal lymph nodes vary in number. Afferent cranial mediastinal lymph vessels come from the muscles and bones of the neck, thorax, abdomen, peritoneal cavity, thyroid

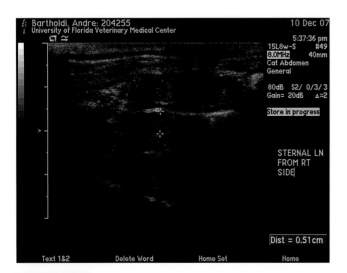

**FIGURE 28.16**    Sagittal ultrasound image of a normal sternal lymph node (between the calipers) in a geriatric cat. The sternal lymph node is isoechoic to the regional cranial mediastinal fat.

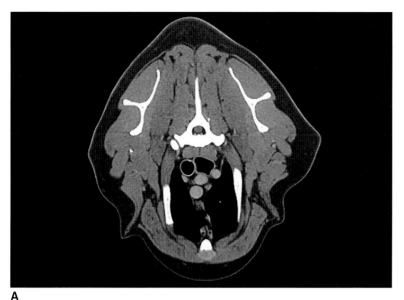
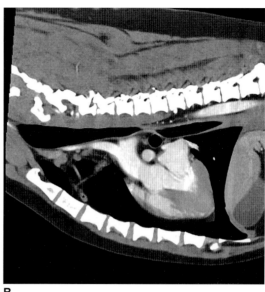

**FIGURE 28.17**  Transverse (**A**) and parasagittal (**B**) plane, soft tissue window CTA images of the thorax of a normal middle-aged dog depicting bilaterally symmetric, soft tissue-attenuating, homogeneously contrast-enhancing, paired sternal lymph nodes (*) within the ventral aspect of the cranial mediastinum, dorsal to the second sternebral segment.

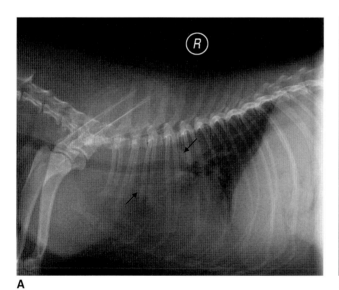
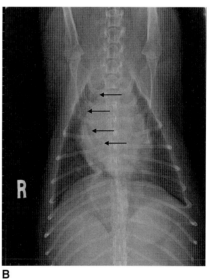

**FIGURE 28.18**  Right lateral (**A**) and ventrodorsal (**B**) radiographs of a geriatric dog with round cell neoplasm of the cranial mediastinum. There is a large, poorly defined soft tissue mass effect of the cranial mediastinum, causing an ill-defined soft tissue mass effect (arrows) on the lateral radiograph and severe rightward displacement of the trachea (arrows) on the ventrodorsal radiograph.

lobes, cranial and middle mediastinal contents (i.e., trachea, esophagus, thymus, mediastinum, heart, and aorta) [1]. Normal cranial mediastinal lymph nodes are difficult to assess on ultrasonography due to reverberation artifact from aerated lung. Normal cranial mediastinal lymph nodes on CT are typically round but can be fusiform, homogeneous, and vary in measurement, depending on the size of the dog or cat (Figure 28.19). Size can be as large as 10 mm for large dogs but usually ranges from 1 to 3 mm in diameter or, more specifically, 3.16 ± 1.09 mm in width and 4.51 ± 1.66 mm in height [24]. In cats, normal cranial mediastinal lymph node size on CT measures 4.02 ± 0.65 mm in width [22].

Lastly, the bronchial lymph nodes are split into two main groups: tracheobronchial and pulmonary. The pulmonary group is often absent. The tracheobronchial lymph nodes are further split into three parts: right, left, and middle (Figure 28.20). The middle tracheobronchial lymph node is the largest of the group when compared to the left and right tracheobronchial lymph nodes. The middle tracheobronchial lymph node lies between the tracheal bifurcation, slightly dorsal to the caudal aspect of the trachea and carina. The left and right tracheobronchial lymph nodes lie to the left and right side of the carina, respectively, best assessed on the VD or DV radiograph. The afferent bronchial lymph vessels come from the bronchi, lungs, cranial

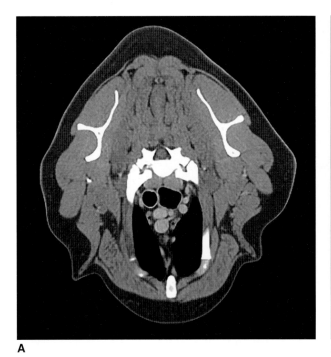 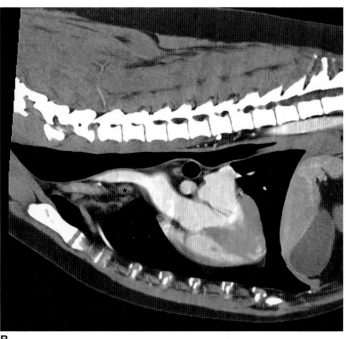

**A**                                    **B**

**FIGURE 28.19** Transverse (**A**) and parasagittal (**B**) plane, soft tissue window, CTA images of the thorax of a normal middle-aged dog depicting a normal, fusiform, soft tissue-attenuating, homogeneously contrast enhancing, cranial mediastinal lymph node (\*) within the dorsal aspect of the cranial mediastinum.

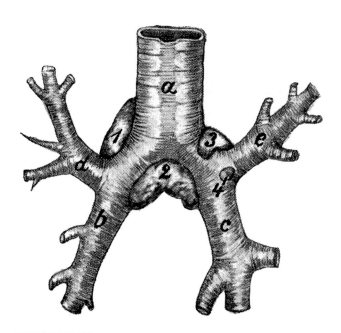

**FIGURE 28.20** Anatomy of bronchial lymph nodes. End of the trachea *a*; left *b* and right *c* main bronchus; left *d* and right *e* cranial bronchus. Left tracheobronchial lymph node *1*; middle tracheobronchial lymph node *2*; right tracheobronchial lymph node *3*; pulmonary lymph node *4*. Source: Dr Hermann Baum (1918). (This work is in the public domain).

mediastinal and middle mediastinal contents (i.e., aorta, esophagus, trachea, heart), and diaphragm [1].

On CT (Figure 28.21), normal left and right tracheobronchial lymph nodes are round and middle tracheobronchial lymph nodes are fusiform and all are homogeneous; the right tracheobronchial lymph node is not always detected on CT, possibly due to overlying vasculature (i.e., azygous vein and caudal vena cava) [24]. The average measurement of normal canine tracheobronchial lymph nodes is 3.17±0.95 mm width of the left, 3.00±1.02 mm width of the right, and 3.06±1.05 mm width of the middle [24]. In cats, normal tracheobronchial lymph nodes on CT measure 3.51±0.62 mm [22].

**Abdomen**   Jejunal lymph nodes are the largest lymph nodes of the abdomen. They are composed of two, or more, and are present along either side of the mesenteric vasculature in the midabdomen. The afferent lymph vessels to the jejunal lymph nodes come from the jejunum, ileum, and pancreas [1].

On abdominal radiographs, mesenteric lymph nodes are difficult to assess as they are soft tissue opaque and are border effaced by intestines and intestinal contents. Mesenteric lymph nodes, specifically jejunal lymph nodes, are best assessed on abdominal ultrasonography. On abdominal ultrasound, jejunal lymph nodes in dogs (Figure 28.22) are slightly lobular, usually mildly hypoechoic but sometimes isoechoic to the mesenteric fat, homogeneous in echogenicity, and with a maximum thickness of 3.9 mm (range 1.6–8.2 mm) and a medial maximum width of 7.5 mm (range 2.6–14.7 mm) [25]. In younger dogs (<6 years of age), the normal jejunal lymph nodes can be heterogeneous in echogenicity (Figure 28.23) [25].

In normal cats, jejunal lymph nodes are located adjacent to the cranial mesenteric artery and origin of the jejunal arteries

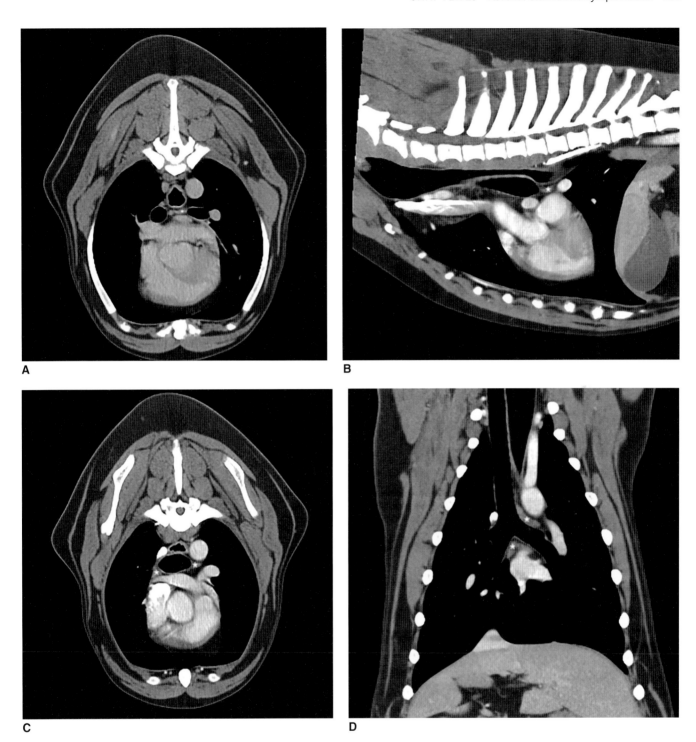

**FIGURE 28.21** Transverse (**A**) and sagittal (**B**) plane, soft tissue window CTA images of the thorax of a normal dog centered over a normal middle tracheobronchial lymph node (*). Transverse (**C**) plane image of the same dog centered over the normal left and right tracheobronchial lymph nodes (*). Dorsal (**D**) plane image of the same dog centered over the normal left and middle tracheobronchial lymph nodes (*).

at the root of the mesentery. Some jejunal lymph nodes can be found along the jejunal vessels in the more distal part of the mesentery, near the jejunum and ileum. On ultrasound, normal jejunal lymph nodes in cats measure 20.1 (11.4–39.0) mm in length and 5.0 (2.8–7.2) mm in diameter, and are hypoechoic, homogeneous, and elongated [26]. The jejunal lymph nodes are usually reactive and enlarged in young dogs and cats up to 1 year of age [2, 3, 27].

On abdominal CT (Figure 28.24), jejunal lymph nodes in dogs and cats are located along the cranial mesenteric artery and vein, and appear elongated, occasionally bilobar, rounded, measuring approximately 42.0 (range 24.0–65.0) mm in length, 9.6 (range 5.0–15.0) mm in width, and 7.1 (range 4.0–12.3) mm in height [28]. On abdominal CT, jejunal lymph nodes in normal cats are fusiform, predominantly homogeneously contrast enhancing, and measure 1.7 (0.3–4.8) cm in length and 0.5 (0.2–1.0) cm in width [29].

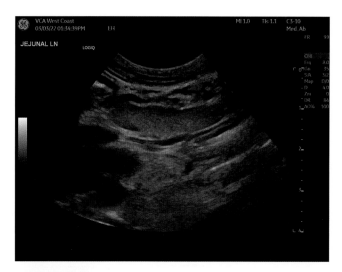

**FIGURE 28.22** Sagittal plane abdominal ultrasound image of a normal jejunal lymph node in a 1-year-old dog. Note the slight lobular margins, peripheral hypoechogenicity, and central isoechogenicity to the mesenteric fat.

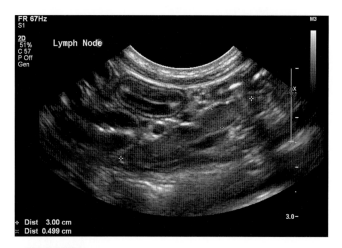

**FIGURE 28.23** Sagittal plane abdominal ultrasound image of a normal jejunal lymph node in a 5-month-old dog. Note the lobular margins and mild heterogeneity.

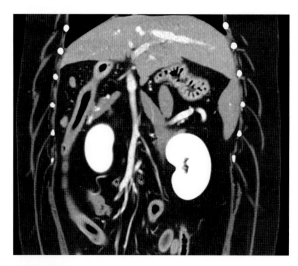

**FIGURE 28.24** Dorsal plane, soft tissue window abdominal CTA image of a dog with normal jejunal lymph nodes (*) located on either side of the mesenteric vasculature in the midabdomen.

In some cats, the left colic lymph nodes (also known as the caudal mesenteric lymph nodes) can be seen on abdominal radiographs and are located dorsal to the mid to caudal aspect of the descending colon, superimposed over the ventral retroperitoneal fat (Figure 28.25). The left colic lymph nodes lie in the caudal part of the descending mesocolon near the pelvic inlet and descending colon. The afferent lymph vessels come from the ileum, cecum, and colon [1].

No published normal left colic lymph nodes measurements have been made on radiographs, but presumed normal left colic lymph nodes in cats are suggested to measure $5.5 \pm 1.7$ mm in height and $10.3 \pm 3.0$ mm in length on lateral radiographs and $6.9 \pm 2.6$ mm in width and $10.1 \pm 3.5$ mm in length on the VD radiograph [30]. In cats, the normal left colic lymph node on ultrasound measures 6.0 mm in length and 2.1 mm in diameter. On CT (Figure 28.26), the left colic lymph nodes in normal dogs are located dorsal to dorsomedial to the descending colon at the level of the trifurcation of the aorta and are usually rounded and measure 8.8 (range 4.5–14.0) mm in length, 6.1 (range 3.8–9.6) mm in width, and 4.5 (range 2.0–6.4) mm in height [28]. On CT, normal left colic lymph nodes in cats are predominantly round, homogeneously contrast enhancing, and measure 0.8 (range 0.1–2.0) cm in length and 0.4 (range 0.1–1.0) cm in width [29].

The iliosacral lymphocenter or sublumbar lymph node is made up of the medial iliac, internal iliac, and sacral lymph nodes. Radiographically, they are located within the caudodorsal retroperitoneal space, ventral to the fifth or sixth lumbar vertebrae (Figure 28.27) [31]. The medial iliac lymph nodes receive afferent lymph vessels from the skin of the dorsal abdominal wall caudal to the last rib, the skin around the pelvis (particularly the anal sacs), base of the tail, thigh, stifle, abdominal and pelvic limb muscles, lumbar muscles, caudal abdominal and intrapelvic intestinal segments (i.e., colon,

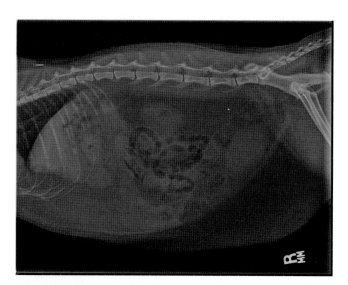

**FIGURE 28.25** Right lateral abdominal radiograph of a normal male cat. Note the fusiform to tubular-shaped soft tissue opacity dorsal to the caudal aspect of the descending colon, superimposed over the retroperitoneal space (asterisk). This soft tissue opacity represents a normal left colic lymph node.

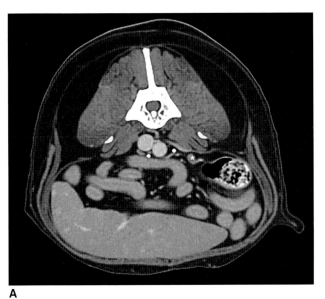

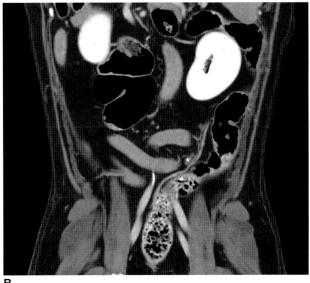

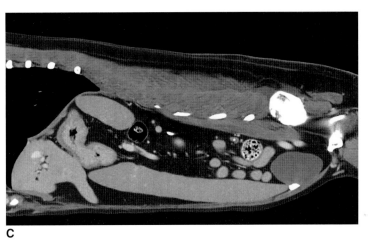

**FIGURE 28.26** Transverse (**A**), dorsal (**B**), and sagittal (**C**) plane, soft tissue window, CTA images of a dog with a normal left colic lymph node (*) located dorsomedial to the descending colon.

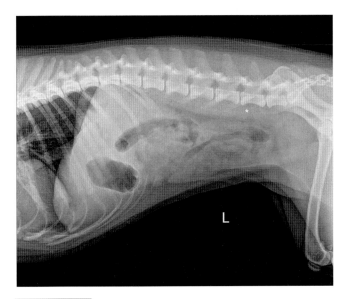

**FIGURE 28.27** Left lateral abdominal radiograph of a normal middle-aged dog. The region of the medial iliac lymph nodes (*) is located ventral to the fifth and sixth lumbar vertebrae.

rectum, anus), caudal reproductive tract (i.e., vagina, vulva, testis, prostate), and caudal urinary tract (i.e., ureter, urinary bladder, urethra) [1].

On abdominal ultrasound (Figure 28.28), normal left and right medial iliac lymph nodes in dogs are found lateral to the aorta and lateral to the caudal vena cava, respectively, at the birfurcation/trifurcation. Medial iliac nodes should be evaluated cautiously for enlargement because their dimensions vary with body size and weight. The medial iliac lymph nodes are isoechoic to hypoechoic to the region fat, fusiform in shape, and measure 1.6±0.5 cm in length, 0.6±0.1 cm in width, and 0.5±0.2 cm in height [32]; other reported measurements for normal right and left medial iliac lymph nodes are 2.22±0.69 cm length, 0.46±0.20 cm height, and 0.61±0.25 cm width and 2.13±0.82 cm length, 0.48±0.18 cm height, and 0.59±0.19 cm width, respectively [33]. If body size and weight are taken into consideration, the mean width of normal left and right nodes is 0.43 and 0.45 cm in small dogs, 0.64 and 0.63 cm in medium-sized dogs, and 0.7 and 0.75 cm in large dogs, respectively.

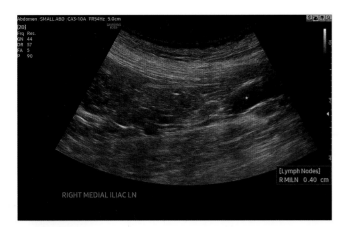

**FIGURE 28.28** Sagittal ultrasound image of a normal right medial iliac lymph node in a dog (between the calipers). Note the lymph node is isoechoic to the surrounding fat. The anechoic tubular structure caudal to this lymph node represents the right external iliac artery (*), branching from the trifurcation of the aorta.

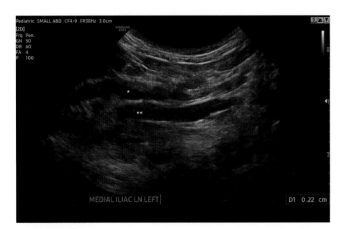

**FIGURE 28.29** Sagittal ultrasound image of a normal left medial iliac lymph node in a dog (between the calipers). Note the lymph node is isoechoic to the surrounding fat. The two anechoic tubular structures ventral to this lymph node are the aorta (*) and caudal vena cava (**).

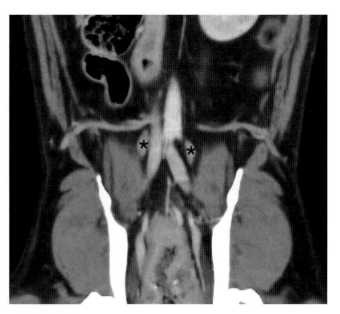

**FIGURE 28.30** Dorsal plane, soft tissue window, CTA image depicting normal left and right medial iliac lymph nodes (*) lateral to the trifurcation, caudal to the deep circumflex iliac vessels.

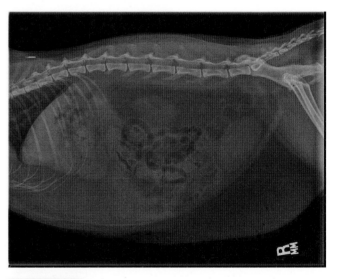

**FIGURE 28.31** Right lateral abdominal radiograph of a normal middle-aged cat. Note the large body habitus with increased subcutaneous fat deposition. In the inguinal region, the inguinal lymph nodes (*) are faintly soft tissue opaque, fusiform, and lobular.

With regard to assessing metastatic medial iliac lymph nodes from anal sac carcinoma, ultrasound identifies more abnormal lymph nodes than abdominal CT [32]. On abdominal ultrasound, the medial iliac lymph nodes in normal cats are infrequently identified (20% of the time) [26]; if seen, they normally measure 13.5 (5.0–23.3) mm in length and 4.5 (1.3–14.0) mm in diameter (Figure 28.29) [26]. On CT, the medial iliac lymph nodes in dogs are located at the level of and/or caudal to the trifurcation of the aorta (Figure 28.30), ventral to L6 and/or L7, immediately caudal to the deep circumflex iliac vessels. These lymph nodes are fusiform in shape and measure 1.4±0.5 cm in length, 0.6±0.2 cm in height, and 0.6±0.2 cm in width [32]. On CT, the medial iliac lymph nodes in normal cats are fusiform in shape, homogeneously contrast enhancing, and measure 1.3 (0.5–2.5) cm in length and 0.4 (0.2–0.9) cm in width [29].

Occasionally, superficial abdominal lymph nodes such as the superficial inguinal lymph nodes can be assessed

radiographically; superficial inguinal lymph nodes are increased in conspicuity in most cats due to the increased volume of fat in the inguinal region (Figure 28.31). These lymph nodes are anatomically located within the subcutaneous tissues of the caudoventral abdominal body wall and medial surface of the thighs. The afferent vessels to the superficial inguinal lymph nodes come from the ventral half of the abdominal wall, including the mammary glands as well as the prepuce and scrotum [1], if present. Other afferent vessels come from the ventral pelvis, tail, and medial aspect of the thigh, stifle joint, and crus [1].

No published normal superficial inguinal lymph nodes have been measured. However, presumed normal superficial

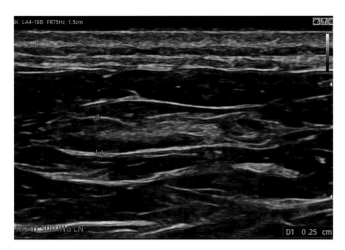

**FIGURE 28.32**   Sagittal ultrasound image of a normal right superficial inguinal lymph node (between the calipers) in a young dog. The superficial inguinal lymph node is isoechoic to the regional subcutaneous fat.

inguinal lymph nodes in cats have been suggested, measuring 5.0 ± 1.5 mm in height and 9.8 ± 3.3 mm in length on the lateral radiograph and 4.3 ± 1.0 mm in width and 10.5 ± 3.4 mm in length on the VD radiograph [30].

On ultrasound, normal superficial inguinal lymph nodes (Figure 28.32) in dogs are hypoechoic to isoechoic to the surrounding tissues, have a corticomedullary or homogeneous echotexture, smooth, clearly defined margins, and fusiform shape; these lymph nodes have a short- to long-axis radiograph <0.5 [33]. On abdominal ultrasound, superficial inguinal lymph nodes in normal cats are homogeneous, with well-defined margins and hilar vascularization, are oval in shape and predominantly hypoechoic [34]; no ultrasonographic normal sizes of superficial inguinal lymph nodes in cats have been reported and are based predominantly on subjective assessment.

There is currently no reported normal superficial inguinal lymph node size in dogs on CT as size criteria have variable efficacy on CT [35]. On CT (Figure 28.33), superficial inguinal lymph nodes in normal cats are fusiform in shape, homogeneously contrast enhancing, and measure 0.9 (0.2–2.0) cm in length and 0.4 (0.1–0.8) cm in width [29].

## Lymphangiogram

Positive-contrast studies of the lymphatic system, including lymphography and lymphangiography, can be used. Lymphography may be used to determine the causes of lymphedema and assess the thoracic duct in dogs and cats with chylothorax. Primary congenital lymphedema (Figure 28.34) has been described in puppies and is due to a dysplasia of vessels and/or nodes. The more common localized form involves one or both distal pelvic limbs; in the less common generalized form, the nose, pinnae, and vulva may also be affected. Tortuosity and dilation of local lymphatics are usually seen and draining lymph nodes are usually absent or small. Causes of lymphedema may also be due to lymphangiosarcoma.

Lymphangiogram is performed to visualize the thoracic duct anatomy, to define location and character of chyle leakage, and to perioperatively plan for thoracic duct ligation. Several methods of performing lymphangiography exist. The more commonly performed method is injecting positive-contrast medium directly into the left and/or right popliteal lymph node(s) [36]. Another method is to inject positive-contrast medium into a mesenteric lymph node [37, 38]. A third method involves injecting positive-contrast medium via the intrametatarsal pad if popliteal and/or mesenteric lymph nodes are difficult to visualize [34]. A fourth and uncommon method is injecting positive-contrast medium subcutaneously in the rectal, vaginal, or perianal tissues [39, 40].

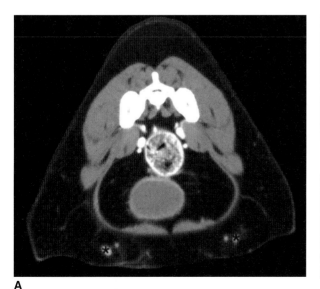

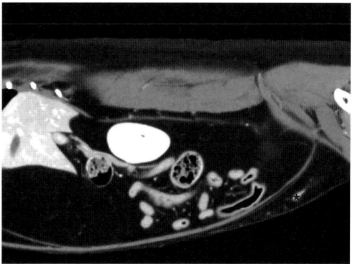

A                                                                 B

**FIGURE 28.33**   Transverse (**A**) and sagittal (**B**) plane, soft tissue window CTA images of a cat with normal, fusiform-shaped, contrast-enhancing inguinal lymph nodes (*).

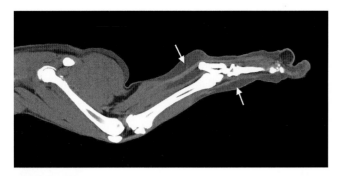

**FIGURE 28.34** Parasagittal plane, soft tissue window, CT image of a 4-month-old golden retriever with pelvic limb lymphedema secondary to popliteal lymph node agenesis; note the increased subcutaneous and deep fascial fluid (arrows) of the crus through pes.

To perform lymphangiography via injection of a lymph node, nonionic iodinated contrast medium is injected directly into a popliteal lymph node or mesenteric lymph node using ultrasound guidance (1 mL/kg of bodyweight) at a rate of 2 mL/min [36]. Thoracic CT or radiography is performed after the thoracic duct is opacified. In some instances, if the popliteal lymph node is used for lymphangiogram, massage of the region of the lymph node to encourage reabsorption of the contrast medium into the lymphatics is recommended if extravasation of contrast is suspected or confirmed. Occasionally, repeated CT or radiographs may be needed if the thoracic duct is not opacified. Thoracic CT is preferred and considered the gold standard over radiography as CT provides multiplanar images,

small tributaries can be identified, and there is no superimposition of regional anatomical structures.

The normal lymphangiogram reveals one or more thoracic duct branches coursing adjacent to the thoracic aorta and entering the cranial vena cava; the thoracic duct is more commonly seen along the right side of the thoracic aorta and less commonly on the left side. Near this junction, a variable number of smaller lymphatic branches are seen that connect with the cranial mediastinal lymph nodes.

To perform lymphangiography using metatarsal pads, nonionic iodinated contrast medium is injected simultaneously by two people into both metatarsal pads. After aseptic preparation, the positive-contrast medium is injected into the adipose tissue at a 45° angle to the surface, at 1 cm depth, using a 22 gauge needle. The injection is completed within 15–30 seconds and followed by massage of the metatarsal pads, legs, tarsal regions, and thighs for 3–4 minutes. A CT is performed 5 minutes after initiating the intrametatarsal pad injection. If the contrast medium fails to opacify, an additional CT scan is performed 5 minutes afterwards. If continued failure of thoracic duct opacification occurs around 30–40 minutes, scanning should be discontinued. As for the intranodal method, a dose of 1 mL/kg body weight of positive-contrast medium is used [41].

In patients with thoracic duct injury or obstruction, extravasated contrast medium may be seen dispersing within the mediastinum and/or pleural space (Figure 28.35). Proliferation of many small lymphatic vessels in the cranial mediastinum is indicative of lymphangiectasia from lymphatic flow

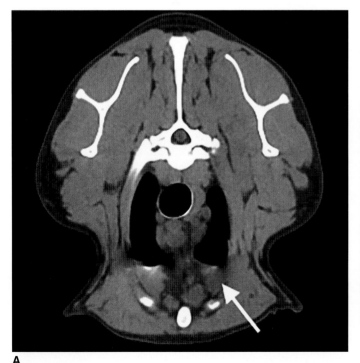 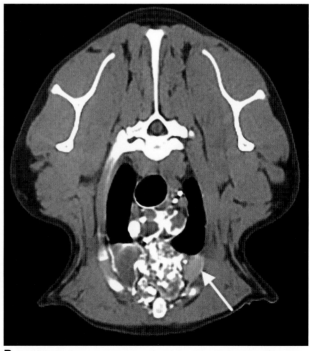

**A**  **B**

**FIGURE 28.35** Transverse plane, soft tissue window, CT images before (**A**) and after (**B**) lymphangiogram in a middle-aged dog diagnosed with chylothorax. Note the numerous, small, tortuous lymphatic vessels in the cranial mediastinum. There is contrast extravasation into the pleural space, best noted in the left pleural space (arrow).

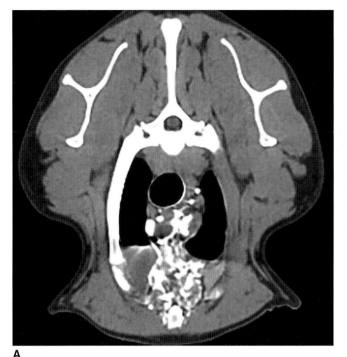

**A**

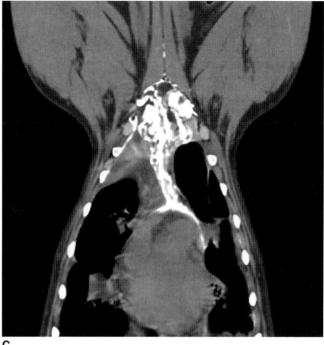

**C**

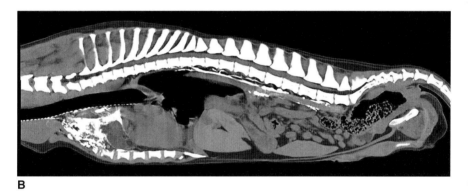

**B**

**FIGURE 28.36**   Transverse (**A**), sagittal (**B**), and dorsal (**C**) plane, soft tissue window, CT images after a lymphangiogram has been performed in a middle-aged dog diagnosed with chylothorax. Note the numerous, small, tortuous lymphatic vessels in the cranial mediastinum.

obstruction (Figure 28.36). The transverse view of the thoracic duct on CT images provides a means of accurately determining the number of parallel branches and their location relative to the aorta in anticipation of surgical ligation.

## Imaging Characteristics of Abnormalities of Lymph Nodes

**Head and Cervical Region**   On lateral cervical radiographs, severe mandibular lymphadenopathy causes a poorly defined soft tissue mass effect ventral to the ramus of the mandible (Figure 28.37). Differentials for this effect include reactive lymphadenopathy, multicentric neoplasia, metastatic mandibular lymphadenopathy, sialocele, sialoadenitis, hemorrhage, edema, abscess, lymphadenitis, or granuloma. On radiographs, severe medial retropharyngeal lymphadenopathy causes a soft tissue mass effect dorsal to the gas-filled pharyngeal region and

ventral to the C1 and C2 vertebrae (Figure 28.38). Other soft tissue changes, including abscesses, of this region may appear similar to medial retropharyngeal lymphadenopathy on radiographs (Figure 28.39). Differentials for soft tissue mass effects of the medial retropharyngeal region include masses associated with the thyroid, vasculature, vertebral or paravertebral structures, esophagus, or trachea.

Ultrasonography and CT are the preferred imaging modalities to assess mandibular and medial retropharyngeal lymph nodes and any mass effect that may be seen on cervical radiographs. Differentiating between metastatic disease and reactive lymphadenopathy, however, is difficult on ultrasound and CT, so cytology or histology is the gold standard.

Reactive lymph nodes are often enlarged to a variable degree and appear homogeneously hypoechoic on ultrasound (Figure 28.40). Loss of definition of the affected lymph node margins is also a common finding and is thought to be caused by edema and cellulitis in those instances in which a regional extranodal inflammatory response is present [43].

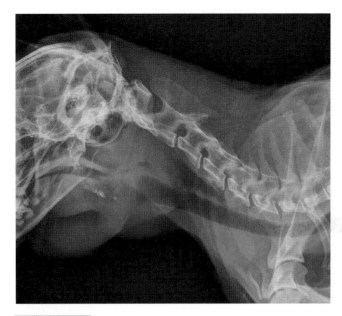

**FIGURE 28.37** Right lateral laryngeal region radiographs of a geriatric cat. There is a large, poorly defined soft tissue mass effect of the ventral cervical and mandibular region as well as the retropharyngeal region ventral to C1–C2, representing mandibular and medial retropharyngeal lymphadenopathy. This cat was diagnosed with mandibular and medial retropharyngeal lymphoma.

Central cavitation of abscessed lymph nodes may also occur and should be differentiated from necrosis and hemorrhage from metastatic lymph nodes from rapid tumor growth causing mixed echogenicity [43–45]. Metastatic mandibular lymphadenopathy is mostly seen ipsilaterally but can be seen contralaterally [46]. On ultrasound, metastatic lymphadenopathy is usually severely enlarged (Figure 28.41).

Similar to ultrasound, the imaging characteristics of reactive and metastatic lymphadenopathy on CT overlap. Reactive lymph

nodes on CT are usually enlarged and rounded with variable contrast enhancement (Figure 28.42). Medial retropharyngeal lymph nodes suggestive of metastatic disease from nasal tumors in cats include lymph node enlargement [47], abnormal lymph node hilus [42], lymph node height asymmetry [42], contrast enhancement [47], and decreased lymph node precontrast heterogeneity (Figure 28.43) [42]. In recent literature, using CT to diagnose metastasis from oral and nasal neoplasia with 12.5% sensitivity, 91.1% specificity, 67.5% accuracy has been reported [48]. MRI can be used to evaluate and differentiate inflammatory and neoplastic medial retropharyngeal lymph nodes in dogs and cats [49, 50].

**Thorax** The sternal lymph nodes drain the cranial abdomen, diaphragm, parietal pleura, ventral and lateral body wall, and, variably, the cranial mammary glands [20, 51, 52]. One might assume that sternal lymph node enlargement is a sign of intrathoracic disease, but it is often secondary to abdominal disease such as abdominal fluid, peritonitis, peritoneal effusion, and neoplastic conditions of the liver, pancreas, duodenum, stomach, spleen (i.e., hemangiosarcoma) [53], and regional lymph nodes.

Neoplastic disease is the most prevalent condition seen in dogs and cats with sternal lymphadenopathy, followed by inflammatory diseases [54]. The most common etiology of sternal lymphadenopathy in dogs and cats is lymphoma [54]. On thoracic radiographs, enlarged sternal lymph nodes are seen as a broad-based soft tissue opacity dorsal to the second sternebra in dogs and dorsal to the third sternebra in cats (Figure 28.44) on lateral radiographs. Sternal lymphadenopathy can occasionally be seen on the VD and DV radiograph as focal mediastinal widening. A mildly enlarged sternal lymph node can appear slightly different in size and shape in the left and right lateral view due to the different orientations with respect to the primary x-ray beam.

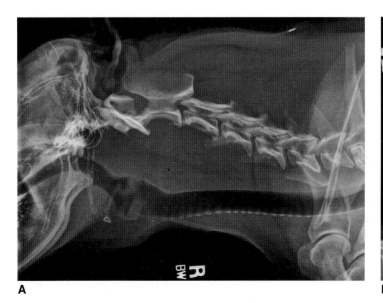

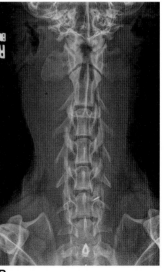

**FIGURE 28.38** Right lateral (**A**) and ventrodorsal (**B**) cervical radiographs of a middle-aged dog with a poorly defined mass effect (*) in the right retropharyngeal region, causing ventral deviation of the gas-filled pharynx. This dog was diagnosed with severe reactive medial retropharyngeal lymphadenopathy.

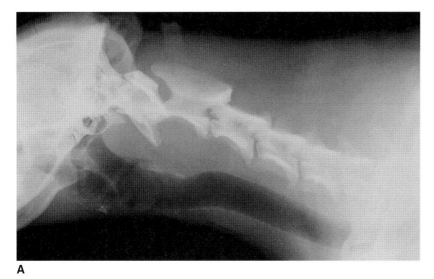 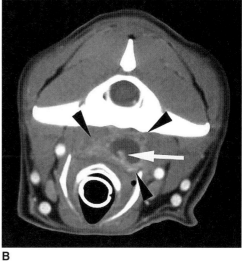

A

B

**FIGURE 28.39** Right lateral cervical radiograph (**A**) of a 3-year-old German shepherd dog with a fusiform soft tissue opaque mass effect of the medial retropharyngeal region; note the focal narrowing of the pharynx and larynx. Transverse plane in soft tissue window after intravenous contrast medium administration of the same dog (**B**) at the level of the retropharyngeal mass effect depicting a rim-enhancing (black arrowheads) abscess with a soft tissue-attenuating retropharyngeal foreign body (white arrow). Source: Courtesy of Dr Elizabeth Huynh (co-author).

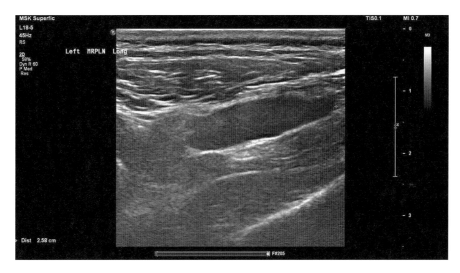

**FIGURE 28.40** Sagittal plane ultrasound image of a mildly enlarged, hypoechoic, reactive lymph node in a middle-aged dog, confirmed with cytology.

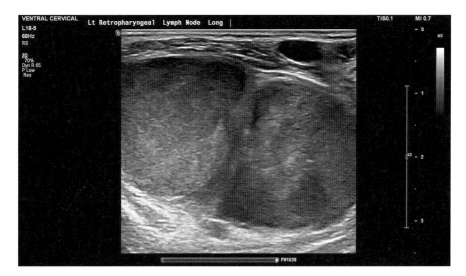

**FIGURE 28.41** Sagittal plane ultrasound image of a severely enlarged, rounded, heterogeneous metastatic lymph node secondary to mast cell tumor in a geriatric dog, confirmed with cytology.

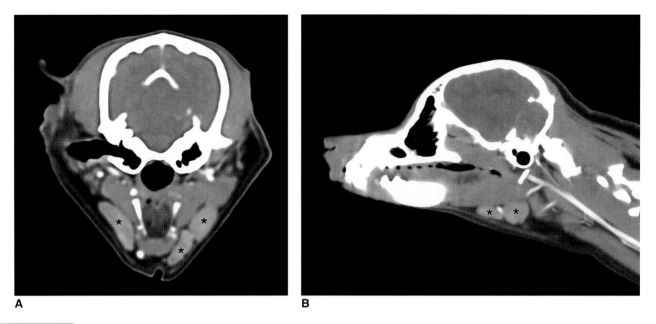

**FIGURE 28.42** Transverse (**A**) and parasagittal (**B**) plane, soft tissue window, CTA images of a young dog with enlarged, rounded, homogeneously contrast-enhancing hyperplastic mandibular lymph nodes (*) confirmed on cytology.

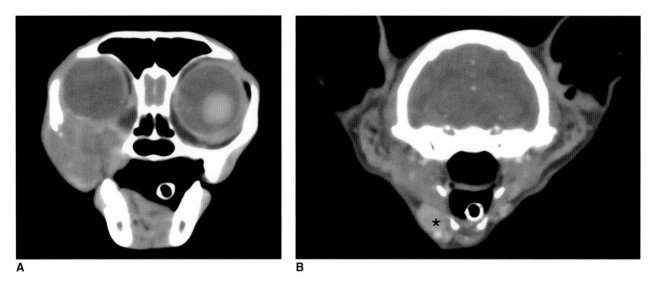

**FIGURE 28.43** Transverse, soft tissue window, CTA images (**A**) centered over a large, aggressive left oral squamous cell carcinoma and (**B**) centered over a large, metastatic, left mandibular lymph node (*) in a geriatric cat.

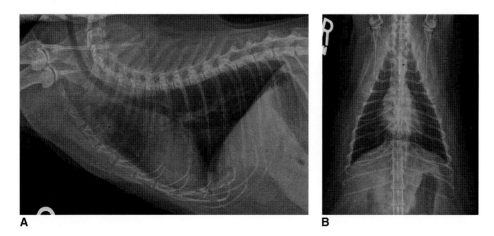

**FIGURE 28.44** Right lateral (**A**) and VD (**B**) thoracic radiographs of a geriatric cat diagnosed with sternal lymphadenopathy secondary to lymphoma. Note the well-defined, lobular, soft tissue mass (*) in the ventral aspect of the cranial mediastinum, dorsal to the third sternebral segment. On the VD projection, this mass causes focal widening of the cranial mediastinal reflection, partially superimposed over the vertebrae.

Sternal lymph nodes can be further assessed using ultrasound and CT although there may an overlap between the appearances of normal, reactive, and metastatic lymph nodes. Reactive sternal lymph nodes may appear enlarged and hypoechoic on ultrasound (Figure 28.45). Malignant lymph

nodes on ultrasound would be enlarged with a short axis >1.73 cm (superficial lymph nodes) [55], hypoechogenicity [56], heterogeneity [57], peripheral or mixed Doppler pattern [55], increased number of vessels [58], and hyperechoic perinodal fat (as seen with lymphoma) [59]. Sternal lymphadenopathy on CT may cause enlargement, variable degrees of contrast enhancement, and heterogeneity (Figure 28.46).

Cranial mediastinal lymphadenopathy also causes cranial mediastinal widening on VD or DV thoracic radiographs. On lateral radiographs, cranial mediastinal lymphadenopathy causes a soft tissue mass effect in the dorsal aspect of the cranial mediastinum, ventral to the trachea and cranial to the cardiac silhouette (Figure 28.47), occasionally dorsally deviating the trachea. In young dogs, the thymus can cause a cranial mediastinal mass effect. The thymus should involute and be inconspicuous in most dogs by 1 year of age. Differentials for cranial mediastinal widening include reactive lymphadenopathy, metastatic disease, thymoma, lymphoma, thymic lymphoma, ectopic thyroid carcinoma, heart base neoplasm, or branchial cyst in cats.

Occasionally, cranial mediastinal lymphadenopathy can be mistaken for cranial pulmonary masses and vice versa [23]. Thoracic CT can be used to differentiate pulmonary masses

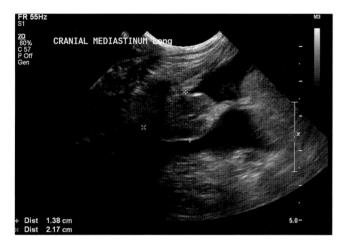

**FIGURE 28.45**  Sagittal plane ultrasound image of a reactive sternal lymph node (between the calipers) in a middle-aged dog diagnosed with anechoic pleural effusion secondary to chylothorax.

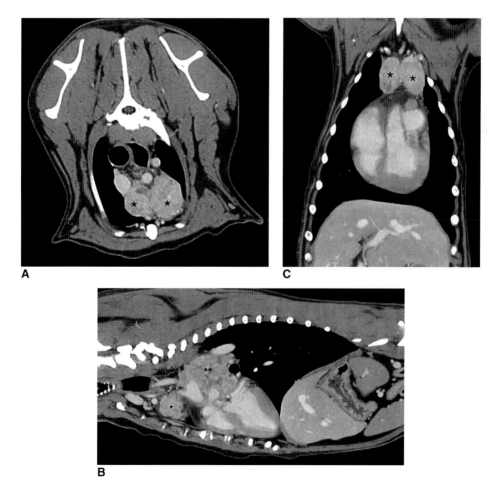

**FIGURE 28.46**  Transverse (**A**), sagittal (**B**), and dorsal (**C**) plane, soft tissue window, CTA images of a geriatric dog with a heart base neoplasm (**\*\***) and enlarged, heterogeneously contrast-enhancing metastatic sternal lymphadenopathy (**\***).

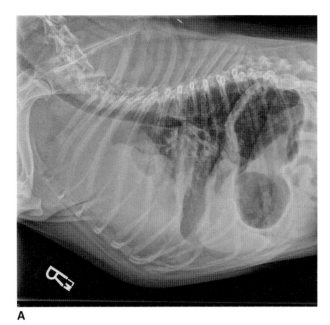 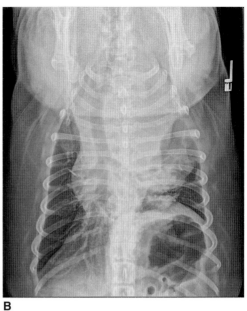

**A**  **B**

**FIGURE 28.47** Right lateral (**A**) and DV (**B**) radiographs of a geriatric dog with cranial mediastinal lymphoma, further characterized by a large, lobular, poorly distinguished, soft tissue mass in the cranial mediastinum, causing caudal displacement of the lungs and cranial mediastinal widening on the DV radiograph.

from cranial mediastinal masses, further characterize the extent of a cranial mediastinal mass, and determine the CT character of a mass to prioritize the differentials. The most common cranial mediastinal masses are lymphoma and thymic epithelial tumors in dogs and cats. In dogs, cranial mediastinal masses with at least two well-defined radiographic margins on a lateral radiograph and causing a rightward shift of the cardiac silhouette on VD or DV radiograph are significantly more likely to be thymic epithelial tumors (Figure 28.48) than lymphoma [60]. On ultrasound (Figure 28.49), mediastinal masses occupy the cranial mediastinum, caudally displacing the lungs, increasing the conspicuity of the mediastinum and mediastinal contents. On CT, mediastinal lymphoma in dogs is more homogeneous and more likely to envelop the cranial vena cava (Figure 28.50) whereas thymic epithelial neoplasms tend to occur in older dogs and are more heterogeneous [61].

The tracheobronchial lymphadenopathy on thoracic radiographs causes a poorly defined soft tissue opaque mass effect, displacing the regional anatomy. Middle tracheobronchial lymphadenopathy produces a soft tissue mass effect dorsal to the carina, causing ventral deviation of the caudal trachea and carina on the lateral radiographs and lateral deviation of the caudal principal bronchi on the VD or DV radiograph (Figure 28.51). Differentials for a poorly defined soft tissue mass effect dorsal to the carina on lateral radiograph include an esophageal foreign body or esophageal mass; a differential for lateral deviation of the caudal principal bronchi on VD or DV radiographs is left atrial enlargement. Therefore, orthogonal radiographs of the thorax are essential to diagnosing tracheobronchial lymphadenopathy.

Tracheobronchial lymphadenopathy is commonly associated with lymphoma (Figure 28.52) and disseminated fungal infection (i.e., coccidioidomycosis and blastomycosis) (Figure 28.53). Of the 110 dogs in a study to establish the cause of tracheobronchial lymphadenopathy, 92 (84%) had neoplasia and 18 (16%) had infectious diseases; the most common of those infectious diseases were attributed to coccidioidomycosis (12/18, 67%) [62]. On CT, differentiating between neoplastic and granulomatous lymphadenopathy is difficult. In one study, the largest tracheobronchial lymph nodes identified had granulomatous lymphadenitis secondary to blastomycosis which can be mistaken for metastatic lymphadenopathy [63]. Tracheobronchial lymph node size and ratios are correlated with metastasis or severe granulomatous lymphadenitis; transverse maximum lymph node diameter of 12 mm or lymph node to thoracic body ratio of 1.05 are proposed cutoffs [63]. Lymph node contrast enhancement pattern is also significantly correlated to disease; a heterogeneous and/or ring pattern is related to metastatic disease (Figure 28.54) [63].

**Abdomen** Mesenteric lymph nodes comprise the jejunal, right colic, middle colic, and left colic lymph nodes [1]. Mesenteric lymphadenopathy is poorly assessed on radiographs as it causes an ill-defined soft tissue opaque mass effect which should be further evaluated and confirmed using abdominal ultrasonography or CT. However, given the degree of superimposed retroperitoneal fat in cats, left colic lymphadenopathy can be appreciated on lateral abdominal radiographs (Figure 28.55), if present.

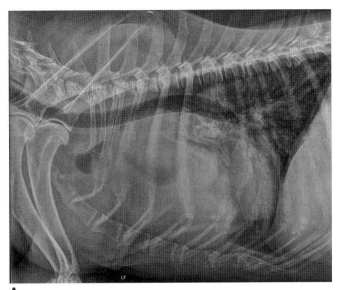
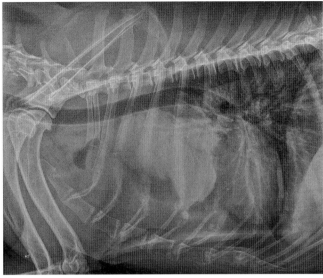

A

B

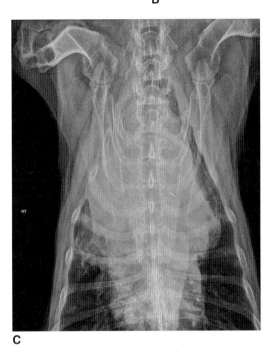

C

**FIGURE 28.48**  Right lateral (**A**), left lateral (**B**), and VD (**C**) thoracic radiographs of a geriatric large-breed dog diagnosed with a thymic epithelial neoplasm (confirmed as thymoma on histopathology); note the well-defined, cranial, caudal, and dorsal margins of this large cranial mediastinal mass. However, this mass does not cause a rightward shift of the cardiac silhouette on the ventrodorsal radiograph.

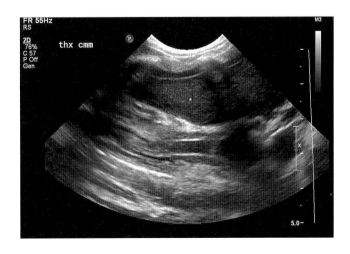

**FIGURE 28.49**  Sagittal plane ultrasound image of a large, homogeneously hypoechoic, cranial mediastinal mass (*) in a geriatric cat diagnosed with cranial mediastinal histiocytic sarcoma.

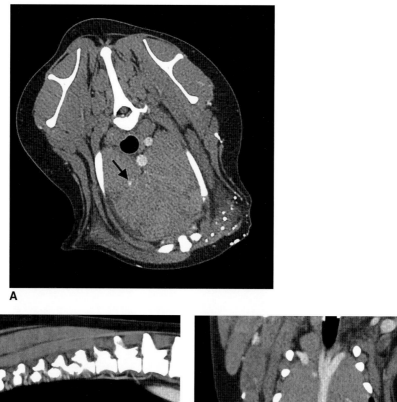

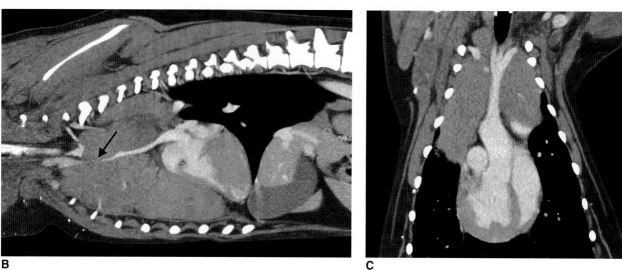

**FIGURE 28.50** Transverse (**A**), parasagittal (**B**), and dorsal (**C**) plane, soft tissue window images of the thorax of a young dog diagnosed with cranial mediastinal lymphoma. Note the compression and envelopment of the cranial vena cava (arrows) by the large, homogeneously contrast-enhancing mass.

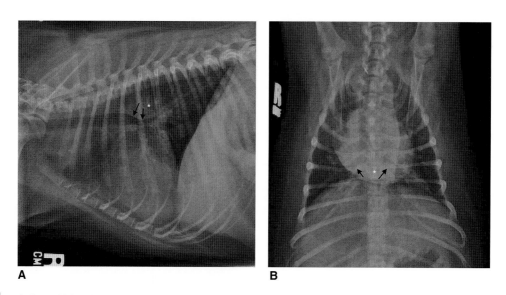

**FIGURE 28.51** Right lateral (**A**) and ventrodorsal (**B**) thoracic radiographs of a geriatric dog diagnosed with tracheobronchial lymphadenopathy secondary to lymphoma. Note the ill-defined soft tissue mass effect (*) dorsal to the carina causing ventral deviation of the caudal intrathoracic trachea and carina (arrow) on the right lateral radiograph and lateral deviation of the caudal principal bronchi (arrows) on the VD radiograph.

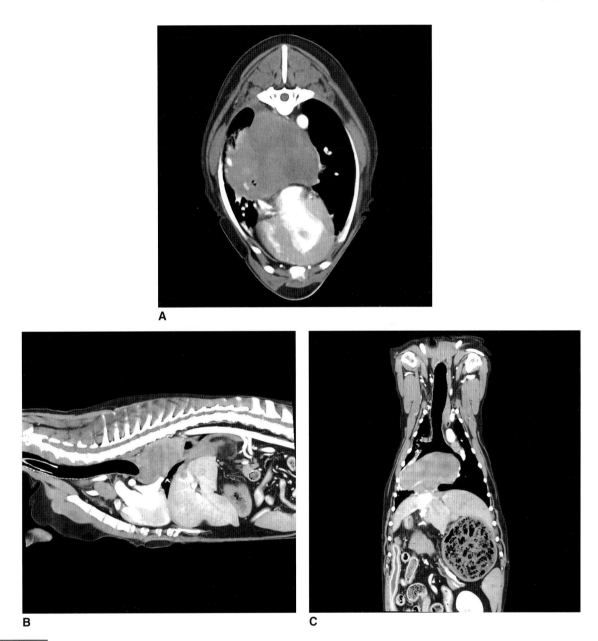

**FIGURE 28.52** Transverse (**A**), sagittal (**B**), and dorsal (**C**) plane, soft tissue window, CTA images centered over the multicentric neoplastic tracheobronchial lymph nodes secondary to lymphoma. Note the severely enlarged, lobular, mildly heterogeneously contrast-enhancing tracheobronchial lymph node masses.

Mesenteric lymphadenopathy on ultrasound in dogs and cats is characterized by enlarged lymph nodes that are usually homogeneous, hypoechoic, and smoothly marginated [64]. Multiple lymph nodes are frequently affected, and a thin hyperechoic capsule is often present. With nodal enlargement, acoustic enhancement is commonly encountered (Figure 28.56), which is an unusual finding in solid organs. Because lymph nodes can be hypoechoic to nearly anechoic, they must be differentiated from cystic or fluid-filled structures. Sometimes lymph nodes can become cystic. As the lymph nodes become larger, they may become distorted, have irregular margins, and develop a heterogeneous echotexture (Figure 28.57); heterogeneity is a feature that has been associated with malignancy in dogs and cats (Figure 28.58). Lymph nodes can occasionally have a "target" lesion where the central area is hyperechoic and the peripheral margin is hypoechoic. Similar to ultrasound, metastatic mesenteric lymphadenopathy on CT can be enlarged, lobular in margination, heterogeneous, sometimes cystic, heterogeneously contrast enhancing, and/or rim enhancing.

Cats with lymphoma often develop a large midabdominal mass that is not associated with a specific intraabdominal organ. This mass frequently originates from mesenteric nodes and may also involve adjacent small intestine. Lymph node enlargement can occur with inflammatory and infectious diseases of the gastrointestinal tract, which cause reactivity of regional nodes (Figure 28.59). Reactive lymphadenopathy on ultrasound and CT is usually typified by less enlargement and shape change than with neoplastic invasion.

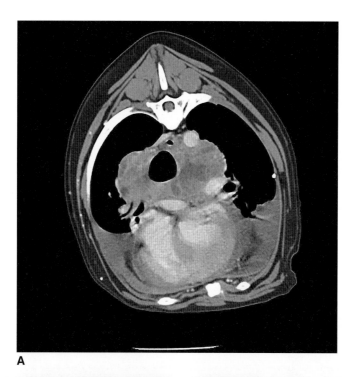

A

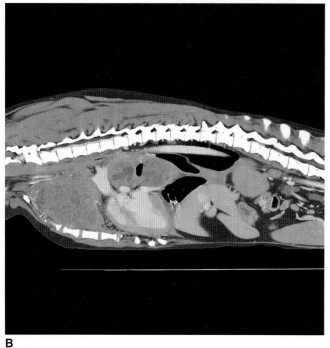

B

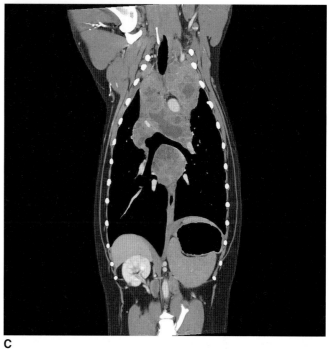

C

**FIGURE 28.53** Transverse (**A**), sagittal (**B**), and dorsal (**C**) plane, soft tissue window, CTA images centered over marked pyogranulomatous inflammation of the tracheobronchial lymph nodes secondary to pythiosis in a middle-aged dog. Note the severely enlarged, coalescing, rim- and heterogeneously contrast-enhancing tracheobronchial lymph node masses. These masses ventrally deviate the principal bronchi and compress the heart on the transverse and sagittal plane images, and laterally deviate the caudal principal bronchi on the dorsal plane image. On the sagittal plane image, there is also pyogranulomatous inflammation of the cranial mediastinal lymph nodes. On the transverse plane, there is moderate bilateral pleural effusion, retracting the lungs from the thoracic body wall.

Sublumbar lymphadenopathy (Figure 28.60) may appear as a soft tissue opaque mass effect within the caudodorsal retroperitoneal space, ventrally deviating the descending colon on lateral radiographs and decreasing the conspicuity of the ventral margin of the iliopsoas muscles [31]. In dogs with apocrine gland adenocarcinoma of the anal sac, the medial iliac lymph nodes are the most common site of metastasis [65].

Early detection of metastatic medial iliac lymphadenopathy is best assessed ultrasonographically (Figure 28.61) as sublumbar lymph nodes measuring >21.5 mm can be seen on

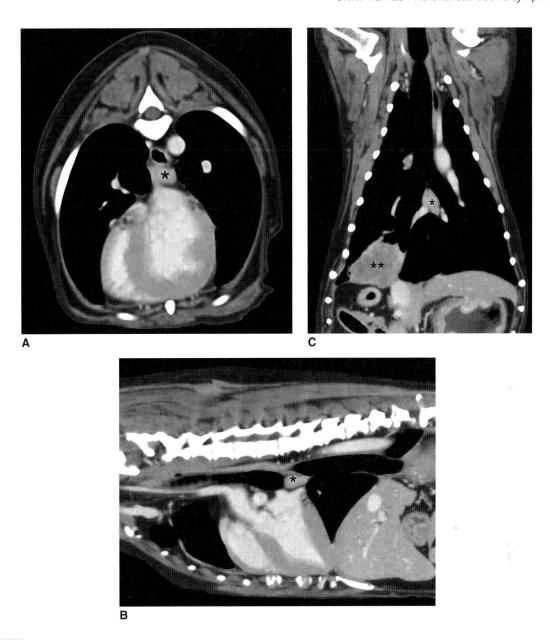

A

C

B

**FIGURE 28.54**   Transverse (**A**), sagittal (**B**), and dorsal (**C**) plane, soft tissue window, CTA images centered over the heterogeneously contrast-enhancing metastatic middle tracheobronchial lymphadenopathy (*) secondary to right caudal pulmonary carcinoma (**).

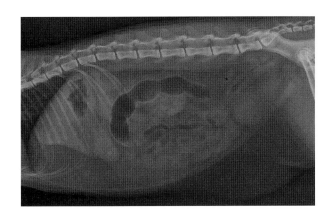

**FIGURE 28.55**   Right lateral abdominal radiograph of a geriatric cat with reactive left colic lymphadenopathy (*).

radiography [31]. In addition, ultrasonography is used to guide needle aspirations to cytologically rule out metastatic disease. An ultrasonographically normal-appearing lymph node does not preclude disease. However, detection of enlarged lymph nodes in the sublumbar regions on ultrasound and CT is a strong indicator of neoplasia, although severe inflammatory disease can result in lymphadenopathy. Again, ultrasound and CT differentiation between benign and neoplastic lymph nodes is difficult because size, echotexture, and shape may be similar; shape, contour, cavitation, and Doppler evaluation of lymph nodes on ultrasound are not useful in differentiating between benign and neoplastic changes (Figure 28.62). Cytologic or histopathologic analysis is needed for further investigation.

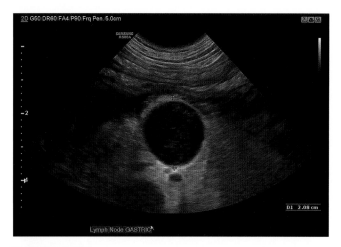

**FIGURE 28.56** Sagittal ultrasound image of a severely enlarged, heterogeneously hypoechoic metastatic gastric lymph node (between the calipers) with distal acoustic enhancement.

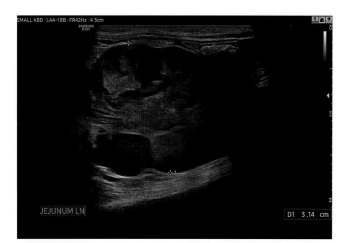

**FIGURE 28.57** Sagittal ultrasound image of a severely enlarged, lobular, moderately heterogeneous jejunal lymph node (between the calipers) in a geriatric cat with malignant hepatic neoplasia (not depicted). Cytolopathologic diagnosis of this lymph node was lymphoid hyperplasia.

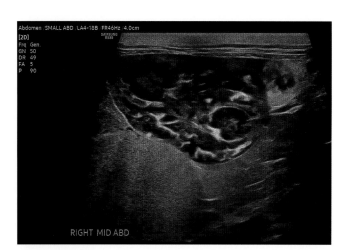

**FIGURE 28.58** Sagittal ultrasound image of a severely enlarged, markedly heterogeneous jejunal lymph node in a geriatric cat. Cytopathologic diagnosis of this lymph node was lymphoma.

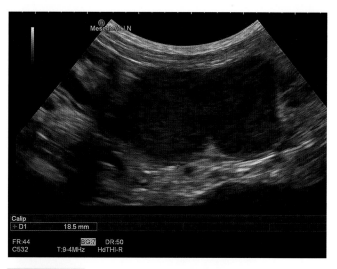

**FIGURE 28.59** Sagittal ultrasound image of a moderately enlarged, lobular, hypoechoic, reactive jejunal lymph node in a middle-aged dog diagnosed with intestinal pythiosis (not depicted).

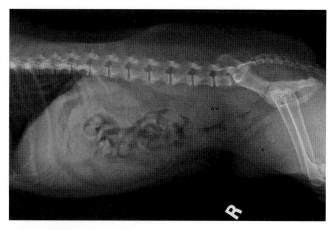

**FIGURE 28.60** Right lateral abdominal radiograph of a geriatric dog with a large, poorly delineated, soft tissue opaque mass effect in the caudodorsal retroperitoneal space, causing ventral deviation of the descending colon, representing severe sublumbar lymphadenopathy (**). Cytopathologic diagnosis of this lymph node was lymphoma. Additionally, there is severe inguinal lymphadenopathy (*), further characterized by an oval soft tissue mass effect, peripherally displacing the adjacent cutaneous margins.

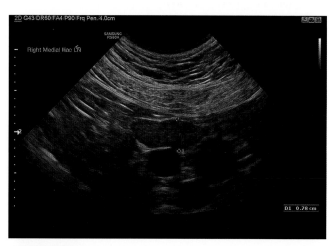

**FIGURE 28.61** Transverse plane ultrasound image of a mildly enlarged, homogeneously hypoechoic, metastatic medial iliac lymph node of a geriatric dog diagnosed with cutaneous mast cell tumor.

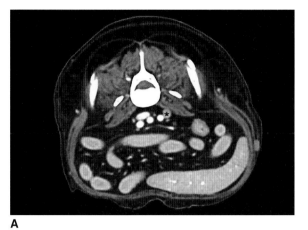
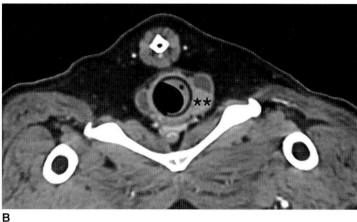

**FIGURE 28.62** Transverse plane, soft tissue window, CTA images centered over a mildly enlarged, rim-enhancing metastatic left medial iliac lymph node (*) (**A**) and a contrast-enhancing left apocrine gland anal sac adenocarcinoma (**) (**B**).

# References

1. Evans, H.E. and de Lahunta, A. (2013). *Miller's Anatomy of the Dog*. St Louis, MO: Elsevier Saunders.
2. Mattoon, J. and Nyland, T. (2015). *Small Animal Diagnostic Ultrasound*. St Louis, MO: Elsevier Saunders.
3. Penninck, D.G. and d'Anjou, M. (2015). *Atlas of Small Animal Ultrasonography*. Hoboken, NJ: Wiley.
4. Grooters, A.M., Biller, D.S., Theisen, S.K., and Miyabayashi, T. (1996). Ultrasonographic characteristics of the adrenal glands in dogs with pituitary-dependent hyperadrenocorticism: comparison with normal dogs. *J. Vet. Intern. Med.* 10: 110–115.
5. Choi, J., Kim, H., and Yoon, J. (2011). Ultrasonographic adrenal gland measurements in clinically normal small breed dogs and comparison with pituitary-dependent hyperadrenocorticism. *J. Vet. Med. Sci.* 73: 985–989.
6. Soulsby, S.N., Holland, M., Hudson, J.A., and Behrend, E.N. (2015). Ultrasonographic evaluation of adrenal gland size compared to body weight in normal dogs. *Vet. Radiol. Ultrasound* 56: 317–326.
7. Combes, A., Pey, P., Paepe, D. et al. (2013). Ultrasonographic appearance of adrenal glands in healthy and sick cats. *J. Feline Med. Surg.* 15: 445–457.
8. Pérez-López, L., Wägner, A.M., Saavedra, P. et al. (2021). Ultrasonographic evaluation of adrenal gland size in two body weight categories of healthy adult cats. *J. Feline Med. Surg.* 23: 804–808.
9. Bertolini, G., Furlanello, T., De Lorenzi, D., and Caldin, M. (2006). Computed tomographic quantification of canine adrenal gland volume and attenuation. *Vet. Radiol. Ultrasound* 47: 444–448.
10. Reusch, C.E. and Feldman, E.C. (1991). Canine hyperadrenocorticism due to adrenocortical neoplasia. Pretreatment evaluation of 41 dogs. *J. Vet. Intern. Med.* 5: 3–10.
11. Penninck, D.G., Feldman, E.C., and Nyland, T.G. (1988). Radiographic features of canine hyperadrenocorticism caused by autonomously functioning adrenocortical tumors: 23 cases (1978–1986). *J. Am. Vet. Med. Assoc.* 192: 1604–1608.
12. Pagani, E., Tursi, M., Lorenzi, C. et al. (2016). Ultrasonographic features of adrenal gland lesions in dogs can aid in diagnosis. *BMC Vet. Res.* 12: 267.
13. Ruppel, M.J., Pollard, R.E., and Willcox, J.L. (2019). Ultrasonographic characterization of cervical lymph nodes in healthy dogs. *Vet. Radiol. Ultrasound* 60: 560–566.
14. Kneissl, S. and Probst, A. (2007). Comparison of computed tomographic images of normal cranial and upper cervical lymph nodes with corresponding E12 plastinated-embedded sections in the dog. *Vet. J.* 174: 435–438.
15. Nemanic, S. and Nelson, N.C. (2012). Ultrasonography and non-contrast computed tomography of medial retropharyngeal lymph nodes in healthy cats. *Am. J. Vet. Res.* 73: 1377–1385.
16. Burns, G.O., Scrivani, P.V., Thompson, M.S., and Erb, H.N. (2008). Relation between age, body weight, and medial retropharyngeal lymph node size in apparently healthy dogs. *Vet. Radiol. Ultrasound* 49: 277–281.
17. Teodori, S., Aste, G., Tamburro, R. et al. (2021). Computed tomography evaluation of normal canine abdominal lymph nodes: retrospective study of size and morphology according to body weight and age in 45 dogs. *Vet. Sci.* 8: 44.
18. Belotta, A.F., Sukut, S., Lowe, C. et al. (2022). Computed tomography features of presumed normal mandibular and medial retropharyngeal lymph nodes in dogs. *Can. J. Vet. Res.* 86: 27–34.
19. Shibata, S.J., Hiramatsu, Y., Kaseda, M. et al. (2006). The time course of lymph drainage from the peritoneal cavity in beagle dogs. *J. Vet. Med. Sci.* 68: 1143–1147.
20. Patsikas, M.N., Karayannopoulou, M., Kaldrymidoy, E. et al. (2006). The lymph drainage of the neoplastic mammary glands in the bitch: a lymphographic study. *Anat. Histol. Embryol.* 35: 228–234.
21. Iwasaki, R., Mori, T., Ito, Y. et al. (2016). Computed tomographic evaluation of presumptively normal canine sternal lymph nodes. *J. Am. Anim. Hosp. Assoc.* 52: 371–377.
22. Thammasiri, N., Thanaboonnipat, C., Choisunirachon, N., and Darawiroj, D. (2021). Multi-factorial considerations for

intra-thoracic lymph node evaluations of healthy cats on computed tomographic images. *BMC Vet. Res.* 17: 59.

23. Ruby, J., Secrest, S., and Sharma, A. (2020). Radiographic differentiation of mediastinal versus pulmonary masses in dogs and cats can be challenging. *Vet. Radiol. Ultrasound* 61: 385–393.

24. Kayanuma, H., Yamada, K., Maruo, T., and Kanai, E. (2020). Computed tomography of thoracic lymph nodes in 100 dogs with no abnormalities in the dominated area. *J. Vet. Med. Sci.* 82: 279–285.

25. Agthe, P., Caine, A.R., Posch, B., and Herrtage, M.E. (2009). Ultrasonographic appearance of jejunal lymph nodes in dogs without clinical signs of gastrointestinal disease. *Vet. Radiol. Ultrasound* 50: 195–200.

26. Schreurs, E., Vermote, K., Barberet, V. et al. (2008). Ultrasonographic anatomy of abdominal lymph nodes in the normal cat. *Vet. Radiol. Ultrasound* 49: 68–72.

27. Krol, L. and O'Brien, R. (2012). Ultrasonographic assessment of abdominal lymph nodes in puppies. *Vet. Radiol. Ultrasound* 53: 455–458.

28. Beukers, M., Grosso, F.V., and Voorhout, G. (2013). Computed tomographic characteristics of presumed normal canine abdominal lymph nodes. *Vet. Radiol. Ultrasound* 54: 610–617.

29. Perlini, M., Bugbee, A., and Secrest, S. (2018). Computed tomographic appearance of abdominal lymph nodes in healthy cats. *J. Vet. Intern. Med.* 32: 1070–1076.

30. Brash, R, Martin-Ambrosio Frances, M, Dominguez, E. (2018). Visibility of presumed normal superficial caudal epigastric and caudal mesenteric lymph nodes in cats on abdominal radiographs. www.evdi-congress.eu/resources/media/Poster_abstracts/Robert_Brash_VISIBILITY_OF_PRESUMED_NORMAL_SUPERFICIAL_CAUDAL_EPIGASTRIC_AND_CAUDAL_MESENTERIC_LYMPH_NODES_IN_CATS_ON_ABDOMINAL_RADIOGRAPHS.pdf

31. Murphy, M.C., Sullivan, M., Gomes, B.J. et al. (2020). Evaluation of radiographs for the detection of sublumbar lymphadenopathy in dogs. *Can. Vet. J.* 61: 749–756.

32. Pollard, R.E., Fuller, M.C., and Steffey, M.A. (2017). Ultrasound and computed tomography of the iliosacral lymphatic centre in dogs with anal sac gland carcinoma. *Vet. Comp. Oncol.* 15: 299–306.

33. Mayer, M.N., Lawson, J.A., and Silver, T.I. (2010). Sonographic characteristics of presumptively normal canine medial iliac and superficial inguinal lymph nodes. *Vet. Radiol. Ultrasound* 51: 638–641.

34. Moraes, N.S. and Borges, N.C. (2021). Sonographic assessment of the normal and abnormal feline mammary glands and axillary and inguinal lymph nodes. *Vet. Med. Int.* 2021: 9998025.

35. Soultani, C., Patsikas, M.N., Mayer, M. et al. (2021). Contrast enhanced computed tomography assessment of superficial inguinal lymph node metastasis in canine mammary gland tumors. *Vet. Radiol. Ultrasound* 62: 557–567.

36. Millward, I.R., Kirberger, R.M., and Thompson, P.N. (2011). Comparative popliteal and mesenteric computed tomography lymphangiography of the canine thoracic duct. *Vet. Radiol. Ultrasound* 52: 295–301.

37. Johnson, E.G., Wisner, E.R., Kyles, A. et al. (2009). Computed tomographic lymphography of the thoracic duct by mesenteric lymph node injection. *Vet. Surg.* 38: 361–367.

38. Kim, M., Lee, H., Lee, N. et al. (2011). Ultrasound-guided mesenteric lymph node iohexol injection for thoracic duct computed tomographic lymphography in cats. *Vet. Radiol. Ultrasound* 52: 302–305.

39. Ando, K., Kamijyou, K., Hatinoda, K. et al. (2012). Computed tomography and radiographic lymphography of the thoracic duct by subcutaneous or submucosal injection. *J. Vet. Med. Sci.* 74: 135–140.

40. Kim, K. and Choen S, Hwang J, Jang M, Yoon J, Choi M. (2018). CT lymphangiography with contrast medium injection into the perianal subcutaneous region in a dog with chylothorax. *J. Vet. Clin.* 35: 299–301.

41. Lin, L.S., Chiu, H.C., Nishimura, R. et al. (2020). Computed tomographic lymphangiography via intra-metatarsal pad injection is feasible in dogs with chylothorax. *Vet. Radiol. Ultrasound* 61: 435–443.

42. Nemanic, S., Hollars, K., Nelson, N.C., and Bobe, G. (2015). Combination of computed tomographic imaging characteristics of medial retropharyngeal lymph nodes and nasal passages aids discrimination between rhinitis and neoplasia in cats. *Vet. Radiol. Ultrasound* 56: 617–627.

43. Ahuja, A., Ying, M., King, W., and Metreweli, C. (1997). A practical approach to ultrasound of cervical lymph nodes. *J. Laryngol. Otol.* 111: 245–256.

44. Ahuja, A., Ying, M., Yang, W.T. et al. (1996). The use of sonography in differentiating cervical lymphomatous lymph nodes from cervical metastatic lymph nodes. *Clin. Radiol.* 51: 186–190.

45. Nyman, H.T., Lee, M.H., McEvoy, F.J. et al. (2006). Comparison of B-mode and Doppler ultrasonographic findings with histologic features of benign and malignant superficial lymph nodes in dogs. *Am. J. Vet. Res.* 67: 978–984.

46. Skinner, O.T., Boston, S.E., and Souza, C.H.M. (2017). Patterns of lymph node metastasis identified following bilateral mandibular and medial retropharyngeal lymphadenectomy in 31 dogs with malignancies of the head. *Vet. Comp. Oncol.* 15: 881–889.

47. Bouyssou, S., Hammond, G.J., and Eivers, C. (2021). Comparison of CT features of 79 cats with intranasal mass lesions. *J. Feline Med. Surg.* 23: 987–995.

48. Skinner, O.T., Boston, S.E., Giglio, R.F. et al. (2018). Diagnostic accuracy of contrast-enhanced computed tomography for assessment of mandibular and medial retropharyngeal lymph node metastasis in dogs with oral and nasal cancer. *Vet. Comp. Oncol.* 16: 562–570.

49. Johnson, P.J., Elders, R., Pey, P., and Dennis, R. (2016). Clinical and magnetic resonance imaging features of inflammatory versus neoplastic medial retropharyngeal lymph node mass lesions in dogs and cats. *Vet. Radiol. Ultrasound* 57: 24–32.

50. Kneissl, S. and Probst, A. (2006). Magnetic resonance imaging features of presumed normal head and neck lymph nodes in dogs. *Vet. Radiol. Ultrasound* 47: 538–541.

51. Raharison, F. and Sautet, J. (2006). Lymph drainage of the mammary glands in female cats. *J. Morphol.* 267: 292–299.

52. Ruberte, J., Sautet, J.Y., Gine, J.M. et al. (1990). Topography of the lymphatic collecting ducts of the mammary glands of the dog. *Anat. Histol. Embryol.* 19: 347–358.

53. Kelsey, J., Balfour, R., Szabo, D., and Kass, P.H. (2022). Prognostic value of sternal lymphadenopathy on malignancy and survival in dogs undergoing splenectomy. *Vet. Comp. Oncol.* 20: 1–7.

54. Smith, K. and O'Brien, R. (2012). Radiographic characterization of enlarged sternal lymph nodes in 71 dogs and 13 cats. *J. Am. Anim. Hosp. Assoc.* 48: 176–181.

55. Belotta, A.F., Gomes, M.C., Rocha, N.S. et al. (2019). Sonography and sonoelastography in the detection of malignancy in superficial lymph nodes of dogs. *J. Vet. Intern. Med.* 33: 1403–1413.

56. Nyman, H.T., Kristensen, A.T., Skovgaard, I.M., and McEvoy, F.J. (2005). Characterization of normal and abnormal canine superficial lymph nodes using gray-scale B-mode, color flow mapping, power, and spectral Doppler ultrasonography: a multivariate study. *Vet. Radiol. Ultrasound* 46: 404–410.

57. Kinns, J. and Mai, W. (2007). Association between malignancy and sonographic heterogeneity in canine and feline abdominal lymph nodes. *Vet. Radiol. Ultrasound* 48: 565–569.

58. Nyman, H.T., Nielsen, O.L., McEvoy, F.J. et al. (2006). Comparison of B-mode and Doppler ultrasonographic findings with histologic features of benign and malignant mammary tumors in dogs. *Am. J. Vet. Res.* 67: 985–991.

59. Davé, A.C., Zekas, L.J., and Auld, D.M. (2017). Correlation of cytologic and histopathologic findings with perinodal echogenicity of abdominal lymph nodes in dogs and cats. *Vet. Radiol. Ultrasound* 58: 463–470.

60. Oura, T.J., Hamel, P.E., Jennings, S.H. et al. (2019). Radiographic differentiation of cranial mediastinal lymphomas from thymic epithelial tumors in dogs and cats. *J. Am. Anim. Hosp. Assoc.* 55: 187–193.

61. Reeve, E.J., Mapletoft, E.K., Schiborra, F. et al. (2020). Mediastinal lymphoma in dogs is homogeneous compared to thymic epithelial neoplasia and is more likely to envelop the cranial vena cava in CT images. *Vet. Radiol. Ultrasound* 61: 25–32.

62. Jones, B.G. and Pollard, R.E. (2012). Relationship between radiographic evidence of tracheobronchial lymph node enlargement and definitive or presumptive diagnosis. *Vet. Radiol. Ultrasound* 53: 486–491.

63. Ballegeer, E.A., Adams, W.M., Dubielzig, R.R. et al. (2010). Computed tomography characteristics of canine tracheobronchial lymph node metastasis. *Vet. Radiol. Ultrasound* 51: 397–403.

64. Pugh, C.R. (1994). Ultrasonographic examination of abdominal lymph nodes in the dog. *Vet. Radiol. Ultrasond* 35: 110–115.

65. Palladino, S., Keyerleber, M.A., King, R.G., and Burgess, K.E. (2016). Utility of computed tomography versus abdominal ultrasound examination to identify iliosacral lymphadenomegaly in dogs with apocrine gland adenocarcinoma of the anal sac. *J. Vet. Intern. Med.* 30: 1858–1863.

Clinic: _____           Date _____

# Musculoskeletal Review Paradigm

Case #: _____          Anatomic Area of Interest: _____

Signalment: Age: _____ yr / mo old; Species: _____; Breed: _____

Immature (physes open)? _____ OR Mature (physes closed or should be)? _____

**Technique:**

Views Available: _____, _____, _____, _____

Special Views: _____ Reason to take? _____

Technique: _____ Poor; _____ OK

Orthogonal radiographs? _____ (minimum of two orthogonal views)

Appropriate collimation and centering: _____ YES; _____ NO (retake - not cat scans or dogo-grams)

Clinical question to be answered? _____

  **I.** ALIGNMENT (and number) of bones

 **II.** BONE - describe changes present. Describe each change as to location (epiphysis, physis, metaphysis, diaphysis)

     a. Periosteum

     b. Cortex

     c. Endosteum

     d. Medullary cavity

**III.** CARTILAGE

    Articular margins/subchondral bone

    Physis specific (immature)

    Apophysis

 **IV.** SOFT TISSUES - diffuse swelling _____; focal swelling _____ – If yes, where centered?

    _____

Summary Sentence (15 words or less without repeating findings):

Important clues:     Aggressive / Nonaggressive (Benign)

                  Monostotic / Polyostotic

                  Articular / Nonarticular

                  Location on Bone - epiphysis, physis, metaphysis, diaphysis (circle all that apply)

Differential Diagnoses(ranked):

1. _____; 2. _____; 3. _____

Review Images - Any other radiographic abnormalities that I should look for OR is there anything I have missed?

Additional tests/procedures/imaging studies?

*Atlas of Small Animal Diagnostic Imaging*, First Edition. Edited by Clifford R. Berry, Nathan C. Nelson, and Matthew D. Winter.

© 2023 John Wiley & Sons, Inc. Published 2023 by John Wiley & Sons, Inc.

Companion website: www.wiley.com/go/berry/atlas

# Thoracic Radiology Checklist

Case, MRN or Accession Number: _____

| Technique | Repeat Films | OK |
|---|---|---|
| 1. Images: LLAT: ☐; RLAT: ☐; VD: ☐; DV: ☐; Special Views: _____ | | |
| 2. Age of patient? _____ years old | | |

| Technique | Repeat Films | OK |
|---|---|---|
| 3. Positioning | ☐ | ☐ |
| 4. Technical (Anatomy included) | ☐ | ☐ |
| 5. Inspiration (Yes or No; If no – repeat) | ☐ | ☐ |

| Interpretation Paradigm | NORMAL | ABNORMAL (Roentgen sign) |
|---|---|---|
| **A. Extrathoracic Structures** | | |
| a. Thoracic Limb | ☐ | ☐ _____ |
| b. Cervical Spine and Soft Tissues | ☐ | ☐ _____ |
| c. Thoracic Spine | ☐ | ☐ _____ |
| d. Ribs and Sternum | ☐ | ☐ _____ |
| e. Diaphragm | ☐ | ☐ _____ |
| f. Cranial Abdomen | ☐ | ☐ _____ |
| g. Thoracic Wall | ☐ | ☐ _____ |
| **B. Pleural Space** | | |
| a. Pleural Fissure Lines? | ☐ | ☐ _____ |
| b. Pneumothorax | ☐ | ☐ _____ |
| c. Pleural Effusion | ☐ | ☐ _____ |
| d. Pleural Mass | ☐ | ☐ _____ |
| e. Extrapleural Sign Present? | ☐ | ☐ _____ |
| f. Diaphragmatic Rupture? | ☐ | ☐ _____ |
| **C. Pulmonary Parenchyma** | | |
| a. Decreased Opacity? | _____ | ☐ _____ |
| i. IF YES, Focal? Lobar? | _____ | ☐ _____ |
| ii. IF YES, Diffuse? | _____ | ☐ _____ |
| iii. IF DIFFUSE, Pulmonary vessels? | _____ | ☐ _____ |
| b. Increased Opacity? | _____ | ☐ _____ |

c. IF YES, then:

    i. Focal (single lobe) ◯; Multifocal ◯ (multiple lobes but not all); Generalized ◯

    ii. Location (anatomic lobes and position in the lobe and in general)?

*Atlas of Small Animal Diagnostic Imaging*, First Edition. Edited by Clifford R. Berry, Nathan C. Nelson, and Matthew D. Winter.
© 2023 John Wiley & Sons, Inc. Published 2023 by John Wiley & Sons, Inc.
Companion website: www.wiley.com/go/berry/atlas

       1.  In general? ☐ cranioventral (pneumonia), ☐ caudodorsal (edema)

       2.  Lung lobes involved and position in the lobe (hilar, mid-zone or peripheral)

_____

_____

   iii.  Mediastinal Shift Present (assumes VD/DV is straight)?

       1.  If YES, Ipsilateral? ◯

       2.  Contralateral? ◯

   iv.  Pulmonary Pattern Present (caveat: can be multiple patterns present; the patterns are presented in order for looking up differentials; different patterns represent different degrees of severity of the same disease)

       1.  Mass present? (solitary, big (> 3 cm), soft tissue opaque or cavitated and round?)

          a.  Lobe involved? _____

       2.  Alveolar pulmonary pattern? (3 out of 5 to call it!)

          a.  Air bronchograms? Yes ◯ OR No ◯

          b.  Uniform soft tissue gray? Yes ◯ OR No ◯

          c.  Border effacement of small vessels in affected area? Yes ◯ OR No ◯

          d.  Border effacement of cardiac silhouette or diaphragm? Yes ◯ OR No ◯

          e.  Lobar sign present? Yes ◯ OR No ◯

       3.  Bronchial pulmonary pattern? Presence of rings and lines – look in periphery

          a.  Generalized? Yes ◯ OR No ◯

          b.  Focal? ◯ Lobar? ◯ Bronchiectasis? ◯

       4.  Vascular pulmonary pattern?

          a.  Pulmonary veins enlarged? Yes ◯ OR No ◯ (left heart failure)

          b.  Pulmonary arteries enlarged? Yes ◯ OR No ◯ (heartworm disease)

          c.  Both pulmonary arteries and veins enlarged? Yes ◯ OR No ◯ (Cats in heart failure or fluid overload)

       5.  Structured interstitial?

          a.  Nodules – variable sizes, soft tissue opacity and random distribution? Yes ☐ OR No ☐?

          b.  Miliary – "Millet seed"; small nodules in peripheral lung fields (thin sections of the lung)? Yes ☐ OR No ☐?

       6.  Unstructured interstitial – BACK DOOR DIAGNOSIS? Yes ☐ OR No ☐? Be sure the films are not expiratory. Never Mild!!

       7.  Severity? Moderate ◯     Severe ◯

## D. Mediastinum

  a.  Cranial Mediastinum

     i.  Pneumomediastinum present? ☐

     ii.  Dilated esophagus? ☐

     iii.  Widened mediastinum on VD? ☐

     iv.  Cranial mediastinal mass? ☐ IF YES, Mass position: Ventral ☐ or Dorsal ☐

     v.  Deviation of the trachea? Yes ☐ OR No ☐; If yes, which direction? Ventral ◯; Lateral ◯ (VD – to which side?); Dorsal ◯

     vi.  Sternal lymph node enlargement? Yes ◯ OR No ◯

  b.  Middle Mediastinum

     i.  Cardiac Silhouette Paradigm

       1.  Cardiac silhouette –

          a.  Normal ◯; Large (Cardiomegaly?) ◯; OR Small ◯; *If LARGE, then*:

          b.  Left Sided? ☐; dorsal elevation of the trachea? ☐

          c.  Right Sided? ☐ (VD radiograph – reverse "D")

          d.  Generalized (round or globoid)? dorsal elevation of the trachea? ☐

          e.  Biatrial enlargement (cat)? ☐; Valentine shape cardiac silhouette on the VD image of the cat? ☐

       2.  Pulmonary circulation

          a.  Normal? ☐

          b.  Pulmonary artery enlarged? ☐; Tortuous? ☐; Blunted? ☐

          c.  Pulmonary veins enlarged? ☐; More than right cranial lobar vein on left lateral radiographic image? ☐

          d.  Overcirculation? ☐; (pulmonary arteries and veins enlarged)

             i.  Generalized? ◯; Lobar? ◯

          e.  Undercirculation? ☐; (small pulmonary arteries and veins)

             i.  Generalized? ◯; Lobar oligemia? ◯

3. Great vessel enlargement?
    a. Aorta? ☐; Presence of ductus diverticulum (left fourth ICS)? ☐
    b. Main pulmonary artery? ☐
    c. Caudal vena cava? ☐ (>2 x descending thoracic aorta diameter on both laterals)
    d. Aortic knob (redundant aorta) (Cat)? ☐ (VD projection)
4. Other considerations for generalized cardiomegaly; Do you believe there is. . . .?
    a. Pericardial effusion? ☐
    b. DiCM? ☐
    c. MV/TV disease in combination? ☐
    d. PPDH? ☐ (differential opacities in the cardiac silhouette)
5. Presence of heart failure?
    a. Left heart failure (pulmonary edema)? ☐
    b. Right heart failure (pleural effusion)? ☐
6. Other cardiac abnormal Roentgen signs?

    _____

7. Do the cardiac abnormalities that I am seeing make sense in combination with each other (all from section b(i))?
    ☐ YES OR NO ☐ (then rethink it!!)
    ii. Tracheobronchial lymph node enlargement? Yes ☐ OR No ☐
        1. Central LN? ◯
        2. Right LN? ◯
        3. Left LN? ◯
    iii. Deviation of the trachea? Yes ☐ OR No ☐
        1. Dorsal? ☐ (Left atrium)
        2. Ventral? ☐ (esophageal or central TB LN enlargement)
        3. Remember central pulmonary masses could push the trachea in either direction, but this is rare
    iv. Esophageal mass, FB or dilation? Yes ☐ OR No ☐
        1. If yes, then which of above? _____
    c. Caudal Mediastinum
    i. Esophageal abnormality?
        1. Dilation? ☐
        2. Fluid distended? ☐
        3. FB or mass? ☐
        4. Hiatal hernia? ☐. Positional? ☐; Single image only? ☐
    ii. Other caudal mediastinal abnormalities?
        1. Pneumomediastinum? ☐
        2. Mass? ☐
        3. Fluid? ☐
    iii. Caudal vena cava visualized? Yes ☐ OR No ☐?
        1. Congenital absence (rare)? ◯
        2. Accessory lung lobe mass or pulmonary pattern border effacement? ◯

**Summary Sentence(s) (should not repeat findings)**

**1.** _____

**2.** _____

**3.** _____

**4.** _____

**5.** _____

**6.** _____

**Can you tie all of these together as one disease process (particularly *important* to think through pathophysiology if *multicompartment* disease; needs to be a known disease – specific name – that occurs in the dog or cat)?**

**DDX or DX?**

1. _____

2. _____

3. _____

4. _____

5. _____

**Next Step (how to get at final answer without necropsy)?**

1. _____

2. _____

3. _____

4. _____

5. _____

# Abdominal Radiology Check List

Case Number: _____

| **Technique** | **Repeat Films** | **OK** |
|---|---|---|
| 1. Images: LLAT RLAT VD DV (circle) | | |
| 2. Age of patient? _____ years old. | | |
| 3. Positioning | _____ | _____ |
| 4. Technical aspects | _____ | _____ |
| 5. Expiration? | _____ | _____ |

| **Interpretation Paradigm** | **NORMAL** | **ABNORMAL (Roentgen sign)** |
|---|---|---|
| **A. Extraabdominal Structures** | | |
|   a. Caudal thorax | _____ | _____ |
|   b. Diaphragm | _____ | _____ |
|   c. Thoracic and lumbar spine | _____ | _____ |
|   d. Pelvis, pelvic limb | _____ | _____ |
|   e. Abdominal wall | _____ | _____ |
|   f. Patient body habitus (description) | _____ | _____ |
| **B. Peritoneal and Retroperitoneal Spaces** | | |
|   a. Peritoneal space | _____ | _____ |
|     i. Pneumoperitoneum | _____ | _____ |
|     ii. Peritoneal effusion | _____ | _____ |
|     iii. Peritoneal mass effect | _____ | _____ |
|     iv. Mineralized structures? | _____ | _____ |
|   b. Retroperitoneal space | _____ | _____ |
|     i. Air within the retroperitoneum? | _____ | _____ |
|     ii. Fluid in the retroperitoneum? | _____ | _____ |
|     iii. Mineralization? | _____ | _____ |
| **C. Gastrointestinal Tract, Liver, Spleen, and Pancreas** | | |
|   a. Stomach | _____ | _____ |
|     i. Normal shape, size? | _____ | _____ |
|     ii. Normal position? | _____ | _____ |
|     iii. Gastric foreign material | _____ | _____ |
|   b. Small Bowel | _____ | _____ |
|     i. Abnormally distended? | _____ | _____ |
|       1. Yes, > 1.5 x L5 mid vertebral body? DOG _____ | | |
|       2. Yes, > 12 mm? CAT _____ | | |
|       3. Yes, Generalized? _____ | | |

*Atlas of Small Animal Diagnostic Imaging*, First Edition. Edited by Clifford R. Berry, Nathan C. Nelson, and Matthew D. Winter.
© 2023 John Wiley & Sons, Inc. Published 2023 by John Wiley & Sons, Inc.
Companion website: www.wiley.com/go/berry/atlas

   4.  Yes, Focal or multifocal? _____
       a.  Sentinel loop? _____
   5.  Radiopaque foreign bodies? Yes _____ OR No _____?
   6.  Plication with abnormal crescent-shaped gas pattern? Yes _____ OR No _____?
c.  Caecum and Colon
   i.    Location normal?
   ii.   Size and shape normal?
   iii.  Luminal contents normal?
   iv.   Pneumocolon indicated? Yes _____ OR No _____?
d.  Liver
   i.    Hepatomegaly? Yes _____ OR No _____?
       1.  Generalized? Yes _____ OR No _____?
           a.  Caudally displaced gastric axis?
       2.  Mass or focal? Yes _____ OR No _____? If so, where? _____
   ii.   Microhepatia? Yes _____ OR No _____?
   iii.  Abnormal mineralizations? Yes _____ OR No _____?
       1.  GB? _____; Biliary? _____; Focal hepatic parenchyma? _____
   iv.   Biliary gas or hepatic abscess formation? _____
e.  Spleen
   i.    Mass lesions? _____
   ii.   Generalized enlargement? Yes _____ OR No _____?
   iii.  Mass effect – mid abdomen? Yes _____ OR No _____?
   iv.   Gas within the splenic parenchyma? _____
f.  Pancreas
   i.    Mass effect/effusion?
       1.  Left Limb location? _____
       2.  Pyloroduodenal angle? _____
       3.  Right limb location? _____

**D. Genitourinary, Adrenals, Lymph Node**
a.  Urinary
   i.    Kidneys?
       1.  Enlarged? _____; Bilateral? _____; Super Big? _____
       2.  Small? _____; Bilateral? _____
       3.  Dystrophic mineralization? _____; renal pelvis? _____; renal diverticulae? _____
       4.  Nephrolithiasis? _____
       5.  Ureteroliths? _____
       6.  Irregular magins? _____
       7.  Retroperitoneal effusion? _____
       8.  EU indicated? _____ (possible ureteral rupture? _____)
   ii.   Ureters
       1.  Ureteroliths? _____
       2.  Enlarged? _____
       3.  EU indicated? _____ (possible rupture or ureteral ectopia)
   iii.  Urinary bladder
       1.  Degree of distention? _____
       2.  Cystolithiasis (mineralized)? _____ (I cann't C. U. – cysteine and urates may not mineralize and will thereby not be visualized on abdominal survey radiographs)
       3.  Gas within the lumen? _____ (cystocentesis or catheterization? _____)
       4.  Gas within the UB wall? _____
   iv.   Urethra/Mass effect? _____
       1.  Mineralization? _____
       2.  Adjacent fluid? _____
       3.  Urethral calculi? _____ (Male dog – caudal perineal evaluation? _____)

  b. Genital
- i. Ovaries?
  - 1. Mass effect? _____
  - 2. Teratoma? _____
- ii. Uterus?
  - 1. Uterine enlargement? _____
    - a. Generalized? _____; Segmentation? _____; Fetal structures? _____
      - i. Evidence of Fetal death? _____
- iii. Prostate?
  - 1. Enlarged? _____
  - 2. Normal size for castration? _____ (not visualized? _____)
  - 3. Mineralization? _____
  - 4. Paraprostatic cysts? _____
- iv. Testes?
  - 1. Scrotal location? _____
  - 2. Abdominal retained testicle with mass effect? _____

  c. Adrenals
- i. Adrenal Mass?
  - 1. Left or right? _____
  - 2. Mineralization? _____
  - 3. Effusion? _____

  d. Lymph node(s)
- i. Medial iliac lymph node?
  - 1. Mass? _____
  - 2. Fluid? _____
- ii. Mesenteric lymph node enlargment? Yes _____
  OR No _____?
  - 1. Mass effect – midabdomen? _____
  - 2. Fluid accumulation? _____

**Summary of Findings:**
**Abnormalities:**


**DDX or Specific DX:**



**Next Step?**

# Index

Page locators in **bold** indicate tables. Page locators in *italics* indicate figures. This index uses letter-by-letter alphabetization.

*Atlas of Small Animal Diagnostic Imaging*, First Edition. Edited by Clifford R. Berry, Nathan C. Nelson, and Matthew D. Winter.
© 2023 John Wiley & Sons, Inc. Published 2023 by John Wiley & Sons, Inc.
Companion website: www.wiley.com/go/berry/atlas